INTERNAL MEDICINE
Just the Facts

D1028594

Editor-in-Chief

Paul G. Schmitz, MD, FACP

Professor of Internal Medicine
Saint Louis University School of Medicine
Department of Internal Medicine
St. Louis, Missouri

Associate Editor

Kevin J. Martin, MB, BCh, FACP

Professor of Internal Medicine
Saint Louis University School of Medicine
Director, Division of Nephrology
St. Louis, Missouri

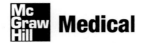 **Medical**

New York   Chicago   San Francisco   Lisbon   London   Madrid
Mexico City   Milan   New Delhi   San Juan   Seoul
Singapore   Sydney   Toronto

The *McGraw-Hill* Companies

INTERNAL MEDICINE
Just the Facts

1 2 3 4 5 6 7 8 9 0   QPDQPD   0 9 8

ISBN 978-0-07-146887-9
MHID 0-07-146887-0

This book was set in Times Roman by International Typesetting and Composition.
The editors were James F. Shanahan and Peter J. Boyle.
The production supervisor was Sherri Souffrance.
Project management was provided by Vastavikta Sharma, International Typesetting and Composition.
Quebecor World Dubuque was printer and binder.

This book is printed on acid-free paper.

Library of Congress Cataloging-in-Publication Data

Internal medicine : just the facts / [edited by] Paul G. Schmitz.
   p. ; cm.
  Includes bibliographical references and index.
  ISBN-13: 978-0-07-146887-9 (soft cover : alk. paper)
  ISBN-10: 0-07-146887-0 (soft cover : alk. paper)   1. Internal medicine—Handbooks, manuals, etc.   I. Schmitz, Paul G.
  [DNLM: 1. Internal Medicine—Handbooks. WB 39 I613   2008]
RC55.I485   2008
616—dc22

2008003649

*To Grandma Pauline for her divine
nurturing of education and spirit*

*And to our patients,
whom we have been given
the privilege of caring for*

INTERNAL MEDICINE
Just the Facts

CONTENTS

Section 6
ENDOCRINOLOGY AND METABOLISM

Section 7
GASTROENTEROLOGY AND LIVER DISEASE

SECTION EDITORS

Cardiovascular Medicine

Frank L. Bleyer, MD
Assistant Professor of Internal Medicine
Division of Cardiology
Department of Internal Medicine
Saint Louis University School of Medicine
St. Louis, Missouri

Assessing the Medical Literature

Thomas E. Burroughs, PhD
Associate Professor of Internal Medicine and
Health Management & Policy
Executive Director, Saint Louis University Center
for Outcomes Research
Saint Louis University
St. Louis, Missouri

Gastroenterology and Liver Disease

Adrian M. Di Bisceglie, MD
Professor of Internal Medicine
Division of Gastroenterology and Hepatology
Department of Internal Medicine
Saint Louis University School of Medicine
St. Louis, Missouri

Endocrinology and Metabolism

George T. Griffing, MD
Professor of Internal Medicine
Division of General Internal Medicine
Department of Internal Medicine
Saint Louis University School of Medicine
St. Louis, Missouri

Psychiatric Disorders

George T. Grossberg, MD
Samuel W. Fordyce Professor
Division of Psychiatry
Department of Neurology and Psychiatry
Saint Louis University School of Medicine
St. Louis, Missouri

Infectious Disease

Donald J. Kennedy, MD
Professor of Internal Medicine
Division of Infectious Diseases
Department of Internal Medicine
Saint Louis University School of Medicine
St. Louis, Missouri

Pulmonary Medicine and Critical Care

George M. Matuschak, MD
Professor of Pharmacological and Physiological
Science
James B. Miller and Ethyl D. Miller Professor
of Internal Medicine
Director, Division of Pulmonary, Critical Care,
and Sleep Medicine
Department of Internal Medicine
Saint Louis University School of Medicine
St. Louis, Missouri

CONTRIBUTORS

Jayant N. Acharya, MD, DM
Associate Professor of Neurology
Division of Neurology
Department of Neurology and Psychiatry
Saint Louis University School of Medicine
St. Louis, Missouri
(Chapter 105)

Alejandro C. Alvarez, MD
Assistant Professor of Internal Medicine
Division of Nephrology
Department of Internal Medicine
Saint Louis University School of Medicine
St. Louis, Missouri
(Chapter 123)

Mona Bahl, MD
Assistant Professor of Internal Medicine
Division of General Internal Medicine
Department of Internal Medicine
Saint Louis University School of Medicine
St. Louis, Missouri
(Chapter 8)

Rama Bandlamudi, MD
Assistant Professor of Internal Medicine
Division of Rheumatology
Department of Internal Medicine
Saint Louis University School of Medicine
St. Louis, Missouri
(Chapter 128)

Krishnamohan R. Basarakodu, MD
Fellow in Hematology and Medical Oncology
Division of Hematology and Medical Oncology
Department of Internal Medicine
Ellis Fischel Cancer Center
Columbia School of Medicine
University of Missouri—Columbia School
of Medicine
Columbia, Missouri
(Chapters 60, 66, 67)

Bahar Bastani, MD
Professor of Internal Medicine
Division of Nephrology
Department of Internal Medicine
Saint Louis University School of Medicine
St. Louis, Missouri
(Chapters 122, 124)

Marla Bernbaum, MD
Clinical Professor of Internal Medicine
Division of Endocrinology
Department of Internal Medicine
Saint Louis University School of Medicine
St. Louis, Missouri
(Chapter 46)

Frank L. Bleyer, MD
Assistant Professor of Internal Medicine
Division of Cardiology
Department of Internal Medicine
Saint Louis University School of Medicine
St. Louis, Missouri
(Chapters 31, 33, 34, 44)

Thomas E. Burroughs, PhD
Associate Professor of Internal Medicine
and Health Management & Policy
Executive Director, Saint Louis University
Center for Outcomes Research
Saint Louis University School of Medicine
St. Louis, Missouri
(Chapters 10–14)

Jeffrey Ciaramita, MD
Fellow in Cardiology
Division of Cardiology
Department of Internal Medicine
Saint Louis University School of Medicine
St. Louis, Missouri
(Chapter 35)

Sara E. Crowder, MD
Assistant Professor of Clinical Obstetrics
and Gynecology
Department of Obstetrics and Gynecology
Columbia School of Medicine
University of Missouri—Columbia School
of Medicine
Columbia, Missouri
(Chapter 80)

Mary Abigail C. Dacuycuy, MD
Fellow in Infectious Diseases
Division of Infectious Diseases
Department of Internal Medicine
Saint Louis University School of Medicine
St. Louis, Missouri
(Chapters 88, 89, 91, 92, 94, 96, 97–99)

Patricia A. Dettenmeier, ANP, MSN
Assistant Professor of Internal Medicine
Division of Pulmonary, Critical Care, and Sleep
Medicine
Department of Internal Medicine
Saint Louis University School of Medicine
St. Louis, Missouri
(Chapter 115)

Adrian M. Di Bisceglie, MD
Professor of Internal Medicine
Division of Gastroenterology and Hepatology
Department of Internal Medicine
Saint Louis University School of Medicine
St. Louis, Missouri
(Chapters 57, 58)

James Drake, MD
Professor of Internal Medicine
Division of General Internal Medicine
Department of Internal Medicine
Saint Louis University School of Medicine
St. Louis, Missouri
(Chapter 6)

Mark S. Dykewicz, MD
Professor of Internal Medicine
Division of Allergy and Clinical Immunology
Department of Internal Medicine
Saint Louis University School of Medicine
St. Louis, Missouri
(Chapters 23, 27, 28)

Joseph Roland D. Espiritu, MD
Assistant Professor of Internal Medicine
Division of Pulmonary, Critical Care, and Sleep
Medicine
Department of Internal Medicine
Saint Louis University School of Medicine
St. Louis, Missouri
(Chapters 112, 117)

Kevin Fitzgerald, MD
Fellow in Cardiology
Division of Cardiology
Department of Internal Medicine
Saint Louis University School of Medicine
St. Louis, Missouri
(Chapter 40)

Joseph H. Flaherty, MD
Associate Professor of Internal Medicine
Division of Geriatric Medicine
Department of Internal Medicine
Geriatric Research, Education and Clinical
Center
St. Louis VA Medical Center
Saint Louis University School of Medicine
St. Louis, Missouri
(Chapter 20)

Michael Forsberg, MD
Assistant Professor of Internal Medicine
Division of Cardiology
Department of Internal Medicine
Saint Louis University School of Medicine
St. Louis, Missouri
(Chapter 41)

Daniel Friedman, MD
Fellow in Cardiology
Division of Cardiology
Department of Internal Medicine
Saint Louis University School of Medicine
St. Louis, Missouri
(Chapter 32)

Julie Gammack, MD
Assistant Professor of Internal Medicine
Division of Geriatric Medicine
Department of Internal Medicine
Geriatric Research, Education and Clinical
Center
St. Louis VA Medical Center
Saint Louis University School of Medicine
St. Louis, Missouri
(Chapter 16)

Mehret Gebretsadik, MD
Resident in Psychiatry
Division of Psychiatry
Department of Neurology and Psychiatry
Saint Louis University School of Medicine
St. Louis, Missouri
(Chapter 107)

Ramaswamy Govindan, MD
Associate Professor of Internal Medicine
Division of Medical Oncology
Alvin J. Siteman Cancer Center
Washington University School of Medicine
St. Louis, Missouri
(Chapter 77)

Stephen L. Graziano, MD
Professor of Medicine
Regional Oncology Center
Upstate Medical University
State University of New York
Syracuse, New York
(Chapter 60)

Miggie Greenberg, MD
Assistant Professor
Director of Adult Psychiatry Inpatient Unit
Division of Psychiatry
Department of Neurology and Psychiatry
Saint Louis University School of Medicine
St. Louis, Missouri
(Chapter 107)

George T. Griffing, MD
Professor of Internal Medicine
Division of General Internal Medicine
Department of Internal Medicine
Saint Louis University School of Medicine
St. Louis, Missouri
(Chapter 52)

George T. Grossberg, MD
Samuel W. Fordyce Professor
Division of Psychiatry
Department of Neurology and Psychiatry
Saint Louis University School of Medicine
St. Louis, Missouri
(Chapters 22, 108, 111)

Sahar Hachem, MD
Fellow in Endocrinology
Division of Endocrinology
Department of Internal Medicine
Saint Louis University School of Medicine
St. Louis, Missouri
(Chapter 46)

Noah M. Hahn, MD
Assistant Professor of Medicine
Division of Hematology and Oncology
Department of Medicine
Indiana University Cancer Center
Indiana University School of Medicine
Indianapolis, Indiana
(Chapter 79)

Matthew T. Haren, PhD
Post Doc Fellow
Division of Geriatric Medicine
Department of Internal Medicine
Geriatric Research, Education and Clinical
Center
St. Louis VA Medical Center
Saint Louis University School of Medicine
St. Louis, Missouri
(Chapter 21)

Ghazala Hayat, MD
Professor of Neurology
Division of Neurology
Department of Neurology and Psychiatry
Saint Louis University School of Medicine
St. Louis, Missouri
(Chapter 103)

Robert M. Heaney, MD
Professor of Internal Medicine
Associate Dean, Graduate Medical Education
Division of General Internal Medicine
Department of Internal Medicine
Saint Louis University School of Medicine
St. Louis, Missouri
(Chapter 4)

Steven C. Herrmann, MD, PhD
Adjunct Assistant Professor
Department of Pharmacological and
Physiological Science
Saint Louis University School of Medicine
St. Louis, Missouri
Director of Cardiovascular Services
Bradford Regional Medical Center
Bradford, Pennsylvania
(Chapter 29)

Margaret Hochreiter, MD, PhD
Associate Professor of Internal Medicine
Division of General Internal Medicine
Department of Internal Medicine
Saint Louis University School of Medicine
St. Louis, Missouri
(Chapter 8)

Christopher N. Hueser, DO, MS
Fellow in Hematology and Oncology
Division of Hematology and Oncology
Department of Internal Medicine
Saint Louis University School of Medicine
St. Louis, Missouri
(Chapter 70)

Syed Huq, MD, MS
Fellow in Hematology and Medical Oncology
Division of Hematology and Medical Oncology
Department of Internal Medicine
Columbia School of Medicine
University of Missouri—Columbia School
of Medicine
Columbia, Missouri
(Chapter 72)

Catherine Iasiello, MD
Fellow in Hematology and Medical Oncology
Division of Hematology and Medical Oncology
Department of Internal Medicine
Ellis Fischel Cancer Center
Columbia School of Medicine
University of Missouri—Columbia School
of Medicine
Columbia, Missouri
(Chapter 59)

Sundeep Jayaprabhu, MD
Resident in Psychiatry
Division of Neurology
Department of Neurology and Psychiatry
Saint Louis University School of Medicine
St. Louis, Missouri
(Chapter 108)

Seema Joshi, MD
Fellow in Geriatric Medicine
Division of Geriatric Medicine
Department of Internal Medicine
Saint Louis University School of Medicine
St. Louis, Missouri
(Chapter 17)

Jeffrey Kao, MD
Resident in Psychiatry
Division of Psychiatry
Department of Neurology and Psychiatry
Saint Louis University School of Medicine
St. Louis Missouri
(Chapter 111)

Donald J. Kennedy, MD
Professor of Internal Medicine
Division of Infectious Diseases
Department of Internal Medicine
Saint Louis University School of Medicine
St. Louis, Missouri
(Chapters 85–100)

C. Daniel Kingsley, MD
Fellow in Hematology and Medical Oncology
Division of Hematology and Medical Oncology
Department of Internal Medicine
Columbia School of Medicine
University of Missouri—Columbia School
of Medicine
Columbia, Missouri
(Chapters 61, 82, 83)

Ganesh C. Kudva, MD, MRCP (UK)
Assistant Professor of Internal Medicine
Division of Hematology and Oncology
Department of Internal Medicine
Saint Louis University School of Medicine
St. Louis, Missouri
(Chapter 63)

Stephen Kuehn, MD
Fellow in Cardiology
Division of Cardiology
Department of Internal Medicine
Saint Louis University School of Medicine
St. Louis, Missouri
(Chapter 42)

Abhay Laddu, MD
Fellow in Cardiology
Division of Cardiology
Department of Internal Medicine
Saint Louis University School of Medicine
St. Louis, Missouri
(Chapter 45)

Jennifer Lash, MD
Fellow in Cardiology
Division of Cardiology
Department of Internal Medicine
Saint Louis University School of Medicine
St. Louis, Missouri
(Chapter 39)

Bahaeldeen A. Laz, MD
Staff Physician, St. John's Hospital
Department of Internal Medicine
Division of Endocrinology
Lake St. Louis, Missouri
(Chapter 51)

Kenneth Patrick L. Ligaray, MD
Fellow in Endocrinology
Division of Endocrinology
Department of Internal Medicine
Saint Louis University School of Medicine
St. Louis, Missouri
(Chapter 47)

Allison Lisle, MD
Resident in Pathology
Department of Pathology
Columbia School of Medicine
University of Missouri—Columbia School
of Medicine
Columbia, Missouri
(Chapter 71)

Christopher R. Longnecker, MD
Assistant Professor of Internal Medicine
Division of Cardiology
Department of Internal Medicine
Saint Louis University School of Medicine
St. Louis, Missouri
(Chapter 37)

Jothika N. Manepalli, MD
Associate Professor of Psychiatry
Division of Psychiatry
Department of Neurology and Psychiatry
Saint Louis University School of Medicine
St. Louis, Missouri
(Chapter 110)

Kevin J. Martin, MB, BCh, FACP
Professor of Internal Medicine
Saint Louis University School of Medicine
Director, Division of Nephrology
St. Louis, Missouri
(Chapter 118)

George M. Matuschak, MD
Professor of Pharmacological and Physiological
Science
James B. Miller and Ethyl D. Miller Professor
of Internal Medicine
Director, Division of Pulmonary, Critical Care,
and Sleep Medicine
Department of Internal Medicine
Saint Louis University School of Medicine
St. Louis, Missouri
(Chapters 112–116)

Deryk McDowell, MD
Fellow in Cardiology
Department of Internal Medicine
Saint Louis University School of Medicine
St. Louis, Missouri
(Chapter 30)

Scott W. McGee, MD
Fellow in Hematology and Medical Oncology
Division of Hematology and Medical Oncology
Department of Internal Medicine
Ellis Fischel Cancer Center
Columbia School of Medicine
University of Missouri—Columbia School
of Medicine
Columbia, Missouri
(Chapters 60, 64)

Nancy F. McKinney, MD
Fellow in Hematology and Medical Oncology
Division of Hematology and Medical Oncology
Department of Internal Medicine
Ellis Fischel Cancer Center
Columbia School of Medicine
University of Missouri—Columbia School
of Medicine
Columbia, Missouri
(Chapters 74, 81)

Gina L. Michael, MD
Assistant Professor of Medicine
Division of General Internal Medicine
Department of Internal Medicine
Saint Louis University School of Medicine
St. Louis, Missouri
(Chapter 8)

Peter Mikolajczak, MD
Fellow in Cardiology
Division of Cardiology
Department of Internal Medicine
Saint Louis University School of Medicine
St. Louis, Missouri
(Chapter 44)

Francis A. Mithen, MD, PhD
Professor of Neurology
Division of Neurology
Department of Neurology and Psychiatry
Saint Louis University School of Medicine
St. Louis, Missouri
(Chapter 102)

Terry L. Moore, MD
Professor of Internal Medicine, Pediatrics, and
Molecular Microbiology and Immunology
Director, Division of Rheumatology and
Pediatric Rheumatology
Department of Internal Medicine
Saint Louis University School of Medicine
St. Louis, Missouri
(Chapters 130, 132)

John E. Morley, MB, BCh
Professor of Internal Medicine
Director, Division of Geriatric Medicine
Geriatric Research, Education and Clinical
Center
St. Louis VA Medical Center
Saint Louis University School of Medicine
St. Louis, Missouri
(Chapters 15, 18)

Joanne E. Mortimer, MD
Professor of Medicine
Deputy Director for Clinical Affairs
Division of Hematology and Oncology
Department of Internal Medicine
Moores Cancer Center
University of California—San Diego School
of Medicine
La Jolla, California
(Chapter 76)

Chinya Murali, MD
Staff Physician, Department of Psychiatry
St. Louis VA Medical Center
St. Louis, Missouri
(Chapter 22)

Rajesh R. Nair, MD
Fellow in Hematology and Oncology
Division of Hematology and Oncology
Department of Internal Medicine
Saint Louis University School of Medicine
St. Louis, Missouri
(Chapter 60)

Ravi P. Nayak, MD
Assistant Professor of Internal Medicine
Division of Pulmonary, Critical Care, and Sleep
Medicine
Saint Louis University School of Medicine
St. Louis, Missouri
(Chapter 113)

Stacy Neff, DO
Resident in Psychiatry
Division of Psychiatry
Department of Neurology and Psychiatry
Saint Louis University School of Medicine
St. Louis, Missouri
(Chapter 109)

Gideon Nesher, MD
Head, Department of Internal Medicine and
Rheumatology Service
Shaare-Zedek Medical Center
Jerusalem, Israel
Clinical Associate Professor of Medicine
Hebrew University Medical School
Jerusalem, Israel
Adjunct Professor
Division of Rheumatology
Department of Internal Medicine
Saint Louis University School of Medicine
St. Louis, Missouri
(Chapter 127)

Robert Neumayr, MD
Fellow in Cardiology
Division of Cardiology
Department of Internal Medicine
Saint Louis University School of Medicine
St. Louis, Missouri
(Chapter 43)

Thomas J. Olsen, MD, FACP
Professor of Internal Medicine
Division of General Internal Medicine
Department of Internal Medicine
Saint Louis University School of Medicine
St. Louis, Missouri
(Chapters 1, 7, 9)

M. Louay Omran, MD
Assistant Professor of Internal Medicine
Division of Gastroenterology and Hepatology
Department of Internal Medicine
Saint Louis University School of Medicine
St. Louis, Missouri
(Chapter 53–56)

Wilman Ortega, MD
Assistant Professor of Internal Medicine
Division of Pulmonary, Critical Care, and Sleep
Medicine
Department of Internal Medicine
Saint Louis University School of Medicine
St. Louis, Missouri
(Chapter 114)

Thomas G. Osborn, MD
Associate Professor of Medicine
Division of Rheumatology
Department of Medicine
Mayo Clinic College of Medicine
Rochester, Minnesota
(Chapter 131)

Rami Owera, MD
Fellow in Hematology and Medical Oncology
Division of Hematology and Medical Oncology
Department of Internal Medicine
Ellis Fischel Cancer Center
Columbia School of Medicine
University of Missouri—Columbia School
of Medicine
Columbia, Missouri
(Chapters 68, 78)

Peri Hickman Pepmueller, MD
Associate Professor of Internal Medicine and
Pediatrics
Division of Rheumatology
Department of Internal Medicine
Saint Louis University School of Medicine
St. Louis, Missouri
(Chapter 129)

Michael C. Perry MD, MS, MACP
Professor of Internal Medicine and Director
Division of Hematology and Medical Oncology
Department of Internal Medicine
Ellis Fischel Cancer Center
Columbia School of Medicine
University of Missouri—Columbia School
of Medicine
Columbia, Missouri
(Chapters 60, 73, 80, 84)

Marian Petrides, MD
Associate Professor of Clinical Pathology
Medical Director, Transfusion Service and
Coagulation Laboratory
Department of Pathology and Anatomical
Sciences
Columbia School of Medicine
University of Missouri—Columbia School
of Medicine
Columbia, Missouri
(Chapter 71)

Paul Petruska, MD
Professor of Internal Medicine
Division of Hematology and Oncology
Department of Internal Medicine
Saint Louis University School of Medicine
St. Louis, Missouri
(Chapter 69)

Marie D. Philipneri, MD, MPH
Assistant Professor of Internal Medicine
Division of Nephrology
Department of Internal Medicine
Saint Louis University School of Medicine
St. Louis, Missouri
(Chapter 121)

Paisith Piriyawat, MD
Assistant Professor of Neurology
Division of Neurology
Department of Neurology and Psychiatry
Saint Louis University School of Medicine
St. Louis, Missouri
(Chapter 101)

Joseph Polizzi, MD
Fellow in Cardiology
Division of Cardiology
Department of Internal Medicine
Saint Louis University School of Medicine
St. Louis, Missouri
(Chapter 38)

Nora L. Porter, MD, MPH
Associate Professor of Internal Medicine
Division of General Internal Medicine
Department of Internal Medicine
Saint Louis University School of Medicine
St. Louis, Missouri
(Chapters 3, 4)

Rizwan A. Qazi, MD
Assistant Professor of Internal Medicine
Division of Nephrology
Department of Internal Medicine
Saint Louis University School of Medicine
St. Louis, Missouri
(Chapters 122, 124)

Osama Qubaiah, MD
Fellow in Hematology and Oncology
Division of Hematology and Oncology
Department of Internal Medicine
Saint Louis University School of Medicine
St. Louis, Missouri
(Chapter 69)

Arun Rajan, MD
Fellow in Hematology and Oncology
Division of Hematology and Oncology
Department of Medicine
Upstate Medical University
State University of New York
Syracuse, New York
(Chapter 60)

Hans-Joachim Reimers, MD, PhD, FAHA
Professor of Internal Medicine
Division of Hematology and Oncology
Department of Internal Medicine
Saint Louis University School of Medicine
St. Louis, Missouri
(Chapter 62)

Timothy Rice, MD
Associate Professor of Internal Medicine
Division of General Internal Medicine
Department of Internal Medicine
Saint Louis University School of Medicine
St. Louis, Missouri
(Chapter 2)

Musab U. Saeed, MD
Fellow in Infectious Diseases
Division of Infectious Diseases
Department of Internal Medicine
Saint Louis University School of Medicine
St. Louis, Missouri
(Chapters 85–87, 90, 93, 95, 96, 100)

Huda Salman, MD
Assistant Professor of Internal Medicine
Division of Hematology and Oncology
Department of Internal Medicine
Saint Louis University School of Medicine
St. Louis, Missouri
(Chapters 60, 75)

Paul G. Schmitz, MD, FACP
Professor of Internal Medicine
Saint Louis University School of Medicine
Department of Internal Medicine
St. Louis, Missouri
(Chapters 119, 125)

Alan B. Silverberg, MD
Professor of Internal Medicine
Division of Endocrinology
Department of Internal Medicine
Saint Louis University School of Medicine
St. Louis, Missouri
(Chapter 50)

Harmeeta K. Singh, MD
Resident in Psychiatry
Division of Psychiatry
Department of Neurology and Psychiatry
Saint Louis University School of Medicine
St. Louis, Missouri
(Chapter 110)

Raymond G. Slavin, MD, MS
Professor of Internal Medicine and Molecular
Microbiology and Immunology
Director, Division of Allergy and Immunology
Department of Internal Medicine
Saint Louis University School of Medicine
St. Louis, Missouri
(Chapters 24, 25, 26)

Richard E. Stewart, MD
Associate Professor of Medicine
Division of Cardiovascular Medicine
Department of Internal Medicine
University of North Texas Health Science
Center
Fort Worth, Texas
(Chapter 36)

Aaron Tang
Senior Medical Student
Saint Louis University School of Medicine
St. Louis, Missouri
(Chapter 45)

Syed H. Tariq, MD
Associate Professor of Internal Medicine
Division of Geriatric Medicine
Department of Internal Medicine
Geriatric Research, Education and Clinical
Center
St. Louis VA Medical Center
Saint Louis University School of Medicine
St. Louis, Missouri
(Chapter 21)

Katherine K. Temprano, MD
Assistant Professor of Internal Medicine
Division of Rheumatology
Department of Internal Medicine
University of Kentucky School of Medicine
Lexington, Kentucky
(Chapter 126)

David R. Thomas, MD
Professor of Internal Medicine
Division of Geriatric Medicine
Department of Internal Medicine
Saint Louis University School of Medicine
St. Louis, Missouri
(Chapter 19)

Florian P. Thomas, MD, MA, PhD
Professor of Neurology and Psychiatry
Associate Professor of Molecular Virology and
Molecular Microbiology and Immunology
Division of Neurology
Department of Neurology and Psychiatry
Associate Chief of Staff, St. Louis VA Medical
Center
Saint Louis University School of Medicine
St. Louis, Missouri
(Chapter 104)

Sri Laxmi Valasareddi, MD
Fellow in Hematology and Medical Oncology
Division of Hematology and Medical Oncology
Department of Internal Medicine
Ellis Fischel Cancer Center
Columbia School of Medicine
University of Missouri—Columbia School
of Medicine
Columbia, Missouri
(Chapter 65)

Vamsidhar Velcheti, MD
Department of Internal Medicine
Division of Oncology
Department of Internal Medicine
Washington University School of Medicine
St. Louis, Missouri
(Chapter 77)

H. Douglas Walden, MD, MPH
Professor of Internal Medicine
Division of General Internal Medicine
Department of Internal Medicine
Saint Louis University School of Medicine
St. Louis, Missouri
(Chapters 3, 5)

Allison P. Wall, MD
Fellow in Hematology and Oncology
Division of Hematology and Oncology
Department of Internal Medicine
Saint Louis University School of Medicine
St. Louis, Missouri
(Chapter 60)

David J. Walsh, MD
Associate Professor of Neurology
Division of Neurology
Department of Neurology and Psychiatry
Saint Louis University School of Medicine
St. Louis, Missouri
(Chapter 106)

Kent R. Wehmeier, MD
Associate Professor of Internal Medicine
Division of Endocrinology
Department of Internal Medicine
Primary Care Service Line
St. Louis VA Medical Center
Saint Louis University School of Medicine
St. Louis, Missouri
(Chapters 48, 49)

Robert M. Woolsey, MD
Professor of Neurology
Saint Louis University
Director, Spinal Cord Injury/Dysfunction
Service
Saint Louis VA Medical Center

Zhiwei Zhang, MD
Assistant Professor of Internal Medicine
Division of Nephrology
Department of Internal Medicine
Renal Section
St. Louis VA Medical Center
Saint Louis University School of Medicine
St. Louis, Missouri
(Chapter 120)

PREFACE

"Just the facts, ma'am." Stan Freburg's parody of the police procedural drama *Dragnet* is instantly recognizable five decades later, even to those who have never seen or heard of the program. *Internal Medicine: Just the Facts* is our effort to provide the student, resident in training, and practicing clinician with objective, practical information through a carefully structured format. Accordingly, this textbook reflects the core information that the busy practitioner, medical student, or resident should master. This text should prove especially useful to healthcare providers preparing for certification and recertification examinations. The structured format necessarily lessens the emphasis on the underlying science of medicine, such as molecular biology, cell biology, and pathophysiology; however, the contributors were careful to include succinct discussions of these pertinent biological principles where appropriate. For an in-depth discussion of the biological basis of disease, the interested reader is referred to standard comprehensive textbooks of internal medicine. One may rightfully think of this book as a high-yield clinical rendering of those standard textbooks.

This textbook covers the totality of internal medicine through 15 unique sections. Each section was designed to maximize the acquisition of practical information involved in the everyday care of patients. Sections 1 through 3 are intrinsically interdisciplinary in nature, and therefore should prove useful to all involved in delivering quality care. The growth of evidence-based medicine provided the stimulus for Section 2, which covers the basic principles vital to the interpretation of the medical literature. Section 3 is devoted exclusively to the unique problems encountered in the older patient. Sections 4 through 15, each expertly written and edited by leaders in the field, cover the subspecialty areas that the practicing physician must comprehend. The references for each section, while short in number, are designed to furnish the healthcare provider with high-impact, evidence-based data or scholarly summaries of the clinical problems likely to be encountered in the practice setting. With the proliferation of information available via the Internet, the authors were compelled to include Web site links, where appropriate. The blueprint for the subspecialty sections was based on an exhaustive review of the medical literature, coupled with extensive feedback from academic faculty, primary care providers, residents, and medical students.

We hope that you enjoy this focused, yet comprehensive approach to the study and practice of internal medicine. To that end, we encourage you, the reader, to let us know what we have done right, and what we could improve on in our commitment to creating an information resource that is useful to the busy practitioner.

Paul G. Schmitz
Kevin J. Martin

ACKNOWLEDGMENTS

The editors wish to thank the many faculty, fellows, residents, and medical students who generously contributed their suggestions and expertise to the chapters for this first edition. Paul wishes to thank his family, Beth, Hannah, and Zachary, for their unwavering support during the preparation of this manuscript and their sublime tolerance of the chaotic nature of academia. He also wishes to thank the many people who have contributed to his growth as an educator and academician, including Morris Davidman, William Keene, Michael O'Donnell, Coy Fitch, and, importantly, his co-editor, Kevin Martin. Many thanks to our colleagues at McGraw Hill, especially Jim Shanahan and Peter Boyle. A special thanks to Diane Goebel for coordinating the overall process from our office in St. Louis. We appreciate her thoughtful attention to detail and willingness to frequently adjust her schedule to accommodate our updates and changes.

INTERNAL MEDICINE
Just the Facts

Section 1
INTERDISCIPLINARY MEDICINE

1 MEDICAL PROFESSIONALISM

Thomas J. Olsen

PHYSICIAN CHARTER

In February 2002, *Medical Professionalism in the New Millennium: A Physician Charter* was published by the European Federation of Internal Medicine, the American College of Physicians, and the American Board of Internal Medicine. This Charter reaffirmed three fundamental and universal principles and values of medical professionalism. The Charter held these to be ideals that should be pursued by all physicians and identified 10 commitments as professional responsibilities of the physician.

DEFINITION OF PROFESSION

A profession is an occupation based on mastery of a complex body of knowledge and skills. It is a vocation in which the practice of an art is used in the service of others. Traditional professions include doctors, teachers, lawyers, and members of the clergy. Members of a profession profess a commitment to competence, integrity and morality, altruism, and promotion of the common good. These commitments form the basis of a contract between the medical profession and society. Society grants the profession the right to autonomy in practice and the privilege of self-regulation.

A physician is a professional who has mastered special knowledge and skills. These include anatomy, physiology, diagnosis, treatment, communication, coordination of care, and knowledge of healthcare systems. Some believe that this knowledge is not proprietary and that the profession holds this knowledge in trust for the good of society. The physician is granted special privileges including interviewing, examining, and treating patients. Physicians probe the body, mind, and spirit of a patient. These special privileges also include prescription of narcotics and dangerous drugs and surgery. Physicians have special responsibilities including placing the interests of the patient and society above their own, caring for the sick and suffering and regulating the behavior of the members of the profession. The American Board of Internal Medicine defines medical professionalism as those attributes and behaviors that serve to maintain patient interest and welfare above physician self-interest. These include altruism, accountability, excellence, duty, service, honor, integrity, and respect for others.

FUNDAMENTAL PRINCIPLES

PRIMACY OF PATIENT WELFARE

The medical profession commits to the education and training of a continuous supply of competent physicians. Laws govern licensure and prescription of medications. The profession oversees training, certification, accreditation, and hospital privileges. Physicians are committed to beneficence and act in the best interest of the patient. They promise nonmaleficence and protect patients from harm. The profession makes a commitment to its members and to society that it will develop systems to identify and treat impaired physicians.

PATIENT AUTONOMY

Physicians demonstrate respect for individual autonomy and foster informed decision making through patient education. Physicians recognize the autonomy of patients to provide informed consent and informed refusal. Physicians should respect informed decisions made by patients and families provided they are ethically sound and do not lead to demands for inappropriate care. Truth telling and confidentiality are fundamental tenets of medical

1

care. The physician respects the privacy of patients, encourages them to seek medical care and discuss their problems candidly and prevents discrimination on the basis of their medical conditions.

SOCIAL JUSTICE

Physicians must be committed to promoting equity in healthcare including improving access to care and a just distribution of finite resources. Physicians must work to eliminate discrimination of healthcare services based on race, gender, socioeconomic status, sexual orientation, ethnicity, or religion.

PROFESSIONAL COMMITMENTS

The Physician Charter identified a set of "definitive professional responsibilities." These are commitments that cross cultural, religious, and national borders. These are the means by which physicians provide for the care of patients and meet the needs of the communities in which they live and work.

Professional competence
Honesty with patients
Patient confidentiality
Maintaining appropriate relations with patients
Improving quality of care
Improving access to care
Just distribution of finite resources
Scientific knowledge
Maintaining trust by managing conflict of interest
Professional responsibilities
Threats to professionalism

Some might ask why a profession that is thousands of years old needs to be reminded of its fundamental principles. Threats to professionalism have come in the form of commodification of healthcare, managed care, and economic market forces, and emphasis on quantity not quality of patient care. In educational settings, emphasis on service over learning and institutional culture can contribute. Technologic advances challenge the ability of the profession to appropriately integrate new treatments in a cost effective and appropriate manner. Inequities in access to medical care affect both individual health and the health of society.

Summary from the Charter on Medical Professionalism

The practice of medicine in the modern era is beset with unprecedented challenges in virtually all cultures and societies. These challenges center on increasing disparities among the legitimate needs of patients, the available resources to meet those needs, the increasing dependence on market forces to transform healthcare systems, and the temptation for physicians to forsake their traditional commitment to the primacy of patients' interests. To maintain the fidelity of medicine's social contract during this turbulent time, physicians must reaffirm their active dedication to the principles of professionalism, which entails not only their personal commitment to the welfare of their patients but also collective efforts to improve the healthcare system for the welfare of society.

BIBLIOGRAPHY

American Board of Internal Medicine, American College of Physicians-American Society of Internal Medicine, European Federation of Internal Medicine. Medical professionalism in the new millennium: a physician charter. *Ann Intern Med.* 2002;136(3):243–246.
Cruess RL, Creuss SR. Teaching medicine as a profession in the service of healing. *Acad Med.* 1997;72:941–952.
Pellegrino E, Thomasma D. *The Virtues in Medical Practice.* New York, NY: Oxford University Press; 1993:35.

2   DERMATOLOGY
Timothy Rice

"These people look, but they don't see, and they hear, but they don't understand." Luke 8:10 (Contemporary English Version of the Bible)

• When examining the skin, the untrained eye can identify a rash without characterizing the salient features. To illustrate this point, visualize your car dashboard or the face of your wristwatch. Without looking, sketch as many details of each item as you can recall. What are the numbers and interval on the speedometer? Does your dashboard have a tachometer and what numbers are on the tachometer or other gauges? Describe the numbers, intervals, and words on the face of your watch. These exercises illustrate the pitfalls of thoroughly examining and describing the features of an item (or skin finding). Accordingly, an accurate description of dermatologic findings requires practice and patience. By carefully examining the skin and describing the features of the lesions in detail the clinician will be prepared to render a plausible diagnosis, or at the least communicate findings to an experienced consultant.

PRIMARY SKIN LESIONS

- An understanding of terminology is essential to accurately describe lesions and recognize morphology. A list of descriptive terms and examples of dermatologic conditions that exhibit these findings is enumerated below:
  - Macule: Flat, <1-cm lesion with a color that differs from the surrounding skin (eg, freckle, flat moles, port-wine stains, rickettsial rash, rubella, measles, vitiligo, tinea versicolor).
  - Patch: Flat >1-cm lesion with a color that differs from the surrounding skin (eg, Café-au-lait).
  - Papule: Solid <1-cm raised lesion, such as a closed comedone, or whitehead, in acne, warts, molluscum contagiosum, psoriasis, syphilitic chancre, urticaria, lichen planus, insect bites, contact dermatitis, seborrheic keratoses, and actinic keratoses.
  - Nodule: Solid 1- to 5-cm raised lesion (eg, dermal nevus, xanthomas, epitheliomas, metastatic cancer).
  - Tumor: Solid, >5-cm raised lesion (eg, mycosis fungoides, small lipomas, fibromas, erythema nodosum, larger epitheliomas).
  - Plaque: Raised, flat-topped >1-cm lesion (eg, eczematous dermatitis, pityriasis rosea, tinea corporis, psoriasis, seborrheic dermatitis, urticaria, condylomata lata of secondary syphilis, gumma of tertiary syphilis, erythema multiforme, lichen simplex chronicus).
  - Vesicle: Clear, fluid-filled <1-cm raised lesion; appears translucent (eg, allergic contact dermatitis, physical trauma, sunburn, thermal burn, herpes, varicella).
  - Bulla: Fluid-filled, >1-cm lesion; often translucent (eg, drug eruptions, pemphigus, dermatitis herpetiformis, erythema multiforme, epidermolysis bullosa, and bullous pemphigoid).
  - Pustule: Pus-filled lesion. Importantly, there are many pustular lesions that are not infectious (eg, impetigo, acne, folliculitis, furuncles, carbuncles, deep fungal infections, hidradenitis suppurativa, kerion, pustular miliaria, and pustular psoriasis of the palms and soles).
  - Cyst: Soft, raised sack filled with semisolid or liquid material. (eg, acne, sebaceous cysts).
  - Wheal: Short-lived, raised, erythematous papule or plaque that migrates to adjacent areas over several hours (eg, urticaria).
- Figure 2–1 schematically depicts several common primary skin lesions.

SECONDARY SKIN LESIONS

- Primary skin lesions can transform after secondary manipulation (scratching) or as a result of superimposed infection.
  - Scale: Shedding of dead epidermal cells (eg, greasy scale-dandruff, dry scale; psoriasis, tinea versicolor, pityriasis rosea).

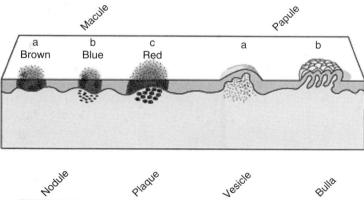
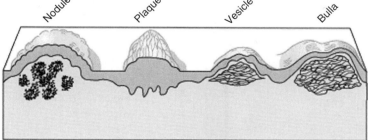

FIG. 2–1 Schematic representation of several common primary skin lesions. Reproduced with permission from Lawley TJ, Yancey KB: Approach to the patient with a skin disorder. In Kasper DL, Braunwald E, Fauci AS, et al. *Harrison's Principles of Internal Medicine.* 16th ed. New York, NY: McGraw-Hill; 2004.

○ Lichenification: Thickening of the skin with accentuated skin-fold markings (eg, atopic dermatitis, lichen simplex chronicus) (Fig. 2–2).

○ Crust: Dried exudate of body fluids—serous (yellow) exudate or hemorrhagic (red) exudate (eg, honey-colored crust is consistent with impetigo; crusts are also seen in scabies, pediculosis, or creeping eruption).

○ Erosion: Loss of the epidermis without loss of the dermis. Erosions heal without scarring (eg, herpes virus lesions and pemphigus).

○ Ulcer: Extension into the dermis which promotes scarring (eg, chancre of primary syphilis, tertiary syphilis, stasis ulcers).

○ Excoriation: Scratching that produces linear, angular erosions (eg, scratched insect bites—scabies).

○ Atrophy: Loss of dermal or subcutaneous tissue produces a skin depression with an intact epidermis. Loss of epidermal tissue produces a shiny, delicate, wrinkled area of the skin.

○ Scar: Fibrous change in the skin caused by trauma or inflammation. Scaring in hair-bearing areas produce hair loss. Scars may be erythematous, hypopigmented, or hypertrophic.

○ Pruritus: Sensation on the skin that induces scratching (eg, atopic dermatitis, allergic contact dermatitis, xerosis, and aged skin). Systemic conditions associated with pruritus, without skin lesions include uremia, cholestasis, pregnancy, malignancy, polycythemia vera, hyperthyroidism, diabetes mellitus, and psychogenic.

○ Fissure: Deep, sharp skin break (eg, tinea pedis, congenital syphilis).

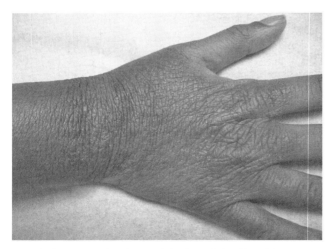

FIG. 2–2 Lichenification. Thickening of the skin with accentuated skin-fold markings in a patient with atopic dermatitis. Photo by Timothy Rice.

SPECIAL SKIN LESIONS

• Milia: 1-mm, firm, white papules filled with keratin (eg, may occur in newborns or in areas of trauma or inflammation).

• Telangiectasia: Small, superficial, dilated vessels (eg, rosacea, scleroderma, long-term topical steroid use, ataxia-telangiectasia, hereditary hemorrhagic telangiectasia, basal cell carcinoma).

• Spider angioma: Red, central punctate arteriole with telangiectatic network of dilated capillaries radiating from the center. On pressure, the lesion disappears and with release of pressure the radiating capillaries fill from the center punctuate arteriole out. This lesion has been described in cirrhosis, hyperestrogenic states (pregnancy), and after oral contraceptive use.

• Burrows: Tunnels in the epidermis (eg, small, short burrows—scabies; or tortuous, long burrows—creeping eruption from hook worm infection).

• Comedone or blackhead: Small, flesh-colored, white, or dark (blackhead) bumps at the opening of a sebaceous follicle (pore) (eg, acne).

DISEASES ASSOCIATED WITH A COMBINATION OF PRIMARY AND SECONDARY SKIN FINDINGS

SCALING PAPULAR DISEASES OR PAPULOSQUAMOUS DISEASES

• These lesions are characterized by sharp margins with no signs of epithelial disruption. Papulosquamous lesions are dry without crusts, fissures, or excoriation. These lesions can be the manifestation of a primary skin condition or can represent the dermatological manifestations of systemic disease. The primary papulosquamous diseases include:
  ○ Tinea
  ○ Psoriasis
  ○ Pityriasis rosea
  ○ Lichen planus
  ○ Pityriasis rubra pilaris

• Systemic diseases that are associated with papulosquamous lesions include:
  ○ Lupus erythematosus
  ○ Cutaneous T-cell lymphoma
  ○ Secondary syphilis
  ○ Reiter disease
  ○ Sarcoidosis

DISEASES ASSOCIATED WITH CRUSTING AND EXCORIATIONS

• Crust and excoriation usually result from infestation:
  ○ Scabies

○ Pediculosis
○ Creeping eruption from hook worm infection

COMMON BENIGN SKIN TUMORS

- Acrochordon (skin tag): Fleshy, brown, tan or skin colored pedunculated skin polyp.
- Cherry angioma: This is a blood-filled papule.
- Dermatofibroma: This is a firm red to brown nodule that produces a depression or *dimple* with lateral compression by the thumb and index finger.
- Epidermal cyst: An epidermal cyst arises when a hair follicle is obstructed with keratin and lipid-rich debris. This is the most common cutaneous cyst.
- Seborrheic keratosis: Seborrheic keratosis lesions are described as *stuck on* brown papules or plaques with a greasy texture. They are the most common of the benign epithelial tumors. These hereditary lesions do not appear until after age 30. New tumors continue to appear throughout the patient's lifetime.

- Lipoma: Soft, rounded tumor that is well-defined and easily movable both against the overlying skin and the underlying structures. Lipomas are the most common subcutaneous tumors.

ALGORITHM FOR EVALUATING SKIN LESIONS

An algorithm for evaluating skin lesions based on location is depicted in Fig. 2–3.

SKIN DISEASES BY LOCATION

The distribution of some common dermatologic diseases and lesions are depicted in Fig. 2–4.
- Scalp
  ○ Seborrhea
  ○ Tinea capitis
  ○ Psoriasis
  ○ Contact dermatitis
  ○ Folliculitis
  ○ Pediculosis

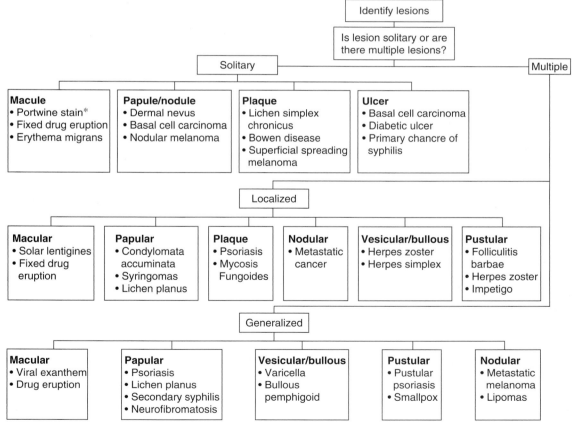

*Conditions labeled with dots are examples.

FIG. 2–3 Algorithm for evaluating skin lesions.
Reproduced with permission from Wolff K, Johnson RA, Suurmond D. *Fitzpatrick's Color Atlas and Synopsis of Clinical Dermatology*. 5th ed. New York, NY: McGraw-Hill; 2001.

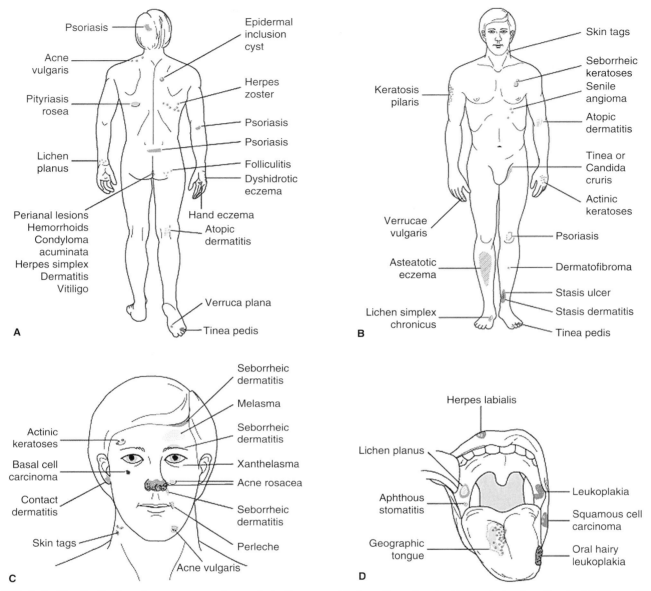

FIG. 2–4 The distribution of some common dermatologic diseases and lesions. Reproduced with permission from Lawley TJ, Yancey KB: Approach to the patient with a skin disorder. In: Kasper DL, Braunwald E, Fauci AS, et al. *Harrison's Principles of Internal Medicine.* 16th ed. New York, NY: McGraw-Hill; 2004.

- Face
  - Acne
  - Rosacea
  - Impetigo
  - Contact dermatitis
  - Lupus erythematosus
- Axillae
  - Contact dermatitis
  - Seborrheic dermatitis
  - Hidradenitis suppurativa
  - Acanthosis nigricans

- Flexural area: cubital and popliteal fossae
  - Atopic eczema
  - Contact dermatitis
  - Bullous pemphigoid
- Extensor area
  - Psoriasis
  - Atopic dermatitis (infants)
  - Dermatitis herpetiformis
- Hands
  - Atopic dermatitis
  - Dyshidrotic eczema

- ○ *Id* reaction from tinea pedis
- ○ Erythema multiforme
- ○ Psoriasis
- ○ Secondary syphilis (palms)
- Feet
  - ○ Tinea pedis
  - ○ Contact dermatitis
  - ○ Atopic dermatitis
  - ○ Dyshidrotic eczema
  - ○ Secondary syphilis (soles)
- Photo/sun exposure distribution
  - ○ Phototoxic dermatitis
    - ▪ Plants containing a furocoumarin (limes, parsley, celery, bishop's weed, and figs)
    - ▪ Drugs include thiazides, sulfonylureas, sulfonamides, tetracyclines, phenothiazines, psoralens, nalidixic acid, and nonsteroidal anti-inflammatory drugs
  - ○ Photoallergic reactions
    - ▪ Thiazides and benzocaine
  - ○ Metabolic disorders
    - ▪ Porphyria cutanea tarda
  - ○ Polymorphous light eruption
  - ○ Solar urticaria
  - ○ Dermatomyositis
  - ○ Porphyria cutanea tarda
  - ○ Systemic lupus erythematosus

SEASONAL DERMATOLOGIC DISEASES

- The following are conditions that occur with seasonal variation.
  - ○ Winter
    - ▪ Acne, folliculitis, psoriasis, atopic eczema, nummular eczema
  - ○ Spring
    - ▪ Actinic keratosis, seborrheic dermatitis, and pityriasis rosea
  - ○ Summer
    - ▪ Contact dermatitis caused by poison ivy, insect bites, and tinea versicolor (apparent increased intensity is sometimes noted because the surrounding skin may be tanned)
  - ○ Fall
    - ▪ Atopic dermatitis, contact dermatitis caused by ragweed and pityriasis rosea
  - ○ Day of the week variation
- Wednesday tends to be the day that patients present with contact dermatitis due to poison ivy. These patients are exposed while working in the yard or garden on Saturday or Sunday. The rash usually appears after 24 to 48 hours.

SKIN FINDINGS IN AILING PATIENTS

- Fever associated with a rash
  - ○ Generalized red rash
    - ▪ Drug eruptions
    - ▪ Viral exanthems
    - ▪ Rickettsial exanthems
    - ▪ Bacterial infections with toxin production
      - • Staphylococcal scalded skin syndrome (SSSS)
      - • Staphylococcal toxic shock syndrome (TSS)
      - • Staphylococcal food poisoning (enterotoxin)
      - • Scarlet fever
      - • Streptococcal TSS
      - • Cutaneous anthrax (usually secondary wound infection with streptococci or staphylococci)
  - ○ Blisters and prominent mouth lesions
    - ▪ Erythema multiforme (major)
  - ○ Generalized pustules
    - ▪ Generalized acute pustular psoriasis
    - ▪ Drug eruptions
  - ○ Generalized vesicles
    - ▪ Disseminated herpes simplex
    - ▪ Generalized herpes zoster
    - ▪ Varicella
  - ○ Generalized purpura
    - ▪ Nonpalpable purpura
      - • Purpura fulminans
    - ▪ Palpable purpura
      - • Bacterial endocarditis
  - ○ Multiple skin infarcts
    - ▪ Meningococcemia
    - ▪ Gonococcemia
  - ○ Facial inflammatory edema
    - ▪ Erysipelas
- Generalized red rash
  - ○ Fever
    - ▪ Drug eruptions
    - ▪ Viral exanthems
    - ▪ Rickettsial exanthems
    - ▪ Bacterial infections with toxin production
  - ○ Blisters and prominent mouth lesions
    - ▪ Erythema multiforme (major)
    - ▪ Toxic epidermal necrolysis
    - ▪ Bullous pemphigoid
    - ▪ Drug eruptions
  - ○ Pustules
    - ▪ Generalized acute pustular psoriasis
    - ▪ Drug eruptions
  - ○ Vesicles
    - ▪ Disseminated herpes simplex
    - ▪ Generalized herpes zoster
    - ▪ Varicella
    - ▪ Drug eruptions

- Generalized wheals and soft tissue swelling
  - Urticaria and angioedema
- Scaling over the entire body
  - Exfoliative erythroderma
- Without redness but with blisters, erosions, and mouth lesions
  - Pemphigus
- Generalized purpura
  - Nonpalpable purpura
    - Thrombocytopenia
    - Purpura fulminans
    - Drug eruptions
  - Palpable purpura
    - Vasculitis
    - Bacterial endocarditis
- Multiple skin infarcts
  - Meningococcemia
  - Gonococcemia
  - Disseminated intravascular coagulopathy
  - Fat embolism syndrome
- Localized skin infarcts
  - Calciphylaxis (calcific uremic arteriolopathy)
  - Atherosclerosis obliterans
  - Atheroembolization
  - Warfarin necrosis
  - Antiphospholipid antibody syndrome
- Facial inflammatory edema with fever
  - Erysipelas
  - Lupus erythematosus

DISTINCTIVE FEATURES OF SKIN AND SOFT TISSUE BACTERIAL INFECTIONS

- Impetigo
  - Honey-colored serous crust is classically described.
  - Variations in impetigo appearance is common, from small vesicles to large bulla.
  - Impetigo is the result of a superficial, cutaneous infection that must be differentiated from ecthyma, an infection that involves the dermis.
  - Impetigo is caused by *Staphylococcus aureus* and group A *Streptococcus pyogenes* (GAS).
  - Treatment for mild localized disease usually involves topical application of mupirocin ointment, although the topical approach is generally less effective than oral antibiotics. In advanced lesions or in patients not responding to topical antibiotics, oral antibiotics should be administered. Cephalexin, 250 mg four times daily; doxycycline, 100 mg twice daily; or cefadroxil 500 mg twice daily. Community-acquired methicillin-resistant *S. aureus* (CA-MRSA) may cause impetigo. In communities with a high incidence of CA-MRSA or MRSA, initial treatment options include trimethoprim-sulfamethoxazole or doxycycline.

- Erysipelas (Fig. 2–5)
  - Sharply marginated, painful, bright red, raised, edematous, indurated plaques with advancing raised borders emanating from the surrounding normal skin. Erysipelas frequently involves the central face.
  - Treatment: Intravenous antibiotics with coverage for group A hemolytic streptococci and staphylococci for 24 to 48 hours. With less severe disease or after initial intravenous (IV) therapy, oral dicloxacillin or cephalexin, 250 to 500 mg is administered four times daily for 7 to 10 days.
- Cellulitis
  - Cellulitis is characterized by lesions that are poorly demarcated, typically flat, erythematous, warm, and tender. The surrounding uninvolved skin appears normal.
  - Treatment: Intravenous antibiotics with activity against group A hemolytic streptococci and staphylococci for 24 to 48 hours. With less severe disease or following the initial IV therapy, oral dicloxacillin or cephalexin, 250 to 500 mg is administered four times daily for 7 to 10 days.
- Folliculitis, furuncles, and carbuncles
  - These three conditions represent a continuum from mild involvement to severe.

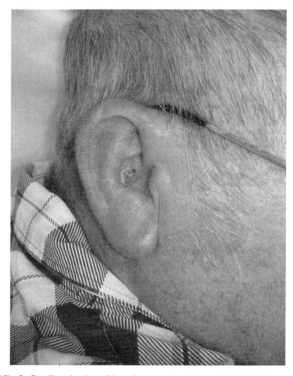

FIG. 2–5 Erysipelas. Sharply marginated, painful, bright red, raised, edematous, indurated plaque with advancing raised borders involving the ear and extending onto the face. Photo by Timothy Rice.

○ Usually caused by methicillin-susceptible *S. aureus*; MRSA infections are increasing in frequency.
○ Folliculitis.
  ▪ Infection of hair follicles
○ Furuncle (boil).
  ▪ Firm, tender, up to 1- to 2-cm nodule with a central necrotic plug
  ▪ Occurs in an area with existing folliculitis
  ▪ If recurrent consider colonization of the nose, perineum, and body folds with *S. aureus*
○ Carbuncles.
  ▪ These large lesions arise from coalescence of several adjacent furuncles.
○ Treatment: Incision and drainage is the mainstay of therapy. For moderate to severe lesions, the patient should also receive oral dicloxacillin or cephalexin, 250 to 500 mg four times daily for 10 days.
• Hidradenitis suppurativa
○ Chronic, recurring infection of the apocrine glands.
○ Usually localized to the axillae, but may also arise in the groin, perianal, and suprapubic area.
○ Treatment: Drainage of the lesions and meticulous hygiene. For severe recurrent hidradenitis, apocrine sweat-bearing skin may be surgically excised.
• Ecthyma
○ A vesicle or pustule that arises from a minor superficial break in the skin from excoriations, insect bites, or minor trauma. Often seen in diabetics, elderly patients (>60 years of age), active military personnel, and alcoholics.
○ Ecthyma progresses rapidly to the crusting stage.
○ Deeper cutaneous infections may occur and extend into the dermis.
○ *S. aureus* and GAS (*S. pyogenes*) are the usual micro-organisms associated with ecthyma.
○ The treatment requires antibiotic administration, usually cephalexin, 250 mg four times daily, doxycycline, 100 mg twice daily, or cefadroxil 500 mg twice daily for 5–7 days. When CA-MRSA or MRSA are suspected, initial antimicrobial treatment options include vancomycin, trimethoprim-sulfamethoxazole, or doxycycline.

CHARACTERISTICS OF CELLULITIS ASSOCIATED WITH SPECIFIC ORGANISMS

• *S. aureus*
○ Focal infection site of entry is usually obvious
• Group A *Streptococcus*
○ The incidence of invasive GAS is increasing
• Group B *Streptococcus* (*Streptococcus* agalactiae)
○ Anogenital cellulitis
○ Puerperal sepsis following childbirth

• *Streptococcus* pneumoniae (Pneumococcus)
○ Bulla, brawny erythema, violaceous hue
• Erysipeloid (*Erysipelothrix rhusiopathiae*)
○ Painful, swollen plaques with sharply defined irregular raised borders at the site of inoculation (eg, finger or hand, spreading to the wrist and forearm)
○ Color characteristics
  ▪ Acute lesions are characterized by purple-red hue
  ▪ With resolution the color changes to brown
○ Enlarges peripherally accompanied by central fading
○ Systemic symptoms are usually absent. In some patients with diffuse eruptions, systemic symptoms including arthritis and endocarditis may occur.
○ Usually develops after exposure to game, poultry, or fish (eg, butchers, veterinarians, or fishermen)
• *Pseudomonas aeruginosa*
○ Ecthyma gangrenosum
  ▪ The lesion begins as an erythematous macule (cutaneous ischemic lesion).
  ▪ Quickly evolving into a blue or gunmetal gray gangrenous plaque with an erythematous halo or frank necrosis.
  ▪ The epidermis overlying the ischemic area develops into a bulla. The epidermis eventually sloughs, resulting in an ulcer.
  ▪ The distribution of the lesion(s) usually involve the intertriginous areas: axilla, groin, perineum.
  ▪ Typically, there is a solitary lesion.
  ▪ Ecthyma gangrenosum has been described in *Pseudomonas septicemia.*
○ Rose spot lesions of *P. aeruginosa*
  ▪ These are characterized by erythematous macules and/or papules on trunk
  ▪ Seen with *Pseudomonas* infection of the gastrointestinal tract
○ Small embolic lesions secondary to *P. aeruginosa*
  ▪ Characterized by multiple painful nodules
  ▪ The lesions may cluster forming vesicular or bullous lesions
• *Haemophilus influenzae*
○ Violaceous erythema hue associated with swelling
○ Involve the cheek and periorbital areas
○ Children are the most susceptible
• *Vibrio vulnificus* and *Vibrio cholerae* (non-01 and non-0139 types)
○ Bulla formation and necrotizing vasculitis
○ Location: extremities; often bilateral
• *Aeromonas hydrophila*
○ The cellulitis occurs after water-associated trauma and usually involves a preexisting wound
○ The lesions are most common in an immunocompromised host
○ The lower leg is the most common site of involvement

- *Capnocytophaga canimorsus*
  - Bites or scratches from dogs in immunosuppressed patients (organ transplantation)
- *Pasteurella multocida B*
  - Bites from cats
- *Clostridium* species
  - Subcutaneous gas and severe systemic toxicity
  - Usually arises from wounds that are contaminated by soil or feces (*Mycobacterium chelonae–Mycobacterium fortuitum* complex)
  - Recent surgery, use of injectables, or following a penetrating wound
- *Cryptococcus neoformans*
  - Produces a red, hot, tender, edematous plaque on the extremity
  - Rarely involves multiple noncontiguous sites
  - Only observed in immunocompromised patients
  - This organism may also be associated with molluscum-like lesions, subcutaneous or mucosal lesions, pustules, and erythematous papules
- Cutaneous *Mucormycosis*
  - Characterized by a single, painful, indurated area
  - Progresses into an ecthyma-like lesion
  - Usually occurs in individuals with uncontrolled diabetes, organ transplantation, or neutropenia

DERMATOLOGIC EMERGENCIES

LIFE-THREATENING CONDITIONS

- Angioedema and urticaria
  - Characterized by swelling of the face, lips, and tongue which may contribute to airway obstruction.
  - Urticaria is a localized process, whereas, angioedema is more extensive and associated with bronchospasm and shock.
- Stevens-Johnson syndrome and toxic epidermal necrolysis
  - Stevens-Johnson syndrome is characterized by severe, intensely painful bullae and mucosal ulcerations with target-like lesions on the trunk.
  - Toxic epidermal necrolysis is characterized by fever, pruritus, pharyngitis, and conjunctivitis.
  - The painful rash usually begins on the upper trunk or face. Affected skin may be erythematous or exhibit bullae. The bullae may erode or the affected skin may slough into large sheets. Pressure on the bulla produces lateral extension of the blister known as Nikolsky sign.
  - The mucous membranes are involved in Stevens-Johnson syndrome and toxic epidermal necrolysis while spared in SSSS.

- Exfoliation and erythroderma
  - There are many underlying diseases that may be associated with these lesions. Psoriasis with its characteristic plaques and/or nail changes may develop erythroderma. Bullous pemphigoid typically presents with tense bullae in addition to erythroderma. Severe drug reactions may be associated with erythroderma. These patients appear acutely ill with fever, malaise, and lymphadenopathy. Other findings in patients with life-threatening erythroderma include leukocytosis with eosinophilia and organomegaly. Hepatic or renal impairment may also occur because of volume contraction, shock, and high-output cardiac failure.
- Staphylococcal scalded-skin syndrome
  - Staphylococcal scalded-skin syndrome may simply be characterized by localized eruption of a few fragile fluid-filled bullae surrounded by normal skin. Conversely, severe manifestations with widespread bullae may develop in some patients. Skin erosions can involve large areas resulting in open, painful lesions. A positive Nikolsky sign is present. The mucous membranes are spared in SSSS.

POTENTIALLY LIFE-THREATENING CONDITIONS

- Cellulitis and erysipelas
  - If untreated, both conditions can result in septicemia, local abscess formation, gangrene, and cavernous sinus thrombosis in patients with facial erysipelas.
- Pustular psoriasis
  - These patients manifest systemic symptoms (fever, chills) accompanied by multiple pustules and large areas of erythema. Pustular psoriasis mainly occurs in patients with pre-existing psoriasis.
  - Treatment involves hospitalization and emergent consultation with a dermatologist.
- Pemphigus vulgaris
  - Pemphigus vulgaris is characterized by superficial blistering initially in the oral mucous membranes, then extending to virtually any mucous membrane area. The lesions are fragile, and easily rupture. The underlying skin may be erythematous. Importantly, the blisters often slough prior to the clinical presentation leaving only ulcerations on examination. Involvement of the lower airway may result in hoarseness. A positive Nikolsky sign is present.
  - Treatment involves hospitalization and consultation with a dermatologist. Antibiotic treatment may be necessary if secondary infection is suspected. Lifelong immunosuppressive therapy may be required in the chronic form of this disease.

COMMON SKIN CONDITIONS

- Intertrigo
  - Intertrigo is an inflammatory condition of two closely opposed skin surfaces (intertriginous area) resulting from heat, moisture, and friction.
  - There are two major categories of intertrigo, one caused by *Candida* infection and a noninfectious category of intertrigo.
  - The lesions are erythematous with macerated plaques and erosions. Fine peripheral scaling and erythematous, papulopustular, satellite lesions may also accompany the primary lesion. The pustules rupture easily, leaving an erythematous base with a surrounding narrow rim of loosened keratin overhanging the edge of the ruptured pustule. The lesions are often pruritic. This condition may be painful especially with significant skin breakdown.
  - Treatment consists of topical antifungal cream as well as avoiding conditions that promote moisture accumulation between skin folds.
- Dermatophyte (tinea) infections of the scalp
  - Tinea capitis
    - Scalp dermatophyte infection is characterized by an erythematous, scaling, well-demarcated patch with hair loss.
    - A kerion is a boggy, elevated, tender nodule that is sometimes associated with tinea capitis.
    - Scalp dermatophyte infection is more common in children.
    - Infected hair stubs (Microsporum canis) fluoresce bright green under a Wood's ultraviolet lamp.
  - Black dot tinea capitis
    - Characterized by an asymptomatic, erythematous, scaling patch on the scalp, which slowly enlarges.
  - Treatment
    - Treatment with topical agents is ineffective.
    - The drug of choice is oral griseofulvin: 500 mg of microsized or 350 mg of ultramicrosized griseofulvin daily with a fatty meal for 6–12 weeks.
    - Terbinafine or itraconazole are alternatives in resistant cases
- Dermatophyte (tinea) infections of the body and feet
  - Tinea pedis (Figs. 2–6 and 2–7) involves the interdigital area in a moccasin-like pattern. The lesions between the digits may appear as dry scaling or moist, macerated pealing areas with fissures between the toes. The moccasin distribution of tinea exhibits hyperkeratotic features with abundant scaling and may be associated with onychomycosis. Other manifestations of tinea pedis include vesicular or bullous lesions on the feet. These features can be associated with autosensitization and an *id* reaction accompanied by vesicular lesions on the hands.

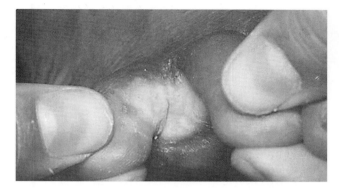

FIG. 2–6 Tinea pedis, interdigital macerated type. The web space between the fourth and fifth toes is hyperkeratotic and macerated in a black individual with plantar keratoderma and hyperhidrosis. The greenish hue is caused by *Pseudomonas aeruginosa* superinfection of this moist intertriginous site. Erythrasma also occurs in the setting of moist intertriginous sites and may occur concomitantly with interdigital tinea pedis or *Pseudomonas intertrigo*. Reproduced with permission from Wolff K, Johnson RA, Suurmond D. *Fitzpatrick's Color Atlas and Synopsis of Clinical Dermatology.* 5th ed. New York: McGraw-Hill; 2001.

- Tinea cruris is a dermatophyte that involves the groin, pubic area, and thighs. Large, well-demarcated plaques with scaling that is prominent at the edge with some central clearing may be noted. These plaques exhibit a dull red, tan, or brown color (Fig. 2–8).
- Tinea corporis (Fig. 2–9) is a dermatophyte that involves the trunk, legs, arms, and/or neck, excluding the feet, hands, and groin. Well-demarcated plaques with scaling at the edge and some central clearing is noted. The peripheral edge of the lesions gradually extends into the surrounding normal skin.

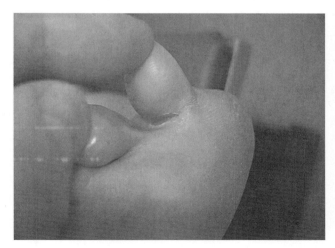

FIG. 2–7 Tinea pedis. The web space between the fourth and fifth toes is mildly hyperkeratotic, some scaling and a fissure. Photo by Timothy Rice.

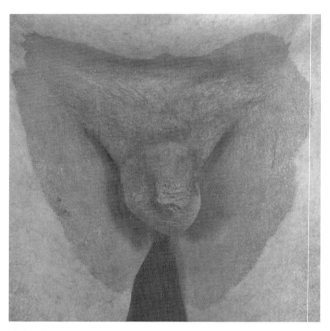

FIG. 2–8 Tinea cruris. Confluent, erythematous, scaling plaques on the medial thighs, inguinal folds, and pubic area. The margins are slightly raised and sharply marginated. Erythrasma should be ruled out by Wood lamp examination. Coral red fluorescence of intertriginous site confirms diagnosis of erythrasma. Reproduced with permission from Wolff K, Johnson RA, Suurmond D. *Fitzpatrick's Color Atlas and Synopsis of Clinical Dermatology.* 5th ed. New York, NY: McGraw-Hill; 2001.

The edge may or may not exhibit fine pustules or vesicles. The lesions may coalesce to produce a gyrate pattern.
○ For tinea infections any of the following agents should be applied twice daily to the involved area for 4 weeks and continued at least 1 week after lesions have completely cleared. Application should extend 3 cm beyond the edge of the lesions.
■ Clotrimazole (Lotrimin, Mycelex)
■ Miconazole (Micatin)
■ Ketoconazole (Nizoral)
■ Econazole (Spectazole)
■ Oxiconazole (Oxistat)
■ Sulconazole (Exelderm)
■ Naftifine (Naftin)
■ Terbinafine (Lamisil)
■ Tolnaftate (Tinactin)
■ Ciclopirox olamine (Loprox)
○ Nystatin is not effective against tinea infections.
• Tinea versicolor (pityriasis versicolor) (Figs. 2–10 and 2–11)
○ Tinea versicolor is a superficial infection of the skin caused by the the yeast *Malassezia furfur* resulting in multiple hypopigmented macules that coalesce into large confluent areas. Patients notice the lesions when the involved skin fails to tan in the summer. The lesions appear in a *rained-down* pattern more extensive on the shoulders and upper chest; lesions are less abundant further down.
○ Topical treatments for this condition include the following: Selenium sulfide (2.5%) lotion or shampoo or ketoconazole shampoo applied daily to the affected areas for 10 to 15 minutes, followed by cleansing (shower), for 1 week. Ketoconazole, econazole, miconazole, or clotrimazole applied daily or twice daily for 2 weeks is also effective.
○ Systemic therapy with ketoconazole 400 mg, fluconazole 400 mg, or itraconazole 400 mg is an alternative in refractory cases. These agents are

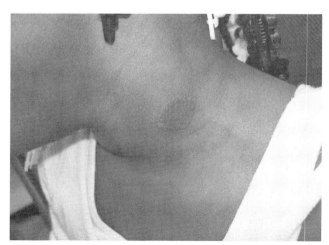

FIG. 2–9 Tinea corporis. Inflammatory annular plaque on a patient's neck with some central clearing. Photo by Timothy Rice.

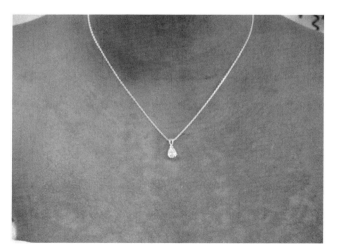

FIG. 2–10 Pityriasis versicolor. Sharply marginated brown macules on the trunk. Fine scale was apparent when the lesions were abraded with the edge of a microscope slide. Photo by Timothy Rice.

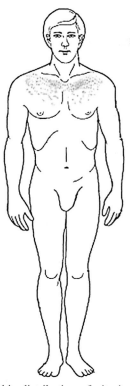

FIG. 2–11 Graphic distribution of pityriasis versicolor. Front and back have similar *rained down* distribution. Drawing by Timothy Rice.

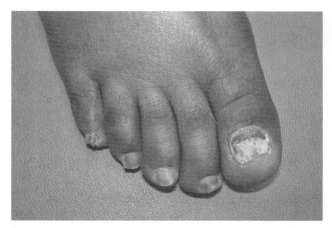

FIG. 2–12 Onychomycosis of toenails. The dorsal nail plate is chalky white. Photo by Timothy Rice.

administered 1 hour prior to exercise which promotes excretion of the antifungal in the sweat.

○ After treatment, the hypo- or hyperpigmentation of the rash may take months to blend in with the surrounding normal skin.

• Onychomycosis (Fig. 2–12)

○ Characterized by a yellowish discoloration of the nail with heaping of keratin resulting in separation of the nail from the nail bed

○ Systemic therapy is of limited benefit, in part because of toxicity (and expense). However, newer oral antifungal drugs (terbinafine and itraconazole) offer shorter treatment periods (oral antifungal medications usually are administered over a 3-month period), higher cure rates, and fewer side effects. Topical therapy is expensive and of limited efficacy (naftifine gel 1% or ciclopirox nail lacquer [Penlac] 8%).

• Differentiation of onychomycosis from onycholysis (psoriasis, trauma, chemicals, certain medications such as tetracycline, hyperthyroidism, and hypothyroidism) is important.

• Pediculosis (Fig. 2–13)

○ Pediculosis infestation presents with pruritus of the scalp and excoriation. Nits are observed on hair shafts and lice may be discovered in the scalp, skin, or clothing.

○ Permethrin 1% cream rinse (Nix) is applied to the scalp and hair and left in place for 8 hours before rinsing. A repeat treatment should be applied in 7 to 14 days. Malathion 0.5% in 78% isopropyl alcohol (Ovide) is an alternative prescription treatment. Malathion binds to the hair providing residual protection against recurrence. A second treatment may be given if live lice are seen a week or more after the first application.

○ Pruritus may persist after treatment but this is rarely a sign of treatment failure. Careful inspection for lice should be carried out to identify treatment failures. Nit removal is not required to cure the infestation.

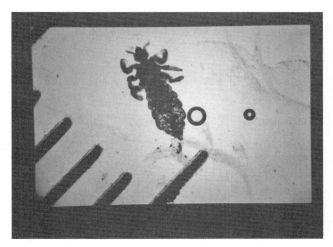

FIG. 2–13 Head lice. Adult louse *Pediculus humanus capitis* next to a millimeter ruler. Photo by Timothy Rice.

ACNE VULGARIS

- The hallmark of acne is the appearance of comedones. Acne may progress to an inflammatory stage with papules and pustules or may become cystic or nodular with subsequent scaring. Treatment of this condition depends on the severity of acne (Table 2–1).
- Comedonal acne
  - Closed comedones or *white heads* are tiny, flesh-colored, noninflamed bumps that give the skin a rough texture and appearance. *Blackheads* or open comedones typically are a bit larger, are noninflamed, and have black material at the ostia (Fig. 2–14).
  - Treatment typically involves the use of a mild soap to avoid irritation of the skin. Diet is not thought to contribute to acne. Treatment may be associated with a disease flair for the first 4 weeks.
  - Topical retinoids are the treatment of choice. Tretinoin 0.025% cream (not gel) twice weekly, increasing in frequency to nightly or as tolerated. If this is not tolerated, adapalene gel 0.1% or a reformulated tretinoin (Renova, Retin-A Micro, or Avita) or tazarotene gel (0.05% or 0.1%) (Tazorac) may be employed. Benzoyl peroxide once or twice daily may be added to topical retinoids. Topical antibiotics decrease the number of comedones.
  - Topical retinoids, tetracycline, minocycline, doxycycline, and isotretinoin are contraindicated in pregnancy.
- Papular inflammatory acne
  - Inflamed papules and pustules represent an advanced inflammatory stage of acne. Begin therapy with topical retinoids, however, antibiotics

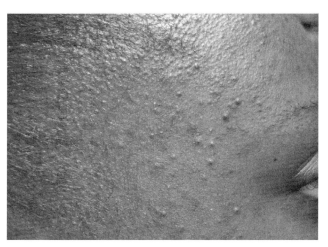

FIG. 2–14 Acne vulgaris. Comedones are keratin plugs in the follicles. Comedones with *white heads* are small or closed ostia. Comedones with large ostia, are referred open comedones or *blackheads*. Photo by Timothy Rice.

(topical and oral) are the mainstay of therapy for severe inflammatory acne. Treatment involves a combination of erythromycin or clindamycin with benzoyl peroxide topical gel. If there is no improvement in 4–6 weeks, oral antibiotics can be added. Antibiotic choices include minocycline, 50 to 100 mg twice daily, or doxycycline, 50 to 100 mg twice daily, which are tapered to 50 mg/day as the acne resolves. Other oral antibiotic choices include tetracycline, 500 mg twice daily, or erythromycin, 500 mg twice daily. These should also be tapered as the inflammatory component of acne improves (2 to 3 months).

TABLE 2–1   Acne Treatment Algorithm

	MILD		MODERATE		
	COMEDONAL	PAPULAR/PUSTULAR	PAPULAR/PUSTULAR	NODULAR	SEVERE, NODULAR
First-line therapy	Topical retinoid	Topical retinoid + BPO or BPO/AB	Topical retinoid + oral antibiotic + BPO or BPO/AB	Topical retinoid + oral antibiotic ± BPO or BPO/AB	Oral isotretinoin
Alternatives	Salicylic acid			Oral Isotretinoin	Oral antibiotic + topical retinoid + BPO or BPO/AB
Alternatives for female patients			Hormonal therapy + topical retinoid ± BPO or BPO/AB	Hormonal therapy + topical retinoid ± BPO or BPO/AB	Hormonal therapy + oral antibiotic + topical retinoid ± BPO or BPO/AB
Maintenance therapy	Topical retinoid ± BPO or BPO/AB		Topical retinoid ± BPO or BPO/AB		Topical retinoid ± BPO or BPO/AB

Reproduced with permission from Zaenglein AL, Thiboutot DM. Expert Committee recommendations for acne management. *Pediatrics* 2006;118;1188–1199.

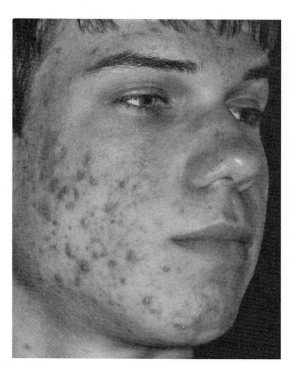

FIG. 2–15 Acne vulgaris. Papulopustular A spectrum of lesions is seen on the face of a 17-year-old male: comedones, papules, pustules, and erythematous macules and scars at site of resolving lesions. The patient was successfully treated with a 4-month course of isotretinoin; there was no recurrence over the next 5 years. Reproduced with permission from Wolff K, Johnson RA, Suurmond D. *Fitzpatrick's Color Atlas and Synopsis of Clinical Dermatology.* 5th ed. New York: McGraw-Hill; 2001.

- ○ Spironolactone (antiandrogen effect) and oral contraceptives with low androgenic activity may be useful in women when other treatments fail.
- • Severe cystic acne (Figs. 2–15 and 2–16)
  - ○ Scarring can occur as a result of large inflammatory cysts and nodules associated with severe cystic acne. A dermatology referral should be considered (Isotretinoin, Accutane treatment) to prevent scarring or if symptoms are not promptly controlled by the above measures.
- • Atopic dermatitis (eczema)
  - ○ Characterized by a pruritic, exudative rash in the antecubital and popliteal folds but may also involve the face, neck, upper trunk, wrists, or hands (Fig. 2–17). The edges of the eruptions do not have discrete margins. With longer duration, the lesions become lichenified from chronic scratching. The eruptions may become chronic or relapsing.
  - ○ Atopic dermatitis has been linked to atopic disease eg, asthma, allergic rhinitis.
  - ○ Instructing the patient to avoid rubbing or scratching the lesions is the first step in improving this condition.

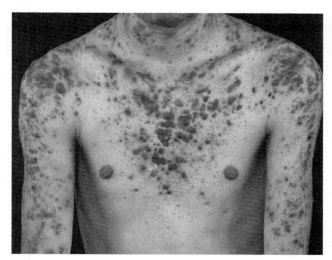

FIG. 2–16 Acne vulgaris: acne conglobata. Inflammatory nodules and cysts have coalesced forming abscesses and even leading to ulceration. There are multiple comedones and many recent red scars following resolution of inflammatory lesions on the upper chest, neck, and arms. Reproduced with permission from Wolff K, Johnson RA, Suurmond D. *Fitzpatrick's Color Atlas and Synopsis of Clinical Dermatology.* 5th ed. New York: McGraw-Hill; 2001.

- ○ Treatment to minimize xerosis consists of hydrating the skin with oil baths or baths with oatmeal powder followed promptly by patting the skin dry and applying a thin film of unscented emollient such as Aquaphor, Eucerin, or Vaseline. Treatment with topical low- to

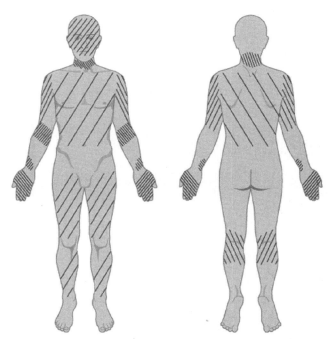

FIG. 2–17 Predilection sites of atopic dermatitis. Reproduced with permission from Wolff K, Johnson RA, Suurmond D. *Fitzpatrick's Color Atlas and Synopsis of Clinical Dermatology.* 5th ed. New York, NY: McGraw-Hill; 2001.

midpotency glucocorticoids should be used if hydration does not control the eruptions. Tacrolimus ointment and pimecrolimus cream are effective, but considered second-line therapies due to concerns over the potential risks of T-cell lymphomas.

○ Special attention should be paid to herpes simplex and to superimposed staphylococcal infection in patients with atopic dermatitis because they are at higher risk for the secondary complications of these infections.

○ Crusted and weeping skin lesions should be treated with oral antibiotics to eradicate *S. aureus.*

  ▪ Patients with eczema may develop a generalized herpes simplex infection referred to as *eczema herpeticum.* This condition is characterized by diffuse, monomorphic vesicles with crusts or erosions. It should be treated with oral acyclovir, 200 mg five times daily for 14–28 days (Fig. 2–18).

• Erythema nodosum

○ Erythema nodosum is characterized by painful red nodules on the anterior aspects of the legs.

○ Erythema nodosum usually lasts approximately 6 weeks and may recur.

○ Erythema nodosum is associated with a variety of micro-organisms including: streptococcus, coccidioidomycosis, other fungi (eg, histoplasmosis, blastomycosis), tuberculosis, syphilis, *Yersinia enterocolitica,* or *Yersinia pseudotuberculosis.*

○ Other conditions which may give rise to erythema nodosum include sarcoidosis, drugs (eg, oral contraceptives), inflammatory bowel disease, Behçet disease, pregnancy, lymphoma, or leukemia.

○ Further evaluation:
  ▪ Careful history for symptoms suggesting infections, pulmonary or gastrointestinal diseases. Rule out offending drugs
○ Further testing:
  ▪ Chest x-ray, partial protein derivative (PPD) testing, and two consecutive anti-streptolysin/anti-DNAase B titers 2 to 4 weeks apart

• Hidradenitis suppurativa (Fig. 2–19)

○ Hidradenitis suppurativa is a chronic, recurring infection of the apocrine glands.

○ It usually involves the axillae but may extend to the groin, perianal, and suprapubic areas.

○ Treatment involves drainage of the pustules and meticulous hygiene. For severe recurrent hidradenitis, apocrine sweat-bearing skin may be surgically excised.

• Lichen planus (Fig. 2–20)

○ Characterized by violaceous, scaly papules with small intersecting white streaks or lines (Wickham striae) that appear at sites of skin trauma or scratches (Koebner phenomenon).

○ Distribution: Flexural area of the wrist and ankles
  ▪ May become generalized and involve the penis or mucous membranes

○ Consider secondary syphilis if pruritus is absent in this condition.

○ Duration: Rash progresses over 2 to 3 weeks and resolves within 6 weeks.

○ Treatment: High-potency topical corticosteroids.

○ Prognosis: May last months or years and may recur.

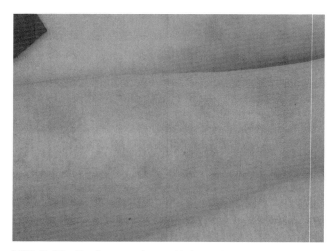

FIG. 2–18 Erythema nodosum. Indurated, very tender inflammatory nodules in the pretibial region. Photo from Timothy Rice and John Alex Holt.

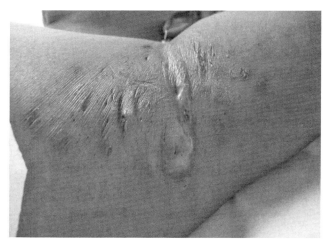

FIG. 2–19 Hidradenitis suppurativa. Axillae photo in a patient with chronic, recurring infection of the apocrine glands. Photo by Timothy Rice.

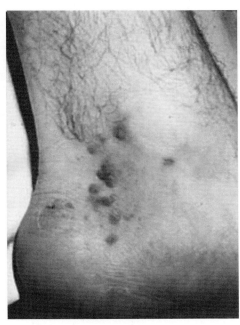

FIG. 2–20 Hypertrophic papular lesions of lichen planus of the ankle. Reproduced with permission from Orkin M, Maibach HI, Dahl MV, eds. *Dermatology*. New York, NY: McGraw-Hill; 1991.

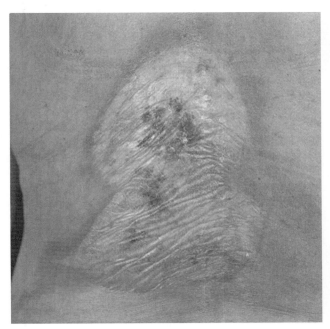

FIG. 2–21 Lichen sclerosus et atrophicus. An ivory-white, indurated but superficially atrophic plaque on the lower back that has arisen from the confluence of multiple whitish papules (best seen on left border). Initially, these papules may show follicular hyperkeratosis; and dry, hyperkeratotic scaling is also evident in the center of this glistening plaque where there is also superficial petechial hemorrhage. The border is surrounded by a hyperpigmented ring of otherwise normal-appearing skin. Reproduced with permission from Wolff K, Johnson RA, Suurmond D. *Fitzpatrick's Color Atlas and Synopsis of Clinical Dermatology.* 5th ed. New York: McGraw-Hill; 2001.

- Lichen sclerosus et atrophicus (Fig. 2–21)
  - Characterized by atrophic, white, sharply demarcated, individual papules that may coalesce to form confluent plaques.
  - These lesions are predominantly located in the anogenital region but occasionally may affect other areas.
  - Females are affected more commonly than males.
  - This dermatologic condition is often mistaken for childhood sexual abuse.
  - Treatment: High-potency topical steroid and a dermatology consultation.
- Psoriasis (Figs. 2–22 and 2–23)
  - Characterized by scaly, erythematous, discrete papular lesions.
  - The psoriatic scale is thick with a stuck-on appearance.
  - Removal of the scale produces punctate bleeding (Auspitz sign).
  - Lesions may appear at areas of skin trauma (Koebner phenomenon).
  - The distribution of the lesions is primarily localized to the scalp and extensor surfaces such as elbows and knees.
  - The fingernails reveal punctate pitting and nail thickening.
  - Psoriatic arthritis
    - Characterized by sausage appearance of the fingers and toes

- Clinical features are similar to those observed with rheumatoid arthritis
- Sacroiliac joint involvement is particularly common
  - Duration: Chronic, with relapses and remissions
  - Treatment of mild to moderate disease
    - Topical steroid cream or ointment or calcipotriene ointment 0.005%, a vitamin D analog or tazarotene gel, a topical retinoid
    - Occlusive dressings alone may eradicate isolated plaques
  - Treatment of extensive disease involves the use of narrow-band ultraviolet B light exposure, oral Methotrexate, psoralen plus ultraviolet A, or oral retinoids (acitretin, and isotretinoin).
  - Scalp involvement may respond to tar shampoo or ketoconazole shampoo in addition to topical steroid solutions.
- Pemphigus vulgaris (Fig. 2–24)
  - Pemphigus vulgaris appears as superficial blistering in the oral mucous membranes, and eventually extends to involve virtually any mucous membrane. This

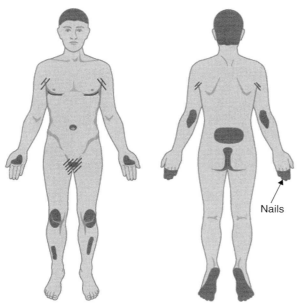

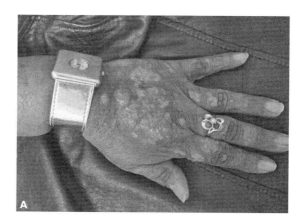

FIG. 2–22 Predilection sites of psoriasis. Reproduced with permission from Wolff K, Johnson RA, Suurmond D. *Fitzpatrick's Color Atlas and Synopsis of Clinical Dermatology.* 5th ed. New York, NY: McGraw-Hill; 2001.

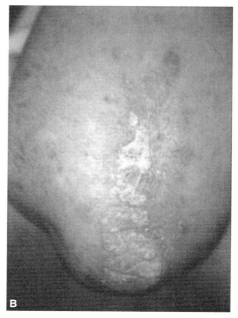

condition is characterized by fragile, easily ruptured, flaccid blister-like lesions. The underlying skin may be erythematous. Importantly, the blisters often slough prior to presentation only leaving ulcerations on examination. Involvement of the lower airway may result in hoarseness. Pressure on the bulla produces lateral extension of the blister (Nikolsky sign).

○ Treatment involves hospitalization and consultation with a dermatologist. Antibiotic treatment is employed if a secondary infection is suspected. Lifelong immunosuppressive therapy may be required in the chronic form of this disease.

FIG. 2–23 Psoriasis of hand (A) and elbow (B). Photos by Timothy Rice.

• Pityriasis rosea (Figs. 2–25 and 2–26)
  ○ Lesions are scaly, oval, discrete, mildly pruritic, and papular.
  ○ Pityriasis rosea is generally localized to the trunk and proximal areas of the extremities, sparing the palms and soles.
  ○ Consider secondary syphilis if pruritus is absent or the palms and soles are involved.
  ○ Distribution tends to be in a *Christmas tree* branching pattern.
  ○ *Herald patch* is a larger lesion preceding the generalized rash by 2 to 10 days and may initially be confused with tinea corporis.
  ○ Duration: The rash progresses over 2 to 3 weeks and resolves within 6 weeks.

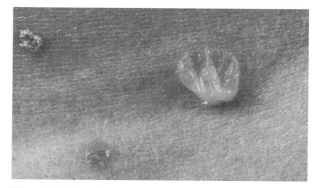

FIG. 2–24 Pemphigus vulgaris. These are the classic initial lesions: flaccid, easily ruptured vesicles and bullae on normal-appearing skin. Ruptured vesicles lead to erosions that subsequently crust. Reproduced with permission from Wolff K, Johnson RA, Suurmond D. *Fitzpatrick's Color Atlas and Synopsis of Clinical Dermatology.* 5th ed. New York, NY: McGraw-Hill; 2001.

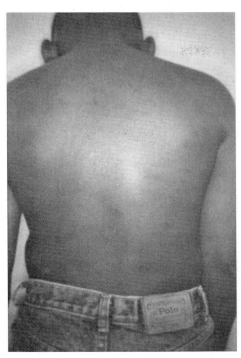

FIG. 2–25 Pityriasis rosea in an African American. Note the "Christmas tree" distribution of lesions. Photo by Timothy Rice.

○ Treatment
  ▪ Oatmeal colloidal (Aveeno) bath every other day
  ▪ Oral antihistamine for pruritus
  ▪ Topical low-potency steroids can be used

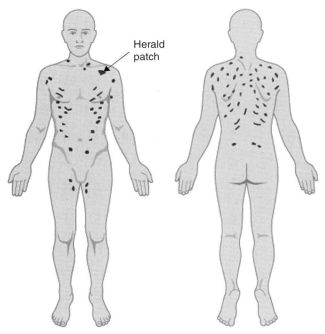

FIG. 2–26 Pityriasis rosea. Distribution *Christmas tree* pattern on the back. Reproduced with permission from Wolff K, Johnson RA, Suurmond D. *Fitzpatrick's Color Atlas and Synopsis of Clinical Dermatology.* 5th ed. New York: McGraw-Hill, 2001.

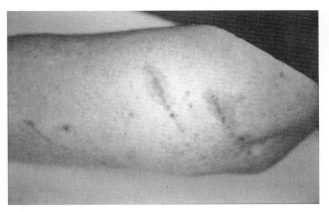

FIG. 2–27 Poison oak. Note the linear, streaking character of the lesions. Photo by Timothy Rice

• Contact dermatitis (Figs. 2–27 to 2–30)
  ○ Contact dermatitis presents as a localized area of erythema and edema with pruritus that often progresses to vesicles and bullae. The location, distribution, and pattern of the rash are strong clues to the etiology of the cutaneous reaction. A linear eruption on exposed skin sparing other areas is a pattern that suggests plant contact dermatitis.
  ○ Causes of contact dermatitis include chemical irritants or an allergen that elicits a type IV (cell-mediated or delayed) hypersensitivity reaction. Tables 2.2–2.4 summarize the myriad causes of contact dermatitis and the signs and symptoms used to differentiate between irritant- and allergen-induced dermatitis.

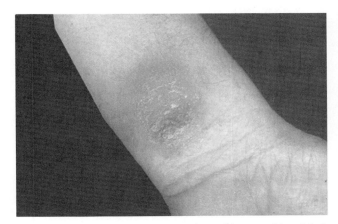

FIG. 2–28 Acute allergic contact dermatitis caused by nickel. This papular erythematous eruption with vesiculation and crusting occurred at the site of contact with the clasp of a watch band. Contact hypersensitivity to nickel was verified by patch testing. Reproduced with permission from Wolff K, Johnson RA, Suurmond D. *Fitzpatrick's Color Atlas and Synopsis of Clinical Dermatology.* 5th ed. New York, McGraw-Hill, 2001.

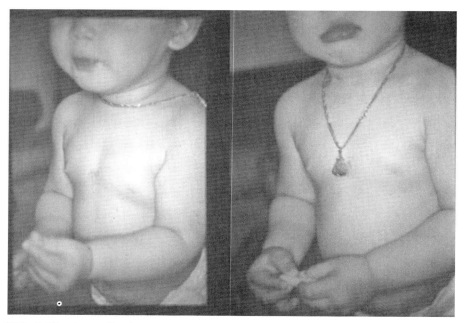

FIG. 2–29   Acute allergic contact dermatitis caused by nickel. This papular erythematous eruption with and crusting occurred at the site of contact with the necklace amulet. Rash resolved with the discontinued use of the necklace. Photo by Timothy Rice.

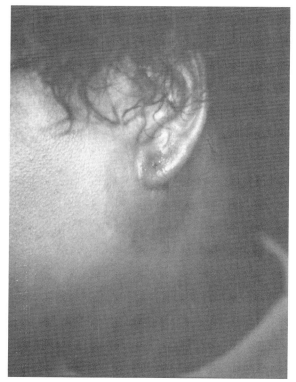

FIG. 2–30   Postinflammatory hyperpigmentation from contact dermatitis caused by nickel in earring. Photo by Timothy Rice.

○ Identifying and removing the offending agent is the cornerstone of management. Symptomatic relief can be achieved with wet bandage dressings applied for 30 to 60 minutes several times a day. Treatment with topical steroids for a maximum of 2 weeks is recommended. Fluocinonide gel, 0.05%, twice or three times daily with compresses, or clobetasol or halobetasol cream twice daily is effective. Oral steroids tapered over 2 weeks can be used for widespread, extensive disease or if there is facial involvement.

• Rosacea
  ○ Facial flushing is the hallmark of this condition.
  ○ Persistent erythema in a butterfly distribution with telangiectasias arise as the disease progresses.
  ○ Later stages are characterized by inflammatory papules, tiny pustules, and nodules.

TABLE 2–2   Most Common Irritant and Toxic Agents

• Soaps, detergents, waterless hand cleaners
• Acids and alkalis*: hydrofluoric acid, cement, chromic acid, phosphorus, ethylene oxide, phenol, metal salts
• Industrial solvents: coal tar solvents, petroleum, chlorinated hydrocarbons, alcohol solvents, ethylene glycol ether, turpentine, ethyl ether, acetone, carbon dioxide, DMSO, dioxane, styrene
• Plants: Euphorbiaceae (spurges, crotons, poinsettias, machineel tree). Ranuculaceae (buttercup), Cruciferae (black mustard), Urticaceae (nettles), Solanaceae (pepper, capsaicin), Opuntia (prickly pear)
• Others: fiberglass, wool, rough synthetic clothing, fire-retardant fabrics, NCR paper

* Lead to chemical burns and necrosis, if concentrated.
DMSO, dimethyl sulfoxide.
Reproduced with permission from Wolff K, Johnson RA, Suurmond D. Fitzpatrick's Color Atlas and Synopsis of Clinical Dermatology. 5th ed. New York, NY: McGraw-Hill; 2001.

TABLE 2–3 Top Ten Contact Allergens (North American Contact Dermatitis Group) and Other Common Contact Allergens

ALLERGEN	PRINCIPAL SOURCES OF CONTACT
Nickel sulfate	Metals, metals in clothing, jewelry, catalyzing agents
Neomycin sulfate	Usually contained in creams, ointments
Balsam of Peru	Topical medications
Fragrance mix	Fragrances, cosmetics
Thimerosal	Antiseptics
Sodium gold thiosulfate	Medication
Formaldehyde	Disinfectant, curing agents, plastics
Quaternium-15	Disinfectant
Cobalt chloride	Cement, galvanization, industrial oils, cooling agents, eyeshades
Bacitracin	Ointments, powder
Methyldibromoglutaronitrile, phenoxyethanol	Preservatives, cosmetics
Carba mix	Rubber, latex
Ethyleneurea melamine-formaldehyde resin	Textile additives
Thiuram	Rubber
p-Phenylene diamine	Black or dark dyes of textiles, printer's ink
Parahydroxybenzoic acid ester	Conserving agent in foodstuffs
Propylene glycol	Preservatives, cosmetics
Procaine, benzocaine	Local anesthetics
Sulfonamides	Medication
Turpentine	Solvents, shoe polish, printer's ink
Mercury salts	Disinfectant, impregnation
Chromates	Cement, antioxidants, industrial oils, matches, leather
Cinnamic aldehyde	Fragrance, perfume

Reproduced with permission from Wolff K, Johnson RA, Suurmond D. *Fitzpatrick's Color Atlas and Synopsis of Clinical Dermatology*. 5th ed. New York, NY: McGraw-Hill; 2001.

- There is also bulbous, greasy hyperplasia of the soft tissue of the nose (rhinophyma).
  - Inflammatory acne can be confused with this condition, however acne is associated with comedone formation, which is not seen in rosacea.
  - Duration: Prolonged course with multiple recurrences.
  - Treatment usually includes topical metronidazole with or without oral antibiotics (usually erythromycin or tetracycline) (Fig. 2–31).
- Herpes simplex
  - Characterized by small vesicles that appear in clusters with a surrounding small rim of erythema. *Rain drops on roses* is the classic description.
  - Herpes simplex lesions arise at the site of primary inoculation, generally on the lips or in the genital region.
  - A primary genital herpes outbreak is usually severe and may be associated with systemic symptoms such as fever. High-dose oral acyclovir, 200 mg orally five times daily (or 800 mg three times daily); Valacyclovir, 1000 mg twice daily; or famciclovir, 250 mg three times daily for 7 to 10 days hastens recovery and reduces the severity of symptoms. Treatment of the primary outbreak has no affect on the rate of recurrent outbreaks.
- Herpes zoster and varicella (Fig. 2–32)
  - Characterized by small vesicles generally appearing in clusters with a small rim of erythema surrounding the lesions. *Rain drops on roses* is the classic appearance of the vesicular rash. Herpes zoster occurs in a dermatomal distribution, but a few lesion may arise outside the primary dermatomal area. Pain in the distribution may precede the appearance of the vesicles.
  - Varicella primary outbreak (chickenpox) is associated with fever and pruritic lesions that appear in different stages over the first 1 to 5 days of the outbreak. Examination early in the course shows newly

TABLE 2–4 Differences Between Irritant and Allergic Contact Dermatitis*

		IRRITANT CONTACT DERMATITIS	ALLERGIC CONTACT DERMATITIS
Symptoms	Acute	**Stinging, smarting** ⇨ **itching**	**Itching** ⇨ **pain**
	Chronic	Itching/pain	Itching/pain
Lesions	Acute	Erythema ⇨ vesicle ⇨ erosion ⇨ crust ⇨ scaling	Erythema ⇨ **papules** ⇨ vesicles ⇨ erosions ⇨ crust ⇨ scaling
	Chronic	Papules, plaques, fissures, scaling, crusts	Papules, plaques, scaling, crusts
Margination and site	Acute	**Sharp, strictly confined to site of exposure**	Sharp, confined to site of exposure **but spreading in the periphery; usually tiny papules; may become generalized**
	Chronic	Ill-defined	Ill-defined, **spreads**
Evolution	Acute	**Rapid** (few hours after exposure)	**Not so rapid** (12 to 72 h after exposure)
	Chronic	Months to years of repeated exposure	Months or longer; exacerbation after every reexposure
Causative agents		**Dependent on concentration of agent and state of skin barrier; occurs only above threshold level**	**Relatively independent of amount applied, usually very low concentrations sufficient but depends on degree of sensitization**
Incidence		**May occur in practically everyone**	**Occurs only in the sensitized**

* Differences are printed in bold.
Reproduced with permission from Wolff K, Johnson RA, Suurmond D. *Fitzpatrick's Color Atlas and Synopsis of Clinical Dermatology*. 5th ed. New York, NY: McGraw-Hill; 2001.

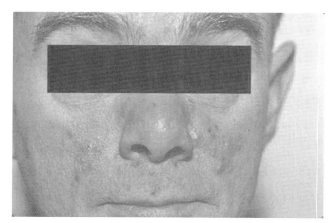

FIG. 2–31 Acne rosacea. Reproduced with permission from Bondi EE, Jegasothy BV, Lazarus GS, eds. *Dermatology: Diagnosis & Treatment.* New York, NY: McGraw-Hill; 1991.

erupting vesicles with older lesions that are crusting and healing. The rash begins centrally and then migrates to involve the extremities.

○ Treatment of varicella with Acyclovir (800 mg by mouth five times daily for 5 to 7 days) is not recommended but should be considered in adolescents or adults with severe disease.

○ Post-exposure immunization against varicella with live attenuated varicella vaccine is effective if given within 72 hours of exposure.

○ Early (<72 hours after appearance) antiviral treatment may reduce the severity and duration of postherpetic neuralgia. Acyclovir, 800 mg five times daily for 7 days, is the recommended treatment. Alternative choices include 7 days of treatment with famciclovir, 500 mg three times daily, or valacyclovir, 1 g three times daily.

• Seborrheic dermatitis (Figs. 2–33 and 2–34)

○ Seborrheic dermatitis is characterized by greasy scales with underlying erythematous patches or plaques located in the eyebrows, eyelids, glabella, nasolabial folds, and scalp; it can also involve the

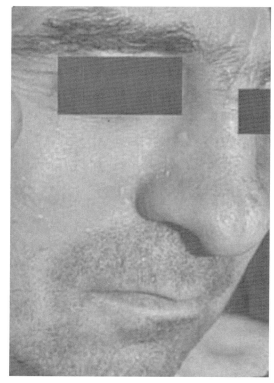

FIG. 2–33 Seborrheic dermatitis. Reproduced with permission from Bondi EE, Jegasothy BV, Lazarus GS, eds. *Dermatology: Diagnosis & Treatment.* New York, NY: McGraw-Hill; 1991.

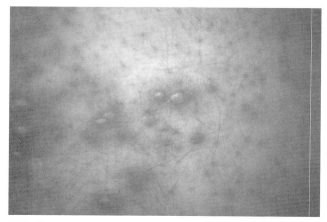

FIG. 2–32 Herpes vesicles in a patient with shingles in a dermatomal distribution the chest wall. Photo by Timothy Rice.

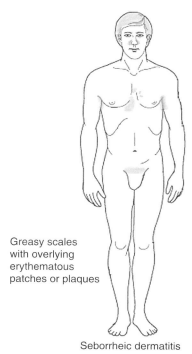

Greasy scales with overlying erythematous patches or plaques

Seborrheic dermatitis

FIG. 2–34 Seborrheic dermatitis distribution front view. Graphic by Timothy Rice.

chest, axilla, groin, submammary folds, and gluteal cleft. This condition may be secondary to an inflammatory reaction to the yeast *M. furfur*.

○ Treatment with a combination of a low-potency topical steroid and a topical antifungal agent is generally effective. Ketoconazole cream or ciclopirox cream coupled with shampoos containing coal tar and/or salicylic acid to treat the scalp and beard areas is effective. Severe involvement of the scalp may respond to high-potency topical steroids (betamethasone or fluocinonide) but these agents should be applied cautiously because they may cause atrophic scaring of the face and are associated with severe flairs when withdrawn.

BIBLIOGRAPHY

Drew GS. Psoriasis. *Prim Care* 2000;27(2):385–406.

Elgart ML. Skin infections and infestations in geriatric patients. *Clin Geriatr Med.* 2002;18(1):89–101, vi.

Feldman SR, Fleischer AB Jr, McConnell RC. Most common dermatologic problems identified by internists, 1990–1994. *Arch Intern Med.* 1998;158(7):726–730.

Hancox JG, Sheridan SC, Feldman SR, Fleischer AB. Seasonal variation of dermatologic disease in the USA: A study of office visits from 1990 to 1998. *Int J Dermatol.* 2004;43(1):6 (doi: 10.1111/j 1365–4632.2004.01828.x).

Salomone JA, Pratt MA. Nontrauma emergencies. In Wolff K, Johnson RA, Suurmond D. *Fitzpatrick's Color Atlas & Synopsis of Clinical Dermatology.* 5th ed.

Sauer GC, Hall JC. *Manual of Skin Diseases.* 7th ed. Lippincott-Raven; 1996:23.

Simpson, EL, Hanifin, JM. Atopic Dermatitis. *Med Clin North Am.* 2006;90:149–167.

Trent JT, Kirsner RS. Identifying and treating mycotic skin infections [review]. *Adv Skin Wound Care.* 2003;16(3):122–129; quiz 130–131.

Wolff K, Johnson, RA, Suurmond D. *Fitzpatrick's Color Atlas & Synopsis of Clinical Dermatology.* 5th ed. McGraw-Hill.

Zaenglein AL, Thiboutot DM. Expert Committee Recommendations for Acne Management. *Pediatrics.* 2006;118;1188–1199.

3 NUTRITION

Nora L. Porter and H. Douglas Walden

BASIC NUTRIENTS AND NUTRITIONAL REQUIREMENTS

• **Calories/Energy**: Basal energy requirements vary with gender, body size, and activity level. Proteins and carbohydrates provide 4 cal/g, fats provide 9 cal/g, and alcohol provides approximately 7 cal/g.

○ **Requirement**: A sedentary adult needs approximately 30 cal/kg of body weight to maintain their weight. Adults who are moderately active need 35 cal/kg, and up to 40 cal/kg are needed for more active individuals. The energy requirement for males are somewhat higher than those for females, but substantial variation exists rendering it difficult to make precise estimates.

• **Protein**: Dietary protein provides essential and nonessential amino acids required for the synthesis of endogenous proteins. Nine of the twenty-one amino acids are essential (cannot be synthesized endogenously) and must be consumed in the diet. Not all protein sources provide all nine essential amino acids. Meat protein is considered to have the highest biologic value in this regard. Although plant and grain proteins do not contain all the essential amino acids, diets rich in plants and grains are associated with a lower risk of cardiovascular disease than those heavy in animal protein sources.

○ **Requirement**: A healthy adult diet should derive about 10% to 15% of calories from protein or approximately 0.8 grams of protein per kilogram of body weight.

• **Carbohydrates**: Carbohydrates are usually classified as either simple carbohydrates which include the monosaccharides (glucose, fructose, and galactose) and disaccharides (sucrose, maltose, and lactose) or complex carbohydrates comprised of polysaccharides (starch and glycogen) and fiber. Whole foods are often higher in complex carbohydrates than processed foods and are preferred as carbohydrate sources.

○ **Requirement**: A healthy adult diet should be comprised of approximately 55% to 65% of calories as carbohydrates, preferably as complex carbohydrates derived from fresh fruit, vegetables, legumes, and whole grains.

• **Fat**: Dietary fats serve important roles as components of cell membranes and substrates for steroid hormone synthesis. In addition, dietary fat insures absorption of the fat-soluble vitamins and serves as an abundant energy reserve in adipose tissue. Diets enriched with saturated fat increase the risk of atherosclerotic disease and certain types of cancer (colon, prostate and breast). *Trans*-saturated fats are associated with an increased risk of atherosclerosis, probably related to their affects on LDL-cholesterol and high-density lipoprotein–cholesterol. Monounsaturated and polyunsaturated fatty acids may be protective from atherosclerosis and are preferable to saturated fat. Consumption of diets enriched with omega-3 fatty acids have been associated with a significant reduction in thromboembolic stroke and heart disease. The omega-3 class of fatty acids possess unique biological properties including an antithrombotic effect, anti-inflammatory effects and triglyceride lowering effect.

○ **Requirement**: A healthy adult diet should contain no more than 30% of calories as fats and less than 7% to 10% of calories as saturated fat. Monounsaturated fats and omega-3 fatty acids may be beneficial. The American Heart Association recommends consumption of omega-3 fatty acids (as fish oil) in patients at risk for coronary artery disease. Trans-saturated fats should be avoided.

• **Fiber**: Dietary fiber is a subset of indigestible carbohydrates found only in plants. It is present in highest quantities in whole grains, vegetables, fruits, and nuts. Fiber is generally classified as insoluble fiber (the fiber that increases water content of the stool and improves bowel motility) and soluble fiber (the fiber that provides the sensation of fullness and slows carbohydrate digestion). Soluble fiber effectively lowers serum glucose and cholesterol levels. In addition, high-fiber diets may be effective in lowering the risk of colon cancer, and possibly lowering all-cause mortality. High-fiber diets are commonly used in patients with diverticulosis, hemorrhoids, irritable bowel syndrome, and constipation.

○ **Requirement**: Experts recommend consumption of approximately 30 g of dietary fiber each day.

• **Water**: Water requirements vary depending on age and the presence of water-depleting states such as fever, diarrhea, vomiting, excessive sweating, renal disease, and extreme environmental conditions. Elderly patients are particularly prone to dehydration because of the frequent presence of a defect in thirst sensation and consumption of medications that promote water loss eg, diuretics.

○ **Requirement**: In the basal state, most individuals require at least 1 mL of water per kcal of energy expended. An increased intake is needed when excessive losses occur.

NUTRITIONAL AND DIETARY ASSESSMENT

• Patients with a variety of medical conditions often have nutritional deficiencies that go unrecognized. A complete nutritional assessment requires historical information, physical examination, and measurement of laboratory markers. A dietary history is a key component of a thorough nutritional assessment. A 24-hour dietary recall or a 3 to 5 day food diary provides valuable information about a patient's eating patterns and nutrient consumption.

• Nutritional assessment should also focus on risk factors that alter nutritional status. For example, past and current medical conditions, surgeries, medication use, alcohol and drug use, a history of recent weight loss or appetite change, functional impairment resulting in difficulty feeding, chewing or swallowing, symptoms of depression, or gastrointestinal symptoms of nausea, vomiting, or diarrhea may all engender risk of nutritional deficiencies. Hospitalized patients may be subjected to starvation because of their underlying medical condition or because testing and procedures require fasting. Information about patients' food preferences and any personal or cultural dietary restrictions may highlight an important risk factor in the development of nutritional disorders, and can prove invaluable in individualizing nutritional education.

• Socioeconomic factors such as poverty and homelessness limit access to nutritious foods.

• The physical examination should focus on the skin, hair, nails, mucous membranes, muscle mass and adiposity, looking for evidence of malnutrition or obesity. Weight and height should be measured on all patients, and body mass index should be calculated:

$$\text{Body mass index (BMI)} = \text{weight (kg)/height (m)}^2$$
$$\text{BMI} = \text{weight (lbs)/height (in)}^2 \times 703$$

• Desirable BMI is 18.5 to 25. BMI, less than 18.5 is considered underweight. A BMI of 25 to 30 is considered overweight, and greater than 30 is considered obese. Specialized measurements such as percent body fat and skin fold thickness may prove useful in some patients.

• The laboratory assessment of nutritional status should include a complete blood count with differential (lymphocyte count), albumin, prealbumin, and transferrin. In patients at risk for deficiencies of specific micronutrients, appropriate blood levels should be measured. Malnourished patients are frequently deficient in magnesium, zinc, and vitamin A.

NUTRITIONAL SUPPORT

• Nutritional support via the gastrointestinal tract (enteral nutrition) or by vein (parenteral nutrition) is available for individuals unable to consume adequate calories by mouth and who are at risk of malnutrition and its complications. It need not be used simply because an individual is unable to eat but should be considered for use when the potential benefits of improving nutritional status outweigh the risks of therapy.

• The enteral route for nutrition is preferred if the gastrointestinal tract is functional. It is generally safer, cheaper, and more physiologic than parenteral feeding. Use of parenteral nutritional support without any enteral nutrition is probably only indicated for selected individuals with advanced bowel or pancreatic disease. Enteral and parenteral nutrition can be provided in both hospital settings and at home.

- Use of oral liquid nutritional support supplements and medications to stimulate appetite (megestrol) are reasonable alternatives to enteral or parenteral nutrition in some situations. Importantly, there is little credible evidence that provision of nutritional support through enteral or parenteral routes improves outcomes for many disease states.
- Evaluation by a nutritionist skilled in nutritional support aids in the design of a nutritional support regimen. The regimen should be tailored to the individual needs of the patient (eg, kidney disease, diabetes, chronic obstructive pulmonary disease [COPD])
  - **Enteral nutrition**: Enteral nutritional support is usually provided by small flexible tubes passed intranasally into either the stomach or jejunum. Feeding tubes can also be surgically placed directly into the jejunum for individuals likely to require enteral nutrition for a prolonged period. Feeding through a tube in the stomach permits bolus feeding but increases the risk of aspiration, particularly in individuals with an impaired ability to protect their own airway. Tubes placed into the duodenum have been found to offer no greater protection against aspiration than those in the stomach. Tubes located in the jejunum protect against aspiration, but bolus feeding cannot be used (feeding by continuous drip infusion must be used). A variety of feeding formulas are available for use and are best selected with the aid of a skilled nutritionist.
  - Complications of enteral nutrition include aspiration, displacement of the feeding tube, wound infection for surgically placed tubes, and diarrhea. Individuals at highest risk for aspiration are those on ventilator support as well as those with delayed gastric emptying, altered mental status, or neurologic dysfunction. Endotracheal and tracheotomy cuffs do not provide adequate protection from aspiration.
  - **Parenteral nutrition**: Parenteral nutritional support can be provided by way of either a peripheral venous or a central venous route. Primarily, peripheral vein use is appropriate as a short-term bridge to enteral feeding in individuals with temporary dysfunction of the gastrointestinal tract. Lipids, dextrose, and amino acids can all be provided through the peripheral route; however, the parenteral provision of adequate carbohydrate calories usually requires use of a central vein where rapid equilibration of the concentrated glucose solutions can take place. For longer-term and more complete nutritional replacement, the central venous route is preferable. Catheters can be peripherally inserted into a central vein. Obtaining consultation from a nutritionist experienced in parenteral nutrition is important and ensures that the patient receives adequate

water and appropriate calories from protein, carbohydrate, and fat sources as well as all of the necessary vitamins and minerals.
  - Complications of parenteral nutrition include mechanical problems with the catheter (placement complications and thrombosis), catheter infection (usually with *Staphylococcus epidermidis* or *Staphylococcus aureus*), and metabolic issues (hyperglycemia, electrolyte abnormalities, and cholestasis). The complications can be substantial, occur with greater frequency in patients most dependent on nutritional support and can lead to death. These complications must be kept in mind as the initial decision for nutritional supplementation is being considered.

VITAMINS AND MINERALS

- Most vitamin and mineral deficiencies (with the exception of vitamin D deficiency) are rare in developed countries. A deficiency of one vitamin or mineral should promote a search for other deficiencies. These nutritional deficiencies are most common in individuals with alcoholism, with malabsorption syndromes, or on parenteral nutrition. Vitamin D deficiency is though to exist in 40%–50% of individuals and has been linked to cancer and cardiac disease. A summary of the sources, possible manifestations of deficiency, and toxicity of vitamins and selected minerals is provided in Table 3–1, Table 3–2, and Table 3–3. The current recommended daily allowance (RDA) for each vitamin and mineral is being revised. Recommended intakes may vary based on gender and age and are often increased in pregnancy and for nursing mothers. Complete information on current US recommendations for intake can be located at www.nal.usda.gov.

NUTRITIONAL NEEDS IN SPECIFIC STATES

- Many chronic medical problems can adversely affect nutritional status and nutritional requirements. Patients with any chronic medical condition should receive an appropriate nutritional assessment and receive dietary education.

ALCOHOLISM

- Patients with alcohol abuse and dependence are at risk for a number of nutritional disorders, including obesity, binge eating, eating disorders, and malnutrition. Dietary intake may be inadequate during binge

TABLE 3–1   Water-Soluble Vitamins

VITAMIN	SOURCES	MANIFESTATIONS OF DEFICIENCY	TOXICITY
Thiamine (B_1)	Yeast, legumes, pork, cereals, rice	Beriberi: High-output congestive heart failure, Wernicke-Korsakoff syndrome, neuropathy	None
Riboflavin (B_2)	Fruits, vegetables, meats, fish, eggs	Pharyngitis, stomatitis, anemia, dermatitis	None
Niacin (B_3)	Fruits, vegetables, meats, cereals	Pellagra: dermatitis, diarrhea, dementia	Flushing, hepatic toxicity (at pharmacologic doses)
Pantothenic acid (B_5)	Egg yolk, liver, kidney, broccoli, milk	Distal paresthesias	None
Pyridoxine (B_6)	Meats, whole grains, vegetables, nuts	Stomatitis, glossitis, irritability, depression	Rare: Sensory neuropathy, dermatitis
Cobalamin (B_{12})	Meat, poultry, fish, dairy products	Megaloblastic anemia, neuropathy, dementia	None
Biotin	Liver, egg yolk, soybean, yeast	Anorexia, nausea, myalgias, mental status changes, paresthesias	None
Folic acid	Fruits, vegetables, legumes, grains	Megaloblastic anemia, neural tube defects	None
Ascorbic acid (C)	Fruits and vegetables	Scurvy: Impaired collagen synthesis (perifollicular hemorrhages, petechiae, purpura, bleeding gums, hemarthroses, impaired wound healing)	Oxalate renal stones

drinking; conversely, overeating may occur during periods of alcohol abstinence. Because alcohol may interfere with vitamin absorption, and because many alcoholics do not have otherwise healthy balanced diets, they may develop deficiencies of vitamins A, C, D, E, K, and the B vitamins. A daily multivitamin and folic acid supplement are recommended for all patients with alcoholism.

CARDIOVASCULAR DISEASE

A number of dietary modifications have been identified which are effective in the prevention of coronary heart disease. The substitution of unsaturated fats, especially polyunsaturated fats, for saturated and *trans*-saturated fats appears to be more effective than lowering the total fat in the diet. Increased consumption of fruits, vegetables, nuts, whole grains, and omega-3 fatty acids from fish oil or plant sources all confer a protective benefit.

DIABETES MELLITUS

• **Prevention**: The Diabetes Prevention Program (DPP) studied the effect of intensive lifestyle modifications in patients at high risk for the development of diabetes. The DPP diet was low in fat and restricted in calories to promote weight loss. Combined with physical activity, this diet was more effective than placebo or metformin

TABLE 3–2   Fat-Soluble Vitamins

VITAMIN	SOURCES	MANIFESTATIONS OF DEFICIENCY	TOXICITY
Retinoic Acid (A)	Liver, kidney, egg yolk, butter, pigmented vegetables	Night blindness, complete blindness, xerophthalmia, dermatitis, immune dysfunction	Dry skin, nausea, headache, fatigue, hypercalcemia, increased intracranial pressure
Calciferol (D)	Fortified milk, fatty fish, eggs	Rickets, osteomalacia	Hypercalcemia
Tocopherol (E)	Vegetables	Neuromuscular disorders, hemolysis	Can increase vitamin K requirements
K	Green leafy vegetables, intestinal bacteria	Impaired coagulation	Interference with anticoagulant therapy

TABLE 3–3   Minerals

MINERAL	SOURCES	MANIFESTATIONS OF DEFICIENCY	TOXICITY
Calcium	Fortified dairy products	Increased risk for osteoporosis	Milk-alkali syndrome, nephrolithiasis
Iron	Meat, chick peas, spinach, figs, apricots	Anemia	Secondary hemochromatosis
Selenium	Meat, egg yolks, poultry, shellfish, tomatoes	Cardiomyopathy, impaired cell-mediated immunity, increased cancer incidence and mortality	Hair loss, nail changes, neuropathy
Chromium	Whole grains, legumes, peanuts, meats	Impaired glucose tolerance, lipid abnormalities	No toxicity from dietary sources
Magnesium	Legumes, nuts, whole grains, green vegetables	Cardiac dysrhythmias, neuromuscular symptoms, hypocalcemia	Diarrhea, abdominal cramps, neurologic changes
Iodine	Fortified salt	Goiter, hypothyroidism, impaired mental function, delayed physical development	Goiter and hypothyroidism, hyperthyroidism
Zinc	Red meat, shellfish, whole grain cereals	Impaired growth and maturation, immune deficiency, sexual dysfunction, skin lesions	Rare: Abdominal pain, diarrhea, nausea, vomiting
Copper	Legumes, meats, nuts	Rare: anemia, neutropenia	Nausea, vomiting, abdominal pain, hepatic necrosis

in preventing the development of diabetes: Risk was reduced 58% in the lifestyle intervention arm compared to a 31% risk reduction in the metformin arm.

• **Medical nutrition therapy**: All patients with diabetes should receive individualized dietary education. The American Diabetes Association has identified a number of goals in the dietary management of patients with diabetes. These include consumption of a healthy, balanced diet; caloric intake to achieve and maintain ideal body weight; management of coexisting risk factors for cardiovascular disease; and glycemic control.

• Because the amount and type of carbohydrates consumed affect glycemic control, monitoring carbohydrates by either carbohydrate counting or use of dietary exchanges is essential for patients with diabetes. Carbohydrates should comprise 45% to 65% of total calories. The use of foods with a low glycemic index may improve glycemic control. Recommended sources of carbohydrates are fruits, vegetables, whole grains, and low-fat dairy products. Sucrose should be counted in the total carbohydrate intake for the day and should be used only in the context of an otherwise healthy, balanced diet. Total carbohydrate requirements depend on weight, physical activity, whether or not weight loss is a goal, and concurrent medication use. Distribution of carbohydrates throughout the day depends on medication, physical activity, and patient preferences. Fat should comprise 25% to 35% of the total calories, with saturated fat contributing less than 7% of total caloric intake, and consumption of *trans*-saturated fat should be minimized. Restriction of protein to (0.8 g/kg), may slow the progression of nephropathy in patients with nephrotic range proteinuria, however recent meta-analysis suggests that this common practice is of marginal benefit. Recommendations for fiber intake for diabetic patients are the same as those for the general population.

DYSLIPIDEMIAS

• Modification of the type of fat consumed has a more favorable affect on serum lipid profiles than simple reduction in total dietary fat. The National Cholesterol Education Program recommends 25% to 35% of total calories from fat, with up to 10% from polyunsaturated fat, up to 20% from monounsaturated fat, and less than 7% from saturated fat. Cholesterol intake should be less than 200 mg/d. Consumption of *trans*-saturated fat should be minimized. Between 50% and 60% of calories should be derived from carbohydrates; recommended sources include whole grains, fruits, and vegetables. Between 20 and 30 g/d of fiber are recommended. The remaining calories, approximately 15%, should come from protein. Total calories should be adjusted to achieve or maintain ideal body weight.

FOOD ALLERGY AND INTOLERANCE

• Adverse reactions to food are common, but only a small percentage of reactions are true food allergies. Food allergy should be suspected when there is a history of an allergic or allergic-like reaction temporally associated with a specific food product, in the absence of anatomic, functional, metabolic, or infectious etiology. Clinical features may include acute severe gastrointestinal symptoms, pruritus, urticaria, angioedema, rhinoconjunctivitis, bronchospasm, eosinophilic esophagitis or gastritis, enteropathy, malabsorption, or anaphylaxis. Food allergy is most common in children younger than age 3 but may occur at any age. The most common foods causing significant food allergy in adults are peanuts, tree nuts, fish, and shellfish. No further testing is indicated following anaphylactic reactions to ingestion of a suspected food. For other reactions, the diagnosis may be confirmed if symptoms resolve with elimination of the food and symptoms recur after an oral challenge. Percutaneous skin testing or serum tests for specific immunoglobulin E are helpful in excluding the diagnosis. Treatment requires elimination of the causal food from the diet.

- The most common food intolerance in the general population is lactose intolerance, which becomes more prevalent with increasing age. Patients develop characteristic symptoms, including abdominal pain, bloating, flatulence, diarrhea, and vomiting after the ingestion of lactose-containing foods. The lactose tolerance test or lactose breath hydrogen test can be used to confirm the diagnosis. Avoidance of lactose-containing foods results in resolution of symptoms. Commercially available lactase enzyme replacements and milk that has been pretreated with lactase are alternatives for patients who wish to continue to consume dairy products. Calcium supplementation may be needed in patients who restrict their consumption of dairy products.

GASTROINTESTINAL DISORDERS

- Gastrointestinal disorders may result in impaired absorption of essential nutrients, necessitating nutritional support or micronutrient supplementation. Conditions that cause fat malabsorption are associated with deficiencies in the fat soluble vitamins A, D, E, and K. Patients with celiac disease, gastrectomy, or short-bowel syndrome may also develop deficiencies of vitamin D, iron, and folic acid. Electrolyte abnormalities such as hypocalcemia, hypomagnesemia, hypokalemia, and hypophosphatemia may also be seen in such patients. Nutritional deficiencies usually resolve when specific therapy for the underlying cause of the malabsorption is initiated (such as pancreatic enzyme supplementation for pancreatic insufficiency or a gluten-free diet for celiac disease). For conditions without specific therapy, monitoring of nutrients and electrolytes and appropriate supplementation are essential.

GOUT

- Obesity and weight gain are risk factors for gout, whereas weight loss reduces the risk of gout. Adjusting caloric intake to achieve and maintain ideal body weight is one approach to decreasing the risk of recurrent gout. The traditional purine-restricted diet may be difficult for patients to follow. A diet with increased protein and complex carbohydrates as well as decreased refined carbohydrates and saturated fat can produce a more substantial reduction in serum urate concentration and may be beneficial. The source of protein may also have an effect on the recurrence of gout. The risk of developing gout increases with increased consumption of meat and fish but decreases with consumption of low-fat dairy products. Increased consumption of organ meats, beer, and distilled spirits may also influence the recurrence of gout, and reduction in dietary intake of these may be helpful.

HYPERTENSION

- One of the most important dietary modifications in the prevention and treatment of hypertension is adjusting caloric intake to achieve and maintain ideal body weight. In addition, specific dietary strategies have been shown to be effective. Several observational studies have documented a lower incidence of hypertension in people following a vegetarian diet, although it is unclear if other lifestyle factors may also play a role in lowering blood pressure. In the Dietary Approaches to Stop Hypertension (DASH) trial, a diet high in fruits, vegetables, and low-fat dairy products produced small but significant reductions in blood pressure compared to a control diet. The DASH diet also included whole grains, poultry, fish, and nuts and restricted red meat, fats, and sugars. The OmniHeart study compared the effect of three different diets low in saturated fat and cholesterol and high in fruits, vegetables, and fiber: a high (58%) carbohydrate diet, a high protein diet (with about half the protein from plant sources), and a high unsaturated fat diet (mostly monounsaturated fat). All three diets had a beneficial effect on lowering blood pressure.

- Dietary intake of specific minerals also has an effect on blood pressure. Sodium restriction (1.6 g/d) in conjunction with the DASH diet resulted in additional blood pressure–lowering benefits. Increased potassium intake has also been associated with decreased blood pressure. Although evidence is insufficient to determine the optimal levels of sodium and potassium intake, expert recommendations suggest an upper limit of 2.3 g/d of sodium and a recommended potassium intake of 4.7 g/d (in patients with normal renal function). Moderation in alcohol intake to no more than 2 drinks per day for most men and no more than 1 drink per day for most women is also an effective approach to lower blood pressure.

LIVER DISEASE

- Patients with liver disease are at increased risk of nutritional deficiencies including protein-energy malnutrition; zinc deficiency; and deficiencies of the fat-soluble vitamins A, D, E, and K. Dietary assessment for intake of these micronutrients as well as total caloric and protein intake is required. Although protein restriction has a role in the management of acute hepatic encephalopathy, it should not be chronically implemented because it increases the risk for protein malnutrition. Because patients with cirrhosis respond poorly to hypoglycemia, their caloric intake should be divided into four to six daily meals, including a late evening snack.

OSTEOPOROSIS

- Adequate calcium intake is necessary for osteoporosis prevention and treatment. The recommended daily intake of calcium is 1000 mg for men and premenopausal women, and 1500 mg for postmenopausal women or those with established osteoporosis. The maximum daily intake is 2000 mg. Many people find it difficult to get enough calcium from diet alone. A serving of dairy (8 oz of milk or yogurt or 1 oz of hard cheese) has approximately 300 mg of calcium. Calcium supplementation should be used in the form of calcium citrate or calcium carbonate to achieve the recommended intake if dietary calcium consumption is inadequate. Vitamin D is also needed. The recommended daily intake is 400 IU for young adults and 800 IU for the elderly or those with malnutrition, intestinal malabsorption, or receiving long-term anticonvulsant or glucocorticoid therapy.

RENAL DISEASE

- **Chronic kidney disease:** Patients with chronic kidney disease are at increased risk for protein-energy malnutrition, a strong predictor of poor clinical outcome. All patients with chronic kidney disease should receive individualized nutritional education and monitoring. Nutritional status in these patients should be periodically monitored by serial measurements of multiple biochemical and anthropometric markers of nutritional status, including serum albumin (and prealbumin for patients on maintenance hemodialysis), cholesterol, transferrin, creatinine, edema-free body weight, assessment of dietary intake, and a standardized subjective global assessment. Energy requirements in patients with chronic kidney disease are similar to those of the general population, approximately 35 kcal/kg/d (30–35 kcal/kg/d for patients older than age 60 years). Low-protein diets may retard the progression of renal failure and decrease the risk of symptomatic uremia, hyperphosphatemia, metabolic acidosis, and hyperkalemia. A diet providing 0.6 to 0.8 g protein/kg/d is adequate to maintain nutritional status in most chronic kidney disease patients.

- **Maintenance dialysis:** The recommendations for nutritional education and assessment of patients with chronic kidney disease apply to those on dialysis as well. Serial measurement of body weight should be obtained postdialysis for hemodialysis patients, and after drainage of dialysate in patients undergoing peritoneal dialysis. Serum bicarbonate should be measured monthly, and maintained at or above 22 mmol/L. Because dialysis removes some amino acids and peptides as well as small amounts of protein and glucose, protein requirements are higher for patients on maintenance hemodialysis. A dietary protein intake of 1.2 to 1.3 g/kg/d is crucial and associated with a reduction in hospitalization rates and overall mortality. Some dialysis patients are unable to meet their increased protein and energy requirements and may require nutritional support. Water-soluble vitamin supplementation is also recommended for chronic dialysis patients. Vitamin A deficiency may develop, so vitamin A levels should be monitored and supplementation initiated if necessary.

BIBLIOGRAPHY

American College of Allergy, Asthma, & Immunology. Food allergy: A practice parameter. *Ann Allergy Asthma Immunol.* 2006;96(3 Suppl 2):S1.

American Diabetes Association. Standards of medical care in diabetes: 2006. *Diabetes Care.* 2006;29(1 Suppl):S4–S42.

American Gastroenterological Association. American Gastroenterological Association medical position statement: Celiac sprue. *Gastroenterology.* 2001;120(6):1522.

American Gastroenterological Association. American Gastroenterological Association medical position statement: Guidelines for the evaluation of food allergies. *Gastroenterology.* 2001;120(4):1023.

American Medical Directors Association. *Altered nutritional status.* Columbia, MD: American Medical Directors Association (AMDA); 2001:32.

American Society for Parental and Enteral Nutrition. Specific guidelines for disease: Adults. *JPEN J Parenter Enteral Nutr.* 2002;26(1 Suppl):61S.

Appel, LJ, MD, MPH; Michael W. Brands, PhD; Stephen R. Daniels, et al. Dietary approaches to prevent and treat hypertension: A scientific statement from the American Heart Association. *Hypertension.* 2006;47:296.

Choi HK, Atkinson K, Karlson EW, et al. Obesity, weight change, hypertension, diuretic use, and risk of gout in men: The health professionals follow-up study. *Arch Intern Med.* 2005;165:742.

Hodgson SF, Watts NB, Bilezikian JP, et al. American Association of Clinical Endocrinologist Medical Guidelines for Clinical Practice for the Prevention and Treatment of Postmenopausal Osteoporosis: 2001 edition, with selected updates for 2003. *Endocr Pract.* 2003;9(6):544.

Hu FB, and Willet W. Optimal diets for prevention of coronary heart disease. *JAMA.* 2002;288(20):2569.

Joint National Committee on Prevention, Detection, Evaluation, and Treatment of High Blood Pressure. The Seventh Report of the Joint National Committee on Prevention, Detection, Evaluation, and Treatment of High Blood Pressure. Hypertension 2003: 42:1206–1246.

National Cholesterol Education Program. Third Report of the NCEP Expert Panel on Detection, Evaluation, and Treatment of High Blood Cholesterol in Adults (Adult Treatment Panel III). *JAMA.* 2001;285:2486–97.

National Kidney Foundation Kidney Disease Outcomes Quality Initiative. Nutrition in chronic renal failure. *Am J Kidney Dis.* 2000;37(1 Suppl 2):S66–70.

Nestle M. *Nutrition in Clinical Practice.* Greenbrae, CA: Jones Medical Publications; 1985.

4 PREVENTIVE MEDICINE

Robert M. Heaney and Nora L. Porter

INTRODUCTION

RATIONALE FOR PREVENTION

Death and disability statistics suggest that preventable conditions are significant contributors to morbidity and mortality. Analysis of underlying causes of death in the population suggests that many of them could be prevented by behavioral changes or simple medical interventions.

Many preventive interventions have been demonstrated to be cost-effective when applied universally or to selected populations. A less tangible but still important benefit of preventive healthcare is the improved quality of life resulting from decreased morbidity.

DEFINITIONS

PREVENTION

Prevention is classified as primary, secondary, or tertiary. *Primary prevention* occurs before the onset of the disease process, with the goal of preventing or delaying development of the disease. *Secondary prevention* occurs after the disease has started but before the onset of symptoms, with the goal of preventing progression to the symptomatic stage. *Tertiary prevention* occurs in an already established disease process, to prevent progression or worsening and to minimize morbidity and disability from the disease process.

SCREENING

Screening is defined as the application of a test to detect a potential disease or condition in a person who has no known signs, symptoms, or test abnormalities. Most screening is secondary prevention, as it is designed to detect disease in the early, asymptomatic stage. Early detection of patients requiring special intervention can minimize the burden of the disease to both the individual and society.

PREVENTION PRACTICES

Practicing clinicians use a number of strategies to provide preventive healthcare to their patients. As the number of preventive interventions can be seemingly endless, a rational approach for determining which patients will benefit most from specific interventions is needed. The clinician should use the patient's medical history and sociodemographic factors to stratify the patient's risk for the development of disease. The history should focus on current and past medical problems; medications; diet; physical activity; alcohol, tobacco, and other substance use; sexual history; and family history. The physical examination should include height and weight (with calculation of the body mass index), and blood pressure. The remainder of the examination can then be customized to focus on the conditions that will be most likely to influence the health and well-being of the individual patient. Appropriate education, screening, immunizations, and medications can then be selected for the patient.

It is not always feasible for patients, especially those with multiple medical problems, to schedule an additional provider visit to address their preventive healthcare needs. For many patients, incorporating preventive components into visits for acute or chronic medical problems can be the most effective way to ensure that patients receive appropriate preventive services.

CRITERIA FOR SCREENING RECOMMENDATIONS

Criteria for screening recommendations seek to ensure clinical efficacy: that is more benefit results than the harm to the patients for whom the screening tests are performed.

- Importance of the screening target. The disease or the condition sought by the screening intervention should have prevalence or incidence or both that warrant the screening. The attributable morbidity or mortality should be significant.

Recommendations have been developed for extremely common conditions with a high morbidity or mortality such as coronary artery disease. They have also been developed for quite uncommon conditions such as testicular carcinoma. It is important to recognize that an intervention which results in a small mortality reduction due to a common condition which affects a relatively large percentage of a population will have greater impact than an intervention with dramatic mortality reduction in condition that is extremely uncommon. For instance a 1% reduction in mortality in the condition that causes 100,000 deaths per year in North America could prevent 1,000 deaths; whereas an intervention that resulted in a 50% mortality reduction from a condition that causes 10 deaths in that same population per year would only prevent 5 deaths.

- Effectiveness of a preventive intervention. Once found, the screening target must be treatable. Although lung cancer is far more common than testicular cancer until recently there was a general recommendation for testicular cancer screening; but very limited indications for lung cancer screening. Lung cancer was usually not curable and a decrease in mortality when the lung cancer is found by a screening test has not yet been demonstrated. This may change as improved imaging and treatment modalities become available.

- Safety. Preventive interventions should be safe and they should be comfortable enough that a reasonable compliance rate with the recommendations can be expected. Before the advent of improved conscious sedation and more flexible endoscopes, it was difficult to convince patients to comply with a second uncomfortable procedure with a low but present perforation rate when making recommendations for screening for colorectal cancer.

- Accuracy and Reliability. For screening intervention to be effective the test itself should be reliable and accurate. Tests should have acceptable sensitivities and specificities. Sensitivity is the ability of the test to detect the disease in all those patients that have the condition being screened. Conversely specificity is the ability of the test to find health (the absence of the disease in question).

- Predictive Value. Sensitivity and specificity are properties of the test; not of the patient. Patients desire to know whether or not they have the disease after the test is performed. Predictive Value, either Positive or Negative, allow clinicians to provide patients with an indication of what a screening test result means for their particular circumstances.

Even a test with good reliability, sensitivity, and specificity can perform relatively poorly. For instance, when screening for a disease condition with a prevalence of 5% in the population, using a test with excellent sensitivity and specificity of 95%; the predictive value of a positive test result is only 50%. On the other hand, the predictive value of a negative test result in this population will be much

better at 99.7% (0.03% likelihood of missing the disease condition at this screening episode because of a false negative test).

It is important to recognize that screening as a secondary preventive intervention has its greatest utility when the likelihood that the patient has the target disease is relatively high. This condition is often not met in routine office practice. The positive predictive values of many screening tests are less than 20% even in research or referral settings. In many practice situations not only are most patients who receive the screening test free of the disease; but most of those with positive tests results are also free of the disease. However, once a screening test is positive; other diagnostics and therapeutics inevitably occur at additional cost and additional risk to the patients.

For these reasons, sequential screening strategies using safe tools as a first step either for general or selective screening, thereby creating relatively higher risk groups (ie, groups with positive stool hemoccults) before applying more expensive or potentially more dangerous screening tests may have some utility while realizing lower costs and better safety profiles in the populations screened.

Recommendations for preventive medical care are dynamic and depend on the diseases prevalent in the communities served, the performance characteristics of tests or interventions to be recommended, and the performance characteristics of the treatments available to the diseases once identified. Recommendations across expert or specialty groups do not always agree; and treating physicians should be familiar with of the evidence that supports recommendations for primary, secondary, and tertiary preventive care.

CANCER SCREENING

The United States Preventive Services Task Force (USPSTF) and numerous specialty organizations make recommendations concerning cancer screening. (Table 4-1). The USPSTF takes an evidence-based approach to the development of clinical practice guidelines, with a focus on conditions with a significant burden to society and potentially effective preventive services available. The USPSTF emphasizes population health, while other organizations' recommendations may be more focused on a single disease or condition. This results in some variation in screening recommendations made by different organizations.

PREVENTION OF LUNG CANCER AND LUNG CANCER RELATED MORBIDITY AND MORTALITY

Lung cancer continues to be the leading cause of cancer death for both men and women in the United States. As such it would expected to be a target for aggressive

TABLE 4-1 Recommendations for Cancer Screening in Patients at Average Risk[a]

CANCER	RISK FACTORS	SCREENING MODALITY	USPSTF RECOMMENDATIONS FOR SCREENING	POTENTIAL RISKS/ COMPLICATIONS	COMMENTS
Breast	Age; family history: first childbirth older than 30 years of age; previous breast biopsy with atypical hyperplasia	Mammography	Every 1–2 years for women age 40 years and older (evidence is best for women ages 50–69 years)	Discomfort of examination; false positive tests; radiation exposure; possible overdetection and overtreatment of carcinoma in situ	AMA, ACR, ACS, ACOG make same recommendation; CTFPHC, AAFP, ACPM recommend beginning screening mammography at age 50 years
Cervical	Early onset of sexual activity, multiple sexual partners, HIV infection; tobacco smoking; atypia or CIN on cervical cytology screening	Cervical cytology screening with Papanicolaou smear	At least every 3 years, beginning at age 21 or within 3 years of onset of sexual activity, whichever is earliest	Discomfort of examination; need for repeat examinations and further testing	
Colorectal	Ulcerative colitis; adenomatous colon polyps; family history of familial polyposis or HNPCC	Multiple options for screening	All men and women age 50 years and older		No evidence of superiority of a single screening modality
		Fecal occult blood testing OR	Annually, with or without flexible sigmoidoscopy (if not having colonoscopy)	Noninvasive; proven mortality benefit; any positive test mandates colonoscopy	
		Flexible sigmoidoscopy OR	Every 5 years (if not having colonoscopy)	Less burdensome bowel preparation and less risk of perforation compared with colonoscopy; does not visualize entire colon	
		Double contrast barium enema OR	Every 5–10 years (if not having colonoscopy or sigmoidoscopy)	Risk of perforation; less sensitive than endoscopic visualization; limited to patients unable to tolerate endoscopy or in whom cecum cannot be visualized endoscopically	
		Colonoscopy	Every 10 years	Burdensome bowel preparation; risk of perforation; requires conscious sedation	
Prostate		DRE, PSA	USPSTF found insufficient evidence to determine whether benefits of PSA testing outweigh harms; no evidence of benefit of DRE. If screening is done is most likely to be beneficial for men ages 50–79 years (beginning at age 45 years in high risk)	False negatives; false positives; adverse effects of biopsies and therapies necessitated by positive test; unclear benefit of early detection	No evidence of benefit of DRE; USPSTF found insufficient evidence to determine whether benefits outweigh harms; ACP, AUA, AAFP, ACS, AMA recommend discussing potential benefits and possible harms with the patient; CTFPHC recommends against routine use of PSA

Testicular cancer	Monthly testicular self examination; clinician-performed testicular examination	No recommendation
Skin cancer	Monthly mole self-examination; clinician-performed examination	No recommendation
Ovarian cancer	Bimanual pelvic examination; CA 125	No recommendation
Lung cancer		No recommendation

AAFP, American Academy of Family Physicians; ACOG, American College of Obstetricians and Gynecologists; ACP, American College of Physicians; ACPM, American College of Preventive Medicine; ACR, American College of Radiology; ACS, American Cancer Society; AMA, American Medical Association; AUA, American Urological Association; CA 125, cancer antigen (125); CIN, cervical intraepithelial neoplasia; CTFPHC, Canadian Task Force on Preventive Health Care; DRE, digital rectal examination; HNPCC, hereditary nonpolyposis colon cancer; PSA, prostate-specific antigen; USPSTF, United States Preventive Services Task Force.

[a]Patients at increased risk may require screening at younger age, increased frequency, or with different modalities.

screening. However, lung cancer is a heterogeneous disease with variable presentations, and wide variations in natural history.

For many decades now screening attempts combining imaging and clinical criteria and laboratory diagnostic tests such as sputum cytology have failed to reveal a significant morbidity or mortality improvement in screened versus unscreened populations. Most recently several authors and groups which studied the use of low dose computerized tomographic studies (LDCT) of the lung have found somewhat conflicting results. The International Early Action Lung Cancer Program reported that low dose CT scan screening resulted in an 88% ten year survival for patients with stage 1 lung cancer. However, another large medical center study assessed the effectiveness of CT scanning found no decrease in advanced lung cancer cases or in lung cancer deaths despite a large increase in the number of new lung cancer cases and a ten-fold increase in lung cancer resection. One of the central problems in any screening methodology and subsequent diagnostic and treatment protocols is the high false positive rate of a screening test, particularly low dose CT. Comparison of studies is difficult when the primary outcome measures vary. Case survival will be strongly effected by early detection biases that have no influence on population based mortality. Lead time bias, length bias, and natural history bias have an impact on all studies to date.

Formulation of screening policy continues to await the rigorous assessment that will be provided by ongoing randomized control trials such as the National Lung Screening Trial and the NELSON Trial. Until data from such trials is available, it is very likely that wide spread adoption of costly screening interventions will cause more harm to patients than good; and not improve the health of populations.

The primary preventive strategy for lung cancer remains the removal of risk factors and the prevention of exposures known to be associated with lung cancer. Of these, cigarette smoking (either passively or actively) continues to be far and away the most important risk factor. The US Preventive Services Task Force has concluded that the evidence is insufficient to recommend for or against screening an asymptomatic person for lung cancer with either low dose computerized tomography, chest x-ray, sputum cytology, or a combination of these methodologies.

SCREENING FOR OTHER DISEASES

Some diseases with high prevalence, significant associated morbidity and/or mortality, and readily available interventions are targeted for universal screening. Screening for other conditions should be considered based on individual patients' risk factors (Table 4–2).

IMMUNIZATIONS

The Advisory Committee on Immunization Practices (ACIP) is an expert panel that develops recommendations regarding indications, contraindications, schedules, and dosages for the routine administration of vaccines (Table 4–3). The overall goal of ACIP is to reduce the incidence of vaccine-preventable diseases while increasing the safe usage of vaccines.

Prior anaphylactic or neurologic reaction to a vaccine or any of its components is an absolute contraindication to future administration of that vaccine. Moderate or severe acute illness is a relative contraindication to all vaccines; however, the severity of the illness should be weighed against the benefit of the vaccine and the risk that the patient might not return for the vaccine after the illness resolves.

TABLE 4–2 Screening Recommendations for Selected Diseases/Conditions in Patients at Average Risk[a]

DISEASE/CONDITION	SCREENING MODALITY	SCREENING RECOMMENDATIONS
Hypertension	Blood pressure check	At least every 2 years
Hypercholesterolemia	Fasting lipid profile	At least every 5 years beginning at 20 years of age
Diabetes mellitus	Fasting glucose	Every 3 years beginning at 45 years of age
Sexually transmitted diseases	Chlamydia, gonorrhea, trichomonas, HIV	Both partners should be tested before initiating sexual intercourse; periodic testing for patients at high risk
Vision problems/glaucoma	Eye examination	Every 1–2 years
Hearing loss	Audiometry	Every 10 years
Thyroid disease	TSH	Women: every 5 years beginning at 35 years of age
Osteoporosis	Bone mineral density	Women 65 years of age

HIV, human immunodeficiency virus; TSH, thyroid-stimulating hormone.
[a]Patients at increased risk may require screening at younger age, increased frequency, or with different modalities.

TABLE 4-3 Recommendations for Vaccinations for Adult Patients

VACCINE	VACCINE TYPE	IMMUNIZATION SCHEDULE	INDICATIONS	SIDE EFFECTS	COMMENTS
Diphtheria/Tetanus	Toxoid	Primary series of three then booster every 10 years (5 years in the event of a tetanus-prone injury)	Universal	Soreness, redness, swelling; anaphylaxis; deep aching pain and muscle wasting in upper arm(s) beginning 2 days to 4 weeks after immunization, lasting months (rare)	Recommended for healthcare workers and others in contact with young children if at least 2 years since diphtheria/tetanus booster.
Diphtheria/tetanus/ acellular tetanus	Toxoid/acellular tetanus	Single dose for all adults as part of primary series or as booster	Universal		
Influenza	Killed virus	Annual before the onset of influenza season (usually beginning in September in the northern hemisphere)	Age older than 65 years; chronic cardiac, pulmonary, renal disease; DM; cirrhosis; immunosuppression; hemoglobinopathy; healthcare workers; residents of chronic care facilities; children aged 6 months to 6 years; women in the 2nd or 3rd trimester of pregnancy during influenza season	Soreness, redness, swelling, aches, fever; anaphylaxis; Guillain-Barré syndrome (1–2 per million doses)	Contraindicated in patients with egg allergy
Pneumococcal	23-valent poly-saccharide	One-time revaccination after 5 years for patients who receive the vaccine for medical indications or if the initial vaccine was given younger than 65 years of age	Age older than 65 years; chronic cardiac, pulmonary, renal or liver disease; functional or anatomic asplenia; DM; immunosuppression; residents of chronic care facilities; Alaskan Natives; certain American Indians	Redness, pain, fever, muscle aches; anaphylaxis (rare)	
Hepatitis B	Recombinant	Series of three vaccines separated by at least 2 months each	Injection drug use; multiple sexual partners; recent STD; MSM; hemodialysis; clotting factor recipients; chronic liver disease; healthcare workers; sexual contacts of patients with hepatitis B; individuals who are institutionalized or in correctional facilities; travelers to countries where hepatitis B is endemic	Soreness, fever; anaphylaxis	
Hepatitis A	Killed virus	Two vaccines separated by at least 6 months	Chronic liver disease; clotting factor recipients; travelers to developing countries; injection drug use; MSM;	Soreness, headache, loss of appetite, tiredness (starts 3–5 days after vaccination, lasts 1–2 days); anaphylaxis (very rare)	Safety during pregnancy unknown; risk of contracting disease should be weighted with the potential risk of the vaccine in pregnant women; may be prudent to delay travel until after delivery if possible

(Continued)

TABLE 4-3   Recommendations for Vaccinations for Adult Patients (Continued)

VACCINE	VACCINE TYPE	IMMUNIZATION SCHEDULE	INDICATIONS	SIDE EFFECTS	COMMENTS
Measles, mumps, rubella[a]	Live attenuated virus	Single dose; second dose separated by 6 months for those at high risk of exposure	Adults born after 1957; second dose for college students; healthcare workers; travelers to countries where measles is endemic; individuals with recent exposure or in an area with a recent outbreak	Fever, rash, lymphadenopathy, parotitis, pain/stiffness in joints, thrombocytopenia	Contraindicated in pregnancy; patients who have received blood products or immunoglobulins in the preceding 11 months; immunocompromised condition except HIV
Varicella[a]	Live attenuated virus	Two vaccines separated by at least 1 month	Healthy adults with no history of or serologic evidence for prior varicella infection; especially those in institutions, colleges, military base; women of child-bearing age; healthcare workers	Soreness, swelling, fever; rash (extremely rarely infectious); pneumonia (very rare)	Contraindicated in pregnancy, patients who have received blood products or immunoglobulins within the preceding 5 months, immunocompromise including HIV; caution should be used in patients using steroids
Meningococcal	Quadrivalent purified capsular polysaccharide	Single vaccine	Universal immunization of adolescents, especially college freshmen who will be living in dormitories; terminal complement deficiencies; functional or anatomic asplenia; travelers to hyperendemic or epidemic areas	Redness, pain, fever	
HPV	Recombinent quadrivalent	Series of 3 vaccines	Females 11–26 years of age	Mild injection site reactions	Serotypes 6, 11, 16, 18 that cause 70% of cervical cance; indicated in women with prior HPV infection; does not eliminate need for routine cervical cancer screening
Zoster	High dose live-attenuated varicella	Single dose	Adults over 60	Soreness, swelling, fever; rash (extremely rarely infectious); pneumonia (very rare)	Contraindicated in pregnancy, patients who have received blood products or immunoglobulins within the preceding 5 months, immunocompromise including HIV; caution should be used in patients using steroids

DM, diabetes mellitus; HIV, human immunodeficiency virus; MSM, men who have sex with men; STD, sexually transmitted disease.

[a]Special considerations for administration of live viruses: measles-mumps-rubella (MMR) and varicella vaccine can be given concurrently. If they are not given concurrently, they should be separated by an interval of 4–6 weeks. Similarly, purified protein derivative (PPD) can be placed at the same time as administration of a live virus vaccine. If not done concurrently, they should be separated by an interval of 4–6 weeks.

HEALTH BEHAVIOR

IMPORTANCE OF BEHAVIORAL CHANGE TO HEALTH AND ILLNESS

There is significant morbidity and mortality attributable to lifestyle factors, with the increasing prevalence of obesity and the metabolic syndrome contributing significantly to heart disease, cerebrovascular disease, and diabetes. As such conditions become increasingly prevalent the importance of lifestyle modification in the prevention and management of chronic diseases cannot be overemphasized. Changes in health behavior can have the biggest impact on the long-term health of individuals and the population as a whole.

A number of behaviors have been directly linked to health outcomes. Dietary factors, tobacco use, excessive alcohol use, drug use, physical inactivity, high-risk sexual behaviors, and excessive sun exposure can all have adverse health consequences. Conversely, adoption of healthier dietary habits, smoking cessation, and use of simple injury prevention interventions such as seat belts and bicycle helmets can have significant health benefits. There is good evidence that physician counseling can motivate patients to make some behavioral changes, including adopting a low cholesterol diet, restricting sodium in the diet, exercising, losing weight, and stopping smoking. Even a brief intervention has been shown to decrease high-risk alcohol consumption.

A number of theoretical models that have been developed for research in health behavior can have practical application in the clinical setting. The Health Belief Model focuses on the individual's perception of four simple constructs: (1) the individual's susceptibility to the condition of interest, (2) the severity of the condition, (3) the benefit of making the suggested behavioral change, and (4) potential barriers to making the change. Exploration of these four factors can help the clinician respond to the patient's specific questions and concerns more effectively. Another commonly used model, the stages of change, holds that all behavior change occurs in a series of predictable steps, from precontemplation (no thought of making a change) through contemplation, preparation, action, and maintenance. By assessing a patient's stage of change, the clinician can provide appropriate counseling to help the individual move to the next stage.

Often, factors beyond the patients' control will have a significant effect on their health. Access to and affordability of nutritious food and appropriate exercise facilities often determine whether patients are able to take advantage of advice about diet and exercise, whereas violence in the home and the community, availability of firearms, and the presence of environmental pollutants can all adversely affect patients' health. Physicians need to be aware of the constraints of a patient's environment in making recommendations for healthy behavioral change, and need to work with the individual patient to develop strategies appropriate to the patient's circumstances. Physicians can also be effective advocates for community change and effective health policy.

HEALTHY PEOPLE 2010

Every 10 years, the United States Department of Health and Human Services establishes a set of disease prevention and health promotion objectives for the nation to achieve over the next decade. The goals of Healthy People 2010 are to increase quality and years of healthy life and to eliminate health disparities. The underlying premise of Healthy People 2010 is that the health of the individual is closely linked to the health of the larger community. Accordingly, a wide variety of focus areas have been selected to address individual and community health needs while promoting broad participation by diverse groups, communities, and government organizations. In addition to specific diseases and conditions, these focus areas encompass preventive services such as immunizations, health behaviors such as physical activity and tobacco use, and healthcare delivery system issues such as access to quality health services, health communication, and public health infrastructure. Healthy People 2010 adopts a systematic approach to health improvement that requires identification of individual and environmental determinants of health in each focus area and evaluation of health status by monitoring leading health indicators.

BIBLIOGRAPHY

Cancer Statistics, 2006. Thun MJ, Jemal A, Siegel R, Ward E, Murray T, Xu J, Smigal C. *In CA Cancer J Clin* 2006;56; 106–130.

"Computed Tomographic Screening and Lung Cancer Outcomes." *JAMA* 297(9): 953, March 7, 2007.

Harris R, Lohr KN. Screening for prostate cancer: An update of the evidence for the U.S. Preventive Services Task Force. *Ann Intern Med.* 2002;137:917.

Harris RP, Helfand M, Woolf SH, et al., for the Methods Work Group Third U.S. Preventive Services Task Force. Current methods of the U.S. Preventive Services Task Force: A review of the process. [*Am J Prev Med.* 2001;20(3S):21]. Rockville, MD: Agency for Healthcare Research and Quality. http://www.ahrq.gov/clinic/ajpmsuppl/harris1.htm.

Hartmann KE, Hall SA, Nanda K, et al. Screening for cervical cancer: systematic evidence review. http://www.ncbi.nlm.nih.gov/books/bv.fcgi?rid=hstat3.chapter 4180.

Humphrey LL, Helfand M, and Benjamin KS, et al. Breast cancer screening: A summary of the evidence for the U.S. Preventive Services Task Force. *Ann Intern Med.* 2002;137:347.

Miller AB, Baines CJ, To T, et al. The Canadian National Breast Screening Study—I. Breast cancer mortality after 11 to 16 years of follow up. *Ann Intern Med.* 2002;137:E305.

Mokdad AH, Marks JS, Stroup DF, et al. Actual causes of death in the United States, 2000. *JAMA.* 2004;291:1238.

Pignone MP, Rich M, Teutsch SM, et al. Screening for colorectal cancer in adults at average risk: a summary of the evidence for the U.S. Preventive Services Task Force. *Ann Intern Med* 2002 137: 132–141.

Somnath S, Hoerger TJ, Pignone MP, Teutsch SM, Helfand M, Mandelblatt JS, for the Cost Work Group of the Third U.S. Preventive Services Task Force. The art and science of incorporating cost-effectiveness into evidence-based recommendations for clinical preventive services [published in *Am J Prev Med.* 2001;20(3S):36]. Rockville, MD: Agency for Healthcare Research and Quality. http://www.ahrq.gov/clinic/ajpmsuppl/saha1.htm. Accessed September 10, 2007.

"Survival of Patients with Stage I Lung Cancer Detected on CT Screening." *NEJM* 355(17): 1763, October 26, 2006.

U.S. Department of Health and Human Services. Centers for Disease Control and Prevention. Recommended adult immunization schedule, http://www.cdc.gov/vaccines/recs/schedules/adult-schedule.htm. Accessed November 14, 2007.

U.S. Department of Health and Human Services. *Healthy People 2010:* Understanding and Improving Health. Washington, DC: U.S. Government Printing Office; www.health.gov/healthypeople. Accessed November 14, 2007.

U.S. Department of Health and Human Services. Office on Women's Health. National Women's Health Information Center. Recommended Screenings and Immunizations for Woman at Average Risk for Most Diseases: www.WomensHealth.gov. Accessed November 14, 2007.

U.S. Department of Health and Human Services. Office on Women's Health. National Women's Health Information Center. Recommended Screenings and Immunizations for Woman with High Risk Factors: www.WomensHealth.gov. Accessed November 14, 2007.

U.S. Department of Health and Human Services. Recommended Screenings and Immunizations for Men: http://www. 4women. gov/screeningcharts/men/men.pdf. Accessed November 14, 2007.

U.S. Preventive Services Task Force. Screening for breast cancer: Recommendation and rationale. *Ann Intern Med.* 2002;137:344.

U.S. Preventive Services Task Force. Screening for cervical cancer: Recommendation and rationale. http://www.ahcpr.gov/clinic/3rduspstf/cervcan/cervcanrr.htm. Accessed November 14, 2007.

U.S. Preventive Services Task Force. Screening for colorectal cancer: Recommendation and rationale. *Ann Intern Med.* 2002; 137:129.

U.S. Preventive Services Task Force. Screening for prostate cancer: Recommendation and rationale. *Ann Intern Med.* 2002; 137:915.

US Preventative Services Task Force "Guide to Clinical Preventative Services, 2006." Recommendations of the U.S. Preventive Services Task Force.

5 PERIOPERATIVE MEDICINE
H. Douglas Walden

Complications of surgical procedures, including myocardial infarction, congestive heart failure, pneumonia, respiratory failure, venous thromboembolism, and delirium, occur in approximately 1 million US patients each year. Surgical complications will likely increase in future years as the population continues to age and surgery is performed on patients with multiple comorbidities. There are significant long-term consequences to perioperative complications, including increased mortality and loss of function, most prevalent in elderly patients.

ROLE OF THE CONSULTANT

The perioperative medical consultant has three primary goals:
1. Evaluate and identify medical conditions to provide an accurate assessment of surgical risk.
2. Formalize recommendations with the surgical team to minimize the patient's perioperative risk.
3. Assist in the comanagement of chronic medical illnesses of the surgical patient.

The preoperative medical consultant can never "clear" a patient for surgery. Surgical risks exist regardless of the procedure or the condition of the patient. A risk assessment can be provided, but should be carefully constructed to avoid suggesting that the procedure is without risk.

Important factors that have been shown to improve compliance with consultant recommendations include each of the following:
1. Provide recommendations within 24 hours of the request.
2. Limit the number of recommendations to five or fewer, if possible.
3. Clearly identify the crucial/critical recommendations.
4. Make specific and relevant recommendations.
5. Be specific with drug dosages, routes, frequency, and duration.
6. Follow up frequently.
7. Discuss recommendations verbally with the requesting physician or team.

Goldman highlighted the role of a medical consultant in his *Ten Commandments for Effective Consultation.* These ten principles appropriately underscore areas of emphasis needed to provide effective consultation.
1. Determine the question.
2. Establish urgency.

3. Look for yourself.
4. Be as brief as appropriate.
5. Be specific and concise.
6. Provide contingency plans.
7. Honor the turf.
8. Teach with tact.
9. Talk is cheap and effective.
10. Follow up.

ANESTHESIA FACTS

Peripheral vasodilatation is a common effect of both general and spinal/epidural anesthetics. All inhaled anesthetics also cause depressed cardiac contractility and diastolic dysfunction. Hypotension, usually transient, is often seen with each method. Many inhaled agents may cause bradycardia and atrioventricular conduction abnormalities.

A decreased tidal volume is commonly seen with both general and spinal/epidural agents and is associated with atelectasis.

The need for invasive hemodynamic monitoring during surgery is controversial, but evidence suggests that it does not lower surgical risk when used routinely. However, its use in selected patients (heart failure) may prove beneficial.

American Society of Anesthesiologists (ASA) Classification

CLASS	DESCRIPTION
I	A normal healthy patient
II	A patient with mild systemic disease
III	A patient with systemic disease that is not incapacitating
IV	A patient with an incapacitating systemic disease that is a constant threat to life
V	A moribund patient who is not expected to survive for 24 hours with or without operation.

Although the anesthesia team will often document the surgical patient's ASA class, it is of limited use to the medical consultant as many surgical patients fall into categories II and III and will require additional measures to optimally determine perioperative risk.

Decisions about the choice and route of anesthesia are best left to the anesthesiologist as little evidence suggests that one agent or route is preferable to another in order to minimize surgical risk.

PREOPERATIVE EVALUATION

HISTORY AND PHYSICAL EXAMINATION

Obtaining a full medical history and performing a careful physical examination are the most important aspects of preoperative evaluation. They may be the only evaluation tools needed in healthy individuals 50 years of age and under, as the operative risk in this patient group is very low.

- Special emphasis should be placed on assessing cardiopulmonary symptoms as well as the patient's functional status and exercise tolerance. Individuals with a poor functional status may require further evaluation to exclude unrecognized disease. Recall that one metabolic equivalent (MET) is an individual's basal oxygen consumption at rest in a sitting position. Four METS is roughly equivalent to walking two blocks on level ground or carrying two bags of groceries up one flight of stairs. Individuals able to generate exercise that exceeds more than four METS in intensity have a lower risk of complications. The absence of cardiopulmonary symptoms in individuals *unable* to perform activities above four METS is not reliable for assessing perioperative risk. These individuals may require additional studies to assess their risk.
- Effort should also be directed toward identifying symptoms of a bleeding disorder (prior excessive surgical blood loss, hemarthroses, unprovoked epistaxis, or unprovoked bruising) that may increase transfusion requirements or require repeat procedures for uncontrollable bleeding. A careful and full medication history is important. Many agents that can affect hemostasis are available without a prescription (aspirin, nonsteroidal anti-inflammatory drugs [NSAIDS], and various herbal preparations) and may not be reported by the patient unless they are questioned specifically about them. Ginseng, garlic, and ginkgo biloba affect platelet function and all herbal products should be discontinued approximately one week prior to surgery. Some consultants also request that patients discontinue vitamin E prior to surgery due to its effects on hemostasis.

MEDICATION MANAGEMENT

All unnecessary medications should be discontinued prior to surgery. Most medications used for chronic medical conditions (hypertension, hypothyroidism, ischemic heart disease, etc) can be continued until the day of surgery and taken with a sip of water on the day of the procedure. Transdermal or intravenous therapy of some agents may be needed if the individual cannot take medications orally. Statins may have favorable effects perioperatively and should be continued throughout the perioperative course.

- Aspirin and clopidogrel are irreversible inhibitors of platelet cyclooxygenase and should be discontinued at least one week prior to surgery if the procedure poses a risk for catastrophic bleeding (central nervous system [CNS] procedures). Despite the possibility of increased surgical blood loss, aspirin need not be discontinued routinely. In peripheral vascular surgery and coronary artery bypass procedures, the benefits of antiplatelet therapy appear to outweigh the possible adverse effects and, therefore aspirin should be continued. Nonsteroidal anti-inflammatory agents inhibit vasodilatory prostaglandins and pose a risk to postoperative renal function. They are best discontinued 1 to 3 days prior to the procedure.

- Perioperative care for patients requiring warfarin therapy due to a history of thromboembolism, atrial fibrillation, or mechanical heart valves can be challenging. For patients undergoing a procedure with a low risk of bleeding (cataract extraction and various dermatological, dental, and gastrointestinal procedures), warfarin can often be continued through the perioperative period without interruption. Discontinuation of warfarin 4 to 5 days before the procedure coupled with bridging anticoagulation therapy using low molecular weight heparin is advisable for patients with an intermediate or high risk for thromboembolism. If anticoagulation with warfarin must be reversed due to bleeding complications or emergent surgery then fresh frozen plasma and/or vitamin K given orally or intravenously is useful. Subcutaneous vitamin K should not be used due to erratic absorption from subcutaneous tissue.
- β-Blockers, clonidine, and benzodiazepines are best continued throughout the perioperative period due to adverse effects of abrupt withdrawal. Administration of these agents through an alternate route (transdermal or intravenous) should be considered if the patient cannot take medications orally.
- The following medications are often held the day prior to surgery based on studies suggesting possible adverse effects in the perioperative period: metformin, diuretics, lipid-lowering agents (other than statins), oral hypoglycemics, and theophylline. Continuation of angiotensin-converting enzyme (ACE) inhibitors and angiotensin II receptor blockers probably pose little risk perioperatively but should be discontinued in patients with volume depletion or hypotension.
- Up to one-third of all surgical patients are taking herbal products. All herbal medications are best stopped prior to surgery. Those thought to have adverse effects in the perioperative period are ginseng, garlic, gingko biloba, echinacea, ephedra, kava, St. John's wort, and valerian.

LABORATORY TESTING

There is little evidence that extensive laboratory testing or imaging studies predict surgical risk or lower complication rates in healthy patients 50 years of age and younger.

- Selective rather than routine testing is recommended. Most laboratory tests are not helpful unless ordered to evaluate a specific sign, symptom, or suspected diagnosis. Unnecessary laboratory tests add to the cost of healthcare and often require additional studies to evaluate false positive results. Evaluation of false positive test results can delay the planned surgical procedure and thus increase risk from the underlying process requiring surgical intervention.
- Tests performed within approximately 6 months of a planned procedure appear to be acceptable if there has been no change in the clinical condition of the patient.
- A chemistry profile may be helpful in healthy patients over age 50 and in patients with diabetes or hypertension or those on diuretics to identify renal disease and electrolyte abnormalities that can be associated with an increased surgical risk.
- Liver function tests should be evaluated in patients with a history of alcohol use. Serum albumin should be analyzed based on its association with pulmonary risk.
- Electrocardiography may be performed on patients older than 50 to detect latent cardiac abnormalities, but the results rarely alter the recommendations.
- Blood counts, urinalysis, coagulation profiles, chest x-rays, and pulmonary function tests should be obtained when signs, symptoms, or history of chronic illness dictate; they offer little benefit when obtained routinely.

CARDIAC RISK ASSESSMENT

The revised cardiac risk index (RCRI) is the best cardiac risk evaluation tool available. It is simple, current, validated, and accurately predicts risk. The six independent predictors of postoperative cardiac complications include:

1. Intrathoracic, intraperitoneal, or infrainguinal vascular surgery
2. History of ischemic heart disease
3. History of congestive heart failure
4. Diabetes mellitus requiring treatment with insulin
5. Serum creatinine >2 mg/dL
6. History of cerebrovascular disease

Each RCRI predictor receives equal weight. The risk of major cardiac complications (myocardial infarction, pulmonary edema, ventricular fibrillation, cardiac arrest, and complete heart block) varies based on the number of predictors present

RISK OF MAJOR CARDIAC COMPLICATIONS BASED ON THE RCRI

None	0.4%
One	0.9%
Two	7.0%
Three or more	11%

Older cardiac risk evaluation tools including those of Goldman (1977), Detsky (1986), and the American College of Physicians (1997) do not reflect current surgical risk and should no longer be used in clinical practice. The 2007 American College of Cardiology/ American Heart Association (ACC/AHA) guidelines on perioperative evaluation for noncardiac surgery provide additional useful recommendations.

Selected patients with severe aortic stenosis, active cardiac ischemia, or decompensated congestive heart failure are also at increased risk. Individuals with asymptomatic aortic stenosis usually tolerate surgical procedures well.

Individuals who are candidates for stress testing, cardiac catheterization, or revascularization regardless of the planned surgery (those with unstable angina, limiting angina, recent myocardial infarction, or previous abnormal cardiac studies) should have the procedures performed prior to planned noncardiac surgery.

If functional status or exercise tolerance cannot be evaluated a negative noninvasive stress test is predictive of a low risk of major cardiac complications.

Use of a dobutamine echocardiogram or a dipyridamole-radionuclide study may be helpful in assessing cardiac risk if an individual is unable to exercise.

CARDIAC RISK REDUCTION

β-Blocker therapy appears to lower cardiac risk in the perioperative period, especially in high-risk patients. This effect appears to be due to a reduction in perioperative ischemia and a reduction in myocardial infarction and death.

The ideal agent, dose, route, and timing/duration of therapy remain unclear. Beginning therapy as soon as possible is reasonable and allows time to monitor treatment. The heart rate should be lowered to 55 to 65 beats per minute; the heart rate achieved in the clinical trials demonstrating benefit. Some β-blockers may be superior to others for this purpose. For example, some evidence suggests that longer-acting agents (atenolol) may be associated with better outcomes than shorter-acting agents (metoprolol).

One retrospective cohort study suggests that individuals with an RCRI of 3 or more benefited from β-blocker therapy whereas those with scores of 0, 1, or 2 failed to benefit or may have been harmed by treatment. Thus, higher-risk patients may obtain a greater benefit from perioperative β-blockade than low-risk individuals.

The ACC/AHA 2006 guideline update on perioperative β-blocker therapy offered these recommendations for use in the absence of contraindications:

1. β-Blockers should be continued in patients undergoing surgery who are receiving β-blockers to treat angina, symptomatic arrhythmias, or hypertension, and to patients undergoing vascular surgery at high cardiac risk with established ischemia on preoperative testing.
2. β-Blockers are probably recommended for patients undergoing vascular surgery in whom preoperative assessment identifies coronary heart disease or high cardiac risk as defined by the presence of multiple clinical risk factors.
3. β-Blockers are probably recommended for patients who are undergoing intermediate or high-risk procedures and in whom preoperative assessment identifies coronary heart disease or high cardiac risk (as defined by the presence of multiple clinical risk factors).
4. β-Blockers may be considered for patients who are undergoing intermediate or high-risk procedures, including vascular surgery, in whom preoperative assessment identifies intermediate cardiac risk as defined by the presence of a single clinical risk factor or for patients undergoing vascular surgery with low cardiac risk who are not currently on β-blockers.

Clonidine, an α_2-agonist, is an alternative to β-blockers for cardiac protection. Studies have demonstrated a significant reduction in mortality and incidence of myocardial infarction with preoperative clonidine as compared to placebo. It can be administered as either the oral or transdermal preparation.

Perioperative statin therapy has been demonstrated to decrease postoperative complications in vascular surgery patients without evidence of increased toxicity in the perioperative period.

Many patients who receive perioperative β-blockers and/or statin therapy are candidates for long-term use and should be continued on these agents at the time of discharge.

Coronary artery revascularization before elective vascular surgery among patients with stable cardiac symptoms does not significantly alter outcome and is not recommended purely as a prophylactic measure. In addition, recent studies have demonstrated an increased risk of cardiac complications and death in patients undergoing surgery within 6 to 8 weeks of receiving intracoronary stents. This may be due to discontinuation of antiplatelet therapy prematurely. Ideally, surgery should be delayed for at least 8 weeks after stent placement.

PULMONARY RISK ASSESSMENT

Pulmonary complications (atelectasis, pneumonia, respiratory failure, and exacerbation of underlying chronic lung disease) are as common as cardiac complications after noncardiac surgery and contribute significantly to morbidity, mortality, and length of hospital stay.

RISK FACTORS FOR PULMONARY COMPLICATIONS

Significant patient-related risk factors for postoperative pulmonary complications include the following:
1. Chronic obstructive pulmonary disease (COPD)
2. Age older than 60
3. ASA class II or greater
4. Functional dependency
5. Congestive heart failure
6. Impaired sensorium
7. Abnormal findings on chest examination
8. Alcohol use
9. Weight loss
10. Serum albumin <3.5 g/dL

Obesity and asthma have not been found to be associated with an increased risk of pulmonary complications.

Procedure-related pulmonary risk factors include the following:
1. General anesthesia
2. Surgery greater than 3 hours duration
3. Surgery of the abdomen, thorax, brain, head and neck, vascular, and aortic sites
4. Emergency procedures

Laboratory and imaging evaluation preoperatively need not be extensive. There is little evidence that spirometry adds to clinical assessment for prediction of pulmonary risk, with the exception of lung resection procedures and determining candidacy for coronary artery bypass. There appears to be no clear spirometric threshold below which surgical risk is unacceptable. Chest radiographs rarely provide information that could not be predicted by history and physical examination; they rarely influence preoperative management. Chest films should be limited to those patients with known cardiopulmonary disease; those older than 50 years of age; and those undergoing upper abdominal, thoracic, or abdominal aortic aneurysm surgery.

Serum albumin (<3.5 g/dL) is the primary laboratory study that predicts pulmonary risk and should be obtained in patients at risk for hypoalbuminemia and those with additional pulmonary risk factors.

STRATEGIES TO REDUCE POSTOPERATIVE PULMONARY COMPLICATIONS

Smoking cessation interventions—Smoking cessation is a reasonable recommendation for patients undergoing surgical procedures. Surprisingly however, there is little evidence that smoking cessation within 8 weeks of surgery actually lessens the pulmonary complication rate. In fact, some studies suggest a slightly higher rate of pulmonary complications in individuals who quit shortly before the procedure. These findings highlight the need for all physicians to regularly assess the smoking habits of their patients and to recommend cessation of smoking regardless of the setting.

Lung expansion modalities—Any modality of lung expansion (incentive spirometry, chest physical therapy, postural drainage, percussion and vibration, suctioning and ambulation, intermittent positive pressure breathing, or continuous positive airway pressure) appears superior to no lung expansion modality at all in patients undergoing abdominal procedures. No modality has been proven superior to another and there appears to be no additive effect of multiple techniques. Therefore, use of incentive spirometry is reasonable for those able to perform it and nasal continuous positive airway pressure is an alternative for those unable to perform incentive spirometry.

Perioperative care—Although malnutrition (and hypoalbuminemia) increases the risk of pulmonary complications there is no evidence that nutritional supplementation (either enteral or parenteral) reduces the complication rate. Pulmonary artery catheter use also does not appear to lower pulmonary complication rates. Evidence does suggest that selective use of nasogastric tubes (only used in patients with postoperative nausea and vomiting, inability to tolerate oral intake, or symptomatic abdominal distension) after surgery significantly lowers the risk of pneumonia and atelectasis.

SELECTED PERIOPERATIVE PROBLEMS

HYPERTENSION

Blood pressures less than 180 mm Hg systolic and less than 110 mm Hg diastolic have not been associated with increased perioperative complications. Hypertension preoperatively, however, is associated with lability of blood pressure intraoperatively. For elective procedures it is reasonable to employ measures to control blood pressure before surgery.

Postoperative hypertension is often due to pain, anxiety, or interruption of previous chronic drug therapy. Attention to these factors is often all that is required. Use of parenteral antihypertensives is rarely needed and can be associated with undesirable hypotension.

FEVER

Fever is very common after surgery and not specific for infection in the postoperative setting. In the first 48 hours postoperatively, fever is due to infection in less than 10% of cases. Release of cytokines, particularly interleukin 6 (IL-6), is thought to mediate fever in the early postoperative setting. Atelectasis has been considered to be a cause of early postoperative fever, but there is no evidence to support this, and this perception should be abandoned.

A careful history and physical examination with special attention to new symptoms suggestive of infection (cough or diarrhea, for example), current medications, history of blood product administration, vascular catheter sites, vital signs, skin, cardiac, and pulmonary examinations are critical. If there are no findings suggestive of infection, routine cultures of blood and urine and chest x-ray have a low yield in the first 48 hours postoperatively and need not be obtained.

Fever developing on or after the fifth postoperative day is due to infection in approximately 90% of cases. The most common causes of infection in this time interval are

1. Urinary tract infection (especially if a urinary catheter has been used)
2. Surgical site infection
3. Pneumonia (especially if COPD) is present or mechanical ventilation is needed)
4. Intravenous catheter-related infection
5. *Clostridium difficile* associated diarrhea

Noninfectious causes of fever that should be considered include venous thromboembolic disease, drug fever, acute adrenal insufficiency, transfusion reactions, gout or pseudogout, malignant hyperthermia, drug/alcohol withdrawal (especially in trauma or emergency surgery), and serotonin syndrome.

CONFUSION

Factors associated with development of postoperative delirium include preoperative alcohol abuse; poor cognitive function; poor physical function status; age older than 70 years; marked abnormalities of serum sodium, potassium, or glucose; and aortic or noncardiac thoracic surgery.

Interventions most helpful in preventing postoperative delirium include early discontinuation of urinary catheters; maintaining normal bowel function; minimizing the use of benzodiazepines, antihistamines, and anticholinergics; and maintaining the hematocrit at or above 30%.

One double-blind placebo-controlled trial demonstrated that administration of haloperidol (0.5 mg three times per day until the third postoperative day) to hip surgery patients older than 70 years of age with intermediate to high risk of postoperative delirium decreased the duration and the length of hospital stay for individuals who actually developed delirium. Haloperidol, however, did not decrease the incidence of delirium in these patients.

RENAL INSUFFICIENCY

Approximately 50% of patients who develop acute renal failure following general, vascular, or cardiac surgery die. Others recover partial function but are at risk for gradual progression to chronic kidney disease and may eventually need some form of renal replacement therapy.

Maintenance of adequate intravascular volume and renal perfusion are keys to prevention of renal complications. Use of dopamine, mannitol, or furosemide has not been effective in preserving renal function. High dose diuretics must be used judiciously to avoid volume depletion and neurohormonal activation. Hemodialysis, hemofiltration, or ultrafiltration should be considered in volume overloaded patients refractory to diuretics.

Individuals on chronic dialysis should undergo dialysis within 24 hours before surgery and should be monitored very carefully for life-threatening hyperkalemia. Dialysis-dependent patients are also at higher risk for bleeding complications, fluid overload, and pulmonary infections.

Adjustments in medication doses must be made if changes in renal function are noted in the postoperative period.

Care should be taken to limit use of intravenous contrast postoperatively in any patient with elevated serum creatinine.

DIABETES MELLITUS

Diabetes mellitus is associated with poor wound healing and an increased frequency of cardiac complications. There is little evidence to guide the optimal management of blood glucose in the perioperative period.

Neutrophil dysfunction occurs, bacterial killing is impaired, and wound infection rates rise when glucose levels exceed 200 mg/dL. Several retrospective analyses have demonstrated a decrease in in-hospital mortality and length of hospital stay with tighter blood glucose control (average 3 day blood glucose less than 150 mg/dL) after coronary artery bypass graft procedures. A large prospective study involving intensive care patients demonstrated that intensive insulin therapy (target blood glucose 100 mg dL) was associated with a lower intensive care unit (ICU) mortality, hospital mortality, ICU days, time on a ventilator, incidence of renal failure, and incidence of infection compared with conventional insulin therapy (target blood glucose 180 to 200 mg/dL). How these studies relate to the typical noncardiac surgical patient is unclear and requires additional investigations. Importantly, attempts at tight glucose control may precipitate hypoglycemia.

For diabetic patients not using insulin preoperatively, the last dose of oral hypoglycemic medication is usually given the night before and held the morning of the surgical procedure. Metformin is usually not continued through the perioperative period because of the risk of lactic acidosis. Other oral agents may be used again after the patient restarts his/her usual diet postoperatively. Insulin may be used in all diabetics and is often preferable for control in the hospital, even in those patients not previously on insulin. Frequent blood glucose monitoring (at least four times daily) is essential.

For diabetic patients using insulin preoperatively, insulin is almost always required postoperatively. It can be provided in a number of ways. Continuing some combination of basal insulin (glargine or neutral protamine Hagedorn [NPH] insulin) with a shorter-acting preparation is appropriate. Glargine insulin can generally be continued throughout the perioperative period without a change in dose because it only rarely causes hypoglycemia. NPH insulin is usually given at a reduced dose (one-half to two-thirds of the usual dose) on the morning of surgery with a dextrose infusion. Frequent blood glucose monitoring both intraoperatively and postoperatively is essential. Small doses of regular insulin can be provided subcutaneously while the patient is taking nothing by mouth to tighten control. An alternate regimen for tight glucose control involves use of an intravenous infusion of regular insulin titrated against a second intravenous infusion of dextrose. Very tight blood glucose control can usually be obtained with this method, although it requires close evaluation and follow-up.

β-Blocker use in diabetic patients must be closely monitored. β-Blockers may mask symptoms and delay recognition and treatment of hypoglycemia. In addition, one large randomized controlled trial of metoprolol initiated the night before surgery in diabetic patients was associated with a higher risk of heart failure in the treated group without a reduction in all-cause mortality or adverse cardiac events.

OTHER ENDOCRINE DISORDERS

Individuals who are taking chronic corticosteroid therapy or who have received the equivalent of 7.5 mg of prednisone daily for a 3- to 4-week period during the previous 12 months may not be able to generate an adequate stress hormone response and are at risk for adrenal insufficiency.

Treatment with intravenous hydrocortisone, 50 to 100 mg every 8 hours, beginning 30 to 60 minutes before surgery should protect adrenally insufficient patients from developing an adrenal crisis. This dose can be continued until the patient resumes a normal diet. Once eating regularly, the patient may resume his/her usual daily steroid dose.

Individuals with asymptomatic or mild hypothyroidism generally tolerate surgery quite well, and most procedures need not be delayed for hormone

replacement. Patients with severe disease should have elective procedures rescheduled after adequate thyroid hormone replacement because of increased risks including heart failure and hypotension.

THROMBOSIS/ANTICOAGULANTS

Surgery increases the risk of deep venous thrombosis (DVT). The incidence of DVT is as high as 25% of patients undergoing general surgical procedures without the use of prophylaxis. Accordingly, prophylaxis is recommended for most surgical procedures.

If bleeding complications pose a very high risk (neurosurgery), a mechanical method of prophylaxis (intermittent pneumatic compression stockings) is preferred.

For many other general surgical procedures, use of heparin (5000 U every 8 hours) or low molecular weight heparin (enoxaparin 40 mg subcutaneously once daily starting 2 hours prior to surgery) is effective.

For hip and knee orthopedic procedures, low molecular weight heparin is preferred (enoxaparin 30 mg every 12 hours subcutaneously). Oral warfarin or subcutaneous fondaparinux (a selective and specific inhibitor of Factor Xa) are alternative anticoagulants in these circumstances, but warfarin is usually more cumbersome to use than low molecular weight heparin. The risk for DVT after hip and knee procedures persists for 4 to 6 weeks after surgery. The American College of Chest Physicians recommends continuation of prophylactic anticoagulation for 28 to 35 days for these orthopedic procedures.

TRANSFUSION

Optimal levels of hemoglobin and hematocrit perioperatively have not been precisely defined. The lower level of accepted hemoglobin may be about 7 g/dL. An increased risk of death has been demonstrated among patients who refused transfusion for cultural reasons when the postoperative hemoglobin fell below 7 g/dL. However, transfusion to hemoglobin levels much higher than this may not be warranted. A strategy to transfuse packed red blood cells only when the hemoglobin fell below 8 g/dL was at least as beneficial as indicated by morbidity, mortality, and patient self-assessment. As a more liberal transfusion strategy provided there was no source of ongoing blood loss. The risks of transfusion, including volume overload and transmission of infectious agents, should be considered in all transfusion decisions.

The American Society of Clinical Oncology recommends that the platelet count be maintained above 40–50,000/μL prior to major invasive procedures. Nonetheless, platelet transfusions may be required if there are other coagulation abnormalities or impaired platelet function. Minor procedures can often be performed at lower platelet counts.

ANTIBIOTIC PROPHYLAXIS

Prophylactic antibiotics have been shown to decrease surgical site infections for many procedures. The antibiotic should be administered prior to the surgical incision. For most surgical sites, a single dose of an appropriate antibiotic given approximately 30 minutes before the surgical incision is adequate. If the surgery is prolonged, one should readminister the antibiotic in order to maintain blood levels in the therapeutic range.

Multiple prophylactic doses through the postoperative period are generally unnecessary even if drains or catheters remain in place. However, extension of the dosing for cardiac surgery through 24 hours postoperatively is recommended. More prolonged antibiotic prophylaxis has not been shown to lower infection rates and may increase antimicrobial resistance and infection with *C. difficile.*

Only elective, nontraumatic surgery that does not involve the respiratory, gastrointestinal, biliary, or genitourinary tract, does not require antibiotic prophylaxis. If surgery involves placement of a foreign material an antibiotic dose is often provided given the consequences of infection of prosthetic material.

The major targets for prophylaxis are common skin organisms (particularly staphylococcus). Cefazolin, 1 to 2 grams intravenously (use of the 2-gram dose is preferable in obese patients), is appropriate for most procedures. Vancomycin may be needed if the patient is a known carrier of methicillin-resistant *Staphylococcus aureus* (MRSA) or if antibiotic resistance patterns indicate a need. Cefotetan or cefoxitin is often provided for uncomplicated appendectomy or colorectal procedures to include anaerobic coverage.

Elimination of nasal carriage of *S. aureus* with topical 2% mupirocin (twice daily for three days) has been shown to lower the risk of surgical site infection in cardiac surgery.

BIBLIOGRAPHY

ACC/AHA 2007 Guidelines on Perioperative Cardiovascular Evaluation and Care for Noncardiac Surgery, Circulation 2007;116(17):1971–1996.

Geerts WH, Pineo GF, Heit JA, et al. Prevention of thromboembolism: the Seventh ACCP Conference on Antithrombotic and Thrombolytic Therapy. *Chest.* 2004;126(3 Suppl):338S–400S.

Goldman L, Lee T, Rudd P. Ten commandments for effective consultation. *Arch Intern Med.* 1983;143(9):1753–1755.

Lee TH, Marcantonio ER, Mangione CM, et al. Derivation and prospective validation of a simple index for prediction of cardiac risk of major noncardiac surgery. *Circulation.* 1999;100:1043–1049.

Medical Consultation *Med Clin North Am.* 2003 Jan;87(1):1–302.

Proceedings of the Perioperative Medicine Summit: Using Evidence to Improve Quality, Safety, and Patient Outcomes. September 22–23, 2005 Cleveland, Ohio. *Cleve Clin J Med.* 2006;73 Suppl 1:S1–120.

Qaseem A, Snow V, Fitterman N, et al. Risk assessment for and strategies to reduce perioperative pulmonary complications for patients undergoing noncardiothoracic surgery: A guideline from the American College of Physicians. *Ann Intern Med.* 2006; 144:575–580.

6   COMMON PROBLEMS IN OTORHINOLARYNGOLOGY
James Drake

PHARYNGITIS

DEFINITION

- An acute upper respiratory tract infection affecting the mucosa of the throat.

EPIDEMIOLOGY

- Pharyngitis is a common condition accounting for approximately 2% of all ambulatory visits in the United States. Although pharyngitis in the adult in secondary to Group A streptococcus, 10% of the time, antibiotics are prescribed in nearly 75% of cases. Therefore, the Centers for Disease Control and Prevention (CDC) has campaigned to discourage physicians from routine antibiotic use.
- Other potentially treatable pathogens include *Neisseria gonorrhea, Mycoplasma pneumoniae,* and *Corynebacterium diphtheriae,* each of which is responsible for less than 1% of cases. Viruses are far more common causes, especially rhinovirus but also coronavirus, adenovirus, respiratory syncytial, and Epstein-Barr (EB) virus.

DIFFERENTIAL DIAGNOSIS

- It is difficult to clinically distinguish bacterial infections from viral. Moreover, the clinician must also exclude life-threatening or systemic conditions that are associated with pharyngitis. For example, epiglottitis, pharyngeal abscess, and diphtheria should be considered in acutely ill patients. In addition, a unilaterally enlarged tonsil suggests that a peritonsillar abscess may be present. The physical examination should exclude the presence of foreign bodies. And finally, the occurrence of multisystem illness should prompt an evaluation for connective tissue disease.

- Group A streptococcus typically exhibits the following features:
  - Fever greater than 38.5°C
  - Tender anterior cervical adenopathy
  - Absence of cough and rhinorrhea
- Influenza typically exhibits the following features:
  - Headaches
  - Myalgias
  - Fever
- EB virus typically exhibits the following features:
  - Posterior cervical adenopathy
  - Often persistent fatigue, weight loss, splenomegaly, hepatitis, and diffuse lymphadenopathy
- Mycoplasma is usually accompanied by acute bronchitis
- Corynebacterium diphtheriae typically exhibits the following features:
  - Gradual onset
  - Low-grade fever
  - Malaise
  - 33% of patients reveal a lightly adhering gray membrane on physical examination of the oropharynx
- *N. gonorrhea* is associated with minimal pharyngeal symptoms
- Human immunodeficiency virus typically exhibits the following features:
  - High-risk behavior 2 to 3 weeks before symptom onset
  - Fever
  - Weight loss greater than 10 lbs
  - Adenopathy/Splenomegaly
  - Decreased peripheral lymphocytes, increased aminotransaminases
- The clinical diagnosis of group A Streptococcus can be presumptively established when three of four of the following clinical manifestations are present: fever, tonsillar exudate, anterior cervical adenopathy, absent cough.
  - These clinical features have a positive predictive value of 40% to 60%.
  - The presence of 0 or 1 of the above manifestations has a negative predictive value of 80%.

LABORATORY DIAGNOSIS

- The gold standard is a throat culture
  - The culture requires 24 to 48 hours to exhibit growth; 1% to 5% of the population are carriers of streptococcus A, thus false-positives are relatively common.
  - The rapid antigen detection test (RADT) requires a throat swab which is used to detect antigen-antibody complexes. It only requires minutes to complete.
    - The sensitivity of the rapid antigen test is 80% to 90%
    - Its specificity is very high (>98%). Thus, when the test is positive the diagnosis is assured.
  - Serology is of little use in establishing the acute diagnosis of pharyngitis. Antistreptolysin titers increase to greater than 300 U/mL within the first week and peak 2 to 3 weeks later.

TREATMENT OBJECTIVES

- Reduce symptoms (resolution occurs 1 to 2 days sooner in patients receiving antibiotic therapy).
- Prevent transmission (more relevant in pediatric patients). The close contact transmission rate is approximately 35%, although this rate is negligible 24 hours after antibiotics are initiated.
- Prevent peritonsillar abscess formation.
- Prevent rheumatic fever (rare in North America, although the data for prevention are robust). In contrast, there are no convincing data to support prophylaxis of acute glomerulonephritis.
- Children younger than age 7 years are at greatest risk for the complications of streptococcal pharyngitis and, thus should be managed more deliberately.
- When all four clinical criteria (some sources accept three of four criteria) are present, the patient should receive antibiotic treatment.
- Patients with a positive RADT coupled with two to three criteria should also be treated .

ANTIBIOTIC THERAPY

- Penicillin 500 mg four times a day for 10 days should be prescribed; the full 10 day course is essential because the relapse rate is high if therapy is discontinued prematurely (50% if discontinued after day 3, 34% if discontinued after day 6 to 7).
- Benzathine penicillin G 900,000 U and procaine penicillin 300,000 U may be administered intramuscularly in noncompliant patients.
- Alternative regimens in penicillin-allergic patients:
  - Cephalosporins
    - Cephalexin 500 mg four times a day for 10 days (avoid these antibiotics if there is a history of a severe immunoglobulin E–mediated reaction to penicillin)
  - Macrolides
    - Erythromycin 500 mg four times a day for 10 days
    - Azithromycin 10 to 12 mg/kg for 5 days
    - Clarithromycin 15 mg/kg for 5 days

EXTERNAL OTITIS

DEFINITION

• External otitis is characterized by an inflammation of the external auditory canal or auricle. The inflammation is usually generalized throughout the ear canal.

EPIDEMIOLOGY

• Approximately 10% of patients develop external otitis during their lifetime.

PATHOGENESIS

• Initiated by degradation of the skin cerumen barrier. The dark, warm, alkaline, and moist ear canal predisposes to bacterial growth. Cerumen possesses natural antibacterial and antifungal properties, in part by promoting an acidic microenvironment. Predisposing factors include skin disorders that extend to the ear canal, swimming, humidity, hearing aids that occlude the ear canal, and mechanical injury (overzealous cleaning or aggressive scratching of the ear canal).

MICROBIOLOGY

• The most common pathogens are constituents of the normal skin flora, including, *Pseudomonas aeruginosa* and *Staphylococcus aureus*. Anaerobic pathogens, especially bacteroides and *Peptostreptococcus,* account for 4% to 25% of infections.

DIAGNOSIS

• The diagnosis typically rests on the classic symptoms of discharge, pruritus, and decreased hearing. Tragal tension usually elicits pain (may be absent in mild cases). Direct visualization of the ear canal reveals an erythematous and edematous canal with debris varying in color (yellow, brown, gray, and white). Severe cases may be accompanied by complete canal obstruction, lymphedema, fever, and periauricular erythema.

TREATMENT

• Gentle ear cleansing with half-strength H_2O_2 removes purulent debris. Careful cleansing with soft wire loops or cotton swabs under direct visualization is acceptable.
• Inflammation and infection require the use of a topical antibiotic. Ideally the preparation should be acidic and contain a steroid, antiseptic, and antibiotic. Ciprofloxacin (Cipro HC) dosed twice daily is the preparation of choice.
• Advanced cases (eg, canal occlusion) require otolaryngology referral for stent placement. Systemic antibiotics may be necessary for severe cases that extend beyond the external ear or in immunocompromised individuals. Amoxicillin, clavulanate, cephalexin, dicloxacillin, or fluoroquinolones are all reasonable antibiotic choices.
• Most patients experience some relief within 36 to 48 hours. The duration of treatment is unclear but should probably be continued for 7 to 14 days. Many patients will discontinue therapy upon complete resolution of signs and symptoms without adverse consequence.

COMPLICATIONS

Necrotizing otitis externa occurs when the infection spreads from skin to soft tissue, cartilage, and bone of the temporal region and basilar skull. These complications most commonly occur in elderly (>65 years of age), diabetics, and immunocompromised individuals. Suspected patients should be promptly referred to an otolaryngologist.

DIFFERENTIAL DIAGNOSIS

• Otomycosis
  ◦ Fungal infections are responsible for 6.5% to 12.5% of external otitis.
  ◦ *Aspergillus niger* and *Candida* are the most common organisms and occur more frequently in tropical and subtropical climates.
  ◦ Intense itching, a sensation of a foreign body within the canal, and discharge are common.
  ◦ The pain is usually intense.
  ◦ Fungal filaments and spores may be identified in the brushings obtained from the canal.
  ◦ Treatment involves meticulous (albeit, gentle) cleaning of the ear canal and administration of topical antifungals such as clotrimazole.
• Contact dermatitis
  ◦ Patients who have persistent edema and erythema of the canal despite ototopical treatment may be experiencing an allergic reaction to one of its components (eg, neomycin, benzocaine, or propylene glycol).
  ◦ Pruritus is the predominant symptom in these settings.
  ◦ Vesicles and erythema may be observed under direct visualization.
  ◦ The treatment includes cleaning the canal and acidification of the ear with a peroxide and steroid based solution.

- Chronic suppurative otitis media
  ○ These patients will have a protracted history of ear problems with frequent otorrhea.
  ○ Polyps and granulation tissue may be observed near the tympanic membrane.
  ○ These patients should be referred to an otolaryngologist for definitive therapy.
- Carcinoma of the external auditory canal
  ○ Carcinoma of the external auditory canal is a rare finding.
  ○ Abnormal tissue growth in the ear canal is observed.
  ○ This should be suspected in patients with recurrent or protracted external otitis despite appropriate therapy.
  ○ Bloody otorrhea, pain and a friable ear canal with surrounding purulence are often noted.
  ○ Referral to an oncologist and otolaryngologist is mandatory as these tumors are usually very aggressive.

ACUTE OTITIS MEDIA

DEFINITION

- An inflammatory condition of the middle ear associated with effusion that is accompanied by rapid onset of signs or symptoms of otitis media (fullness, pain, hearing loss, and vertigo).

EPIDEMIOLOGY

- Peak incidence occurs between 6 and 24 months of age, although it may occur at any age.
- Risk factors:
  ○ Family history (based on a recent meta-analysis of 22 studies)
  ○ Genetics (twin studies suggest a higher incidence in monozygotic versus dizygotic twins)
  ○ Ethnicity (especially Native Americans and Eskimos)
  ○ Tobacco smoke (poorly understood)
  ○ Day care (direct spread of pathogenetic organisms)
  ○ Pacifier use
- Less likely if breast fed, which appears to decrease bacterial colonization.
- Increased incidence in the fall and winter.
- Associated with allergic rhinitis and impaired host defenses.

PATHOGENESIS

- Upper respiratory infection or allergic symptoms precede many cases. Congestion of the nose, nasopharynx, eustachian tube isthmus (negative pressure in eustachian tube) may promote stasis in the middle ear.

Accordingly, secretions accumulate in the middle ear and viruses and bacteria proliferate.

MICROBIOLOGY

- *Streptococcocus pneumonia*, *Haemophilus influenzae* (most are nontypeable), and *Moraxella catarrhalis* are the most common pathogens.
- Rarely *S. aureus* and gram-negative bacilli may be involved.
- Many viruses have been implicated in otitis media including respiratory syncytial virus, rhinovirus, influenza, and adenovirus.

CLINICAL FEATURES

- Ear pain, hearing loss, and vertigo are quite common. Examination of the external ear may also reveal swelling and discharge. Nonspecific symptoms include: fever, headache, vomiting, and diarrhea

DIAGNOSIS

- Otoscopic examination demonstrates a tympanic membrane that is erythematous, bulging, and immobile. Cloudiness of the membrane is usually noted.

TREATMENT

- Pain control with medication such as ibuprofen and acetaminophen and antibiotic administration.
  ○ Resolution generally occurs without antibiotics. However, antibiotics may hasten resolution of symptoms and may slightly improve cure rates. Amoxicillin is generally the first choice if no antibiotic has been administered in the preceding month. If the patient is penicillin allergic (but did not exhibit a type 1 reaction), a cephalosporin such as cefuroxime may be substituted. If antibiotics have been administered in the preceding 1 month, amoxicillin-clavulanic acid or a cephalosporin are used. Macrolides such as erythromycin, azithromycin, or clarithromycin are generally acceptable alternatives. Although more expensive, fluoroquinolones are also very effective. Trimethoprim-sulfamethoxazole generally is avoided because of multidrug-resistant pneumococci.
- Duration of therapy
  ○ Usually 10 days, but shorter courses (eg, azithromycin 500 mg orally every day for 3 days or 500 mg for 1 day followed by 250 mg for 4 days) may be effective.
- Antihistamine and decongestants are not of proven efficacy unless an associated allergy is present.

COMPLICATIONS

- Treatment failure or resistance is likely if there is no improvement in symptoms by 48 to 72 hours (this should suggest resistance to β-lactam antibiotics).
- Hearing loss (if it occurs) is most commonly conductive and may persist as long as the middle ear effusion is present.
- Vestibular and balance dysfunction may occur but usually resolve as the infection improves. Perforation of the tympanic membrane may occur but generally heals spontaneously; however, it may require evaluation by an otolaryngologist.
- Mastoiditis can accompany acute otitis because of the anatomic proximity and connection to the middle ear. Rarely, it persists after resolution of acute otitis media. Intracranial complications such as meningitis, epidural abscess, cavernous sinus thrombosis, and brain abscess are rare in developed countries.

HEARING LOSS IN ADULTS

CLASSIFICATION

- Sensorineural: Involves the inner ear, cochlea, or auditory nerve.
- Conductive: Any condition that inferes with the transmission of sound to the inner ear.
- Mixed: Combination of the above.

ETIOLOGY

- Outer ear disease is associated with conductive loss.
  - Congenital: Atresia of the external auditory canal; unilateral > bilateral. Associated with diminished hearing since childhood.
  - Infection: External canal occlusion caused by accumulation of debris, edema, or inflammation.
  - Trauma: Penetrating trauma to the external auditory canal or meatus (eg, bullet, knife).
  - Tumor involving the canal or adjacent structures: Squamous cell > basal cell or melanoma
  - Benign bony growth: exotosis, osteoma.
  - Dermatologic: Desquamation, debris, edema: psoriasis or eczema within the canal.
- Middle ear
  - Congenital: Atresia or malformation of the ossicular chain: present since childhood.
  - Eustacean tube dysfunction: Seen with allergies, upper respiratory infection, high-altitude. Often resolves with resolution of the underlying condition.

- Infection: Otitis media—fluid accumulation in the middle ear space prevents the typanic membrane from vibrating. Usually resolves after 4 to 6 weeks.
- Tumors: Malignant—rare-squamous cell, Langerhans cell histocytosis.
- Tumors: Benign
  - Cholesteatoma: a growth of desquamated epithelium within the middle ear space. Can erode into nearby structures. Otosclerosis—bony overgrowth of the foot plate of the stapes.
- Tympanic membrane perforation: Location and size predict hearing loss. Small anterior/inferior quadrant perforations cause the least deficit; large or posterior/superior quandrant perforations cause the greatest hearing loss.
- Barotrauma: Occurs when a patient is exposed to a sudden, large change in ambient pressure (often diving or flying). If the eustachian tube is unable to equilibrate with the ambient pressure (upper respiratory infection, anatomic variations, pregnancy), the relative negative pressure of the middle ear can lead to accumulation serous fluid or blood or rupture of the tympanic membrane.
- Vascular-glomus tumor: Benign. Arise from the dome of the jugular bulb or the promentory of the middle ear.
- Inner ear
  - Hereditary: Sensorineural hearing loss inherited as an autosomal dominant or recessive trait.
  - Congenital malformation of the inner ear: Most common is a malformation, Mondini malformation, whereby the normal 2 1/2 turns of the cochlea is replaced by 1 1/2 turns.
  - Presbycusis: Sensorineural hearing loss associated with aging. Tinnitus is often also present. Patients may note an inability to hear or understand speech in a crowded or noisy enviroment.
  - Infection: Meningitis in children and viral cochleitis in adults are the most common. The latter usually manifests as sudden sensorineural hearing loss.
  - Ménière's disease: Consists of episodes of vertigo lasting for hours, tinnitus, aural fullness, and sensorineural hearing loss. The hearing loss usually recovers over 12 to 24 hours but may become progressive with repeated attacks.
  - Noise exposure: A short burst of 120 to 155 decibels of noise or protracted lower levels (as low as 85 decibels for greater than 8 hours) may lead to profound sensorineural hearing loss. OSHA has guidelines for noise exposure and hearing protection.
  - Barotrauma: Caused by sudden, large change in ambient pressure (eg. diving or flying). Sudden pressure differences between inner and middle ear may lead to rupture of the round or oval window.

- Trauma-penetrating trauma: Usually causes sensorineural or mixed hearing loss. Blunt trauma with concussive forces to the inner cochlear fluids leads to sensorineural hearing loss.
- Tumors: Generally benign. Most common is an acoustic neuroma, which originates from the vestibular portion of the eighth cranial nerve. Can be associated with unilateral tinnitus, disequilibrium, or facial hyperesthesia and muscle twitching.
- Autoimmune: Bilateral, asymetric, sensorineural hearing loss, which may fluctuate or be progressive in nature. A cochlear antibody may be present.
- Iatrogenic: Secondary to drugs including aminoglycosides or other antibiotics such as tetracycline or vancomycin, chemotherapeutic agents such as 5-Flouracil, ciesplatinum, or bleomycin. Aspirin and antimalarials can induce reversible hearing loss.
- Neurogenic: Cerebrovascular accidents or multiple sclerosis.
- Miscellaneous: Diabetes, anemia, hypo- or hyperthyroidism, and syphilis have been reported to cause sensorineural loss.

EVALUATION

- History: Onset and progression
- Trauma—noise or barotrauma
- Prior ear surgery
- Pain or drainage from the affected ear(s)
- Associated tinnitus, vertigo
- Family history of hearing loss
- Exam: Simple hearing loss
- Weber and Rinne to distinguish conductive from sensorineural hearing loss.
- Ear examination including pneumoscopy
- Formal audiologic assessment: Includes pure tone, air, and bone conduction testing speech audiometry; and impedence tympanography.
- Laboratory tests: Complete blood count, glucose, thyroid function tests, and serology for syphilis. Magnetic resonance imaging or CT in patients with progressive asymetric sensorineural hearing loss.

TREATMENT

After ruling out diabetes, thyroid dysfunction, central nervous system syphilis, or other infectious etiologies, and anatomic (vascular, neoplhastic, and traumatic disorders) disorders, patients may benefit from hearing amplification.
- Hearing aids: Appropriate candidates must be identified based on audiology. Patients with poor results on audiometric word discrimination may not benefit. In general, appropriate application of a hearing aid device will improve hearing by 50%.

- Binaural: Most benefit with these devices but they are expensive. They promote balanced hearing, sound localization, directional hearing, improved speech recognition, and noise discrimination.
- Single: Two single hearing aids may suffice for patients with financial contraints or the hearing loss is minimal.
- Bone conductive hearing devices: Used in patients for whom air conduction (conventional) hearing devices are not indicated, such as patients with congenital atresia of the ear canal, chronic infection of the middle or outer ear that is exacerbated by standard hearing aids, single-sided deafness following removal of an acoustic neuroma, trauma, viral or vascular insult. An implantable device is superior to an external one.
- Cochlear implants: Surgically implanted devices that use electrical stimulation to stimulate hearing. Candidates for this procedure have profound bilateral sensorineural hearing loss with little or no benefit from hearing aid use after 6 months.

REFERENCES

Cook JA, Hawkins DB. Hearing loss and hearing aid treatment options. *Mayo Clin Proc.* 2006;81:234.
Durant JD, Lovrinic, JH. *Basis of Hearing Science*, 2nd ed, Baltimore, MD: Williams & Wilkins; 1984.
Kleen AJ, Weber PC. Hearing aids. *Med Clin North Am.* 1999;83:139
Prasher D. New strategies for prevention and treatment of noise-induced hearing loss. *Lancet.* 1998;352:1240.
Ruben, RR Diseases of the inner ear and sensory neural deafness. In: *Pediatric Otolaryngology*, Bluestone CD, Stool SE, eds, Philadelphia, PA; WB Sanders; 1990. p547.

BIBLIOGRAPHY

Bisno, AL, Gerber MA, Gwoltney JM, et al. Practice guidelines for the diagnosis and management of group A streptococcal pharyngitis. *Clin Infect Dis.* 2002;35:113.
Casey JR, Pichichero ME. Changes in frequency and pathogens causing acute otitis media in 1995–2003. *Pediatr Infect Dis J.* 2004;23:824.
Clark WB, Brook I, Bicani D, Thompson DH. Microbiology of otitis externa. *Otolaryngol Head Neck Surg.* 1997;116:23.
Cooper RJ, Hoffman JR, Bartlett J, et al. Principles of appropriate antibiotic use for acute pharyngitis in adults: Background. *Ann Intern Med.* 2001;134:509–517.
Heibben T, Thent M, Chonmaitree T. Prevalence of various respiratory viruses in the middle ear during acute otitis media. *N Engl J Med.* 1999;340:260.
Humair J, Revaz SA, Bovier P, Stedler H. Management of acute pharyngitis in adults. *Arch Intern Med.* 2006;166:640–644.

Rosenfeld RM, Brown L, Cannon DR, et al. Clinical practice guideline: Acute otitis externa. *Otolaryngol Head Neck Surg.* 2006;134:S4.

Rosenfeld RM, Singer M, Wassermen JM, Stinnett SS. Systemic review of topical anti-microbial therapy for Acute otitis externa. *Otolaryngol Head Neck Surg.* 2006;134:S24.

Russel JD, Donnelly M, McShane DP, et al. What causes acute otitis externa? *J Laryngol Otol.* 1993;107:898.

Subcommittee on Management. American Academy of Pediatrics and American Academy of Family Physician. Diagnosis and management of acute otitis media. *Pediatrics.* 2004;113; 1351,1451.

Tabata GS, Chan LS, Shebelle P, et al. Evidence assessment of management of acute otitis Media. *Pediatrics.* 2001;108:239.

Uhari M, Mantysarri K, Niemela M. A meta-analytic review of the risk factors for acute otitis media. *Clin Infect Dis.* 1996;22: 1079.

7 COMMON PROBLEMS IN OPHTHALMOLOGY

Thomas J. Olsen

INTRODUCTION

The eye is part of a complex neurologic system that allows an individual to perceive and function optimally in the environment. Loss of vision is a dreaded disability. Sight interacts with and optimizes the other senses. Visual problems can arise from the eye itself, surrounding structures such as the orbit or extraocular muscles, the optic tract, or the visual cortex. Careful examination of the eye can aid in the diagnosis of common conditions and alert the clinician to potentially serious problems. The primary care physician should be able to assess common complaints and triage emergent problems to ophthalmologists for definitive care.

ANATOMY

- The lids are skin folds lined with conjunctiva providing protection to the eye and a mechanism for distribution of tears.
- The conjunctiva is the mucous membrane covering the anterior surface of the eye, reflecting onto the lids.
- The cornea is the transparent anterior portion of the eye, which is contiguous with the sclera.
- The iris is a diaphragm with a pupillary opening in the center; it contracts and dilates to adjust light entry.

- The lens is the refracting body in the eye, located posterior to the iris.
- The ciliary muscle changes the shape of the lens by contracting and relaxing.
- Aqueous humor is the fluid produced by the ciliary body, filling the anterior and posterior chambers.
- The retina lines the sclera in the posterior portion of the eye and is comprised of light-sensitive rods and cones.
- The optic nerve contains the ganglion cell axons of the retina. The nerve exits at the optic disc. The optic vessels enter the eye at the optic disc.

VISUAL ACUITY

Visual acuity is usually assessed using the Snellen chart at 20 feet; testing the eyes independently. Patients should wear their glasses to determine corrected acuity. If corrective lenses are not available, a pinhole can be used in with good lighting conditions. This focuses images on the retina regardless of the refractive error. The Rosenbaum card can also be used at a distance of 14 inches. Patients with visual acuity worse than 20/40 should be referred for evaluation and correction.

- Myopia: nearsightedness; caused by image focus anterior to the retina
- Hyperopia: farsightedness; caused by image focus posterior to the retina
- Presbyopia: requiring magnification for reading because of loss of accommodation with age

DISEASES OF THE LIDS

BLEPHARITIS

- Definition: inflammation of the eyelid
- Symptoms: itching or irritation of the lids, can be seen in association with other skin complaints
- Signs: crusting, scaling on lashes, erythema of the lids
- Etiology: rosacea, seborrhea, contact dermatitis
- Treatment:
  ○ Local bacterial infections should be treated with topical antimicrobials
  ○ Lid scrubs
  ○ Avoidance if caused by contact dermatitis as with cosmetics
  ○ Tends to be a chronic recurring condition requiring ongoing lid care

CHALAZION

- Definition: painless granulomatous inflammation of the lid, reflecting a local response to duct obstruction
- Symptoms: bump on the lid

- Signs: nodule on the lid
- Treatment
- Warm compresses and massage
  - Referral for incision and drainage or injection if it persists or is bothersome; consider neoplasm

HORDEOLUM

- Definition: infection of accessory glands of the lids, often caused by Staphylococcus organisms
- Symptoms: painful lump on the lid which may drain
- Signs: erythematous, painful nodule on lid, spontaneous drain age
- Treatment
- Warm compresses
  - Occasionally an oral antibiotic
  - Local lid care
  - Treat underlying skin disorders

CONJUNCTIVITIS

- Allergic
  - Symptoms: itching of the eyes, tears; often with nasal congestion and sneezing
  - Signs: hyperemia, chemosis, lid edema, mucosal discharge, and tearing
  - Etiology: seasonal or perennial allergies
  - Treatment
  - Avoidance/environmental control of animal dander, dust, mold, pollen
    - Oral antihistamines can reduce the symptoms of itching and watery eyes.
    - First-generation antihistamines are limited by their sedative effects; mast cell stabilizers, such as cromolyn, nonsteroidal anti-inflammatory medications, such as ketorolac, and antihistamines such as olopatadine, are available as ocular preparations.
- Infectious-Viral
  - Symptoms: mild pain; mild decrease in visual acuity, foreign body sensation, possible recent respiratory infection
  - Signs: mild photophobia, conjunctival injection; can be unilateral or bilateral, watery discharge, can develop blepharitis
  - Etiology: usually adenoviral; less commonly herpes or coxsackievirus; a rapid detection system for adenovirus is currently in development
  - Treatment
  - Lid care
    - Avoid spread through contact by careful handwashing. Viral conjunctivitis is self-limiting.

- Infectious-bacterial
  - Symptoms: mild pain, mild decrease in acuity or blurring, crusting on the lids, and discharge
  - Signs: conjunctival injection, mucopurulent discharge, crusting on lids; can have blepharitis, little change in visual acuity
  - Etiology: often staphylococcus, but many other bacteria have been described
  - Treatment
  - Lid scrubs
    - Hand washing
    - Broad-spectrum ocular antibiotics (aminoglycosides, sulfacetamide, or fluoroquinolones)

THE RED EYE

ACUTE ANGLE CLOSURE GLAUCOMA

- Symptoms: abrupt onset of unilateral painful eye, clouded vision: can have systemic symptoms of nausea, vomiting, and headache; can have had previous episodes
- Signs: marked reduction in acuity, injection of vessels more prominent in the area of the limbus, firm globe by palpation with patient's eyes closed; sluggish or fixed pupil.
- Etiology: blockage of flow of aqueous humor by the iris because of a shallow anterior chamber causing increased intraocular pressure
- Diagnosis: measure intraocular pressure
- Treatment: emergent referral, topical β-blockers, miotic agents, and acetazolamide

SUBCONJUNCTIVAL HEMORRHAGE

- Symptoms: none
- Signs: bright red bulbar conjunctival hemorrhage that appeared suddenly
- Etiology: bleeding from conjunctival vessel associated with minor trauma, sneezing, cough, or Valsalva maneuver; can be associated with antiplatelet or anticoagulation therapy
- Diagnosis: normal eye examination
- Treatment: reassurance; can take several weeks to resolve

FOREIGN BODY

- Symptoms: gritty sensation in eye, pain, tearing, and redness
- Signs: decreased vision, conjunctival injection
- Etiology: damage caused by foreign body often under the lid, often occupational exposure

- Diagnosis: assess visual acuity; evert eyelid and inspect; fluorescein stain with cobalt blue lamp
- Treatment: remove foreign body if present under lid
  - Refer for rust ring (corneal staining from some metallic foreign bodies) or corneal abrasion
  - Artificial tears

ACUTE ANTERIOR UVEITIS

- Symptoms: gradual onset of painful eye, photophobia, and often decreased vision
- Signs: can have reduced visual acuity, injection of vessels more prominent in the area of the limbus; constricted pupil
- Etiology: none found in 60% to 80% of patients; can be associated with ankylosing spondylitis, Reiter syndrome, sarcoidosis, inflammatory bowel disease or juvenile rheumatoid arthritis; can be seen postoperatively; can occur with herpes, syphilis, or Lyme disease
- Diagnosis and Treatment: referral as this condition requires a slit-lamp examination to detect inflammatory changes in the anterior chamber
  - Assess intraocular pressure
  - Ophthalmologist can prescribe topical steroids
  - Evaluate and treat underlying infection or inflammatory condition

GLAUCOMA

- Definition: prolonged elevation of intraocular pressure resulting in damage to the optic nerve and irreversible loss of vision. The most common etiology is primary open angle glaucoma caused by decreased outflow of aqueous from the anterior chamber.
- Symptoms: usually none; gradual visual loss might be reported as the process progresses.
- Signs: elevated intraocular pressure, peripheral visual field loss with preserved central vision, increase in optic cup to disc ratio, and a deep cup.
- Risk factors: Advancing age, African American descent, family history, hypertension.
- Treatment: Importantly, the goal is to detect elevated intraocular pressure prior to any visual loss by screening.
  - If the disease is already present, treatment is directed at prevention of further visual field loss.
  - Serial evaluation of visual fields with special equipment and serial observation and measurement of changes in the optic disc are used to monitor glaucoma and response to treatment.
  - Several classes of medications are prescribed to lower intraocular pressure and have proven effective in preventing visual loss.

- β-Blockers decrease aqueous production. Prostaglandin analogues increase aqueous outflow. Carbonic anhydrase inhibitors reduce production of aqueous. Laser trabeculectomy involves treatment of the trabecular network with a laser. This improves outflow of aqueous and reduces intraocular pressure. Most patients need to continue medications indefinitely. The pressure can increase overtime and, therefore monitoring intraocular pressure is essential.

CATARACTS

- Definition: The lens consists of a capsule surrounding a soft outer cortical material and a central nucleus. Cataracts are characterized by opacification of the lens causing impairment of vision. Cataracts can exist without interefering with vision. Associated diseases can produce changes in vision in patients with cataracts.
- Risk factors include ultraviolet B radiation (cortical, posterior subcapsular cataracts), diabetes, corticosteroids (posterior subcapsular location).
- Symptoms: decreased visual acuity and color perception.
- Signs: Opacification of the lens when examined with a penlight or ophthalmoscope and visual impairment.
- Treatment: Referral if there is impairment of visual acuity.
  - Nonsurgical interventions include revising corrective prescriptions, using bifocals, ensuring appropriate lighting, and serial examinations to assess changes in acuity and functional impairment.
  - Surgical interventions include extracapsular cataract extraction (ECCE) or phacoemulsification. ECCE involves an incision at the side of the cornea that allows extraction of the cataract in a single piece. Phacoemulsification is a process by which the lens nucleus is broken up via an ultrasound probe and then aspirated. Following one of these procedures, an intraocular lens is implanted. Complication rates are low and vision is effectively restored.

AGE-RELATED MACULAR DEGENERATION

- Definition: This form of macular degeneration is typically a disease affecting individuals older than 60 years of age. It is characterized by changes in the macula, including accumulation of drusen under the retinal pigment, atrophy of the retina, and choroidal neovascularization. Drusen is accumulated debris possibly related to inflammation. The visual impairment primarily involves central vision and affects reading and recognition. Neovascularization accounts for approximately 10% of the cases of age-related macular degeneration. However, vision loss is caused by atrophy of the fovea in 20% of cases and neovascularization in 80% of cases. Exudative or wet macular degeneration is caused by neovascularization with bleeding or retinal detachment because of leaking. Atrophic or dry macular degeneration involves the retinal epithelium and light sensitive elements.

- Risk factors: Age, family history, and smoking are definitely associated with increased risk. Age-related macular degeneration (AMD) is seen in less than 0.1% of those younger than 50 years of age and more than 10% in those older than 80 years of age. Hypertension, obesity, and hyperlipidemia are associated. Several genes have been identified that are associated with AMD (many cases are associated with a positive family history).
- Symptoms: distortion of vision especially central vision; acute changes or loss of central vision should prompt urgent referral; vision can deteriorate rapidly. Risk factors for progression include a large accumulation of drusen, large sized drusen, hyperpigmentation, and hypertension.
- Treatment: Patients require regular eye examinations with attention to changes in the retina. Magnification and use of appropriate lighting can help with adaptation to central loss.
  - Antioxidants and zinc. Treatment for 7 years with zinc and vitamins A, C, and beta-carotene retard progressive visual loss in patients with moderate macular degeneration.
  - Laser treatment: used to photocoagulate neovascular lesions to reduce the risk of severe visual loss. One study revealed that laser treatment decreased visual loss from 65% to 47% at 5 years.
  - Surveillance is necessary to detect recurrence.
  - Use of photosensitizers is indicated in some patients with neovascularization.
  - A recent study found that intravitreal ranibizumab prevented visual loss and improved acuity with low rates of serious side effects. Ranibizumab is a recombinant, humanized monoclonal antibody fragment that binds vascular endothelial growth factor A (VEGF A).
    - VEGF A is thought to play a role in the development of neovascularization in AMD.

BIBLIOGRAPHY

Arroyo JG. A 76-year-old man with macular degeneration. *JAMA.* 2006;295:2394–2406.

De Jong PT. Age-related macular degeneration. *N Engl J Med.* 2006;355:1474–1485.

Khaw PT, Shah P, Elkington AR. Glaucoma-1:Diagnosis. *Br Med J.* 2004;328:97–99.

Khaw PT, Shah P, Elkington AR. Glaucoma-2:Treatment. *Br Med J.* 2004;328:156–58.

Kunimoto DY, Kanitkar KD, Makar MS. *Willis Eye Manual: Office and Emergency Room Treatment of Eye Disease.* Philadelphia, PA: Lippincott Williams & Wilkins; 2004.

Leibowitz HM. The red eye. *N Engl J Med* 2000;343:345–351.

Naradzay J, Barish RA. Approach to ophthalmologic emergencies. *Med Clin North Am.* 2006;90:305–328.

Rosenfeld PJ, Brown DM, Heier JS, et al., for the MARINA Study Group. Ranibizumab for neovascular age-related macular degeneration. *N Engl J Med.* 2006;355:1419–1431.

Sapira, JD. *The Art and Science of Bedside Diagnosis.* Baltimore, MD: Urban and Schwarzenberg; 1990.

Schwartz K, Budenz D. Current management of glaucoma. *Curr Opin Ophthalmol.* 2004;15:119–126.

Shingleton BJ, O'Donoghue MW. Blurred vision. *N Engl J Med.* 2000;343:556–562.

Singh A. Medical therapy of glaucoma. *Ophthalmol Clin North Am.* 2005;18:397–408.

8 SELECTED TOPICS IN MEN'S HEALTH

Gina L. Michael, Margaret C. Hochreiter, and Mona Bahl

BENIGN PROSTATIC HYPERPLASIA

- Benign prostatic hyperplasia (BPH) is the most common benign neoplasm in American men. There is no definitive diagnostic test for BPH, and thus clinical diagnosis depends on symptoms and physical examination. The pathologic diagnosis is based on histology and prostate gland weight. BPH accounts for significant healthcare expenditure and reduced quality of life, predisposes the elderly (>65 years of age) to urinary tract infection and sepsis, and is an indirect cause of mortality.

EPIDEMIOLOGY AND NATURAL HISTORY

- The prevalence of prostatic hyperplasia at autopsy increases linearly from 8% in men aged 31 to 40 years, to more than 80% in men older than age 80 years.
- Using an American Urological Association (AUA) Symptom Index score of 7 (Table 8–1), in a population based study the clinical prevalence of BPH was 26%, 33%, 41%, and 46% in men in the fifth, sixth, seventh, and eighth decades of life, respectively.
- BPH was the primary or secondary reason for more than 12 million office visits in 2000.

TABLE 8–1   American Urological Association Benign Prostatic Hyperplasia Symptom Score

	NEVER	LESS THAN 1 TIME IN 5	LESS THAN HALF THE TIME	ABOUT HALF THE TIME	MORE THAN HALF THE TIME	ALMOST ALWAYS
Over the past month, how often have you had a sensation of not emptying your bladder completely after you finished urinating?	0	1	2	3	4	5
Over the past month, how often have you had to urinate again less than 2 hours after you finished urinating?	0	1	2	3	4	5
Over the past month, how often have you found you stopped and started again several times when you urinated?	0	1	2	3	4	5
Over the past month, how often have you found it difficult to postpone urination?	0	1	2	3	4	5
Over the past month, how often have you had a weak urinary stream?	0	1	2	3	4	5
Over the past month, how often have you had to push or strain to begin urination?	0	1	2	3	4	5
	none	1 time	2 times	3 times	4 times	5 or more times
Over the past month, how many times did you most typically get up to urinate from the time you went to bed at night until the time you got up in the morning?	0	1	2	3	4	5

Total symptom score (circle the answer for each question and calculate the sum)
SOURCE: AUA Practice Guidelines Committee. AUA guideline on management of benign prostatic hyperplasia (2003). Chapter 1: Diagnosis and treatment recommendations. *J Urol.* 2003;170:530–547.

- Direct costs for office visits and surgery for BPH were estimated at $1.1 billion dollars in 2000, and outpatient prescriptions for BPH accounted for an additional $194 million in annual spending.

PATHOPHYSIOLOGY

- Anatomically, BPH is the result of an increase in stromal tissue in the transitional (periurethral) zone of the prostate gland. The stromal tissue consists of collagen and smooth muscle cells, which are responsive to α-blockers. Epithelial cells are also increased, but to a lesser degree. Epithelial cells constitute glandular tissue and may be responsive to 5-alpha-reductase inhibitors.
- Development of BPH depends on the presence of androgen, in particular dihydrotestosterone. The exact relationship is unclear and may depend on the number or type of androgen receptors present in the gland.
- In addition to age, risk factors for the development of BPH include a positive family history as well as white or African American race, with rates lower in Asians.

Sexual activity, vasectomy, smoking, and diet have *not* been shown to play an etiologic role.
- Benign prostatic hyperplasia symptoms, as well as more objective measures such as urinary flow rates and prostate gland size, tend to show progression of BPH with age in most men; but some may have stabilization or even improvement.
- Continued resistance to urine flow can lead to bladder distension with detrusor dysfunction and uninhibited bladder contractions, causing urgency and incontinence.

DIAGNOSIS

- The diagnosis of BPH is largely clinical, based on lower urinary tract symptoms (LUTS). Symptoms can be divided into obstructive (hesitancy, straining, decreased force of stream, sensation of incomplete emptying, and postvoid dribbling) and irritative (urgency, frequency, and nocturia). The AUA Symptom Score (see Table 8–1) identifies patients who will benefit from treatment.

TABLE 8–2 Differential Diagnosis of Lower Urinary Tract Symptoms

CATEGORY	CAUSE OF LUTS	COMMENTS/EVALUATION
Malignant	Carcinoma of the prostate, bladder, or penis	Digital rectal examination. PSA testing should be offered to men with life expectancy of 10 or more years. Microscopic or gross hematuria should be evaluated with urine cytology and renal imaging. Consider cystoscopy.
Infectious	Cystitis, prostatitis, sexually transmitted diseases (*Chlamydia, Gonorrhea*)	Urinalysis. Urine culture and postprostatic massage specimen if indicated. STDs may cause urethral stricture or scarring.
Neurologic	Spinal cord injury, stroke, diabetic autonomic neuropathy, Parkinson disease, multiple sclerosis, Alzheimer disease	Neurologic diseases cause detrusor weakness and/or uninhibited detrusor contractions. Alzheimer can cause functional urinary incontinence.
Medical	Poorly controlled diabetes mellitus, diabetes insipidus, congestive heart failure, obstructive sleep apnea	
Iatrogenic	Prostatectomy, cystectomy, traumatic ureterocystoscopic procedures, radiation cystitis	Surgery may cause neurologic impairment, scarring, or strictures.
Anatomic	Ureteral and bladder stones	Microscopic or gross hematuria should be evaluated with urine cytology and renal imaging. Consider cystoscopy.
Behavioral	Polydipsia, excessive alcohol, or caffeine consumption	Consider assessing serum sodium. Consider a voiding diary.
Pharmacologic	Diuretics, sympathomimetics, anticholinergics, OTC decongestants	Diuretics cause urinary frequency, sympathomimetics increase urethral resistance, and anticholinergics decrease detrusor contractility.
Other	Overactive bladder	Urodynamic studies may be helpful.

LUTS, lower urinary tract symptoms; OTC, over-the-counter; PSA, prostate-specific antigen; STD, sexually transmitted disease.
SOURCE: Adapted with permission from Beckman TJ, Mynderase LA. Evaluation and medical management of benign prostatic hyperplasia. *Mayo Clin Proc.* 2005;80:1356.

○ Although BPH is the primary cause of LUTS in men aged 50 years and older, the differential diagnosis of LUTS includes other significant urinary tract pathology (Table 8–2); thus it is important to assure that the symptoms are caused by BPH.

○ The history should elucidate previous urologic disease or surgery, neurologic disease, or prostate and bladder cancer. Medications should be reviewed to identify agents which can affect bladder function (sympathomimetics, anticholinergics, and over-the-counter medications).

○ Although the diagnosis of BPH is based on history, the physical examination is also important in ruling out other causes of LUTS. The examination should look for evidence of autonomic neuropathy and other neurologic disorders.

○ A digital rectal examination and prostate examination should be performed, noting anal sphincter tone, prostate size, consistency, and nodules. Prostatic size correlates poorly with LUTS in part because the predominant site of hyperplasia, the transition zone, is centrally located and not palpable.

○ Laboratory evaluation should include a urinalysis to exclude infection or hematuria. Serum prostate-specific antigen (PSA), although elevated in 25% of men with BPH, can help determine if further testing for prostate cancer is indicated in men with a life expectancy of greater than 10 years. Measurement of serum creatinine is optional. Urine cytology may be considered in patients with predominantly irritative symptoms.

○ Imaging of the kidneys with ultrasound, computed tomography (CT) scan, or intravenous pyelogram need only be performed in patients with renal insufficiency, hematuria, or a history of stones.

○ Cystometrics, measurement of post void residual bladder volume, either by catheterization or suprapubic ultrasound, and determination of urinary flow rates may be helpful in difficult cases, but are usually not necessary unless surgical treatment is being considered.

COMPLICATIONS

- Benign prostatic hyperplasia can lead to acute urinary retention, recurrent urinary tract infections, bladder stones, hydronephrosis, and renal failure. Obstructive uropathy caused by BPH must be ruled out as a treatable cause in men with acute renal failure.
- Benign prostatic hyperplasia is *not* believed to increase the risk of prostate cancer.

THERAPEUTIC APPROACH

- The decision to treat BPH is established on the basis of the AUA Symptom Score (see Table 8–1). Watchful waiting is advised for those with mild symptoms (score 0–7). For patients with moderate (8–19), and severe (20–35) symptom score, medical therapy should be considered. The current medical therapy consists of α-adrenergic blockers, 5-alpha-reductase inhibitors, combination therapy, or phytotherapy.

α-ADRENERGIC BLOCKING AGENTS
- α-Blockers are the most commonly prescribed medication for LUTS secondary to BPH.
- The tone of the prostatic periurethral smooth muscle is increased by α-adrenergic receptors, and blockade of these receptors promotes urethral dilation. α-receptors in the spinal cord or other extraprostatic areas may also be involved.
- The efficacy of all the α-blocking agents are similar and generally result in a 30% to 40% decrease in symptom score and an increase in urinary flow rate. Side-effect profiles, however, are different and are discussed below.
- Nonselective α₁-blocking agents, approved for the treatment of BPH, exhibit a long half-life (terazosin, doxazosin), and are dosed once daily. Side effects derive from their actions on the systemic circulation, and include orthostatic hypotension (4%–6%) and dizziness (13%–15%). Other common side effects include rhinitis, headache, and fatigue (asthenia). Initial titration of these drugs with low starting doses and bedtime dosing are recommended.
- Tamsulosin is specific for the α₁-A-subtype receptor concentrated in the prostate and bladder neck. This drug is less likely to produce symptomatic hypotension (3%) and does not require titration. However, the other side effects, with the exception of asthenia, are equal to or greater than the nonselective agents. Studies have also shown a 10% incidence of retrograde ejaculation with tamsulosin.
- Alfuzosin is another uroselective α-blocker widely used in Europe but just recently approved in the United States. It appears to have similar efficacy but less side effects than the other agents.
- Clinicians should be aware that phosphodiesterase 5 inhibitors, commonly used to treat erectile dysfunction, can cause profound hypotension when combined with α-blocking agents. Physicians should consult the manufacturer's recommendations when prescribing these medications together (see Erectile Dysfunction below).

5-ALPHA-REDUCTASE INHIBITORS
- By inhibiting the conversion of testosterone to dihydrotestosterone, these agents reduce the size of the prostate gland, specifically decreasing the epithelial glandular tissue in the transitional zone of the prostate.
- Efficacy studies show a 20% reduction in prostate gland size, an improvement in LUTS symptom score, decreased incidence of acute urinary retention, and a 64% reduction in the need for prostate surgery in men with enlarged prostate glands (>40 cm³). These medications are ineffective in men with normal prostate size and require 6 to 12 months to exert an effect.
- PSA correlates with prostate gland size; and therefore, after exclusion of prostate cancer, an elevation of PSA can be used as a proxy for increased prostate gland size and an indicator of patients who may have a greater response to therapy with a 5-alpha-reductase inhibitor.
- The 5-alpha-reductase inhibitors currently available include finasteride and dutasteride. Their side-effect profiles are similar and include an initial increased rate of erectile dysfunction (ED) that returns to baseline after the first year of treatment, decreased libido, and decreased ejaculate volume.
- These agents induce a 50% reduction in the PSA level, therefore the PSA should be measured before initiating treatment in appropriate candidates. This effect should be adjusted for in the subsequent monitoring of PSA by multiplying the PSA value by a factor of 2.

COMBINATION THERAPY
- The combination of an α-blocker and 5 alpha-reductase inhibitor has been studied and found to be more successful than either drug alone. In the Medical Therapy of Prostatic Symptoms study, the reduction in clinical endpoints using combination therapy was additive.

PHYTOTHERAPY
- The plant derivative *saw palmetto* has been widely used over-the-counter as a treatment for LUTS symptoms. A 1-year randomized, controlled trial of 225 men, published in 2006, showed no significant difference between saw palmetto and placebo in BPH symptom scores or urinary flow rates. Previously, several studies showed

effectiveness when compared with placebo. Poor study design or lack of standardization of this unregulated over-the-counter agent may account for the disparity in results.

UROLOGIC REFERRAL

- Referral to a urologist for consideration of surgical intervention for BPH is indicated for those with refractory LUTS, refractory urinary retention, persistent gross hematuria, renal insufficiency caused by BPH, recurrent urinary tract infections, and bladder stones.

PROSTATITIS

- Infection and/or inflammation of the prostate gland is a common problem in men, resulting in 2 million medical office visits per year. Prevalence estimates range from 9% to 16% of the general population.

ACUTE BACTERIAL PROSTATITIS

- Acute prostatitis is usually easily diagnosed by primary care providers.

PATHOPHYSIOLOGY AND MICROBIOLOGY

- Bacteria migrate into the prostatic ducts from the urethra or infected urine in the bladder; concomitant infection may occur in the bladder or epididymis.
- Common bacterial pathogens are the same organisms that cause urinary tact infections, and include gram-negative rods, such as *Escherichia coli, Proteus, Enterobacter,* and the gram-positive *Enterococcus.* Less commonly, *Staphylococcus, Gardnerella vaginalis,* and *Haemophilus influenzae* are isolated.
- Risk factors for the development of acute prostatitis include urethral catheterization, urethral stricture, trauma to the perineum, and human immunodeficiency virus (HIV) infection.

DIAGNOSIS

- Patients present with acute onset of fever, chills, myalgias, and lower back pain, which may radiate to the scrotum, perineum, or rectum. Dysuria and cloudy urine may be present. The patient may also have other LUTS such as hesitancy or urgency.
- Physical examination reveals an edematous and tender prostate gland. Prostate massage should not be done because of the risk of inducing bacteremia; moreover the findings have little effect on the management.
- Urinalysis and urine culture should be obtained. A positive urine culture is consistent with the clinical

diagnosis of prostatitis and can guide antibiotic choice.
- Prostate-specific antigen screening should not be done during an episode of acute prostatitis, because the PSA value is transiently elevated.

THERAPEUTIC APPROACH

- Patients who are immunocompromised, have acute urinary retention, have multiple comorbidities, or in whom there is a concern of sepsis, and have extreme discomfort should be hospitalized for intravenous antibiotics with broad spectrum coverage until culture results are available.
- Fluoroquinolones have become the recommended class for empiric oral treatment of prostate infections because of their superior penetration of the prostate, which results in higher drug concentration in prostatic tissue than in plasma. Trimethoprim-sulfamethoxazole has also been used.
- Duration of treatment is 4 weeks.
- Complications can include sepsis, the development of chronic prostatitis, and prostatic abscess; the latter is more common in patients with HIV infection.

CHRONIC PROSTATITIS

- In contrast to acute prostatitis, chronic prostatitis is more difficult to diagnose, more difficult to treat, and more common. The National Institutes of Health (NIH) standardized the definitions of prostatitis in 1999, dividing chronic prostatitis into chronic bacterial prostatitis, chronic prostatitis/pelvic pain syndrome (CP/CPPS), and asymptomatic inflammatory prostatitis.

CHRONIC BACTERIAL PROSTATITIS

- Chronic bacterial prostatitis frequently presents as relapsing urinary tract infections with the same organism. Symptoms are variable, ranging from dysuria and LUTS to asymptomatic bacteruria. Vague pelvic, suprapubic, or perineal pain is a frequent complaint. Ejaculatory pain and hematospermia may occur.
- The prostate gland may be tender or enlarged on examination, or it may be normal.
- Urine culture and urinalysis should be obtained. A diagnostic *two-glass test* is recommended, in which a midstream urine specimen is collected, followed by a 1-minute prostatic massage and then collection of a second urine specimen. The midstream urine specimen reflects inflammation and pathogens present in the bladder, whereas the postmassage urine reflects inflammation and pathogens present in the prostate.
- Patients with recurrent urinary tract infections should undergo imaging of the kidneys and have measurement

of postvoid residual bladder volume, to rule out structural and functional abnormalities of the kidneys.

- The organisms causing chronic bacterial prostatitis include gram-negative rods, with *E. coli* responsible 80% of the time. Studies have failed to show an association with sexually transmitted bacteria, including *Chlamydia trachomatis* (CT). Prostatic calculi may play a role by entrapping bacteria.
- Therapy with fluoroquinolones has produced 60% to 80 % cure rates. Trimethoprim-sulfamethoxazole has also been used, but the cure rates are lower. Duration of treatment is 4 to 6 weeks for fluoroquinolones and 90 days for Trimethoprim-sulfamethoxazole.
- Recurrences are common. Treatment with a different antibiotic and/or longer duration should be considered as well as culturing for and treating *Chlamydia* with doxycycline or azithromycin. For persistent relapses, long-term, low-dose antibiotic suppression may be indicated.

CHRONIC PROSTATITIS/PELVIC PAIN SYNDROME

- Representing more than 80% of the cases of diagnosed *prostatitis,* CP/CPPS is more common than acute and chronic bacterial prostatitis. Surveys demonstrate that patients with CP/CPPS have increased healthcare expenditure and reduced quality of life.
- The presentation of CP/CPPS is similar to chronic bacterial prostatitis except that pelvic pain is the predominant symptom and is present for at least 3 months. The pain localized to the suprapubic area, between the rectum and testicles, and/or in the testicles. Pain is also frequently reported with ejaculation, and also less commonly with urination. Physical examination of the prostate reveals tenderness in one-third of patients.
- There is no definitive diagnostic test for CP/CPPS. Using the traditional *four-glass test,* patients with CP/CPPS have negative cultures of urine and expressed prostatic secretions. The CP/CPPS category has been further divided into two groups, with type IIIA being inflammatory, as defined by the presence of leukocytes in expressed prostatic secretions, postprostatic massage urine, or semen. Type IIIB is noninflammatory, with an absence of leukocytes in these fluids.
- The etiology or etiologies of CP/CPPS are unknown. Bacterial infections have been suspected, but evidence from cultures and polymerase chain reaction analysis of prostate biopsy material suggest that the etiology may be noninfectious. It is also uncertain if inflammation of the prostate is responsible for symptoms or if the prostate itself is even the anatomic focus of the pain; thus the NIH-coined the term, *chronic pelvic pain syndrome.* Obstruction of the ejaculatory duct may play a role in

some men with postejaculatory pain. Muscle spasm may also be involved, because uroflow studies have shown increased contraction in the striated muscles of the pelvic floor and/or spasm of the internal urinary sphincter in 30% of patients.

- Chronic prostatitis/pelvic pain syndrome is a diagnosis of exclusion. Differential diagnosis includes other causes of pelvic pain including urogenital cancer, acute prostatitis (indicated by a markedly tender prostate gland), hernia, or rectal mass. Patients with hematuria or an elevated PSA should be referred to a urologist for evaluation. Patients with significant abdominal pain should have an abdominal CT scan performed. Patients with testicular pain should receive an ultrasound of the scrotum.
- Treatment of CP/CPPS remains a focus of investigation. Several randomized trials have shown no benefit from antibiotics; however, patients are commonly offered a 4- to 6-week course, preferably with a fluoroquinolone, but trimethoprim-sulfamethoxazole is also an option. Repeated courses of antibiotics are not recommended. α-Blockers have been shown to reduce symptoms in those with higher initial symptom scores in studies lasting 12 to 14 weeks, but not 6 weeks, and should be tried. Nonsteroidal anti-inflammatory medications are also frequently used to reduce symptoms, but a randomized controlled trial did not show statistical significance. Patients with postejaculatory pain may warrant a transrectal ultrasound, to rule out looking for obstruction of the ejaculatory duct, and consideration of correction if found.

ASYMPTOMATIC INFLAMMATORY PROSTATITIS

- Asymptomatic inflammatory prostatitis is an investigational category established by the NIH for research purposes. This category includes men who are asymptomatic but found to have prostatic inflammation on biopsy or other study. It will not be discussed further.

CYSTITIS

PATHOPHYSIOLOGY AND MICROBIOLOGY

- Urinary tract infections in men are viewed as complicated, because they are frequently associated with anatomic or functional abnormalities.
- Additional risk factors for urinary tract infection in men include age > 65, disabled, uncircumcised, instrumentation of the genitourinary tract, sexual activity, and the presence of HIV infection.
- Gram-negative bacilli cause 80% of the cases with *E. coli* as the causative organism in more than half. Gram-positive organisms, such as *Enterococcus* and *Staphylococcus,* are responsible for the remainder.

- Asymptomatic bacteruria is not predictive of future symptomatic infection, so screening is unnecessary.

DIAGNOSIS

- The diagnosis is established on a urinalysis and urine culture. Because the risk of contamination is less in men than in women, a colony count of >1000 is thought to indicate the presence of bacteria.
- A digital rectal examination should be performed. An exquisitely tender, boggy prostate gland should raise consideration of acute bacterial prostatitis; and patients should be treated as such.
- Although most men with a urinary tract infection have a demonstrable abnormality on imaging studies and/ or urodynamic studies, the clinical relevance of these abnormalities is unclear; and they have not been found to alter the clinical management. Therefore, imaging studies are usually only performed when there is a treatment failure, recurrence, or pyelonephritis is suspected.

THERAPEUTIC REGIMEN

- If the prostate is not tender, amoxicillin, trimethoprim-sulfamethoxazole, or a fluoroquinolone can be administered for 7 to 14 days. Single-dose and short-course therapy have not been shown to be effective in men.
- Recurrences with the same bacterial pathogen should raise suspicion for chronic bacterial prostatitis, and therefore a 4- to 6-week course of a fluoroquinolone should be considered.

URETHRITIS

EPIDEMIOLOGY

- Urethritis is defined as an inflammation of the urethra and is most commonly caused by sexually transmitted infections. *C. trachomatis* (CT) and *Neisseria gonorrhoeae,* or gonococcus (GC), are the main causative pathogens.
- The centers for Disease Control and Prevention (CDC) data from 2000 through 2004 reported that the CT infection rate in men increased by 48%. This increase is due in part to more widespread availability of nucleic acid amplification testing (NAAT).
- During the same time period, the GC infection rate in men decreased by 16%.
- Minorities have higher infection rates. In 2004, the CT infection rate was 11 times higher in African American males compared with white males. The GC rate was 17 times higher.

- Aside from minority status, other risk factors include age 20 to 24 years and a history of multiple sexual partners with early onset of sexual activity.

ETIOLOGY

- Comprised of main categories: gonococcal urethritis (GU) and nongonococcal urethritis (NGU). In GU gram-negative intracellular diplococci typical of GC can be identified on urethral smear. NGU includes all other causative infectious pathogens.
- CT is the most common cause of NGU in the United States, accounting for up to 50% of cases. It is also the most common cause of urethritis overall.
- *Ureaplasma urealyticum* and *Mycoplasma genitalium* account for up to one-third of NGU cases. It is not recommended they be tested for as they are difficult to isolate, and isolation does not generally alter therapy.
- Less common causes of NGU include herpes simplex virus 2 and *Trichomonas vaginalis,* which should be suspected if the history and physical examination suggest their presence.
- Rare causes of NGU include adenovirus and herpes simplex virus 1 in men practicing oral sex as well as enteric pathogens such as *E. coli* in men practicing anal sex.
- Noninfectious etiologies include tumor, trauma, and chemical irritants. Systemic diseases like Wegener's granulomatosis and Stevens-Johnson syndrome may also cause urethritis.

CLINICAL MANIFESTATIONS

- Urethral discharge is common. When present, it may be clear, mucopurulent, or grossly purulent. Characterization of the discharge cannot predict the causative organism.
- Other symptoms include dysuria, which is typically worse with first morning micturition, and itching or pain of the penis/urinary meatus. Hematuria/ hematospermia may also be present.
- Some men are asymptomatic and seek care because of known partner exposure. They should be evaluated and, if indicated, treated to eradicate potential carrier status.

DIAGNOSIS

- Urethritis may be confirmed if any one of the following three criteria is present: (1) mucopurulent or purulent urethral discharge, (2) Gram stain of urethral smear with at least 5 white blood cells (WBCs) per oil immersion field, and (3) first-void urine specimen with either 10 or more WBCs per high-power field on microscopy or positive leukocyte esterase test.

- Of the aforementioned criteria, obtaining a Gram stain of the urethral smear is preferred because it is sensitive and specific in documenting both the presence/absence of pyuria *and* the presence/absence of GC.
- If GC is diagnosed by Gram stain, a culture should also be sent to obtain antibiotic sensitivity information. Sensitivity testing for GC is important due to growing emergence of quinolone-resistant gonorrheal strains.
- CT cannot be diagnosed by Gram stain. The preferred methods of testing for CT are nucleic acid amplification testing (NAAT) such as polymerase chain reaction and ligase chain reaction (given their higher sensitivity rates), but traditional cultures may also be used.
- NAAT can be performed on first-void urine samples or urethral smears. Oral and anal specimens require traditional cultures. More costly than cultures, NAAT should not be used for GC testing because antibiotic sensitivity information cannot be obtained.

TREATMENT

GENERAL GUIDELINES
- Patients should only be treated with antimicrobials if they have objective evidence of urethritis or a confirmed infection. The exception is the patient who is unlikely to follow up; in this instance presumptive treatment for GC and CT should be initiated.
- Patients should refrain from sexual intercourse for 7 days after the start of treatment and should refer all sexual partners from the preceding 60 days for evaluation. All patients should be offered testing for HIV and syphilis.
- Healthcare providers should report communicable diseases to appropriate health authorities in their area.
- Because coinfection is likely, all patients who are treated for GU should also be treated for NGU.

GONOCOCCAL URETHRITIS
- Single-dose intramuscular ceftriaxone is the preferred treatment. It allows for directly observed therapy (DOT) and, compared with single-dose oral cefixime, provides a higher and more sustained bactericidal level against GC.
- Treatment with quinolones is less desirable because of emerging resistance patterns. The CDC recommends consultation with the local health department about resistance patterns before using these agents to treat GC. In addition, men who have sex with other men and patients who may have acquired infections outside the United States, or in Hawaii or California, should *not* be treated with quinolones.

NONGONOCOCCAL URETHRITIS
- The preferred treatment agents for NGU are either single-dose azithromycin or a 7-day course of doxycycline. Treatment with azithromycin allows for DOT.

PERSISTENT URETHRITIS
- If symptoms persist after treatment, patients should be retested for the presence of urethritis. Treatment should not be initiated in symptomatic patients who have no objective evidence or signs of urethritis. Patients who are noncompliant with the original treatment regimen should be retreated with the same regimen.
- If signs of urethritis are present, the CDC recommends obtaining a urethral culture or first-void urine specimen for *T. vaginalis*. It is also recommended that patients be treated with metronidazole or tinidazole to cover for *T. vaginalis* infection and with erythromycin to cover for possible tetracycline-resistant *U. urealyticum.*

COMPLICATIONS OF URETHRITIS

- Potential complications of urethritis include epididymitis, prostatitis, urethral stricture, and reactive arthritis (Reiter's Syndrome).

EPIDIDYMITIS

- Epididymitis is characterized by inflammation or infection of the epididymis; a collection of efferent tubules on the posterior aspect of each testis. In most cases, epididymitis is caused by retrograde spread of bacteria from the bladder or urethra by way of the vas deferens. Advanced cases may spread to the ipsilateral testis to produce epididymoorchitis.

ETIOLOGY

- In sexually active men younger than 35 years, the most common causative pathogens are GC and CT.
- In older men over the age of 35, sexually transmitted organisms are also possible, but urinary pathogens such as *E. coli* are the most common cause. Risk factors include conditions that predispose this population to bacteruria (eg, lower urinary tract obstruction secondary to BPH and prostate cancer).
- Less common causes of epididymitis include tuberculous and fungal infections. Amiodarone therapy and certain vasculitides can cause noninfectious epididymitis.

CLINICAL MANIFESTATIONS

- Patients commonly complain of scrotal pain, dysuria, fever, and chills.
- On examination, there is tenderness of the epididymis and scrotal erythema. With epididymoorchitis, the adjacent testis may be tender and a reactive hydrocele may be present.

DIAGNOSIS

- It is imperative to distinguish epididymitis from testicular torsion. Distinction must be made quickly to preserve testicular viability. Ultrasound studies may aid in diagnosis but emergent urologic consultation should not be delayed if there is any suspicion.
- Once torsion is excluded, testing should include urinalysis with culture, urethral swab for Gram stain and culture, and a complete blood count. Other tests are directed by the history and physical examination.

TREATMENT

- General measures include supportive care with analgesia, local ice packs, and scrotal support to help facilitate lymphatic drainage.
- For epididymitis presumed secondary to sexual transmission, GC and CT should be covered with single-dose ceftriaxone plus a 10-day course of doxycycline.
- Epididymitis presumed secondary to common urinary pathogens should be treated with a 10-day course of ofloxacin or levofloxacin. Additionally, evaluation of the urinary tract for structural abnormalities should be considered.

COMPLICATIONS

- Potential complications include chronic epididymitis, testicular/epididymal abscess, and testicular infarction.

ORCHITIS

- Isolated orchitis is most commonly caused by the hematogenous spread of viruses that selectively attack the testis.
- Mumps virus is the most clinically significant pathogen.
- Mumps orchitis generally occurs in postpubertal males. Most patients present with the sudden onset of testicular pain and fever and give a history of preceding mumps parotitis.

- As with epididymitis, testicular torsion must be excluded. Additionally, mumps serology may be ordered for confirmatory testing.
- Treatment is supportive (analgesia, scrotal support, and ice packs).
- Although the most worrisome complication of mumps orchitis is infertility, it is a rare consequence and generally occurs in severe, bilateral cases. With the advent of the measles-mumps-rubella vaccine, infertility rates are generally lower than 5%.

ERECTILE DYSFUNCTION

- The National Institutes of Health Consensus Conference on Impotence (December 7–9, 1992) defined ED as "the inability to achieve or maintain an erection sufficient for satisfactory sexual performance."

PHYSIOLOGY OF ERECTION

- Normal erectile function is the result of complex interactions between vascular, neurologic, hormonal, and psychologic factors.
  - In the resting, flaccid state the arteries and arterioles of the penis are contracted as are the sinusoids of the corpus cavernosum.
  - During erection, dilatation of the arteries and arterioles occurs, along with expansion of the sinusoids. As blood flow increases, the penis expands until limited by the capacity of the tunica albuginea. Expansion of the sinusoids against each other and against the tunica compresses the subtunical venous plexus. The tunica itself compresses the emissary veins preventing egress of blood from the penis.
  - The penile erectile state is under control of adrenergic, cholinergic, and nonadrenergic, noncholinergic (NANC) neurons. The baseline vascular and smooth muscle tone of the flaccid penis is maintained by tonic sympathetic stimulation.
  - After sexual stimulation, erection occurs when parasympathetic discharge overcomes the tonic sympathetic stimulation.
  - Increased parasympathetic tone results in decreased norepinephrine release, acetylcholine release from cholinergic nerve terminals, and an increase in the activity of nitric oxide synthase (NOS).
  - Nitric oxide (NO) is produced by parasympathetic NANC neurons and the endothelium. Increased NO production results in increased generation of cyclic guanosine monophosphate (cGMP), which decreases intracellular calcium levels ultimately causing a relaxation of the corporeal smooth muscle of the penis as well as the arteries and arterioles.

○ Withdrawal of sexual stimulation results in a return of sympathetic tone, decrease in NO production, and decreased production and then degradation of cGMP primarily by phosphodiesterase type 5 (PDE5).

EPIDEMIOLOGY

• Worldwide estimates for the prevalence of ED range from less than 5% for men younger than age 40 years to 86% for men older than age 80.
  ○ The Massachusetts Male Aging Study (MMAS), which studied men aged 40 to 70 years, found the total prevalence of mild to severe ED to be 52%
  ○ Estimates based on the MMAS indicate approximately 30 million men with this problem in the United States alone with 600,000 to 700,000 new cases each year.
• Once considered an inevitable consequence of aging, ED is now recognized in association with many chronic medical conditions, medications, and lifestyle factors.

PATHOPHYSIOLOGY

• ED can occur as a result of vascular, neurologic, or psychogenic problems, either alone or in combination. More than 80% of cases have an organic basis. The recognition of the importance of intact endothelial function for production of NO helps explain the association of ED and many of the epidemiologically established risk factors.
  ○ Atherosclerosis accounts for up to 80% of organically based cases. Mechanisms of injury include endothelial damage, cellular migration, and vascular smooth muscle proliferation. The effect of decreased blood flow is compounded by decreased NO production caused by the damaged endothelium.
  ○ Diabetes mellitus: In the MMAS, ED was three times more common in diabetics than in nondiabetics. Diabetes has multiple deleterious effects on erectile function, including neuropathy, accelerated atherosclerosis, and increased concentrations of glycosylated end products in tissues resulting in locally decreased NO concentrations.
  ○ Studies have demonstrated that ED is associated with increased levels of glycosylated hemoglobin (HbA_{1C}), but no longitudinal studies exist that show a correlation between improvement in glycemic control and amelioration of ED.
  ○ Hyper- and hypothyroidism: The mechanisms by which abnormal thyroid status cause ED are currently unknown.
  ○ Hyperprolactinemia, whether idiopathic, drug-induced, or tumor-related, is a rare cause of ED. It accounted

for only 0.76% of cases in a compilation of seven large series of ED patients. Elevated prolactin levels inhibit pulsatile secretion of luteinizing hormone (LH), thus decreasing secretion of testosterone, and interfere with conversion of testosterone to dihydrotestosterone.
  ○ Low testosterone levels: Although androgen levels correlate with libido and the presence of nocturnal erections, a causal relationship between low levels of androgens and ED has not yet been proven. Androgens have been shown in animal studies to be important in maintenance of normal levels of NOS in erectile tissue and of the enzymes (PDE5) responsible for the degradation of cGMP. This suggests a central role overall for androgens in the erectile process and also provides a possible explanation for the clinical observation that PDE5 inhibitors work less well in untreated hypogonadal ED than in ED of other causes.
  ○ LUTS, independent of age and other comorbidities: Mechanistic studies using a rabbit model of partial bladder outlet obstruction, a common cause of LUTS, suggest an increase in basal smooth muscle tone in the corpora cavernosa of affected individuals.
  ○ Peyronie disease occurs in 3% of men 30 to 80 years of age. More than half have ED. The inelastic scar tissue characteristic of the disease restricts expansion of the corpus cavernosum decreasing rigidity.
  ○ Treatment for prostate cancer
    ▪ With modern surgical techniques, potency rates after unilateral nerve-sparing surgery range from 18% to 58% and for bilateral nerve-sparing surgery from 31% to 82% in previously potent men.
    ▪ ED increases steadily in the months after external beam radiation to the prostate. Estimates of potency range from 20% to 86%. The likelihood of ED correlates with the radiation dose.
    ▪ Retained potency after permanent brachytherapy is reported as 50% after 3 years and 29% after 4 years in longitudinal studies.
    ▪ Hormonal deprivation therapy: ED is related to a decrease in androgen levels.

EVALUATION OF THE PATIENT WITH ERECTILE DYSFUNCTION

• The initial evaluation of men with a complaint of ED involves a complete medical, sexual, and psychosocial history; physical examination; and laboratory testing.

HISTORY
• A goal of the history is to establish the nature of the sexual problem, to make sure that it is in fact ED and

not another aspect of sexual dysfunction such as decreased libido or an ejaculatory disorder. The International Index of Erectile Function (IIEF)-5 (Table 8–3) is a brief, self-administered questionnaire, which can be used to establish the diagnosis of ED and assess its severity. The International Society for Sexual Medicine (ISSM) recognizes three types of ED: (1) organic, (2) psychogenic, and (3) mixed. Further questioning by the clinician and possibly specialized testing beyond the IIEF-5 is necessary to distinguish among these.

- The medical history should also identify:
  - Risk factors for coronary artery disease. Erectile dysfunction shares risk factors with coronary artery disease and may predate the development of overt coronary artery disease by several years. Presentation with ED may provide an opportunity for initiation of risk factor modification for coronary artery disease.
  - Symptoms associated with endocrinopathies.
  - Symptoms suggestive of LUTS or a history of pelvic surgery or trauma. A history of prostate cancer or Peyronie disease precludes certain treatments for ED.
  - Frequent bicycle riding: Can cause excessive pressure on the pudendal arteries.
  - Operative repair of certain lower limb fractures: can damage the pudendal nerves.
  - Symptoms of neurological disease such as stroke, seizure disorder, Parkinson disease, dementia, and neuropathy.

- A list of the patient's medications. Many medications including antihypertensives, neuroleptics, anticonvulsants, lipid-lowering drugs, gastrointestinal medications, and opioids may contribute to ED. The use of specific medications may preclude certain therapies for ED.
- Lifestyle and habits. Smoking, the use of recreational drugs and alcohol, and activity levels should be explored because they have potential causative implications, may offer opportunities for goal-directed therapies, or may indicate a need for further assessment before ED can be addressed.

PHYSICAL EXAMINATION

- A physical examination should be performed on every patient presenting with ED. Even though the physical is unlikely to determine the cause of ED, the presence or absence of key findings may suggest further evaluation.
- Elements of the physical examination include:
  - Body habitus, body hair, and fat distribution. Obesity per se is a risk factor for ED. The examination may suggest obstructive sleep apnea or an endocrinopathy.
  - Cardiovascular system. Evidence of organic heart disease, congestive heart failure, and the presence of bruits indicative of peripheral vascular disease.
  - Breast examination: Gynecomastia may be suggestive of an endocrinopathy, liver disease, or use of illicit drugs.

TABLE 8–3 The International Index of Erectile Function 5 Questionnaire

OVER THE PAST
SIX MONTHS

1. How do you rate your **confidence** that you could get and keep an erection?	Very low 1	Low 2	Moderate 3	High 4	Very high 5
2. When you had erections with sexual stimulation, how often were your erections hard enough for penetration?	Almost never/never 1	A few times (much less than half the time) 2	Sometimes (about half the time) 3	Most times (much more than half the time) 4	Almost always/always 5
3. During sexual intercourse **how often** were you able to maintain your erection after you had penetrated (entered) your partner?	Almost never/never 1	A few times (much less than half the time) 2	Sometimes (about half the time) 3	Most times (much more than half the time) 4	Almost always/always 5
4. During sexual intercourse **how difficult** was it to maintain your erection to completion of intercourse?	Extremely difficult 1	Very difficult 2	Difficult 3	Slightly difficult 4	Not difficult 5
5. When you attempted sexual intercourse, how often was it satisfactory for you?	Almost never/never 1	A few times (much less than half the time) 2	Sometimes (about half the time) 3	Most times (much more than half the time) 4	Almost always/always 5

The IIEF-5 score is the sum of the ordinal responses to the five items; thus the score can range from 5 to 25.
Severe ED is classified as a total score of 5–7; moderate 8–11; mild to moderate 12–16; mild 17–21; and no ED 22–25.
ED, erectile disfunction; IIEF, International Index of Erectile Function.
SOURCE: Reprinted with permission from Nature Publishing Group from Rosen RC, Cappelleri JC, Smith MD, et al. Development and evaluation of an abridged, 5-item version of the International Index of Erectile Function (IIEF-5) as a diagnostic tool for erectile dysfunction. *Int J Impot Res.* 1999; 11:319.

○ Neurologic examination: In particular, evaluation of cutaneous sensation in the perineum may be of value in investigating potential neurologic causes of ED.

○ A complete genitourinary evaluation including the penis, the scrotum and its contents, and a digital rectal examination of the prostate. Relevant findings include testicular atrophy, Peyronie's disease or prostatic disease such as BPH, prostatitis, or nodules suggestive of cancer.

LABORATORY TESTING

• The goal of initial laboratory testing is to screen for the presence of common systemic disorders that may cause ED. ISSM recommendations include a fasting blood glucose, HbA_{1C}, fasting cholesterol panel, and morning testosterone level. The AUA also recommends that a PSA blood test be offered to all men older than age 50 years with a life expectancy of at least 10 years.

○ Low testosterone levels on initial screening require further testing. A morning level of bioavailable testosterone should be checked to verify hypogonadism and to exclude low levels related to reduced sex hormone-binding globulin.

• Further blood tests may be indicated as a result of information uncovered in the history, physical, or initial laboratory testing. These include but are not limited to:

○ Thyroid function tests

○ Complete blood count

○ Prolactin level

○ Leuteinizing hormone (LH) level

○ Follicle-stimulating hormone level

• Occasionally, before consideration of any treatment of ED, additional diagnostic testing or expert consultation may be advisable.

○ For the patient requiring cardiovascular evaluation, the algorithm provided by the Second Princeton Consensus Conference on Sexual Dysfunction and Cardiac Risk (Figure 8–1) may be followed.

○ Referral to a specialist should be considered for the situations summarized in Table 8–4.

MEDICAL MANAGEMENT OF ERECTILE DYSFUNCTION

• The advent of the PDE5 inhibitors in 1998 has catapulted primary care physicians as the principal providers of care for patients with this condition. Urologists are involved in the care of difficult patients, including those requiring combination therapy or who are candidates for surgery.

ORAL THERAPY

• Phosphodiesterase type 5 inhibitors are the only oral medications approved in the United States for treatment of ED. Apomorphine is a centrally acting agent sold as a sublingual preparation outside the United States. It is moderately effective but has significant potential side effects and interactions.

• Three PDE5 inhibitors are available: (1) sildenafil (Viagra), (2) vardenafil (Levitra), and (3) tadalafil (Cialis). They work by inhibiting the enzymes that degrade cGMP.

○ Sildenafil and vardenafil are similar in speed of onset (30–60 min) and duration of action (4 h), but sildenafil requires an empty stomach for optimal absorption. Tadalafil has a similar onset of action but a much longer duration of action (up to 36 h).

○ Side effects common to the three drugs are headache, flushing, stomach upset, and nasal stuffiness. Also in July 2005, the US Food and Drug Administration (FDA) reported an increased incidence of irreversible unilateral blindness attributed to nonarteritic anterior ischemic optic neuropathy in men taking PDE5 inhibitors.

○ Sildenafil is unique in its effects on color vision, producing blue-tinged vision in some individuals caused by its greater affinity for PDE6 in the retina. Because of its greater effects on the QTc interval in the electrocardiogram, a precaution exists for prescribing vardenafil for patients also taking class 1A or class 3 antiarrhythmics or patients with congenital long QTc intervals. Tadalafil is associated with complaints of back ache and myalgia.

○ A contraindication for all PDE5 inhibitors is organic nitrate therapy, because these agents cause a synergistic drop in blood pressure (BP) to dangerously low levels. If an individual who has taken one of these drugs suffers an acute coronary syndrome (ACS), nitrates should be withheld for 24 hours after the most recent ingestion of sildenafil or vardenafil or 48 hours after the last use of tadalafil. Otherwise, standard protocols for ACS can be used.

○ Caution should be exercised in prescribing PDE5 inhibitors for patients with unstable BP or who are taking α-blocking agents such as terazosin or prazosin because of significant drops in standing BP. Patients should be warned not to take these drugs simultaneously with PDE5 inhibitors.

○ Dosing should be initiated in the middle of the therapeutic range and adjusted according to effectiveness and side effects.

○ Overall approximately 60% to 65% of ED patients in the large clinical trials preceding FDA approval of these drugs responded to therapy, but it should be noted that many studies showed a response to placebo in up to 25% to 30% of participants.

○ Special patient populations such as men with diabetes, spinal cord injury, and multiple sclerosis, as

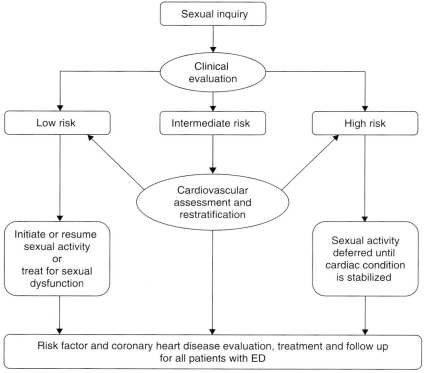

Low-risk patients:
    Asymptomatic, <3 cardiovascular risk factors; controlled hypertension; mild stable angina pectoris; postrevascularization; post-MI (>6 to 8 weeks); mild valvular disease; LV dysfunction (NYHA Class I).

High-risk patients:
    Unstable or refractory angina pectoris; uncontrolled HTN; CHF (NYHA Classes III or IV); recent MI (<2 weeks); high-risk arrhythmia; obstructive hypertrophic cardiomyopathy; moderate to severe valvular disease particularly aortic stenosis.

Intermediate- or Indeterminate-risk patients:
    Asymptomatic, ≥3 risk factors excluding gender; moderate stable angina pectoris; history of MI (>2 weeks, <6 weeks); CHF (NYHA Class II); noncardiac sequellae of atherosclerotic disease.

FIG. 8–1 Princeton Sexual Dysfunction and Cardiac Risk Assessment.
CHF, chronic heart failure; ED, erectile dysfunction; HTN, hypertension; LV, left ventricle; MI, myocardial infarction; NYHA, New York Heart Association.
SOURCE: Reprinted from with permission from Elsevier.

TABLE 8–4 Indications for Referral to a Specialist

Primary ED
Urologic problems
    Trauma
    Congenital/acquired structural abnormalities interfering with ability to have erection such as Peyronie disease, buried penis
Pelvic or perineal trauma or surgery
Complex endocrinological problem
Neurologic disease
Suspected psychogenic ED
Relationship difficulties
Vascular problems
Treatment failure
Patient preference

ED, erectile disfunction.
SOURCE: Adapted from Rosen R, Hatzichristou D. Clinical evaluation and symptom scales: Sexual dysfunction assessment in men. In: Lue TF, Bosson R, Guiliano F, Khoury S, Montorsi F. *Sexual Medicine: Sexual Dysfunction in Men and Women.* Paris: Health Publications; 2004:173–220. Available at http://www.issm.info/. Accessed September 2, 2006.

well as those with a history of treated prostate cancer have a good response to PDE5 inhibitors.

○ For the approximately 35% of men who have no or a poor initial response to PDE5 inhibitors, it is important to ensure that an adequate trial has been given, including dosage adjustments and trials of more than one drug. Additionally, the patient must clearly understand that the drugs cannot work without adequate sexual stimulation. With proper dosing adjustments and reeducation, up to 40% of initial nonresponders became responders.

○ Nonresponders should also have comorbid conditions addressed. Potential improvement in ED may be a motivating factor for patients to make lifestyle changes, such as those aimed at weight loss and smoking cessation, which help ameliorate risk factors for ED. Randomized controlled trials of weight loss in obese men and of a Mediterranean diet in men with the metabolic syndrome showed improvement in ED in the treatment groups over time.

○ Hypogonadal men should be considered for testosterone replacement therapy in the absence of contraindications. It is not recommended that testosterone be prescribed to men with normal testosterone levels. Clinical trials have indicated that PDE5 inhibitors exhibit enhanced effectiveness in hypogonadal men treated with testosterone.

○ Referral for sex therapy and marital counseling may be indicated in some cases.

PARENTERAL THERAPY

• For patients in whom PDE5 therapy fails or is contraindicated, drug treatment options include an intraurethral drug suppository or penile injection therapy. Many primary practitioners may consider referral to a urologist or other specialist in sexual medicine at this time.

• Alprostadil (prostaglandin E_1) induces erection by relaxation of trabecular smooth muscle and dilation of cavernosal arteries.

○ When it is provided in the form of an intraurethral suppository, alprostadil produces an erection sufficient for intercourse in about 40% of ED patients.

○ Men who are prescribed alprostadil must be taught how to administer it. The first dose should be administered in the physician's office because of the occurrence of systemic hypotension or syncope in approximately 3% of patients. Medicated urethral system for erection (MUSE) is available in four dosages, and titration should be done under direct supervision of a physician.

○ Approximately 50% of patients experience genital discomfort with alprostadil, with 7% withdrawing from controlled trials during the in-office titration phase.

○ Alprostadil is contraindicated in patients with an increased likelihood of priapism such as those with sickle cell anemia, polycythemia, or a previous episode of priapism. Patients should be warned that a prolonged erection is a medical emergency and to immediately seek medical attention for any erection lasting more than 4 hours. MUSE should *not* be used by those whose partner is pregnant or attempting to become pregnant.

○ There is insufficient evidence to recommend combining PDE5 inhibitors and MUSE.

○ Additionally, there is concern about hypotension from the combination.

○ Alprostadil delivered into the corpus cavernosum by way of injection is an effective drug treatment for ED. Alprostadil is the only drug approved by the FDA for injection treatment of ED. Up to 70%

of patients in controlled trials responded in both the in-office titration and at-home phases, whereas response to placebo injections was rare. Injection therapy carries the highest risk of priapism of any of the therapies currently approved by the FDA.

○ Treatment should be initiated at the lowest available dosage, typically 2.5 μg. The patient must remain in the office until tumescence has completely subsided because of the risk of priapism (approximately 1%). The physician must have a plan for prompt and effective treatment of the condition if it occurs. Subsequent dose titration must also be done under direct in-office supervision.

○ Injectable alprostadil should not be used by patients with Peyronie's disease, who have a penile implant, or who are at increased risk of priapism. Caution should also be exercised in prescribing for patients on anticoagulants or aspirin.

○ The most common side effect of penile injection therapy is localized pain. In a study that looked at effects on BP of injection therapy with alprostadil, no significant treatment-related changes in BP were found.

• Injection therapies with drug combinations including alprostadil, phentolamine, and papaverine are used and are highly effective; but only the alprostadil component is approved for injection treatment of ED by the FDA. Some studies suggest an increased incidence of penile fibrosis attributed to the papaverine component and also an increased incidence of priapism compared with the use of alprostadil alone.

• Combinations of PDE5 inhibitors and injectable therapy have not been adequately studied, so there are no definite recommendations available about their use.

NONMEDICAL THERAPIES FOR ERECTILE DYSFUNCTION

• A variety of devices are available for treatment of ED. The vacuum erection device (VED) is available with or without a prescription. Patient satisfaction is variable but generally higher in older men in stable relationships. It is important that only devices with a vacuum limiter be used to avoid injury to the penis. Patients on anticoagulants and antiplatelet agents should exercise caution in use of VEDs. Although trials of VED use with either injectable alprostadil or a PDE5 inhibitor have been completed and the results indicate improved patient satisfaction with combination therapy, there is insufficient follow-up data to recommend this approach to treatment by the primary care provider.

• The use of other nonmedical therapies for ED requires referral to a urologist. Penile implants should be considered only when other treatments have failed.

Patients must appreciate the irreversible effects of this therapy including possible changes in penile appearance and the fact that if the device is removed for any reason, other erectile therapies are less effective.

- Whether arterial or venous, vascular surgery has a very limited place in treatment of ED. It should be considered only in healthy individuals with recently acquired, often traumatic, ED secondary to a focal arterial occlusion and in the absence of generalized vascular disease. The AUA does not currently recommend surgery for treatment of venous causes of ED.

OTHER THERAPIES AND FUTURE DIRECTIONS

- Many other therapies have been used to manage ED, including a wide variety of herbal compounds.
  - Yohimbine is a drug that has traditionally been used although the evidence is inconclusive except possibly for psychogenic ED. It is currently not recommended because of side effects and safety concerns. Yohimbine can cause increased heart rate and blood pressure, increased motor activity, irritability, and tremor.
  - Korean red ginseng has shown limited effectiveness in recent small trials but cannot be recommended because of ongoing concerns about the safety of herbals and potential interactions with other medications.
  - Drugs targeted at other areas of the cascade of physiologic reactions necessary to achieve an erection may become available for treatment in the future. These include activators of guanylate cyclase and inhibitors of the rho kinase signaling pathway.

BIBLIOGRAPHY

Alexander RB, Propert KJ, Schaeffer AJ, et al. Ciprofloxacin or tamsulosin in men with chronic prostatitis/chronic pelvic pain syndrome. *Ann Intern Med.* 2004;141:581.

American Urological Association. The management of erectile dysfunction: An update. Erectile dysfunction erectile Dysfunction guideline. http://www.auanet.org/guidelines/. Published May 2006. Accessed July 9, 2006.

AUA Practice Guidelines Committee. AUA guideline on management of benign prostatic hyperplasia (2003). Chapter 1: Diagnosis and treatment recommendations. *J Urol.* 2003;170:530.

Beckman TJ, Mynderse LA. Evaluation and medical management of benign prostatic hyperplasia. *Mayo Clin Proc.* 2005;80:1356.

Bent S, Kane C, Shinohara K, et al. Saw palmetto for benign prostatic hyperplasia. *N Engl J Med.* 2006;354:557.

Berger RE, Lee JC. Sexually transmitted diseases: The classic diseases. In Walsh PC, Retik AB, Vaughan ED, et al, eds. *Campbell's Urology.* 8th ed. Philadelphia, PA: Saunders; 2002:678–680.

Bhasin S, Glenn R, Cunningham FJ, et al. Testosterone therapy in adult men with androgen deficiency syndromes: An Endocrine Society Clinical Practice Guideline. *J Clin Endocrinol Metab.* 2006–2010;91:1995.

Bradshaw CS, Tabrizi SN, Read TR, et al. Etiologies of non-gonococcal urethritis: Bacteria, viruses and the association of orogenital exposure. *J Infect Dis.* 2006;193:336.

Centers for Disease Control and Prevention. *Sexually Transmitted Disease Surveillance, 2004.* Atlanta: U.S. Department of Health and Human Services; September 2005.

Workowski KA, Berman SM. Centers for Disease Control and Prevention sexually transmitted diseases treatment guidelines, 2006. *MMWR Recomm Rep.* 2006;55(RR-11):1–94.

Collins MM, Fowler FJ, Elliott DB, et al. Diagnosing and treating chronic prostatitis: Do urologists use the four-glass test? *Urology.* 2000;55:403.

Hua VN, Schaeffer AJ. Acute and chronic prostatitis. *Med Clin North Am.* 2004;88:483.

Junnila J, Lassen P. Testicular masses. *Am Fam Physician.* 1998; 57:685.

Kodner C. Sexually transmitted infections in men. *Prim Care.* 2003;30:173.

Kostis JB, Rosen RC, eds. A symposium: Sexual dysfunction and cardiac risk. The Second Princeton Consensus Conference. *Am J Cardiol.* 2005;96(suppl 12B):85M–93M.

Lipsky BA. Prostatitis and urinary tract infection in men: What's new; what's true? *Am J Med.* 1999;106:327.

Lue TF. Male sexual dysfunction. In Tanagho EA and McAninch JW, eds. *Smith's General Urology.* 16th ed. McGraw-Hill; 2004: 592–611.

Luzzi GA, O'Brien TS. Acute epididymitis. *BJU Int.* 2001;87:747.

McConnell JD, Roehrborn CG, Bautista OM, et al. The long-term effect of doxazosin, finasteride, and combination therapy on the clinical progression of benign prostatic hyperplasia. *N Engl J Med.* 2003;349:2387.

McCormack WM, Rein MF. Urethritis. In Mandell GL, Douglas RG Jr, Bennett JE, eds. *Principles and Practice of Infectious Diseases.* 6th ed. New York: Churchill-Livingstone, 2005: 1347–1355.

NIH Consens Statement. *Impotence.* 1992;10(4):1–31.

Philip J, Selvan D, Desmond AD. Mumps orchitis in the non-immune post-pubertal male: A resurgent threat to male fertility? *BJU Int.* 2006;97:138.

Rosen RC, Cappelleri JC, Smith MD, et al. Development and evaluation of an abridged, 5-item version of the International Index of Erectile Function (IIEF-5) as a diagnostic tool for erectile dysfunction. *Int J Impot Res.* 1999;11:319–326.

Rosen R, Hatzichristou D. Clinical evaluation and symptom scales: sexual dysfunction assessment in men. In Lue TF, Bosson R, Guiliano F, Khoury S, Montorsi F. *Sexual Medicine: Sexual Dysfunction in Men and Women.* Paris: Health Publications; 2004:173–220. Available at http://www.issm. info/. Accessed September 2, 2006.

Schaeffer AJ, Landis JR, Knauss JS, et al. Demographic and clinical characteristics of men with chronic prostatitis: The National Institutes of Health Chronic Prostatitis Cohort Study. *J Urol.* 2002;168:593.

Schaeffer AJ. Chronic prostatitis and the chronic pelvic pain syndrome. *N Engl J Med.* 2006;355:1690.

Wei JT, Calhoun E, Jacobsen SJ. Urologic diseases in America project: Benign prostatic hyperplasia. *J Urol.* 2005;173:1256.

Weidner W. Treating chronic prostatitis: Antibiotics no, alpha-blockers maybe. *Ann Intern Med.* 2004;141:639.

9 WOMEN'S HEALTH

Thomas J. Olsen

The medical care of women overlaps with the health-care of men in a variety of areas (see also Chap. 8, Selected Topics in Men's Health). There are specific areas of medical importance to women that are covered elsewhere in this book, including: osteoporosis, cancer screening (Pap smears and mammography), sexually transmitted diseases, and breast and uterine cancer. This chapter will deal with management of the abnormal Pap smear, abnormal vaginal bleeding, menopause, and vulvovaginitis.

MANAGEMENT OF THE ABNORMAL PAP SMEAR

Results of cervical cytology specimens are reported using the 2001 Bethesda System. The report includes several components:

- Specimen type (conventional smear, liquid based)
- Specimen adequacy (satisfactory for evaluation, rejected or unsatisfactory)
- General categorization (negative for lesion or cancer, epithelial cell abnormality, other)
- Automated review (if examined by automated device)
- Ancillary testing (describe additional tests and results)
- Interpretation/Result (negative for malignancy, organisms [trichomonas, etc.], other nonneoplastic findings [atrophy, inflammation])
- Other (endometrial cells in a woman over 40 years of age)
- Epithelial Cell Abnormalities (type of cell and degree of atypia)
- Other malignant neoplasms

UNSATISFACTORY SPECIMEN

These specimens must be repeated.

LACK OF TRANSFORMATION ZONE

Endocervical cells were not obtained when the Pap smear was taken. If the smear is otherwise normal the smear can be repeated in 12 months. Women who are immunocompromised, have HPV, or who have had previous smears with atypical squamous cells of undetermined significance (ASCUS) should have the smear repeated sooner (usually 6–8 months).

ENDOMETRIAL CELLS OUT OF PHASE

Endometrial cells that are reported as abnormal on a Pap smear from a woman over 40 years of age must be considered in relation to the last menses. If the smear was not obtained in close proximity to the last menses, the woman should be referred to a gynecologist for further evaluation.

ASCUS

If reflex testing for HPV DNA was not obtained at the time the Pap smear was done, the smear should be repeated with testing for HPV DNA. If high-risk serotypes are present, the patient should be referred for colposcopy. If high-risk HPV serotypes are not present, the smear and HPV DNA testing should be repeated in 6 to 12 months.

NEGATIVE FOR INTRAEPITHELIAL LESION OR MALIGNANCY BUT POSITIVE FOR HIGH-RISK HPV DNA

These women should be informed of the presence of the infection. They should be counseled about the role of smoking, stress, healthy lifestyle, and nutrition in the natural history of the infection. The smear should be repeated with HPV testing every 6 months until the infection clears. Most infections clear in 2 years.

LOW-GRADE SQUAMOUS INTRAEPITHELIAL LESION (LGSIL) OR HIGH-GRADE SQUAMOUS INTRAEPITHELIAL LESION (HGSIL)

These women should be referred for further evaluation by colposcopy.

ABNORMAL VAGINAL BLEEDING

Disorders of menstruation can present as reduced bleeding, excessive bleeding, or bleeding at unpredictable times. These conditions can be associated with hormonal disturbances, anatomical abnormalities (fibroids), or in some cases, both.

Menorrhagia: prolonged or excessive bleeding occurring at predictable intervals.

Metrorrhagia: menstrual bleeding occurring at irregular intervals or bleeding between periods.

Menometrorrhagia: prolonged or excessive bleeding occurring at irregular intervals for irregular duration.

Perimenopausal bleeding: variation in length of the menstrual cycle can occur as well as noncyclic bleeding.

Postmenopausal bleeding: uterine bleeding that occurs more than 12 months after cessation of menses.

DISORDERS OF MENSTRUATION

Common causes of noncyclic uterine bleeding include the following:
- Anovulation
- Fibroids
- Endometrial polyps, hyperplasia, or cancer
- Cervical or vaginal neoplasm
- Endometriosis
- Adenomyosis
- Pregnancy
- Postpartum state
- Coagulopathy
- Medications

ANOVULATORY BLEEDING

This is the most common cause of noncyclic uterine bleeding. The approach to evaluation and treatment of a patient is based on an understanding of the underlying causes of anovulation.
- Physiologic
  - Adolescence
  - Pregnancy
  - Lactation
  - Perimenopausal
- Hormonal causes
  - Polycystic ovary syndrome
  - Hypothyroidism
  - Hypothalamic dysfunction as occurs in anorexia nervosa
  - Premature ovarian failure (<40 years of age)
  - Pituitary disease
- Iatrogenic causes
  - Post radiation
  - Chemotherapy

EVALUATION AND MANAGEMENT

Evaluation of abnormal uterine bleeding begins with a thorough history. The age of the patient should suggest specific diagnostic possibilities (eg, anorexia). Recent changes in weight, stress, and treatment for other medical conditions should be explored. Symptoms of hypothyroidism should be assessed. The physical examination should include measurement of the body mass index (BMI), assessment for signs of goiter, and galactorrhea. A speculum examination and bimanual pelvic examination including rectovaginal examination and Pap smear may reveal an anatomic cause.

A pregnancy test, thyroid-stimulating hormone (TSH), and prolactin level should be obtained. If the pregnancy test is negative, a progestogen challenge can be performed. Medroxyprogesterone 10 mg daily for 5 to 10 days may result in a menses. This confirms anovulation as the cause of abnormal bleeding. The patient may be managed with a progesten on a periodic basis. Low dose oral contraceptives will restore menstrual cycles to normal.

If the patient does not have withdrawal bleeding from the medroxyprogesterone, or if a structural abnormality is uncovered, referral to a gynecologist for further evaluation is indicated. Patients with hypothyroidism or hyperprolactinemia require treatment of the underlying disorder.

VULVOVAGINITIS

This is an extremely common condition and is often seen by the primary care physician. Knowledge of the symptoms and signs of the common infectious causes of vaginitis will allow effective treatment for the majority of patients. Lactobacilli and other bacteria constitute normal vaginal flora. Lactobacilli produce lactic acid and maintain a mildly acidic vaginal pH. Disruption of the normal vaginal flora can be caused by antibiotic use, stress, diabetes, or elevated estrogen levels (pregnancy, oral contraceptives, estrogen therapy.)

The three most common causes of vaginitis are bacterial vaginosis, candidal vulvovaginitis, and trichomonas vaginitis. Symptoms, findings on examination, nature of the discharge, and microscopic findings help differentiate the causes and guide treatment.

BACTERIAL VAGINOSIS

Symptom/Signs: vaginal discharge and odor
Discharge: thin, white, malodorous
pH: high
Microscopic examination: white blood cells (WBCs),

bacteria laden epithelial cells (clue cells), negative potassium hydroxide (KOH) test.
Treatment: metronidazole 500 mg twice daily for 5 to 7 days, or metronidazole 0.75% gel, one applicator intravaginally once daily for 5 days.
Recurrent infection: therapy can be extended beyond 7 days; antibiotic can be changed to clindamycin 300 mg twice daily for 7 days

VULVOVAGINAL CANDIDIASIS

Symptom/Signs: vaginal discharge, vulvar pruritus and burning, vulvar erythema and edema, vaginal erythema
Discharge: thick, white, adherent
pH: normal
Microscopic examination: WBCs and red blood cells (RBCs) on wet prep, hyphae on KOH.
Treatment: over-the-counter preparations are available: single dose oral treatment with fluconazole 150 mg once daily, or topical imidazole creams or suppositories for 1, 3, or 7 days depending on the preparation.
Recurrent infection: obtain vaginal cultures which may reveal nonalbicans yeast, consider a longer initial course, maintenance therapy is sometimes required.

TRICHOMONAS VAGINITIS

Symptoms/Signs: vaginal discharge, erythema of the vaginal mucosa.
Discharge: copious, thin
pH: high
Microscopic examination: wet prep shows WBCs and motile trichomonads
Treatment: metronidazole 2 gm as a single dose, or metronidazole 500 mg twice daily for 7 days
Recurrent infection: confirm the diagnosis, the partner should be evaluated, repeat the initial course.

MENOPAUSE

Women transition into menopause over a period of time. A woman who has had 12 consecutive months of amenorrhea is menopausal. Symptoms may begin in the transition period and continue into the postmenopausal period. Common problems in women at this stage of life include vasomotor symptoms, atrophic vaginitis, and postmenopausal bleeding.

VASOMOTOR SYMPTOMS

Vasomotor symptoms include hot flashes and night sweats. Women commonly report a sensation of warmth that spreads throughout the body and is associated with sweating. These symptoms can begin in the transition period and are associated with lower relative estrogen levels. In some women these episodes occur multiple times during the day and night. They may subside in 1 to 2 years but may persist for 5 to 10 years in others. Alcohol, caffeine, or spicy food may trigger hot flashes.

Treatment of moderate to severe vasomotor symptoms is the main indication for postmenopausal estrogen therapy or combined estrogen-progestogen therapy. Hormonal therapy is used at the lowest effective dose for the shortest duration possible (<5 years). Preparations include oral conjugated equine estrogen 0.3 to 0.625 mg daily and oral estradiol 0.5 to 1.0 mg daily. Combined estrogen-progestogen preparations are also available.

Soy products, black cohosh, evening primrose, and dong quai have not been consistently proven in clinical trials. Antidepressants including selective serotonin reuptake inhibitors (SSRIs) and serotonin-norepinephrine reuptake inhibitors (SNRIs) have yielded mixed results in clinical trials, as has the α-blocker clonidine.

ATROPHIC VAGINITIS

Vaginal dryness may be a symptom early in the menopause transition. Over time the lining of the vagina is thinned and vaginal secretions decrease. Dyspareunia, burning on urination, vaginal discharge, urinary incontinence, or urinary tract infections may be associated with atrophic vaginitis.

Examination reveals loss of vaginal rugae, a thinned mucosa, scant secretions, friability of the mucosa, and edema of the vaginal mucosa or labia.

Mild symptoms may respond to water-based lubricating jelly or vaginal moisturizers. All hormonal preparations are approved for treatment of severe vaginal atrophy and are effective. Topical preparations are preferred. These include conjugated equine estrogen cream 1 gm vaginally nightly for 2 weeks then 1 or 2 days weekly, estradiol 1 gm vaginally nightly for 2 weeks then 1 or 2 days weekly, or estradiol ring every 90 days.

POSTMENOPAUSAL BLEEDING

Postmenopausal vaginal bleeding can be caused by many of the same factors as abnormal bleeding earlier in life. The cause is more likely to be structural than hormonal in a postmenopausal woman. Endometrial carcinoma and vaginal atrophy are common causes. Infection and trauma can cause bleeding. As a woman ages, fibroids are less likely to be the cause of bleeding.

The physical examination should include a complete pelvic examination and Pap smear. The absence of atrophy and trauma are important.

Women with undiagnosed vaginal bleeding should be referred to a gynecologist. Transvaginal ultrasound and endometrial biopsy can facilitate the assessment of endometrial atrophy or endometrial carcinoma.

BIBLIOGRAPHY

American College of Obstetricians and Gynecologists. *ACOG Practice Bulletin.* Management of anovulatory bleeding. 2000;14:909–916.

American College of Obstetricians and Gynecologists. *ACOG Practice Bulletin.* Use of botanicals for management of menopausal symptoms. 2001;28:945–955.

Eckert L. Acute vulvovaginitis. *N Engl J Med.* 2006;355(12): 1244–1252.

Grady D. Management of menopausal symptoms. *N Engl J Med.* 2006;355(22):2338–2347.

Estrogen and progestogen use in peri- and postmenopausal women: March 20007 position statement of the North American Menopause Society. *Menopause.* 2007;14(2):168–182.

Solomon D, Davey D, Kurman R, et al. The 2001 Bethesda System: terminology for reporting results of cervical cytology. *JAMA.* 2002;287(16):2114–2119.

Section 2
ASSESSING THE MEDICAL LITERATURE

10 THE BASICS OF STATISTICS
Thomas E. Burroughs

INTRODUCTION

Statistics can be defined as the *science of classifying, organizing, and analyzing data*. Biostatistics can be thought of as a set of tools used to summarize and analyze key questions in the biologic sciences, including medicine. The list of research questions where biostatistics could be used is endless, but examples would include the following:

- What is the direction and strength of the association between cyclooxygenase-2 (COX-2) inhibitors and the frequency of cardiovascular events?
- Does a new medication for type 2 diabetes result in improved blood glucose levels?
- What baseline patient characteristics are associated with the survival of patients with colon cancer?
- What is the national prevalence of acquired immunodeficiency syndrome (AIDS)?
  There are two primary branches in biostatistics:
  1. *Descriptive statistics* simply describe characteristics of data. These statistics include measures of central tendency (eg, the mean, median, and mode), variability (eg, range, variance, standard deviation) and association (eg, the correlation).
  2. *Inferential statistics* are used to draw conclusions about relationships in a population based on data from a sample. Inferential statistics can be used for either estimation or hypothesis testing.
- Estimation is used to *estimate* population values, such as the prevalence of hepatitis C or the incidence of breast cancer. Hypothesis testing is used to test hypotheses (eg, drug A has fewer side effects than drug B or a new triaging procedure reduces emergency room wait times).

BASIC TERMINOLOGY

There are fundamental terms and symbols that must be defined to comprehend biostatistical analysis. These include:
- *Variable*. A variable is any factor in a study that can vary from observation to observation.
- *Population* versus *sample*. A population is the complete set of observations about which the investigator wishes to draw conclusions. A sample is any subset of that population.
- *Parameter* versus *statistic*. A parameter is any numerical index (eg, median, range) for the entire population. A statistic is a numerical index for a sample. Greek symbols are used for parameters. Roman letters are used for statistics.
- *Independent* versus *dependent* variable. An independent variable is one that is hypothesized to cause or influence a dependent variable.

THE FOUR SCALES OF MEASUREMENT

The scale of measurement for a variable determines the type of analyses that can be conducted for that variable.
1. *Nominal variables* are mutually exclusive categories such as gender, primary diagnosis, and blood type.
2. *Ordinal variables* are ordered categories that allow one to rank them in terms of an absolute amount of some characteristic such as Olympic medals (gold, silver, bronze), hospital rankings (first place, second place, etc), or stage of cancer but do not tell one how much the rankings differ. For example, first place versus second place in a race discloses the winner but does not disclose by how many seconds they won.
3. *Interval variables* are ones where the distance between values has the same meaning anywhere along the scale. For example, the difference between 32 degrees and 38 degrees means the same thing as the difference between 50 and 56 degrees.

4. *Ratio variables* have all the characteristics of an interval variable and also have an absolute zero point (0 indicates the complete absence of whatever is being measured). As an example, there is still thermal motion present at 0 degrees celsius (interval scale), but there is no such motion present at 0 degrees Kelvin (ratio scale).

THE MEANING OF SIGNIFICANCE

The word "significant" has very different meanings depending on the context. In a clinical context, the phrase "clinically significant" refers to something that is clinically important. In statistics, the word "significant" refers to a numeric result that is reasonably unlikely to be caused by random chance.

- Sometimes a tiny numeric difference reaches statistical significance (because of very precise measurement or a very large sample size), but this difference is not nearly large enough to be clinically important. For example, with a large enough sample size, it might be possible to find that a blood glucose level of 80 is statistically different than a blood glucose level of 83. It would prove difficult, however, to argue that this 3-point difference is clinically significant.

Do statistics lie? Mark Twain and Benjamin Disraeli (prime minister of England for three terms beginning in 1868) are both given credit for saying "There are three kinds of lies . . . lies, damn lies, and statistics." Statistics are used as the basis for making critical decisions, but they cannot lie. They can certainly be incorrectly chosen, inaccurately interpreted, or be generalized far beyond what is appropriate. The users of statistics can lie, but statistics themselves cannot.

In medicine, it is important to have a basic understanding of statistics, so that one can be an informed consumer. It is important to be a competent judge of the appropriateness of the statistical analysis and to identify situations whereby the author misleads (intentionally or unintentionally) the reader through carefully designed graphics, excluding pertinent results, or overemphasis of specific results.

BIBLIOGRAPHY

Dawson-Saunders, B, Trapp, RG. *Basic & Clinical Biostatistics,* 2nd ed. Appleton & Lange, Connecticut 1994.

GraphPad Software, InStat guide to choosing and interpreting statistical tests, 1998, GraphPad Software, Inc., San Diego California USA, www.graphpad.com (accessed 11/15/2007)

Shott, S. *Statistics for Health Professionals,* WB Saunders, Philadelphia 1990.

11 DESCRIBING AND DISPLAYING DATA

Thomas E. Burroughs

When conducting research or reporting the results of a study, researchers use descriptive statistics to summarize the variables and findings. Measures of central tendency are used to describe the *average* for the variables. Measures of variability are used to indicate how much *spread* or *dispersion* there is among the observations. Frequency distributions, along with their graphical counterparts, are used to display the actual observation. Each provides unique information that is important for the reader to appreciate.

FREQUENCY DISTRIBUTIONS

A frequency distribution is a table that divides the observations for a variable into intervals and shows the frequency and percentage of observations that occur within each interval, and the cumulative frequency and percentage of observations that occur from the upper limit of each interval through the lowest interval.

- Frequency distributions can utilize multiple columns to summarize the data in slightly different ways (see Table 11–1).
  1. *Interval* or *category* (first column) divides the range of actual values into intervals of the same width.
  2. *Frequency* or *count* (second column) is the *number* of observations within a specific interval.
  3. *Cumulative frequency* or *cumulative count* (third column) reflects the total *number* of observations that are included in the specified interval and all intervals below.
  4. *Relative frequency* or *percent* (fourth column) shows the *percentage* of observations within a specific interval are included in the specified interval and all intervals below.
  5. *Cumulative percent* or *cumulative relative frequency* (fifth column) reflects the *percentage* of observations that are derived from the specified interval and all intervals below.

GRAPHICAL DISPLAYS OF FREQUENCY

The information contained in a frequency distribution can also be displayed through several graphical methods.

1. A *histogram* is used to display the number or percentage of observations for a continuous variable such as temperature, height, weight, or high-density lipoprotein

TABLE 11–1 Frequency Distribution

		POSTPRANDIAL BLOOD GLUCOSE LEVELS		
CATEGORY	COUNT	CUMULATIVE COUNT	PERCENT	CUMULATIVE PERCENT
351–400	14	300	5%	100%
301–350	29	286	10%	95%
251–300	78	257	26%	86%
201–250	69	179	23%	60%
151–200	53	110	18%	37%
101–150	27	57	9%	19%
51–100	22	30	7%	10%
0–50	8	8	3%	3%

(HDL) concentration. There is one bar for each interval or category in the frequency distribution (eg, 61–80 lb, 81–100 lb, 101–120 lb). The height of each bar represents the number or percentage of cases in each interval. A histogram can also be constructed for the cumulative frequency or cumulative percent.

2. A *bar chart* is used to display the number or percentage of observations for a categorical variable such as gender, primary diagnosis, or type of surgery. There is one bar for each category and the height of each bar represents the number or percentage of cases in each interval. A bar chart for a categorical variable is analogous to a histogram for a continuous variable.

3. A *frequency polygon or line graph* is similar to a histogram. The only difference is that connected lines are used to display the data values instead of bars. Frequency polygons or line graphs should not be used with categorical variables, as the lines imply continuity across the different categories or intervals.

4. A *box-and-whisker plot* is a graph that displays the distribution for a set of observations. The plot is comprised of a box in the middle and one line (whisker) emerging from each side of the box (Fig. 11–1). The left side of the box is placed at the 25th percentile for the variable, and the right side of the box is at the 75th percentile for the variable. In the middle of the box is a vertical line representing the median. The corresponding actual values for these percentiles and median are placed immediately above or below their respective positions on the box. The "whiskers" extend to the minimum value on the left side and the maximum value on the right side.

5. A *stem and leaf plot* is a means of showing the exact value of each observation (Fig. 11–2). The left column shows the first digits *(stems)* of each observation. The

right column shows the final digit *(leaf)* of each observation. For example, for the number 102, the stem would be 10, and the leaf would be two. For the number 107, the stem would be 10 and the leaf would be 7.

MEASURES OF CENTRAL TENDENCY

Measures of central tendency describe the *average* for a specific variable. There are three basic measures of central tendency.

1. *Mode* represents the most frequent value among the observations.
   - The mode reflects the number at the highest point along the frequency curve, and can help define the shape of a distribution. A bimodal distribution has two modes or peaks; a trimodal distribution has three modes or peaks. The mode is the only measure of central tendency that can be used to describe discrete data.

2. *Median* represents the value that is at the 50th percentile of the distribution. This is the number below and above which half of the observations fall.
   - The median is usually reported for highly skewed data. The median is not influenced by the actual values of the observations above and below it. For example, when measuring blood glucose levels in 100 patients an increase in the upper 3 observations by 80 points each will have no effect on the median but the mean will rise considerably.

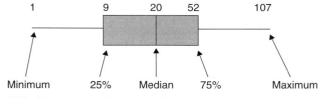

FIG. 11–1 Box and whisker plot.

ED WAIT TIMES	F	STEM	LEAF
100–109	2	10	2,7
90–99	1	9	3
80–89	0	8	
70–79	1	7	8
60–69	1	6	5
50–59	1	5	2
40–49	3	4	2,4,5
30–39	2	3	5,7
20–29	1	2	0,9
10–19	7	1	2,2,4,4,7,19
1–9	6	0	1,2,5,8,8,9

FIG. 11–2 Stem and leaf plot (F = number of observations).

3. *Mean* (μ, $\overline{X}$) is the arithmetic average of all of the observations.
   - The mean is the most consistent of the three measures, but is highly influenced by outliers (unusually high or unusually low values).
     ○ Basic symbols and formula

$$\overline{X} = \frac{\sum X}{n}$$

   - ▪ $\overline{X}$ is the sample mean
   - ▪ X represents each raw score
   - ▪ n refers to the sample size
   - ▪ μ is the population mean
   - ▪ Σ is the summation sign

MEASURES OF VARIABILITY

Measures of variability are used to describe the amount of dispersion, spread or scatter of scores for a variable.
- Understanding variability is a critical element in statistical analysis. There is variability in nearly everything, including patient characteristics and clinical outcomes. Identification of the factors that underlie variability in outcomes, facilitates improvements in patient care and outcomes.
- There are five basic measures of variability.
  1. The *range* is the difference between the highest and lowest scores.
  2. The *semi-interquartile range* (IQR) is the difference between the score at the 25th percentile and the score at the 75th percentile, eg, essentially the range after eliminating the top 25% and bottom 25% of the data. This is used to control for outliers or extreme values.
  3. The *variance* (σ^2, s^2) is the average of the squared deviations of the individual observations around their mean. These deviations are squared so that the positive and negative values do not cancel one another out (a property of the mean which is theoretically important for statistical tests).
  4. The *standard deviation* (σ, s) is simply the square root of the variance. This adjusts the variance into the same scale as the original values.
  5. The *coefficient of variation* (CV) is used to standardize the variance so that variables with different scales can be directly compared across or within studies. CV is expressed as a percentage and reveals the amplitude of variability relative to the mean.
     ○ Basic symbols and formula

$$s^2 = \frac{\sum (X - \overline{X})^2}{n-1}$$

$$s = \sqrt{s^2}$$

$$\sigma^2 = \frac{\sum (X - \mu)^2}{n-1}$$

$$\sigma = \sqrt{\sigma^2}$$

$$CV = 100\sqrt{\frac{s}{\overline{X}}}$$

- ▪ X represents the raw scores
- ▪ $\overline{X}$ is the sample mean
- ▪ s^2 is equal to the sample variance
- ▪ s is equal to the sample standard deviation
- ▪ σ^2 is equal to the population variance
- ▪ σ is equal to the population standard deviation
- ▪ n is equal to the sample size
- ▪ Σ is the summation sign

CHARACTERISTICS OF A DISTRIBUTION

The distributional characteristics of a variable determine the type of analysis that can be conducted. Most statistical tests have very specific distributional requirements, such as requiring that the data be normally distributed. If these requirements are not met the results of the analysis will not be accurate.
- A *symmetric distribution* is one in which the right and left side are mirror images of one another. A normal curve is an example of a symmetric distribution. In a symmetric distribution, the mean, median, and mode equal one another.
  ○ An *asymmetric* or *skewed distribution* is one where the right and left sides are not mirror images of one another. If the left tail of the distribution extends farther to the left than the right tail, the distribution is negatively skewed. If instead the right tail extends farther than does the left tail, the distribution is positively skewed. Skewed distributions are not normally distributed, and, therefore are less amenable to analysis via conventional statistical tests.
    ▪ *Pearson's skewness coefficient* measures the amount of skew by determining how many standard deviations the median is above the mean.
      - Skewness coefficient = $\frac{\overline{X} - Mdn}{s}$. Positive values indicate positive skew. Negative values indicate negative skew. A value of 0 indicates a symmetric distribution. Values greater than 0.2 or less than -0.2 suggest severe skewness.
    ▪ *Fisher's skewness measure* converts the measure of skew into a z-score that can be statistically evaluated. Fisher's skewness measures greater than 1.96 or less than -1.96 suggest statistically significant skew.
      - *Kurtosis* is a measure of how flat or peaked the curve is.

TABLE 11–2. Interpreting *r* (for Positive or Negative Correlations)

0.00 to 0.25	little if any correlation
0.26 to 0.49	low
0.50 to 0.69	moderate
0.70 to 0.89	high
0.90 to 0.99	very high
1.00	perfect

For *Fisher's measure of kurtosis,* a value of 0 indicates a perfectly normal curve. Values greater than zero indicate that a distribution is too peaked to be normal, and values lower than zero indicate that a distribution is too flat to be considered normal. Measures of kurtosis are only meaningful for symmetric data.

MEASURES OF ASSOCIATION

Measures of association, such as the correlation coefficient, are used to quantify the magnitude and direction of relationships among two or more variables. There are a number of different measures of association that are designed to handle different types of data and relationships.

- A correlation can *never* be used to establish a cause-and-effect relationship. A strong correlation does not mean that one variable necessarily causes another. A carefully controlled experiment is required to establish causal relationships.
- Measures of association typically range from -1 to $+1$, with a value of 0 indicating that there is no relationship between the variables.
- There are two aspects to any measure of association.
  1. *Strength* indicates the magnitude of the association (see Table 11–2). The closer the association is to zero the weaker the association, regardless of whether the correlation is positive or negative. The farther away from zero, the stronger the correlation.
  2. *Direction* indicates the nature of the relationship between the variables. A positive correlation indicates that both variables move in the same direction (eg, height and weight in children). A negative correlation is an inverse relationship where the two variables move in opposite directions (weight of automobile and miles per gallon)

- To test whether a correlation is significantly different than 0, a specific t-test can be employed.
- There are several measures of association that can be employed for different analytic situations.
  - *Pearson product moment correlation* (*r*) is used to quantify the association between two continuous variables, and is the most commonly used measure of association.

$$r = \frac{\sum XY - (\sum X \sum Y)/n}{\sqrt{(SS_x)(SS_y)}}$$

$$SS_x = S_x^2(n-1)$$

$$SS_y = S_y^2(n-1)$$

  - *Covariance* is a measure of association that is in the same scale as the original variable, and has not been standardized.
  - *Coefficient of determination* (r^2), often described as the measure of "meaningfulness," is used to indicate the amount of variation shared between two variables. It is calculated by squaring the correlation coefficient.
  - *Multiple correlation* (R^2) is used to quantify the association between a single dependent variable and a set of independent variables. For regression analysis and analysis of variance, R^2 is used to report how much variance in the dependent variable is accounted for by the independent variables.
  - *Partial* and *semi-partial correlation* (part correlation) are used to examine the relationship between two variables after statistically adjusting for (controlling for, partialling out) the influence of a third variable. The two approaches are quite similar.
    1. A partial correlation ($r_{12.3}$) is the correlation between variables 1 and 2, after the effect of variable 3 is removed from both variables 1 and 2.
    2. A semi-partial correlation ($r_{1(2.3)}$) is the correlation between variables 1 and 2, after the effect of variable 3 is removed from both variables 1 and 2.
- A variety of other correlation measures are used to quantify the relationships when one or both of the variables are not continuous. These are summarized in Table 11–3.

TABLE 11–3. Correlation Measures for Noncontinuous Variables

TYPE OF CORRELATION	VARIABLE 1	VARIABLE 2
Spearman rank order (p or rho)	Rank of X (ordinal)	Rank of Y (ordinal)
Kendal's tau	Ordinal	Ordinal
Goodman and Kruskal Gamma		
Biserial	Continuous reduced to dichotomous	Continuous
Tetrachoric	Continuous reduced to dichotomous	Continuous reduced to dichotomous
Point biserial	Continuous	Dichotomous
Phi-coefficient	Dichotomous	Dichotomous
Contingency coefficient	Discrete (at least 2 levels)	Discrete (at least 3 levels)
Eta	Continuous	Continuous

BIBLIOGRAPHY

Dawson-Saunders, B, Trapp, RG. *Basic & Clinical Biostatistics,* 2nd ed, Appleton & Lange, Connecticut 1994.

Guyatt, GH; Drummond R. *Users' Guides to the Medical Literature: Essentials of Evidence-based Clinical Practice* Chicago, IL: AMA Press, 2007.

Sonnad S.S. Describing data: statistical and graphical methods. Radiology 2002; 225:622–628

12 OVERVIEW TO INFERENTIAL STATISTICS: ESTIMATION AND HYPOTHESIS TESTING

Thomas E. Burroughs

- Inferential statistics is the second primary branch of statistics (the first being descriptive statistics) and is used to infer characteristics or relationships about a population on the basis of data from a sample. Inferential statistics are used to test questions such as whether a new drug has better efficacy than an old drug, whether increased nurse staffing is associated with higher patient satisfaction, and to estimate rates such as the incidence of congestive heart failure in the US population. Inferential statistics are typically used to answer the primary research questions in a clinical trial or research study.
- There are two basic objectives of inferential statistics:
  1. *Estimation* is used to estimate population parameters based on a sample; for example, to identify the prevalence of hepatitis C or to determine the incidence of new acquired immune deficiency syndrome cases annually in men younger than 25 years old.
  2. *Hypothesis testing* is used to test hypotheses about specific relationships in the population. For example, do COX-2 Inhibitors and NSAIDs have different rates of cardiovascular events?
- Inferential statistics include tests such as *t* tests, *z* tests, analysis of variance (ANOVA), and regression analysis,

just to name a few. Any test that produces a *p* value comes from inferential statistics.

BASIC PRINCIPLES

- Hypothesis testing determines whether an observed difference (eg, between Drug A and Drug B) is larger than what is expected from random chance alone.
- Mathematical distributions are used to characterize what these data would look like because of chance alone. There are many such distributions including the normal distribution, *t* distribution, *F* distribution, gamma distribution, exponential, and Weibull distribution.
- Most variables of interest follow a normal distribution.
- The *central limit theorem* allows researchers to conduct traditional parametric statistics even when the original data is not normally distributed. This theorem argues that even if the original data is not normally distributed, the means derived from this data become normally distributed as the sample size increases. This observation permits use of the normal curve for many statistical tests, regardless of the shape of the original data.
- In the simplest terms, the normal curve is used to display what one would expect if the result were simply caused by random chance alone (Fig. 12–1). For example, suppose that one is testing whether the intelligence quotient (IQ) for medical students is significantly different than the national norm of 100. In this case, the normal curve depicts the distribution of IQs if they were not different than 100. Accordingly, the analysis involves collecting a sample of IQ data from medical students and comparing the results to the normal curve to determine whether or not the sample of IQs is significantly different than 100. If the observed result falls far enough in the tails of the distribution, the result is unlikely to be caused by chance alone.
- Thus, the normal curve is constructed to determine whether a result is significant or whether it is caused by chance alone. If the observed result falls in the middle of the distribution, it is likely caused by chance alone. If instead the result falls in one of the tails of the distribution, the result is unlikely to be caused by chance alone and instead is deemed significant.

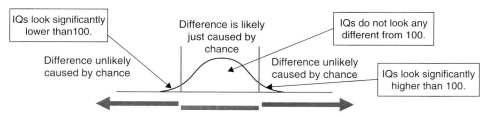

FIG. 12–1 Example depicting the normal distribution of IQs. If IQs fall within the tails, the results are considered significant.

○ Suppose we would like to test whether two diabetes drugs result in lower glycated hemoglobin values for patients with type 2 diabetes. In this case, we can simply examine the difference in HbA1c between Drug A and Drug B $(\bar{x}_A - \bar{x}_B)$. If the result falls in the middle of the curve, we conclude that the difference between the drugs is indistinguishable from zero. If the observed result falls in the right tail, we conclude that it is significantly different than zero (more specifically, that Drug A is associated with higher glycated levels than Drug B). If it falls in the left tail, we conclude that the Drug A is associated with significantly lower glycated levels than Drug B.

A fundamental issue is exactly where to place the threshold values (eg, p-values) beyond which an observed effect is deemed to be statistically significant and not caused by chance alone. Generally, statisticians have determined that a result is not *significant* unless the likelihood of it being caused by chance alone is less than 5% ($\alpha < 0.05$). As we move the p-values closer to the tail of the normal distribution curve, confidence increases that the result is statistically significant, and *not* caused by chance alone.

HYPOTHESIS TESTING

- *Hypothesis*: a statement we want to statistically test.
  ○ Two possible outcomes for each hypothesis statement:
  1. *Null hypothesis* (Ho): A claim that there is *no* difference between the population mean (μ) and the hypothesized value (μo). Examples include the following: There is no difference between medical student IQs and the national norm of 100; or there is no difference in diabetic complications for patients on intensive insulin therapy compared to traditional insulin therapy.
  2. *Alternative hypothesis* (Ha): A claim that disagrees with the null hypothesis. Examples include the following: Medical student IQs are significantly higher than the national norm of 100; or patients on intensive insulin therapy have significantly fewer diabetic complications than those on traditional insulin therapy.
- Investigators typically expect to reject the null hypothesis and, thus state that there is a significant difference between Groups.

STATISTICAL SIGNIFICANCE

- *Alpha* (α) is the area/proportion of the normal curve that lies outside the vertical (threshold) bars (in the tails of the curve) (see Fig. 12–1). If the result for our sample falls within the tail area, we conclude that it is unlikely to be caused by chance alone; and we declare the result *statistically significant.*
  ○ α-levels must be set far enough into the tails of the curve so that there is a very small chance that the results are caused by chance alone. Typically, statisticians consider a finding significant if the likelihood of a result caused by chance alone is less than 5% ($\alpha < 0.05$).
  ○ The farther into the tails the result falls (hence, the smaller α is), the smaller the chance that the result is caused by chance alone ($\alpha = .0001$ is further out than $\alpha = .001$, which is further out than $\alpha = .01$, and so on). In other words, when the alpha is set at .05, any result within the tail occurs 5% of the time based on chance alone. Conversely, when the $\alpha = .05$, we may erroneously conclude that there is a significant difference 5% of the time. This is referred to as the type I error rate.
- A *P* value is the exact probability of the observed result. This indicates the exact likelihood that the observed result is caused by chance alone. In contrast, α indicates how far in the tail the observed result must be to reach significance. The *p* value represents how far into the tail the observed result actually reached, eg, a *p* value of .03 indicates that the result passed the 5% cutoff but didn't quite reach the 1% cutoff. In the literature, a result could be said to be significant at $\alpha = .05$ or could be said to have a *p* value of .03. Both descriptions are statistically equivalent.
- **1-sided versus 2-sided tests** (1-tail versus 2-tail test). A 1-sided test is conducted when the investigator is interested in testing for significant differences in only one direction. A 2-sided test is conducted when the investigator is testing for differences in both directions. For example, if we are only interested in examining whether the IQs of physicians are significantly higher than 100, a 1-sided test is appropriate. If instead we want to examine whether the IQs of physicians are *different* than 100 (higher or lower), a 2-tail test is used.
- A **Type I error** (or false positive) occurs whenever the investigator concludes that a result is significantly different from chance when in fact it is not. The type I error rate is exactly equal to the α-level. Thus, at an α of 0.05, the investigator inaccurately concludes that something is significant (when in fact the result is simply caused by chance) 5% of the time. When the α is less than 0.01, the type I error rate drops to 1%.
- A **Type II error** (or false negative) is said to occur when the results fail to reject the null hypothesis ($p > 0.05$) even though a significant difference exists.
- **Power** is the probability of accurately rejecting a null hypothesis (eg, rejecting a null hypothesis that is false). Power is also thought of as the likelihood that *significant differences* are real and do not represent a Type I or II

error. Power analysis is conducted to determine what size the sample must be to ensure adequate statistical power (and, hence a low likelihood of a type I or II error).

- **Confidence intervals** (CI) for specific statistics (means, correlation) indicates the range of values around the results where we expect the *true* population data to be located.
- *95% CI* indicates the range in which we expect the true population statistic to fall 95% of the time.
- **Basic symbols used in inferential statistics**:
  ○ Ho = null hypothesis (no significant difference exists).
  ○ Ha = alternative hypothesis (a significant difference exists).
  ○ μ = population mean.
  ○ σ = population standard deviation.
  ○ *n* = sample size.
  ○ *t* or *z* = specific statistical significance tests.
  ○ α = level of significance (typically .05 or .01); smaller values increase confidence that the result is *not* caused by chance alone. At α = .05, 5 times out of 100 the result, which we would mistakenly call significant, would be caused by chance. This also reflects a type I error.
- There is a wide range of statistical tests that can be used in hypothesis testing. The choice of test depends on the specific question being addressed, the number of groups being compared, the number of covariates/variables being examined, and the distributional characteristics of the variables.

T TEST AND *Z* TEST

- These tests are used to test for significant differences in means for one and two groups.
- The independent variable must be continuous (interval or ratio), and the dependent variable must be categorical (nominal or ordinal).
- The distinction between a *z* test and a *t* test is straightforward. If the standard deviation for the entire population is known, use a *z* test. If the population standard deviation is *not* known, use a *t* test and estimate the standard deviation from the sample data.
- The *t* distribution is slightly different than the *z* distribution (*the normal curve*) and looks increasingly like a normal curve as the sample size increases. Once the sample size reaches 20, the *t* and *z* curves are nearly identical.
- In this context, the term *degrees of freedom* (df) is used to determine the exact shape of a *t* distribution or *f* distribution used for a specific statistical test. The df is a measure of the number of independent pieces of information on which a parameter estimate is based. The df for an estimate is the number of observations minus the number of additional parameters estimated in that calculation. As more parameters are estimated, the df available decrease.

Furthermore, df can also be thought of as the number of observations which may vary given the additional parameters estimated.

- Specific types of *t* tests and *z* tests:
  ○ **Single-mean *z* test** is used to examine whether a result for a single variable differs significantly from a prespecified value. The population standard deviation *must* be known to conduct a *z* test. Example research questions include the following:
    ▪ Are glycated hemoglobin levels at hospital A significantly different from 6.5?
    ▪ Is the average length of stay for bypass patients significantly different from 4 days?
  ○ In each case, we must know the population standard deviation. If this is unknown, use a *t* test.
  ○ **Single-mean *t* test** is used to test whether a result for a variable differs significantly from some prespecified value and the population standard deviation is *unknown*. The examples listed earlier for the single-mean *z* test all work here if the population standard deviation is unknown. If the sample size is large enough, the two tests provide the same information.
  ○ **Two-mean *t* test** is used to test whether the means of two groups differ from one another (and the population standard deviations are unknown). Examples include the following:
    ▪ Are glycated hemoglobin levels significantly different for patients on intensive insulin therapy than those on traditional insulin therapy?
    ▪ Is the average length of stay for bypass surgery significantly different for patients at an academic medical center compared to a community hospital?
  ○ **Dependent means *t* test (paired or matched *t* test)** is used to test whether the means of two groups differ when the members of the two groups are related through repeated measures or matching. For example, do T4 cell counts differ for patients on Drug A and Drug B, after matching patients based on age and gender?
  ○ **Independent means *t* test** is used to test whether the means of two groups which are independent of one another differ. For example: Do T4 cell counts differ for patients on Drug A and Drug B, with patients randomly assigned to Drug A or Drug B?

BASIC SYMBOLS AND FORMULAS

$$z = \frac{\bar{x} - \mu}{\sigma / \sqrt{n}}$$

$$t = \frac{\bar{x} - \mu}{s / \sqrt{n}}$$

- *t* = result of a *t* test
- *z* = result of a *z* test
- μ = population mean

- $\overline{X}$ = sample mean
- σ = population standard deviation
- s = sample standard deviation
- *n* = sample size

ANALYSIS OF VARIANCE

- The ANOVA is used to test for differences among the means of three or more groups and to simultaneously examine the affect of additional independent variables on the dependent variable.
- There are several advantages to ANOVA over multiple *t* tests.
  - The ANOVA limits the type I error rate. Remember that type I errors are *false positives* (indicating a result is significant when in fact the result is caused by random chance). At α = .05, a test has a 5% chance of a type I error. At α = .01, there is a 1% chance of a type I error. When multiple tests are conducted, the type I error rate is calculated by adding all the individual type I error rates together. If two tests are conducted at α = .05, there is a .05 + 05 or 10% chance of a type I error. If four tests are conducted at α = .05, there is a 20% chance of a type I error. To compare four groups, we would have to conduct six *t* tests, creating a type I error rate of 30% at α = .05. By employing *ANOVA* the type I error rate at 5%.
  - The ANOVA also allows the investigator to examine more than one independent variable in a single analysis and to examine interactions among independent variables. With a *t* test one can determine whether two drugs differ in their control of cholesterol levels. With ANOVA one can examine multiple drugs as well as the simultaneous affects of additional factors such as cholesterol, age, gender, and body mass index. One can also test for interactions, such as the joint affect of statin type and age on cholesterol levels.
  - When multiple variables are examined in a single analysis, it is possible to calculate for *main effects* as well as *interactions*. A main effect occurs whenever a significant difference is explained by a single independent variable. An interaction exists whenever two independent variables combine to produce a significant difference.
- ANOVA employs the *F distribution* to test for significance = F is a two-parameter distribution with two types of degrees of freedom, *df between groups* (number of groups − 1) *and df within groups* (*n* − number of groups + 1). For example a research paper might report the result of an analysis as follows: $F_{3,35} = 9.37, p < .001$. This indicates that the investigator calculated the F statistic, using four groups (4 − 1 = 3), 38 participants (38 − 4 + 1), and significant differences at α = .01.

- The F test is an overall test and determines whether or not there is at least one significant difference across all the compared groups. The F test does not determine specifically which of the groups are different from one another.
  - *Post-hoc tests* or *multiple comparison tests* are used to determine exactly which pair(s) of means is significantly different from one another. There are a number of different multiple comparison tests, including the Scheffé test, the Tukey honest significance difference test, the Student-Newman-Keuls test, the Duncan test, and the Fisher least significant difference test. The choice among these tests depends on the specific analyses and variables being examined.
- There are several types of ANOVAs:
  - *1-Way* ANOVA only has one independent variable (or *factor*), such as type of drug. For example, do T4 cell counts differ among Drug A, Drug B and placebo?
  - *2-Way* ANOVA has two independent variables.
  - *Factorial* ANOVA has two or more independent variables. For example, do T4 cell counts differ among Drug A, Drug B, and placebo, and do T4 cell counts differ by decade of patient age?
  - *Repeated measures* ANOVA includes repeated observations for a single individual. For example, do T4 cell counts differ across three drugs as measured weekly for 8 weeks?
  - *Analysis of covariance* (ANCOVA) is similar to ANOVA, except that it also allows the investigator to control for one or more continuous variables before examining the effect of the categorical factors. For example, ANCOVA tests whether T4 cell counts differ by drug (Drug A, Drug B, placebo), gender, and ethnicity after controlling for age.

STATISTICAL POWER

- *Power* can be defined as the probability that a test can correctly detect a statistical difference and not caused by random chance.
- Power analysis is a statistical approach used for the following:
  - Determining how large a sample size is needed to accurately conclude that there is a significant difference.
  - Calculating the exact probability of identifying a true significant difference between groups.
- To use power analysis, the investigator must know type of statistical test is being used, the effect of size, and an estimate of variability for the dependent variable(s).
- There are a number of factors that influence statistical power:
  - The specific type of statistical test being used. Some tests are inherently more powerful than others.
  - In general, power increases as sample size increases, eg, smaller samples have less power than larger samples.

- The larger the difference (effect size), the larger the power needed to detect a real difference.
- The likelihood of error in the analysis. Measurement error acts like *noise* that can bury the *signal* of true experimental effects.
- Performing power analysis is an important component in designing a research study; because without such calculations, the sample size chosen may be inappropriate (to high or to low). Clearly, if the chosen sample size is too large, the investigator is consuming more time and resources than necessary. Conversely, if the sample size is too small, the study will be insufficiently powered to detect a statistically significant difference.
- There are a series of formulas employed for power analysis, based on the specific type of statistical test conducted. If the study involves an array of statistical tests, it is ideal to conduct power analysis for all the tests to ensure an accurate picture of the needed sample size. Thus, by conducting power analysis for only one dependent variable, the power might be inadequately powered for other variables.

NONPARAMETRIC ANALYSIS

- Statistical tests can be divided into *parametric* and *nonparametric analyses.* Parametric methods estimate at least one population parameter using a specific distribution such as the normal curve, *t* distribution, F distribution, gamma, or Weibull. Nonparametric methods, in contrast, do not use any mathematical distribution in testing for differences across groups. All the tests described up to this point were parametric tests.
- Nonparametric methods, unlike parametric tests, do not make assumptions about the distribution of the data. These analyses are used in the following circumstances:
  - Dependent variable is nominal or ordinal.
  - Assumptions for parametric tests aren't met (normality, homogeneity of variance, linearity).
  - Sample size is very small.
- Nonparametric tests examine the ranks of individual data, rather than the actual numeric values. When subjected to a mathematical transformation, these ranks become normally distributed.

- Nonparametric analyses, in general, are not as robust as parametric methods, rendering it less likely for the results to reach statistical significance.
- There are nonparametric equivalents for almost every type of parametric test (Table 12–1).
- The *Chi-square test* (χ^2) tests for associations between two categorical variables such as the relationship between Drug (A or B) and mortality (alive or dead).
  - Data are typically displayed in a contingency table where one variable defines the columns and the second variable defines the rows. For the previous example, we would construct a 2 × 2 table (two rows and two columns), where the two rows represent drug, and the two columns represent mortality, creating four cells.
  - The number of actual observations and the number expected by chance alone are calculated for each of the four cells. The observed and expected values are then compared to determine whether or not the observed values are significantly different than that expected values. If they are significantly different, one can conclude that there is a significant relationship between the two variables.
  - Chi-square results can be compared to a chi-square distribution to determine of significance.
  - The chi-square distribution changes considerably depending on the number of outcomes for each variable (eg, two levels: mortality; three levels: urban/suburban/rural) being examined. As a result, there are multiple configurations of the chi-square distribution. The *df* are used to determine which specific chi-square configuration is employed. The df for χ^2 is defined as follows:

(number of rows − 1) × (number of columns − 1)

$$\chi^2 = \frac{\Sigma\,(Observed - Expected)^2}{Expected}$$

SELECTING THE RIGHT STATISTICAL TEST

- A central issue in conducting or interpreting statistics is determining the correct test or procedure to use. Table 12–2 outlines appropriate tests based on the

TABLE 12–1 Choice of Statistical Test Based on Measurement Scale and Type of Comparison

NUMBER OF GROUPS	INDEPENDENT OR DEPENDENT GROUPS	NOMINAL	ORDINAL	INTERVAL/RATIO
1	—	Chi-square goodness of fit	—	—
2	Independent	Chi-square test	Mann-Whitney *U* test	*t* test
3+	Independent	Chi-square test	Kruskal-Wallis test	ANOVA
2	Dependent	McNemar test	Wilcoxon signed-ranks test	Paired *t* test
3+	Dependent	Cochran *Q* test	Friedman test	Repeated measures ANOVA

ANOVA, analysis of covariance.

TABLE 12–2 Choice of Statistical Test Based on Measurement Scale and Study Group

SCALE OF MEASUREMENT	TWO TREATMENT GROUPS OF DIFFERENT INDIVIDUALS	THREE OR MORE TREATMENT GROUPS OF DIFFERENT INDIVIDUALS	TWO TREATMENTS FOR SAME OR MATCHED INDIVIDUALS	MULTIPLE TREATMENTS ON THE SAME INDIVIDUALS	ASSOCIATION BETWEEN TWO VARIABLES
Interval or Ratio (*Assumes Normality*)	Unpaired *t* test Independent means *t* test	Analysis of variance	Paired *t* test Dependent means *t* test	Repeated-measures analysis of variance	Pearson product-moment correlation Linear regression
Ordinal	Mann-Whitney rank sum	Kruskal-Wallis	Wilcoxon signed-rank	Friedman statistic	Spearman rank correlation
Nominal	Chi-square	Chi-square	McNemar	Cochrane *Q*	Relative risk or odds ratio

scale of measurement for the dependent variable and the type of comparisons that are planned. It is important to recognize that the table does not list every appropriate test, but instead focuses on those that are most commonly used for each situation.

13 REGRESSION AND SURVIVAL ANALYSIS

Thomas E. Burroughs

THE BASICS OF REGRESSION ANALYSIS

Regression analysis is used for two primary purposes: (1) to examine the relationships between a set of independent variables and a single dependent variable, and (2) to develop models that can be used to predict a dependent variable based on input of the independent variables. For example, regression analysis could be utilized to examine the strength of relationships between glycosylated hemoglobin (HbA_{1c}) levels and patient age, type of diabetes, and frequency of physician encounters. Second, regression models could be created to predict the HbA_{1c} level of a new patient based on his or her age, type of diabetes, and frequency of physician encounters.

Linear regression analysis is used for dependent variables that are continuous, and logistic regression is used for dependent variables that are dichotomous or binary. When researchers refer to "regression" they typically imply linear regression. Logistic regression is usually referred to in its entirety. These two regression methods share some similarities but should be considered as unique mathematical models with inherent advantages and disadvantages.

LINEAR REGRESSION

Simple regression examines a single independent variable (also called a predictor variable) to predict a single dependent variable. *Multiple regression* extends this to cases in which there is more than one independent variable. Generally speaking, as more independent variables are introduced, the regression model is more likely to predict the dependent variable. For both simple and multiple regression, the dependent variable must be continuous. The independent variable can be either continuous or categorical.

- In the simplest terms, regression analysis calculates the mathematical construct between the two variables being correlated. The general formula used is

$$\hat{y} = \beta_0 + \beta_1 X_1 + \beta_1 X_2 + \ldots + \beta_n X_n,$$

where $\hat{y}$ is the predicted value of y, X_i denotes the independent variables, and β_i denotes the individual beta weights (also called standardized regression coefficients) for each independent variable.

- The *beta weights* or *standardized regression coefficients*, (β_n), determine the relative importance of their corresponding independent variable. It is also possible to calculate and report unstandardized regression coefficients, but these are difficult to directly compare to the weights of other variables. Standardized weights are said to have a mean of 0.0 and a standard deviation of 1.0, making interpretation straightforward.

- To assess the statistical significance of individual beta weights, *t tests,* and their corresponding *P values,* are used.

- An *F test*, interpreted identically to that in an *analysis of variance (ANOVA),* assesses the overall fit of the entire regression equation. Larger *F values* indicate a higher level of fit between the regression equation and the original data.

- The *squared multiple correlation, R^2,* is used to assess the amount of variation in the dependent variable that is explained jointly by all of the independent variables.

- *Method of variable selection and entry:* For most regression analyses, there is a fair amount of variance in the dependent variables that is shared across more than one independent variable. In these cases, it is difficult to determine which independent variable is responsible for this shared variance. The variable that is deemed responsible will reach a higher level of significance because its predictive strength will increase. There are five methods of introducing variables into a regression model:

1. *Simultaneous entry* is an approach where all independent variables are entered into the equation simultaneously. Each is given credit for the unique variance it shares with the dependent variable. None of the independent variables are given credit for overlapping variance. This variance is used in the calculation of *R* and in the overall prediction of *y*.

2. *Stepwise entry* is a regression approach where the variables in the equation are entered based on which variable has the greatest association with the dependent variable at the affiliated step. This method is often criticized as there is no theoretical rationale for determining which variables get credit for shared variance. There are two basic types of stepwise entry: (1) forward and (2) backward.

3. *Forward selection* is a form of stepwise regression where the independent variables are entered into

the equation one at a time. In the first step, the independent variable with the largest bivariate correlation with the dependent variable (DV) is entered, and then the overall fit of the equation, *R*, and the bivariate correlations for the remaining IVs are recalculated. In the second step, the IV that has the largest bivariate correlation with the remaining variance is entered next. This process continues until there are no IVs that are significantly associated with the remaining variance.

4. *Backward deletion* is a form of stepwise regression where all of the variables are placed into the equation using simultaneous entry, and then variables are removed from the equation one at a time, until the removal does not lead to a significant decline in the predictive strength of the equation, as assessed by *R*.

5. *Hierarchical regression* occurs when independent variables are entered into the equation in blocks with the order determined by the researcher based on conceptual or theoretical reasoning. At each block, simultaneous entry is conducted for those variables in that block. The next block is then entered to determine the extent to which they can predict the remaining variance. This process continues until all blocks, defined by the research, have been entered.

- Continuing with the earlier example examining the relationships between HbA_{1c} for persons with diabetes and gender, age, type of diabetes (type 1, type 2), and frequency of physician encounters; HbA_{1c} is the dependent variable ($\hat{y}$); gender (X_1), age (X_2), type of diabetes (X_3), and frequency of physician encounters (X_4) are the independent variables. In this case, the regression equation would be

$$\hat{y} = \beta_0 + \beta_1 X_1 + \beta_2 X_2 + \beta_3 X_3 + \beta_4 X_4$$

- Assuming that a regression equation is calculated on the basis of 100 patients with diabetes, the following model emerges:

$$\hat{y} = 1.20 + 0.653(age) - 0.366(diabetes\_type) - 0.637(docotor\_frequency).$$

- By comparing the size of the beta weights (β), the age has the strongest relationship with HbA_{1c} (eg, as age increases, HbA_{1c} increases), the frequency of physician encounters has the next strongest relationship (eg, as frequency of visits increases, HbA_{1c} decreases [note the negative sign preceding the beta weight]), and the weakest relationship is with the type of diabetes (patients with type 2 diabetes have higher HbA_{1c} levels than patients with type 1).

- This example can also illustrate how a regression equation can be employed in a clinical setting (diabetes clinic) to predict the HbA_{1c} of new diabetic patients. Thus, simply enter each new patient's age, type of diabetes, and frequency of physician encounters into the model and solve the equation.

LOGISTIC REGRESSION

Logistic regression is a type of regression analysis that can be used with dichotomous dependent variables. The independent variables can be either categorical or continuous. Many of the most important variables in medicine, such as alive/dead, disease/no disease, and infection/no infection, are binary. Logistic regression, like linear regression, can be used to predict outcomes for an individual, and to quantify the relationship between a single dependent variable and a set of independent variables. For example, the "chance of dying" will be used to illustrate logistic regression.

- In logistic regression, the dependent variable is based on the probability or odds of the binary outcome, either of which are, conveniently, continuous rather than dichotomous. The odds of dying, for example, would be the chances of dying divided by the chances of not dying.

- Odds can range from 0 (no chance of dying) to 1 (a 50:50 chance of dying) up to infinity (it is certain that the patient will die).

- Logistic regression uses the log odds (also called *logit*), rather than the log alone, as the dependent variable. This transforms the odds into a variable that ranges from minus infinity to plus infinity.

- The logit is calculated as

$$Log \frac{p}{1-p},$$

where *p* is the probability that the variable is coded as 0 (not dying), and $p - 1$ is the probability that the variable is coded as 1 (dying).

- The structure of the logistic regression equation is similar to that described for multiple regression and can be interpreted similarly. Accordingly, the essential logistic equation is

$$Log \frac{p}{1-p} = b_0 + b_1 X_1 + b_2 X_2 \ldots b_n X_n,$$

where *b* denotes the individual beta weights, and *X* denotes the independent variables.

- In logistic regression, the maximum likelihood estimation is used to estimate the *individual beta weights (b_i)* that best fit the data. These are computed to be those that have the highest likelihood of producing the observed set of data in the study. This method is different than the least-squares approach used in linear regression.

- Each *b* can be converted into an odds ratio by exponentiating it (e^b), which reveals how much the odds increase multiplicatively with a one-unit change in the independent variable. A *t* test can be calculated to determine whether an individual beta weight is significant.
- There are four related measures that are typically used to assess the overall fit of the regression model.
  - *−2 Log likelihood* (*−2 LL*) tests the *likelihood* of obtaining the observed results given the parameter estimates (*beta weights*) calculated for the model. *−2 LL* is used, however, to test the overall fit of the model. Multiplying the likelihood by *−2 log* is performed to adjust for the very small likelihood number. Small values derived from *−2 LL* suggest a robust model. Significance can be tested with a chi-square (χ^2). When the χ^2 is significant ($P < 0.05$), it indicates that the model does *not* fit the data.
  - The *chi-square model* represents the difference between *−2 LL* when only the constant term is used in the model (eg, no predictor variables are included) minus *−2 LL* with all the predictor variables included in the model. A significant *chi-square model* ($P < 0.05$) indicates that adding the predictor variables to the model significantly improves its fit.
  - *Improvement* is characterized by the change in model fit between successive stages of model building, eg, this is the change in *−2 LL* from the previous stage.
  - *Goodness of fit statistics* compare the observed probabilities to those predicted by the model. The difference in these probabilities is the *residual,* which follows a chi-square distribution. A nonsignificant result suggests a model that fits well.

In summary, in a good model, *−2 LL* and *goodness of fit* will be nonsignificant ($P > 0.05$), and the *chi-square model* and *improvement* will be significant ($P < 0.05$).

SURVIVAL ANALYSIS

Survival analysis is a commonly used statistical method in medicine. It is a means of examining "time to an event" such as death, disease relapse, pregnancy, or need for additional treatment when the period of observation differs across participants.

- In addition to examining time-to-event, survival analysis can be used to test whether groups differ in terms of time-to-event and can be used to predict time-to-event on the basis of group membership and other covariates.
- Survival analysis is used in longitudinal research such as clinical trials, during which scientists seek to determine whether or not a proposed treatment was successful. In such studies, the period of observation can vary across subjects. Some subjects can enroll in the study later than others, and some subjects will drop out for various reasons.
- With other statistical methods, participants who drop out of the study or enroll late would typically be treated as missing values in the analysis. This would eliminate a lot of useful data from the analysis.
- In survival analysis, these cases, which contain only partial information, are called *censored* cases and are not treated as missing values.
- There are several terms that must be understood to appreciate survival analysis.
  - *Survival function* is the probability of an individual in the population surviving beyond time *t*.
  - *Survival curve* is a graphical distribution of the survival function (on *y*-axis) over time (*x*-axis) (Fig. 13–1).
  - *Median survival time* is the time at which half of the population is alive, and half is dead.
  - *Censored observation* is an observation for which the duration of study is limited in time. This occurs whenever subjects enter the study late or drop out of the study prior to completion.
  - *Hazard rate* is the probability (per unit of time) that a case that has survived to the beginning of a respective interval will fail in that interval.
  - *Number of cases at risk* is the number of cases that entered a time interval minus half of the cases that died or were censored.
  - *Proportion failing* is the number of cases that failed/died divided by the number at risk in that interval.
  - *Proportion surviving* is 1 minus the proportion failing
  - *Probability density* is the probability of failing/ dying in a specific interval per unit of time.

All of the terminology described above can be employed with all three methods of survival analysis.

There are three commonly used approaches to survival analysis: (1) life table method, (2) Kaplan-Meier product-limit method, and (3) Cox proportional-hazards modeling.

LIFE TABLE METHOD

The life table method is the most basic of the three types of survival analysis. It can be used to estimate the underlying survival function, but it cannot be used to compare the survival distributions of two or more groups or to integrate covariates into the prediction of survival times.

- The life table method calculates the survival function by dividing the actual survival data into a defined number of intervals and then calculates and/or plots the cumulative proportion of cases that survive through each interval.

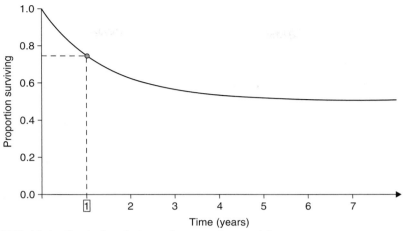

FIG. 13–1   Survival analysis graph: proportion surviving.

- Within each interval, the number and proportion of cases that entered the interval "alive" (proportion surviving), the proportion that failed/died in the interval (proportion failing), and the number of cases that were lost or censored in the interval are calculated.
- The survival function is calculated by multiplying the proportions surviving from all of the previous intervals.
- The theoretical survival function is estimated using a least-squares regression algorithm.
- Goodness of fit test (chi-square) compares the likelihood of the actual data under the estimated survival function to the likelihood of the actual data under the null model (allows the hazard to change in each interval). If the chi-square is statistically significant, then the estimated theoretical distribution fits the data significantly worse than the null model, and the estimated distribution as a model for the actual data is rejected.

KAPLAN-MEIER PRODUCT-LIMIT METHOD

The Kaplan-Meier product-limit method uses a different method of estimating the underlying survival distribution and allows for testing differences among groups. It does not integrate covariates into the prediction of survival times, however.

- Rather than dividing the survival times into a certain number of intervals, the Kaplan-Meier method divides the survival times into very narrow windows that contain only a single observation.
- The survival function produced with the Kaplan-Meier method is referred to as the *product limit estimator* because predicted survivals are estimated by multiplying all the survival proportions from previous "windows."
- Note that traditional statistical methods could be used to test these differences, but these methods would not

take advantage of the information that is provided by the censored observations. Instead they would be eliminated from the analysis and treated as missing values.
- There are several tests that can be used to test for group differences with the Kaplan-Meier method. These tests include the Gehan generalized Wilcoxon test, the Cox-Mantel test, the Cox *F* test , the log-rank test, and the Peto and generalized Wilcoxon test. Most of these tests involve a transformation into a *z*-score for statistical testing.
- The chi-square test, as described for the life table method, is used to evaluate overall model fit.

COX PROPORTIONAL-HAZARDS MODELING

Cox proportional-hazard modeling is the third primary type of survival analysis. It can calculate and plot a survival distribution(s) for one or more groups and will allow for statistical testing of survival across these groups. This approach also examines the relationship between covariates (risk factors) and survival.
- This method is the most commonly used of the regression-based approaches to survival analysis.
- Cox proportional-hazards methods are used to determine whether categorical or continuous covariates are associated with survival times. Traditional regression methods are not appropriate because: (1) survival times are not normally distributed (they typically follow a Weibull or exponential distribution), and (2) the traditional methods cannot use censored data.
- The Cox proportional-hazards model makes no assumptions about the shape or nature of the underlying survival distribution, but does require that the hazard distribution for the groups being compared are proportional over time.

- Like regression, Cox proportional-hazards modeling uses multiple methods for determining the order in which variables are entered into the regression model: forward selection, backward selection, stepwise selection, and best subset selection.
- The chi-square test, as described for the life table method, is used to evaluate overall model fit.
- Beta weights, just like in linear regression, are used to quantify the relationship between the predictor and dependent variables. In this case, the beta weight indicates the amount that the log of the hazard rate changes when the predictor variable increases by one unit. Positive values indicate that as the value of the covariate increases, the hazard increases, and the prognosis worsens. A negative coefficient, in contrast, suggests that decreases in the covariate correspond to improvements in survival.

BIBLIOGRAPHY

Motulsky H, Intuitive Biostatistics. Oxford University Press, September, 1995.Shott, S. Statistics for Health Professionals, WB Saunders, Philadelphia, 1990.
Stanton A. Glantz, Bryan K. Slinker, and Brian K. Slinker, *Primer of Applied Regression and Analysis of Variance*. McGraw-Hill Professional, 1990.

14 EPIDEMIOLOGY AND STUDY DESIGN

Thomas E. Burroughs

Epidemiology can be defined as "the comparative study of the distribution and determinants of disease in human populations." This discipline focuses on the rates with which diseases occur, the etiology and prevention of disease, and the allocation of resources in communities and healthcare facilities. From a methodological perspective, epidemiology is very closely related to both biostatistics and clinical research. Many of the same statistical techniques and research methods are used across both areas. The primary distinction between them is the type of questions being examined. Clinical research typically focuses on issues involving the evaluation of different treatments and the course of disease. Epidemiology, in contrast, focuses on disease patterns in the natural population.

BASIC DEFINITIONS

- *Count* is the number of events.
- *Odds* are the number of events divided by the number of nonevents.
- *Odds ratio* is the odds of an event divided by the odds of a nonevent.
- *Proportion* is the number of events divided by the population from which it came.
- *Rate* is the number of events divided by the number at risk during a specific period of time.

PREVALENCE AND INCIDENCE RATES: QUANTIFYING THE BURDEN OF DISEASE

Prevalence and incidence rates are both used to quantify the magnitude or frequency of disease or condition in a specific population during a specific period of time. There are several types of incidence and prevalence rates, which differ primarily in two ways: 1) who is included in the denominator or total number of people at risk, and 2) what time interval is used in calculating the rate.

- *Prevalence rates* are used to describe the proportion of individuals who have a specific disease, regardless of whether these are new or existing cases.
  - *Prevalence rate* is the (number with a disease)/(number at risk for disease)
  - *Period prevalence rate* refers to the prevalence rate during a specific time period.
  - *Point prevalence rate* refers to the prevalence rate at a specific point in time.
- *Incidence rates* describe the rate at which new cases (eg, of disease, infection) arise in the population. Incidence explicitly examines the proportion of *new* cases, where prevalence includes both new and existing cases.
  - *Incidence rate* is the (number of new cases of disease)/(total number at risk).
  - *Instantaneous incidence rate* (also referred to as the incidence density or hazard rate) is the incidence rate at a single point in time.
  - *Cumulative incidence* is the incidence rate for a longer time window (eg, 5 years, 10 years).
  - *Mortality rate* is the proportion of people dying (due to a specific cause or due to all causes) during a specific period of time
  - *Case fatality* rate refers to the proportion of people with a specific disease who die from that disease.

COMPARING RATES

Clinical research often examines whether two rates are significantly different from one another. For example, does the incidence of lung cancer differ for smokers compared to people who have never smoked? There are several methods of comparing rates.

- *Relative risk* (RR) (*risk ratio* or *rate ratio*) is a measure of how exposure to a risk factor changes the risk of a specific outcome. This is calculated as the incidence of disease in the exposed group divided by incidence of disease in the unexposed group.
  - A relative risk (RR) of 1 indicates that disease is equally likely in the exposed and unexposed groups; RR greater than 1 indicates that disease is more common in the exposed group; RR less than 1 indicates that disease is less common in the exposed group.
- *Attributable risk* is the rate of a disease in exposed individuals that can be attributed to the exposure. This is obtained by subtracting the incident rate of disease among unexposed persons from the incidence rate among exposed individuals.
- *Odds ratio* (OR) is the odds of disease in exposed individuals divided by the odds of a disease in unexposed individuals.
  - An OR of 1.0 indicates that disease is equally likely in both populations; an OR greater than 1 indicates that disease is more common in the exposed population and an OR less than 1 indicates that disease is less common in the exposed group.

BASIC STUDY DESIGNS

In epidemiology, there are a number of study designs that are used to answer research questions about disease frequency, risk factors for disease, and the impact of these diseases on society.

- These study designs are not limited to epidemiology. The same designs are used in a wide variety of disciplines where basic statistical and economic analyses are performed. The most commonly employed study designs can be grouped into three major categories: (1) descriptive studies, (2) analytic studies, and (3) experimental studies.
- *Descriptive studies* characterize the development and magnitude of a disease without an emphasis on hypothesis testing.
  - *Case reports* are a detailed clinical description of the characteristics of a new disease or condition in a single patient.
  - *Correlational* or *ecological* studies correlate disease rates with specific characteristics within a population. For example, a study might examine the association between lung cancer rates and cigarette consumption, age, gender, and family history of lung cancer.

- *Cross-sectional* or prevalence studies compare disease prevalence among different exposed groups in a population. An example would be comparing respiratory symptoms in a cross section of workers in a hazardous job compared to those in a job that was not hazardous.
- *Analytic studies* examine relationships and risk factors to determine the magnitude of disease *and* possible etiology of disease.
  - *Case-control studies* compare the frequency of exposure in a group with the disease (cases) to the frequency of exposure in a group without the disease (noncases or controls). Cases, whenever possible should be incident cases (new), not prevalent cases (existing). Controls should either be randomly selected or, better, matched with cases with respect to key confounding factors. The number of controls should not exceed four per case.
  - *Cohort studies* are longitudinal studies of a defined population, initially without disease, to identify factors associated with the development of disease.
- Experimental studies
  - *Randomized control trials (RCT)* are studies where participants are randomized to an intervention and then monitored for outcomes. These are considered the *gold standard* for clinical research.
  - *Factorial Designs* are studies designed to test the effect of a set of categorical variables on a categorical outcome (disease/no disease) when all the factors are at fixed levels that are controlled by the experimenter.
- The phases of trials generally required for FDA approval include
  - *Phase 1*: toxicity study to examine biological activity of a new drug (and safety).
  - *Phase 2*: small scale studies to quantify dose: response and frequency of adverse events.
  - *Phase 3*: examines the effectiveness of a drug (at a specific dose range) after the drug is shown to be safe.
  - *Phase 4*: large scale studies conducted to monitor the safety and efficacy of the drug after it has gone to market.

BIBLIOGRAPHY

Hebel JR and RJ McCarter. *A Study Guide to Epidemiology and Biostatistics* (6th Edition), Jones and Bartlett, 2006, Boston MA.

GERIATRIC MEDICINE

15 GERIATRIC ASSESSMENT

John E. Morley

- Numerous studies have demonstrated that a comprehensive geriatric assessment (CGA) in older persons can improve outcomes (Table 15–1).
- These improved outcomes include reduced hospitalizations (approximately 12%), decreased mortality (14–22%), improved physical function (20–70%), enhanced cognition (47%), and increased likelihood of the older person staying at home (26–45%).
- The CGA can be done at home, in an outpatient setting, in a hospital, or in a nursing home.
- CGA focuses on physical as well as psychologic, social, and functional aspects related to the older persons aging and disease processes. It also identifies resources in the person's family and community that can help the older person.
- Generally, the CGA is carried out by a multidisciplinary team that includes at least a physician, nurse, and social worker. It may also include other individuals such as a pharmacist, physical therapist, dietitian, and occupational therapist.
- Recently, there has been an emergence of virtual teams where the team discussion is carried out on an intranet.
- It is important to recognize that a CGA has no benefits unless the recommendations are carried out.

GERIATRIC ASSESSMENT DETERMINES HOSPITAL OUTCOMES

- In persons older than 70 years of age, a body mass index of 21 or less and a loss of one of the basic activities of daily living (transfer, toileting, washing, dressing, and eating) strongly determines whether a person will die or be institutionalized both during a concurrent hospital admission or within the next 6 months.

WHO SHOULD GET A GERIATRIC ASSESSMENT

- Geriatric assessments complement a thorough medical assessment.
- The elderly who benefit most are those who are vulnerable but not so profoundly impaired that nothing can be done for them.
- A CAG is recommended for the following persons:
  - Whose health has deteriorated from good to fair or poor in the last 6 months
  - Who cannot lift 10 pounds or walk a quarter of a mile without stopping
  - Who need help with managing money or shopping
  - With new onset of memory problems
  - Who have lost 5% of their body weight anytime in the past year
  - Who are having new onset of falls
  - Who are sad
  - With urinary incontinence
  - On seven or more medications
  - With uncontrolled pain

HEALTH MAINTENANCE IN THE OLDER PERSON

- The busy clinician often has insufficient time to fully assess the health maintenance needs of the older adult and, therefore we developed the Saint Louis University Health Maintenance Questionnaire (SLUMS) that allow the older person to track their own health maintenance needs (Fig. 15–1, Fig. 15–2).
- Additional common geriatric assessment tools are as follows:
  - Androgen Deficiency in Aging Males (ADAM) (Fig. 15–3)
  - Activities of daily living (ADLs)

TABLE 15-1   Components of the Geriatric Assessment

DIMENSION	SCREENING TEST	ASSESSMENT TESTS
Advanced directives	Do you have an advanced directive or living will?	Detailed discussion. Document the patients wishes in chart. Discuss ventilation separately from cardiac resuscitation. Discuss feeding tube placement. Discuss long-term plans if the person becomes cognitively impaired. Assess the persons ability to make appropriate decisions.
Affective	Are you sad?	Geriatric Depression Scale
Alcohol abuse	Do you drink alcohol?	CAGE Michigan Alcohol Screening Test
Blood pressure	In older persons all blood pressures must be measured sitting and standing.	Check for postural hypotension at 1 and 3 minutes after standing. If the person falls, is dizzy, syncopal or has a stroke or myocardial infarction within 2 hours of a meal, check for postprandial hypotension. Both orthostatic and postprandial hypotension are more common in the morning. Because of atherosclerotic occlusion of vessels older persons often have a higher blood pressure in one arm than the other. Always treat the higher blood pressure. Arteriosclerosis can lead to pseudohypotension. This can be screened for by the Osler maneuver; but because it has poor sensitivity and specificity, intra-arterial blood pressure measurement should be considered. *White coat* hypertension is common, therefore always obtain home blood pressures. A wide pulse pressure portends a poor prognosis in older persons.
Caregiver burden	Is the caregiver having problems coping?	Geriatric Depression Scale. Caregiver Burden Inventory looks at time, developmental needs, social burden, and emotional burden.
Dehydration	How much fluid do you drink each day?	Check serum osmolality Remember elevated BUN-to-creatinine ratio occurs with renal failure, liver disease, heart failure, and gastrointestinal bleeding.
Delirium	Is the person confused? Does the level of confusion fluctuate?	Confusion Assessment methodology (acute onset; fluctuates; lack of attention; disorganized thinking including illusions, delusions, and hallucinations; hyperalert or lethargic)
Dental	Do you have false teeth? Do you have sores in your mouth or gum disease? Do you often have bad breath?	DENTAL screening tool
Dizziness	Do you get dizzy or does your head spin around?	Check for postural hypotension Dix-hallpike Maneuver for BPPV Hemoglobin Geriatric Depression Scale
Driving assessment	Do you drive? How do you meet your transportation needs?	If poor vision, cognition or motor function refer to a driving rehabilitation specialist to test the patient in a driving simulator or on-road. This may include monitoring driving when alone using a GPS device. If the patient refuses the physician must report the patient to the Department of Motor Vehicles as unsafe to drive.
Economic	Do you have enough money to pay your bills and purchase medicines and food?	Health Insurance Medicare Part D. Can a cheaper drug replace a more expensive one?
Fatigue	Are you easily exhausted (tired)?	Bioavailable testosterone (in males) C-Reactive Protein, hemoglobin, TSH, and vitamin B_{12} Epworth Sleep Inventory for Sleep Apnea Fried Frailty Test (see Chap. 18)
Function	Do you need help at home?	Barthel Index. Katz ADL. Lawton IADL. More sophisticated testing involves giving a person a medicine bottle and asking them how they would take their medicines, opening and shutting a variety of small doors, putting beans in a tin can, putting on a jacket, or buttoning a shirt. Social activities inventory.

TABLE 15–1   Components of the Geriatric Assessment (Continued)

DIMENSION	SCREENING TEST	ASSESSMENT TESTS
Hearing	Do you have trouble hearing, especially in a noisy environment?	Hearing Handicap Inventory for the Elderly Audioscope Remove cerumen Consider hearing frequency testing
Incontinence	Do you wet yourself?	Urine for cells and culture. Does it occur when coughing, sneezing (stress). Do you get the urge to go and have to go immediately (urge)? Urodynamics.
Insomnia	Do you have trouble sleeping? Are you tired during the day? Does your partner say that you stop breathing when sleeping?	Full sleep history including daytime napping, pain at night, nocturia, time that the patient retires and the sleep environment. Consider overnight sleep test for sleep apnea.
Masked renal failure	Loss of muscle mass leads to normal serum creatinine levels in the face of severe renal failure	Use Cockcroft-Gault formula or measure serum Cystatin-C
Memory	Do you have problems remembering anything or do any of your family or friends think you are having problems?	SLUMS If positive, obtain a TSH, vitamin B$_{12}$, and homocysteine level Consider MRI in some cases
Mobility/balance	Do you have trouble walking or lose your balance? Have you had a fall? Do you have a fear of falling?	Get up and walk from a chair (consider having the patient hold a glass of water). Measure gait speed over 10 m. Stand on one foot with eyes open and shut. Observe the patient turning or dance with the patient. This should also be done while distracting the patient. Measure stride length and variability.
Nutrition	Have you lost weight? SNAQ	Body mass index Mini-Nutritional Assessment Use Meals on Wheels mnemonic to identify treatable causes
Osteoporosis	What was your height when 25 years old? Compare it to measured height currently.	Bone mineral density: All women should have a DEXA at 50 years and men by 65 years of age. If results are borderline it should be repeated in 2 years during the same season. 25-OH vitamin D levels should be >30 ng/dL. All persons with a hip fracture should have calcium, vitamin D and bisphosphonates, unless contraindicated (eg, renal failure).
Pain	Do you hurt? Does your medicine relieve your pain?	Pain scale (faces better than Likert Scale) Full pain history If muscle pain check ESR for polymyalgia rheumatica If temporal headache check neck muscles for cramping
Polypharmacy	Are you on 7 or more medications? Is the person on any inappropriate medicines using the Beers Criteria?	Add history of herbal and over the counter medications. Ask why they are taking all medications, are they compliant, who prescribed them, and are there any side effects? Check for orthostasis.
Prostate	Do you have difficulty initiating your urine stream or dribble afterwards?	International Prostate Symptom Score Rectal examination Prostate-specific antigen
Sexuality	Are you having sexual relations? Do you want to have sex? How is your sexual desire? Then only: Are you impotent?	For women: Ask about dyspareunia (pain on intercourse) Poor vaginal lubrication, itching, or burning. Are intimacy needs being met? For men: ADAM questionnaire for low testosterone; if positive, obtain a bioavailable testosterone level. Discuss erectile dysfunction including soft erections. For both: Does the patient or partner health interfere with sex Are they using appropriate protection from sexually transmitted diseases?
Skin assessment	Do you have any new sores, rashes, or growths on your body? Are you itching? Are any of your moles growing?	Full body examination Braden Scale to determine risk of pressure ulcers

(Continued)

TABLE 15–1 Components of the Geriatric Assessment (Continued)

DIMENSION	SCREENING TEST	ASSESSMENT TESTS
Social support	Who lives with you? Who helps you?	Older American Resources and Services questionnaire (OARS) OARS Social Resources Scale explores fully the available helpers and strength of relationships
Spells	Do you have spells? Have you fainted (lost consciousness)? Have you fallen recently?	Orthostasis (if present, obtain BUN, glucose, creatinine, sodium, and hemoglobin) Carotid sinus massage Echocardiography Holtor Event Monitor ECG Consider partial complex seizures (often missed in the elderly) and if suspected, obtain an EEG
Vaccinations	Have you been vaccinated for flu, pneumonia, and tetanus?	Influenza: yearly Pneumonia: every 5 years Tetanus: every 10 years Herpes zoster: once
Vision	Do you have trouble seeing?	Snellen eye chart Useful field of vision Dark adaptation Fundus examination

ADAM, Androgen Deficiency in Aging Males; ADL, activities of daily living; BPPV, benign paroxysmal positional vertigo; BUN, blood urea nitrogen; CAGE, cut down (on drinking), annoyance, guilt (about drinking), (need for) eyeopener (Ewing & Rooss four-question alcohol screening); ECG, electrocardiogram; EEG, electroencephalogram; ESR, erythrocyte sedimentation rate; GPS, Global Positioning System; OARS, Older American Resources and Services Questionnaire; MRI, magnetic resonance imaging; SLUMS, Saint Louis University Health Maintenance; SNAQ, Simplified Nutrition Assessment Questionnaire; TSH, thyroid-stimulating hormone

○ Cut down (on drinking), annoyance, guilt (about drinking), (need for) eyeopener (Ewing & Rooss four-question alcohol screening, CAGE)
○ Cockcroft-Gault Formula
○ DENTAL (see section in the following text for a full description)
○ Epworth Sleepiness Questionnaire
○ Geriatric Depression Scale
○ Dix-Hallpike maneuver
○ Instrumental activities of daily living (IADLs)
○ Mini-Simplified Nutrition Assessment Questionnaire (SNAQ)
○ Mini-Nutritional Assessment (MNA) scale
○ Osler maneuver
○ SLUMS and the Saint Louis University Dental Status Exam
○ Social Activities Inventory

ACTIVITIES OF DAILY LIVING AND INSTRUMENTAL ACTIVITIES OF DAILY LIVING

Basic ADLs	**Instrumental ADLs**
Bathing	Using the telephone
Dressing	Shopping
Toileting	Food preparation
Transfers	Housekeeping
Continence	Laundry
Feeding	Transportation
Managing	Taking medicine
	Money
ADLs Score:___/16	IADLs Score: ___/8

CAGE QUESTIONS

1. Have you ever felt you should **C**ut down on your drinking?
2. Have people **A**nnoyed you by criticizing your drinking?
3. Have you ever felt **G**uilty about your drinking?
4. Do you take a drink first thing in the morning (**E**ye opener)

Two affirmative answers may be suggestive of alcoholism.

COCKCROFT-GAULT ASSESSMENT OF CREATININE CLEARANCE

$$C_{cr} = \frac{(140 - \text{age}) \times (\text{body weight})}{72 \times \text{serum creatinine}}$$

C_{cr} = creatinine clearance. In women multiply by 0.85.

DENTAL

- Screening assessment for dental conditions that may interfere with proper nutritional intake and possibly dispose a person to involuntary weight loss.
  ○ **D**ry mouth (2 points)
  ○ **E**ating difficulty (1 point)
  ○ **N**o recent dental care (1 point) (within 2 years)
  ○ **T**ooth or mouth pain (2 points)
  ○ **A**lterations or change in food selection (1 point)
  ○ **L**esions, sores or lumps in mouth (2 points)
- A score of *greater than* 3 points could indicate dental problems. These patients should be evaluated by a dentist.

Saint Louis University
Mental Status (SLUMS) Examination

Name _____   Age _____

Is patient alert? _____   Level of education _____

__/1	❶ 1. What day of the week is it?
__/1	❶ 2. What is the year?
__/1	❶ 3. What state are we in?

4. Please remember these five objects. I will ask you what they are later.

    Apple   Pen   Tie   House   Car

5. You have $100 and you go to the store and buy a dozen apples for $3 and a tricycle for $20.

  ❶   How much did you spend?

__/3 ❷   How much do you have left?

6. Please name as many animals as you can in one minute.

__/3   ❶ 0-4 animals ❶5-9 animals ❷10-14 animals ❸15+ animals

__/5 7. What were the five objects I asked you to remember? 1 point for each one correct.

8. I am going to give you a series of numbers and I would like you to give them to me backwards. For example, if I say 42, you would say 24.

__/2   ❶ 87   ❶ 649   ❶ 8537

9. This is a clock face. Please put in the hour markers and the time at ten minutes to eleven o'clock.

  ❷ Hour markers okay

__/4 ❷ Time correct

__/2 ❶ 10. Please place an X in the triangle.

  ❶   Which of the above figures is largest?

11. I am going to tell you a story. Please listen carefully because afterwards, I'm going to ask you some questions about it.

Jill was a very successful stockbroker. She made a lot of money on the stock market. She then met Jack, a devastatingly handsome man. She married him and had three children. They lived in Chicago. She then stopped work and stayed at home to bring up her children. When they were teenagers, she went back to work. She and Jack lived happily ever after.

❷ What was the female's name?	❷ What work did she do?
❷ When did she go back to work?	❷ What state did she live in?

__/8

_____   **TOTAL SCORE**

Department of Veterans Affairs

SAINT LOUIS UNIVERSITY

SCORING		
HIGH SCHOOL EDUCATION		**LESS THAN HIGH SCHOOL EDUCATION**
27-30	Normal	20-30
20-26	MCI	15-19
1-19	Dementia	1-14

FIG. 15–1   Saint Louis University Mental Status (SLUMS) Examination. MCI,

SOURCE: WA Banks and JE Morley. Memories are made of this: recent advances in understanding, cognitive impairment, and dementia. *J Gerontol Med Sci.* 2003; 58A:314–21.

EPWORTH SLEEPINESS QUESTIONNAIRE (SCREENING FOR SLEEP DISORDERS)

• How likely are you to doze off or to fall asleep in the following situations, in contrast to just feeling tired? This refers to your usual way of life in recent times.

0 = Would never doze

1 = Slight chance of dozing

2 = Moderate chance of dozing

3 = High chance of dozing

Situations:

Sitting and reading

Watching TV

Sitting inactive in a public place

As a passenger in a car for an hour

Saint Louis University Division of Geriatrics
Passport to Aging Successfully*

Please complete this questionnaire before seeing your physician and take it with you when you go.

SAINT LOUIS
UNIVERSITY

NAME _____ **AGE** _____

BLOOD PRESSURE laying down: _____ standing: _____

WEIGHT now: _____ 6 months ago: _____ change: _____

HEIGHT at age 20: _____ now: _____

CHOLESTEROL LDL: _____ HDL: _____

VACCINATIONS ☐Influenza (yearly) ☐Pneumococcal ☐Tetanus (every 10 years)

TSH Date: _____ **FASTING GLUCOSE** Date: _____

Do you SMOKE? _____

How much ALCOHOL do you drink? _____ per day

Do you use your SEATBELT? _____

Do you chew TOBACCO? _____

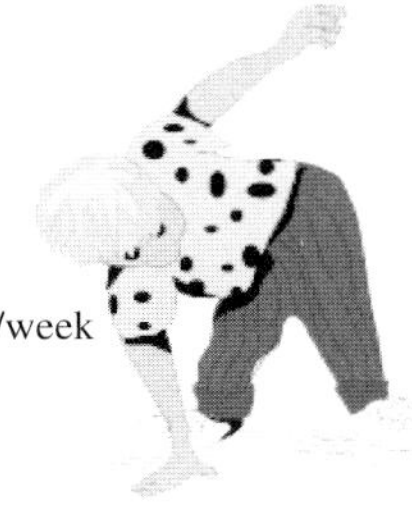

EXERCISE: How often do you...

do endurance exercises (walk briskly 20 to 30 minutes/day or climb 10 flights of stairs)_____ /week

do resistance exercises?____ /week   do balance exercises? _____ /week

do posture exercises? _____ /week   do flexibility exercises? ____ /week

Can you SEE ADEQUATELY in poor light? _____

Can you HEAR in a noisy environment? _____

Are you INCONTINENT? _____

Have you a LIVING WILL or durable POWER OF ATTORNEY FOR HEALTH? _____

Do you take ASPIRIN daily (only if you have had a heart attack or have diabetes)? _____

Do you have any concerns about your PERSONAL SAFETY? _____

When did you last have your STOOL TESTED for blood? _____

When were you last screened for OSTEOPOROSIS? _____

Are you having trouble REMEMBERING THINGS? _____

Do you have enough FOOD? _____

Are you SAD? _____

Do you have PAIN? _____

If so, which face best describes your pain?

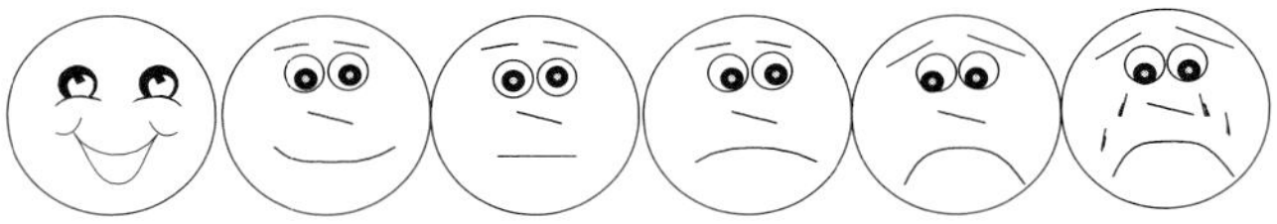

0   1   2   3   4   5

MALES
Do you have trouble passing urine? _____
Have you discussed PSA testing with your doctor? _____
What is your ADAM score? _____

FEMALES
When was your last pap smear? _____
When was your last mammogram? _____
Do you check your breasts monthly? _____
Are you satisfied with your sex life? _____

Now, please answer the four questionnaires on the next page.

*This questionnaire is based on the health promotion and prevention guidelines developed by Gerimed® and Saint Louis University Division of Geriatric Medicine.

FIG. 15–2 Passport to Aging Successfully. ADAM, Androgen Deficiency in Aging Male; HDL, high-density lipoprotein; LDL, low-density lipoprotein; PSA, Prostate-specific antigen.

Lying down to rest in the afternoon
Sitting and talking to someone
Sitting quietly after lunch without alcohol
In a car while stopped for a few minutes
Scoring: Out of 24; the higher the number, the more likely the patient has a sleep disorder.

GERIATRIC DEPRESSION SCALE (SHORT FORM)

1. Are you basically satisfied with your life?
2. Have you dropped many of your activities and interests?
3. Do you feel that your life is empty?

SAINT LOUIS UNIVERSITY
ADAM QUESTIONNAIRE
ANDROGEN DEFICIENCY IN AGING MALES

1. Do you have a decrease in libido (sex drive)? _____

2. Do you have a lack of energy? _____

3. Do you have a decrease in strength and/or endurance? _____

4. Have you lost height? _____

5. Have you noticed a decreased "enjoyment of life"? _____

6. Are you sad and/or grumpy? _____

7. Are your erections less strong? _____

8. Have you noted a recent deterioration in your ability to play sports? _____

9. Are you falling asleep after dinner? _____

10. Has there been a recent deterioration in your work performance? _____

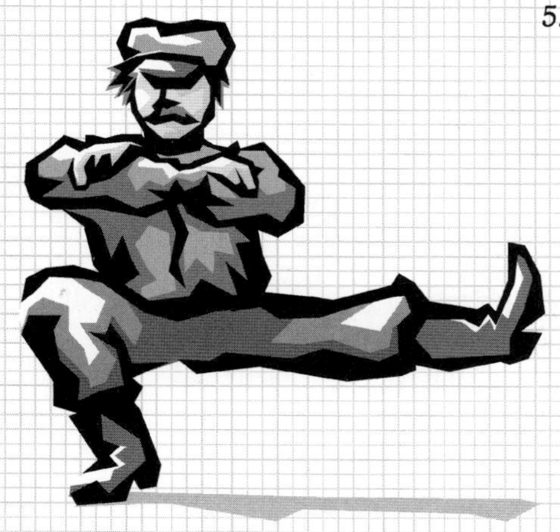

This questionnaire was developed by John E. Morley, M.B., B.Ch. It is to be used solely as a screening tool to assist your physician in diagnosing androgen deficiency.

FIG. 15–3 ADAM Questionnaire.

4. Do you often get bored?
5. Are you in good spirits most of the time?
6. Are you afraid that something bad is going to happen to you?
7. Do you feel happy most of the time?
8. Do you often feel helpless?
9. Do you prefer to stay at home rather than going out and doing new things?
10. Do you feel you have more problems with memory than most?
11. Do you think it is wonderful to be alive now?
12. Do you feel pretty worthless the way you are now?
13. Do you feel full of energy?
14. Do you feel your situation is hopeless?
15. Do you think that most persons are better off than you?

- Scoring: Score one point for each *depressed* answer (no for #1, 5, 7, 11, 13; yes for #2, 3, 4, 6, 8, 9, 10, 12, 14, 15). A score greater than 5 suggests probable depression.

DIX-HALLPIKE MANEUVER

- With the patient sitting, turn his or her head to 45 degrees on one side. Hold the head at this angle while rapidly lowering the patient so that the head is 30 degrees below the level of the examining table. Observe for nystagmus that develops within a few seconds after lowering them, lasts less than 30 seconds, and decreases with repeated testing. Also ask if their symptoms are reproducible.

SIMPLIFIED NUTRITION ASSESSMENT QUESTIONNAIRE

1. My appetite is
A. Very poor
B. Poor
C. Average
D. Good

E.   Very good
2.   When I eat
A.   I feel full after eating only a few mouthfuls.
B.   I feel full after eating about a third of a meal.
C.   I feel full after eating over half a meal.
D.   I feel full after eating most of the meal.
E.   I hardly ever feel full.
3.   Food tastes
A.   Very bad
B.   Bad
C.   Average
D.   Good
E.   Very good
4.   Normally I eat
A.   Less than one meal a day
B.   One meal a day
C.   Two meals a day
D.   Three meals a day
E.   More than three meals a day

- Instructions: Complete the questionnaire by circling the correct answers and then tally the results based upon the following numerical scale: A = 1, B = 2, C = 3, D = 4, E = 5
- Scoring: If the mini-SNAQ is less than 14, there is a significant risk of weight loss.

THE MINI-NUTRITIONAL ASSESSMENT SCALE

See Fig. 15–4 for the MNA.

OSLER MANEUVER FOR PSEUDOHYPERTENSION

- Inflate the blood pressure cuff until there is no longer a pulse. Run your finger along the artery. At this stage, it should have collapsed. If you can still feel the artery, this is suggestive of arteriosclerosis sufficient to produce pseudohypertension.

SAINT LOUIS UNIVERSITY SOCIAL ACTIVITIES ASSESSMENT

1.   How often do you go out socially?
A.   Daily
B.   Twice a week or more
C.   Weekly
D.   Monthly
E.   Rarely
2.   How often do you garden?
A.   At least an hour daily
B.   Less than 1 hour daily
C.   Twice or week or more

D.   Weekly
E.   Rarely
3.   How often do you go to church/synagogue/mosque?
A.   More than once a week
B.   Weekly
C.   At least once a month
D.   Only on religious holidays
E.   Never
4.   How often do you talk to friends or family on the telephone?
A.   More than once a day
B.   Daily
C.   Two to four times a week
D.   Weekly
E.   Rarely
5.   How often do you go to a restaurant to eat?
A.   Daily
B.   Twice a week or more
C.   Weekly
D.   Monthly
E.   Rarely
6.   How often do you go for a walk?
A.   Daily
B.   Twice a week or more
C.   Weekly
D.   Monthly
E.   Rarely
7.   How often do you go dancing?
A.   Daily
B.   Twice a week or more
C.   Weekly
D.   Monthly
E.   Rarely
8.   How often do you go to a concert/theater/movie?
A.   Daily
B.   Twice a week or more
C.   Weekly
D.   Monthly
E.   Rarely
9.   How often do you play with your grandchildren?
A.   Daily
B.   Twice a week or more
C.   Weekly
D.   Monthly
E.   Rarely
10. How satisfied are you with the time spent and quality of your social activities?
A.   Extremely satisfied
B.   Very satisfied
C.   Satisfied
D.   Somewhat satisfied
E.   Not at all satisfied

Mini Nutritional Assessment
MNA®

Last name:		First name:	Sex:	Date:
Age:	Weight, kg:	Height, cm:	I.D. Number:	

Complete the screen by filling in the boxes with the appropriate numbers.
Add the numbers for the screen. If score is 11 or less, continue with the assessment to gain a Malnutrition Indicator Score.

Screening

A Has food intake declined over the past 3 months due to loss of appetite, digestive problems, chewing or swallowing difficulties?
  0 = severe loss of appetite
  1 = moderate loss of appetite
  2 = no loss of appetite ☐

B Weight loss during the last 3 months
  0 = weight loss greater than 3 kg (6.6 lbs)
  1 = does not know
  2 = weight loss between 1 and 3 kg (2.2 and 6.6 lbs)
  3 = no weight loss ☐

C Mobility
  0 = bed or chair bound
  1 = able to get out of bed/chair but does not go out
  2 = goes out ☐

D Has suffered psychological stress or acute disease in the past 3 months
  0 = yes   2 = no ☐

E Neuropsychological problems
  0 = severe dementia or depression
  1 = mild dementia
  2 = no psychological problems ☐

F Body Mass Index (BMI) (weight in kg) / (height in m²)
  0 = BMI less than 19
  1 = BMI 19 to less than 21
  2 = BMI 21 to less than 23
  3 = BMI 23 or greater ☐

Screening score (subtotal max. 14 points) ☐ ☐
12 points or greater Normal – not at risk – no need to complete assessment
11 points or below   Possible malnutrition – continue assessment

Assessment

G Lives independently (not in a nursing home or hospital)
  0 = no   1 = yes ☐

H Takes more than 3 prescription drugs per day
  0 = yes   1 = no ☐

I Pressure sores or skin ulcers
  0 = yes   1 = no ☐

Ref. Vellas B, Villars H, Abellan G, et al. Overview of the MNA® - Its History and Challenges. J Nut Health Aging 2006;10:456-465.
Rubenstein LZ, Harker JO, Salva A, Guigoz Y, Vellas B. Screening for Undernutrition in Geriatric Practice: Developing the Short-Form Mini Nutritional Assessment (MNA-SF). J. Geront 2001;56A: M366-377.
Guigoz Y. The Mini-Nutritional Assessment (MNA®) Review of the Literature - What does it tell us? J Nutr Health Aging 2006; 10:466-487.

J How many full meals does the patient eat daily?
  0 = 1 meal
  1 = 2 meals
  2 = 3 meals ☐

K Selected consumption markers for protein intake
  • At least one serving of dairy products (milk, cheese, yogurt) per day   yes ☐   no ☐
  • Two or more servings of legumes or eggs per week   yes ☐   no ☐
  • Meat, fish or poultry every day   yes ☐   no ☐
  0.0 = if 0 or 1 yes
  0.5 = if 2 yes
  1.0 = if 3 yes ☐ . ☐

L Consumes two or more servings of fruits or vegetables per day?
  0 = no   1 = yes ☐

M How much fluid (water, juice, coffee, tea, milk…) is consumed per day?
  0.0 = less than 3 cups
  0.5 = 3 to 5 cups
  1.0 = more than 5 cups ☐ . ☐

N Mode of feeding
  0 = unable to eat without assistance
  1 = self-fed with some difficulty
  2 = self-fed without any problem ☐

O Self view of nutritional status
  0 = views self as being malnourished
  1 = is uncertain of nutritional state
  2 = views self as having no nutritional problem ☐

P In comparison with other people of the same age, how does the patient consider his/her health status?
  0.0 = not as good
  0.5 = does not know
  1.0 = as good
  2.0 = better ☐ . ☐

Q Mid-arm circumference (MAC) in cm
  0.0 = MAC less than 21
  0.5 = MAC 21 to 22
  1.0 = MAC 22 or greater ☐ . ☐

R Calf circumference (CC) in cm
  0 = CC less than 31   1 = CC 31 or greater ☐

Assessment (max. 16 points) ☐ ☐ . ☐

Screening score ☐ ☐

Total Assessment (max. 30 points) ☐ ☐ . ☐

Malnutrition Indicator Score
17 to 23.5 points   at risk of malnutrition ☐
Less than 17 points   malnourished ☐

FIG. 15–4 The Mini-Nutritional Assessment (MNA) Scale.

BIBLIOGRAPHY

Cohen, HJ, Feussner JR, Weinberger M, et al. A controlled trial of inpatient and outpatient geriatric evaluation and management. *N Engl J Med.* 2002;346:905.

Flaherty JH, Morley JE, Murphy DJZ, Wasserman MR. The development of outpatient glidepaths. *J Am Geriatr Soc.* 2002; 50:1886.

Fleck DM, Cooper JW, Wade WE. Updating the Beers criteria for potentially inappropriate medication use in older adults. *Arch Intern Med.* 2003;163:2716.

Stuck AE, Siu AL, Wieland GD, Adams J, Rubenstein LZ. Comprehensive geriatric assessment: a meta-analysis of controlled trials. *Lancet.* 1993; 342:1032.

16 GERIATRIC SYNDROMES: THE "I'S" OF GERIATRICS

Julie Gammack

INTRODUCTION

What makes care of the elderly different from that of young adults is a specific focus on geriatric syndromes, or the "I's" of geriatrics (Table 16–1). Also termed the *giants of geriatrics*, these conditions are common but frequently overlooked during traditional medical encounters. Geriatric syndromes are defined as diseases or conditions of decreased functional capacity, often of multifactorial etiology, which are commonly observed in the aging population. Geriatric syndromes can have a significant impact on quality of life, independence, and overall health. It is therefore important to screen for these syndromes to reduce the risk of functional decline and disability. Many tools are available to screen for geriatric syndromes and take only a short time to administer.

This chapter provides a brief overview of 10 common geriatric syndromes, some of which are covered in detail elsewhere in this textbook. Each syndrome is first defined and described. Common screening tools are then listed (Table 16–2), and management strategies are provided. For each syndrome, several landmark articles or well-written reviews are referenced for further reading on the topic in the bibliography.

INSTABILITY (FALLS)

DEFINITION

A fall results when the body comes to rest inadvertently on the ground or at a lower level.

OVERVIEW

- Thirty-three percent of people older than 65 years of age fall each year.
- Five to ten percent of falls result in fracture (200,000/y).
- Fifty percent of fallers do so repeatedly. Risk factors for falling include: advanced age, delirium, medical illnesses, dizziness, fear of falling, female gender, functional dependence, fall history, impaired

TABLE 16–1   The I's of Geriatrics

Instability
Immobility
Incontinence
Inanition
Intellectual impairment
Incoherence
Isolation
Iatrogenesis
Insomnia
Impoverishment

mobility, musculoskeletal dysfunction, incontinence, polypharmacy, medication change, and vitamin D deficiency.

SCREENING TOOLS

- The Tinetti gait and balance test is a two-part screening tool to identify risk of falling. A score of <19/28 requires a comprehensive fall assessment.
  - Gait assessment includes step length/height, step symmetry, step continuity, path, trunk sway, walk stance.
  - Balance assessment includes sitting balance, rising attempts, standing balance, nudge, eyes closed, 360 degree turn, sit down.
- The Get Up and Go assessment identifies those at risk for mobility impairment.
  - To perform the test: rise from a seated position, walk 10 feet, turn around, return, and sit down.
  - Normal adult performance is <10 seconds; frail elders score 11 to 20 seconds, and abnormal is >20 seconds.
- Orthostatic blood pressure (BP)
  - Measurement is made by establishing supine BP and heart rate (HR) after a 3-minute rest. Move to sitting position and remeasure BP and HR after 3 minutes, repeat with standing after 3 minutes. Abnormal response is >20 beat increase in HR, a 20 mm Hg drop in systolic BP, or 10 mm Hg drop in diastolic BP when moving from supine to sitting or standing.

MANAGEMENT

- Treat underlying medical conditions that cause cardiac, vascular, orthopedic, and neurologic conditions.
- Reduce polypharmacy, especially medications active in the central nervous system.
- Inquire about falls annually for all elders.
  - Those with a single fall should be screened with the Get Up and Go test for gait and balance impairment with further fall evaluation if indicated.
  - Those with multiple falls require a comprehensive fall evaluation.

TABLE 16–2   Screening for Geriatric Syndromes and Related Nutritional Concerns

GERIATRIC GIANT	CLINICAL CONDITIONS	SCREENING TOOL
Instability	Falls	Up and go test
		Tinetti gait and balance test
Immobility	Functional impairment	Comprehensive geriatric assessment
	Frailty	Interdisciplinary assessment
		Frailty scale
Incontinence	Incontinence	Voiding diary
		American Urological Association symptom index
Inanition	Weight loss	Body mass index
	Malnutrition	Mini-Nutritional Assessment
		MEALS ON WHEELS
		Simplified Nutritional Appetite Questionnaire (SNAQ)
Intellectual impairment	Dementia	Mini-Mental State Examination
	Mild cognitive impairment	St. Louis University mental state examination
		Clock drawing task
Incoherence	Delirium	Confusion Assessment Method
Isolation	Depression	Geriatric Depression Scale
	Bereavement	Cornell Scale for Depression in Dementia
	Losses	Hamilton Dementia Rating Index
Iatrogenesis	Polypharmacy restraints	Beers criteria
		Number of medications
Insomnia	Primary sleep disorders	Epworth Sleepiness Scale
	Secondary sleep disorder	Sleep Disorders Center: sleep apnea risk
		Pittsburgh Sleep Quality Index
Impoverishment	Sensory loss	Snellen chart
	Financial loss	Audiometry
	Safety	

- A comprehensive fall evaluation includes medication modifications, exercise and physical therapy, environmental modifications, behavioral and educational programs, and assessment for assistive devices.
- Falls can be reduced by 20% to 40% through multifactorial and interdisciplinary interventions.
- To reduce fall risk, encourage patients to engage in exercise activities in the core physical domains of balance (eg, Tai Chi), flexibility, endurance, and strength.
- Identify safety risks during a home safety evaluation including loose carpets, clutter, exposed cords/wires, poor lighting, unsafe stairways, slippery shower/tub, inadequate grab bars, and damaged/inadequate assistive devices.
- Consider hip protectors that can reduce fracture rates by up to 50%.

IMMOBILITY (FUNCTIONAL IMPAIRMENT)

DEFINITION

Functional Impairment is the inability of an individual to participate in everyday tasks, or the need for support from another person or assistive device to perform daily activities.

OVERVIEW

- The primary scales for measuring functional status are the activities of daily living (ADL) and the instrumental activities of daily living (IADL).
  ○ The ADL include bathing, dressing, transferring, toileting, grooming, feeding, and mobility.
  ○ The IADL include using the telephone, preparing meals, managing finances, taking medications, doing laundry, doing housework, shopping, and managing personal transportation.
- Age-related physiologic changes can lead to a cascade of frailty, functional decline, disability, hospitalization, institutionalization, and death.
  ○ Frailty is identified if three or more of the following criteria are present: (1) 12-month weight loss >10 lb, (2) physical exhaustion, (3) grip weakness, (4) slow walking speed, and (5) low physical activity.
- The annual incidence of frailty among older women is 5%, and the prevalence is 15%.

SCREENING TOOLS

The comprehensive geriatric assessment (CGA) is administered by an interdisciplinary team (physician, nurse, social worker, dietician, pharmacist, and therapist).

- A CGA includes review and management of illnesses and comorbid conditions, functional impairments, psychiatric disorders, social networks, and financial resources.

MANAGEMENT

CGA goals include identifying and addressing functional deficits or risks for functional decline, restoring function, improving quality of life, and preventing further disability.

The interdisciplinary components of functional evaluation and management are:
- Management of contributing medical illnesses
- Screening for and managing geriatric syndromes
- Dietary evaluation and treatment of nutritional deficits
- Speech and language therapy for communication, swallowing, or cognitive rehabilitation
- Medication evaluation and counseling
- Occupational therapy for upper extremity evaluation, IADL assessment, mobility aids, orthotic and prosthetic devices, and splints
- Physical therapy for lower extremity/trunk evaluation, bed mobility, transfers, walking, mobility aids, and wheelchair training.
- Identifying social service needs, eligibility, and resources available in the home or community
  Using appropriate mobility, safety, and assistive equipment
- Orthotics are exoskeletons designed to assist, resist, align, and stimulate function across a native joint or limb.
- Prosthetics are artificial devices used to replace an absent or dysfunctional body part.
- Install grab bars near the toilet and in the tub/shower.
- Use raised toilet seats and bathtub benches to facilitate safe transfers in the bathroom.
- A cane supports 15% to 20% of body weight, and the support increases with increased number of tips.
- A walker supports one lower extremity but not full body weight and requires upper body strength and coordination.
- Wheelchairs (manual or electric) and scooters provide trunk and leg support, can be adjusted for arm and legs, and can accommodate physical disabilities.

INCONTINENCE (URINARY)

DEFINITION

The involuntary loss of urine

OVERVIEW

Urinary incontinence (UI) is common in older adults but is *not* normal aging.
- Fifteen to thirty percent of the geriatric community and more than 50% of nursing home patients have UI.
- Risk factors include impaired cognition and mobility, neurologic disorders (stroke, Parkinson disease, dementia), diabetes, congestive heart failure, severe constipation, benign prostatic hyperplasia, atrophic vaginitis/urethritis, multiparity, and certain medications.

Detrusor innervation (parasympathetic nerves S2–S4) and urethral sphincter innervation (sympathetic S2-S4 and cholinergic stimulation) coordinate bladder filling and emptying. Urine storage is under sympathetic control via detrusor relaxation and sphincter contraction. Voiding is under parasympathetic control via detrusor contraction and sphincter relaxation.

AGING RELATED CHANGES

- Involuntary detrusor contractions or overactivity.
- Decreased detrusor contractility during micturition leading to poor urine flow, decreased bladder capacity, decreased estrogen levels resulting in urethral mucosal atrophy and urethritis, eg, predisposing to urge incontinence.
- Benign prostatic hyperplasia

TYPES OF INCONTINENCE

- Urge incontinence is the most common form of UI with abrupt urgency, frequency, and nocturia with small or large volume loss.
  ○ Precipitants include age-related bladder and urethral changes, CNS disease, and bladder irritation (bladder stones, infection, inflammation, tumors).
- Stress incontinence is the second most common form of UI. Episodic, stress-related (sneeze, cough, laugh) urine is lost when intra-abdominal pressure exceeds sphincter closure pressure.
  ○ Risks for stress incontinence include impaired pelvic supports (multiparity, pelvic surgery) and decreased sphincter tone (prostatectomy, sphincter surgery).
- Overflow incontinence is caused by bladder outlet obstruction (benign prostatic hyperplasia [BPH], urethral stricture) or detrusor underactivity (peripheral neuropathy, spinal cord injury).
  ○ Leakage is small, continual, and associated with large postvoid residual urine volume (>200–300 cc).

○ Symptoms include dribbling, weak urinary stream, intermittency, hesitancy, frequency, and nocturia.
• Functional incontinence describes the leakage of urine in the setting of normal urinary structure and function.
  ○ Potential causes include impaired cognition, impaired mobility, inaccessible urinal, and lack of caregivers.

SCREENING TOOLS

• A voiding diary should include at least 24 hours of voids and include the frequency of incontinence, quantity of urinary leakage, impact of urinary leakage on everyday life, fluid consumed, activities preceding incontinence episodes, and time/volume of continent voids.
• The American Urological Association BPH Symptom Index should be used to determine the severity of BPH symptoms.

MANAGEMENT

• Lifestyle interventions include managing fluid intake, reducing caffeine and alcohol, treating constipation, and managing contributing medical illnesses.
• Behavioral therapies include:
  ○ Bladder training uses progressively longer timed bladder emptying for urge incontinence.
  ○ Prompted voiding uses toileting on a fixed schedule, regardless of sensation of fullness.
  ○ Pelvic muscle exercises (Kegel) are useful for stress incontinence. This involves repeated contraction of the pelvic muscles: three sets of 8 to 10 contractions held for 6 to 8 seconds; start 3 to 4 times per day. The contractions are held for progressively longer times, up to 10 seconds if possible.
• Nonpharmacologic and surgical therapies include biofeedback, pessaries, electrical stimulation, weighted vaginal cones, colposuspension, slings, periurethral collagen injection, and artificial sphincter replacement.
• Stress incontinence:
  ○ Topical estrogen can reduce atrophic vaginitis and urethritis, but the impact on stress incontinence is unclear. Vaginal devices (pessaries) and surgical resuspension surgeries are used when other measures fail.
• Overflow treatment:
  ○ Relieve underlying obstruction, reduce drugs that impair detrusor contractility, treat constipation, use intermittent clean catheterization versus indwelling catheter.
• Pharmacologic therapy for urge incontinence:
  ○ Oxybutynin immediate-release (IR) (2.5–5 mg twice daily to four times daily), extended-release (ER), or topical (3.9 mg twice per week)

○ Tolterodine IR (1–2 mg twice daily) and ER (2–4 mg/d)
○ Trospium chloride (20 mg twice daily): must take on empty stomach and adjust for renal insufficiency, cytochrome P34A interactions
○ Darifenacin hydrobromide(7.5–15 mg/d): cytochrome P34A interactions
○ Solifenacin succinate (5 –10 mg/d): cytochrome P34A interactions, possible QTc prolongation

INANITION (MALNUTRITION)

DEFINITION

Significant weight loss is defined as an unintentional 5% in 1 month or 10% in 6 months loss in body weight.

OVERVIEW

• Most unintentional weight loss is *not* caused by the presence of malignancy.
• Older adults lose more muscle relative to fat with unintentional weight loss.
• Weight loss and anorexia are independent predictors of falls, functional disability, and mortality.
• Weight loss is usually multifactorial in etiology and associated with chronic medical conditions, medication side effects, malignancies, and psychosocial conditions.
• The physiologic, age-related reduction in appetite and energy intake has been termed *the anorexia of aging*.
• Up to 15% of community dwelling, 60% of hospitalized, and 85% of nursing home residents suffer from protein-energy malnutrition (PEM). PEM is a strong independent predictor of mortality in elderly people and leads to sarcopenia (muscle mass more than two standard deviations below young-normal). Sarcopenia is present in up to 6% to 15% of people older than 65 years of age.

SCREENING TOOLS

• Body mass index (BMI) (BMI = weight in kg/height in m^2) increases throughout adult life until approximately 50 to 60 years of age, then declines. BMI <18.5 is underweight, and BMI >25 is overweight.
• The Mini-Nutritional Assessment (MNA) is a commonly used tool to assess nutritional status (Chap. 15). This tool has been used to predict mortality and weight loss, however it is fairly time consuming.

- MNA includes anthropometric, dietary, general, and self assessments.
- Scoring: 18 questions, 30 points; <17/30 indicates malnourishment.
- The MEALS ON WHEELS mnemonic is a useful tool to recall potentially reversible causes of weight loss in older adults (see Table 19–4).

The Simplified Nutritional Assessment Questionnaire (SNAQ) is a four-item (20 point) survey. A score of 14 points or less predicts 5% weight loss over 6 months in community dwelling or institutionalized elders.

The mnemonic SCALES predicts risk for undernutrition with a score of four or more points.

S Sadness: Geriatric Depression Scale (GDS) = 10–14 (1) or >15 (2)

C Cholesterol <160 mg/dL (1)

A Albumin = 3.4–4 mg/dL (1), <3.5 mg/dL (2)

L Loss of weight 1 kg/1 m (1), 3 kg/1 m (2)

E Eat: needs assistance (1)

S Shopping: needs assistance (1)

MANAGEMENT

Educate patients and families on the risks of weight loss in older adults.

- Address factors that cause undernutrition in older people:
  - Address social factors of poverty, inability to shop, prepare meals or feed self, and lack of a social support network.
  - Social isolation is associated with decreased appetite.
  - Elders tend to consume substantially more food when sharing a meal with others.
- Screen for psychologic factors associated with weight loss:
  - Depression, dementia, alcoholism
- Manage medical factors that reduce appetite or increase metabolic requirements:
  - Cardiac failure, chronic obstructive pulmonary disease (COPD), infection, cancer, poor dentition, dysphagia, malabsorption syndromes, gastrointestinal symptoms, hypermetabolism, and medications.
- Provide additional calories through nutritional supplements, home-delivered meals, or community-based meal programs.
- Avoid specialized diets (low salt, low cholesterol), which result in decreased dietary intake and weight loss, especially in long-term care.
- Consider appetite-augmenting medications such as megestrol acetate, mirtazapine (if depressed), testosterone (in deficient men), or dronabinol.

IMPAIRED COGNITION (DEMENTIA)

DEFINITION

- Dementia is a gradual but progressive decline in memory and at least one other cognitive domain (aphasia, apraxia, agnosia, executive function) causing impaired daily functioning.
- Mild cognitive impairment (MCI) is memory loss without deficits in other domains or functional impairment. MCI progresses to dementia at a rate of 10% per year.
- Pseudo-dementia is cognitive impairment caused by other psychiatric or medical illnesses that is potentially reversible (delirium, depression, infection, thyroid/endocrine, metabolic disease).

OVERVIEW

- The prevalence of dementia in individuals older than 65 years of age is 10%, and for those older than 85 years of age, it is 40% to 50%.
- Risk factors include increasing age, family history, head injury, low education, female gender, apolipoprotein E4 allele, and chromosome 1, 14, and 21 mutations.
- Life expectancy is 8 to 10 years after dementia symptoms begin. The etiology of memory loss is Alzheimer disease (65–75%), vascular (multi-infarct) (10–20%), Lewy body dementia (15–25%), and other (5%).
- Clinical features include memory impairment, behavior and mood changes, impaired physical motor functioning, difficulty learning, disorientation, impaired judgment, delusions, hallucinations, aggression, and wandering.

SCREENING TOOLS

- Mini-Mental State Examination (MMSE): 30-point test of multiple cognitive functions; score of <24 suggests cognitive impairment and need for further evaluation.
- St. Louis University mental status examination: 30-point test of multiple cognitive functions; scoring is stratified by level of education and categories of MCI and dementia
- Clock drawing task: Rapid and simple test with several scoring scales.
  - Ask the patient to draw a clock face, place all the numbers on the clock, and place the hands on the clock to read, "ten to eight."

○ Score 1 point each for: closed circle, all numbers present, numbers in correct positions, hands at correct time. A score of 2 or less is abnormal.

MANAGEMENT

Goals include enhancing quality of life, maximizing function, stabilizing cognition, and treating mood or behavioral disturbances.

- Pharmacologic strategies:
  ○ Titrate to maximal tolerated dose over weeks to months.
    ▪ Cholinesterase antagonists (donepezil 10 mg/d, galantamine 12 mg twice daily, rivastigmine 6 mg twice daily)
    ▪ N-methyl-D-aspartate (NMDA) receptor antagonists (memantine 10 mg twice daily)
- Nonpharmacologic strategies:
  ○ Behavioral management includes maintaining consistent daily activities, reorientation, redirection, ensuring safety, providing sensory aids, and environmental modifications.
  ○ Social management includes individual and group psychotherapy, screening for caregiver burnout, establishing a will, power of attorney, advance directives, and estate planning before decision making capacity is lost, developing financial and caregiving plans, and educating family/caregivers about disease.

INCOHERENCE (DELIRIUM)

DEFINITION

Delirium is an acute disturbance of attention and cognition with fluctuating levels of consciousness and disorganized thinking.

OVERVIEW

- Delirium affects 10% to 20% of all hospitalized adults, and 30% to 40% of hospitalized elders.
- Delirium presents with hyperactive (25%), hypoactive (50%), or mixed (25%) behaviors.
- Delirium is associated with a 10-fold risk of death in hospital and a three- to fivefold risk of hospital complications.
- Delirium predicts poor functional recovery and eventual nursing home placement.
- Risk factors include increasing age, cognitive and functional impairment, medical comorbidity, male gender, alcohol history, and surgical interventions.

- Predisposing factors include infections, hypoxia, pain, medications, indwelling devices, restraints, electrolyte and cardiac disturbances, stool impaction, urinary retention, and bed rest.
- Delirium has been associated with an increase in anticholinergic activity, serotonin imbalance, or cytokine excess.

SCREENING TOOLS

Confusion Assessment Method (CAM): Delirium is present with criteria 1 and 2 plus either 3 or 4.
1. Acute change in mental status with fluctuating course
2. Inattention
3. Disorganized thinking
4. Altered level of consciousness

MANAGEMENT

- Reversing delirium requires identification and treatment of the underlying cause and precipitating factors.
- Treatment requires an interdisciplinary effort by physicians, nurses, therapists, and family.
- A multifactorial approach includes minimizing medications, eliminating restraints, providing protective environment, treating pain and other distressing symptoms, providing proper hydration and nutrition, providing sensory aids, and reorienting the patient.
- Avoid benzodiazepines as these frequently worsen confusion.
- Use antipsychotics only in severe circumstances with small frequent doses of intravenous (IV) or oral (PO) haloperidol.

ISOLATION (DEPRESSION AND LOSS)

DEFINITION

Depression is a psychiatric disorder characterized by depressed mood *or* anhedonia, plus any five of these additional features: change in appetite, sleep disturbance, psychomotor agitation or retardation, loss of energy, feelings of worthlessness or guilt, difficulty concentrating, thoughts of suicide or death.

OVERVIEW

- Minor depression is present in up to 15% of older persons.
- Major depression is present in only 1% to 2% of healthy community dwellers.

- Elders are more likely to present atypically with apathy, social withdrawal, weight loss, agitation, confusion, somatic symptoms, and fatigue than with depressed mood.
- Psychotic depression is more common in older adults with paranoia, delusions, and psychosis.
- Older age is associated with increasing risk of completed suicides. Risks include first depressive episode, age >75 years, physical illness, living alone, male gender, and alcoholism.

SCREENING TOOLS

- The GDS Short Form is a 15-question survey that can be self-administered. Six or more *positive* responses suggest depression.
- The Hamilton Depression Rating Scale is a 17-item mood assessment administered by a trained interviewer. Scoring is a 0 to 1–2 and a 0 to 1–2 to 3–4 point scale with a total >17 points indicating moderate to severe symptoms.
- Cornell Scale for Depression in Dementia is a 19-point caregiver report of mood and behavior. Scoring is a 0 to 1–2 scale with 12 or more points suggesting depression.

MANAGEMENT

- Effective treatments in the elderly include psychotherapy, pharmacotherapy and electroconvulsive therapy (ECT).
- Pharmacotherapy is often selected based on depression cosymptoms and drug properties and side effects.
- Sixty to eighty percent of patients respond to appropriate treatment. Relapse rates are 30% to 40% within 1 year.
- Response to serotonin selective reuptake inhibitors (SSRIs) and serotonin-norepinephrine reuptake inhibitors (SNRIs) is similar to tricyclic antidepressants (TCAs) but with fewer side effects.
  - ○ Recommended TCAs include nortriptyline 50 to 75 mg/d and desipramine 100 to 150 mg/d.
  - ○ Recommended SSRIs include citalopram, escitalopram oxalate, and paroxetine (10–40 mg/d), sertraline (50–150 mg/d).
    - Side effects include headache, nausea, dizziness.
    - Fluoxetine is usually avoided because of a very long half-life and risk of agitation.
- Mixed serotonin (S), dopamine (D), or norepinephrine (NE) receptor activity.
  - ○ Bupropion (150–300 mg/d; D, NE) can increase anxiety and lower seizure threshold.

- ○ Venlafaxine (75–225 mg/d; S, NE) can increase blood pressure and nausea.
- ○ Duloxetine (15–60 mg/d; S, NE) acts through cytochrome P450 pathway and can increase transaminases.
- ○ Mirtazapine (15–45 mg/d; S, NE) is associated with weight gain, increased appetite, sedation.
- ECT is highly effective with 70% response rates and is the first-line treatment for patients at high suicide risk, inability to eat, or for psychotic depression.

LOSSES

Older adults experience many forms of loss as they age. These losses can contribute to the development of mood disorders.

Loss of work (retirement)
Finances (fixed income)
Family (geographic distance)
Friends (death)
Health and function
Independence (driving, mobility)
Spouse (death or disability)
Social importance (contribution to community)
Freedom (structured housing communities)
Safety (personal and family)

Bereavement is the psychological and physical process of grieving a loss (traditionally a death).

- Uncomplicated bereavement is not associated with marked functional impairment and does not mandate pharmacologic treatment.
- Most severe symptoms of grief (the feeling of sorrow) improve over several months.
- Bereavement is a risk factor for the subsequent development of depression.

IATROGENESIS (POLYPHARMACY AND RESTRAINTS)

DEFINITIONS

- Inappropriate medication use (often termed broadly as *polypharmacy*) is defined as the overuse, underuse, and inappropriate use of medication in elderly adults.
- Adverse drug reactions (ADRs) are defined by the World Health Organization as "any noxious, unintended drug reaction that occurs at doses normally prescribed."
- Restraints are any physical or chemical measure used with the purpose of limiting voluntary or involuntary movements or mobility.

OVERVIEW

- Overuse of medications includes the use of medications without clear ongoing medical need (eg, proton pump inhibitors, iron sulfate).
- Underuse of medication includes failure to titrate medications to appropriate and effective doses or failure to prescribe medications known to be beneficial (eg, antidepressants, pain medications).
- Inappropriate prescribing includes use of a high-risk medication when a *safer* alternative could be used (eg, nonsedating rather than sedating antihistamine). Inappropriate prescribing also includes drug-drug, drug-disease, and drug-food interactions.
- Older adults are more sensitive to medication effects and more likely to experience ADRs because of physiologic changes of aging such as:
  ○ Altered drug distribution caused by increased body fat and decreased water mass
  ○ Decreased renal clearance
  ○ Altered drug absorption caused by achlorhydria and sicca symptoms
  ○ Blunted cardiovascular responsiveness (autonomic insufficiency): decreased stress-induced tachycardia and increased orthostatic hypotension
- Thirty-five percent of ambulatory older adults have experienced an ADR, and 29% required healthcare services for this reaction.

SCREENING

Evaluate medication list and medical history for high-risk factors:
- Six or more concurrent chronic conditions
- Twelve or more doses of drugs per day
- Nine or more medications (the Centers for Medicare and Medicaid Services has established a threshold of nine medications as a potential state of medication overuse)
- Prior adverse drug reaction
- Low body weight or low BMI
- Age 85 years or older
- Estimated creatinine clearance (CrCl) <50 mL/min
  The Beers criteria and the Canadian criteria are the two most commonly cited references for inappropriate medication use in older adults. Beers and colleagues identified:
- Forty-eight individual medications or classes of medications to avoid in older adults
- Twenty diseases-drug combinations to be avoided in older adults
  Multiple revisions and versions have been published including prescribing in long-term care, outpatient, and hospital settings.

MANAGEMENT

- For all medication prescribing, the mantra "start low, go slow" should be employed when initiating and titrating medication in the elderly.
- Reduce the number, dose, and frequency of medication whenever possible.
- Screen the medication list for potential problems and revisions at every encounter.
- Avoid medications known to cause more frequent or severe ADRs in older adults.
- Review the purpose, proper use, and ongoing need for each medication at every encounter.

RESTRAINTS

- When a dosing schedule, dose, or medication is selected to intentionally interfere with a person's ability to be alert, interactive, and mobile, this constitutes a restraint. Antipsychotics used in long-term care can be considered a restraint if the purpose is not for the safety of patient or others or for disease-specific symptom management.
- Physical restraints include vests, waist, wrist or ankle belts, geriatric chair, or wheelchair with fixed tray table. Side rails that prevent movement out of a bed when desired are considered restraints.
- Other medical devices can hinder the mobility, normal functioning, and recovery of an older adult. Such devices include indwelling urinary catheters (without medical indication), IV fluids, and oxygen if not medically necessary.
- The use of restraints is associated with an increased risk of falls, injuries, and deaths. The removal of restraints has not been shown to increase the risk of injuries, and thus the gold standard in nursing homes is a *restraint-free environment*.

INSOMNIA

DEFINITION

Insomnia is the subjective report of insufficient or nonrestorative sleep despite adequate opportunity to sleep.

OVERVIEW

- Sleep problems are not normal aging symptoms.
- The annual incidence is 5%, and prevalence is 30% to 60%.

- Men and women are equally affected, but men older than 85 years of age are at the highest risk.
- Consequences of poor sleep include physical and mental fatigue, anxiety, accidents and falls, decreased memory, and poor concentration.
- Aging-related sleep changes include:
  - Sleep phase is advanced (earlier to bed, earlier to rise). Increased sleep fragmentation, time in bed, sleep latency.
  - Decreased total sleep time, slow wave sleep, and sleep efficiency.
  - Time spent in rapid eye movement (REM) sleep is not changed.
  - Insomnia etiology: primary sleep disorders, physical illnesses, behavioral patterns, environmental disturbances, stimulating medications.

SCREENING TOOLS

- Epworth Sleepiness Scale: 8 questions, 24 points; 10+ points suggests sleepiness
- Sleep Disorders Center: sleep apnea risk
- Pittsburgh Sleep Quality Index

MANAGEMENT

- Review the 24-hour sleep pattern and sleep diary.
- Interview the bed partner.
- Institute sleep hygiene and nonpharmacologic approaches.
- Institute pharmacologic approaches.
- Consider a sleep center referral if primary sleep disorders are suspected.

NONMEDICATION MANAGEMENT: SLEEP HYGIENE

- Adjust light, temperature, ventilation, and noise.
- Reserve the bed for sleep and sex.
- Minimize caffeine, cigarettes, stimulants, alcohol, daytime napping.
- Use behavioral strategies to reduce stress and maladaptive sleep habits.
- Increase daytime exercise, sunlight.
- Keep a regular sleep schedule.

MEDICATION MANAGEMENT

Use lowest effective dose, intermittent dosing, short-term prescribing, and medications with shorter half-lives.

Medications to avoid:
- Benzodiazepines are associated with hangover effect, physical dependence, dizziness, and falls.
- Antihistamines (diphenhydramine, doxylamine) cause significant anticholinergic effects, daytime sedation, and orthostatic hypotension.
- TCAs have significant anticholinergic properties, risk for altered cardiac conduction, and daytime sedation. Medications to consider:
- Zolpidem: 5–10 mg; has physical dependence and abuse potential without tolerance.
- Zaleplon: 5–20 mg; short half-life, with no tolerance or rebound.
- Eszopiclone: 1–3 mg; Food and Drug Administration (FDA) approved for long-term use; no rebound or tolerance.
- Trazodone: 50–150 mg; sedating non–tricyclic antidepressant; improves sleep continuity and deep sleep without addiction or tolerance; has potential for oversedation and orthostatic hypotension.
- Ramelteon: 8 mg; melatonin receptor agonist without abuse potential but unpredictable metabolism.

IMPOVERISHMENT (SENSORY, FINANCIAL, AND SAFETY CHALLENGES)

SENSORY CHALLENGES

- Presbyopia (age-related loss in near vision) is caused by gradual hardening of the lens and decreased muscular effectiveness of the ciliary body.
- Presbycusis is aging-related hearing loss caused by sensorineural loss, usually symmetrical, that progresses over time and is worsened by noise injury.

OVERVIEW

- Visual impairment (acuity <20/40): increases with age and affects 20% to 30% older than age 75. Blindness (acuity <20/200) affects 2% older than age 75.
- The most common causes of vision loss in older adults is macular degeneration (most common cause), glaucoma (most common in African Americans), and cataracts.
- Aging changes in the eye include yellowing of the cornea and lens, impaired contrast sensitivity, reduced visual acuity, and slower light-dark adaptation.
- Aging changes of the ear include drier cerumen, loss of cochlear hair cells and neurons, and stiffening of the basilar membrane.

SCREENING TOOLS

- Visual acuity can be tested with a standard Snellen chart, however, professional ophthalmologic evaluation is recommended every 1 to 2 years for older adults.
- Audiometry screens for hearing loss is performed at selected frequencies (0.5, 1, 2, and 4 KHz) and at two intensity levels (25 and 40 dB HL).
- The Hearing Handicap Inventory for the Elderly includes 10 questions; 3 or more positive responses suggest hearing impairment.

MANAGEMENT

- Cataracts are best treated by surgical removal and replacement with a prosthetic lens.
- Macular degeneration is treated with laser photocoagulation of neovascularized areas or intravitreal endothelial growth factors (wet form) and oral antioxidant supplementation (dry form).
- Glaucoma is treated with topical medication (β-blockers, prostaglandin analogs, sympathomimetics, carbonic anhydrase inhibitors) or surgical interventions (trabeculoplasty, trabeculectomy).
- Use a hearing aid, amplification device, or visual and/or vibrational alarms for hearing impaired.
- Improve the listening environment by eliminating background noise, facing the listener, and speaking with lower pitch voice.

SAFETY AND ELDER ABUSE

"Abuse is any intentional action that causes harm, creates serious risk for harm, or fails to protect from harm, vulnerable elders by a caregiver or other involved person." (US National Academy of Sciences.)

OVERVIEW

- Forms of abuse include physical, psychological, neglect, financial exploitation, and abandonment.
- Neglect, especially self-neglect, is the most common form of elder abuse.
- The annual incidence of elder abuse is 450,000, and approximately 4% of those aged 65 years and older are affected.

SCREENING

- Assess caregiver stress, caregiver skills, and caregiver cognitive capacity (if indicated).
- Identify high-risk situations: family history of abuse, alcohol or drug use, financial stress, and isolation.
- Evaluate patient for clean and appropriate clothing, proper hygiene, nutritional status/weight stability, contractures, skin rash or ulcers, bruises or other injuries, and anxiety/depression.
- Evaluate caregiver for impatience, irritability, or demeaning statements, ambivalence to medical and personal care requirements, overuse of sedatives or other inappropriate medication.

MANAGEMENT

- All healthcare providers (not just physicians) have an obligation to report any suspicion of any form of elder abuse.
- Document findings and provide a supportive environment for the victim.

FINANCIAL CHALLENGES

- Ninety percent of seniors older than age 65 receive Social Security benefits (accounting for 41% of the total income of the elderly).
  - The average monthly benefit was $1007 ($12,084 annual) in 2006.
- In 2006, the federal poverty level for an individual was $9080 per year. Most states set the Medicaid eligibility income at or below the poverty level.
  - In 2004, nearly 15% of seniors received Medicaid benefits.
- At age 65, elders are eligible for Medicare Part A and B health benefits.
  - Eighty percent of US senior citizens are eligible for Medicare.
  - Medicare Part A covers hospital, nursing home, home health, and hospice services at an annual deductible of $912.
  - Medicare Part B covers physicians, nurse practitioners, psychologists, social workers, rehabilitation therapists, laboratory tests, and medical equipment with a monthly premium of $78, annual deductible of $110, and 20% copay on these services.
  - Medicare Part D is a voluntary medication benefit that began January 1, 2006. Enrollees pay a monthly premium (average $32 per month), $250 deductible, and then 25% of the cost of prescription drugs until $2250 is spent. The next $1350 in medication is

paid entirely by the enrollee. After spending $3600, medication costs revert to a flat 5% or $2 to $5 per prescription. At $100 per month ($1200 annual) in medication usage, an enrollee with Medicare Part D pays approximately $810. At $200 per month ($2400 annual) the enrollee pays $1210.

- Medigap supplemental insurance plans cover Medicare Part A and Part B deductibles and coinsurance costs. The basic plan costs $40 to $125 per month.
- Medicare HMOs offer basic Medicare A and B services and additional benefits such as medications, preventive medicine, and vision coverage.
  ○ Enrollees must continue to pay their monthly Medicare Part B premiums and must obtain their healthcare from the HMO's provider network.
  ○ Each year, the HMOs can change their premiums, benefits, and provider networks.

CONCLUSION

As the US population ages, a greater percentage of individuals will be living into their eighth and ninth decades of life. Many of these individuals will develop functional and cognitive impairments. Caring for the elderly will increasingly require a focus on functional status with the goal to promote wellness, maintain independence, and prevent decline. A comprehensive approach using screening tools and an interdisciplinary team best meets the complex care needs of this population.

BIBLIOGRAPHY

Iatrogenesis

Fick DM, Cooper JW, Wade WE, et al. Updating the Beers criteria for potentially inappropriate medication use in older adults: results of a US consensus panel of experts. *Arch Intern Med.* 2003 Dec 8–22;163(22):2716–2724.

Gurwitz JH, Field TS, Harrold LR, et al. Incidence and preventability of adverse drug events among older persons in the ambulatory setting. *JAMA.* 2003;289(9):1107–1116.

Hanlon JT, Schmader KE, Ruby CM, et al. Suboptimal prescribing in older inpatients and outpatients. *J Am Geriatr Soc.* 2001;49(2):200–209.

Inouye SK, Bogardus ST Jr, Charpentier PA, et al. A multicomponent intervention to prevent delirium in hospitalized older patients. *N Engl J Med.* 1999;340(9):669–676.

Immobility

Fleming KC, Evans JM, Weber DC, et al. Practical functional assessment of elderly persons: a primary-care approach. *Mayo Clin Proc.* 1995;70(9):890–910.

Fried LP, Tangen CM, Walston J, et al; Cardiovascular Health Study Collaborative Research Group. Frailty in older adults: evidence for a phenotype. *J Gerontol A Biol Sci Med Sci.* 2001;56(3):M146–156.

Wells JL, Seabrook JA, Stolee P, et al. State of the art in geriatric rehabilitation. Part I. review of frailty and comprehensive geriatric assessment. *Arch Phys Med Rehabil.* 2003;84(6): 890–897.

Impoverishment

Gorbien MJ, Eisenstein AR. Elder abuse and neglect: an overview. *Clin Geriatr Med.* 2005;21(2):279–292.

Social Security Administration, Office of Policy Data. Fast facts & figures about Social Security, 2006. http://www.ssa.gov/policy/docs/chartbooks/fast_facts/2006/index.html. Published September 2006. Accessed November 19, 2006.

US Department of Health and Human Services. Prescription drug coverage. http://www.medicare.gov/pdphome.asp. Published October 13. Accessed November 19, 2006.

Inanition

Morley JE. Nutrition in the elderly. *Curr Opin Gastroenterol.* 2002;18(2):240–245.

Morley JE. Anorexia and weight loss in older persons. *J Gerontol A Biol Sci Med Sci.* 2003;58(2):131–137.

Reuben DB, Hirsch SH, Zhou K, et al. The effects of megestrol acetate suspension for elderly patients with reduced appetite after hospitalization: a phase II randomized clinical trial. *J Am Geriatr Soc.* 2005;53(6):970–975.

Wilson MM, Thomas DR, Rubenstein LZ, et al. Appetite assessment: simple appetite questionnaire predicts weight loss in community-dwelling adults and nursing home residents. *Am J Clin Nutr.* 2005;82(5):1074–1081.

Incoherence

Inouye SK. Delirium in older persons. *N Engl J Med.* 2006;354(11): 1157–1165.

Inouye SK, van Dyck CH, Alessi CA, et al. Clarifying confusion: the confusion assessment method. A new method for detection of delirium. *Ann Intern Med.* 1990;113(12):941–948.

Schor JD, Levkoff SE, Lipsitz LA, et al. Risk factors for delirium in hospitalized elderly. *JAMA.* 1992;267(6):827–831.

Incontinence

American College of Obstetricians and Gynecologists. Urinary incontinence in women. *Obstet Gynecol.* 2005;105(6): 1533–1545.

Ouslander JG, Schnelle JF. Incontinence in the nursing home [review]. *Ann Intern Med.* 1995;122(6):438–449.

Wilson MM. Urinary incontinence: selected current concepts [review]. *Med Clin North Am.* 2006;90(5):825–836.

Insomnia

Kamel NS, Gammack JK. Insomnia in the elderly: cause, approach, and treatment. *Am J Med.* 2006;119(6):463–469.

Montgomery P, Dennis J. A systematic review of non-pharmacological therapies for sleep problems in later life. *Sleep Med Rev.* 2004;8(1):47–62.

Instability

Alexander NB. Gait disorders in older adults. *J Am Geriatr Soc.* 1996;44(4):434–451.

American Geriatrics Society, British Geriatrics Society, and American Academy of Orthopaedic Surgeons Panel on Falls Prevention. Guideline for the prevention of falls in older persons. *J Am Geriatr Soc.* 2001;49(5):664–672.

Tinetti ME. Clinical practice. Preventing falls in elderly persons. *N Engl J Med.* 2003;348(1):42–49.

Intellectual Impairment

Grossberg GT. Diagnosis and treatment of Alzheimer's disease. *J Clin Psychiatry.* 2003;2006;64(suppl 9):3–6.

Joshi S, Morley JE. Cognitive impairment. *Med Clin North Am.* 2006;90(5):769–787.

Tariq SH, Tumosa N, Chibnall JT, et al. Comparison of the Saint Louis University mental status examination and the mini-mental state examination for detecting dementia and mild neurocognitive disorder—a pilot study. *Am J Geriatr Psychiatry.* 2006;14(11):900–910.

Isolation

Gebretsadik M, Jayaprabhu S, Grossberg GT. Mood disorders in the elderly. *Med Clin North Am.* 2006;90(5):789–805.

Yesavage JA, Brink TL, Rose TL, et al. Development and validation of a geriatric depression screening scale: a preliminary report. *J Psychiatr Res.* 1982–1983;17(1):37–49.

17 THE CONFUSED PATIENT
Seema Joshi

INTRODUCTION

- Misdiagnosis and inappropriate management of confusional states can be associated with serious adverse effects on outcome including: increased mortality, impaired functional status, increased length of hospital stay, and institutionalization. Cognitive dysfunction reflects the level of consciousness (arousal) or the content of consciousness (cognition).
- Cognitive dysfunction may further be characterized by disorientation, learning impairment, hallucinations, delusions, labile emotions, and aphasia.
- Altered mental status is a common admitting diagnosis in the elderly. The confused patient should undergo an extensive evaluation for delirium, which is often reversible following treatment of the underlying disorder.
- Importantly, the clinical features and subsequent diagnosis of delirium is frequently missed by physicians (32% to 66%) and nurses (69%).[1]

- Unlike delirium, dementia is characterized by cognitive dysfunction that is more gradual in onset and progression and associated with a clear sensorium. This chapter will focus on two of the most common causes of confusion in the elderly: dementia and delirium.

EPIDEMIOLOGY

- Approximately 10% to 20% of community dwelling persons and 48% of nursing home residents have cognitive impairment.[2,3]
- Dementia is a common cause of cognitive impairment in the elderly. Worldwide it is estimated that 24.3 million people have dementia today, with 4.6 million new cases of dementia every year (one new case every 7 seconds). The number of people affected is projected to double every 20 years to 81.1 million by 2040.[4]
- Epidemiological studies indicate that Alzheimer disease is the most common cause of dementia worldwide. It is responsible for 75% of all dementias and affects 5% of the population older than 65 years of age and 30% of patients older than 85 years.[5]
- The prevalence of delirium on admission to hospitals ranges from 10% to 31%.[6]
- The incidence of delirium increases progressively after the fourth decade of life.[7]
- The mortality rates among hospitalized patients with delirium range from 22% to 76%; similar to the mortality rates among patients with acute myocardial infarction or sepsis.[8]

DELIRIUM AND DEMENTIA

- Delirium is a complex syndrome in the elderly. It is characterized by the acute or subacute onset of altered consciousness and cognition. The cognitive status is typically reversible and usually fluctuates during the day.
- The *Diagnostic and Statistical Manual of Mental Disorders, 4th Edition, Text Revision (DSM-IV-TR)* defines the diagnostic criteria used to establish a diagnosis of delirium.
- The Confusion Assessment Method (CAM) is a screening tool for delirium and was derived from the *Diagnostic and Statistical Manual of Mental Disorders, 3rd edition, Revised (DSM-III-R);*[9] it requires a brief structured assessment of key features to establish the diagnosis of delirium. Its four key elements include:
  - Acute change in mental status and fluctuating course
  - Inattention
  - Disorganized thinking
  - Altered level of consciousness

- Based on the *DSM-III-R* and *DSM-IV* criteria, the essential feature of dementia is impairment in short and long-term memory, associated with impairment in abstract thinking, impaired judgment, other disturbances of higher cortical function, or personality change. The disturbance is severe enough to interfere significantly with work or social activities or relationships with others.
- It is important to differentiate delirium from dementia because of its reversible nature. Table 17–1 summarizes the clinical differences between delirium and dementia.

ETIOLOGY AND RISK FACTORS

- Precipitating factors in the presence of existing predisposing factors (Table 17–2) result in the development of delirium.
- The mnemonic DELIRIUMS permits identification of most of the underlying (precipitating) causes of delirium. However, it does not address pain as a cause of delirium. Pain should always be considered as a cause of delirium especially in the postoperative period.
  Drugs (Table 17–3)
  Emotional (acute psychotic and depressive episodes)
  Low oxygen states (anemia, pulmonary embolus, myocardial infarction, stroke)
  Infection
  Retention of urine and feces
  Ictal states, especially partial complex seizures
  Under nutrition and dehydration
  Metabolic (organ failure, thyroid disease, vitamin B12 deficiency)
  Subdural hematoma
- Dementia is mostly irreversible; however there are a number of important reversible causes of dementia which can be classified using the mnemonic DEMENTIA.
  Drugs (any drug with anticholinergic activity)
  Emotional—depression
  Metabolic (hypothyroid states)

TABLE 17–2   Predisposing Factors for Delirium

Age >65 years
Male sex
Cognitive impairment
Sensory impairment
Polypharmacy
Functional impairment
Multiple coexisting medical conditions

  Eyes and ears (declining function)
  Normal pressure hydrocephalus
  Tumor or other space-occupying lesion
  Infection (syphilis, AIDS)
  Anemia (vitamin B_{12} or folate deficiency)
  The irreversible causes of dementia include Alzheimer disease, vascular dementia, Parkinson disease, frontotemporal dementia, dementia with Lewy bodies, prion disease, and Huntington disease.

PATHOPHYSIOLOGY

- The pathophysiologic mechanisms underlying the development of delirium are not well understood. Nonetheless, acetylcholine is believed to play an important role in the development of delirium in a variety of settings. For example, administration of anticholinergic agents can induce delirium in healthy patients. This effect is amplified in patients with underlying medical conditions.
- Serum anticholinergic activity in elderly patients with delirium is elevated even in the absence of anticholinergic medications. Thus, medical conditions that precipitate delirium have been shown to inhibit the synthesis of acetylcholine in the brain.

TABLE 17–1   Features Differentiating Delirium from Dementia

FEATURES	DELIRIUM	DEMENTIA
Level of consciousness	Hyperalert/Hypoactive	Alert
Orientation	Disorganized	Disoriented
Course	Fluctuating	Slow decline
Onset	Acute or Subacute	Chronic
Attention	Impaired	Usually normal

TABLE 17–3   Medications Associated with Delirium and Confusion in the Elderly

MEDICATIONS	EXAMPLES
Antiarrhythmics	Amiodarone, digoxin
Antibiotics	Penicillins, ciprofloxacin
Anticholinergics	Benztropine, oxybutynin
Anticonvulsants	Phenytoin, carbamazepine, barbiturates
Antidepressants	Amitriptyline, doxepin, imipramine
Antihistamines	Diphenhydramine
Antihypertensives	Atenolol, methyldopa
Antiparkinson agents	Amantadine, levodopa, benztropine
Antipsychotics	Clozapine, haloperidol, thioridazine
Benzodiazepines	Diazepam, flurazepam, triazolam, alprazolam, chlordiazepoxide
Corticosteroids	Prednisone, prednisolone
H_2 blockers	Cimetidine, famotidine
Narcotic analgesics	Meperidine, oxycodone, codeine
Miscellaneous	Lithium, alcohol

- Other neurotransmitters that may be involved in the genesis of delirium include dopamine, norepinephrine, serotonin, γ-aminobutyric acid, glutamate, and melatonin. Cytokines such as interleukin-1, interleukin-2, interleukin-6, tumor necrosis factor-α (TNF-α), and interferon may also play a role in the pathogenesis of delirium.
- Chronic hypercortisolism may also be involved in the pathogenesis of delirium secondary to its effects on serotonin receptors.
- There is growing evidence that accumulation of β-amyloid plays a central role in the pathogenesis of Alzheimer disease. The hereditary forms of Alzheimer appear to accelerate accumulation of amyloid in the extracellular space. The accumulation of amyloid-β peptide impairs memory, produce tissue oxidative damage and promotes cell death.[10] A recent report suggests that inhibiting the synthesis of β-amyloid in a transgenic mice model reduced the generation of neurofibrillary tangles that have been linked to nerve cell death.

DIAGNOSTIC APPROACH

- Both delirium and dementia are largely clinical diagnoses (although laboratory data may be essential to exclude other remediable causes). An algorithm that can be used to evaluate the confused patient is depicted in Fig. 17–1.
- The evaluation of the patient with confusion should focus on:
  - A detailed history, including an informant (someone who knows the patient, usually a family member) based history to assess pre-existing cognitive and functional status.
  - A thorough physical and neurological examination
  - Evaluation of cognitive, behavioral, and functional status using the Mini-Mental State Examination (MMSE) and Confusion Assessment Method (CAM).
  - Appropriate laboratory and imaging studies guided by the mnemonic DELIRIUMS
  - Polypharmacy and adverse drug reactions are a major cause of confusion in the elderly. A review of

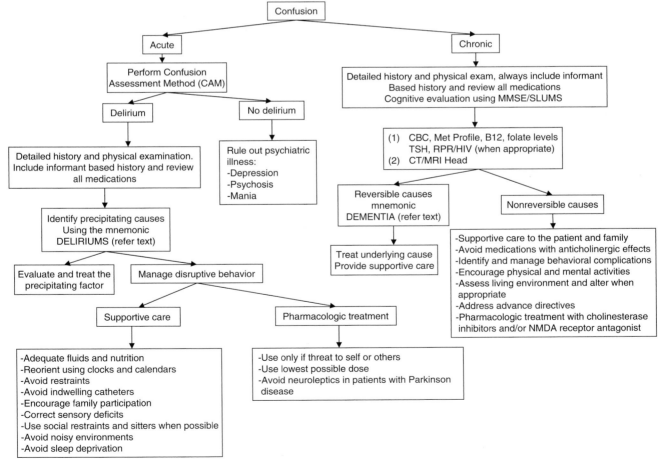

FIG. 17–1 Diagnostic approach to the confused patient.

the patient's medications is an essential part of the history. Some commonly used medications, including over-the-counter preparations, that can induce delirium are listed in Table 17–3.

MANAGEMENT

Management of the confused patient is guided by the underlying diagnosis, eg, delirium or reversible causes of dementia. The management of delirium should be guided by the following principles:

> ***Identifying and treating the underlying causes***
> ***Managing disruptive behaviors***
> ***Providing supportive care and rehabilitation***

- Disruptive behaviors can be managed with nonpharmacologic and pharmacologic interventions. Nonpharmacologic approaches are summarized in Table 17–4. These strategies are designed to promote a calm and comfortable environment, correct sensory deficits, and provide orienting stimuli.
- Nonpharmacologic approaches should always be employed. Pharmacologic management may be considered if the patient's behavior becomes a safety threat.
- Physical restraints should not be used in the treatment of delirium. Restraints are associated with an increased risk of serious injuries.
- Physical activity should be initiated early to prevent deconditioning.
- There is limited evidence on the use of pharmacologic agents in the treatment of delirium.
- Medications only treat the symptoms of delirium and do not address the underlying causes.
- Current data on the use of antipsychotics in delirium are based on a single randomized control trial comparing neuroleptic agents to benzodiazepines in hospitalized patients with AIDS, having a mean age of 39.2 years.[11]
- Haloperidol is the most widely used antipsychotic agent. It has been recommended by the American Psychiatric Association (APA) for the treatment of delirium.[12] The optimal dose of an antipsychotic has not been established. Haloperidol may be administered at a starting dose of 0.25 to 1.0 mg orally or parenterally (intravenous use is not FDA approved). It may be used as often as every 20 to 30 minutes, not to exceed a maximum dose of 3 to 5 mg in 24 hours.
- Lorazepam may be used in patients with contraindications to neuroleptic agents such as Lewy body dementia and Parkinson disease. It may be administered orally or parenterally at a dose of 0.5 to 1.0 mg and is repeated every 2 hours (maximum of 3 mg in 24 hours) as needed.
- There are no truly effective therapies for treating dementia. Acetylcholinesterase inhibitors have been approved by the FDA for the treatment of mild to moderate AD. Clinical trials demonstrated efficacy with small improvements in cognitive and global functions in mild to moderate disease with the duration of benefit persisting as long as 36 months for some patients.[13]
- Memantine has been recently approved for the treatment of moderate to severe dementia. It seems to be beneficial alone or in combination with donepezil in moderate to severe dementia.
- An increased risk for all-cause mortality was seen with vitamin E supplementation in a recent meta-analysis.[14] Based on current data, it would be prudent to avoid high-dose vitamin E supplementation.
- Consumption of fish and intake of omega-3 polyunsaturated fatty acids has been associated with a reduced risk for cognitive decline. Leisure-time physical activity at midlife is associated with a decreased risk for dementia and AD later in life. Regular physical activity may reduce the risk or delay the onset of dementia and AD, especially among genetically susceptible individuals.[15,16]
- Atypical antipsychotics are used frequently for the treatment of behavioral symptoms that are associated with advanced AD. The FDA issued a public health advisory on April 11, 2005, which indicated that mortality was increased in patients receiving atypical antipsychotic drugs.

TABLE 17–4 Nonpharmacologic Approach to the Treatment of Delirium

Correct sensory deficits—Use eyeglasses and hearing aids appropriately
Use orienting stimuli—clocks, calendars
Ensure adequate fluid and nutrient intake
Optimize medications—Eliminate unnecessary medications
Mobilize as soon as possible
Avoid isolation
Avoid physical restraints—Use social restraints
Encourage family participation
Prevent sleep deprivation
Prevent constipation
Treat urinary retention
Avoid sedatives
Avoid indwelling devices such as urinary catheters

PRECAUTIONS

- Neuroleptics may be associated with extrapyramidal symptoms, prolonged corrected QT interval, hyperglycemia, and ketoacidosis.
- Benzodiazepines may cause paradoxical excitation, respiratory depression, and oversedation.

SUMMARY

The elderly are particularly vulnerable to developing delirium during an acute illness. Delirium is associated with adverse outcomes, and the diagnosis is often missed by healthcare professionals. Delirium and dementia often coexist. Dementia is a major risk factor for delirium. Therefore, successful treatment of confusion in the elderly requires a multicomponent approach using nonpharmacologic treatment and, when necessary, judicious use of pharmacologic agents.

REFERENCES

1. Inouye SK. Delirium in hospitalized older patients: recognition and risk factors. *J Geriatr Psychiatry Neurol.* 1998:11(3): 118–125.
2. Unverzagt FW, Gao S, Baiyewu O, et al. Prevalence of cognitive impairment: data from the Indianapolis Study of Health and Aging. *Neurology.* 2001;57(9):1655–1662.
3. Magaziner J, German P, Zimmerman SI, et al. The prevalence of dementia in a statewide sample of new nursing home admissions aged 65 and older: diagnosis by expert panel. Epidemiology of Dementia in Nursing Homes Research Group. *Gerontologist.* 2000;40(6):663–672.
4. Ferri CP, Prince M, Brayne C, et al. Global prevalence of dementia: a Delphi consensus study. *Lancet.* 2005;366(9503): 2112–2117 .
5. Nourhashemi F, Sinclair AJ, Vellas B. Clinical aspects of Alzheimer's Disease. *Principles and Practice of Geriatric Medicine.* 4th ed. Chichester, UK: John Wiley and Sons; 2006.
6. Siddiqi N, House AO, Holmes JD. Occurrence and outcome of delirium in medical in-patients: a systematic literature review. *Age Ageing.* 2006;35(4):350–364.
7. Tueth MJ, Cheong JA. Delirium: diagnosis and treatment in the older patient. *Geriatrics.* 1993;48(3):75–80.
8. Inouye SK. Delirium. In: Cassel CK, ed. *Geriatric Medicine: An Evidence Based Approach*, 4th ed. New York: Springer; 2003.
9. Inouye SK, vanDyck CH, Alessi CA, et al. Clarifying confusion: the confusion assessment method: a new method for detection of delirium. *Ann Int Med.* 1990;113(12): 941–948.
10. Flood JF, Morley JE, Roberts E. An amyloid beta-protein fragment, a beta[122–8], equipotently impairs post-training memory processing when injected into different limbic system structures. *Brain Res.* 1994;663(2):271–276.
11. Breitbart W, Marotta R, Platt M. A double blind trial of haloperidol, chlorpromazine and lorazepam in the treatment of delirium in hospitalized AIDS patients. *Am J Psychiatry.* 1996;153(2):231–237.
12. American Psychiatric Association. Practice guidelines for the treatment of patients with delirium. *Am J Psychiatry.* 1999;156(5 Suppl):1–20.
13. Raskind MA, Peskind ER, Truyen L, et al. The cognitive benefits of galantamine are sustained for at least 36 months; a long term extension trial. *Arch Neurol.* 2004;61:252–256.
14. Miller ER, Paster-Barriuso R, Dalal D, et al. Meta-analysis: high dose vitamin E supplementation may increase all cause mortality. *Ann Int Med.* 2005;142:37–46.
15. Kalmijn S, Van Boxtel MPJ, Ocke M, et al. Dietary intake of fatty acids and fish in relation to cognitive performance at middle age. *Neurology.* 2004;62:275–280.
16. Rovio S, Kåreholt I, Helkala EL, et al. Leisure-time physical activity at midlife and the risk of dementia and Alzheimer's disease. *Lancet Neurol.* 2005;4:705–71.

18 FRAILTY

John E. Morley

DEFINITION

- Many older persons live successfully at home but are extraordinarily vulnerable to developing a marked deterioration in their ability to continue to function alone at home when exposed to a stressor, such as a urinary tract infection or a hip fracture. Persons such as this are considered frail.
- Frailty is a form of predisability and should be distinguished from functional impairment.
- Objectively, frailty is defined as having five components:
  1. Weight loss of 10 lb or more
  2. Physical exhaustion by self-report
  3. Weakness as measured by grip strength
  4. Decline in walking speed
  5. Low physical activity
- Frailty represents a condition where early intervention and appropriate prevention can prevent the onset of disability.
- The vulnerability of frail elders (>65 years of age) requires the physician to choose therapeutic interventions carefully and to avoid overtreatment, which can be disastrous.

EPIDEMIOLOGY

- Frailty occurs in 6.9% of persons older than 70 years of age.
- Frailty is more common in women than in men of the same age.
- Frailty is associated with a cascade that results in deterioration of function, hospitalization, institutionalization, and death.

CAUSES OF FRAILTY

- The major causes of frailty are as follows:
  - Sarcopenia
  - Protein energy undernutrition
  - Pain
  - Decline in executive function (cognitive decline)
  - Limited activity
  - Chronic diseases
  - Polymyalgia rheumatica
  - Apathetic presentation of endocrine disorders such as hyperthyroidism, hypothyroidism, and Addison disease (hypoadrenalism)

SARCOPENIA

- Sarcopenia is defined as age-related loss of muscle mass. In some persons there is excessive loss of muscle, similar to the excessive loss of bone that occurs in osteoporosis.
- Sarcopenia is measured by dual-energy radiograph absorptiometry and calculated as follows: appendicular skeletal mass/height^2. A person whose muscle mass is two standard deviations below the level of the sex-specific mean in adults ages 20 to 40 years is considered to have a critical level of sarcopenia. By this definition 12% of persons 60 to 70 years of age have sarcopenia.
- Fatty infiltration of muscle leads to myosteatosis and a decline in muscle power. Patients with sarcopenic obesity (also known as the *fat frail*) have the highest risk of developing future functional disability and an early death. Active obese persons tend to have a lower propensity to develop disability than obese persons who are housebound.
- There are multiple factors involved in the pathogenesis of sarcopenia. These include genetic factors. For example, persons with a single or double I allele for angiotensin-converting enzyme (ACE) generate more power than persons with the D allele. Small babies have been shown to have less strength when they reach 70 years of age than do large babies.
- The major factors in the development of sarcopenia are lack of exercise and excess production of cytokines. Interleukin-6 (the geriatric cytokine) and tumor necrosis factor-α result in activation of the muscle cell *death chamber* (ubiquitin-proteasome system) resulting in muscle atrophy, decreased strength, and functional decline.
- Anabolic steroids increase protein synthesis, inhibit the ubiquitin-proteasome system, and stimulate satellite cell production from precursor cells while inhibiting production of adipocytes. A number of highly selective androgen-receptor molecules are being developed to specifically treat sarcopenia.
- In older persons, the incorporation of amino acids into muscle protein is reduced. Older persons need higher levels of leucine and creatinine for protein synthesis than do younger persons.
- Insulin resistance leads to increased incorporation of fat into muscle and a decrease in protein synthesis. High levels of angiotensin II seen in diabetic patients stimulate the breakdown of actin and myosin in muscle. Diabetes mellitus is associated with decreased muscle strength, increased falls, and a decline in function.
- Low levels of vitamin D are associated with decreased muscle mass, increased falls, and functional deterioration. 25-hydroxyvitamin D levels in older persons should be greater than 30 ng/dL.

TREATMENT OF SARCOPENIA

- Exercise (should include all five forms of exercise):
  1. Endurance
  2. Resistance
  3. Balance
  4. Posture
  5. Flexibility
- Water exercise is particularly effective for persons with arthritis. Older persons should be encouraged to increase their spontaneous physical activity, such as getting out of the house once a day and parking as far away from their destination as possible.
- Anabolic steroids (eg, testosterone, nandrolone in males with low testosterone levels).
- Vitamin D at least 800 IU daily. Levels of 25-hydroxyvitamin D need to be measured; and if lower than 30 ng/dL, higher doses of vitamin D should be given.
- Encourage adequate caloric intake with adequate amounts of protein (1.2 g/kg/d) enriched with leucine (whey protein) and creatine (meat protein). Supplements may be necessary to obtain sufficient amounts of protein and specific amino acids.
- Assess for peripheral vascular disease (Doppler assessment of the ankle-brachial index) and aggressively treat.
- Advise on the use of a cane or walker to reduce the incidence of falls.
- If the patient has hypertension, congestive heart failure, or diabetes mellitus, use an ACE inhibitor, because these agents appear to increase muscle strength.

POLYMYALGIA RHEUMATICA

- An inflammatory condition of older persons presenting with proximal muscle weakness and muscle pain. It is associated with an elevated erythrocyte sedimentation rate and C-reactive protein. May be associated with weight loss and depression.
- May be associated with temporal arteritis. Accordingly, visual problems associated with muscle weakness require a temporal artery biopsy.
- Treatment includes prednisone 15 to 20 mg daily. Always administer vitamin D and bisphosphonate to prevent bone loss.

ANEMIA AND FRAILTY

- Anemia is associated with fatigue, orthostasis, cognitive impairment, mobility impairment, functional deterioration, and falls in older persons.
- All older persons with a hemoglobin of 12 g/dL or less must have their anemia fully evaluated.
- If the corrected reticulocyte count is elevated, either hemolysis or hemorrhage is a cause for the anemia. If the corrected reticulocyte count is not elevated, there is either a nutritional cause (iron deficiency, vitamin B_{12} deficiency, folate deficiency, or protein deficiency) or bone marrow failure (myelodysplasia, infiltration, anemia of chronic disease, or anemia of chronic kidney failure).
- Myelodysplasia presents with only a low hemoglobin in 50% of persons. This condition can be successfully treated with a combination of granulocyte colony-stimulating factor, recombinant human granulocyte-macrophage colony-stimulating factor, and recombinant erythropoietin along with supportive therapy.
- Many instances of anemia in older persons are associated with chronic kidney disease. This type of anemia is highly responsive to erythropoietin or darbepoietin alpha. Kidney failure is often missed in older persons because of *masked renal failure*. This is caused by loss of muscle mass leading to pseudonormalization of the serum creatinine level. Thus, the creatinine clearance should be calculated in all persons older than 70 years of age.

ENDOCRINE CAUSES OF FRAILTY

- Apathetic hyperthyroidism presents with blepharoptosis (hooded eyes), proximal weakness, atrial fibrillation, weight loss, and depression. The supersensitive thyroid-stimulating hormone (TSH) level may be normal and the diagnosis requires measuring a free thyroxine by dialysis.

TABLE 18–1   Frailty Mnemonic for the Management of Frailty

Food intake maintained/avoid weight loss
Resistance exercises
Atherosclerosis prevention
Isolation avoidance/treat depression
Limit pain, use morphine if necessary
Tai Chi or other balance exercises
Yearly check for vitamin D deficiency

- Addison's disease can present with weakness, weight loss, abdominal pain, and fatigue. These patients have low or low-normal sodium, a mildly elevated potassium, and eosinophilia. The diagnosis is established with a cosyntropin stimulation test and measuring the cortisol at 30 minutes compared to the baseline value.
- Hypothyroidism can present insidiously as a frailty syndrome, and a TSH should be obtained in all frail persons.
- Vitamin B_{12} deficiency can present as frailty without anemia in the older person.

FRAILTY MANAGEMENT

- The management of frailty is complex. The general strategies to prevent frailty are outlined in Table 18–1. Management of frailty includes appropriate treatment of underlying diseases but the physician must take care to avoid polypharmacy resulting in side effects caused by drug-drug interactions. The key to preventing functional loss is aggressive treatment of pain (with opiates if necessary), as well as depression (with electroconvulsive therapy if necessary). Prevention of hip fracture with calcium, vitamin D, and bisphosphonates and the judicious use of hip pads when the person is having recurrent falls is also essential to limit disability in frail persons.

BIBLIOGRAPHY

Fried LP, Ferrucci L, Darer J, et al. Untangling the concepts of disability, frailty, and comorbidity: implications for improved targeting and care. *J Gerontol A Biol Sci Med Sci*. 2004;59:255.

Fried LP, Tangen CM, Walston J, et al. Frailty in older adults: evidence for phenotype. *J Gerontol A Biol Sci Med Sci*. 2001; 56A:M146.

Morley JE, Baumgartner RN, Roubenoff R, et al. Sarcopenia. *J Lab Clin Med*. 2001;137:231.

Morley JE, Haren MT, Rolland Y, et al. Frailty. *Med Clin North Am*. 2006;90:837.

19 NUTRITION IN OLDER ADULTS

David R. Thomas

TABLE 19–1   **Causes of Anorexia in Older Persons**

Adverse drug effects
Anorexia resulting from the physiologic changes of aging
Decrease in taste or smell
Alterations in the neurotransmitter regulators of food intake
Terminal anorexia of malnutrition

INTRODUCTION

- Nutrition is essential at every stage of life. Importantly, certain characteristics of aging account for more observed nutritional problems in older persons.
- First, adequate nutrition is influenced by physiologic changes in older persons, including slower gastric emptying, altered hormonal responses, decreased basal metabolic rate, and altered taste and smell. Anorexia, a failure of appetite regulation, is a chief cause of decreased nutrient intake in older persons (Table 19–1). Other factors such as marital status, income, education, socioeconomic status, diet-related attitudes and beliefs, and convenience play a role as well.
- Second, adequate nutrition is affected by comorbid conditions in older persons. Coexisting medical diseases and psychologic factors have a tremendous impact on appetite and weight loss (Table 19–2).
- Third, physicians often fail to assess and address nutrition in older persons.

EPIDEMIOLOGY

- The nutritional status of older adults living at home is poor. Persons older than the age of 70 years consume one-third less calories compared to younger persons. Energy intakes of older men range from 2100 to 2300 calories per day compared to younger men who consume 2700 calories per day. Ten percent of older men and 20% of older women have intakes of protein below the U.S. recommended daily allowance (RDA), and one-third consume fewer calories than the RDA. Fifty percent of older adults have intakes of minerals and vitamins less than the RDA, and 10% to 30% have subnormal levels of minerals and vitamins. Of community-dwelling elderly persons, 16% to 18% consume less than 1000 kcal daily.
- Undernutrition reportedly occurs in 5% to 12% of community-dwelling older persons. In higher risk populations, such as sheltered housing, the proportion increases to 20%. Thirty percent to 40% of men and women older than 75 years of age are at least 10% underweight. Up to 11% of adults attending a medical outpatient clinic are undernourished.[1]
- Acute illness is characterized by a spontaneous decrease in food intake, occurring both before and during hospitalization. In the month before hospitalization, 65% of

the men and 69% of the women had an insufficient energy intake, and undernutrition was present in 53% of men and 61% of women by the time of admission to the hospital.
- The prevalence of undernutrition ranges between 32% to 50% in hospitalized persons. The reasons for this high prevalence include poor recognition and monitoring of nutritional status, and inadequate intake of nutrients for days at a time. Moreover, older persons are often discharged from the hospital with a poor nutritional status.
- More than 90% of older persons admitted to a skilled-care facility after hospitalization have undernutrition or are at high risk of undernutrition.[2] Prevalence rates for protein-energy malnutrition in nursing home residents range from 23% to 85%.
- In medical outpatients, up to 11% of older persons are undernourished, and 90% have reversible causes of undernutrition, which are often overlooked.
- These data suggest that a large number of older adults are undernourished, with prevalence increasing to over one-half of older adults in selected populations.

DEFINITIONS

- *Starvation* is caused by a lack of food. Historically, starvation has been divided into *kwashiorkor*, a relatively greater reduction in dietary protein compared to calories, and *marasmus*, a more balanced lack of both protein and calories in the diet. A key part of the definition of starvation requires that the deficit can be reversed solely by the administration of food.
- *Sarcopenia* is an age-related decrease in skeletal muscle mass. This decline in skeletal muscle mass is thought to be mediated by physical inactivity, hormonal influences, or extreme dieting. Although weight loss is not always present, older persons with sarcopenia often exhibit signs of muscle wasting. The deficit is not related to food intake and cannot be reversed by feeding.
- *Cachexia* is a wasting syndrome of both fat and muscle mass that is related to the cytokine-induced effects of disease. Cachexia has been associated with a number of chronic disease conditions, including cancer, acquired immunodeficiency syndrome, renal failure, chronic obstructive lung disease, chronic heart failure, and rheumatologic diseases.[3] A hallmark of

TABLE 19–2 Medical Conditions Associated with Protein Energy–Undernutrition

MEDICAL CONDITION	INCREASED METABOLISM	ANOREXIA	MECHANISM SWALLOWING DIFFICULTIES	MALABSORPTION
Cardiac disease	X	X		X
Cancer	X	X	X	X
Pulmonary disease	X	X		X
Infection(s)		X		X
AIDS	X	X	X	X
Tuberculosis	X	X		
Esophageal candidiasis		X	X	
Alcoholism	X	X		X
Rheumatoid arthritis	X	X	X	X
Gallbladder disease		X		
Malabsorption syndromes				X
Hyperthyroidism/ hyperparathyroidism	X	X		
Parkinson disease	X			
Essential tremors	X			

AIDS, acquired immunodeficiency syndrome.

the cachexia syndrome is that it is remarkably resistant to correction by hypercaloric refeeding.

- Clinicians frequently confuse the effect of cytokine-induced acute-phase reactants on biochemical variables with undernutrition. However, these biochemical markers are not specific for nutritional status. For example, hypoalbuminemia occurs in disease states such as hepatic disease, renal disease, congestive heart failure, stress, and even occurs after 8 hours of bed rest. Most hepatic proteins, such as transthyretin, transferrin, and retinol-binding protein, which are often used in the diagnosis of undernutrition are also negative acute-phase reactants. Cachexia must be clearly distinguished from starvation (Table 19–3).

DIAGNOSIS

- There is no gold standard for the diagnosis of undernutrition. Historically, the combination of a decrease in hepatic proteins, such as albumin, and a loss of body mass has been used to diagnose undernutrition.
- Body weight is easily measured and a critical first sign of undernutrition. Body weight can be adjusted for height by calculating the body mass index (BMI) (BMI = weight in kilograms divided by height in meters squared). Age and gender-adjusted BMIs below 19 in men and 19.4 in women have been used to define undernutrition. An increased risk of death has been shown to begin at a body mass index <23.5 in men and <22.0 in women. In hospitalized adults with serious illness, excess mortality within 6 months has been demonstrated when the body mass index is <20. The increase in mortality is linear—the lower the BMI, the greater the risk.

- Several screening instruments have been developed for use in assessing undernutrition. The first type aims at identifying persons at risk for malnutrition but is not used to diagnose clinical malnutrition. The Nutritional Screening Initiative is an example of this type of instrument.
- Other instruments have been developed to diagnose malnutrition. The Mini-Nutritional Assessment (MNA) was developed to assess malnutrition in older populations. Using the validated cutoffs of adequate nutritional status (MNA score ≥24), at-risk for malnutrition (MNA score between 17 and 23.5), and malnutrition (MNA score <17), the sensitivity is 96%, and

TABLE 19–3 Distinguishing Starvation from Cachexia

	STARVATION	CACHEXIA
Appetite	Suppressed in late phase	Suppressed in early phase
Body mass index	Not predictive of mortality	Predictive of mortality
Serum albumin	Low in late phase	Low in early phase
Transthyretin	Low in late phase	Low in early phase
Transferrin	Low	Low
Retinol binding protein	Low	Low
Cholesterol	May remain normal	Low
Total lymphocyte count	Low, responds to refeeding	Low, unresponsive to refeeding
C-reactive protein	Little data	Elevated
Inflammatory disease	Usually not present	Present
Response to refeeding	Reversible	Resistant

specificity is 98%, with a positive predictive value of 97% for undernutrition.[4]

- The Subjective Global Assessment instrument was developed to assess the risk of hospital complications in patients undergoing gastrointestinal surgery. The Subjective Global Assessment is useful in predicting surgical complications. The likelihood ratios for major complications, septic complications, and pneumonia was 0.53 in the well nourished group, 0.69 in the mildly to moderately malnourished group, and 1.8 in the severely malnourished group.

- The Simplified Nutritional Assessment Questionnaire (SNAQ) is a four-question instrument to assess appetite in older persons. Scores on the SNAQ prospectively predict weight loss in older persons.[5]

TREATMENT

- Management of undernutrition should first be directed to assessing risk factors and removing obvious causes.

- Anorexia can be associated with illness, drugs, dementia, or mood disorders. Decreased food intake can result from dysphagia, chewing problems, nausea, vomiting, diarrhea, pain, or fecal impaction. Increased metabolic requirements can be precipitated by fever, infection, or the presence of acute wounds. Treatment of these conditions can restore appetite and body weight.

- A mnemonic, MEALS ON WHEELS, is useful in considering the potential treatable causes of malnutrition (Table 19–4).[6] The SCALES (Sadness, Cholesterol, Albumin, Loss of weight, Eat, and Shopping) mnemonic is a useful test in an outpatient setting where albumin and cholesterol levels are available.

- Inappropriate restriction of an older persons diet (low salt, calorie restriction, no concentrated sweets) should be avoided. Unpalatability because of overly restrictive diets can cause decreased intake.[7]

- Depression is a major cause of weight loss in long-term care settings, accounting for up to 36% of residents with weight loss. An evaluation for depression, using the Geriatric Depression Scale, should be obtained on all patients with anorexia.

- Delirium caused by acute illness and/or pain can be a reversible cause of decreased dietary intake. Reversal of delirium can result in resumption of appetite.

- Drugs have been found to be a cause of weight loss in long-term care residents. All drugs potentially aggravating anorexia should be discontinued.

- Certain causes of malnutrition can be irreversible. Palliative care, including orexigenic drugs, enteral or parenteral feeding, consistent with the person's wishes, should be considered.

TABLE 19–4 The Meals on Wheels Mnemonic

Medications (eg, digoxin, theophylline, antipsychotics)
Emotional problems (depression)
Anorexia tardive (nervosa/alcoholism)
Late-life paranoia
Swallowing disorders

Oral problems
Nosocomial infections (tuberculosis, *Helicobacter pylori, Clostridium difficile*)

Wandering and other dementia-related behaviors
Hypertheyroidism/hypercalcemia/hypoadrenalism
Eenteric problems (malabsorption)
Eating problems
Low-salt, low-cholesterol diets
Stones (cholelithiasis)

- A management algorithm for the management of undernutrition in older adults has also been developed.[8]

- True starvation responds to refeeding. In starvation, provision of adequate calories and protein will reverse the wasting syndrome and restore the older person to health. Increased nutrient intake can be achieved through the use of calorie-dense foods. Exercise can increase dietary intake. Nutritional supplementation can increase dietary intake and produce weight gain. Nutritional supplementation must be given between meals so as not to substitute for calorie intake at meals. Reasonable nutritional requirements are summarized in Table 19–5.

- In persons who cannot consume adequate nutrition because of impaired swallowing enteral feeding through a percutaneous gastrostomy can be life saving. When the enteral route cannot be utilized total parenteral nutrition can be life saving, but is associated with an increase in infectious complications. Total parenteral nutrition should not initiated for persons with a limited life expectancy (less than 3 months).

- Cachexia is remarkably resistant to hypercaloric refeeding. In cachexia, the primary goal is to control the cytokine excess caused by the underlying medical condition.

- Observational data have shown that a number of pharmacologic agents can improve appetite and produce weight gain.[9] The effect on body weight can be caused by modulating the effects of excessive cytokine levels.

TABLE 19–5 Calculating Nutritional Requirements

	CLINICAL CONDITION	AMOUNT
Protein	Maintenance	1.2 to 1.5 g/kg/d
	Stress[a]	1.5 to 2.0 g/kg/d
Calories	Maintenance	25–30 kcal/kg/d
	Stress	30–35 kcal/kg/d
Free water		30–35 mL/kg/d

[a]Stress generally refers to persons with burns, wounds, cancer, infections, and other similar conditions.

REFERENCES

1. Wilson MM, Vaswani S, Liu D, Morley JE, Miller DK. Prevalence and causes of undernutrition in medical outpatients. *Am J Med.* 1998;104;56–63.
2. Thomas DR, Zdrowski CD, Wilson MM, et al. Malnutrition in subacute care. *Am J Clin Nutr.* 2002;75:308–813.
3. Thomas DR. Distinguishing starvation from cachexia. *Geriatric Clinics of North America.* 2002;18:883–892.
4. Guigoz Y, Vellas B. The mini-nutritional assessment for grading the nutritional state of elderly patients: presentation of the MNA, history and validation. Nestle Nutrition Workshop Series: Clinical & Performance Programme; no. 1. Denges, Switzerland; 1998:1–2.
5. Wilson MM, Thomas DR, Rubenstein LZ, et al. Appetite assessment: simple appetite questionnaire predicts weight loss in community-dwelling adults and nursing home residents. *Am J Clin Nutr.* 2005;82(5):1074–1081.
6. Morley JE, Silver AJ. Nutritional issues in nursing home care. *Ann Intern Med.* 1995;123:850–859.
7. Tariq S, Thomas DR, Morley JE, et al. The use of a no–concentrated-sweets diet in the management of type 2 diabetes in the nursing home. *J Am Diet Assoc.* 2001;101(12):1463–1466.
8. Thomas DR, Ashmen W, Morley JE, Evans JE. Nutritional management in long-term care: development of a clinical guideline. *Journal of Gerontology: Medical Sciences.* 2000;55: 725–734.
9. Thomas DR. Guidelines for the use of orexigenic drugs in long-term care. *Nutr Clin Pract.* 2006;21(1):82–87.

20 GEROPHARMACOLOGY

Joseph H. Flaherty

PRINCIPLES AND CHALLENGES OF GEROPHARMACOLOGY

- The principles of geropharmacology are based on the appropriate use of drugs to produce the greatest *benefit* to older persons while avoiding or decreasing the *risks* of adverse drug reactions (*ADRs*) and adverse drug events (*ADEs*).
- The challenge prescribers face when caring for older persons is that the patients often are afflicted by several chronic conditions that are amenable to FDA approved *medications*, accordingly = increasing the *number of medications* seems to be unavoidable. The conundrum is highlighted by studies that reveal a higher incidence ADRs and ADEs in patients receiving multiple drugs.

- When faced with this challenge, an evaluation of risks versus benefits supersedes indications.

EVALUATION OF BENEFITS

EVALUATION OF BENEFITS: COMPREHENSIVE GERIATRIC ASSESSMENT, LIFE EXPECTANCY, AND PRIORITIZING OUTCOMES

- Studies using comprehensive geriatric assessment (CGA) with the proper interventions have been shown to improve or maintain function, improve quality of life, and prevent institutionalization. Since evaluation of the benefits of drug therapy for older persons involves more than just whether or not the drug is indicated (eg, bisphosphonates improve bone density), the prescriber can employ the CGA to guide decisions regarding benefits that are most applicable or important to the individual patient (see Chap. 15, Geriatric Assessment). The CGA can also aid in identifying patients at risk for certain ADRs and ADEs (eg, the CGA is more accurate than a conventional medical evaluation in identifying patients at risk for falls or those with a baseline cognitive problem who might be at risk for central nervous system side effects of a drug).
- Life expectancy should be used to facilitate decisions about therapeutic versus preventive drug therapy (Table 20–1). If certain drugs require years to exert a beneficial effect, the benefit is likely outweighed by the risk of side effects. In addition, one should utilize the CGA to identify patients who are frail and have a shortened life expectancy.
- Outcomes or benefits that are important to older persons are similar to those of younger persons, (eg, mortality), but *prioritization* of the outcomes may change, and outcomes related to maintaining or improving physical function (eg, as measured by activities of

TABLE 20–1 Life Expectancy Table

MEN	YEARS STILL TO LIVE					
At age Health Status	70	75	80	85	90	95
Healthy	18.0	14.2	10.8	7.9	5.8	4.3
Average	12.4	9.3	6.7	4.7	3.2	2.3
Frail	6.7	4.9	3.3	2.2	1.5	1.0
WOMEN	YEARS STILL TO LIVE					
At age Health Status	70	75	80	85	90	95
Healthy	21.3	17.0	13.0	9.6	6.8	4.8
Average	15.7	11.9	8.6	5.9	3.9	2.7
Frail	9.5	6.8	4.6	2.9	1.8	1.7

SOURCE: Modified using: Centers for Disease Control; www.cdc.gov/nchs/datawh/statab/unpubd/mortlabs/lewk3.htm

daily living) or cognitive function and prevention of institutionalization (eg, nursing home admission) become more important for persons who are frail, have dementia, or are at the end of life.

- Benefits may also be measured using a calculation of the number needed to treat (NNT). Since many studies do not report this number, knowing how to calculate NNT may prove especially useful: NNT = 1/ARR (absolute risk reduction).

EVALUATION OF RISKS

- Risks or side effects of drugs that are associated with or can lead to a decline in physical or cognitive function should be given special consideration by the prescriber (Table 20–2).
- ADRs are defined by the World Health Organization (WHO) as "noxious or unintended reactions, which occur at doses used for prophylaxis, diagnosis or therapy." These can be idiosyncratic and unexpected, or may be listed as side effects of the drugs. These do not include occurrences arising out of a dosing error, eg, such events would be described as ADEs.
- ADEs are further defined as an injury resulting from medical intervention relating to a drug. For example, an injury may include a fracture secondary to a fall precipitated by orthostatic hypotension. Moreover, orthostatic hypotension leading to a fall may, in turn, engender a fear of falling, with subsequent loss of physical function and requirement for nursing home placement. As many as 30% of hospital admissions among older patients may be linked to ADEs. In one study, 35% of ambulatory older patients had an ADE and 29% required a physician visit, emergency department visit, or hospitalization.[1]
- Although there is overlap in the use of the terms *ADR*, *ADE*, and medication *side effects*, (eg, constipation from a narcotic could be considered any of the three), the most important concerning geropharmacology is ADE; ADEs encompass the broadest scenarios that may affect older persons, and ADEs are seen as more preventable than ADRs and side effects. It also encourages

TABLE 20–2 Risks or Side Effects of Medications of Special Importance for the Elderly

Falls
Weakness
Fatigue
Cognitive changes such as delirium or depression
Anorexia
Weight loss
Urinary frequency or incontinence
Lightheadedness or dizziness

the prescriber to be more vigilant and suspicious of drugs that are prescribed.

- Risks may also be measured using a calculation of the number needed to harm (NNH). NNH = 1/ARR of having a side effect. Although NNH may be helpful to predict the subsequent risk of ADRs, it is not useful in predicting the risk of ADEs.
  ○ Clinical example: An 85-year-old woman lives in her own home and is independent in her activities of daily living (ADLs) but partially dependent in her instrumental activities of daily living (IADLs). She is frail with several comorbidities including congestive heart failure and diabetes, with a life expectancy of less than 4 years. She is already on seven medications, including aspirin, calcium supplements, and vitamin D. She has never had any fractures, but her bone mineral density (BMD) is consistent with osteoporosis. Should she take a bisphosphonate? Answer: If the bisphosphonate has only been shown to improve BMD over 4 years but *not* decrease the risk of a fracture, which might otherwise lead to institutionalization (more important outcome), the risks of side effects (which could lead to a decline in function) may be greater than the less important outcome (improved BMD). Thus, although there is a clear *indication* for the use of the bisphosphonate, the evaluation of *risks versus benefits supersedes* this.

PRACTICAL APPROACHES TO AVOIDING OR DECREASING RISKS

- In order to avoid or decrease the risk of ADRs and ADEs, the most important factors for prescribers to consider are
  Number of medications
  Specific medications which are considered potentially inappropriate for use among older persons
  Pharmacodynamics and pharmacokinetics of drugs
- Age as an *absolute number* is the least important factor because as people age, variation (standard deviation) increases. However, because there are some well-recognized age-related changes (as noted below) and because the older population has a higher prevalence of chronic diseases, frailty, and functional disabilities compared to the younger population, this group is at higher risk for ADRs and ADEs. It is in this sense that age is a factor when prescribing drugs.
- Number of medications
  ○ Depending on where older patients reside or are receiving their healthcare, the number of medications vary. On average, community-dwelling older persons take approximately five medications, patients requiring

home care services take six, nursing home residents take seven to nine, and hospitalized patients receive 10.[2]

○ An increased number of drugs is associated with

Increased risk of ADRs/ADEs

Severity of ADRs/ADEs

Poor compliance

Medication errors

Increased risk for hospitalization

- An exponential relationship exists for ADRs, so that for patients on two to three drugs, the risk is 10%; with five to six drugs the risk is 20% to 30%, but with 10 or more drugs, the risk of adverse effects approaches 100%.[3]

- Compliance is the second most common reason for hospitalization associated with polypharmacy.[4]

- As many as 50% of discharged patients will encounter a medication error, and patients on five or more drugs discharged from the hospital have medication error rates as high as 70%.[5]

- In a study of patients receiving home care, patients taking 10 or more medications doubled the risk of hospitalization, despite similar illnesses.[2]

- Importantly, reducing the number of medications in order to reduce the risk of ADRs/ADEs and improve compliance has been shown to be safe and effective.

- For example, one study of older patients (age ≥65 years) showed that in the medication reduction group ($n = 70$, average number of drugs = 13, range 10–26), reducing the average number of drugs to 8, compared to the usual care group ($n = 50$, average number of drugs = 13, range 10–21; no change in average number of medications), resulted in fewer hospitalizations (38/70, 54% vs 42/50, 84%; respectively, $P <0.05$) and fewer (not statistically significant) number of deaths (7/70, 10% vs 10/50, 20%; respectively, $P = NS$).[6]

- A practical approach to proper medication use and medication reduction is described by the mnemonic AVOID TOO MANY.

Alternatives: When possible, use *nonmedication* interventions instead of a medication.

Vague symptoms: Avoid treating vague symptoms with drugs, such as vague gastrointestinal symptoms with proton pump inhibitors.

Over-the-counter (OTC) medications: These count as drugs.

Interaction: Always look for these. Notorious offenders for drug-drug interactions include antihistamines, seizure medications, some antibiotics, and warfarin.

Duration: The physician and patient need to determine and discuss how long a drug will be used. This is primarily related to *symptomatic* medications.

Therapeutic versus preventive: Especially for frail older patients or those with shortened life expectancy,

priority should be given to treating illnesses that are already present, before focusing on preventive medications.

Once-a-day drugs: These can simplify medication regimens, but once-a-day medications are often more expensive than the twice, thrice, or four times a day drugs.

Other prescribers: A reminder to be careful when referring patients to multiple specialists. Specialists often feel obligated to "do something" and that something often results in another medication or two.

Money: Buying medications is an issue for most patients. Persons on numerous medications often will buy the ones that are more affordable instead of the ones that are most important.

Adverse effects: Adverse effects or side effects of other drugs should rarely be treated with the addition of other drugs. Exception: constipation with narcotics.

Need: The prescriber should ask him or herself, "Does my patient really need this medication—will it make a difference in my patient's quality of life, life expectancy, functional status, or some other aspect of life?"

Yes/No: before prescribing new drugs or adjusting the current regimen, find out if the patient is actually taking the existing drugs, and if not, why not (eg, due to side effects, costs).

- Nonprescription drug use (OTC medications) among the elderly is sevenfold that of the general adult population compared to twofold for prescription drugs.[3] Some OTC drugs can be as dangerous as prescription drugs.

○ Commonly used drugs in this category include pseudoephedrine containing preparations, nonsteroidal anti-inflammatory drugs (NSAIDs), H2 blockers, and sleeping aids.

SPECIFIC MEDICATIONS WHICH ARE POTENTIALLY INAPPROPRIATE FOR USE AMONG OLDER PERSONS

- The Beers Criteria for potentially inappropriate medication use among older persons was developed using a modified Delphi method (a set of procedures and methods for formulating a group judgment or consensus on a subject for which precise data are lacking). The latest revision and update covered two types of inappropriate medication use: (1) medications or classes of medications that should generally be avoided in persons >65 years of age because they are either ineffective or they pose unnecessary risks and safer alternatives are available (48 individual medications or classes of medications were identified in this category), (2) medications that

should not be used in older persons known to have specific medical conditions (20 individual medications or classes were identified in this category).[7]
- Tables 20–3 and 20–4 include a partial list of the above.

PHARMACODYNAMICS AND PHARMACOKINETICS[8]

- Table 20–5 describes important pharmacologic changes associated with aging and the resultant clinical effects.
- Pharmacodynamics relates to the responsiveness or sensitivity to a particular drug at a given concentration. Although pharmacodynamics is less extensively studied than pharmacokinetics, three generalizations can be made.
  - Sensitivity to drugs may increase (eg, with sedatives or narcotics) or decrease with age (eg, less sensitive to drugs affecting β-adrenergic receptors).
  - The response of older persons to any given medication is variable, so knowledge of common side effects and minimizing use of drugs is essential.
  - Age-related changes, underlying diseases, or frailty (see Chap. 18, Frailty) may increase sensitivity to drugs. Examples include
    - Increased risk of orthostatic hypotension because of age-related changes in the autonomic nervous system and decreased baroreceptor function.
    - Increased risk for acute cognitive changes (such as delirium) in persons with dementia, both vascular and Alzheimer type, who are given any centrally acting drug.
    - Because frail patients have diminished reserve, even minor side effects such as constipation or urinary frequency can lead to poor outcomes, such as decreased function or falls.
- Pharmacokinetics is the study of drug absorption, distribution, metabolism and elimination.
  - Absorption
    - Although there are age related changes in gastric motility and blood flow (usually a decrease) and pH (usually an increase), drug absorption is not typically affected, unless there are other underlying gastrointestinal problems (eg, diabetic gastroparesis). There is little information in the elderly concerning absorption of delayed-release, transdermal, or transbronchial formulations to formulate guidelines concerning these types of drugs.

TABLE 20–3   Potentially Inappropriate Medication Use in Older Adults Independent of Diagnosis

DRUG	CONCERN
Propoxyphene (Darvon) and combination products (Darvon with ASA, Darvon-N, Darvocet-N)	Offers few analgesic advantages over acetaminophen, yet has the adverse effects of other narcotics
Indomethacin	Of all available NSAIDs, this drug produces most CNS adverse effects
Muscle relaxants and antispasmodics: methocarbamol (Robaxin), carisoprodol (Soma), Chlorzoxazone (Paraflex), metaxalone (Skelaxin), cyclobenzaprine (Flexeril), oxybutynin (Ditropan)	Most muscle relaxants and antispasmodics are poorly tolerated by elderly patients, since these engender anticholinergic adverse effects, sedation and weakness. Additionally, their effectiveness at doses tolerated by the elderly is questionable
Amitriptyline (Elavil), Chlordiazepoxide-amitriptyline (Limbitrol), and perphenazine-amitriptyline (Triavil)	Because of its strong anticholinergic and sedation properties, amitriptyline is rarely the antidepressant of choice for elderly
Doses of short-acting benzodiazepines (BDZ): doses greater than lorazepam (Ativan), 3 mg; oxazepam (Serax), 60 mg; alprazolam (Xanax), 2 mg; temazepam (Restoril), 15 mg; triazolam (Halcion), 0.25 mg	These drugs have a long half-life in the elderly, producing sedation and increasing risk for falls. Short- and intermediate-acting BDZs are preferred if a BDZ is required
Digoxin (Lanoxin) (should not exceed >0.125 mg/day except when treating atrial arrhythmias)	Decreased renal clearance may lead to increased risk of toxic effects
Meperidine (Demerol)	Not an effective oral analgesic in doses commonly used, may cause confusion and has many disadvantages compared to other narcotics
Ketorolac (Toradol)	Immediate and long-term use should be avoided
Daily fluoxetine (Prozac)	Long half-life and risk of producing excessive side effects, sleep disturbance, and increasing agitation. Safer antidepressants available.
Short acting nifedipine (Procardia, Adalat)	Potential for hypotension
Clonidine (Catapres)	Potential for CNS adverse effects
Estrogens only (oral)	Evidence of carcinogenic effects and lack of cardioprotection

BDZ, benzodiazepine; CNS, central nervous system; NSAID, nonsteroidal anti-inflammatory drug

SOURCE: Fick DM, Cooper JW, Wade WE, et al. Updating the Beers Criteria for potentially inappropriate medication use in older adults: results of a US consensus panel of experts. *Arch Intern Med.* 2003;163(22):2716–2724.

TABLE 20–4 Potentially Inappropriate Medication Use in Older Adults: Considering Diagnoses or Conditions

DISEASE OR CONDITION	DRUG	CONCERN
Hypertension	Phenylpropanolamine HCl, pseudoephedrine, diet pills, amphetamines	May produce elevation of blood pressure
Gastric and duodenal ulcers	NSAIDs and aspirin (>325 mg) (coxibs excluded)	May exacerbate ulcers or produce new ones
Bladder outflow obstruction	Anticholinergics and antihistamines, GI antispasmodics, muscle relaxants, anticholinergics, antidepressants	May decrease urinary flow, leading to urinary retention
Arrhythmias	Tricyclic antidepressants	Proarrhythmic effect and ability to produce QT interval prolongation
Insomnia	Decongestants, theophylline, methylphenidate, amphetamines	Concern about CNS stimulation
Parkinson disease	Metoclopramide, conventional antipsychotics	Concern about anticholinergic/dopaminergic effect
Cognitive impairment	Barbiturates, anticholinergics, antispasmodics, muscle relaxants	Concern about CNS altering effects
Depression	Long-term BDZ use, sympatholytic agents (methyldopa, reserpine)	May exacerbate depression
Anorexia and malnutrition	CNS stimulants, fluoxetine, methylphenidate	Concern due to appetite suppressing effect
Syncope/falls	Short-to intermediate-acting BDZs, tricyclic antidepressants	May induce ataxia, impaired psychomotor activity
SIADH/hyponatremia	Fluoxetine, citalopram, fluvoxamine, paroxetine, sertraline	May cause SIADH
Seizure disorder	Bupropion (Wellbutrin), clozapine (Clozaril)	May lower seizure threshold
COPD	Long-acting BDZs, propranolol	May induce respiratory depression
Chronic constipation	TCAs, anticholinergics, calcium channel blockers	May exacerbate constipation

BDZ, benzodiazepine; CNS, central nervous system; COPD, chronic obstructive pulmonary disease; GI, gastrointestinal; NSAID, nonsteroidal anti-inflammatory drug ; SIADH, syndrome of inappropriate antidiuretic hormone secretion; TCA, tricyclic antidepressant
SOURCE: Fick DM, Cooper JW, Wade WE, et al. Updating the Beers Criteria for potentially inappropriate medication use in older adults: Results of a US consensus panel of experts. *Arch Intern Med.* 2003;163(22):2716–2724.

- It is also important to recognize whether a drug is better absorbed with food (eg, megestrol acetate) or without food (eg, levodopa/carbidopa).
- Distribution
  - Two concepts to remember concerning drug distribution in the elderly are protein binding and volume of distribution.
    - Serum albumin is a major drug-binding protein. This protein declines in hospitalized patients due to cytokine excess and malnutrition. Accordingly, highly protein-bound drugs will have a higher than expected free drug level in the body, often resulting in toxicity.
      - Commonly used drugs in this category include: phenytoin, warfarin, NSAIDs.
  - When ordering serum drug levels in older patients, therapeutic ranges routinely reported may not be an appropriate guide to determine toxicity or efficacy because these ranges have typically been studied in younger people and do not usually take into account protein binding.

TABLE 20–5 Age-Related Changes Pertinent to Geropharmacology

PARAMETER	AGE-RELATED CHANGES	CLINICAL EFFECT
Tissue sensitivity	Alteration in receptor number and affinity	Patients may be more or less sensitive to a drug
Absorption	Gastric motility and blood flow (decrease) Gastric pH (increase)	Insignificant, unless there are other underlying gastrointestinal diseases
Distribution	Total body water and lean body mass (decrease → Vd decrease) Total body fat (increase → Vd increase)	Water-soluble drugs → higher plasma concentration Fat-soluble drugs → longer half-life
Metabolism	Reductions of hepatic blood flow and decline in phase I drug metabolism	Decreased clearance of drugs metabolized by liver; first-pass metabolism also affected
Excretion	Renal blood flow reduced and renal clearance declines	Longer half-life and/or higher serum concentrations

SOURCE: Cepeda OA, Morley JE. Polypharmacy, is it another disease? In: Pathy MS, Sinclair AJ, Morley JE, eds. *Principles and Practice of Geriatric Medicine. 4th ed.* London: John Wiley & Sons, Ltd; 2006:215–221.

- Vd is a virtual space in a given patient which a particular drug occupies. Two common changes that occur with age which affect Vd are:
  - Decrease in total body water and lean body mass → Decreases Vd
  - Increase in total body fat → Increases Vd
- If Vd is decreased, then drugs that distribute into this compartment (eg, water-soluble drugs), will distribute less effectively resulting in a higher plasma concentration, placing patients at increased risk for side effects.
  - Drugs with a decreased Vd in the elderly include digoxin, aminoglycosides and other antibiotics, atenolol, sotalol, theophylline, hydrochlorothiazide, lithium, and several sedative-hypnotics. Alcohol is also included in this category.
- If the Vd for a drug is increased, (eg, fat-soluble drugs) the drug will have a significantly longer half-life, thus, increasing the risk for side effects.
  - Commonly used drugs with an increased Vd in the elderly include amiodarone, desipramine, diazepam, haloperidol
- Elimination
  - Predicting risks of ADRs and ADEs related to drug elimination is dependent on clearance and half-life, as described by the following relationship:

$$t1/2 = 0.693 \times Vd/Clearance$$

  - If clearance is decreased, $t1/2$ is increased, and the patient is clearly at higher risk for side effects.
- The two major sites of drug clearance are the liver and kidneys, with lung and the gastrointestinal track playing a lesser role. Hepatic drug metabolism
  - Most drugs that are metabolized by the liver will become inactive compounds.
  - Occasionally, a drug is metabolized to an active compound, (eg, codeine is metabolized to morphine)
  - Liver size may decline with age, and reductions of hepatic blood flow of 25% to 47% have been reported in persons between 25 and 90 years of age.
  - Drugs that undergo "first-pass" metabolism by the liver depend on hepatic blood flow. If hepatic blood

flow is decreased, it may lead to increased bioavailability of the drug, thus increasing the risk for side effects. Unfortunately, there are no simple methods to quantitate hepatic blood flow in the elderly.

- Commonly used drugs which are hepatically metabolized include many of the antipsychotics, narcotic analgesics, propranolol, tricyclic antidepressants (TCAs), theophylline.
  - Hepatic biotransformation (or metabolism) of drugs can involve either phase I or II reactions (see below). Most studies support an age-related decline in phase I drug metabolism, which is more prominent for men than women. Phase II metabolism is less affected or not affected by age.
  - The cytochrome P450 (CYP) system of the liver is the main enzyme responsible for phase I reactions. Approximately 1000 CYP enzymes are known, but only 50 are functionally active in humans. The clinician should be aware of 5 of these enzymes (see Table 20–6). The prescriber should also know if a drug is a substrate, inducer, or inhibitor of the specific enzyme. Substrates are those agents that are metabolized by a particular P450 enzyme. Inhibitors impair the ability of specific P450 enzymes to metabolize their target substrates, thus producing increased blood levels of those substrates. Conversely, inducers cause an increase in the production of P450 enzymes, leading to increased metabolism of the substrates of that P450 enzyme.
  - When considering if the metabolism of certain drugs are affected by the CYP enzymes one should have a high index of suspicion. This is underscored by the sixfold difference observed in the normal population in the rates of CYP drug metabolism (see Genetic Polymorphism below) and that any given drug may be metabolized by different CYP enzymes or may be inducers of one enzyme while serving as a substrate of others. Thus, even if a patient has been on a certain drug for some time without side effects, addition of a new drug may alter the CYP metabolism of the existing drug, resulting in a side effect.

TABLE 20–6 Practical Tool to Identify Drugs That Interact with Cytochrome P450 Enzymes Resulting in Higher Risk of Side Effects

CYP ENZYMES	SUBSTRATES	INHIBITORS	SUBSTRATE SIDE EFFECTS
1A2			
2C9			
2C19			
2D9			
3A4			

Insert known substrates and inhibitors in each column to determine the likelihood of substrate-specific side effects (see practical example that follows)

Drug A Substrate + Drug B Inhibitor of same CYP enzyme → ↓metabolism/clearance, ↑ risk of side effects of Drug A

- Example: An 82-year-old man in the hospital for acute myocardial infarction given haloperidol for agitation

Metoprolol (CYP2D6 Substrate) + Haloperidol (CYP2D6 Inhibitor) →

↓ metabolism/clearance, ↑ risk of side effects of metoprolol such as bradycardia or other arrhythmia

- A useful tool to examine these potential interactions involves filling in the columns of Table (20–6) using the patient's medication list and information about how the drug is metabolized from a medical formularly. A more thorough method is to use a website such as http://www.genemedrx.com/ where the prescriber can enter all the drugs a patient takes (as well as results of genetic testing, if available); the program details the drug-drug interactions based on metabolism.
- Example: A 75-year-old woman who lives independently at home with a history of diabetes, urinary incontinence, chronic muscle spasms of her neck, one previous non-ST elevation myocardial infarction a year ago, and hyperlipidemia is admitted for new-onset atrial fibrillation. Her medications prior to admission are glyburide, losartan, cyclobenzaprine, oxybutynin (extended release), simvastatin, metoprolol, and aspirin, all at appropriate doses, and all of which she has taken for over one year. During her hospitalization, it is decided to start amiodarone and clopidogrel. On discharge, she is in normal sinus rhythm and has no complaints. Within 2 weeks, she has developed two episodes of hypoglycemia, has become more lethargic and fallen twice, has lower than her usual blood pressure, has developed constipation and dry mouth, and muscle aches. By employing Table 20–6, the clinician can readily identify several potential substrate related side-effects:

CYP ENZYMES	SUBSTRATES	INHIBITORS	SUBSTRATE SIDE EFFECTS
1A2	Cyclobenzaprine	Amiodarone	
2C9	Glyburide	Amiodarone	Falls, lethargy
		Clopidogrel	Hypoglycemia
2C19			
2D9	Metoprolol	Amiodarone	Myopathy
	simvastatin	Amiodarone	Low blood
3A4	Losartan		pressure
	cyclobenzaprine		falls, lethargy
	simvastatin		myopathy
	oxybutynin		dry mouth,
			constipation

- Importantly, the clinician can now determine the likely cause of her symptoms and formulate an alternative strategy to minimize the likelihood of

drug-drug interactions. For example, metformin and pravastatin are not metabolized by the CYP enzymes; trospium is a drug used for urinary incontinence that is not metabolized by the CYP system; and nonpharmacological strategies can be offered in lieu of cyclobenzaprine, a poor choice for the elderly.
  - Commonly used drugs that are not metabolized by the CYP system include pravastatin, metformin, citalopram, escitalopram, gabapentin, atenolol, and azithromycin.
- Renal excretion of drugs
  - Renal blood flow is reduced by about 1% per year in persons older than 50 years of age, and average clearance declines by 50% from 25 to 85 years of age.
  - Although the effects of age on renal function are somewhat more predictable than that of liver function, the prescriber must go beyond the use of blood urea nitrogen (BUN) and creatinine as sole markers to determine if clearance of a drug might be affected as these are affected by diet and muscle mass.
  - The Cockcroft and Gault formula can be used to estimate creatinine clearance (CrCl) but even this formula has limitations in the elderly.

$$CrCl = (140\text{-age}) \times weight\ (kg)/70 \times serum\ Cr$$
For women, multiply $\times 0.85$

  - If more than 60% of a drug is excreted by the kidneys, a reduction in renal function can result in significantly longer half-life and attendant higher blood levels. If a drug which is primarily eliminated by the kidney must be used, the prescriber can increase the interval between doses, decrease the dose, or both, depending on the situation.
    - Commonly used drugs which require significant renal elimination include atenolol, sotalol, digoxin, lithium, amphotericin, allopurinol, many of the H2 blockers, many antibiotics, many narcotics. Although the active metabolite of morphine, morphine-6-glucuronide, is excreted by the kidney, it can still be used in the elderly with impaired renal function. However, when initiating morphine, the prescriber should administer test doses and monitor the effect before determining the maintenance dose and interval.
    - Normeperidine (the metabolite of Meperidine) has potent anticholinergic properties and may precipitate seizures in the elderly. Therefore, meperidine should not be used in the elderly.
- The P-glycoprotein (P-gp) transporter does not affect drug metabolism or excretion directly, but rather drug bioavailability. P-gp is found in cancer cells as well as the liver, kidney, gut lumen and the blood-brain barrier. It removes P-gp substrates from the cytosol of enterocytes and returns them back into the gut lumen or from the capillaries of the blood-brain barrier back

into the bloodstream. P-gp inhibitors antagonize this process and lead to retention of P-gp substrates. P-gp inducers increase the amount of active P-gp, thus leading to extrusion of P-glycoprotein substrates.[9]

- P-gp inhibitors are being investigated in clinical trials to overcome the intrinsic or acquired multidrug resistance of human cancers, but this area applies to geropharmacology because inhibition of the transporting function of P-gp can cause clinically significant drug interactions, and can increase the brain penetration and accumulation of drugs. This will become important in the future and may help explain some of the instances whereby some patients develop an acute reaction to a particular drug, while most others do not (eg, lorazepam).

PHARMACOGENETICS

- Expression of genes may influence the metabolism of drugs, the availability of drugs at their site of action and how drugs bind to their target receptors. Thus, an individual's genetic profile could affect the clinical efficacy of a drug, the required dose of drugs, the choice of drugs, and the risk of side effects of drugs.
- In the next few decades, pharmacogenetic approaches will become available in the clinical setting and will undoubtedly aid prescribers in determining the probability that an individual patient will respond to a specific drug, or develop a specific side effect.
- Large-scale CYP2D6 phenotyping studies have shown that 5% to 10% of whites and about 1% of Asians are of the slow metabolizer phenotype. Since some cardiovascular drugs, psychoactive drugs, and morphine derivatives are CYP2D6 substrates, prescribers could theoretically identify those who are slow metabolizers, and avoid these drugs, thus, preventing ADRs and ADEs.[10]
- There are several apolipoprotein (APO) E2 and E4 polymorphisms. Those with the APO E2 polymorphism may have a greater lipid-lowering response to statin therapy compared to those with APO E4.

References

1. Hanlon JT, Schmader KE, Kornkowski MJ, et al. Adverse drug events in high risk older outpatients. *J Am Geriatr Soc.* 1997;45(8):945–948.
2. Flaherty JH, Perry HM 3rd, Lynchard GS, et al. Polypharmacy and hospitalization among older home care patients. *J Gerontol A Biol Sci Med Sci.* 2000; Oct;55(10):M554–559.
3. Nolan L, O'Malley K. Prescribing for the elderly: part 1. Sensitivity of the elderly to adverse drug reactions. *J Am Geriatr Soc.* 1988;36:142–149.
4. Col N, Fanale JE, Kronholm P. The role of medication non-compliance and adverse drug reactions in hospitalizations of the elderly. *Arch Intern Med.* 1990;150:841–845.
5. Omori DM, Potyk RP, Kroenke K. The adverse effects of hospitalization on drug regimens. *Arch Intern Med.* 1991;151(8):1562–1564.
6. Ireland GA, Morley JE. Health care consequences of medication reduction in the older patient. *J Invest Med.* 1995.
7. Fick DM, Cooper JW, Wade WE, et al. Updating the Beers Criteria for potentially inappropriate medication use in older adults: Results of a US consensus panel of experts. *Arch Intern Med.* 2003;163(22):2716–2724.
8. Cepeda OA, Morley JE. Polypharmacy, is it another disease? In: Pathy MS, Sinclair AJ, Morley JE, eds. *Principles and Practice of Geriatric Medicine. 4th ed.* London, John Wiley & Sons, Ltd, 2006:215–221.
9. Tanigawara Y. Role of p-glycoprotein in drug disposition. *Ther Drug Monit.* 2000;22:137–140.
10. Beyth RJ, Shorr RI. Epidemiology of adverse drug reactions in the elderly by drug class. *Drugs Aging.* 1999;14:231–239.

21 ANDROPAUSE

Syed H. Tariq and Matthew T. Haren

EPIDEMIOLOGY

- The prevalence of hypogonadism has been estimated to be between 2% to 5% at 40 years of age and 30% to 70% by 70 years of age.[1] It is estimated that at least 5 million males in the United States have hypogonadism, with less than 10% receiving hormone replacement.
- Longitudinal studies have shown that total testosterone declines at a rate of 0.4% per year after the age of 30 years. Bioavailable and free testosterone decline, and sex hormone-binding globulin (SHBG) increases, at rates of approximately 1% to 1.2% per year.

PATHOPHYSIOLOGY

- In young persons, the most common form of hypogonadism is testicular failure characterized by a fall in testosterone and a rise in luteinizing hormone (LH).
- In older persons, testosterone levels fall but rarely to the levels seen in primary hypogonadism in young men.
- This fall is associated with a small increase in LH, except late in life.
- The causes of late-life hypogonadism are multifactorial. Defects have been shown to occur at the level of the gonadotrophin-releasing hormone (GnRH) pulse generator in the hypothalamus, the pituitary, and the testes.

- With aging, there is a decrease in Leydig cells and the testicular response to stimulation with human chorionic gonadotrophin.
- The negative feedback of testosterone at the pituitary level increases with aging.
- There is a decreased pulse generation of GnRH with the pulses being generated more chaotically.
- It is the combination of these factors that leads to the age-related decline in testosterone level (Fig. 21–1).
- Testosterone circulates in a free form and bound to albumin and SHBG.
- In general, it is believed that the testosterone that is free and bound to albumin is available to tissues (bioavailable), whereas that bound to SHBG has limited ability to enter tissues.
- The exception to this is reproductive tissues where SHBG receptors (SHBG-R) can bind unliganded SHBG at the cell surface. Testosterone can then bind to the SHBG/SHBG-R complex to stimulate signaling events within the cell.
- Testosterone may also enter the cell as the membrane receptor complex via transport mechanisms involving the membrane transporter megalin, a low-density lipoprotein receptor-related protein.
- After entering cells, either testosterone or dihydrotestosterone bind to the androgen receptor (AR) in the cytoplasm. This receptor then dimerizes and is translocated to the nucleus.
- The testosterone-receptor complex then binds to androgen response elements on DNA with its action being modulated by a number of coactivators and corepressors.
- Binding to the DNA results in generation of messenger RNA and proteins.
- AR function is regulated by the number of cytosine-adenine-guanine CAG repeats.

- When there are a large number of CAG repeats, the receptor functions less well than when there are less CAG repeats.
- Finally, testosterone also has a number of nongenomic, membrane-mediated effects that involve, among others, signaling molecules such as Src, Pi3K, and Akt.
- The effects of aging on these complex intracellular actions of testosterone have not been studied.

DEFINING ANDROPAUSE

- The diagnosis of andropause in older males requires the presence of any number of a constellation of signs and symptoms as well as a demonstrated low biochemical measurement of serum testosterone (total, free, or bioavailable).

BIOCHEMICAL DETERMINATION OF TESTOSTERONE

- Although the measurement of testosterone is relatively simple, the development of a large number of kits for platform assays has created considerable confusion.
- There is a large variability in the values for each assay. This makes it essential that normal values, and not the manufacturers values, are determined for each laboratory.
- This entails obtaining three pooled values in the morning on at least two occasions from at least 40 healthy men between the ages of 20 and 40 years of age. Most laboratories use a value between 250 and 350 ng/dL as the lower limit of normal.
- Many authorities believe that especially with the older person, free or bioavailable (albumin bound + free) testosterone should be obtained. Most laboratories offer an analog-free testosterone assay, which is generally believed to be of no value. Salivary testosterone provides a reasonable approximation of free testosterone levels.

SYMPTOM COMPLEX

- A number of questionnaires have been developed to help screen for andropause and to provide an objective measure of treatment response.
- Two questionnaires have excellent specificity: the Saint Louis University Androgen Deficiency in Aging Males questionnaire and the Aging Male Survey. Unfortunately, neither has very good sensitivity.

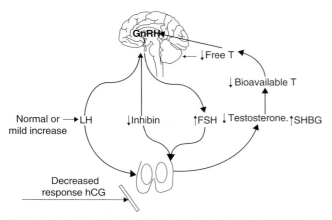

FIG. 21–1 Effect of aging on hypothalamic-pituitary-gonadal axis. FSH, follicular stimulating hormone; GnRH, gonadodotropin-releasing hormone; hCG, human chorionic gonadotropin; LH, luteinizing hormone; SHBG, sex hormone-binding globulin.

Andropause is Likely with an Answer of Yes to Question 1 or 7 or Any 3 Other Questions.
(Circle one)

Yes No 1. Do you have a decrease in libido (sex drive)?
Yes No 2. Do you have a lack of energy?
Yes No 3. Do you have a decrease in strength and/or endurance?
Yes No 4. Have you lost height?
Yes No 5. Have you noticed a decreased enjoyment of life?
Yes No 6. Are you sad and/or grumpy?
Yes No 7. Are your erections less strong?
Yes No 8. Have you noticed a recent deterioration in your ability to play sports?
Yes No 9. Are you falling asleep after dinner?
Yes No 10. Has there been a recent deterioration in your work performance?

FIG. 21–2 Saint Louis University Androgen Deficiency in Aging Male (ADAM) Questionnaire.

- Nevertheless, they are both considered a reasonable approach to symptom identification.
- A simplified algorithmic approach to diagnosing andropause is presented in Fig. 21–2. This approach is compatible with recent consensus recommendations.[2,3]

TESTOSTERONE REPLACEMENT THERAPY

BENEFITS

SEXUAL FUNCTION

- Testosterone replacement leads to a marked increase in libido, but this effect can also be seen with placebo.
- A meta-analysis has confirmed that testosterone increases enthusiasm for sex and sexual activity.[4]
- Treatment does not have an effect on erectile function, but it does improve the response to sildenafil (Viagra).
- Furthermore, a meta-analysis of the usefulness of androgen replacement for erectile dysfunction showed that testosterone-treated patients improve significantly more than placebo-treated patients and that patients with primary testicular failure respond better to treatment than those with secondary testicular failure.[5]

MUSCULOSKELETAL SYSTEM

Muscle

- Testosterone replacement in young hypogonadal men and supraphysiological treatment in eugonadal young men have been shown to increase muscle mass and strength.

- In older men with low bioavailable testosterone or low-normal total testosterone levels, intramuscular testosterone increases muscle mass and strength.
- However, numerous studies of oral and transdermal testosterone in older men with low to normal total testosterone levels show significant increases in lean mass without improvements in muscle strength.[6]
- Intramuscular testosterone increases muscle insulin like growth factor-1 (IGF-1), messenger RNA and transdermal testosterone increases serum IGF-1.
- Oral testosterone undecanoate has no effect on serum IGF-1 levels.[6]
- The muscle response to testosterone is related to dose.[7]

Bone

- A number of studies have shown that testosterone treatment can increase bone mineral density.[8,9]
- This effect of testosterone is not blocked by 5-α-reductase inhibition.
- It would seem that aromatization of testosterone to estrogen is the major cause of the positive effects of testosterone on bone. This has been clearly demonstrated in people with congenital aromatase deficiency.
- Testosterone also appears to directly increase the activity of osteoblasts.

COGNITIVE FUNCTION

- Some studies have demonstrated that testosterone replacement may improve visuospatial cognition.[10] However, this has not been a universal finding.[11]
- Testosterone replacement has been shown to produce small improvements in cognition in persons with Alzheimer disease.[12,13]

CARDIOVASCULAR SYSTEM

- Testosterone produces coronary artery vasodilation and increased brachial artery flow.
- Testosterone decreases angina and decreases ST-segment depression on the ECG during exercise testing.
- The ability of testosterone to reduce myocardial ischemia has been suggested but is not yet well established.
- Testosterone decreases total and low-density lipoprotein cholesterol. There is increased hepatic lipase activity with testosterone administration, resulting in increased cholesterol clearance.

HEALTH-RELATED QUALITY OF LIFE

- Eight trials (involving 390 patients) have examined the effect of testosterone on the quality of life of older men.
- Of these, four studies (193 patients) showed positive effects using various health-related quality of life scales.

SIDE EFFECTS

- The major side effect of testosterone is an excessive increase in hematocrit. When the hematocrit increases above 55, testosterone therapy should be withheld.
- Testosterone can also be associated with worsening sleep apnea and the development of gynecomastia related to the aromatization of testosterone to estrogen.
- Parenteral testosterone administration has minimal deleterious effects on the liver.
- Testosterone can cause a slight decrease in serum high-density lipoprotein cholesterol levels.
- Testosterone therapy increases prostate-specific antigen levels slightly. Testosterone may increase prostate size, which worsens benign prostate hypertrophy. The effects of testosterone on the development or the acceleration of prostate cancer are uncertain. There is a need for a large study to determine these effects.
- At present, the prudent physician should follow prostate-specific antigen levels and conduct a rectal examination every 6 to 12 months.

NOVEL THERAPEUTICS

- Oral (testosterone undecanoate) and injectable testosterone therapies have been used for an extended period with minimal side effects. Gooren[14] published a 10-year safety study for testosterone undecanoate.
- A new injectable testosterone undecanoate is now available and maintains testosterone levels for 3 to 4 months. Similarly prolonged testosterone effects can be obtained with subcutaneous pellet implantation.
- Trans-scrotal and transdermal patches have a high degree of skin irritation and are less commonly used today. Subcutaneous gels have become very popular in the United States because they provide physiologic levels of circulating testosterone with minimal inconvenience and only a small amount of skin irritation.
- To date, buccal administration of testosterone has been poorly accepted by patients. Sublingual and inhalation forms of testosterone are under development.
- There is interest in developing selective androgen-receptor modulators that will not have effects on the prostate.[15] Although potentially exciting, the role of these agents remains to be determined.

NEED FOR A MEN'S HEALTH INITIATIVE

- Increasingly, older males are receiving testosterone therapy for an ephemeral condition known as the *andropause.*

- At present, there is no adequate definition of andropause, no agreement on how to diagnose it, and no information on the long-term effects of testosterone in older males.
- Testosterone appears to be predominantly a quality of life drug, which should only be used if it produces symptomatic improvement; this is alarming, considering the lack of efficacy for measurable improvement in quality of life using current standard approaches.
- Andropausal symptoms are particularly responsive to the placebo effect.
- To clearly define the positive and negative effects of testosterone in older males requires a large study (7,000–16,000 men) for 5 to 7 years, similar to the Women's Health Initiative. Until such a study is completed physicians should utilize the above information to best determine the appropriate use of testosterone in older males.

REFERENCES

1. Morley JE, Perry HM III. Andropause: an old concept in new clothing. *Clin Geriatr Med.* 2003;19:507–528.
2. Nieschlag E, Swerdloff R, HM Behre, et al. Investigation, treatment and monitoring of late-onset hypogonadism in males. *Aging Male.* 2005;8:56–58.
3. Nieschlag E, Swerdloff R, Behre HM, et al. International Society of Andrology (ISA). International Society for the Study of the Aging Male (SSAM). European Association of Urology (EAU). Investigation, treatment and monitoring of late-onset hypogonadism in males, ISA, ISSAM, and EAU recommendations. *Eur Urol.* 2005;48:1–4.
4. Isidori AM, Elisa Giannetta, Daniele Gianfrilli, et al. Effects of testosterone on sexual function in men: results of a meta-analysis. *Clin Endocrinol (Oxf).* 2005;63:601–602.
5. Jain P, Rademaker AW, McVary KT. Testosterone supplementation for erectile dysfunction: results of a meta-analysis. *J Urol.* 2000;164(2):371–375.
6. Wittert GA, Ian M Chapman, Matthew T Haren, et al. Oral testosterone supplementation increases muscle and decreases fat mass in healthy elderly males with low-normal gonadal status. *J Gerontol A Biol Sci Med Sci.* 2003;58(7):618–625.
7. Bhasin S, Woodhouse L, Storer T W, et al. Testosterone dose-response relationships in healthy young men. *Am J Physiol Endocrinol Metab.* 2001;281(6):E1172–E1181.
8. Benito M, Vasilic B, Wehrli FW, et al. Effect of testosterone replacement on trabecular architecture in hypogonadal men. *J Bone Miner Res.* 2005;20:1785–1791.
9. Aminorroaya A, Kelleher S, Conway AJ, et al. Adequacy of androgen replacement influences bone density response to testosterone in androgen-deficient men. *Eur J Endocrinol.* 2005;152:881–886.
10. Cherrier HH, Craft S, Matsumoto AH. Cognitive changes associated with supplementation of testosterone

or dihydrotestosterone in mildly hypogonadal men: a preliminary report. *J Androl.* 2003;24(4):568–576.

11. Haren MT, Wittert GA, Chapman IM, et al. Effect of oral testosterone undecanoate on visuospatial cognition, mood and quality of life in elderly men with low-normal gonadal status. *Maturitas.* 2005;50:124–133.

12. Cherrier MM, Matsumoto AM, Amory JK, et al. Testosterone improves spatial memory in men with Alzheimer disease and mild cognitive impairment. *Neurology.* 2005;64:2063–2068.

13. Tan RS, Pu SJ. A pilot study on the effects of testosterone in hypogonadal aging male patients with Alzheimer disease. *Aging Male.* 2003;6:13–17.

14. Gooren LJ. A ten-year safety study of the oral androgen testosterone undecanoate. *J Androl.* 1994;15:212–215.

15. Chengalvala M, Oh T, Roy AK. Selective androgen receptor modulators. *Expert Opinion on Therapeutic Patents.* 2003;13: 59–66.

22 DEPRESSION IN THE ELDERLY

Chinya Murali and George T. Grossberg

INTRODUCTION

Depression is a very common illness causing morbidity and mortality in all age groups but particularly so in the elderly (>65 years or older). The incidence is reported to be 1% in the general population but under-reporting is likely. An epidemiologic catchment area (ECA) study estimated a 1-year prevalence of major depressive disorder at 0.9% and a lifetime prevalence at 1.4%.[1]

In the Cache County, Utah, study, point prevalence of major depression was estimated at 4.4% in women and 2.7% in men with a lifetime prevalence of 20.4% for women and 9.6% for men.

EPIDEMIOLOGY

The population of the United States is aging; according to the data from the 2000 U.S. census, there were 35 million elderly (>65 years of age) in 2000 constituting 12.5% of the population, These numbers are projected to double to 71.5 million by 2030 constituting 20% of the population.

DIAGNOSIS OF DEPRESSION

The diagnosis of depression is established using the American Psychiatric Association *Diagnostic and Statistical Manual, Fourth Edition, Text Revision (DSM-IV-TR)*; the criteria for a major depressive disorder is listed in Table 22–1.

Depression is an episodic illness with wide variation in its presentation; low-grade chronic symptoms lasting more than 2 years are classified as *dysthymia*.

Several studies and surveys point to depression being under-recognized in the elderly, and even sub-syndromal depression (SSD) affects the overall well being of the elderly individual. In one study, 24% of SSD subjects progressed to a major depressive disorder (MDD) or dysthymia over a 3-month period.

TABLE 22–1 Criteria for Major Depressive Episode

A. Five (or more) of the following symptoms have been present during the same 2-week period and represent a change from previous functioning; at least one of the symptoms is either (1) depressed mood or (2) loss of interest or pleasure. **Note:** Do not include symptoms that are clearly caused by a general medical condition, or mood-incongruent delusions or hallucinations.
   1. Depressed mood most of the day, nearly every day, as indicated by either subjective report (eg, feels sad or empty) or observation made by others (eg, appears tearful). Note: In children and adolescents, can be irritable mood.
   2. Markedly diminished interest or pleasure in all, or almost all, activities most of the day, nearly every day (as indicated by either subjective account or observation made by others).
   3. Significant weight loss when not dieting or weight gain (eg, a change of more than 5% of body weight in 1 month), or decrease or increase in appetite nearly every day. **Note:** In children, consider failure to make expected weight gains.
   4. Insomnia or hypersomnia nearly every day.
   5. Psychomotor agitation or retardation nearly every day (observable by others, not merely subjective feelings of restlessness or being slowed down).
   6. Fatigue or loss of energy nearly every day.
   7. Feelings of worthlessness or excessive or inappropriate guilt (which can be delusional) nearly every day (not merely self-reproach or guilt about being sick).
   8. Diminished ability to think or concentrate, or indecisiveness, nearly every day (either by subjective account or as observed by others).
   9. Recurrent thoughts of death (not just fear of dying), recurrent suicidal ideation without a specific plan, or a suicide attempt or a specific plan for committing suicide.
B. The symptoms do not meet criteria for a mixed episode.
C. The symptoms cause clinically significant distress or impairment in social, occupational, or other important areas of functioning.
D. The symptoms are not caused by the direct physiologic effects of a substance (eg, a drug of abuse, a medication) or a general medical condition (eg, hypothyroidism).
E. The symptoms are not better accounted for by bereavement, ie, after the loss of a loved one, the symptoms persist for longer than 2 months or are characterized by marked functional impairment, morbid preoccupation with worthlessness, suicidal ideation, psychotic symptoms, or psychomotor retardation.

SOURCE: American Psychiatric Association. *Diagnostic and Statistical Manual.* 4ᵗʰ ed. Washington, DC: American Psychiatric Association; 1994. American Psychiatric Association. *Diagnostic and Statistical Manual.* 4ᵗʰ ed, text rev. Washington, DC: American Psychiatric Association; 2000.

History of post-traumatic stress disorder increases the likelihood of comorbid depression and anxiety.

In elderly patients, depressed mood may not be prominent, whereas decreased energy and disturbed sleep and appetite (vegetative symptoms) are more likely to be present. In addition, there are certain unique presentations of depression including dementia, somatic symptoms, failure to thrive, and medical comorbidities.

Targeted screening for depression of elderly at higher risk is indicated in the following situations:[2]

- Recent bereavement
- Social isolation
- Persistent complaints of memory difficulties
- Chronic disabling illness
- Persistent sleep difficulties
- Significant somatic concerns or recent-onset anxiety
- Refusal to eat or neglect of personal care
- Recurrent or prolonged hospitalization
- Diagnosis of dementia, Parkinson disease, or stroke
- Recent placement in a nursing or long-term care (LTC) home

The often used screening scale is the Geriatric Depression Scale (GDS), which is a 30-point scale; a score of 10 or more is an indication for treatment. A 15-point abbreviated scale is also in use (Table 22–2).

UNIQUE PRESENTATIONS

DEMENTIA OF DEPRESSION

Elderly patients with subclinical cognitive problems who develop dementia over the next 3 years have a higher incidence of depressive symptoms. Depression can be an early symptom of dementia. Cognitive decline with depressive symptoms frequently causes diagnostic confusion, retarded depression similar to apathy is often noted in frontal-lobe dementia. There is generally improvement in the level of functioning, concentration, memory and energy level with adequate treatment of depression sometimes termed *pseudodementia*. Reliance on caregiver reports is very important in addition to patient examination to better assess the situation.

TABLE 22–2   Geriatric Depression Scale (GDS)

Patient_____

Examiner_____ Date_____

Directions to Patient: Please choose the best answer for how you have felt over the past week.

Directions to Examiner: Present questions VERBALLY. Circle answer given by patient. Do not show to patient.

1. Are you basically satisfied with your life? . . . . yes / no (1)
2. Have you dropped many of your activities and interests? . . . . yes (1) / no
3. Do you feel that your life is empty? . . . . yes (1) / no
4. Do you often get bored? . . . . yes (1) / no
5. Are you hopeful about the future? . . . . yes / no (1)
6. Are you bothered by thoughts you can t get out of your head? . . . . yes (1) / no
7. Are you in good spirits most of the time? . . . . yes / no (1)
8. Are you afraid that something bad is going to happen to you? . . . . yes (1) / no
9. Do you feel happy most of the time? . . . . yes / no (1)
10. Do you often feel helpless? . . . . yes (1) / no
11. Do you often get restless and fidgety? . . . . yes (1) / no
12. Do you prefer to stay at home rather than go out and do things? . . . . . yes (1) / no
13. Do you frequently worry about the future? . . . . yes (1) / no
14. Do you feel you have more problems with memory than most? . . . . .yes (1) / no
15. Do you think it is wonderful to be alive now? . . . . .yes / no (1)
16. Do you feel downhearted and blue? . . . . .yes (1) / no
17. Do you feel pretty worthless the way you are now? . . . . .yes (1) / no
18. Do you worry a lot about the past? . . . . yes (1) / no
19. Do you find life very exciting? . . . . yes / no (1)
20. Is it hard for you to get started on new projects? . . . . yes / no (1)
21. Do you feel full of energy? . . . . yes / no (1)
22. Do you feel that your situation is hopeless? . . . . yes (1) / no
23. Do you think that most people are better off than you are? . . . . yes (1) / no
24. Do you frequently get upset over little things? . . . . .yes (1) / no
25. Do you frequently feel like crying? . . . . yes (1) / no
26. Do you have trouble concentrating? . . . . yes (1) / no
27. Do you enjoy getting up in the morning? . . . . yes / no (1)
28. Do you prefer to avoid social occasions? . . . . .yes (1) / no
29. Is it easy for you to make decisions? . . . . yes / no (1)
30. Is your mind as clear as it used to be? . . . . .yes / no (1)

TOTAL: Please sum all bolded answers (worth one point) for a total score _____/30.

Scores: 0–9 Normal, 10–19 Mild Depressive, 20–30 Severe Depressive

SOURCE: Geriatric Depression Scale. http://www.stanford.edu/~yesavage/GDS.html.

SOMATIC PRESENTATION

The presentation can include worsening of arthritis, chronic anxiety, and focus on bowel function (constipation/diarrhea).

The number of patients with depression who reported only somatic symptoms has been reported between 45% to 95% of all depression. One-half of depressed patients reported multiple unexplained somatic symptoms, and 11% denied psychologic symptoms of depression on direct questioning.

Depression can present as failure to thrive or failure to rehabilitate eg, following major surgery (hip or back) and during recovery from major medical illness (myocardial infarction, stroke, and sepsis).

Psychotic symptoms are more likely in elderly persons with depression, predominant among them are delusions of guilt, persecution, and sometimes jealousy.

MEDICAL COMORBIDITIES

Depression is known to accompany many general medical conditions including chronic obstructive pulmonary disease (COPD); Parkinson disease; cerebrovascular accident (CVA); diabetes mellitus; myocardial infarction; osteoarthritis; and cancers of the pancreas, colon, and brain.

DEPRESSION AND MALNUTRITION

Depression reduces the appetite and alters normal sleep patterns more severely in elderly patients leading to significant weight loss and dehydration. It is very important to monitor the patient's weight and hydration as there is risk of severe morbidity and mortality secondary to electrolyte abnormalities. Not surprisingly, electroconvulsive therapy (ECT) is undergoing a resurgence in the elderly as it has been associated with earlier and more effective symptom resolution compared to medications.

LONG-TERM CARE FACILITIES

Depression is often seen in patients placed in a long-term care facility.

Older adults (>65 years or older) with any of the above risk factors have a higher incidence of depression, therefore, healthcare providers must be familiar with the physical, psychological, and social risk factors that precipitate depressive disorders.

SITUATIONAL OR REACTIVE DEPRESSION

Negative life events including social isolation, financial problems, poor physical health, and retirement are some of the significant stressors that precipitate depression.

Complicated bereavement includes depression lasting more than 2 months, presence of psychotic symptoms, and severe guilt with thoughts of suicide.

GRIEF/BEREAVEMENT

The elderly are more likely to face losses such as death (eg, spouse, children, friends, pets), retirement, disability (eg, loss of eyesight, hearing, ability to walk, drive a vehicle).

Grieving elders describe themselves as being sad, mourning the loss of loved ones, experiencing sleep problems, having no or low appetite, and experiencing brief periods of auditory hallucinations, eg, hearing loved ones talking to them.

Grief can continue for longer than 1 year. Different dimensions to coping with loss include feelings of shock, disbelief, and denial, followed by a period of reorganization and recovery.

There is wide variation in the intensity and sequence in which these stages manifest. Some authors have speculated that grief is channeled into somatic symptoms.

SUICIDE IN THE ELDERLY

The incidence of self-harm increases with advancing age with the highest risk in white males, unmarried or widowed. The ratio of nonlethal self-harm to completed suicide in the adult (>20 years of age) population is 20:1, whereas in the elderly (>65 years of age) it is 4:1. The lethal potential increases with age so healthcare providers should be vigilant and screen patients. The corelation of mood disorders with suicidal ideation is significant. The risk factors for suicidal ideations are similar to that of depression mentioned earlier in this chapter. In addition, particular attention should be given to the following:[3]

• Recently bereaved individuals with unusual symptoms (eg, active suicidal ideation, guilt not related to the deceased, psychomotor retardation, mood congruent delusions, marked functional impairment after 2 months of the loss, reaction that seems out of proportion to the loss) and persistent bereavement 3 to 6 months after the loss
• Presence of psychotic symptoms
• Recent major physical illness (eg, within 3 months)

- Significant somatic concerns or recent onset anxiety or akathisia because of medications
- Recent initiation of antidepressant medications
- Recent placement in a nursing or LTC home
  Hospitalization is necessary to maintain a safe environment and for comprehensive evaluation and treatment.

BIPOLAR DISORDER

Bipolar disorder (BPD) can occur at any age with the first episode being depression in the majority of patients. As people get older, depressive episodes outnumber hypomania/mania; episodes can occur with increasing frequency and are more likely to be treatment resistant. Among patients with BPD who meet criteria for recovery, 5% of patients relapse each month, and 80% of relapses are characterized by depression.

Misdiagnosis of BPD as unipolar depression is common. In one survey, 60% of patients with BPD were diagnosed with unipolar depression; 26% were diagnosed with anxiety disorder. As misdiagnosis and comorbidity are common, clinicians should look at individual and family histories very carefully.

Treating with an antidepressant alone in BPD can cause a rapid switch to hypomania or mania, increased mood lability, and a tendency toward rapid cycling illness. It is very important to first treat with mood stabilizers alone and then cautiously add an antidepressant if necessary.

TREATMENT

The main aim of treatment is to
1. Achieve remission
2. Prevent recurrence
3. Prevent relapse

NONPHARMACOLOGIC TREATMENT

- Psychotherapy
  - There is more data available for the effectiveness of cognitive behavior therapy in the elderly, interpersonal therapy, and supportive therapy rather than psychodynamic psychotherapy.
  - Bright light therapy has been very effective for seasonal affective disorder (SAD); this has also been viewed as an adjunct to treatment in nonseasonal affective disorders. Bright light is produced by light boxes (can vary between 6000–10000 lux); patients are exposed to light for approximately 0.5 to 1 hour with adequate protection for the eyes.
  - Short-term studies looking at using bright light as adjunctive treatment to drug therapy in depression noted that treatment response in the bright light group was improved, but the results did not achieve statistical significance. When morning light treatment was used in addition to sleep deprivation, mood improved significantly; albeit, hypomania was more common in this group compared to the control group.
  - Exercise, particularly aerobic exercise, is thought to release endorphins with an attendant sense of well-being. In one meta-analysis of randomized controlled trials, exercise was effective in reducing symptoms in the short term in the elderly with minor or major depression.

PHARMACOTHERAPY

- Different classes of antidepressants may be effective in the elderly. Importantly, the "start slow, go slow" approach is critical as elderly patients are exquisitely sensitive to many drugs and tend to develop side effects or toxic symptoms at much lower drug levels.[4]
- Drug therapy may require 6–8 weeks for optimum results, however, if there is no evidence of any benefit by 4 weeks most clinicians will change drug therapy.
- The major effects of antidepressants are thought to be mediated through serotonin and norepinephrine. There are five major classes of antidepressants: selective serotonin reuptake inhibitors (SSRIs), serotonin-norepinephrine reuptake inhibitors (SNRIs), tricyclic antidepressants (TCAs), monoamine oxidase inhibitors (MAOIs) and miscellaneous drugs. The dosages, benefits, and side-effects are listed in Table 22–3.
- Of the different classes, SSRIs are the most widely prescribed drugs; the benefits include better tolerability, efficacy, relative safety, and minimal interaction with other drugs. However, recently there are increasing data that SSRIs and other antidepressants can increase the risk of impulsive acts including suicide.
  - In 2004, the Food and Drug Administration (FDA) ordered strong warnings for suicidal tendencies in pediatric patients on antidepressants, and it was extended to all age groups.
  - Recent information from a meta-analysis of 372 studies involving approximately 100,000 patients on 11 different antidepressants suggests increased risk among adults between the ages of 18 to 25 years; effects were mixed in adults age 25 to 64 years, but in elderly patients, the risk of suicidal thoughts was slightly lower. An FDA psychopharmacologic drugs advisory committee will be reviewing the information shortly and issuing further recommendations.
  - One study followed postadmission elderly patients for a suicidal attempt for 10 years; the proportion of

TABLE 22–3 Pharmacologic Therapy for Major Depression

MEDICATIONS	STARTING DOSAGE (MG)[a]	AVERAGE DOSAGE (MG)	MAXIMUM DOSAGE (MG)	BENEFITS	MAJOR SIDE EFFECTS
Selective serotonin reuptake inhibitors (SSRIs)					
Citalopram HBr (Celexa)	10–20 daily	20–60 daily	60 daily	Less activating, minimal interaction at P450, works well for anxiety	Sedation, GI upset, serotonin syndrome, sexual dysfunction
Escitalopram (Lexapro)	5–10 daily	10–20 daily	20 daily		
Fluvoxamine (Luvox)	50–100 daily	100–200 daily	300 daily	Effective for OCD, anxiety	Sexual dysfunction, serotonin syndrome
Fluoxetine HCl (Prozac)	10–20 daily	20–40 daily	60–80 daily	Nonsedating, increases energy level, long half-life	GI upset, serotonin syndrome, sexual dysfunction
Paroxetine HCl (Paxil)	10–20 daily	20–30 daily	60 daily	Effect on anxiety, short half-life, increases appetite	GI upset, serotonin syndrome, sexual dysfunction
Sertraline HCl (Zoloft)	25–50 daily	50–150 daily	200 daily	Minimal interaction at P450, works for anxiety	GI upset, serotonin syndrome, sexual dysfunction
Other antidepressants					
Bupropion HCl (Wellbutrin)	75 BID	100 TID	150 TID	Nonsedating, smoking cessation, improves attention	Lowers seizure threshold, increasing anxiety, sleep disturbance, increases anxiety
Bupropion HCl (Wellbutrin SR)	100–150 daily	150–200 BID	200 BID		
Mirtazapine (Remeron)	7.5–15 QHS	15–45 QHS	45 QHS	Improves sleep, appetite, works well for anxiety, soluble form available	Sedation, weight gain
Serotonin-norepinephrine reuptake inhibitors (SNRIs)					
Duloxetine (Cymbalta)	20–30 daily	30 daily	60–120 daily	Helps chronic pain	Liver toxicity
Venlafaxine (Effexor)	18.75 BID	75–225 (split BID)	75–375 (split BID)	Effective for hard to treat depression, anxiety disorders, slow titration possible	GI upset, sexual dysfunction, increased blood pressure at higher doses, serotonin syndrome
Venlafaxine XR (Effexor XR)	37.5 daily	75–225 daily	225–300 daily		
Selected tricyclic antidepressants (TCAs)					
Amitriptyline HCl (Elavil)	25–50 QHS	150–200 QHS	150–300 QHS	Sedating, helps with chronic pain at lower doses, proven effectiveness	Constipation, sedation, Orthostasis, dry mouth, Urinary hesitancy, mild cognitive disturbance, tachycardia
Nortriptyline HCl (Pamelor, Aventyl HCl Pulvules)	10–25 QHS	75–100 QHS	75–150 QHS		
Desipramine HCl (Norpramin)	25–50 daily	150–200 daily	150–300 daily		Prolonged QT interval (lethal in overdose) Generally avoided in the elderly
Monoamine oxidase inhibitors (MAOI)					
Selegiline [transdermal] (Emsam)	6 mg/24 h	12 mg/24 h	12 mg/24 h	Helpful for hard to treat depression, Lower risk of tyramine interaction with 6 mg patch	Minimal GI effects, insomnia, irritability, agitation, restlessness, suicidal ideations, hypertensive crises
Tranylcypromine	10 BID	30 daily	30 daily	Useful in drug-resistant depression, severe anxiety	Insomnia, irritability, agitation, aggressiveness, severe restlessness, mania, suicidal ideations, Avoid tyramine-containing food, risk of hypertensive crises Interaction with SSRIs, TCAs, narcotics, antihistamines Generally avoided in the elderly
Isocarboxazid	10 BID	60 daily	60 daily		
Phenelzine	15 TID	60 daily	90 daily		

BID, twice daily; GI, gastrointestinal; HBr , hydrobromic acid; OCD, obsessive-compulsive disorder; QHS, at bedtime; TID, three times daily.

[a]Maximum allowable based on manufacturers' package inserts information in *Physicians' Desk Reference*. 60th ed. Montvale, NJ: Thomson Healthcare.

elderly patients exposed to antidepressants were at reduced risk of attempting suicide.

- Transdermal selegiline
  - This agent is a selective, reversible MAO-B inhibitor at lower doses, but nonselective MAO inhibitor at higher doses (a tyramine-free diet must be instituted). Recently a transdermal delivery system for selegiline was approved by the FDA for the treatment of depression with less onerous dietary restrictions. This might increase the use of this drug class for treatment-resistant patients.
- Adjunctive therapies
  - Augmentation strategies are employed for treatment-resistant depression; commonly used combinations include SSRIs with bupropion, addition of lithium, or thyroid hormone.
  - More recent augmentation strategies involves the use of atypical antipsychotics because of their effects on the 5-hydroxytryptamine (5-HT) (serotonin) system.[5]
  - St. John's wort has not been shown to be effective for use in the elderly, however, some studies have shown a response in mild depression in adults.

OTHER SOMATIC THERAPIES

ELECTROCONVULSIVE THERAPY

ECT has been shown to be highly effective in depression, moreover, patients with *refractory depression* are more likely to respond to it.[6] The basic principle of ECT has remained unchanged since its introduction; advances in anesthesiology, neuromuscular blockage with succinylcholine, pulse generation machines, and careful patient selection have greatly improved the safety and tolerability of ECT. Response rates in treatment-resistant patients range from 50% to 90% based on different studies.

ECT works best with depression complicated by psychotic symptoms or associated with suicidal ideations.

Since the elderly are very sensitive to medications and medications require lengthy titration, ECT is now used more frequently in the elderly. It is associated with faster recovery times, thereby decreasing the morbidity, hospital stays, and facilitating a return to baseline.

ECT has been shown to reduce suicide-attempt rates and reduce overall mortality rates in depressed patients over 3 years of follow-up. Despite its potential benefits, ECT still has significant risks and side effects including post-ictal confusion, short-term memory loss, and cardiopulmonary complications.

Bitemporal ECT remains the gold standard in terms of efficacy however, cognitive side effects including retrograde and anterograde amnesia and confusion are not uncommon. Although ECT is effective for acute symptoms, it is associated with a high relapse rate, hence the need for medications to maintain the improvement.[7]

The mechanism of action of ECT is incompletely understood, however is may act through effects on monoaminergic systems (including dopamine, serotonin), by reducing corticotropin-releasing factor (CRF) or by as yet unknown effects on other neurotrophic factors.

VAGAL NERVE STIMULATION

In this therapy, a stimulator is surgically attached to the left vagus nerve and is connected to a programmable pulse generator that is implanted subcutaneously in the patient's chest. The stimulator can be programmed to deliver electrical pulses to the nerve at various frequencies and currents.

Side effects of vagal nerve stimulation (VNS) are generally mild, surgical complications are rare; a common side effect is incisional pain; less common side effects include infections, hoarseness of voice, dysphagia, and coughing.

Typically, stimulation parameters involve delivering electrical pulses of 0.25 milliamperes at 20 to 30 Hz, with a cycling ratio of 30 seconds every 3 to 5 minutes.

VNS is FDA approved for treatment of drug-resistant epilepsy. Interestingly, it was also shown to improve mood symptoms.

A single open study of VNS in 60 nonepileptic patients with treatment-resistant depression found a 31% response rate and 15% remission rate after 10 weeks. These response and remission rates were sustained at 1 year and improved at 2 years after surgery.

A sham-controlled study failed to show statistically significant antidepressant effects for active VNS; at the end of the initial 10-week evaluation period, response rate was 15% with VNS and 10% with sham. These patients were continued in an open phase study on active VNS for up to 1 year; the response rate increased to 27% and the remission rate was 16%.[8]

VNS is now FDA approved for treatment-resistant depression.

RAPID TRANSCRANIAL MAGNETIC STIMULATION

In transcranial magnetic stimulation (TMS), a bank of capacitors is rapidly discharged into an electric coil to produce a magnetic field, which induces an electric field in the underlying region of the cerebral cortex to depolarize cortical neurons, which, in turn, generate action potentials that exert biologic effects (reference 9). For example, TMS applied to the left motor cortex causes action potentials that propagate through the corticospinal tract leading to twitches in contralateral skeletal muscles.

TMS applied to the left prefrontal cortex has been shown to increase release of dopamine in the ipsilateral caudate nucleus. TMS may also directly alter gene expression patterns.

High-frequency or *fast* rapid TMS (rTMS) stimulation is delivered at a rate >1 Hz; low-frequency or *slow* rTMS refers to stimulation rates <1 Hz. No anesthesia is needed with rTMS.

Most studies of TMS use are small; however, in a review of studies that measured clinical remission of depressive symptoms, 41% of 139 patients treated with high-frequency rTMS to the left prefrontal cortex achieved a 50% decrease in their Hamilton depression scale scores.

Recent studies suggest that longer treatment courses, more frequent magnetic pulses, or increased field intensity could increase the likelihood of treatment success.

The FDA is reviewing these data, and no decision regarding its use has been formalized.

DEEP BRAIN STIMULATION

Deep brain stimulation (DBS) involves stimulating the brain structures using a small electrical stimulator implanted in a defined brain location such as the subcortical area and connected to a programmable subcutaneous pulse generator. It has been FDA approved for the treatment of Parkinson disease; bilateral DBS of the subthalamus or globus pallidus is generally accepted treatment for refractory Parkinson disease.

DBS has also been noted to have an effect on mood state.

Patients with resistant depression not responding to the other modalities of treatment (multiple medications, psychotherapy, and electroconvulsive therapy) may benefit from deep brain stimulation. One recent study looked at stimulation of the subgenual cingulate region (Brodmann area 25) in treatment-resistant depression; four out of six patients showed remarkable improvement; however, two patients failed to show a sustained antidepressant response. These results suggest that disrupting focal pathologic activity in limbic-cortical circuits using electrical stimulation of the subgenual

cingulate white matter can effectively reverse symptoms in otherwise treatment-resistant depression.[10]

This method of treatment is still considered experimental.

CONCLUSION

Depression is a very common illness in the elderly, and various modalities of treatment are available, none of which is curative. The goal is to achieve and maintain remission, decrease morbidity and mortality, and provide the best possible quality of life.

REFERENCES

1. Robins LN, Regier DA. *Psychiatric disorders in America: the epidemiologic catchment area study*. New York, NY: The Free Press; 1991.
2. Canadian Coalition of Senior's Mental Health. National Guidelines for Senior's Mental Health: Assessment and Treatment of Depression. Toronto, ON; 2006.
3. Canadian Coalition of Senior's Mental Health. National Guidelines for Senior's Mental Health: The Assessment of Suicide Risk and the Prevention of Suicide. Toronto, ON; 2006.
4. Holtzheimer PE III, Nemeroff CB. Advances in the treatment of depression *NeuroRx*. 2006 Jan;3:42–56.
5. Meltzer HY. The mechanism of action of novel antipsychotic drugs. *Schizophr Bull*. 1991;17:263–287.
6. UK ECT Review Group. Efficacy and safety of electroconvulsive therapy in depressive disorders: a systematic review and meta analysis. *Lancet*. 2003;361:799–808.
7. American Psychiatric Association. Practice guideline for the treatment of patients with major depressive disorder (revision). *Am J Psychiatry*. 2000;157(4 suppl):1–45.
8. Rush AJ, Sackeim HA, Marangell LB, et al. Effects of 12 months of vagus nerve stimulation in treatment-resistant depression: a naturalistic study. *Biol Psychiatry*. 2005;58:355–363.
9. Holtzheimer PE III, Russo J, Avery DH. A meta-analysis of repetitive transcranial magnetic stimulation in the treatment of depression [erratum 2037:2005, 2003]. *Psychopharmacol Bull*. 2001;35:149–169.
10. Mayberg HS, Lozano AM, Voon V, et al. Deep brain stimulation for treatment-resistant depression neuron. *Neuron*. Mar 2005;45:651–660, 03v.

23 ASTHMA

Mark S. Dykewicz

OVERVIEW AND PATHOPHYSIOLOGY

Asthma is a chronic airway disorder that is sometimes fatal and can cause significant impairment of daily life.

- The chronic airway inflammation is associated with airway hyperresponsiveness that leads to recurrent episodes of wheezing, dyspnea, chest tightness, and coughing, particularly at night or in the early morning.
- There is typically widespread but variable airflow obstruction within the lung that is often reversible either spontaneously or with treatment.
- The immunohistopathologic features of asthma include inflammatory cell infiltration.
  - The inflammatory cascade of asthma may involve neutrophils (especially in patients with more severe asthma or sudden-onset, near-fatal asthma exacerbations), eosinophils, lymphocytes, mast cell activation, and epithelial cell injury.
- Factors that influence the development and expression of asthma include the following:
  - Host factors: genetic inheritance predisposing to allergy and airway hyperresponsiveness, obesity, gender (male sex is a risk factor for asthma in children, but by adulthood the prevalence of asthma is greater in women than in men).
  - Environmental factors: allergens, occupational sensitizers, tobacco smoke (passive and active exposure), outdoor/indoor air pollution.
- Adults with asthma have accelerated loss of lung function compared to age-matched controls.

INITIAL NONEMERGENT ASSESSMENT AND DIAGNOSIS

MEDICAL HISTORY

- Symptoms helpful in establishing the diagnosis.
  - Is there a history or presence of episodic symptoms of airflow obstruction (wheezing, chest tightness, dyspnea, cough)?
  - Are symptoms triggered by cold air (a useful question for distinguishing asthma from patients who are deconditioned without asthma), exercise, acute allergen exposure (eg, pets, molds, house dust mites [from vacuuming, dusting], seasonal pollens), airborne irritants (eg, cleaning solutions, smoke)?
  - Patient's upper respiratory infections "go to the chest" or take more than 10 days to clear up.
- Environmental assessment: ask about home environment (presence of pets, cockroaches), work exposures, passive cigarette smoke exposure.
- Tobacco abuse.
- Presence of risk factors for asthma: family history of asthma or allergic disease, personal history of allergic disease (eg, rhinitis, sinusitis), gastroesophageal reflux.

PHYSICAL EXAMINATION

- Lung auscultation may detect wheezing and prolonged expiration, but may be normal.
- Dysphonia, inspiratory stridor, and monophonic wheezing loudest over the central airway suggest vocal cord dysfunction, upper airway foreign bodies, epiglottitis, organic diseases of the larynx, and extrinsic and intrinsic tracheal narrowing.
  - When upper airway obstruction suspected, refer for laryngoscopy. Flow-volume curves may also demonstrate flattening of the inspiratory phase.

SPIROMETRY

- Perform upon initial assessment, and periodically during follow-up (see Chronic Management: Interval Assessment and Monitoring below).
- More sensitive than physical examination for detecting airway obstruction, but may be normal, particularly in milder asthma or *cough variant asthma,* in which patients may have a cough that responds to asthma medication such as bronchodilators.
- Cough variant asthma must be distinguished from eosinophilic bronchitis, in which patients have cough and produce sputum eosinophils but have normal indices of lung function when assessed by spirometry and airway hyperresponsiveness.
- Establish airflow obstruction: forced expiratory volume at 1 second (FEV-1) <80% predicted if forced vital capacity (FVC) normal; FEV-1/FVC ≤0.70 (70%), valid even if FVC below 80%.
- For chronic management, establish if airflow obstruction is reversible (either by acute bronchodilator response or an interval assessment before and after introduction of treatment, eg, inhaled corticosteroids).
- Spirometry and other asthma endpoints including symptoms do not always track together.

PEAK FLOW MEASUREMENTS

- Although not as sensitive as spirometry for detecting obstruction, may be more useful for assessing control (see Chronic Management below)

ALLERGY TESTING

- If there is persistent asthma, allergic sensitivity should be assessed by skin testing or in vitro testing for specific IgE. Always assess the clinical significance of positive tests in the context of medical history.

CHEST X-RAY

- Should ideally be performed on initial diagnosis to rule out other causes of respiratory symptoms.

SEVERITY ASSESSMENT

- The intensity of asthma before therapeutic intervention is used to determine initial severity (Table 23–1).
  ○ The level of severity should be determined based on the most severe category in which any feature appears.
- Severity assessment can be divided into two domains: (1) *impairment* (including symptoms, impact on quality of life), and (2) *risk* of future morbidity or impairment (eg, exacerbations, progressive loss of lung function, death).
  ○ Inquire about nocturnal awakenings; the need for rescue medication; missed days of work or school; the ability to engage in normal daily activities, or desired activities, including exercise; and general quality-of-life assessments.

TABLE 23–1 Classification of Asthma Severity by Clinical Features Before Treatment

INTERMITTENT

Symptoms less than once a week
Brief exacerbations
Nocturnal symptoms not more than twice a month
- FEV_1 or PEF ≤80% predicted
- PEF of FEV_1 variability <20%

MILD PERSISTENT

Symptoms more than once a week or less than once a day
Exacerbations may affect activity and sleep
Nocturnal symptoms more than twice a month
- FEV_1 or PEF ≥80% predicted
- PEF or FEV_1 variability <20–30%

MODERATE PERSISTENT

Symptoms daily
Exacerbations may affect activity and sleep
Nocturnal symptoms more than once a week
Daily use of inhaled short-acting β_2-agonist
- FEV_1 or PEF 60–80% predicted
- PEF or FEV_1 variability >30%

SEVERE PERSISTENT

Symptoms daily
Frequent exacerbations
Frequent nocturnal asthma symptoms
Limitation of physical activities
- FEV_1 or PEF ≤60% predicted
- PEF or FEV_1 variability >30%

FEV_1, forced expiratory volume at 1 second; PEF, peak expiratory flow
SOURCE: Global Initiative for Asthma (GINA), National Heart, Lung, and Blood Institute. Pocket guide for asthma management and prevention, revised 2006. Bethesda, MD: Medical Communications Resources, Inc., 2006.

ROUTINE CHRONIC MANAGEMENT

ASSESSMENT

- Periodic assessment of asthma control is recommended at 1-month to 6-month intervals to determine if goals of therapy are being met, and if any therapy adjustments are needed.
- Asthma control should be assessed (Table 23–2).
  ○ Control is the degree to which therapy minimizes the same parameters used to assess severity. The control assessment is used to determine adjustments in therapy.
    ■ Therapies may produce responsiveness in one domain (impairment) without producing responsiveness in the other domain (risk).
      • Example: Substituting a long-acting β-agonist (LABA) for an inhaled corticosteroid might maintain control of symptoms and function but not reduce the risk of exacerbations.
  ○ Clinical assessment and patient self-report are the primary methods for monitoring asthma control.
- Recommended assessments at each visit include the following:

TABLE 23–2 Levels of Asthma Control

CHARACTERISTIC	CONTROLLED (ALL OF THE FOLLOWING)	PARTLY CONTROLLED (ANY MEASURE PRESENT IN ANY WEEK)	UNCONTROLLED
Daytime symptoms	None (twice or less/week)	More than twice/week	Three or more features of partly controlled asthma present in any week
Limitations of activities	None	Any	
Nocturnal symptoms/ awakening	None	Any	
Need for reliever/ rescue treatment	None (twice or less/ week)	More than twice/week	
Lung function (PEF or FEV$_1$)‡	Normal	<80% predicted or personal best (if known)	
Exacerbations	None	One or more/year*	One in any week†

Any exacerbation should prompt review of maintenance treatment to ensure that it is adequate.
†*By definition, an exacerbation in any week makes that an uncontrolled asthma week.*
‡*Lung function is not a reliable test for children 5 years or younger.*
SOURCE: Global Initiative for Asthma (GINA), National Heart, Lung, and Blood Institute. Pocket guide for asthma management and prevention, revised 2006. Bethesda, MD: Medical Communications Resources, Inc., 2006.

- Signs and symptoms of asthma
  - Interval history should include frequency of daytime asthma symptoms and use of rescue medications (eg, short-acting bronchodilators), nocturnal awakening from asthma symptoms, exercise-induced symptoms.
- Quality-of-life and functional status assessments
  - Control level of impairment can be rapidly assessed by some validated standardized questionnaires (Asthma Control Test, Asthma Control Questionnaire, and Asthma Therapy Assessment Questionnaire).
  - Use of some questionnaires has been shown to have good predictive value for exacerbations.
- History of exacerbations since last assessment.
- Level of pharmacotherapy (including adherence to therapy and potential adverse events from medication).
- Patient-provider communication and patient satisfaction.
  - Teach patients to recognize symptoms that indicate inadequate asthma control.
- Pulmonary function tests
  - Spirometry is recommended at the first assessment, after treatment has been initiated and symptoms and peak expiratory flow (PEF) have stabilized, during periods of prolonged loss of asthma control, and at least every 1 to 2 years to assess the maintenance of airway function.
  - Importantly, patients may report few symptoms but have severely reduced FEV-1.
- Peak flow monitoring
  - Peak flow is not reliable for assessing severity, but may be useful in assessing control on an ongoing basis.
  - Use if moderate-to-severe persistent asthma, or if a patient has a history of having poor subjective perception of bronchospasm.

- Measure peak flow on awakening before taking a bronchodilator. As a comparative benchmark, it is generally preferable to use *personal best* peak flow once established, rather than predicted peak flow.
- Use the same peak flow meter over time; different brands of peak flow meters may give different readings.
- Check peak flows during exacerbations.
- Peak flow <80% of personal best indicates the need for additional medication.

GOALS OF ASTHMA THERAPY

- Prevent chronic/troublesome symptoms.
- Maintain (near-) *normal* lung function.
- Maintain normal activity levels (eg, exercise).
- Prevent recurrent exacerbations and minimize the need for emergency department visits or hospitalizations.
- Provide optimal pharmacotherapy with minimal or no adverse effects.
- Meet patient/family expectations for asthma care.
- Action plan
  - Patients should know asthma goals, be taught how to recognize asthma exacerbations, and have an action plan (preferably written) that provides instructions on steps to be taken if asthma worsens (see Acute Exacerbations, ahead).
- Ultimately, the level of control should guide treatment, which may include maintaining the current treatment, stepping up, or stepping down. Adherence, environmental control, and comorbid conditions should always be considered, however, before stepping up therapy.

MEDICATIONS

- Medications for chronic therapy should be based upon the initial severity and subsequent level of control achieved with intervention (Fig. 23–1).
- Medications are commonly classified into two groups:
  1. Controllers: inhaled and oral corticosteroids, leukotriene modifiers, long-acting β agonists, theophylline, cromolyn, nedocromil
  2. Relievers: short-acting β-agonists (SABA), short bursts of oral corticosteroids.

PREVENTION

- Influenza vaccine annually.
- Avoidance of deleterious airborne exposures.
  - Perennial allergens: house dust mites, pets, cockroaches, molds.
  - Reasonable avoidance measures to recommend if sensitivity is present.
    - For house dust mites: Wash bed linens and blankets weekly in hot water, encase pillows and mattresses in airtight covers, replace carpets with hard flooring, especially in sleeping rooms. (If possible, use vacuum cleaner with filters).
    - For animals with fur, removal of animals is optimal, but may consider removing the animal from sleeping areas, installing air filters, washing the pet.
    - For cockroach allergy, use pesticides: remove patient from home when spraying occurs.
- Outdoor pollen and mold allergens
  - Close windows and doors and remain indoors when pollen and mold counts are highest.
    - Indoor mold allergens: reduce dampness in the home; clean any damp areas frequently.
    - Tobacco smoke: avoidance of passive smoke exposure

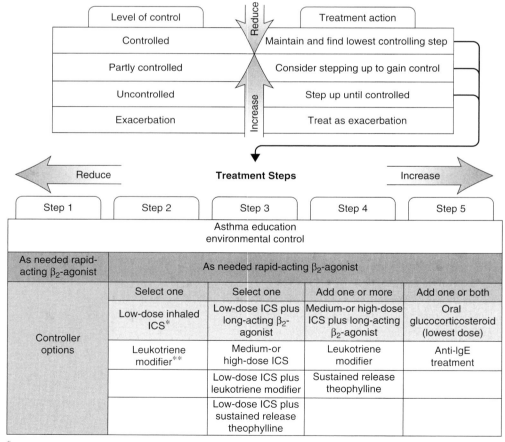

For Children Older than 5 years, Adolescents, and Adults

Level of control	Treatment action
Controlled	Maintain and find lowest controlling step
Partly controlled	Consider stepping up to gain control
Uncontrolled	Step up until controlled
Exacerbation	Treat as exacerbation

Reduce ← **Treatment Steps** → Increase

	Step 1	Step 2	Step 3	Step 4	Step 5
	Asthma education environmental control				
As needed rapid-acting β₂-agonist	As needed rapid-acting β₂-agonist				
		Select one	Select one	Add one or more	Add one or both
Controller options		Low-dose inhaled ICS*	Low-dose ICS plus long-acting β₂-agonist	Medium-or high-dose ICS plus long-acting β₂-agonist	Oral glucocorticosteroid (lowest dose)
		Leukotriene modifier**	Medium-or high-dose ICS	Leukotriene modifier	Anti-IgE treatment
			Low-dose ICS plus leukotriene modifier	Sustained release theophylline	
			Low-dose ICS plus sustained release theophylline		

* ICS-inhaled glucocorticosteroids
** Receptor antagonist or synthesis inhibitors

Alternative reliever treatments include inhaled anticholinergics, short-action oral β₂-agonists, some long-acting β₂-agonists, and short-acting theophylline. Regular dosing with short-and long-acting β₂-agonist is not advised unless accompanied by regular use of an inhaled glucocorticosteroid.

FIG. 23–1 Management approach based upon control.

- Occupational sensitizers: reduce or, preferably, avoid exposure to these agents.
- Drugs: avoid aspirin and NSAIDs if there is a history of respiratory exacerbations from these agents or severe asthma is present.
  - Up to 28% of adults with asthma have sensitivity to aspirin or NSAIDs, *aspirin-exacerbated respiratory disease* (AERD). AERD may be associated with nasal polyps. The diagnosis can only be confirmed by aspirin challenge.

MANAGEMENT OF ACUTE EXACERBATIONS

- Early treatment of asthma exacerbations is essential.

TREATMENT AT THE PATIENT'S HOME

- As part of routine asthma care, educate patients to recognize early indicators of an exacerbation, and what actions should be taken.
  - A written asthma action plan to guide patient self-management of an exacerbation is especially important for patients who have moderate or severe asthma and for any patient with a past severe exacerbation.
  - For patients who have difficulty perceiving the severity of their symptoms, a peak-flow–based plan may be particularly useful.
- An action plan should include thresholds for the following
  - Stepped up therapy including increased use of SABAs and, if appropriate, adding a short course of oral corticosteroids (see Management in an Urgent Care Setting below).
  - When the patient should communicate with the clinician (eg, significant deterioration of symptoms or peak flow, decreased responsiveness to SABAs, or decreased duration of benefit from them).
- Removal or withdrawal from environmental factors contributing to the exacerbation.

MANAGEMENT IN AN URGENT CARE SETTING

ASSESSMENT (SEE TABLE 23–3)
- General appearance
  - During acute exacerbations, the following suggest a severe, or life-threatening episode.
    - Tachypnea (respiratory rate >30/min), tachycardia, decrease in systolic blood pressure >15 mm Hg during inspiration (pulsus paradoxus), alteration in

consciousness, diaphoresis, and use of accessory (intercostal, subcostal, and sternocleidomastoid) muscles.
- Absence of these findings does not necessarily preclude a life-threatening exacerbation.
- Initial brief physical examination should
  - Assess overall patient status, including level of alertness, fluid status, and presence of cyanosis, respiratory distress, and wheezing.
    - Importantly, severe obstruction may be accompanied by a *silent chest*.
- Identify possible complications (eg, pneumonia, pneumothorax, or pneumomediastinum).
  - Assess for presence of subcutaneous emphysema or unequal breath sounds.
- Rule out upper airway obstruction.
  - Both intrathoracic and extrathoracic central airway obstruction can cause severe dyspnea and may be misdiagnosed as asthma.
  - Causes of central airway obstruction include upper airway foreign bodies, epiglottitis, organic diseases of the larynx, vocal cord dysfunction, and extrinsic and intrinsic tracheal narrowing.
  - Clues to the presence of alternative reasons for dyspnea include dysphonia, inspiratory stridor, monophonic wheezing loudest over the central airway, normal Po_2, and unexpectedly complete resolution of airflow obstruction after intubation.
  - Flow-volume loops may prove useful in the diagnosis of upper airway obstruction. If suspected, the patient should be referred for emergent laryngoscopy.
- Laboratory studies
  - Complete blood count (CBC) is not required routinely but may be appropriate in patients who have fever or purulent sputum.
    - Modest leukocytosis is common in asthma exacerbations and corticosteroid treatment will increase circulating polymorphonuclear leukocytes within 1 to 2 hours of administration.
  - Serum electrolyte measurements should be considered in patients who have been taking diuretics regularly and in patients who have coexistent cardiovascular disease.
    - Frequent SABA administration can cause transient decreases in serum potassium, magnesium, and phosphate.
  - Consider arterial blood gas (ABG) measurement for evaluating arterial carbon dioxide tension (Pco_2) in patients who have suspected hypoventilation, severe respiratory distress, and those who have FEV-1 or PEF (25% of predicted after initial treatment.
    - In such settings, a $Pco_2 \geq 40$ mm Hg indicates severe airflow obstruction and increased risk of respiratory failure. Emergent intubation should be considered in these patients.

TABLE 23–3 Severity of Asthma Exacerbations

PARAMETER	MILD	MODERATE	SEVERE	RESPIRATORY ARREST IMMINENT
Breathless	Walking Can lie down	Talking Infant-softer, shorter cry; difficulty reading Prefer sitting	At rest infant stops feeding Hunched forward	
Talks in	Sentences	Phrases	Words	
Alertness	May be agitated	Usually agitated	Usually agitated	Drowsy or confused
Respiratory rate	Increased	Increased	Often >30 min	
	Normal rates of breathing in awake children: Age — Normal rate <2 months — <60/min 2–12 months — <50/min 1–5 years — <40/min 6–8 years — <30 min			
Accessory muscles and suprasternal retractions	Usually not	Usually	Usually	Paradoxical thoraco-abdominal movement
Wheeze	Moderate, often only and expiratory	Loud	Usually loud	Absence of wheeze
Pulse/min	<100	100–120	>120	Bradycardia
	Guide to limits of normal pulse rate in children: Infants — 2–12 months — –Normal rate <160/min Preschool — 1–2 years — –Normal rate <120/min School age — 2–8 years — –Normal rate <110/min			
Pulsus paradoxus	Absent <10 mm Hg	May be present 10–25 mm Hg	Often present >25 mm Hg (adult) 20–40 mm Hg (child)	Absence suggests respiratory muscle fatigue
PEF after initial bronchodilator % predicted or % personal best	Over 80%	Approx 60–80%	<60% predicted or personal best <100L/min adults or response lasts <2 h	
PaO_2 (on air)* and/or $PaCo_{21}$	Normal test not usually necessary <45 mm Hg	>60 mm Hg <45 mm Hg	<60 mm Hg Possible cyanosis >45 mm Hg Possible respiratory failure (see text)	
SaO_2% (on air)†	>95%	91–95%	<90%	

hypercapnia (hypoventilation) develops more readily in young children than in adults and adolescents.

*Note: The presence of several parameters, but not necessarily all, indicates the general classification of the exacerlsation.

†Note: Kilopascals are also used internationally, conversion would be appropriate in this regard.

SOURCE: Global Initiative for Asthma (GINA), National Heart, Lung, and Blood Institute. Pocket guide for asthma management and prevention, revises 2006. Bethesda, MD: Medical Communications Resources, Inc., 2006.

○ Measure serum theophylline concentration in patients receiving theophylline to exclude toxicity.
  ▪ Consider additional tests if other comorbid conditions exist that may complicate the treatment of asthma exacerbations (eg, diabetes, cardiovascular disease, pneumonia).
• Lung function tests
  ○ Repeated FEV-1 or PEF measuremenst at presentation to the ED and 1 hour after treatment are the strongest single predictor of hospitalization among adults who present to the ED with an asthma exacerbation.

○ A predicted FEV-1 or PEF >70% is usually associated with a favorable outcome and, accordingly, such patients may be safely discharged from the ED.
  ▪ Note that this threshold differs from the ≥80% predicted FEV-1 or PEF desired for long-term asthma control.
○ There is limited value of pulmonary function measures in severe exacerbations.
• Chest radiography
  ○ Not recommended routinely, but may prove useful to exclude other comorbid conditions such as congestive

heart failure, pneumothorax, pneumomediastinum, pneumonia, or lobar atelectasis.

- Electrocardiogram (ECG)
  - Not required routinely, but a baseline ECG and continual monitoring of cardiac rhythm are appropriate in patients >50 years of age and in those who have documented heart disease or chronic obstructive pulmonary disease (COPD).
  - A pattern of right ventricular strain may reverse promptly with treatment of airflow obstruction.

TREATMENT

- Oxygen to relieve hypoxemia (in moderate or severe exacerbations).
  - Administer supplemental oxygen to maintain a Sao_2 >90% (>95% in pregnant women and in patients with coexistent heart disease).
- SABAs
  - Repetitive or continuous administration of SABAs is the most effective means of reversing airway obstruction.
  - Three successive treatments of SABA every 20 to 30 minutes can be given safely as initial therapy.
    - Subsequently, the frequency of administration varies according to the improvement in airflow obstruction and associated symptoms as well as the occurrence of side effects.
    - Continuous administration of SABA may be more effective in severely obstructed patients.
  - In mild to moderate exacerbations, equivalent bronchodilation can be achieved either by high doses (4–12 puffs) of a SABA via metered-dose inhaler (MDI) with a valved holding chamber under the supervision of trained personnel or by nebulizer therapy. Nebulizer therapy may be preferred in patients who are unable to effectively use an MDI.
- Inhaled ipratropium bromide
  - Can provide additive benefit to SABA in severe exacerbations.
  - For ongoing hospital management, ipratropium bromide is no longer recommended.
- Systemic corticosteroids
  - These agents hasten resolution of airflow obstruction, reduce the relapse rate, and may reduce hospitalizations. Some benefit may occur within 1 hour, although the full benefit may require several days.
  - Prescribe in moderate or severe exacerbations for patients who fail to respond promptly and completely to a SABA.
  - For patients who receive oral corticosteroids chronically, give supplemental doses of oral corticosteroids for exacerbations, even if only mild.
  - Oral prednisone has effects equivalent to intravenous (IV) methylprednisolone.
  - Prednisone dose (or equivalent): 40 to 60 mg/ day as single dose or 2 divided doses for 3 to 10 days.
- Consider adjunctive treatments, such as IV magnesium sulfate or heliox driven nebulization of inhaled β-agonists, in severe exacerbations unresponsive to initial treatments.
  - IV magnesium sulfate (2 g in adults, and 25 to 75 mg/kg [up to 2 g] in children) added to conventional therapy reduces hospitalization rates in ED patients who present with severe asthma exacerbations (PEF <40%).
- The following treatments are NOT recommended
  - Methylxanthines
    - Methylxanthines provide no additional benefit to optimal therapy in the ED or hospital, and increase the risk for adverse effects.
  - Antibiotics
    - Not generally recommended for the treatment of acute asthma exacerbations except as needed for comorbid conditions.
    - Reserved for patients who have fever and purulent sputum, if evidence of pneumonia, or bacterial sinusitis strongly suspected.
  - Mucolytic agents (eg, potassium iodide, acetylcysteine) may worsen cough or bronchial obstruction.
  - Sedation is not generally recommended.
    - Hypnotic and anxiolytic drugs are respiratory depressants and are contraindicated in severely ill asthma patients.
- Repeat assessment
  - Response to initial treatment in the ED is a better predictor of the need for hospitalization than the severity of an exacerbation on presentation. Evaluate the patient's subjective response; physical findings; FEV-1 or PEF; and pulse oximetry or ABG.
- Intubation considered if there are:
  - Signs of impending respiratory failure including inability to speak, altered mental status, intercostal muscle retraction, worsening fatigue, and a Pco_2 of ≥42 mm Hg.
- Hospitalization is a consideration based on
  - The duration and severity of symptoms, severity of airflow obstruction, response to ED treatment, severity of prior exacerbations, medication use at the time of the exacerbation, access to medical care and medications, adequacy of support and home conditions, and presence of underlying psychiatric illness.
- Disposition at discharge
  - Before hospital discharge, prevent relapse of the exacerbation or recurrence of symptoms by providing: follow-up within 1 to 4 weeks; simple action plan with instructions for medications prescribed at discharge

and for increasing medications or seeking medical care if asthma worsens; review of inhaler techniques, and whenever possible; consider initiating inhaled corticosteroids.

BIBLIOGRAPHY

Baren JM, Boudreaux ED, Brenner BE, et al. Randomized controlled trail of emergency department interventions to improve primary care follow-up for patients with acute asthma. *Chest.* 2006;129(2):257–265.

Blitz M, Blitz S, Hughes R, et al. Aerosolized magnesium sulfate for acute asthma: a systematic review. *Chest.* 2005;128(1): 337–344.

Camargo CA Jr, Smithline HA, Malice MP, et al. Continuous versus intermittent beta-agonists in the treatment of acute asthma. *Cochrane Database Syst Rev.* 2003b;(4): CD001115.

Cates CC, Bara A, Crilly JA, et al. Holding chambers versus nebulisers for beta-agonist treatment of acute asthma. *Cochrane Database Syst Rev.* 2003;(3):CD000052.

Edmonds ML, Camargo CA Jr, Pollack CV Jr, et al. Early use of inhaled corticosteroids in the emergency department treatment of acute asthma. *Cochrane Database Syst Rev.* 2003(3): CD002308.

Krishnan JA, Riekert KA, McCoy JV, et al. Corticosteroid use after hospital discharge among high-risk adults with asthma. *Am J Respir Crit Care Med.* 2004;170(12):1281–1285.

Manser R, Reid D, Abrahmson M. Corticosteroids for acute severe asthma in hospitalised patients. *Cochrane Database Syst Rev.* 2001;(1):CD001740.

National Heart, Lung, and Blood Institute, National Asthma Education and Prevention Program, Expert Panel Report 3: Guidelines for the Diagnosis and Management of Asthma, Full Report 2007, U.S. Department of Health and Human Services; National Institutes of Health; National Heart, Lung, and Blood Institute, Accessed November 8, 2007 at http://www.nhlbi.nih.gov/guidelines/asthma/.

Rodrigo GJ, Rodrigo C, Hall JV. Acute asthma in adults: a review. *Chest.* 2004;125(3):1081–1102.

Rowe BH, Bota GW, Fabris L, et al. Inhaled budesonide in addition to oral corticosteroids to prevent asthma relapse following discharge from the emergency department: a randomized controlled trial. *JAMA.* 1999;281(22):2119–2126.

Zeiger RS, Heller S, Mellon MH, et al. Facilitated referral to asthma specialist reduces relapses in asthma emergency room visits. *J Allergy Clin Immunol.* 1991;87(6): 1160–1168.

Global Initiative for Asthma (GINA), National Heart, Lung, and Blood Institute. *Pocket Guide for Asthma Management and Prevention,* revised 2006. Bethesda, MD: Medical Communications Resources, Inc., 2006.

24   IMMUNOLOGIC LUNG DISEASES

Raymond G. Slavin

- The lung is a superb immunologic shock organ. It has ready access to a vast array of potent aeroallergens, contains resident immunologically competent cells including mast cells and lymphocytes, and finally has a rich blood supply that can recruit inflammatory cells and cytokines from other areas.
- The Gell and Coombs classification of immunologic diseases can be applied to pulmonary disorders. Type I, which is mediated by immunoglobulin E (IgE), is best exemplified by bronchial asthma. Type II, or autoimmunity, is exemplified by Goodpasture syndrome in which antibody is directed toward a basement membrane antigen in the lung. Type III immune complex disease includes several drug reactions causing serum sickness, which may affect the lung. Type IV disease mediated by sensitized lymphocytes includes infectious processes such as tuberculosis.
- This chapter examines two unique lung diseases each of which is mediated by two of these immunologic responses: allergic bronchopulmonary aspergillosis (ABPA), which manifests types I and III, and hypersensitivity pneumonitis, which demonstrates types III and IV.

ALLERGIC BRONCHOPULMONARY ASPERGILLOSIS

- This condition is an example of the pulmonary infiltrate with eosinophilia syndrome (ie, pulmonary infiltrates with peripheral blood and sputum eosinophils). Initially thought to be rare in the United States, it is being increasingly reported in this country.

CLINICAL CHARACTERISTICS

- Usually, ABPA patients are atopic and have a history of bronchial asthma.[1]
- Complaints include anorexia, headache, mild temperature elevation, production of solid sputum plugs, and acute attacks of wheezing dyspnea.

LABORATORY CHARACTERISTICS

- Peripheral blood eosinophils are generally >1000/mm^3.
- Fungal mycelia and large number of eosinophils are seen in sputum.

TABLE 24–1   Diagnostic Criteria for Allergic Aspergillosis

MAJOR CRITERIA	MINOR CRITERIA
1. Episodic bronchial obstruction	1. Aspergillus fumigatus positive sputum culture
2. Peripheral blood eosinophilia	2. History of expectorating brown plugs or flecks
3. Positive immediate skin reactivity	3. Arthus (late) skin reactivity
4. Serum precipitating antibodies	
5. Elevated serum IgE	
6. Elevated IgG and IgE anti-Aspergillus antibodies	
7. History of pulmonary infiltrates	
8. Central bronchiectasis	

IgE, immunoglobulin E; IgG, immunoglobulin G.
Slavin RG. Allergic bronchopulmonary aspergillosis. In Fireman P, Slavin RG, eds. *Atlas of Allergies*. 2nd ed. London: Mosby-Wolfe 1996:131–139.

• A positive, immediate skin test to aspergillus is seen in 100% of patients.
• Serum immunoglobulin G (IgG) precipitating antibody is found in two-thirds of patients.
• Serum IgE levels are markedly elevated, being significantly higher than in uncomplicated bronchial asthma, on the order of >1000 IU/mL.

IMAGING STUDIES

• A large homogenous shadow on plain films of the chest is most common, which frequently shifts from one side to another.
• Atelectasis caused by mucous plugging is often seen.
• Bronchiectasis is a frequent complication of ABPA and is best seen in high-resolution computed tomography.

PULMONARY FUNCTION TESTING

• During an acute clinical flare, there is a significant decline in total lung capacity, vital capacity, forced expiratory volume at 1 second (FEV-1), and diffusing capacity of lung for carbon monoxide (DLCO).
• A decrease in DLCO is caused by accompanying bronchiectasis and is an important index of disease severity.

LUNG BIOPSY

• A marked inflammatory process is present, which is largely bronchocentric.[2]
• Large numbers of eosinophils and major basic protein are evident.

DIAGNOSIS

• The diagnostic criteria for ABPA are shown in Table 24–1. It has been suggested that the presence of the first seven major criteria makes the diagnosis of ABPA highly likely, whereas all eight makes it certain.

• A practical approach to the diagnosis of ABPA is seen in Figure 24–1. First, evaluate any patient with a history of pulmonary infiltrates and asthma with an aspergillus skin test. If this is positive, serum should be checked for a total IgE level and precipitins. If the total serum IgE is less than 500 IU/mL, ABPA is highly unlikely. If the IgE is higher than 500 IU/mL anti-*Aspergillus* IgE and IgG should be determined irrespective of precipitins. If these are elevated, a high-resolution computed

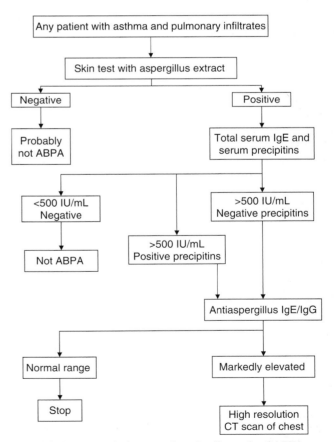

FIG. 24–1   A practical approach to the diagnosis of ABPA

tomography of the chest should be obtained to determine the extent of lung involvement.

PATHOGENESIS

- There is generally no clear relationship between exposure to an environment rich in *Aspergillus* spores and the development of ABPA. This tends to indicate that specific host susceptibility is more important to the development of ABPA than the extent of exposure to the organism.
- A cardinal feature of ABPA is that the organism is actively growing in the respiratory tract and continually shedding antigens into the tissues. Antigens released from the mycelia combine with IgE and IgG antibodies to set in motion a chain of immunological reactions culminating in bronchial wall damage and the surrounding pulmonary eosinophilic consolidation.

ASSOCIATION WITH CYSTIC FIBROSIS

- The incidence of ABPA is markedly increased in patients with cystic fibrosis (CF), on the order of 7% to 10%.[3] Because CF patients have a high degree of atopy, the diagnosis of ABPA may be particularly difficult. The Cystic Fibrosis Foundation has recently recommended that all CF patients have yearly determination of total serum IgE.

TREATMENT

- The basic aim of therapy in ABPA is to break the vicious cycle in which fungus, trapped in viscid secretions contained in the constricted asthmatic airway, continues to provide large quantities of antigenic and enzymatic material. The clinical presentation of ABPA may be quite subtle and a paucity of symptoms may be associated with profound tissue damage. Therefore, early and vigorous treatment is important to prevent the inexorable consequences of bronchiectasis, pulmonary fibrosis, and cor pulmonale.
- The cornerstone of treatment is systemic corticosteroids. Once the diagnosis of ABPA is made, corticosteroids must be given in a large enough quantity over a sufficient period of time. A daily dose of prednisone, 60 mg/kg body weight in divided doses, is frequently required to clear the chest radiograph completely in the adult. After radiographic clearing, a single daily dose of 0.5 mg/kg of body weight is given for 2 weeks. At this point, there is a gradual taper to 0.25 mg/kg body weight over a 6-week period. The dose is then switched to 0.5 mg/kg body weight every other day for another 6 weeks, and then gradually tapered over a 3-month period. In total, the steroid treatment is given over approximately a 7-month period. During this period,

monthly serum IgE levels are obtained. A decrease from the initial, markedly elevated level is always seen but generally does not return to normal levels. A rise in the serial IgE level, subsequently tested on a monthly basis, should prompt an increase in steroid therapy.
- There have been promising reports on the effectiveness of itraconazole, an oral antifungal agent, on decreasing the fungal burden in ABPA. In one study of nine patients treated with prednisone, the addition of itraconazole at a dose of 400 mg daily resulted in a decrease in recurrence of radiographic shadows and a reduction in oral steroid requirement. An open study showed that this approach reduced recurrence of flare-ups, reduced IgE levels and blood eosinophils, and improved FEV-1. In a study of clinically stable ABPA patients, 400 mg daily of itraconazole alone resulted in reduction in sputum eosinophils and eosinophilic cationic protein, total serum IgE, specific IgG to aspergillus, and requirement of oral steroids for respiratory symptoms.[4]

HYPERSENSITIVITY PNEUMONITIS

INTRODUCTION

- Hypersensitivity pneumonitis (HP) has several synonyms, including *pulmonary hypersensitivity syndrome* and *extrinsic allergic alveolitis.* The last term seems particularly appropriate, because it graphically describes the condition. *Extrinsic* meaning it comes from an outside source, *allergic* denoting a hypersensitivity basis, and *alveolitis* referring to that part of the lung most affected by the disease. Whatever name is used, it refers to the same basic process: a hypersensitivity reaction of the lung to inhalation of an organic dust.
- Three factors determine how one responds to inhalation of an organic dust:
  1. *Basic immunologic reactivity of the host.* An atopic individual characteristically responds with production of IgE antibody. A nonatopic person is more likely to produce IgG.
  2. *Nature and source of the antigen.* Is it small enough to reach the distal part of the lung? Is its temperature requirement such that it will grow in the respiratory tract?
  3. *Nature and circumstances of the exposure.* Is the exposure intense and intermittent or is it low-grade and chronic?
- Table 24–2 shows the nature of the disease related to the exposure. An intermittent short-term extensive exposure such as that experienced by a pigeon breeder cleaning out the coops manifests acute reversible disease. A pet store employee who has intermittent, lower grade but long-term exposure, develops a subacute form, which is usually reversible. Finally, a long-term, low-grade

TABLE 24–2 Nature of Disease Related to Exposure

EXPOSURE	EXAMPLE	DISEASE
Intermittent, short term	Pigeon breeder	Acute: reversible
Intermittent, long term	Pet store employee	Subacute: usually reversible
Long term	Parakeet owner	Chronic: irreversible

exposure experienced by a parakeet owner may result in chronic irreversible disease.

CAUSES

- Table 24–3 places the causes of HP into four categories.[5] The first example of HP was farmer's lung caused by a thermophilic organism. These are unicellular branching organisms that resemble true bacteria. A previously common occupational form of HP was bagassosis or Louisiana sugarcane workers disease. Mold can also cause HP: in maple bark strippers disease, developing in loggers that strip the tree bark and, thus, are exposed to cryptostroma corticale, and malt workers lung, developing in brewery workers exposed to aspergillus clavatus present in the moldy barley on brewery floors. Probably the most common cause of HP today is avian antigen. Birds are becoming an increasingly popular pet and serve as a potent source of antigens responsible for HP. Finally, an example of a chemical source is toluene di-isocyanate, which may cause disease in bathtub refinishers.

CLINICAL FEATURES

ACUTE
- Chills, fever, and shortness of breath seen 4 to 6 hours after exposure.
- Physical examination reveals only crackling rales in the lower lung fields. Hypersensitivity pneumonitis is an example of interstitial pneumonitis in which disparity is seen between symptoms and physical findings.
- Chest radiograph shows nodular densities and a *ground glass* appearance in the lower lung fields.

TABLE 24–3 Causes of Hypersensitivity Pneumonitis

ANTIGENS	DISEASES
Thermophilic actinomycetes	
Micropolyspora faeni	Farmer lung
Thermoactinomyces sacchari	Bagassosis
Molds	
Cryptostroma corticale	Maple bark disease
Aspergillus clavatus	Malt-worker lung
Animals	
Ox or pig	Pituitary snuff-taker lung
Pigeon	Pigeon-breeder disease
Chemicals	
Toluene di-isocyanate	Bathtub finisher lung

- Serum IgG precipitating antibody is an immunologic hallmark for HP.
- Early on PFTs show no sign of airway obstruction, but there is evidence of alveolar capillary block and DLCO is the first parameter to decrease.

CHRONIC
- This insidious form may be difficult to differentiate from chronic obstructive pulmonary disease.
- Shortness of breath, productive cough, and airway obstruction progressing to pulmonary fibrosis is seen.

IMMUNOPATHOGENESIS

- The following scenario has been suggested.[6] Inhaled antigen acts on alveolar macrophages to activate and release enzymes and reactive oxygen (O_2) metabolites resulting in parenchymal inflammation and damage leading to interstitial fibrosis. Interstitial fibrosis is also produced by macrophage release of fibronectin and fibroblast growth factor. Inhaled antigen also acts on alveolar lymphocytes, which have also been stimulated by interleukin-1 produced by alveolar macrophages. This results in interleukin-2 production leading to further T-cell proliferation and lymphokine release.
- Activated alveolar lymphocytes also produce mononuclear cell chemotactic factors, which results in granuloma formation and, together with B cells, induces hyperglobulinemia in the alveolar lining fluid.

DIAGNOSIS

- The condition should be suspected in any case of recurrent pneumonia, interstitial pneumonitis, or pulmonary fibrosis.
  - Typical history is characterized by signs and symptoms 4 to 6 hours after exposure.
  - Chest radiograph shows a ground glass appearance in the lower lung field with nodular densities suggesting alveolar pneumonia.
  - PFT reveal a restrictive pattern with DLCO decreasing first.
  - Serum IgG precipitating antibody is present on double- gel diffusion testing.
  - Bronchoalveolar lavage shows hyperglobulinemia with an increase in CD8+ T-suppresson cells.
  - Lung biopsy reveals significant increase in lymphocytes, plasma cells, and foamy histocytes. In advanced cases, fibrosis is seen with thickening of the alveolar capillary wall and obliteration of the alveolar spaces.[7]

TREATMENT

- In the acute form, simple removal from the offending agent generally suffices. If symptoms are severe, start the patient on a tapering dose of prednisone beginning with 60 mg/d. Supportive measures would include O_2, antitussives, and antipyretics.

- For the repeated, acute, or subacute form, decrease exposure as much as possible coupled with the administration of long-term corticosteroids, emphasizing alternate-day therapy.
- The chronic form can be treated with long-term corticosteroids but only if radiographic findings and physiologic changes indicate a response.

PREVENTION

- It is vital that the antigen responsible for HP be determined so that appropriate environmental control measures can be carried out. Several measures can decrease the antigenic burden:
  - Chemicals can be added to prevent growth. A good example is propionic acid which, when added to sugar cane, eliminates the growth of the thermophilic organism responsible for bagassosis.
  - Water should be changed frequently in humidification or air conditioning units.
  - Storage dryers decrease the growth of mold and thermophilic organisms in hay and straw.
  - Crops should be harvested when the moisture content is low.
- There are many ways to decrease exposure to organic dust:
  - Mechanically handle dusty materials within closed spaces.
  - Effective ventilation removes dust from the ambient air.
  - Personal respirators or masks may be used.
  - When the aforementioned measures have failed, remove the worker from the disease-producing environment.[8]

REFERENCES

1. Rosenberg M, Patterson R, Mintzer R, et al. Clinical and immunologic criteria for the diagnosis of allergic bronchopulmonary aspergillosis. *Ann Intern Med.* 1977;86:405–414.
2. Slavin RG, Bedrossian CW, Hutcheson PS, et al. A pathologic study of allergic bronchopulmonary aspergillosis. *J Allergy Clin Immunol.* 1988;81:718–725.
3. Stevens DA, Moss RB, Kurup VA, et al. Allergic bronchopulmonary aspergillosis in cystic fibrosis—State of the Art: Cystic Fibrosis Foundation Consensus Conference. *Clin Infect Dis.* 2003;37(suppl 3):S225–S264.
4. Wark PAB, Hensley MJ, Saltos N, et al. Anti-inflammatory effect of itraconazole in stable allergic bronchopulmonary aspergillosis: a randomized controlled trial. *J Allergy Clin Immunol.* 2003;111:952–957.
5. Fink JN, Zacharisen MC. *Hypersensitivity Pneumonitis in Middleton's Allergy Principles and Practice.* 6th ed. Philadelphia: Mosby; 2003:1373–1390.
6. Stankus RP, deShazo RD. In *Interstitial Lung Disease.* Schwartz MI, King TE, eds. Philadelphia: BC Decker; 1988:111–122.
7. Temprano J, Knutsen AP, Slavin RG. Hypersensitivity pneumonitis. *Curr Pediatr Rev.* 2005;1:265–281.
8. Slavin RG. *Hypersensitivity Pneumonitis in Current Therapy in Allergy, Immunology, and Rheumatology.* 5th ed. Philadelphia: Mosby; 1996:261–263.

25 ALLERGIC RHINITIS

Raymond G. Slavin

Allergic rhinitis is an allergic inflammatory response in the nose. It can be classified as seasonal or perennial, depending on the allergens triggering the reaction.

EPIDEMIOLOGY

- Allergic rhinitis is the most common atopic disease in the United States.
- It affects 24 million Americans—an estimated 8% of the population—with an equal distribution between males and females.
- The prevalence of allergic rhinitis varies by age: 32% of patients are 17 years of age or younger, 43% are 18 to 44 years of age, 17% are 45 to 64 years of age, and only 8% are 65 years of age or older.
- Indirect costs of treating allergic rhinitis including lowered productivity and time lost from work or school are substantial. The total direct healthcare cost of treating allergic rhinitis is estimated at $3.4 billion.[1]

PATHOPHYSIOLOGY

The airborne allergens responsible for allergic rhinitis can be divided into seasonal (trees, grass, weeds, and mold) and nonseasonal or perennial (house dust mites, pets, and insects).

- The allergic or immunologic process begins when inhalants are deposited on the nasal mucosa. They are processed by antigen-presenting cells, most notably dendritic cells, and are then presented to helper T-cells. In individuals who are genetically predisposed, this interaction promotes the generation and release of cytokines that induce B cells to produce antigen-specific immunoglobulin E (IgE). The IgE attaches to high avidity receptors on mast cells and basophils, and the patient is thereby sensitized.

• On subsequent exposure, the inhaled allergen bridges IgE molecules resulting in release of mediators, most notably, histamine. Histamine causes increased epithelial permeability, vasodilation, and stimulation of a parasympathetic reflex. As a result, acetylcholine is released, resulting in marked hypersecretion of mucous and increased blood flow. Activation of centers in the central nervous system results in sneezing.

DIAGNOSIS

CLINICAL MANIFESTATIONS

Symptoms of allergic rhinitis can include paroxysms of sneezing, nasal congestion, clear rhinorrhea, and itching of the nose and palate. Distinct temporal patterns of symptom production can aid diagnosis. For example, seasonal allergic rhinitis symptoms typically appear during a specific time of the year when aeroallergens are abundant in the outside air. Symptoms of rhinitis that occur whenever the patient is exposed to a pet with fur suggest IgE-mediated sensitivity to that species. Allergic rhinitis can result in fatigue and significant disability.[2]

PHYSICAL EXAMINATION

The patient with allergic rhinitis can appear uncomfortable, exhibiting mouth breathing. Children in particular can have so-called *allergic shiners* (dark rings under the eyes). Allergic shiners develop because the edematous nasal tissue compresses the veins that drain the eyes, leading to pooling of blood under the orbits. On the bridge of the nose, an allergic crease may be present—a result of continued upward rubbing of the tip of the nose (the so-called *allergic salute*). On nasal examination, the mucosa typically appears pale and swollen, with a bluish-gray appearance when the mucosal edema is severe. Many patients have a normal examination, although they are often sneezing and have rhinorrhea with mucosal edema. The other physical findings tend to be present in the more severely affected patients.

LABORATORY TESTING

Although a careful history is the most important step toward the diagnosis of allergic disease, skin testing can be useful in pinpointing the offending allergen. The simplicity, ease and rapidity of performance, low cost, and high sensitivity of skin testing make such tests preferable to in vitro testing such as a radioallergosorbent assay test (RAST).

DIFFERENTIAL DIAGNOSIS

The two nasal conditions most commonly confused with allergic rhinitis are infectious rhinitis and perennial nonallergic rhinitis (vasomotor rhinitis).[3]

• Infectious rhinitis is characterized by constitutional symptoms and purulent rhinorrhea. A nasal smear shows a preponderance of neutrophils, whereas in allergic rhinitis, eosinophils predominate.

• Perennial nonallergic rhinitis is more frequent in women and is precipitated by such nonspecific factors as changes in temperature, humidity, and barometric pressure; strong odors; alcohol; and cigarette smoke. Nasal congestion frequently shifts from side to side and is often alleviated by exercise.

TREATMENT

Therapy for allergic rhinitis comprises three elements: first, minimizing contact with the allergen (environmental control); second, pharmacotherapy; and third, immunotherapy, which is reserved for selected patients. Together, these treatments ensure an excellent prognosis for allergic rhinitis (Table 25–1).[4]

ENVIRONMENTAL CONTROL

Reducing or completely avoiding the offending allergen is a vital part of allergy management. In the case of seasonal allergies, keeping the doors and windows closed and the air conditioning on will reduce the aeroallergen burden manyfold. Measures to avoid house dust mites should focus on the patient's bedroom and include encasing the mattress, box spring, and pillows in occlusive covers; weekly washing of bedding at 54°C (130°F) or hotter, dehumidification to less than 50%; and removal of reservoirs, such as carpeting. Removal of

TABLE 25–1 Management of Allergic Rhinitis

Environmental Control
Air conditioning for seasonal inhalants
House dust mite avoidance measures
Pet avoidance
Pharmacotherapy
Nonsedating antihistamines
Decongestants
Topical nasal sprays
Corticosteroids
Antihistamines
Immunotherapy (allergy shots)

pets is the optimal approach for pet-sensitive patients. If the patient will not part with the pet, weekly washings of the animal will reduce airborne levels of allergen. Also, patients with allergic rhinitis appear to be more sensitive to nonspecific irritants, such as cigarette smoke.

PHARMACOTHERAPY

Oral antihistamines are effective in reducing itching, sneezing, and rhinorrhea from allergic rhinitis. A major limitation of the first-generation (classic) antihistamines has been sedation. The second-generation antihistamines, cetirizine (Zyrtec), fexofenadine (Allegra), and loratadine (Claritin) and its metabolite desloratadine (Clarinex), produce significantly less sedation. In patients with nasal congestion, an antihistamine-decongestant combination can be used. An intranasal antihistamine spray azelastine (Astelin) has also proved to be efficacious. In severe cases, a short course of oral corticosteroids might be needed.

The most effective medications for controlling symptoms of allergic rhinitis are nasally inhaled corticosteroids. They include beclomethasone (Beconase), budesonide (Rhinocort), fluticasone propionate (Flonase), mometasone (Nasonex), and triamcinolone (Nasacort). These agents are generally not associated with significant systemic side effects. Local side effects (eg, nasal irritation and a burning sensation) are minimized if patients are instructed to direct the spray toward the ear and away from the septum.

Leukotriene receptor antagonists have been approved for use in allergic rhinitis and can be considered as a component of combination therapy, particularly if there is associated asthma.

Omalizumab (Xolair) is a recombinant, humanized, monoclonal anti-IgE antibody for treatment of moderate to severe asthma. It has been shown to significantly reduce serum IgE and to have beneficial effects on allergic rhinitis. However, it is costly and has only been approved for use in asthma by the Food and Drug Administration, thus, precluding its routine use in allergic rhinitis.

IMMUNOTHERAPY

Allergen immunotherapy is highly effective in controlling symptoms of allergic rhinitis. It should be considered in patients with severe symptoms that cannot be controlled by other treatment modalities and in those with comorbid conditions such as asthma. Immunotherapy may prevent worsening of asthma or possibly prevent its development. The effectiveness of symptomatic medications, particularly intranasal corticosteroids, has made immunotherapy less necessary than in the past.

COMPLICATIONS

In addition to the discomfort and decrease in quality of life experienced by patients with allergic rhinitis, this condition can result in complications. There is good evidence that poorly managed allergic rhinitis can result in otitis media and sinusitis. Rhinitis and asthma frequently coexist. Moreover, rhinitis appears to be a risk factor for development of asthma, and treatment of rhinitis can improve coexisting asthma. Prevention of asthma is an especially important goal in patients with a family history of asthma or atopic disease and early sensitization to aeroallergens.[5]

REFERENCES

1. Low AW, Reed SD, Sundy JS, et al. Direct costs of allergic rhinitis in the United States: estimates from the 1996 medical expenditure panel survey. *J Allergy Clin Immunol.* 2003;111:296.
2. Dykewicz MS, Fineman S. Executive summary of Joint Task Force Practice Parameters on diagnosis and management of rhinitis. *Ann Allergy Asthma Immunol.* 1998;81:463.
3. Zeiger RS. Allergic and non-allergic rhinitis. Classification and pathogenesis (pt 1 & 2). *Am J Rhinol.* 1989;3:21,113.
4. Howarth PH. Allergic and nonallergic rhinitis. In Adkins NF Jr, Yunginger JW, Busse WW, et al, eds. *Allergy: Principles and Practice.* 6th ed. Philadelphia, PA: Mosby; 2003:1391.
5. Skoner DP. Complications of allergic rhinitis. *J Allergy Clin Immunol.* 2000;105:S605.

26 SINUSITIS
Raymond G. Slavin

DEFINITION

Sinusitis is defined as inflammation of one or more of the paranasal sinuses. It has been suggested that the term rhinosinusitis may be more accurate for the following reasons: rhinitis typically precedes sinusitis; sinusitis without rhinitis is rare: the mucosa of the nose and sinuses are contiguous and symptoms of nasal obstruction and nasal discharge are prominent in sinusitis.[1] Rhinitis associated with sinusitis can be allergic, bacterial, viral, or perennial nonallergic.

Sinusitis can be classified as follows:
• Acute—Symptoms for less than 4 weeks
• Subacute—Lasting from 4 to 8 weeks
• Chronic—Persistent sinus inflammation longer than 8 weeks

EPIDEMIOLOGY

Rhinosinusitis is the most frequently reported chronic disease in the United States, affecting 16% of the adult population.

Chronic rhinosinusitis accounts for 11.6 million physician office visits a year, and the overall direct cost in the United States is estimated to be $4.3 billion annually.

In one study of patients with rhinosinusitis, a 36-item health survey showed significant worsening in several domains, including bodily pain, general health, vitality, and social functioning. Comparison with other chronic diseases (eg, chronic obstructive pulmonary disease, heart failure, angina, and back pain) revealed significantly worse bodily pain and social functioning in patients with sinusitis.[2]

PATHOGENESIS

The paranasal sinuses are composed of the ethmoid, frontal, maxillary, and sphenoid sinuses. Microorganisms, pollutants, irritants, and other foreign particles that escape the filtering apparatus of the nose are trapped in the mucus of the sinuses. The steady beating of the cilia that line the sinuses moves mucus out of the sinuses and into the nasal passages via the drainage ostia. This ongoing clearance of the sinuses is important for maintaining health.

The key factors that predispose an individual to rhinosinusitis are local (Table 26–1). The most common of these are viral upper respiratory infections (URIs) and allergic rhinitis. Edema of the nasal mucosa, which is characteristic of acute infectious or allergic rhinitis, results in obstruction of the ostia, decreased ciliary action in the paranasal sinuses, and increased mucus volume and viscosity. The subsequent accumulation of mucus in the sinus provides an environment for secondary bacterial infection and the conversion of mucus to mucopus.

TABLE 26–1 Factors Predisposing to Sinusitis

Intrinsic (local)	Allergic rhinitis
	Anatomic variants
	Septal deviation
	Haller cells (infraorbital ethmoid cells)
	Hypertrophied adenoids
	Nasal polyps, chronic mucosal thickening
	Nasal or sinus tumors
	Cigarette smoke
	Swimming and diving; barotraumas
	Rhinitis medicamentosa
	Cocaine abuse
	Nasal intubation
	Periapical abscess in a protruding tooth
	Dental extraction or injections
Extrinsic (systemic)	GERD
	Immune deficienc

GERD, gastroesophageal reflux disease

A recently described cause of sinusitis is gastroesophageal reflux disease (GERD).

- pH probe monitoring of both children and adults with chronic sinusitis shows a high incidence of both esophageal and nasopharyngeal reflux.
- Medical treatment of GERD in children and adults has been shown to result in significant improvement in sinusitis symptoms.
- In patients with sinusitis refractory to medical therapy, treatment of associated GERD should be considered before surgical intervention.

In cases of sinusitis resistant to usual medical therapy, immunodeficiency is a possibility.

- The majority of immunodeficiency patients with recurrent sinusitis have defects in humoral immunity. However, other types of immunodeficiencies, including AIDS, can present with recurrent sinusitis as one of their clinical features.
- Appropriate laboratory studies in patients with recurrent or chronic sinusitis can include quantitative immunoglobulin measurement (IgG, IgA, and IgM), specific antibody responses (tetanus toxoid and pneumococcal vaccine), and measurement of T-cell number and function (delayed hypersensitivity skin tests and flow cytometric enumeration of T cells).

Cultures from both adults and children with acute sinusitis grow predominantly aerobic organisms, with the heaviest yield being *Streptococcus pneumoniae, Haemophilus influenzae,* and *Moraxella* (formerly *Branhamella*) *catarrhalis.* Although the role of viruses and bacteria in causing actual infectious sinusitis is well established, the role of microbial infection in chronic sinus disease is much less clear. It was once believed that anaerobic organisms were responsible for instances of chronic sinusitis, but aerobes have now been implicated as the major cause. A noninfectious form of chronic rhinosinusitis, sometimes referred to as chronic hyperplastic eosinophilic rhinosinusitis, is marked by a preponderance of eosinophils and mixed mononuclear cells and by a paucity of neutrophils. It is often associated with nasal polyps, asthma, and aspirin sensitivity.[3]

Fungal sinusitis can take one of three forms: allergic fungal sinusitis, mycetoma, or fulminant invasive disease. There is an evolving literature of the potential for non-IgE immunologically mediated reactions to fungi that results in an inflammatory process in the sinuses.

DIAGNOSIS

CLINICAL MANIFESTATIONS

- Acute sinusitis: The most important clinical clue to the diagnosis of acute sinusitis is the failure of symptoms to resolve after a typical cold. The previously clear nasal discharge becomes yellow or green. Fever persists and chills may develop. Pain is often felt in the cheek, or it may be referred to the forehead. The discomfort is often worse on bending over or straining. If the ostium of the maxillary sinus is blocked, pain may be severe and felt in the teeth.

On physical examination, thick, purulent, green or deep yellow secretions are seen in the nose on the side of the diseased sinus. Because the maxillary sinus is most frequently involved, purulent secretions will be seen most often in the middle meatus, which is the drainage site of the maxillary sinus. The middle meatus may be hidden by the middle turbinate; as a result, it may be necessary to shrink the turbinate with a topical decongestant. Once this is accomplished, the nose, particularly the middle meatus, can be examined thoroughly not only for pus but also for underlying problems, such as nasal septal deviation, spurs, and polyps. Frequently, a streak of pus is visible along the lateral wall of the oropharynx. When the diagnosis of sinusitis is in doubt, referring the patient to an otolaryngologist for fiberoptic nasopharyngoscopy can be helpful, because this technique affords a better opportunity for visualization of the drainage ostia of infected sinuses.

- Chronic sinusitis: If mucopus is not evacuated, acute sinusitis may enter a subacute or chronic phase. Chronic maxillary sinusitis may exist alone, but it is usually associated with chronic ethmoid and frontal sinusitis. The lack of pain or systemic symptoms makes chronic sinusitis difficult to diagnose on history alone. A patient may complain of dull pressure in the face or head. Chronic sinusitis generally presents as persistent, sometimes unilateral, nasal stuffiness, hyposmia, purulent nasal and postnasal secretions, sore throat, fetid breath, and malaise. The secretions often pool in the hypopharynx at night, and the patient complains of increasing postnasal drainage with resultant cough and, sometimes, wheezing. On physical examination, a patient with chronic sinusitis may display an edematous and hyperemic nasal mucosa bathed in mucopus. Nasal polyps may accompany chronic sinusitis.

NASAL SMEAR AND SINUS CULTURE

Nasal culture does not give an adequate picture of the organisms responsible for sinusitis. Microscopic examination of nasal secretions, however, may be of great diagnostic value. In instances of sinusitis, one sees sheets of polymorphonuclear neutrophils and bacteria. This is unlike viral URIs, in which polymorphonuclear neutrophils are scanty, or allergic rhinitis, in which a high percentage of eosinophils may be seen. Antral puncture provides a true specimen of the microbiology of the sinus cavity and is generally performed by an otolaryngologist when it is important to determine the pathogen (eg, if fungal infection is suspected). There is recent evidence that aspiration of sinus contents through a fiberoptic rhinoscope may also yield good sinus specimens.

RADIOLOGY

Two imaging modalities are used for the diagnosis of sinusitis: plain x-rays and computed tomography (CT). In adults, plain films of the sinuses that show mucosal thickening greater than 8 mm, an air-fluid level, or opacification have been shown to correlate with positive bacterial cultures on antral punctures. Conventional radiographs can depict changes of acute sinusitis in maxillary, ethmoid, frontal, and sphenoid sinuses; but they cannot delineate the status of individual ethmoid air cells or the ostiomeatal complex, nor can they accurately show the extent of inflammatory disease in affected patients.

For these reasons, CT is the radiographic modality of choice for examining the paranasal sinuses. Coronal CT scans demonstrate the ostiomeatal complex and detect subtle disease that is not shown on plain films. The cost of CT scans used to be prohibitive, but through improved technology and the use of limited slices, the price has been reduced to the point where it is quite close to that of plain films in most centers. A limited four-slice coronal CT scan of the sinuses provides much more information than plain films do; and compared with full CT, four-slice coronal CT provides the increased information at a much reduced radiation dose and cost.[4]

Transillumination and ultrasonography are used in the diagnosis of sinusitis. Both are subject to great error, however, and cannot be recommended at the present time.

DIFFERENTIAL DIAGNOSIS

The condition most often misdiagnosed as rhinosinusitis is a viral URI, which is the most important predisposing cause of acute rhinosinusitis. Rhinosinusitis is probably present if the URI symptoms do not resolve in 3 to 6 days; if the secretions, particularly postnasal secretions, turn yellow or green and persist throughout the day; and if the patient notes fullness of the head and discomfort in the face and teeth.

ASSOCIATED CONDITIONS

- Otitis media
  - Many similarities exist between otitis media and sinusitis including histology, pathogenesis, and rash factors.
  - Otitis media and sinusitis frequently coexist.
  - In patients with acute bacterial sinusitis, one should look for the presence of otitis media. The converse is also true.

- Asthma
  - The association between sinusitis and asthma is extremely high.
  - A causal relationship appears to exist but no direct factor has yet been found.
  - Studies in both adults and children suggest that medical and surgical management of sinusitis results in objective and subjective improvement of asthma.[5]

TREATMENT

Concern has been raised about the overdiagnosis of rhinosinusitis and unnecessary treatment with antibiotics of uncomplicated viral upper respiratory infection. More strict criteria for the use of antibiotics are symptoms for 10 to 14 days or severe symptoms, such as fever with purulent nasal discharge, facial pain or tenderness, and periorbital swelling.

The antibiotic of choice for treatment of acute sinusitis is ampicillin or amoxicillin. An appropriate dosage of amoxicillin for acute sinusitis in the adult is 875 mg twice daily for 10 to 14 days. In patients with penicillin sensitivity, trimethoprim-sulfamethoxazole (one double-strength tablet twice a day) is an adequate alternative. β-Lactamase-producing organisms are being increasingly recognized. In penicillin-resistant sinusitis, recommended antibiotics include amoxicillin with clavulanic acid (Augmentin), and the quinolones (eg, levofloxacin [Levaquin]). Antibiotic treatment for chronic sinusitis should be continued for at least 2 weeks. If the patient reports feeling better by the last day of the regimen but still has purulent nasal discharge, the antibiotic can be continued for another 5 to 7 days.

Ancillary treatments for sinusitis, including oral decongestants and mucus thinners, have been advocated, but there are no controlled studies showing their effectiveness. The addition of intranasal corticosteroids may be modestly beneficial in the treatment of patients with recurrent acute or chronic rhinosinusitis.

In some cases of chronic resistant sinusitis, surgical treatment must be considered. A wide array of surgical procedures is available, but functional endoscopic sinus surgery (FESS) has emerged as the technique of choice.

COMPLICATIONS

Complications of sinusitis have decreased in incidence since the introduction of antibiotics. The complications most commonly encountered are cellulitis, abscess, and cavernous sinus thrombosis (all involving the orbit); epidural or subdural abscess; mucocele formation; and osteomyelitis.

PROGNOSIS

The prognosis for patients with sinusitis should be excellent if the diagnosis is made accurately and promptly, and an appropriate antibiotic is administered for a sufficient period of time. Consultation with a specialist should be sought in the following situations
- If there is a need to clarify the allergic or immunologic basis for sinusitis
- If sinusitis is refractory to the usual antibiotic treatment
- If sinusitis is recurrent
- If sinusitis is associated with unusual opportunistic infections
- If sinusitis significantly affects performance and quality of life

Consultation is also appropriate when concomitant conditions are present that complicate assessment or treatment, including chronic otitis media, bronchial asthma, nasal polyps, recurrent pneumonia, immunodeficiencies, aspirin sensitivity, allergic fungal disease, granulomas, and multiple antibiotic sensitivities.

REFERENCES

1. Slavin RG, Spector SL, Bernstein IL. The diagnosis and management of sinusitis: a practice parameter update. *J Allergy Clin Immunol.* 2005;116(suppl):S15–S29.
2. Gliklich RE, Metson R. The health impact of chronic sinusitis in patients seeking otolaryngological care. *Otolaryngol Head Neck Surgery.* 1995;113:104–115.
3. Hamilos D. Chronic sinusitis. *J Allergy Clin Immunol.* 2000; 106:213–220.
4. Wippold FJ, Levitt RG, Evens RG, et al. Limited coronal CT: an alternative screening examination for sinonasal inflammatory disease. *Allergy Proc.* 1995;16:165–173.
5. Borish L. Sinusitis and asthma: entering the realm of evidence–based medicine. *J Allergy Clin Immunol.* 2002;109:606–612.

27 ANAPHYLAXIS

Mark S. Dykewicz

DEFINITION

- Anaphylaxis is an acute, allergic systemic reaction, during which all or some of the following are present: urticaria/angioedema, upper airway obstruction, bronchospasm, and hypotension. In some cases, these manifestations may be accompanied by cardiovascular and/or gastrointestinal disturbances. Anaphylaxis can be fatal without evidence of cutaneous involvement.

TERMINOLOGY

- Several schemes have been used to classify anaphylaxis into several broad categories.
  - Classic:
    - Anaphylaxis: immunoglobulin E (IgE) antibody mediated.
    - Anaphylactoid: non–IgE antibody mediated.
    - The clinical presentations and acute treatment of both types of reactions are similar, but prevention strategies may differ.
  - Recently, the term *anaphylactoid* has been abandoned in favor of the following terminology:
    - Anaphylaxis immunologic: IgE (eg, from penicillin) or non-IgE (eg, infusion of aggregates of heterologous immunoglobulin that cause complement activation).
    - Anaphylaxis nonimmunologic (eg, radiocontrast media).

INCIDENCE AND SEVERITY

- The incidence of anaphylaxis is likely underestimated because of misdiagnosis. It is estimated that anaphylaxis is responsible for 500 to 1000 deaths in the United States each year.

CAUSES OF ANAPHYLAXIS

- The principal causes of anaphylaxis are foods, drugs (eg, antibiotics, nonsteroidal antiinflammatory drugs [NSAIDs], vaccines), insect stings, latex, exercise, and idiopathic.

FOOD-INDUCED ANAPHYLAXIS

- Prevalence/incidence:
  - Approximately 35% to 55% of anaphylaxis cases are caused by food allergies.
  - The incidence of food allergies and anaphylaxis is increasing.
  - Accidental food exposures are common and unpredictable.
- Common triggers:
  - Eight foods are responsible for approximately 90% of all allergic reactions to foods.
    - In both children and adults, peanuts, tree nuts, shellfish, and fish are common triggers. Allergic sensitivity to these foods tends to persist throughout life.
    - In children, other common triggers include milk, eggs, soy, and wheat. Sensitivity to these foods tends to disappear with advancing age.
  - It is a common misconception that food anaphylaxis occurs after ingestion of *new* foods.
  - However, anaphylaxis reactions occur to many foods that had been previously ingested with impunity but have induced an IgE antibody response (ie, a latent period of sensitization).
  - Once food anaphylaxis has developed, reingestion of that the offending food almost always results in a recurrent reaction.
  - Fatalities from food-induced anaphylaxis most commonly occur in patients with a history of systemic allergic reactions yet have no epinephrine available for use at the time of their reaction.

INSECT VENOM–INDUCED ANAPHYLAXIS

- Incidence:
  - It is estimated that 0.5% to 5%, or 1.36 to 13 million, Americans are sensitive to one or more insect venoms of the Hymenoptera order (bees; wasps; yellow jackets; hornets; and in the southern United States, fire ants. At least 40 to 100 deaths occur each year in the United States.
  - The incidence is increasing perhaps because of an increase in the population density of fire ants and Africanized bees.
  - Immunotherapy is 98% to 99% effective at preventing anaphylaxis from stinging insect venom. In a patient presenting with anaphylaxis from a stinging insect, the *use of epinephrine alone may not prevent fatality.* Therefore, refer sensitized or susceptible adults for skin testing and immunotherapy.
  - Patients at risk for anaphylaxis should carry self-injectable epinephrine and be counseled on avoidance.

EXERCISE-INDUCED ANAPHYLAXIS

- The mechanism is uncertain. There is an inconsistent relation to exercise intensity, and anaphylaxis may occur only episodically.
- There are *cofactor dependent* exercise-induced anaphylaxis syndromes, in which both exercise and a cofactor must be present for an episode to occur. These include the following:
  - Specific food; IgE-dependent exercise anaphylaxis: a particular food must be eaten before or during exercise.

○ Nonspecific food; non-IgE dependent, postprandial exercise anaphylaxis: exercise in the postprandial state causes a reaction.
○ Aspirin/NSAID-dependent exercise anaphylaxis.

IDIOPATHIC ANAPHYLAXIS

- There is no associated immunologic abnormality or triggering event, but coexistent allergic disease or pre-existing urticaria/angioedema are frequent.
- The number of mast cells are not increased or only mildly increased in skin, and not increased in the bone marrow. This is in contrast to systemic mastocytosis, which is associated with elevated numbers of mast cells in most tissues.
- Histamine and tryptase are increased in acute episodes but not between.
- For frequent episodes, prophylactic treatment regimens are used (eg, antihistamines, prednisone, and oral adrenergic agents).

PATHOPHYSIOLOGY

- For IgE-mediated anaphylaxis, prior exposure to the allergen promotes specific IgE antibodies to the allergen during a sensitization period which is not usually associated with clinical symptoms. After a sufficient amount of allergen-specific IgE becomes bound to membranes of mast cells and basophils, reexposure to an allergen results in crosslinking of adjacent IgE antibodies and activation of inflammatory mediators.
  ○ IgE-mediated food anaphylaxis does *not* occur after ingestion of a *new food,* but rather after ingestion of a food to which there has been prior (and often repeated) exposure.
- Histamine is the most important mediator of these reactions, acting through both H_1 and H_2 histamine receptors (Table 27–1).
- Other mediators include leukotrienes, tryptase (sometimes used for diagnosis, as discussed below), prostaglandins, heparin, and chymase.

TABLE 27–1 Roles of H_1 and H_2 Histamine Receptors in Anaphylaxis

H_1 ONLY	H_2 ONLY	H_1 AND H_2
Coronary artery vasoconstriction	Coronary vasodilation	Pulse
Bronchial constriction	Ventricular inotropy	Pulse pressure
	Ventricular chronotropy	Fall in diastolic pressure
	Atrial chronotropy	Headache

- Because the integrity of the vascular endothelium is disrupted by the effects of histamine and other mediators, loss of intravascular volume via third spacing can play a major role in the development of hypotension.

CLINICAL PRESENTATION

CLINICAL MANIFESTATIONS OF ANAPHYLAXIS

- The most frequent signs and symptoms of anaphylaxis in adults are urticaria and angioedema, upper airway edema, dyspnea/wheezing, flushing, hypotension, and gastrointestinal symptoms.
- In children, respiratory symptoms are the most common manifestations.
- In severe cases of anaphylaxis, neurological manifestations including seizures are common, and cutaneous manifestations may be conspicuously absent.

TEMPORAL COURSE

- Immediate:
  ○ Anaphylaxis may develop within minutes of exposure to parenteral allergens, but it may have an onset more than an hour after ingestion of oral allergens.
  ○ The more rapidly anaphylaxis develops, the more likely the reaction is to be severe and potentially life threatening.
- Biphasic reactions:
  ○ In biphasic reactions, patients seem to have fully recovered when a severe recurrence suddenly develops (eg, 4–6 hours after an initial reaction), usually with the same manifestations as were present during the initial reaction. Bronchospasm during these recurrences is typically refractory to standard therapy and often requires intubation and mechanical ventilation.
  ○ Biphasic reactions may occur in up to one-third of patients with food induced fatal or near fatal reactions and are more likely if there is a severe immediate reaction (eg, hypotension), a delay of 30 minutes or more after antigen exposure before the onset of symptoms, an ingested antigen, or a delay in administration of epinephrine.

DIFFERENTIAL DIAGNOSIS

- Vasodepressor/vasomotor/vasovagal reactions
  ○ More likely present if there is diaphoresis and blanching (rather than flushing), rapid improvement of hypotension with recumbency, and bradycardia with hypotension.
- Syndromes associated with flushing (eg, metastatic carcinoid)

- Postprandial syndromes (eg, scombroid poisoning from spoiled fish)
- Systemic mastocytosis
- Psychiatric disorders that can mimic anaphylaxis, such as panic attacks or vocal cord dysfunction syndrome
- Angioedema (eg, hereditary angioedema)
- Other causes of shock (eg, cardiogenic)

DIAGNOSIS

- The diagnosis of anaphylaxis is usually based upon history and physical examination that have the constellation of symptoms and signs typical for this disorder (discussed earlier).
- When the diagnosis is in doubt, (for example, hypotension without cutaneous manifestations), elevated serum tryptase levels may prove useful to differentiate anaphylaxis from other clinical conditions.
  - Tryptase elevation is less likely in IgE-mediated food anaphylaxis. The absence of elevated tryptase levels does not rule out anaphylaxis by mast cell mechanisms. Tryptase is not elevated in anaphylactoid reactions without mast cell activation (eg, complement activation).
  - Ideally, serum tryptase should be drawn 1 to 2 hours after the onset of anaphylaxis, but it remain elevated as long as 5 hours after the event. Under ideal conditions the positive predictive value of a serum tryptase is 92.6%, but the negative predictive value is only 52%.
  - Elevated tryptase levels can be detected in samples stored at room temperature for days and in frozen samples for months or years. Accordingly, if stored serum samples were collected at an appropriate time after the event, it may be possible to retrospectively diagnose anaphylaxis.

ACUTE MANAGEMENT

- Immediately place the patient in the recumbent position and elevate the feet.
- Assess airway, breathing, circulation, and level of consciousness (altered mentation should suggest the presence of hypoxia).
- Epinephrine: Administer epinephrine, the treatment of choice for anaphylaxis. Aqueous epinephrine 1:1000 dilution (1 mg/mL), 0.2 to 0.5 mL (0.01 mg/kg in children, maximum 0.3-mg dosage) intramuscularly every 5 minutes, as necessary, should be used to control symptoms and increase blood pressure.
  - Prompt recognition of signs and symptoms of anaphylaxis is crucial. If there is any doubt, it is generally better to administer epinephrine. Caution is warranted when administering epinephrine to patients > 65 years of age or those with known cardiac disease.
  - More than one dose of epinephrine is required in most patients with anaphylaxis. If the clinician deems it appropriate, the 5-minute interval between injections can be liberalized to permit more frequent injections.
  - Intramuscular epinephrine injections into the thigh have been reported to provide more rapid absorption and higher plasma epinephrine levels in both children and adults than intramuscular or subcutaneous injections administered in the arm.
  - Intravenous (IV) epinephrine, 1:10,000 dilution 1 to 3 mL, can be administered over several minutes and repeated as necessary in cases of anaphylaxis not responding to intramuscular epinephrine and volume resuscitation.
  - Alternatively, an epinephrine infusion can be prepared by adding 1 mg (1 mL) of a 1:1000 dilution of epinephrine to 250 mL of 5% dextrose in water to yield a concentration of 4.0 mg/mL. This solution is infused at a rate of 1 to 4 mg/min (15 to 60 drops per minute with a microdrop apparatus [60 drops per minute = 1 mL = 60 mL/h]), increasing to a maximum of 10.0 mg/min.
- Oxygen: Administer oxygen to patients with anaphylaxis who have prolonged reactions, have preexisting hypoxemia or myocardial dysfunction, receive inhaled β-agonists as part of therapy for anaphylaxis, or require multiple doses of epinephrine. Continuous pulse oximetry and/or arterial blood gas determination (where available) should guide oxygen therapy where hypoxemia is a concern.
- Intravenous fluids: Normal saline should be administered via a large bore catheter for fluid replacement and stabilization of blood pressure. Crystalloid volumes in excess of 10–20 L may be necessary in adults. Small children should receive up to 30 mL/kg in the first hour.
- H_1 antihistamines: Consider diphenhydramine, 1 to 2 mg/kg or 25 to 50 mg per dose (parenterally).
- H_1 antihistamines are considered second-line therapy to epinephrine and should never be administered alone in the treatment of anaphylaxis.
- H_2 antagonists: Consider ranitidine, 50 mg in adults and 12.5 to 50 mg (1 mg/kg) in children, which can be diluted in 5% dextrose and injected intravenously over 5 minutes. Cimetidine (4 mg/kg) can be administered intravenously to adults, but no pediatric dosage in anaphylaxis has been established.
  - In treating hypotension, the combination of a H_1 and H_2 antagonist is superior to an H_1 antagonist alone. Whether alone or in combination, these agents are second-line therapy to epinephrine.
- Inhaled β-agonist: In bronchospasm resistant to parenteral epinephrine, consider an inhaled β-agonist (eg, nebulized albuterol, 2.5–5 mg in 3 mL of saline) and repeat as necessary.

- Vasopressors: In hypotension refractory to volume replacement and epinephrine injections, consider a continuous infusion of vasopressors. For example, dopamine (400 mg in 500 mL of 5% dextrose) can be infused at 2 to 20 mg/kg/min and titrated to maintain systolic blood pressure of greater than 90 mm Hg.
- Glucagon: Consider infusion when concomitant β-adrenergic blocking agent is present, thus impairing the response to epinephrine. Glucagon dosage is 1 to 5 mg (20 to 30 mg/kg [maximum dose, 1 mg] in children) administered intravenously over 5 minutes and followed by an infusion (5–15 mg/min) titrated to clinical response.
- Systemic glucocorticosteroids: Consider for patients with a history of idiopathic anaphylaxis or asthma and patients who experience severe or prolonged anaphylaxis. Usually, glucocorticosteroids are not acutely helpful but may prevent recurrent or protracted anaphylaxis.
- Because of the risk for biphasic reactions, patients with severe anaphylaxis should be monitored in a medical setting for a minimum of 6 to 8 hours.
- Drugs that may complicate treatment or make patients more resistant to treatment include β-blockers, angiotensin-converting enzyme inhibitors and angiotensin II receptor blockade agents.

PREVENTION

- General measures useful in all patients:
  - Obtain a thorough history for medication, food, insect sting, and latex allergies.
  - Avoid cross-reacting drugs and use oral instead of parenteral drug administration when possible.
  - Monitor patients in the office for 20 to 30 minutes after injections of offending drugs or allergen immunotherapy.
- Measures for patients at specific risk:
  - Consider an allergy consultation to verify the risk, administer testing, counseling regarding avoidance, hidden allergens, cross-reactions to various allergens, unforeseen risks during medical procedures, and when and how to use self-administered epinephrine.
  - Instruct patient to wear and carry appropriate medical alert identification about anaphylaxis risk.
  - Teach self-injection of epinephrine using autoinjectors, and counsel patients on carrying epinephrine whenever there is any possibility of exposure.
  - If considering administration of a drug to which the patient would be at high risk of anaphylaxis, use a non-crossreactive drug or consider an allergy consultation for formal desensitization or administer an appropriate medication pretreatment regimen (eg, for patients sensitive to radiocontrast media).
  - The effect of medication desensitization persists as long as the offending medication is continued.

- Patients with food-induced anaphylaxis should have food sensitivities identified and receive instruction regarding avoidance of those foods.
- Patients with stinging insect–induced anaphylaxis should be instructed on avoidance measures (eg, keep outdoor areas free of garbage, avoid using scented products or wearing bright colors outdoors during the day, wear closed shoes, and avoid drinking from open cans when the contents are not visible). Patients should also be evaluated for insect venom immunotherapy.
- For latex-sensitive patients:
  - Instruct the patient to use latex-free products; alert employers, healthcare providers, and school personnel about the need for latex-free products and equipment; and instruct on possible cross-sensitivity to certain foods (eg, banana, avocado, kiwi, chestnut, etc.).

BIBLIOGRAPHY

Chiu AM, Kelly KJ. Anaphylaxis: drug allergy, insect stings, and latex. *Immunol Allergy Clin North Am.* 2005;25(2):389–405.

Dohl M, Suko M, Suglyama H, et al. Food dependent exercise-induced anaphylaxis: a study on 11 Japanese cases. *J Allergy Clin Immunol.* 1991;87:34.

Douglas DM, Sukenick E, Andrade WP, et al. Biphasic systemic anaphylaxis: an inpatient and outpatient study. *J Allergy Clin Immunol.* 1994;93:977–985.

Joint Task Force on Practice Parameters; American Academy of Allergy, Asthma and Immunology; American College of Allergy, Asthma and Immunology; Joint Council of Allergy, Asthma and Immunology. The diagnosis and management of anaphylaxis: an updated practice parameter. *J Allergy Clin Immunol.* 2005; 115; 3:S483–S523.

Kemp SF, Lockey RF, Wolf BL, Lieberman P. Anaphylaxis: a review of 266 cases. *Arch Intern Med.* 1995;155:1749–1754.

Kemp SF, Lockey RF. Anaphylaxis: a review of causes and mechanisms. *J Allergy Clin Immunol.* 2002;110:341–348.

Lang DM, Alpern MB, Visintainer PF, et al. Elevated risk for anaphylactoid reaction from radiographic contrast media associated with both beta blocker exposure and cardiovascular disorders. *Arch Intern Med.* 1993;153:2033–2040.

Lin RY, Curry A, Pesola G, et al. Improved outcomes in patients with acute allergic syndromes who are treated with combined H₁ and H₂ antagonists. *Ann Emerg Med.* 2000;36:462–468.

Pumphrey RSH. Lessons for management of anaphylaxis from a study of fatal reactions. *Clin Exp Allergy.* 2000;30:1144–1150.

Sicherer SH, Leung DY. Advances in allergic skin disease, anaphylaxis, and hypersensitivity reactions to foods, drugs, and insects. *J Allergy Clin Immunol.* 2006;118(1):170–177.

Simons FER, Gu X, Simons KJ. Epinephrine absorption in adults: intramuscular versus subcutaneous injection. *J Allergy Clin Immunol.* 2001;108:871–873.

Webb LM, Lieberman P. Anaphylaxis: a review of 601 cases. *Ann Allergy Asthma Immunol.* 2006;97(1):39–43.

28 DRUG ALLERGIES

Mark S. Dykewicz

OVERVIEW

- Most adverse drug reactions result from nonimmunologic or unknown mechanisms (eg, toxic overdose, toxic side effects, intolerance).
- Patients with a history of immunologically mediated drug reactions (eg, drug rash) are at greater risk than the general population for developing allergic reactions to structurally distinct, non–cross-reactive drugs.
- Diagnosis of immune-mediated drug allergy is usually based on clinical presentation.
- There are a limited number of skin tests and in-vitro tests that have good predictive value for identifying drug hypersensitivity.
- Drug reactions to many nonprotein drugs result from immune responses to chemically reactive drug metabolites that bind to self-protein carriers, rather than to the parent drug. Testing with a parent drug may not identify sensitivity to reactive intermediate products.

CLASSIFICATION OF DRUG REACTIONS

Classifying drug reactions on the basis of either the temporal relation between drug exposure and adverse manifestations or the presumptive immunologic mechanisms aids evaluation and management.

CLASSIFICATION BY TEMPORAL RELATION BETWEEN DRUG EXPOSURE AND REACTION

- Temporally, drug reactions are classified as immediate, accelerated, or delayed.
  - Immediate reactions occur within 1 hour of administration and include anaphylaxis. These can be immunoglobulin E (IgE)-antibody mediated.
  - Accelerated reactions, such as urticaria and angioedema, occur within 72 hours of administration. These may be mediated by IgE or other mechanisms.
  - Delayed reactions occur 72 hours or more after administration, and can include urticarial and nonurticarial skin rashes; serum sickness–like reactions; fever; and a variety of cardiopulmonary, hematologic, hepatic, renal, and vasculitic effects. These are not mediated by IgE.

GELL AND COOMBS CLASSIFICATION SYSTEM

- This classification defines four basic immunologic mechanisms and clinical patterns. Some clinical presentations can involve several mechanisms, but not all presentations conform to the Gell and Coombs classification.
  - Type I: IgE
    - Mechanism: Drug antigen cross-linking of IgE bound to mast cells or basophils.
    - Time course: (immediate (within 1 hour) or accelerated (up to 72 hours).
    - Presentation: Variable—any manifestation of anaphylaxis (eg, urticaria, pruritus, bronchospasm) or isolated cardiogenic shock.
    - Mediators: Histamine, leukotrienes, tryptase (peaks after 30–60 min).
    - Common causes: Antibiotics, vaccines, allergen extracts.
    - Testing: The only immune mechanism identified by immediate skin testing (albeit limited agents are available that have high predictive value).
    - IgE-mediated reactions occur only if there has been prior production of IgE antibody from exposure to the drug or cross-reactive drugs or agents. However, non-IgE mediated, anaphylactic (anaphylactoid) reactions, for example, from radiocontrast agents, can occur on first exposure to a drug.
  - Type II: cytotoxic
    - Mechanism: Cellular lysis from interaction between IgG or immunoglobulin M (IgM) antibodies, complement, and drug antigen associated with cell membranes.
    - Time course: Days to weeks after beginning course of drug.
    - Presentation: Neutropenia, thrombocytopenia, anemia.
    - Common causes: Antibiotics, heparin
      - Heparin-induced thrombocytopenia mediated by antibodies directed against antigen complexes of heparin and platelet factor 4 on the surface of platelets
    - Testing
      - For suspected hemolytic anemia, check tests to confirm hemolysis (eg, lactate dehydrogenase [LDH], bilirubin), and immune process (Coombs, indirect Coombs).
      - For suspected heparin-induced thrombocytopenia, confirm with anti-heparin antibodies.
  - Type III: immune complex
    - Mechanisms: Formation of immune complexes between drug antigen and antibodies, the deposition of which in tissues causes end organ damage.

- Time course: Usually 1–4 weeks after onset of drug exposure, although can occur within several days if prior drug exposure.
- Serum sickness is the prototype of a type III reaction. Any of its manifestations can be present in type III reactions. These include skin lesions (eg, urticaria, angioedema, maculopapular or morbilliform rash, palpable purpura), arthralgias and arthritis, lymphadenopathy, fever, nephritis, and hepatitis.
  - Treatment should include corticosteroids and regular (*not* as needed [PRN]) dosing of antihistamines, the latter to prevent histamine-induced disruption of vascular endothelium that can promote greater deposition of immune complexes into tissues.
- Drug-induced lupus syndromes are also type III reactions.
  - Renal involvement is rare, as is the presence of anti–double-stranded DNA antibodies (in contrast to systemic lupus erythematosus).
  - Clinical presentation and associated autoantibodies can vary depending on the type of causal drug.
    - Hydralazine and procainamide are usually associated with serositis but not rash, and with anti-histone antibodies.
    - Minocycline is more likely to cause serositis than rash, and presence of perinuclear antineutrophil cytoplasmic antibody (P-ANCA) is more characteristic.
    - Thiazides, angiotensin-converting enzyme (ACE)- inhibitors, calcium channel blockers, and statins are associated with subacute cutaneous lupus erythematosus, a photosensitive rash with skin sensitizing (SS)-A and/or SS-B antibodies.
    - Depending on the suspected causal drug, there should be testing for not only antinuclear antibody (ANA), but the specific type of autoantibody associated with lupus from the drug.
- Type IV: delayed lymphocyte hypersensitivity
  - Mechanisms: In a recent expansion of this classification, reactions are mediated by one or more of four types of sensitized CD4+ or CD8+ T cells.
  - Time course: Onset generally several days or weeks after exposure.
  - Cutaneous reactions are the predominant presentation.
    - Allergic contact dermatitis is a classic example and typically develops 24 to 72 hours after topical exposure.
    - Other presentations include eczema, and maculopapular, bullous, and pustular exanthema.

CLINICAL PRESENTATIONS

DERMATOLOGIC REACTIONS

- Mechanisms: Gell and Coombs types I, III, IV, others.
- The time course conforms to time course of the underlying mechanism. Late rashes can occur several weeks after drug cessation.
- Manifestations
  - Presentation can be variable ranging from maculopapular and morbilliform rashes to urticaria, angioedema, erythema multiforme, erythema nodosum, bullous eruptions, and exfoliations.
  - Eruptions are typically symmetrical, involve the trunk, and can be accompanied by pruritus, fever, and, occasionally, eosinophilia.
  - Palm and sole involvement suggests a viral exanthem rather than a drug reaction.
  - Photosensitive drug rashes can be either phototoxic or photoallergic.
    - Phototoxic reactions are nonimmunologic. They generally appear as sunburn 4 to 8 hours after light exposure and often occur with the first exposure to the drug (eg, tetracycline).
    - Photoallergic reactions are immunologic and are typically eczematous rashes that occur after days or months of exposure (eg, sulfonamide antibiotics).
    - Neither type of photosensitive reaction predicts risk for other nonphotosensitive types of adverse reactions to a drug.
  - Bullous exanthema
    - Includes erythema multiforme minor, erythema multiforme major, Stevens-Johnson syndrome, and toxic epidermal necrolysis (TEN).
    - Bullous exanthema from drugs are lymphocyte mediated. Viral infections have also been implicated as causes of bullous exanthema.
    - Erythema multiforme minor and major.
      - *Target* lesions of skin are characteristic (Fig. 28–1). Erythema multiforme minor presents without involvement of mucous membranes, whereas erythema multiforme major also has mucous membrane lesions.
    - Stevens-Johnson syndrome and TEN
      - Recent terminology distinguishes Stevens-Johnson syndrome from erythema multiforme major; the former having blistering *purpuric macules* of face, trunk, and extremities, the latter having *target lesions*. In Stevens-Johnson syndrome, mucous membrane lesions are present by definition, often accompanied by high fever and severe constitutional symptoms.
      - Both Stevens-Johnson syndrome and TEN are potentially fatal, with TEN having greater mortality.

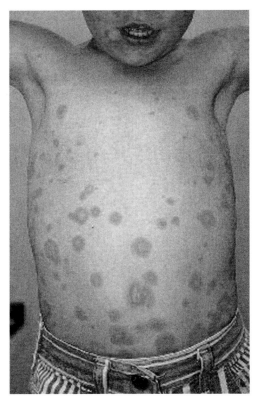

FIG. 28–1 Erythema multiforme.
SOURCE: Michael Redman, PA-C. © DermAtlas, http://www. DermAtlas.org.

- Skin biopsies demonstrate separation of skin at dermoepidermal junction: <10% epidermal detachment in Stevens-Johnson syndrome, ≥30% epidermal detachment in TEN. Stevens-Johnson syndrome can evolve into TEN.
- TEN can have the appearance of "scalded skin," with a positive Nikolsky sign (lesions or blisters spread easily and are rubbed off when pressed with a sliding motion).
- There is controversy about whether early use of corticosteroids in Stevens-Johnson syndrome is helpful, although corticosteroids are contraindicated in TEN because of an associated increased risk of infection and sepsis. There are conflicting data about whether intravenous immunoglobulin (IVIG) is beneficial in Stevens-Johnson syndrome.

DRUG FEVER

- This may or may not be associated with other allergic manifestations, for example, rash.

- It usually occurs 7 to 10 days into a treatment course, with prompt defervescence within 48 hours of cessation of the responsible agent.

OTHER SYSTEMIC MANIFESTATIONS

- Drug reactions can result in systemic involvement involving multiple internal organs, even in the absence of concomitant cutaneous reactions.
- Examples include renal disease (eg, interstitial nephritis), hepatic reactions (eg, hepatocellular, cholestatic, granulomatous), myocarditis, and vasculitis.
- Lung involvement can present as part of a syndrome consisting of malaise, nonproductive cough, chest discomfort, and migratory infiltrates, without or with peripheral eosinophilia (Löffler syndrome).
- Long-term treatment with penicillin, sulfonamides, or phenytoin can result in generalized lymphadenopathy.
- Drug rash with eosinophilia and systemic symptom (DRESS) is a potentially fatal disorder associated with antiseizure drugs that presents with cutaneous reactions, eosinophilia, fever, and internal organ dysfunction.
- Aseptic meningitis can occur from nonsteroidal anti-inflammatory drugs (NSAIDs), radiocontrast media, and other agents. Cerebrospinal fluid (CSF) studies may resemble findings of viral meningitis or demonstrate minimal elevation of neutrophils.

REACTIONS TO SPECIFIC DRUGS

ACE INHIBITORS

- Mechanism: Nonimmunologic adverse effects of angiotensin-converting enzyme (ACE) inhibitors are thought to stem from an accumulation of bradykinin and other vasoactive peptides.
- Presentation
  - The most frequently documented adverse reactions include cough (10% to 25%) and angioedema (0.1% to 0.2%). ACE-inhibitor induced cough and angioedema generally do not occur in the same individuals.
  - Onset of cough can occur from 1 day to up to many months after starting these drugs and can be persistent. Cough usually resolves within several weeks after drug cessation but can persist for more than a month.
  - Angioedema can occur within several weeks of commencing a drug course but may develop after many months of use.
    - Angioedema usually involves the face and oropharyngeal tissue and can result in life-threatening upper airway obstruction.

- For patients with ACE-inhibitor–induced angio-edema that is unresponsive to usual measures, fresh frozen plasma administration has been reported to be beneficial in case reports.
- Visceral angioedema can cause abdominal pain.
- Patients with idiopathic angioedema and urticaria are susceptible to more severe and frequent episodes when given ACE inhibitors.
  ○ Intolerance to one ACE inhibitor usually predicts intolerance to all drugs of this class.
  ○ The angiotensin II receptor blockers are generally well tolerated in patients who develop cough from ACE-inhibitors and in most patients who develop ACE-inhibitor–induced angioedema.

ANTIBIOTICS

- β-Lactam antibiotics
  ○ Penicillins
    - Most deaths from anaphylaxis to penicillins occur in patients with no history of penicillin allergy.
    - Patients tend to lose their sensitivity over time if penicillin is avoided.
      • By 5 years after an immediate reaction to penicillin, more than 90% of patients have negative results on skin testing.
    - Nonimmunologic rashes can occur from some penicillins (ampicillin or amoxicillin) in association with concomitant viral infections, allopurinol administration, chronic lymphocytic leukemia, or hyperuricemia. Typically nonpruritic, these rashes are not associated with an increased risk of future intolerance of penicillin antibiotics.

- Most immunologic reactions to penicillins are directed against central β-lactam core determinants (in contrast to some other β-lactams such as cephalosporins), although reactions to side-chain determinants of semi-synthetic penicillins can occur.
  • Less than 5% of a penicillin dose is metabolized to the penicillin core *minor determinants* (eg, benzyl penicillin G, penicillates, and benzylpenicilloylamine), but IgE antibodies to these minor determinants most commonly are responsible for severe immediate-type reactions to penicillin. Approximately 95% of a penicillin dose is metabolized to the *major determinant*, the benzylpenicilloyl moiety, but this antigen is less commonly responsible for severe immediate reactions.
  • Skin testing with a commercially available major penicillin determinant preparation can identify at least 90% of patients at risk for immediate reaction to penicillin. The negative predictive value of penicillin skin testing is significantly increased by the addition of a minor determinant mixture, but that test is not currently commercially available.

CEPHALOSPORINS

- Cephalosporins and penicillins have analogous bi-cyclic β-lactam structures and amide side chains (Fig. 28–2). Unlike penicillins, immunologic reactions to cephalosporins are more frequently related to the side chain rather than β-lactam core determinants.

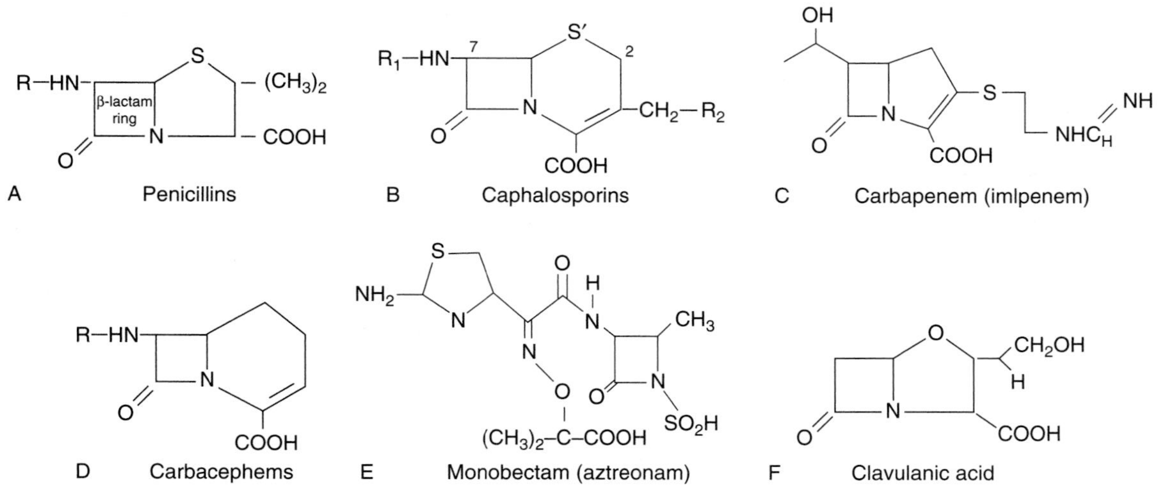

FIG. 28–2 Note the common structural features of various penicillin and caphalosporin antibiotics, in particular, the beta-lactam ring and side-chain (R-).

- The degree of immunologic cross-reactivity between cephalosporins and penicillins is controversial. Although patients with penicillin allergy are more likely than the general population to have a reaction to cephalosporins, immunologic cross-reactivity alone does not sufficiently explain this increased risk.
  - Ideally, cephalosporins should be avoided in patients who have a history of an immediate-type reaction to penicillin.
  - Cephalosporin skin testing has uncertain negative predictive value, but a patient should be presumed allergic in the presence of a positive cephalosporin skin test (performed at a nonirritating concentration).
  - There is a lower incidence of immediate-type reactions to third-generation cephalosporins than to the first- and second-generation compounds.

OTHER β-LACTAMS

- Carbapenems (imipenem) and carbacephem (loracarbef) contain bi-cyclic β-lactam rings that are associated with significant cross-reactivity to penicillin.
- Reactions to monobactams (eg, aztreonam) are typically directed against side-chain determinants rather than the monocyclic β-lactam nucleus. Generally there is no immunologic cross-reactivity with other β-lactams that have bi-cyclic core structures, except for cross-reactivity between aztreonam and ceftazidime, which contain an identical side chain.

SULFONAMIDES

- Rashes from sulfonamide (sulfa) antibiotics occur in 2% to 10% of the general population, but the incidence in patients with acquired immunodeficiency syndrome (AIDS) is substantially greater.
- Allergic reactions to sulfonamide (sulfa) antibiotics are generally directed against reactive metabolites derived from arylamine cyclic moieties.
  - Slow acetylators are more likely to metabolize sulfa antibiotics through oxidative pathways that generate reactive metabolites.
  - There is significant immunologic cross-reactivity among sulfa antibiotics.
  - There is no immunologic cross-reactivity between sulfonamide antibiotics and nonantibiotic agents that have sulfonamide moieties (eg, thiazides, celecoxib, glyburide, triptans), as the latter agents do not contain arylamine moieties.
    - Nonetheless, patients with a prior history of allergic reactions to sulfonamide or penicillin antibiotics are at increased risk for developing reactions to nonantibiotic sulfonamides, likely reflecting a greater tendency to mount allergic reactions to multiple, unrelated drugs.

- The sulfapyridine moiety of sulfasalazine is responsible for most nonurticarial skin rashes from that agent.
  - A graded-challenge protocol performed over 1 month generally is successful at inducing tolerance to sulfasalazine in patients who require this agent.
- Desensitization protocols for sulfonamide antibiotics can frequently permit the use of these agents for *Pneumocystis carinii* pneumonia (PCP) prophylaxis in AIDS, toxoplasmosis, and other infections for which there are no good alternatives.
  - Desensitization protocols should not be attempted in patients with a history of severe drug reactions, such as Stevens-Johnson syndrome or TEN.

VANCOMYCIN

- Vancomycin infusions are commonly associated with the red man syndrome (skin flushing, erythema, pruritus, hypotension, and pain or muscle spasms of the chest and back).
  - These reactions are caused by non–IgE-mediated histamine release that is more likely with rapid infusion rates (>10 mg/min).
    - Tolerance of readministration is promoted by reduction of the infusion rate and pretreatment with H_1 (but not H_2) antihistamines.
- Rarer IgE-mediated reactions to vancomycin (anaphylaxis) can be identified by immediate type skin tests.

ASPIRIN AND NONSTEROIDAL ANTIINFLAMMATORY DRUGS

- Three basic patterns of sensitivity reactions occur: respiratory reactions, skin reactions (ie, urticaria and/or angioedema only), and generalized anaphylaxis.
  - An individual patient with aspirin sensitivity typically presents with only one pattern of sensitivity.
    - Respiratory reactions: aspirin-exacerbated respiratory disease
      - Caused by abnormal arachidonic acid metabolism with increased leukotriene production. Mast cell activation can also occur.
      - Patients generally develop dose-dependent reactions to aspirin or structurally distinct NSAIDs that are significant inhibitors of cyclooxygenase-1 (COX-1).
      - Patients often tolerate agents that have less effect on COX-1 (eg, salsalate, acetaminophen, sodium or magnesium salicylate) or selective COX-2 inhibitors (eg, celecoxib).

- Patients can present with concomitant asthma, nasal polyps, and aspirin sensitivity, the *aspirin triad*.
  - Between 30% and 40% of patients with nasal polyps and sinusitis and approximately 10% to 21% of adults with asthma have positive bronchial responses to aspirin.
- If required, patients generally can be desensitized to aspirin over 2 to 3 days using published protocols at experienced centers.
  - Patients with the aspirin triad who undergo desensitization have been reported to have more favorable long-term courses with both asthma and upper respiratory (ie, nasal polyps, sinusitis) disease.
- Aspirin-exacerbated respiratory disease patients desensitized to aspirin can tolerate other structurally distinct NSAIDs (eg, ibuprofen).
- As with all desensitization protocols, once desensitization has been achieved, there must be continued administration of the agent.
- Urticaria and/or angioedema reactions
  - Patients fall into two subsets.
  - Some patients will develop reactions with aspirin and structurally distinct NSAIDs that are significant inhibitors of COX-1.
    - Typically these patients have a history of idiopathic urticaria.
    - Desensitization is often unsuccessful.
  - Some patients will react only to a particular NSAID or aspirin but tolerate structurally dissimilar agents.
    - Typically these patients do *not* have a history of idiopathic urticaria.
    - Cautious graded challenge can assess whether sensitivity to a structurally dissimilar agent is present. This can identify patients who otherwise are needlessly denied the benefit of all NSAIDs.
    - When there is sensitivity specific for aspirin, desensitization (performed with different protocols than those used for aspirin-exacerbated respiratory disease) is usually successful.
    - Despite apparently specific immunologic sensitivity, immediate type skin testing is not useful.
- Anaphylaxis
  - Patients usually have anaphylaxis only to aspirin or a particular NSAID but tolerate structurally dissimilar agents.
  - Immediate type skin testing is not useful for identifying sensitivity.
  - Cautious graded challenge to a structurally dissimilar agent can be considered.

LOCAL ANESTHETIC AGENTS

- Most adverse reactions to local anesthetics are toxic, non–IgE-antibody mediated responses from rapid absorption, inadvertent intravenous administration, overdose, or anxiety.
- In severe cases, hypotension, convulsions, and cardiorespiratory failure can occur.
  - Concurrent administration of epinephrine can be responsible for tachycardia and tremulousness.
- Allergic contact dermatitis and some large local reactions do occur through delayed-type immunologic responses.
- Local anesthetics are either benzoic acid esters (type I [eg, procaine, benzocaine]) or non-esters and amides (type II [eg, lidocaine, bupivacaine, mepivacaine]).
  - There is no immunologic cross-reactivity between the two classes, but type I agents cross-react with each other.
- Management of suspected local anesthetic allergy includes subcutaneous graded-challenge dosing with a local anesthetic without epinephrine.

RADIOGRAPHIC CONTRAST MEDIA

- These agents can cause either vasomotor/vasovagal reactions (eg, bradycardia with hypotension and nausea) or non–IgE-mediated anaphylactic reactions (eg, tachycardia with hypotension, urticaria, bronchospasm).
  - There are very rare cases of IgE-antibody mediated reactions to newer, lower osmolar contrast agents.
- Although asthma and allergies generally can be associated with a mild increase in reaction risk, it is a common misconception that shellfish allergy confers a special increased risk for anaphylactic reactions to contrast media.
  - Anaphylaxis and other allergic reactions to shellfish occur from IgE-mediated reactions to shellfish proteins, but there are no shellfish proteins in contrast media.
- A previous anaphylactic reaction to contrast media at any time is predictive of a lifelong increased risk of a repeat anaphylactic reaction, even though the patient may have tolerated contrast in the interim.
- The risk for most anaphylactic reactions to contrast media cannot be predicted by immediate-type skin testing, and test dosing is not reliable for preventing reactions.
- The use of nonionic contrast media and medication pretreatment can reduce the risk of a reaction.
  - Pretreatment generally consists of corticosteroids (prednisone, 50 mg, given 13 hours, 7 hours, and 1 hour before contrast administration), H_1 antihistamines (diphenhydramine, 50 mg orally, 1 hour before administration), and oral adrenergic

agents (ephedrine, 25 mg; or albuterol, 4 mg, orally, 1 hour before administration). H_2 receptor blockers are sometimes added.
  ○ Despite an adequate pretreatment regimen, reactions can occur.
  ○ Corticosteroids administered alone 1 to 2 hours before administration of contrast do not reliably prevent reactions.

MANAGEMENT

ACUTE EVALUATION OF SUSPECTED DRUG HYPERSENSITIVITY REACTION

• Diagnosis
  ○ The diagnosis of drug allergy depends largely on the clinical presentation and its timing in relation to drug use.
  ○ Obtain a complete history of manifestations and establish the time course of the suspected reaction.
    ▪ Does the presentation fit with a known pattern/mechanism of reaction?
    ▪ Which drug(s) were introduced in an appropriate time frame for the presenting pattern?
    ▪ Recently introduced drugs are more likely culprits, whereas drugs used with impunity for prolonged periods (months, years) are rarely responsible.
      • Exceptions: ACE inhibitors, drugs associated with cutaneous lupus
    ▪ Is the suspect reaction characteristic of a particular drug (eg, angioedema from ACE inhibitors)?
    ▪ For late drug rashes, review all drugs used in the past month, as the causal drug already may have been discontinued.
    ▪ If several drugs are suspected based on the timing of administration, which drug is most likely the "bad actor"?
      • Example: Phenytoin is more likely to cause a drug rash than a benzodiazepine.
  ○ Perform a complete physical examination; a drug reaction can cause skin and mucous membrane lesions, lymphadenopathy, hepatosplenomegaly, joint, and other manifestations.
    ▪ Although urticaria can sometimes be difficult to distinguish from maculopapular rashes, individual lesions of urticaria are transient and can resolve within hours (and usually within 24 hours) whereas nonurticarial skin lesions are more persistent.
  ○ Laboratory testing
    ▪ For suspected anaphylaxis, obtain a serum tryptase level (see Chap. 27, Anaphylaxis).

    ▪ For delayed-type reactions (eg, drug rash), consider obtaining complete blood count (CBC), liver and renal studies, and urinalysis that can identify blood abnormalities or internal organ involvement.
    ▪ Consider skin biopsy (eg, if Stevens-Johnson syndrome, TEN, cutaneous lupus suspected).

ACUTE TREATMENT

• Stop suspect drugs and substitute non–cross-reactive drugs.
• For anaphylaxis, use epinephrine and adjunctive agents.
• For late drug rashes, prescribe the following:
  ○ Antihistamines: These generally should be prescribed with scheduled dosing for patient comfort, although they will not alter the course (with certain exceptions such as serum sickness).
  ○ Corticosteroids: Consider if systemic symptoms are present (eg, fever, arthralgias) or the rash is severe or progressive (unless TEN is suspect). Several weeks of administration might be required.

PREVENTION

• Avoid prescribing cross-reactive drugs if there is previous history of hypersensitivity to a drug.
• Test the patient to identify if a patient is at increased risk for a reaction.
• When feasible, use oral rather than parenteral administration to reduce the risk for anaphylaxis.
• Immediate-type skin testing
  ○ Immediate-type skin testing (read approximately 20 minutes after application) can only identify risk for IgE-mediated, immediate-type reactions, not for non–IgE-mediated reactions such as late, nonurticarial skin rashes.
  ○ Antihistamines but not corticosteroids blunt immediate-type skin test responses and should be withheld for 48 to 72 hours before testing. (Note: Corticosteroids do blunt delayed-type skin testing such as purified protein derivative [PPD] testing.) Phenothiazines and tricyclic antidepressants can also impair immediate-type skin testing.
  ○ Immediate skin testing can have good predictive value for immediate-type reactions from protein agents and a limited number of small-molecular-weight drugs with allergenic metabolites that have been identified and made available for skin testing (eg, penicillin).
  ○ Testing requires knowledgeable personnel and use of appropriate concentrations (ie, high enough to

provoke a positive response but low enough to avoid causing a systemic allergic response or nonspecific local irritant responses).

- In-vitro testing
  - ○ There are a limited number of in-vitro tests for detection of IgE antibodies against drugs, including β-lactam antibiotics and anesthetic agents.
  - ○ Generally, in-vitro testing for drug-specific IgE is less sensitive than skin tests but can be useful in certain cases in which skin testing is not possible (eg, in patients with severe, generalized eczema or in those who must take medications that can suppress skin-test responses).
- Drug challenges
  - ○ When the probability of a true drug allergy is low, a graded challenge can be used to more safely administer a drug.
  - ○ The patient is given a test dose at a dose lower than would likely cause a serious reaction. Several subsequent doses are then escalated in large increments, and the patient is observed between doses (eg, 30 minutes for parenteral administration, 2 hours for oral administration when immediate reactions are of concern) to assure tolerance before administering higher doses.

DESENSITIZATION

- If the probability of a drug allergy is high and drug administration is essential, one may consider desensitization, in which the drug is administered in increasing doses in small increments.
- As discussed earlier, different protocols can be applicable depending on the type of drug and reaction. Desensitization when there is high risk for IgE-mediated anaphylaxis should be performed in monitored settings with emergency therapy available.
- Because of the risk of adverse reactions, experienced physicians should perform desensitization.

- Once desensitization is achieved, the drug must be continued; otherwise, desensitization will be lost.

BIBILIOGRAPHY

Dykewicz MS. Drug allergy. In Slavin RG, Reisman RE, eds. *An Expert Guide to Allergy and Immunology*. Philadelphia, PA: American College of Physicians; 1999:127.

Greenberger PA. Drug allergy. *J Allergy Clin Immunol*. 2006; 117:S464.

Gruchalla RS, Pirmohamed M. Antibiotic allergy. *N Engl J Med*. 2006;354:601.

Joint Task Force on Practice Parameters, and the Joint Council of Allergy, Asthma and Immunology. Executive summary of disease management of drug hypersensitivity: a practice parameter. *Ann Allergy Asthma Immunol*. 1999;83:665. www.jcaai.org.

Kelkar PS, Li JT. Current concepts: cephalosporin allergy. *N Engl J Med*. 2001;345:804.

Pichler WJ. Delayed drug hypersensitivity reactions. *Ann Intern Med*. 2003;139:683.

Romano A, Gueant-Rogriguez RM, Viola M, et al. Cross-reactivity and tolerability of cephalosporins in patients with immediate hypersensitivity to penicillins. *Ann Intern Med*. 2004; 141:16.

Solensky R. Drug desensitization. *Immunol Allergy Clin North Am*. 2004;24:425.

Srivastava M, Rencic A, Diglio G, et al. Drug-induced, Ro/SSA-positive cutaneous lupus erythematosus. *Arch Dermatol*. 2003;139:45.

Stevenson DD, Szczeklik A. Clinical and pathologic perspectives on aspirin sensitivity and asthma. *J Allergy Clin Immunol*. 2006;118:773.

Strom BL, Schinnar R, Apter AJ. Absence of cross-reactivity between sulfonamide antibiotics and sulfonamide nonantibiotics. *N Engl J Med*. 2003;349:1628.

Warrier MR, Copilevitz CA, Dykewicz MS, et al. Fresh frozen plasma (FFP) in the treatment of resistant ACE inhibitor (ACE-I) angioedema. *Ann Allergy Asthma Immunol*. 2004;92:573.

CARDIOVASCULAR MEDICINE

29 CARDIAC STRUCTURE AND BASIC PHYSIOLOGY

Steven C. Herrmann

CARDIAC ULTRASTRUCTURE

- Myocytes comprise more than 75% of the total heart volume, but constitute less than 30% of the total number of cells in the heart (Fig. 29–1).
- Each myocyte is approximately 100 µm in length and 20 µm in diameter.
- A myofiber is composed of a group of myocytes embedded within a collagenous matrix which, in turn provides structural support and contributes to the compliance/elasticity of cardiac tissue.
- Cardiac myocytes contain contractile proteins (myofibrils) that are involved in cardiac contraction and relaxation.
- The myocytes are surrounded by a complex, invaginating membrane known as the sarcolemma.
- The sarcolemma communicates with the extracellular space through the transverse tubule (T-tubule) system. Recent studies have suggested that the structure and function of the T-tubules are more complex than previously believed. Many of the proteins involved in cellular Ca^{2+} cycling are concentrated at the T-tubule.
- The myocytes are endowed with abundant mitochondria to supply the energy (ATP) for cellular contraction.

MYOFIBRIL STRUCTURE

- Myofibrils contain thick filaments composed of myosin and thin filaments composed of actin (Fig. 29–2).
- The cardiac sarcomere is defined as the region of the myofilament between two Z-lines from which thin (actin) filaments emanate.

- The optimal sarcomere length (for contraction) is approximately 2.0 µm.
- Sarcomere lengths significantly below or above 2.0 are associated with decreased cardiac contractile force (Frank-Starling mechanism).
- The I-band contains only thin filaments and is bisected by the Z-line.
- The A-band contains overlapping thin and thick filaments.
- Titin is a large, flexible protein that attaches the thick filament to the Z-line. Titin is a major determinant of the length-tension relationship in cardiac muscle.
- Thick filaments (myosin) possess a globular head that contains ATPase activity.
- The thin and thick filaments interact during cardiac contraction.

REGULATION OF CELLULAR CONTRACTION

- The troponin complex is the major regulatory protein involved in cardiac contraction and consists of three subunits; troponin I (inhibitory), troponin C (calcium receptor), and troponin T.
- Troponin T is bound to another regulatory protein known as tropomyosin which is closely associated with the thin filaments and inhibits actin and myosin binding through troponin I.
- When cellular levels of calcium increase, calcium binds to troponin C which strengthens the interaction between troponin T and troponin C, thus, disinhibiting troponin I and tropomyosin and altering the conformation of the complex. The change in conformation allows the thick and thin filaments to interact (contraction).
- The myosin head pulls the actin molecule, shortening the distance between the two Z-lines as the sarcomere shortens and contracts.
- ATP is required to inhibit actin-myosin binding and produce cardiac relaxation.

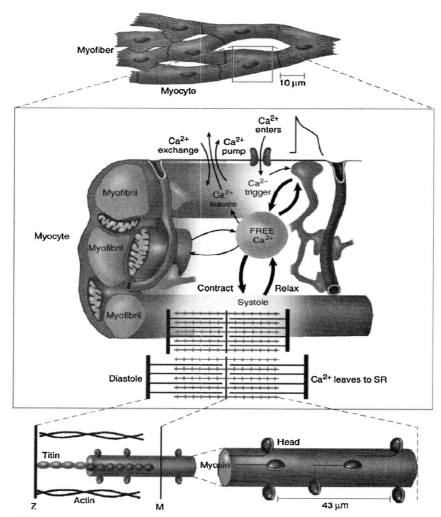

FIG. 29–1 Cardiac ultrastructure.

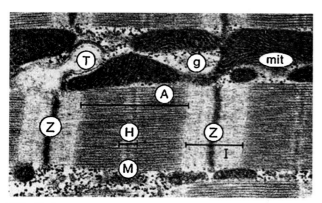

FIG. 29–2 Myofibril structure. T, T-tubules; G, glycogen granules; I, I band containing only actin; Z, Z-line; H, clear zone of only myosin; A, actin myosin overlap.
SOURCE: With permission: Zipes, et al, Mechanisms of cardiac contraction and relaxation. In: Braunwald E, Zipes DP, eds. *A Textbook of Cardiovascular Medicine.* 7th ed. Philadelphia: Elsevier Saunders; 2005.

EXCITATION CONTRACTION COUPLING

• Calcium ions enter the myocyte during phase II (plateau) of the cardiac action potential through L-type calcium channels.

• The calcium that enters the myocyte during the plateau phase causes release of additional calcium, stored in the sarcoplasmic reticulum, which binds to troponin C.

• The calcium signal is cycled down by active sequestration of calcium via the sarcoplasmic reticulum protein SERCA.

• The efficiency and speed of uptake of calcium by SERCA is involved in myocardial relaxation.

LENGTH-TENSION RELATIONSHIP

- Preload reflects the extent of stretch on the ventricle/myocytes at the end of the cardiac filling phase (diastole) just before the contraction phase (systole) begins. In physiologic terms, preload reflects the wall tension in the ventricular myocytes at the end of diastole (Fig. 29–3).
- Preload can be estimated clinically as the end-diastolic volume or end-diastolic pressure.
- As end-diastolic pressure/volume increases, the force of contraction and stroke volume increases. In the clinical setting, preload, is estimated from the pulmonary capillary wedge pressure using a pulmonary artery catheter (Swan-Ganz catheter).
- The Frank-Starling relationship is partly explained by the maximum overlap of the thin and thick filaments, which occurs at a sarcomere length of approximately 2.2 μm. At longer sarcomere lengths, overlap is reduced and generated force and stroke volume is decreased.
- At very short sarcomere lengths, there is buckling of actin and myosin, and the force of contraction and stroke volume is reduced.
- Titin alters the length-tension relationship; at longer sarcomere lengths, titin is stretched which increases its elastic recoil, leading to an increase in stroke volume.
- As the myocytes are stretched, the calcium sensitivity of troponin C increases. As calcium interacts with troponin C, additional cross bridges are formed and the force of contraction/ stroke volume is increased.

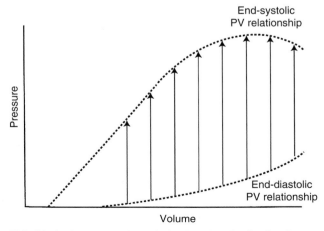

FIG. 29–3 Length-tension relationship. Per the Starling law, as the ventricular end diastolic volume increases the pressure generated by the ventricle increases until the optimal sarcomere length is reached and then once exceeded the ventricular pressure generated declines. PV, pressure-volume (analogous to tension-length) SOURCE: Katz, 2006. With permission Lippincott Williams & Wilkins)

- The Frank-Starling mechanism provides the physiologic rationale for volume resuscitation of a hypotensive patient; by increasing preload, stroke volume, and cardiac output.

CARDIAC AFTERLOAD

- Cardiac afterload can be thought of as the resistance to ejection of blood into the aorta.
- Afterload can be estimated from the aortic compliance, aortic blood pressure, and the aortic valve resistance.
- Wall stress (which is technically equivalent to afterload), is calculated as the wall tension divided by the wall thickness. As myocardial radius increases, wall stress (and afterload) tends to increase (the Laplace relationship). However, an increase in myocardial thickness (hypertrophy) will attenuate wall stress and afterload. Importantly, the changes in ventricular geometry observed with sustained hypertension (hypertrophy) normalize wall stress and afterload.
- The inverse relationship between afterload and stroke volume provides the physiologic rationale for the treatment of systolic heart failure with vasodilator therapy.

CARDIAC CONTRACTILITY

- Contractility represents the inotropic state of the heart and is unique to cardiac muscle. Changes in inotropy result in changes in force generation, which are independent of preload.
- A variety of factors can alter the intrinsic inotropy (contractility) of the heart. For example activation of β_1 receptor with catecholamines increases contractility. Digoxin promotes an increase in contractility *in vitro* by augmenting intracellular calcium flux.
- Contractility is decreased in the presence of cardiac ischemia, hypoxia, or metabolic acidosis.
- Clinically, a change in contractility is calculated as an increase in the pressure developed by the ventricle as a function of time, or dP/dt.
- Contractility can be increased by a variety of pharmacological agents including dobutamine and milrinone.

RHYTHM EFFECTS ON CARDIAC FUNCTION

- As the frequency of contraction increases, the force of contraction also increases. This is known as the treppe/Bowditch effect.
- A premature contraction, followed by a pause, results in an increase in the force of contraction

(which patients may describe as a "pounding" sensation.

- The increased force of contraction is thought to be secondary to the compensatory pause which promotes an increase venous return or preload.

THE CARDIAC CYCLE

- The relationship between pressure and flow on the right or left side of the heart can be depicted using the Wiggers diagram (see Fig. 29–4).

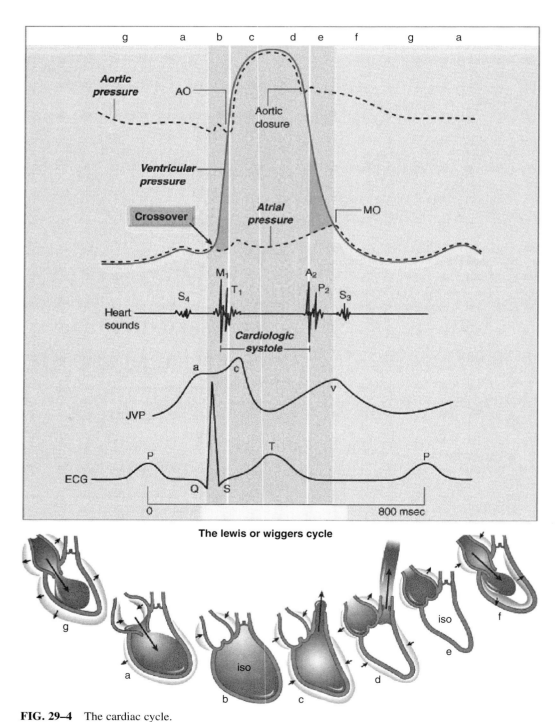

FIG. 29–4   The cardiac cycle.
Source: With permission: Zipes, et al, Mechanisms of cardiac contraction and relaxation. In: Braunwald E, Zipes DP, eds. *A Textbook of Cardiovascular Medicine.* 7th ed. Philadelphia: Elsevier Saunders; 2005.

- On the Wiggers diagram, the atrioventricular valves open when the atrial pressure exceeds ventricular pressure and close when ventricular pressure exceeds atrial pressure (g through b).
- The aortic valve opens when ventricle pressure exceeds aortic pressure and closes when aortic pressure is greater than ventricular pressure (c through e).
- Atrial pressure increases during ventricular diastole as blood flows passively from the pulmonary veins (e).
- Atrial contraction, as denoted by the P-wave on the electrocardiogram, results in an increase in atrial pressure (f). On the Wiggers diagram (and at the bedside), this reflects the *a* wave on the left atrial pressure tracing (or observed during a careful neck vein examination). This active component of diastole is equivalent to the mitral *a* wave observed with Doppler interrogation of the heart.

- Ventricular contraction is represented electrically by the QRS complex on the surface electrocardiogram. Electrical activation precedes mechanical activation.
- After the QRS complex, the pressure in the ventricle begins to rise, and the mitral valve closes when ventricular pressure exceeds atrial pressure. Closure of the mitral valve results in the first heart sound.
- Ventricular pressure continues to rise after mitral valve closure. While the aortic valve is closed, this phase is referred to as isovolumetric contraction.
- When the ventricular pressure exceeds aortic pressure, the aortic valve opens and blood is ejected into the aorta. Left ventricular pressure exceeds aortic pressure by only a millimeter or two during the normal cardiac cycle.
- The compliance of the aorta stores the kinetic energy of the ejected blood and propels it forward as the aorta recoils after accommodating the stroke volume.

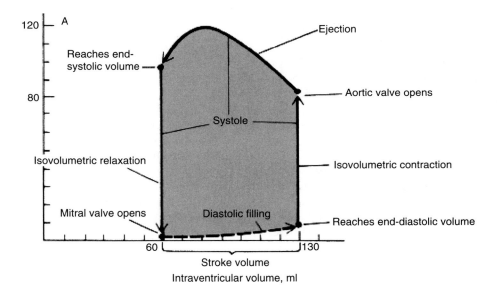

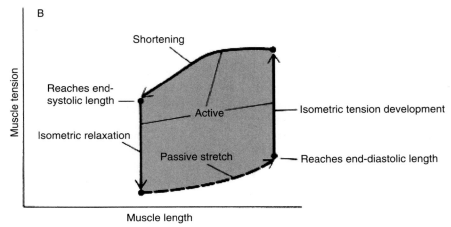

FIG. 29–5 The ventricular loop diagram.
Source: With permission McGraw-Hill, Mohrman DE, Heller LJ. *Cardiovascular Physiology.* 6th ed. McGraw-Hill; 2006.

- As the ventricle relaxes (electrically characterized as the T wave on the electrocardiogram), the pressure in the ventricle begins to fall. When left ventricular pressure falls below aortic pressure, the aortic valve closes creating the second heart sound.
- After aortic valve closure, the pressure in the ventricle falls rapidly. The ventricular pressure still exceeds atrial pressure, however and the mitral valve remains closed. This phase of relaxation, when both the mitral and aortic valve are closed, is referred to as isovolumetric relaxation.
- When left ventricular pressure falls below atrial pressure, the mitral valve opens and blood passively flows from the atrium into the ventricle. This phase of diastole is characterized by an E-wave via Doppler interrogation.
- The filling patterns on the right side of the heart mirror those on the left side, but under normal conditions the pressures are less.

THE VENTRICULAR LOOP DIAGRAM

- The Wiggers diagram or cardiac cycle can also be depicted as a flow-volume relationship, eg, the ventricular loop diagram (Fig. 29–5).
- On the ventricular loop diagram, the abscissa (x-axis) represents ventricular volume and the ordinate (y-axis) is ventricular pressure.
- Diastole is defined on the bottom of the loop, traveling from left to right as filling occurs, increasing ventricular volume.
- The slope of the ventricular filling curve is related to compliance of the ventricle; the stiffer the ventricle, the steeper the diastolic filling curve, leading to an increase in end-diastolic pressure.
- Preload is depicted as the bottom right point of the loop diagram eg, end-diastolic volume (EDV).
- Isovolumetric contraction occurs at the bottom right of the loop diagram and is represented as a vertical line (no change in volume).The peak of the vertical line (pressure) is roughly equivalent to afterload.
- When the ventricular pressure exceeds aortic pressure the aortic valve opens and blood is ejected into the aorta. Accordingly during this phase, ventricular volume decreases until the isovolumetric relaxation period begins, defined as a vertical line on the left hand side of the loop diagram.
- Mitral valve opening occurs at the bottom of the isovolumetric relaxation line, and the cycle repeats.
- Stroke volume is defined as the volume difference between isovolumetric contraction and isovolumetric relaxation.
- The relationship between volume and pressure shown on the loop diagram is termed lusitropy. An increase in

afterload, represented by an increase in the height of the isovolumetric contraction line, will result in a narrowing of the ventricular loop, reducing stroke volume, assuming that preload remains unchanged.

BIBLIOGRAPHY

Guyton AC, Hall JE, eds. *Guyton Textbook of Medical Physiology.* 11th ed. Philadelphia: Saunders; 2005.
Mohrman DE, Heller LJ. *Cardiovascular Physiology.* 6th ed. McGraw-Hill; 2006.

30 CARDIAC DIAGNOSTIC TESTING
Deryk McDowell

INTRODUCTION

- Cardiac diagnostic testing is an integral part of the evaluation of cardiac patients. These tests are important in guiding both conservative medical management as well as the invasive treatment of many cardiac problems. These techniques are expensive and carry a modest but real risk to the patient, so they should not be used indiscriminately. Therefore, a thorough knowledge of the indications and risks of each test is expected of the physician who recommends these tests to the patient.

EXERCISE STRESS TESTING

DESCRIPTION

- The exercise stress test (EST) is most commonly used to diagnose coronary artery disease in low- to intermediate-risk patients.
- The EST is also used to assess exercise capacity and functional reserve in patients with known coronary artery disease.
- The test employs physical exercise (treadmill, stationary bicycle, or arm crank) in a controlled environment coupled with continuous telemetry monitoring and serial electrocardiographs (ECGs) to evaluate for evidence of myocardial ischemia. Serial hemodynamic measurements are also obtained to determine the physiologic response to exercise.

- Stress testing is often performed in conjunction with an imaging modality to increase the sensitivity for detecting coronary artery disease.
- The treadmill is the most common exercise modality used in clinical practice today. There are several different standardized protocols used in clinical practice ranging from the more strenuous (Bruce) to less strenuous (asymptomatic cardiac ischemia project protocol).

INDICATIONS

- To diagnose coronary artery disease (CAD) in adult patients with an intermediate pretest probability of CAD on the basis of gender, age, and symptoms.
- To risk stratify or determine functional exercise capacity in patients with known CAD.
- To evaluate a change in functional status in patients with known CAD.
- To risk stratify patients with low-risk unstable angina who have been free of active ischemia or symptoms of heart failure 8 to 12 hours following their initial clinical presentation.
- To establish activity parameters, determine prognosis, and assess the efficacy of medical treatment either prior to discharge or early after discharge following an acute myocardial infarction (MI).
- To evaluate exercise capacity and functional status in patients with valvular heart disease and equivocal or no symptoms.

CONTRAINDICATIONS

- Absolute contraindications to stress testing include the following:
  ○ Acute MI (within 2 days)
  ○ High-risk unstable angina
  ○ Uncontrolled cardiac arrhythmias
  ○ Symptomatic severe aortic stenosis
  ○ Decompensated heart failure
  ○ Acute pulmonary embolus
  ○ Acute myocarditis or pericarditis
  ○ Acute aortic dissection
- Relative contraindications to stress testing include:
  ○ Known left main coronary artery stenosis
  ○ Moderate stenotic valvular heart disease
  ○ Electrolyte abnormalities
  ○ Severe arterial hypertension (systolic blood pressure [SBP] >200 or diastolic blood pressure [DBP] >100)
  ○ Tachyarrhythmias or bradyarrhythmias
  ○ Hypertrophic cardiomyopathy
  ○ High-grade atrioventricular (AV) block
  ○ Exercise intolerance

- If confounding baseline ECG abnormalities exist, exercise stress testing alone should not be performed because it lacks sufficient sensitivity to detect myocardial ischemia. Such abnormalities include:
  ○ Left bundle-branch block
  ○ Ventricular paced rhythm
  ○ Pre-excitation (Wolff-Parkinson-White) syndrome
  ○ >1 mm of resting ST segment depression with or without signs of left ventricular hypertrophy
  ○ ST segment abnormalities caused by drugs, eg, digoxin

ELECTROCARDIOGRAPHIC FINDINGS

- The hallmark electrocardiographic finding of myocardial ischemia is characterized by horizontal or downsloping ST segment depression. This typically occurs during peak exercise; but in a small percentage of patients, the ST segment abnormalities only occur during the recovery phase. This emphasizes the importance of continuous monitoring until the heart rate (HR) has returned to normal.
- A stress test is considered abnormal when there is >1 mm of horizontal or downsloping ST segment depression that persists 80 msec after the J point in three consecutive beats. There is no correlation between the site of ST segment depression and myocardial territory that is ischemic or the coronary artery that is involved.
- ST segment elevation can also occur during exercise and in the absence of pathologic Q waves, this is a marker of transmural ischemia. There is a significant correlation between the ECG site of ST segment elevation and the coronary artery involved.
- Upsloping ST segment depression associated with J point depression is a normal finding and not sensitive or specific for obstructive CAD.

OTHER FINDINGS

- Exercise capacity is reported as the number of metabolic equivalents (METs) achieved. One MET is equal to the amount of oxygen consumed in 1 minute in the resting state. Normal daily activity requires approximately 3 to 4 METs, whereas light exercise requires 5 to 7 METs and heavy aerobic exercise requires >8 METs.
- The expected blood pressure response to exercise is an increase in the SBP to a peak of 160 to 200 mm Hg while maintaining a near normal or slightly increased DBP. Exercise-induced hypotension (failure to increase the SBP >120 mm Hg or a decrease in SBP lower than baseline) is a marker of severe heart failure

or three-vessel CAD. Exertional hypertension (SBP >210 mm Hg in men and >190 mm Hg in women) is not associated with increased mortality.

- For an exercise stress test to be considered maximal the patient must achieve at least 85% of the age-predicted maximum HR, which is calculated as (220 − age) × 85%. A HR that increases rapidly at low work loads is a sign of deconditioning, hypovolemia, anemia, or decreased left ventricular (LV) function. Chronotropic incompetence is defined as the failure to achieve 85% of age-predicted maximum HR in the absence of β-blockade. Importantly, chronotropic incompetence is a marker of increased mortality. A prolonged HR recovery time (defined as failure of the HR to fall by more than 12 beats per minute during the recovery phase) is also associated with increased mortality.

ACCURACY

- A recent meta-analysis, that included more than 24,000 patients, evaluated the accuracy of stress testing when compared to angiography for diagnosing CAD. The sensitivity was 68% and the specificity was 77%.
- Diagnostic accuracy improves with increasing severity of CAD. The sensitivity of patients with one-vessel disease is as low as 25%, whereas patients with three-vessel disease or left main disease have a sensitivity as high as 86%.

DISCONTINUING A TEST

- Absolute indications for discontinuing an exercise test include the following:
  ○ Decrease in SBP >10 mm Hg from baseline when accompanied by other evidence of ischemia
  ○ Moderate to severe angina
  ○ Development of central nervous system abnormalities (ie, ataxia, dizziness)
  ○ Clinical indicators of poor perfusion (ie, cyanosis or pallor)
  ○ Technical difficulty in monitoring the ECG or blood pressure
  ○ Sustained ventricular tachycardia
  ○ ST elevation >1 mm in any lead without significant Q waves
- Relative indications for stopping an exercise test include the following:
  ○ Decrease in SBP >10 mm Hg from baseline in the absence of other evidence of ischemia
  ○ >3 mm of ST segment depression or marked QRS axis shift

○ Arrhythmias other than sustained ventricular tachycardia
○ Fatigue, shortness of breath, leg cramps, or claudication
○ Development of a bundle-branch block that cannot be distinguished from sustained ventricular tachycardia
○ Increasing chest pain
○ Hypertensive response to exercise

PROGNOSIS

- In addition to diagnostic information, an exercise treadmill test also provides prognostic information.
- The Duke treadmill score is calculated as follows:

$$\text{Exercise time} - (5 \times \text{ST deviation in mm}) - (4 \times \text{angina index})$$

- The angina index is 0 in the absence of angina, 1 for nonlimiting angina, and 2 for exercise limiting angina.
- A Duke score of greater than +5 indicates a low-risk population with a 5-year survival of 97%, whereas high-risk patients with a score of less than −11 have a 5-year survival of 72%.

NUCLEAR IMAGING

- Nuclear myocardial perfusion imaging is occasionally obtained in conjunction with stress testing to further aid diagnostic accuracy. This is especially useful in patients with baseline ECG abnormalities.
- The technique involves injection of a radioactive isotope (technetium 99m [^{99m}Tc] sestamibi or ^{99m}Tc tetrofosmin), that is extracted from plasma by viable myocardium. The images are acquired with a special camera that captures radioactive emissions. The intensity of the image is proportional to the perfusion of the myocardium.
- Exercise is the preferred stress modality; however, in patients who are unable to achieve a minimum level of exercise, a vasodilator is infused in concert with the nuclear tracer injection. Both dipyridamole and adenosine are safe and effective in achieving coronary hyperemia. Contraindications to the usage of vasodilators include the presence of bronchospastic airway disease, theophylline use, or caffeine intake on the day of the test.
- Images are acquired both at rest and after peak-exercise or vasodilator infusion. The images are then compared, and stress-induced perfusion defects identified. The defects correlate with the presence of epicardial coronary artery disease.
- The use of myocardial perfusion imaging increases the accuracy of stress testing for diagnosing coronary artery disease. In one meta-analysis involving more

than 1000 patients, the sensitivity of perfusion imaging was 88% and the specificity was 77%.

ECHOCARDIOGRAPHY

DESCRIPTION

- Echocardiography is a noninvasive modality that utilizes reflected sound waves to image the heart and define both its structure and function.
- Two-dimensional echocardiography is used to assess cardiac structure, left ventricular function, valvular integrity and function, and the pericardium. It also permits calculation of chamber dimensions, areas, and volumes.
- The Doppler principle, as it applies to echocardiography, states that the frequency of ultrasonic reflection increases as the reflecting object moves closer to the transducer and decreases as the reflecting object moves further away from the transducer. By applying this principle to echocardiographic analysis, the velocity of flow can be measured, which can then be utilized to calculate stroke volume, intracardiac pressure gradients, and cross-sectional areas within the heart (ie, valve areas).
- Color flow imaging is an adjunct to Doppler imaging that arbitrarily assigns different colors to blood that is moving toward the transducer (red) and away from the transducer (blue). It is used to detect abnormal flow such as valvular regurgitation, intraventricular shunts, and obstruction of flow within or between the cardiac chambers.
- Tissue Doppler interrogation measures the velocity and direction of the myocardium itself (especially the mitral annulus) and is used to assess diastolic function.
- Contrast echocardiography employs echo reflectors such as agitated saline or commercially developed perfluorocarbons to opacify various cardiac chambers. Agitated saline bubbles are too large to traverse the pulmonary capillary bed and thus only opacify the right-sided cardiac structures when injected intravenously. If they are visible in the left-sided chambers, an intracardiac or extracardiac right to left shunt exists. The commercially based perfluorocarbon bubbles are much smaller in size and capable of crossing the pulmonary capillary bed. They are used to assess wall motion.

INDICATIONS

Echocardiography provides indispensable and comprehensive cardiac information noninvasively, and therefore is the most commonly ordered cardiac diagnostic test.

- Evaluation of murmurs and valvular heart disease:
  - Any murmur associated with cardiorespiratory symptoms.
  - Asymptomatic patients with a murmur suggestive of structural heart disease.
  - Assessing the severity of established valvular heart disease and concomitant ventricular size and function.
  - Evalution of patients with established valvular heart disease and new or progressive cardiac symptoms. Also sometimes used in the serial evaluation of asymptomatic patients with moderate to severe valvular heart disease. Serial echocardiographic data can be used to determine optimal timing of medical and/or surgical interventions.
  - Detection of vegetations, myocardial abscesses, or shunts in patients with known or suspected bacterial endocarditis. In addition, serial studies may prove useful in patients with a complex clinical course.
  - Evaluation of prosthetic heart valves in patients with new or progressive cardiac symptoms (sometimes useful in asymptomatic patients).
- Chest pain and suspected ischemic heart disease:
  - Evaluation of chest pain in patients with suspected MI, suspected aortic dissection, suspicion of valvular or pericardial disease, or in patients with hemodynamic instability.
  - Measurement of baseline left ventricular function in the setting of an acute MI.
  - Assessment for mechanical complications of an MI such as papillary muscle rupture or ventricular septal defect.
  - Assessment of left ventricular function in patients with chronic ischemic heart disease.
- Left ventricular function, pericardial disease, and miscellaneous structural abnormalities:
  - Excellent test to assess left ventricular function in patients with signs and symptoms of congestive heart failure (dyspnea or edema).
  - Patients with suspected pericardial disease, a pericardial friction rub, or suspicion of bleeding into the pericardial space (ie, trauma). The echocardiogram is also useful as a follow-up study to assess resolution of pericardial pathology.
  - Used to identify cardiac masses, tumors, and thrombi as well as a tool to assess recurrence following excision of masses (particularly those at high risk for recurrence, ie, myxoma).
- Pulmonary disease:
  - To evaluate patients with suspected pulmonary hypertension
  - To follow pulmonary pressures in patients treated for pulmonary hypertension
- Hypertension:

○ Assessment of LV function, hypertrophy, or remodeling in patients with longstanding hypertension or in patients with changing clinical status
• Neurologic or vascular events:
  ○ To evaluate for a cardiac source of emboli in patients with abrupt occlusion of a major peripheral artery
  ○ To evaluate for a cardiac source of embolus in patients younger than age 45 years with a stroke or in any patient with a stroke and no evidence of cerebrovascular disease
• Arrhythmias and palpitations:
  ○ Evaluation of structural heart disease in patients with documented atrial or ventricular arrhythmias
  ○ Evaluation of patients with a family history of a genetically transmitted cardiac disease that may predispose to arrhythmias such as hypertrophic obstructive cardiomyopathy or tuberous sclerosis
• Syncope:
  ○ To evaluate syncope in patients with exertional syncope or in patients with suspected structural heart disease
  ○ Evaluation of syncope in patients working in a high-risk setting (ie, pilots)
• Routine screening:
  ○ Patients with a family history of genetically transmitted heart disease
  ○ In potential donors for cardiac transplantation
  ○ To evaluate patients with phenotypic features of Marfan syndrome
  ○ At baseline and then routine reevaluation of patients undergoing chemotherapy with cardiotoxic agents such as doxorubicin (Adriamycin)
• Critically ill or injured patients:
  ○ Echocardiography is indicated in any patient who is hemodynamically unstable with no obvious explanation.
  ○ To evaluate cardiac function in a patient with serious blunt or penetrating trauma, especially when the patient is hemodynamically unstable.
  ○ Evaluation of suspected iatrogenic injury from venous catheters, guidewires, pacemaker leads, or pericardiocentesis needles regardless of tamponade symptoms.
• Adults with congenital heart disease:
  ○ To evaluate patients with suspected congenital heart disease based on signs and symptoms such as a murmurs, cyanosis, unexplained arterial desaturations, an abnormal ECG, or an abnormal chest x-ray.
  ○ Follow-up examinations in patients with known congenital heart disease, especially when there has been a change in clinical course.
  ○ Routine echocardiograms are indicated in patients with known congenital heart disease to follow

ventricular function, valvular function, or pulmonary artery pressures.

TRANSESOPHAGEAL ECHOCARDIOGRAPHY

• A similar study to a surface echocardiogram, however, the ultrasound probe is passed into the esophagus to examine the cardiac structures in close proximity. Transesophageal echocardiography offers superior assessment of cardiac anatomy and physiology because of the proximity of the probe.
• The most common indications for a transesophageal echocardiographic (TEE) examination are:
  ○ Evaluation for left atrial appendage thrombus prior to elective cardioversion of atrial fibrillation or atrial flutter
  ○ Examine the valves for vegetations
  ○ Evaluation of prosthetic valve function
  ○ Evaluation for a thrombus in patients with a stroke or other embolic phenomenon
  ○ Evaluation of aneurysm or dissection of the aorta
  ○ Evaluation for intracardiac masses, tumors, or thrombi
  ○ Evaluation of congenital heart disease
• A TEE is a relatively safe procedure. The most common adverse events are related to the mechanical effects of the probe in the esophagus and include retching, vomiting, and transient hypoxia.
• Contraindications to performing a TEE examination are related to esophageal pathology and include the following:
  ○ Esophageal stricture or malignancy
  ○ Esophageal ulcer or varices, especially with recent hemorrhage
  ○ Zenker diverticulum
  ○ Altered mental status or an uncooperative patient
  ○ History of dysphagia or odynophagia

STRESS ECHOCARDIOGRAPHY

• Echocardiography is often used as an imaging modality to increase the sensitivity and specificity of exercise stress tests for the detection of CAD. Stress echocardiography also assesses myocardial viability in patients with known CAD and in whom revascularization is being considered.
• The hallmark of an abnormal stress echocardiogram is loss of contractile function as HR and, consequently, myocardial oxygen demand increase. Both physical exercise (ie, treadmill) and pharmacologic stress (dobutamine) are used to achieve the appropriate

workload, which is 85% of the age predicted maximum HR.

- Vasodilators (ie, adenosine, dipyridamole) that are used with nuclear myocardial perfusion imaging (see above) are usually not helpful in stress echocardiography because they lack sensitivity.
- Indications for stress echocardiography include the following:
  ○ The detection of coronary artery disease in intermediate-risk patients presenting with chest pain, ECG abnormalities, or prior to noncardiac surgery especially when baseline ECG abnormalities render treadmill testing insensitive.
  ○ For risk stratification in patients with known CAD or who are post-MI.
- Contraindications to stress echocardiography include the following:
  ○ Uncontrolled arrhythmias
  ○ Acute MI
  ○ Unstable angina
  ○ Hemodynamically significant left ventricular outflow tract obstruction
  ○ Severe aortic stenosis
  ○ Aortic dissection
- The exercise echocardiography exhibits a sensitivity between 79% and 85% and a specificity of 80% to 87%. As with treadmill stress testing, the diagnostic accuracy improves as the coronary disease severity increases. Dobutamine stress echocardiography has a sensitivity of 80% and a specificity of 84% to detect coronary ischemia.
- The accuracy of stress echocardiography is limited in patients with a left bundle-branch block or ventricular paced rhythm because baseline wall motion abnormalities are induced by abnormal ventricular depolarizations. In these patients nuclear perfusion scans are more likely to provide useful information. In patients who have poor acoustic windows, the stress echocardiogram is usually nondiagnostic.

CARDIAC CATHETERIZATION

DESCRIPTION

- Cardiac catheterization and coronary angiography are the most common invasive diagnostic and therapeutic procedures performed by cardiologists.
- These procedures involve insertion of a specialized catheter into the systemic circulation (usually via femoral artery puncture) and advancement into individual coronary arteries or retrograde advancement across the aortic valve and into the LV. In addition, a catheter can be placed through the venous system into the right sided chambers and pulmonary circulation.

- Following placement of the catheter in the desired location, hemodynamic data can be acquired, and angiography can be performed by injection of radiocontrast dye and fluoroscopic image acquisition.
- Catheterization is primarily used to diagnose obstructive coronary artery disease, assess its severity, and design the optimal medical and/or surgical treatment.
- Alternate uses of cardiac catheterization include the following:
  ○ To exclude CAD as a cause of left ventricular systolic dysfunction
  ○ To quantify the severity of left ventricular systolic dysfunction
  ○ To differentiate myocardial restriction from pericardial constriction
  ○ To assess the severity of valvular regurgitation
  ○ To detect active myocarditis or acute transplant rejection by means of endomyocardial biopsy

INDICATIONS

- Asymptomatic patients or stable angina:
  ○ Patients with high-risk findings on a noninvasive test regardless of symptoms
  ○ Patients with class III to IV angina that persists despite medical therapy or any patient with class I to II angina who is intolerant of medical therapy
  ○ Individuals in a high-risk occupation that affects the safety of others
  ○ Patients successfully resuscitated from sudden cardiac death
- Unstable angina:
  ○ Patients who are refractory to initial medical stabilization are subjected to emergent catheterization.
  ○ Patients who have high-risk characteristics (heart failure, rhythmic instability, etc) undergo urgent catheterization.
  ○ Patients with high-risk features on noninvasive testing
- Acute MI:
  ○ For primary revascularization in patients with an acute MI who present within 12 hours of symptom onset or at any time if symptoms persist (angina, heart failure, or electrical instability)
  ○ In patients younger than 75 years of age who suffer an acute MI complicated by cardiogenic shock within 36 hours
  ○ Patients in the post-MI setting with spontaneous ischemia or ischemia provoked by low level exertion or any patient with high-risk features on a postdischarge stress test

- Postrevascularization ischemia:
  - Suspected abrupt closure or subacute stent thrombosis after revascularization
  - Recurrent ischemia 9 months after percutaneous coronary intervention (PCI) or 12 months after bypass surgery
- Preoperative evaluation prior to noncardiac surgery:
  - Patients with high-risk findings on preoperative noninvasive evaluation
  - Any high-risk clinical patient with equivocal noninvasive test findings
  - Stable or unstable angina that is not responsive to adequate medical therapy
- Valvular heart disease:
  - Prior to valvular surgery to assess the coronary arteries
- Congenital heart disease:
  - Prior to surgical correction in patients with symptoms suggestive of ischemia or in patients with congenital abnormalities that are associated with coronary anomalies
- Congestive heart failure:
  - Patients with systolic dysfunction and chest pain or reversible ischemia on noninvasive testing
  - Patients with unexplained systolic dysfunction
- Other conditions:
  - Patients with any disease affecting the aorta when knowledge of coronary anatomy might affect management (ie, aortic dissection)
  - Prospective cardiac transplant donors who are at risk for CAD
  - Asymptomatic patients with Kawasaki disease to identify coronary artery aneurysms

CONTRAINDICATIONS

- The only absolute contraindication to cardiac catheterization is refusal of the patient to undergo the procedure.
- Relative contraindications include the following:
  - Electrolyte abnormalities
  - Febrile illness
  - Acute renal failure
  - Decompensated heart failure
  - Severe allergy to radiographic contrast agents
  - Bleeding disorder or anticoagulated state
  - Severe, uncontrolled hypertension
  - Pregnancy
- In some emergent situations, a cardiac catheterization may be indicated despite the presence of one or more of these relative contraindications.

COMPLICATIONS AND SAFETY

- Cardiac catheterization is a relatively safe procedure; however, like all invasive procedures it does carry risk.
- The risk of death, MI, or cerebrovascular accident is approximately 1 in 1000 procedures. The two major factors that have been associated with an adverse outcome include disease of the left main coronary artery and severe aortic stenosis.
- Vascular access site complications (ie, retroperitoneal hemorrhage, hematoma, pseudoaneurysm, distal embolization) occur in approximately 1 in 100 procedures.
- Contrast-induced nephropathy characterized by a transient elevation of the serum creatinine secondary to iodinated contrast. Diabetic renal disease (creatinine > 2.0 mg/dl) is most commonly associated with this complication. Several strategies have been employed to prevent contrast-induced nephropathy including hydration, mannitol, diuresis, dopamine, fenoldopam, *N*-acetyl cysteine, bicarbonate, and hemofiltration. In addition, the physicochemical properties of the contrast agent is associated with contrast-induced nephropathy.
  - Currently accepted strategies for minimizing risk of contrast-induced nephropathy include limiting contrast volume, utilizing low-osmolar contrast, aggressive hydration (usually involving isotonic fluids or bicarbonate containing fluids), and avoidance of nephrotoxins such as NSAIDs in the periprocedural period. The use of *N*-acetyl cysteine can be considered although its efficacy is controversial.
- Importantly, the risk of renal atheroembolic disease is significant in patients with advanced large vessel atherosclerosis. Atheroemboli can induce digital ischemia and progressive renal dysfunction (often slowly over a period of months). Once established, renal atheroembolic disease is generally considered irreversible.

CORONARY COMPUTED TOMOGRAPHY ANGIOGRAPHY AND CARDIAC MAGNETIC RESONANCE IMAGING

- Coronary computed tomography (CT) angiography is a developing technology that permits noninvasive assessment of the coronary artery anatomy. Images are acquired following a single injection of iodinated contrast.

- Patients may receive an intravenous β-blocker to achieve a HR of 60 to 70 at the time of the test. Irregular or rapid heart rhythms reduce image quality.
- As a relatively new technology, the utility of CT angiography in clinical practice is undergoing investigation. Currently it has been suucessfully used to identify focal coronary artery lesions as well as the origin and proximal course of anomalous coronary arteries.
- Cardiac magnetic resonance imaging (CMR) is another relatively new technology that provides high resolution, highly detailed images of the heart and its surrounding structures.
- Like coronary CT angiography, the clinical application of CMR remains incompletely understood. Nevertheless, CMR has been used in the:
  - Diagnosis and assessment of diseases of the aorta
  - Diagnosis of dilated cardiomyopathy and determination of an ischemic or nonischemic etiology
  - Diagnosis of other cardiomyopathies including sarcoidosis, hemochromatosis, Chagas disease, arrhythmogenic right ventricular cardiomyopathy, and hypertrophic cardiomyopathy
  - Determination of restrictive versus constrictive physiology
  - Determination of myocardial viability
  - Evaluation of LV thrombus formation
- Disadvantages of CMR are prolonged image acquisition time and technical limitations in patients with implantable medical devices such as pacemakers or defibrillators.

BIBLIOGRAPHY

Cheitlin MD, et al. ACC/AHA/ASE 2003 guideline update for the clinical application of echocardiography. *J Am Coll Cardiol.* 2003;42:954.

Gibbons RJ, et al. ACC/AHA 2002 guideline update for exercise testing. *Circ.* 2002;106:1883.

Murphy JG. *Mayo Clinic Cardiology Review.* 2nd ed. Philadelphia, PA: Lippincott, Williams, and Wilkins; 1999.

Scanlon PJ, et al. ACC/AHA guidelines for coronary angiography: a report of the American College of Cardiology/American Heart Association task force on practice guidelines. *J Am Coll Cardiol.* 1999;33:1756.

Zipes DP, Libby P, Bonow R, Braunwald E. *Braunwald's Heart Disease: A Textbook of Cardiovascular Medicine.* 7th ed. Philadelphia, PA: WB Saunders; 2004.

31 ELECTROCARDIOGRAM BASICS

Frank L. Bleyer

INTRODUCTION

- The 12-lead electrocardiogram (ECG) is a recording that reflects the heart's electrical activity. Electrical signals are detected on the surface of the body by electrodes attached to the extremities and chest wall. The ECG machine amplifies the signal and records it on special graph paper (Fig. 31–1).
- The graph paper plots electrical voltage on the vertical axis and time on the horizontal axis.
- Heavy horizontal lines are 5-mm apart and light horizontal lines are 1-mm apart. Vertically, the lines are 1-mm apart and represent 0.1 mV.
- The normal ECG paper speed is 25 mm/sec, therefore the heavy lines are 0.2 seconds apart and the light lines are 0.04 seconds apart.
- The electrocardiogram is comprised of several characteristic waveforms that reflect different components of the cardiac cycle.

WAVES AND INTERVALS

P WAVE

- The P wave represents left and right atrial depolarization (Fig. 31–2).

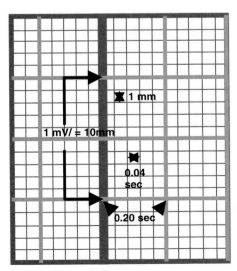

FIG. 31–1 ECG graph paper.

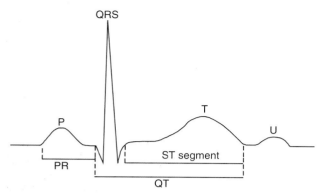

FIG. 31–2 ECG waveforms.

- The duration of the P-wave is between 0.08 and 0.11 seconds.
- Its amplitude is less than 0.25 mV.
- In sinus rhythm the P-wave is always upright in limb leads I and II, inverted in lead aVR, and variable in lead II and aVL. In any of the limb leads it may be notched.

PR INTERVAL

- The PR interval is measured from the beginning of the P wave to the beginning of the QRS complex.
- The PR-interval reflects the duration of conduction through the atrioventricular node and His-Purkinje system. A short interval may reflect preexcitation or an accessory pathway.
- The normal interval ranges between 0.14 and 0.25 seconds (shortens with increased heart rates).
- The PR segment reflects the distance between the end of the P wave and the beginning of the QRS complex.

QRS COMPLEX

- The QRS complex reflects the electrical activity generated from right and left ventricular depolarization.
- Normal QRS width is between 0.06 and 0.1 seconds.
- QRS voltage varies among different leads.

ST SEGMENT

- The ST segment is the distance between the end of the QRS complex and the beginning of the T wave.
- Although it is usually isoelectric in the limb leads, minimal ST elevation can be seen in otherwise healthy patients in leads III and aVF. Minor ST segment depression of up to 0.5 mm can also be seen in the limb leads of healthy individuals.

- In the precordial leads, ST elevation is seen in almost all healthy patients, typically in V_2 and V_3, and may be as high as 3 mm in these leads. In V_5 and V_6, ST elevation is rare except in pathologic states. ST segment depression in the precordial leads is considered abnormal.

T WAVE

- The T wave reflects ventricular repolarization.
- The T wave is usually asymmetric with a broad slow upstroke and a relatively brisk return to the baseline.

QT INTERVAL

- The QT interval is measured from the beginning of QRS complex to end of the T wave.
- It varies with heart rate and ranges between 0.35 and 0.46 seconds.

U WAVE

- The U wave is a low-frequency deflection that appears after the T wave.
- It is upright in all leads, except aVR and its amplitude is 5% to 25% of the T wave amplitude. The U wave is not always seen and is thought to reflect repolarization of the Purkinje system of the papillary muscles. Electrolyte disorders, drugs, and some antiarrhythmic agents have been associated with U waves.

STEPWISE APPROACH TO INTERPRETING THE ELECTROCARDIOGRAM

RATE

- The heart rate in resting healthy patients is between 60 and 100 beats per minute.
- If the rhythm is regular, the QRS complexes allow the heart rate to be readily calculated. For example, if the QRS complexes are one large box apart, the heart rate is 300 beats per minute; if two, then 150 beats per minute, and so forth (Fig. 31–3).

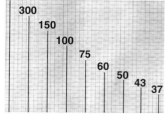

FIG. 31–3 Horizontal lines reflect the number of large boxes between successive QRS complex starting with 1. Thus, 1 box width = 300 beats per minute and 4 box width = 75 beats per minute.

- If the rhythm is irregular, an average heart rate can be determined by counting the number of QRS complexes in 6 seconds, which is 30 large boxes, and then multiplying by 10.

RHYTHM

- First, determine if the rhythm is regular.
- Identify the P waves. Are they upright in I and II, indicating a sinus rhythm? If negative P waves are observed in leads II, III, and aVF, consider an ectopic atrial rhythm or junctional rhythm. Are all the P waves of the same morphology? If not, consider a multifocal atrial arrhythmia.
- Determine if every P wave is associated with a QRS complex. If not, are there more or less P waves than QRS complexes? Note if the P wave occurs before or after each QRS complex.
- Determine the PR interval.
- Determine the width of QRS complex. Is it narrow (<0.125 seconds) or wide (>0.125 seconds)?
- By obtaining this information, the rhythm can be correctly classified (see below).

AXIS

- The hexaxial reference system, which is used to calculate the heart's electrical axis in the frontal plane, is comprised of leads I, II, III, aVR, aVL, and aVF.
- Limb lead I reflects a 0 degree dipole (right arm compared to left arm), lead II reflects a 60 degree dipole (right arm and left leg), and lead III a 120 degree dipole (left arm and left leg). The augmented leads utilize Einthoven's law to create unipolar leads by combining the standard limb leads (I-III) and referencing them as 0. This allows different electrical vectors to be assessed with the standard limb leads eg, aVF reflects a 90 degree pole, aVR a 150 degree pole, and aVL a 30 degree pole (Fig. 31–4).
- Examine the QRS complex in leads I and aVF and determine if the QRS is positive or negative in each of these leads. The vector quadrant can then be determined (Table 31–1).
- Next, examine the QRS complexes to determine which lead is isoelectric (or closest to isoelectric). The QRS vector is directed 90 degrees from this lead toward the vector quadrant identified in Table 31–1.
  - For example, a QRS complex which is upright in I and aVF and isoelectric in aVL indicates that the vector is 90 degrees from aVL toward the normal quadrant; and thus the heart's axis is 60 degrees.

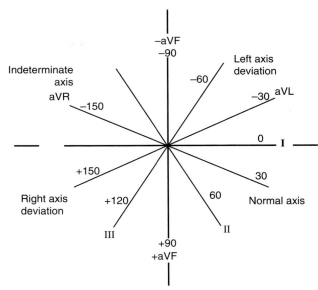

FIG. 31–4 Hexaxial reference system used to calculate the heart's electrical axis (see text for discussion). aVF, augmented voltage unipolar left foot lead, aVL, augmented voltage unipolar left arm lead; aVR, augmented voltage unipolar right arm lead.

INTERVALS, VOLTAGE, AND OTHER MISCELLANEOUS ECG FINDINGS

- Determine the PR interval, QRS width, and QT interval.
- Evaluate the amplitude and direction of the P, QRS, and T waves.
- Determine if there are pathologic Q waves.
- Review the ST segment, noting if there is elevation or depression.

CHAMBER ENLARGEMENT

LEFT ATRIAL ENLARGEMENT CRITERIA

- The terminal portion of the P wave in V_1 is ≥0.04 mm/sec (ie, 1 box).
- Notched P waves that exceed 0.12 seconds.

TABLE 31–1 Heart Axis Evaluation Using Leads I and aVF

	aVF POSITIVE	aVF NEGATIVE
I Positive	0 to +90 Normal	0 to −90 Left axis Deviation
I Negative	+90 to +180 Right axis deviation	−90 to −180 Indeterminant

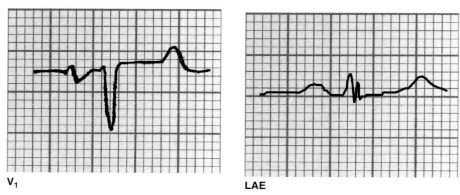

FIG. 31–5 The P wave in lead II (right) is broad and substantially notched, while V1 (left) reveals a deeply inverted (negative) P wave. LAE, left atrial enlargement.

- Leftward shift of the P wave axis to +15 degrees or less (Fig 31–5).

RIGHT ATRIAL ENLARGEMENT CRITERIA

- Characterized by tall P waves with a height ≥2.5 mm in leads II, III, and aVF (Fig. 31–6). Axis is 75 degrees or greater
- Positive deflection of the P wave is observed in lead V_1 or V_2 (≥1.5 mm)

ECG CRITERIA FOR LEFT VENTRICULAR HYPERTROPHY

- Limb leads
  - R wave in lead I + the S wave in lead III exceeds 25 mm
  - R wave in aVL is > 11 mm
  - R wave in aVF is >20mm
  - S wave in aVR is >14 mm

- Precordial leads
  - R wave in V_5 or V_6 is >26 mm
  - R wave in V_5 or V_6 + S wave in V_1 is > 35 mm
  - Largest R wave + largest S wave is >45 mm
- Cornell criteria
  - R wave in aVL + the S wave in V_3 exceed 20 mm (females) or 28 mm (males) (Fig. 31–7, Table 31–2).

ECG CRITERIA FOR RIGHT VENTRICULAR HYPERTROPHY

- Right axis deviation that is >100
- R/S ratio in V_1 is >1
- R wave in V_1 is ≥7 mm
- S wave in V_1 is <2 mm
- QR pattern present in V_1
- RSR –V_1 exceeds 10 mm
- R wave in V_1 + S wave in V_5 or V_6 >10.5 mm
- R/S ratio in V_5 or V_6 is ≤1

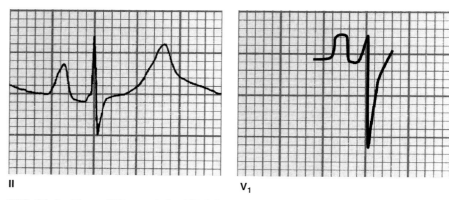

FIG. 31–6 Note tall P-wave in lead II (left) and the large positive deflection of the P-wave in V_1 (right).

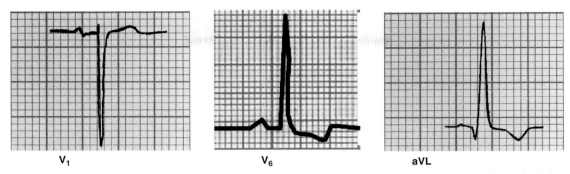

| V₁ | V₆ | aVL |

FIG. 31–7 Note the large R-waves in the precordial leads, V1 and V6 and the limb lead, aVR. Various criteria has been shown to correlate with echocardiographic evidence of LVH (also see Table 31–2). aVL, augmented voltage unipolar left arm lead.

- ST depression and T wave inversion in the right precordial leads (Fig. 31–8).

ECG CRITERIA FOR BUNDLE-BRANCH AND FASCICULAR BLOCKS

LEFT BUNDLE-BRANCH BLOCK

- QRS duration exceeds 0.12 seconds
- Broad monophasic R waves in limb lead 1, aVL and precordial leads V_5, and V_6
- Absence of Q waves in limb lead I and precordial leads V_5 and V_6

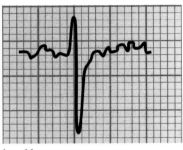

Lead I

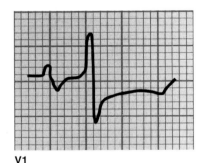

V1

TABLE 31–2 Point Score System Used to Classify LVH

Amplitude	Scoring
Any of the following:	3 points
Largest R or S wave in limb leads >20 mm	
S wave in V_1 or V_2 ≥30 mm	
R wave in V_5 or V_6 ≥30 mm	
ST-T segment changes (typical pattern of LV strain with STT segment vector shifted in direction opposite to the mean QRS vector)	
Without digitalis	3 points
With digitalis	1 point
Left atrial involvement	3 points
Terminal negative deflection of the P wave in V_1 is 1 mm or more in depth with a duration of 0.04 seconds or more	
Left axis deviation −30 degrees or more	2 points
QRS duration ≥0.09 seconds	1 point
Intrinsicoid deflection in V_5 and V_6 ≥0.05 seconds	1 point

3 points, possible LVH; 4 points, probable LVH; 5 points, definite LVH; LV, left ventricle; LVH, left ventricular hypertrophy

V6

FIG. 31–8 Lead 1 reveals right axis deviation. Note that the R/S in V1 exceeds 1 consistent with right ventricular hypertrophy. Note R/S ratio in V6 is less than 1 and associated ST-T wave changes.

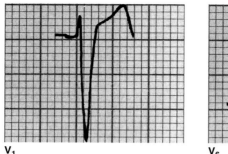

FIG. 31–9 Note the prolonged QRS duration in V1 and V6 with broad monophasic R-waves.

• Displacement of the ST segment and T wave in a direction opposite to the major deflection of the QRS complex (Fig. 31–9).

RIGHT BUNDLE-BRANCH BLOCK

• Prolongation of QRS duration (>0.12 seconds)
• Secondary R wave (R1) in the right precordial leads with an R_1 > the initial R wave
• Delay in the onset of the intrinsicoid deflection in the right precordial leads (>0.5 seconds)
• Wide S wave in limb lead I and the precordial leads V_5 and V_6 (Fig. 31–10)

LEFT ANTERIOR HEMIBLOCK

• The axis is between −30 and −90 (left axis deviation)
• Presence of a QR or R wave in leads I and aVL as well as an RS complex in leads II, III, and aVF
• Normal or slightly prolonged QRS duration (Fig. 31–11)

LEFT POSTFASCICULAR BLOCK

• QRS axis is between +90 and +180 degrees (right axis deviation, RAD)

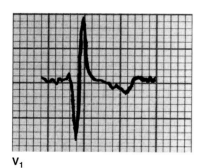

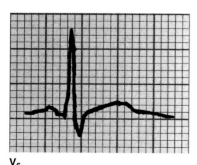

FIG. 31–10 Note the secondary R wave in V1 and the wide S wave in V6.

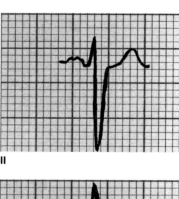

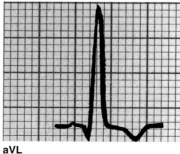

FIG. 31–11 Note the left axis deviation and the RS complex in lead II and the QR wave in lead aVL.

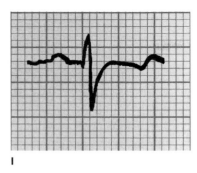

I

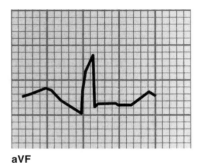

aVF

FIG. 31–12   Note the deep S wave in lead 1 and prolonged QRS duration in aVF.

- Exhibits an S1 Q3 pattern (deep S wave in lead I and a Q wave in lead III)
- Normal or slightly prolonged QRS duration (0.08–0.15 seconds)
- No other factors responsible for RAD (Fig. 31–12)

TABLE 31–3   Q Wave and ST Segment Lead Involvement Depending on the Area of Infarct

ANATOMIC AREA OF INFARCT	LEADS
Anterior wall	Elevation $V_1 - V_4$
Anterolateral wall	Elevation $V_1 - V_6$ + I and aVL
High Lateral wall	Elevation I and aVL
Inferior wall	Elevation II, III, and aVF
Posterior wall	Depression $V_1 - V_3$, upright T wave
Right ventricular infarct	Elevation RV_4

aVF, augmented voltage unipolar left foot lead; aVL, augmented voltage unipolar left arm lead.

ECG CRITERIA FOR ACUTE MYOCARDIAL INFARCTION

EVOLUTIONARY QRS AND ST CHANGES

1. Hyperacute T wave which are short lived
2. R wave increases in amplitude
3. ST elevation >1 to 2 mm in 2 or more contiguous leads, usually with upwardly convex configuration (see Table 31–3)
4. Loss of the R wave
5. Loss of the Q wave with development of new Q waves in 6–9 hours
6. Loss of ST elevation and termination of T wave inversion

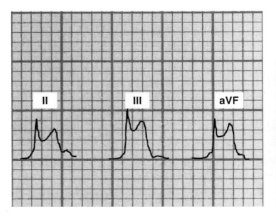
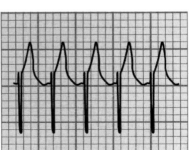
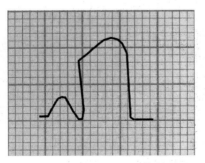

FIG. 31–13   Note the concave morphology of the ST segment elevation (left) and hyperacute T wave changes (middle). The right panel reveals marked ST segment elevation.

BIBLIOGRAPHY

O'Keefe JH, Hammill SC, Freed MS. *The Complete Guide to ECGs.* 2nd ed. Physicians Press; 2002.

Surawicz B, Knilans TK. *Chaus Electrocardiography in Clinical Practice.* WB Saunders; 2001.

Wagner GS. *Practical Electrocardiography.* 10th ed. Lippincott Williams & Williams; 2000.

32 ARRHYTHMIAS

Daniel Friedman

INTRODUCTION

- The molecular basis of cardiac arrhythmogenesis has grown immeasurably in the past decade.
- Drug therapies have been developed which selectively alter the ion currents responsible for each phase of the cardiac action potential. Importantly, some of these agents have been shown to alter the natural history of arrhythmias.
- Technological advances in catheter-based ablation have afforded a potential cure for a large number of clinical arrhythmias.
- Pacemaker devices and the implantable cardioverter-defibrillators have revolutionized the treatment of bradyarrhythmias and life-threatening arrhythmias.

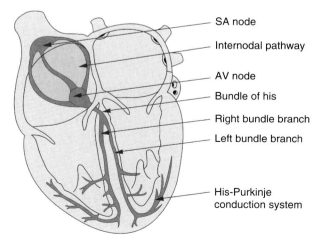

FIG. 32–1 Anatomy of the cardiac conduction system. AV, atrioventricular; SA, sinoatrial.

SOURCE: Reprinted with permission from Hurst JW, et al. *The Heart.* 11th ed. McGraw-Hill; 2004

THE CARDIAC CONDUCTION SYSTEM

- The initial cardiac electrical impulse originates in the sinoatrial node (sinus node) located near the junction of the superior vena cava and the right atrium (Fig. 32–1).
  - Normal sinus rhythm is characterized by an electrocardiographic tracing that reflects impulse propagation that originates from the sinoatrial node.
  - The blood supply to the sinoatrial node is derived from either the left or right coronary arteries.
  - The sinoatrial node is innervated by the autonomic nervous system (both adrenergic and cholinergic inputs) that may influence the rate of sinoatrial node impulse genesis.
  - The sinoatrial node impulse propagates to the right and left atria, respectively and then the atrioventricular node (the AV node). The AV node allows passage of the impulse to the ventricles and therefore regulates the timing of contraction between the atria and ventricles.
- The AV node is anatomically located in the anteromedial portion of the right atrium anterior to the coronary sinus ostium and extends to the central fibrous body of the heart (Fig. 32–1).
  - The AV node is a complex structure with multiple anatomical zones and functional electrical inputs. The AV junctional area is believed to be comprised of four areas or zones: (1) the transitional zone (comprised of transitional cells which bridge normal atria and the AV node proper), (2) the AV node proper (specialized nodal cells sometimes referred to as the compact node), (3) lower nodal zone, and (4) the penetrating AV bundle (bundle of His).
  - The atrioventricular node is innervated by the autonomic nervous system (adrenergic and cholinergic inputs) that can affect the rate of impulse propagation to the ventricles.
  - The blood supply to the AV node is usually derived from the right coronary artery, although the left coronary artery provides the principle blood supply in 15% to 20% of patients. The AV node is less apt to sustain ischemic damage than the sinoatrial node (likely because of collateral flow).
- The electrical impulse exits the AV node in the central fibrous body to the specialized ventricular conduction system within the muscular interventricular septum known as the His-Purkinje system (Fig. 32–1).
  - The His bundle rapidly conducts the impulse to the ventricles via a bifascicular (right and left bundle branches) or a trifascicular (right bundle branch, left bundle branch, and septal branch) network of fibers.
  - The His-Purkinje system is relatively insensitive to changes in autonomic tone and ischemic injury.
  - The right bundle branch is well organized as it courses to the apex of the heart, however, the left bundle branch bifurcates into an anterior fascicle and a posterior fascicle.

BASIC ELECTROPHYSIOLOGY PRINCIPLES

- Electrical impulses in the heart are initiated by action potentials (depolarizations) that are propagated sequentially from cell to cell. The action potential is initiated when the resting membrane potential reaches the threshold for the cardiac myocyte.
- Changes in the membrane potential of the cardiac myocyte result from the movement of ions across ion channels within the myocyte membrane (Fig. 32–2).
- Sodium, potassium, calcium, and chloride ion channels are the major channels involved in generation of the cardiac action potential.
- The cardiac action potential consists of five phases:
  - Phase 0: Rapid membrane depolarization that is the result of sodium entry into the cells via a sodium channel. This phase of the cardiac action potential is initiated by partial depolarization that reaches the threshold potential of the cell.
  - Phase 1: Early rapid repolarization of atrial and ventricular cells due to efflux of potassium ions and closure of sodium channels.
  - Phase 2: Plateau phase due to slow influx of calcium ions via an L-type calcium channel, which is counterbalanced by the efflux of potassium ions.
  - Phase 3: Repolarization of the cell due to inactivation of the calcium and sodium channels, as the efflux of potassium through open potassium channels continues.
  - Phase 4: Diastolic or recovery phase of the action potential. This phase is relatively flat in atrial and ventricular cells and is due to the action of the Na-K-ATPase pump. In the sinoatrial and atrioventricular node, the action potential is characterized by relatively slow conduction (flatter phase 0) and delayed repolarization. The action potential in nodal tissue is chiefly dependent on L-type calcium channels.
- Thus, the cardiac action potential varies in shape and height depending on the tissue.
  - The sinoatrial and atrioventricular cells slowly depolarize between action potentials resulting in a pacemaker-like action (also referred to as automaticity). The sinoatrial node usually has a higher automaticity than the rest of the heart. The mechanism responsible for the slow depolarizations between action potentials is the result of an inward calcium current.
  - Atrial and ventricular action potentials lack spontaneous depolarizations between action potentials and therefore do not exhibit pacemaker activity. However, the duration of atrial and ventricular action potentials differs.
- Collectively, these unique cardiac action potentials produce the characteristic waves, segments, and intervals traced on the surface electrocardiogram.

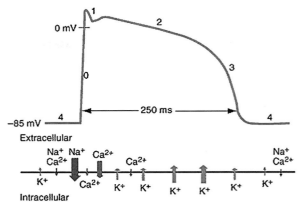

FIG. 32–2 Cardiac action potential and the associated ion flux. Source: Reprinted with permission from Kasper, et al, *Harrison's Principles of Internal Medicine.* McGraw-Hill; 2004:213.

- The mechanisms underlying most arrhythmias are broadly classified into three categories: (1) disorders of impulse generation, (2) disorders of impulse propagation, or (3) a mixture of both. Importantly arrhythmias may be initiated by one mechanism, but maintained by another.
- Disorders of impulse generation:
  - Slow depolarization occurs during phase 4 of the action potential in cells that have intrinsic automaticity such as the sinoatrial and atrioventricular node.
  - Disturbances in automaticity are usually characterized by increased automaticity in cells with intrinsic pacemaker activity or ectopic automaticity arises in cells that normally do not have pacemaker activity.
  - Clinical examples of arrhythmias that occur as the result of abnormal automaticity include: sinus tachycardia, ectopic atrial tachycardia, and accelerated idioventricular rhythm.
  - Triggered arrhythmias are a relatively rare cause of tachycardias, usually drug-induced. Triggered arrhythmias are due to early or delayed afterdepolarizations eg, depolarizations which occur before the next action potential of the cell.
    - If the afterdepolarization occurs before phase 4 of the cardiac action potential, it is called an early afterdepolarization (EAD). Early afterdepolarizations are believed to be responsible for the ventricular tachycardia known as torsade de pointes.
    - If the afterdepolarization occurs during phase 4 of the cardiac action potential, it is called a delayed afterdepolarization (DAD). Delayed afterdepolarizations appear to precipitate the arrhythmias secondary to ischemic injury, digitalis toxicity, hypokalemia, hypercalcemia, and catecholamines.
- Disorders of impulse propagation (reentry):
  - Arrhythmias due to reentry are more common than those due to abnormal impulse formation.

○ Reentry is defined as a continuous repetitive propagation of an excitatory wave traveling in a circular path, returning to its site of origin to reactivate that site. Reentry requires that three conditions be met:

- Adjacent pathways with differing electrophysiological properties must be joined proximally and distally (forming a loop). Examples of these pathways include accessory atrioventricular connections, dual AV nodal pathways, and strategically localized scar formation after myocardial infarction.

- Unidirectional block must be present in one pathway (thus, allowing propagation in only one direction or pathway).

- Conduction velocities of the two pathways must differ. Accordingly, one pathway must be sufficiently slow to allow recovery of the previously blocked pathway, which in turn allows propagation of the signal in a retrograde direction.

○ Reentry occurs when an impulse travels through the slow pathway and blocks antegrade propagation through the fast pathway. When the impulse reaches the distal portion of the slow pathway, it activates the fast pathway (which is now recovered) in the retrograde direction. The impulse travels in the retrograde direction along the fast pathway to the proximal portion of the pathway where the slow pathway is once again activated in the antegrade fashion.

○ Examples of arrhythmias whose mechanism is believed to depend on reentry include atrial flutter, atrioventricular nodal reentry tachycardia, sinus nodal reentry tachycardia, atrioventricular reentry tachycardia, and ventricular tachycardia (perhaps from myocardial scarring after an infarction).

ANTIARRHYTHMIC MEDICATIONS

- Antiarrhythmic medications are classified according to the modified Vaughan Williams classification system. This system assumes that the drugs have a predominant mechanism of action. While technically an oversimplification this system remains clinically useful.

- Class I agents block sodium channels and are further classified according to their relative ability to block the sodium channel.

  ○ Ia agents include quinidine, procainamide, and disopyramide. These drugs slow conduction throughout the His-Purkinje system, atria, and ventricles and prolong the refractory state of these tissues. These agents can also block potassium channels and therefore may prolong the QT interval as well as the QRS duration. Torsade de pointes (polymorphous ventricular tachycardia, PVT) is an important potential side effect of these agents.

  ○ Ib agents include lidocaine and mexiletine. These agents are relatively weak antagonists of sodium channels.

  ○ Ic agents include propafenone and flecainide. These agents are potent antagonists of cardiac sodium channels. They widen the QRS and produce bradycardia. They usually prolong the PR interval, and can induce ventricular tachycardia at high heart rates.

- Class II antiarrhythmic agents include the β-adrenergic blocking medications. These medications decrease sinus nodal and atrioventricular nodal conduction.

- Class III antiarrhythmic agents primarily inhibit potassium channels and prolong the refractory state of cardiac tissue (decrease automaticity).

  ○ These medications include sotalol, amiodarone, bretylium, ibutilide, and dofetilide.

  ○ Sotalol has β-adrenergic blocking properties in addition to its effects on potassium channels.

  ○ Amiodarone inhibits β-adrenergic receptors, α-adrenergic receptors, sodium channels, and calcium channels. The long-term administration of amiodarone has been associated with multiple organ system dysfunction (thyroid disease, liver injury and pulmonary fibrosis).

  ○ Ibutilide is often used to chemically cardiovert patients with atrial fibrillation or atrial flutter.

  ○ Dofetilide is a highly selective potassium channel antagonist.

  ○ All of these agents prolong the QT interval and may cause torsade de pointes.

- Class IV antiarrhythmic medications are comprised of the calcium channel antagonists, diltiazem, and verapamil. These agents delay conduction in the sinoatrial and atrioventricular nodes.

- Other commonly used antiarrhythmic medications include adenosine and digoxin.

  ○ Adenosine is an α-1 agonist, which decreases conduction through the AV node and SA node . The biological half-life of adenosine is measured in seconds. Adenosine is widely considered the drug of choice to terminate supraventricular tachycardias.

  ○ Digoxin is used as an antiarrhythmic agent primarily to control the ventricular rate in atrial fibrillation or atrial flutter.

    - Digoxin exerts its effects via the autonomic nervous system as a vagotonic medication. It therefore slows the sinoatrial node rate, slows atrioventricular nodal conduction, and shortens atrial refractoriness.

    - At toxic levels, digoxin can induce a variety of arrhythmias including AV block, accelerated junctional rhythm, ectopic atrial tachycardia, fascicular tachycardia, and ventricular tachycardia.

    - In addition to withholding the drug, treatment for digoxin toxicity usually includes administering digoxin-specific Fab antibody.

SPECIFIC CARDIAC ARRHYTHMIAS

PREMATURE ECTOPIC BEATS

- Ectopic complexes or beats (premature atrial complexes or premature ventricular complexes) are complexes that originate from areas of the heart other than the sinoatrial node. Premature beats are a frequent cause of an irregular heart rate or pulse.
- Ectopic complexes may occur in structurally normal or abnormal hearts, but are more frequent in diseased hearts.
- Premature atrial complexes may result in a compensatory pause, may reset the sinoatrial node, or may be interpolated on the electrocardiogram.
- Premature atrial complexes do not necessarily require specific treatment. A search for an underlying pathologic process is generally advisable if the premature complexes are frequent or new. Underlying pathologic processes include ischemia, infection, inflammation, and stimulants such as caffeine, tobacco, and alcohol.
- Premature atrial complexes may be a harbinger of supraventricular tachycardia. These complexes may initiate atrial fibrillation, atrial flutter, and other reentry tachycardias.
- If patients with premature atrial complexes are symptomatic, medications such as β-adrenergic blockers and calcium channel blockers may be used to decrease the frequency of the premature complexes.
- Premature junctional complexes or beats originate near the atrioventricular node. They may arise in patients with underlying His-Purkinje disease, although many are insignificant. There is no specific treatment for premature junctional complexes.
- Premature ventricular beats are commonly seen in structurally normal hearts as well as diseased hearts. The incidence of premature ventricular beats increases with age and underlying heart disease.
- Frequent premature ventricular beats may lead to symptoms of palpitations. Underlying processes include ischemia, infection, inflammation, electrolyte disorders, and stimulants. Treating the underlying process can reduce or eliminate premature ventricular complexes. If not, symptomatic complexes can be treated with antiarrhythmic medications such as β blockers and type Ib /Ia antiarrhythmic drugs.

BRADYARRHYTHMIAS

- Sinus node dysfunction is comprised of the following arrhythmias: sinus bradycardia, sinoatrial exit block, sinoatrial arrest, and tachycardia-bradycardia syndrome or sick sinus syndrome.
- Sinus node dysfunction is usually idiopathic and associated with fibrosis and fatty infiltration of the SA node as patients age. Other causes of sinus node dysfunction include medications, electrolyte abnormalities, autonomic disturbances, and intrinsic heart disease.
- Evaluation of sinus node disorders should include a 12-lead ECG, ambulatory Holter monitoring to correlate symptoms with ECG findings, and tilt table testing. Any medications that might interfere with function of the sinoatrial node should be discontinued.
- Insertion of a transvenous pacemaker is the treatment of choice for sinus node dysfunction. Atropine boluses or insertion of a temporary pacemaker are used to acutely manage patients with sinus node dysfunction and hemodynamic instability.
- The tachycardia-bradycardia syndrome is characterized by sinus node dysfunction and paroxysmal supraventricular tachycardia (most commonly atrial fibrillation). These patients may require medication to reduce the heart rate during the tachycardia phase and a permanent pacemaker to prevent bradyarrhythmias.
- Acquired atrioventricular block is classified as first, second, or third (complete) degree block.
  ○ First-degree atrioventricular block is characterized by a prolonged (>200 msec) PR interval which remains fixed. (Fig. 32–3). The incidence of first-degree atrioventricular block increases with age and is most commonly due to degenerative conduction system disease.

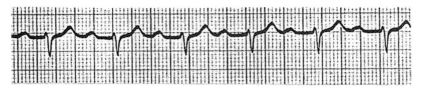

1st degree AV block (PR = 280 ms)

FIG. 32–3 First-degree atrioventricular block. AV, atrioventricular.
SOURCE: Reprinted with permission from Frank G. Yanowitz, MD http://library.med. utah.edu/kw/ecg/

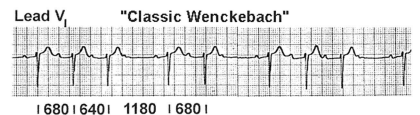

FIG. 32–4 Second-degree atrioventricular block, Mobitz type I.
SOURCE: Reprinted with permission from Frank G. Yanowitz, MD http://library.med.utah.edu/kw/ecg/

○ There is no treatment for first-degree atrioventricular block and it usually does not cause symptoms.

• Second-degree atrioventricular block is classified as either Mobitz type I (Wenckebach phenomenon) or Mobitz type II.

○ Second-degree atrioventricular block Mobitz type I (Fig. 32–4) is characterized by an prolonged PR interval that increases from one beat to the next until there is a nonconducted P wave. The PR interval following the nonconducted P wave is short. Other characteristics include group beating and a progressively shorter RR interval with successive beats. Patients with Mobitz type I second-degree atrioventricular block usually do not require a pacemaker unless symptoms are present.

○ Second-degree atrioventricular block Mobitz type II (Fig. 32–5) is characterized by a prolonged PR interval (which is fixed) with an occasional nonconducted P wave. These patients often have additional signs of conduction system disease such as bundle-branch block and usually require a permanent pacemaker to prevent life-threatening bradyarrhythmias.

• Third-degree atrioventricular block or complete heart block (Fig. 32–6) is characterized by dissociation between the atrial and ventricular electrical impulses during which the atrial rate is typically higher than the ventricular rate. An escape rhythm, which is either junctional or ventricular, is usually present. These patients are nearly always symptomatic and require permanent pacemaker implantation.

• Atrioventricular nodal block is sometimes associated with an inferior or anterior MI.

○ Block associated with inferior infarction is often temporary and, therefore, if necessary, need only be treated with a temporary pacemaker.

○ However, block associated with an anterior infarction is often permanent and generally requires permanent pacemaker implantation.

• A small number of patients with chronic bifascicular or trifascicular block will eventually progress to complete heart block.

○ These patients may also experience syncope and rarely sudden death.

○ A permanent pacemaker is indicated in patients with chronic bifascicular or trifascicular block who have syncope with intermittent third-degree atrioventricular block or when other remediable causes have been excluded.

• Atrioventricular dissociation is not a primary rhythm disturbance but can occur in association with a rhythm disturbance.

○ Atrioventricular dissociation is characterized by independent electrical activity of the atria and ventricles.

○ By definition it exists in third-degree heart block. It may also arise in ectopic rhythms that usurp control of the ventricles.

• Neurocardiogenic syncope or pre-syncope is a commonly encountered cause of syncope, particularly in a younger patient.

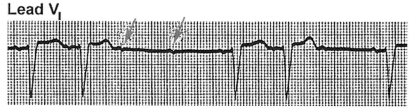

FIG. 32–5 Second-degree atrioventricular block, Mobitz type II.
SOURCE: Reprinted with permission from Frank G. Yanowitz, MD http://library.med.utah.edu/kw/ecg/

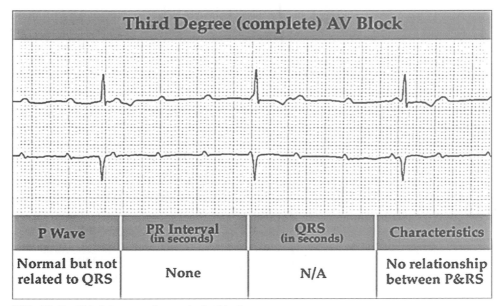

FIG. 32–6 Third-degree atrioventricular block.
Source: Reprinted with permission from Frank G. Yanowitz, MD http://library.med.utah.edu/kw/ecg/

○ This condition is a subtype of autonomic nervous system dysfunction that is characterized by vasodepressor or cardioinhibitory signs and symptoms induced by tilt-table testing.

○ Therapy with a permanent pacemaker may be indicated in patients with recurrent syncope without clear, provocation or with a hypersensitive cardioinhibitory response. In addition, a permanent pacemaker may be indicated in patients with recurrent neurocardiogenic syncope associated with bradycardia.

○ Therapy for patients with neurocardiogenic syncope with a vasodepressor response includes β-blockers (controversy exists regarding the effectiveness of these agents), disopyramide, theophylline, selective serotonin reuptake inhibitors, midodrine, and salt loading or fludrocortisone. Patient should be instructed to avoid prolonged standing, to utilize compression stockings while walking, and to maintain adequate hydration.

• Carotid sinus hypersensitivity is a cause of sinus arrest and syncope.

○ Pressure on the carotid sinus from tight fitting neck garments or rapid head swivelling can provoke the cardioinhibitory response.

○ Carotid sinus massage is typically performed during tilt-table testing to test for carotid sinus hypersensitivity.

○ If carotid sinus pressure induces ventricular asystole for longer than 3 seconds in the absence of AV or SA nodal blocking medications, a permanent pacemaker should be inserted.

PACEMAKERS

• Pacemaker systems consist of a pulse generator that contains the battery and circuitry and one, two, or three pacemaker leads that are affixed to the heart.

• The pulse generator is generally implanted in the infraclavicular region of the chest wall on either the left or right side of the body. It is placed between the prepectoral fascia and the subcutaneous tissue.

• The lead system can contain one lead (single chamber lead placed in the right atrium or right ventricle), two leads (dual chamber leads placed in the right atrium *and* right ventricle) or three leads (biventricular pacemaker with leads placed in the right atrium, right ventricle, and a cardiac vein—to pace the left ventricle).

• The nomenclature for describing the mode of pacing is standardized according to the NASPE/BPEG generic code which is comprised of a series of letters.

○ Most pacemaker modes can be described using a combination of the first four letters.

  ▪ The first letter represents the chamber(s) paced.

  ▪ The second letter represents the chamber(s) sensed.

  ▪ The third letter indicates the response to sensing.

  ▪ The fourth letter indicates whether rate modulation is turned on.

• Biventricular pacemakers are also called cardiac resynchronization devices because they are used in patients with heart failure that have dyssynchrony between the walls of their ventricles.

- The pacemaker resynchronizes the timing of the contraction of the walls of the left ventricle to improve cardiac output.
- This therapy has shown to reduce morbidity and mortality in some heart failure patients.
- The pacemaker lead threshold is the smallest impulse (voltage potential over time) required to capture and pace the cardiac chamber.
  - High pacemaker lead thresholds are a sign of pacemaker lead malfunction or movement of the position of the tip of the pacemaker lead. Interrogation of the pacemaker for dysfunction should be scheduled regularly.
  - Pacemaker leads pace the heart in unipolar or bipolar mode.
    - Unipolar mode required that the pulse generator serve as one pole and the tip of the lead as the opposite pole. This circuit produces a large stimulus artifact on the surface ECG.
    - Bipolar pacing involves the ring of the lead as one pole and the tip of the lead as the opposite pole. This circuit causes a smaller stimulus artifact on the surface ECG.

TACHYARRHYTHMIAS

- Supraventricular tachycardias are commonly encountered tachyarrhythmias that originate from the atria.
  - The ECG of a supraventricular tachycardia is characterized by a narrow (<120 msec in duration) QRS complex tachycardia (rate >100 bpm). However if there is aberrant conduction in the ventricles, the QRS complex may not be narrow.
  - Importantly, the relationship between the P wave and the QRS complex is crucial to correctly differentiate among the various supraventricular tachycardias.
- Sinus tachycardia occurs when the sinoatrial node discharges at a rate that exceeds 100 bpm.
  - The P wave morphology and axis in sinus tachycardia should be identical to the P wave morphology and axis observed with normal sinus rhythm.
  - Sinus tachycardia may be secondary to an underlying physiologic process (dehydration) or it may be pathologic (pulmonary embolus).
    - The onset and termination of sinus tachycardia is usually gradual. Increasing vagal tone by carotid sinus massage or vagal maneuvers will slow sinus tachycardia temporarily.
    - Several underlying processes that may lead to sinus tachycardia include hypovolemia, hypotension, anemia, fever, medications, illicit drug use, heart failure, infectious and/or inflammatory conditions, thyrotoxicosis, caffeine or other stimulants, and alcohol or drug withdrawal.

- Inappropriate sinus tachycardia is sometimes seen in young healthy patients and may merely represent a variation of normal automaticity of the sinoatrial node or could reflect an ectopic atrial tachycardia focus near the sinoatrial node.
- There is no specific treatment for a physiologic compensatory sinus tachycardia. Management of the underlying condition decreases the heart rate.
- Inappropriate sinus tachycardia is sometimes treated with β-adrenergic blockers, calcium-channel blockers, digoxin, or catheter based ablation.
- Atrial flutter is a common atrial tachycardia whose mechanism almost always involves a macroreentry circuit (Fig. 32–7).
  - Atrial flutter is commonly seen in patients who also have atrial fibrillation. The symptoms produced by atrial flutter as well as the risk for thromboembolic complications are similar to those seen with atrial fibrillation.
  - The macroreentrant circuit in atrial flutter usually rotates around the tricuspid annulus in a counterclockwise direction (type 1 or isthmus-dependent). Occasionally the circuit rotates around the annulus in a clockwise direction (type 1 reverse or clockwise flutter). The flutter circuit usually travels through the cavotricuspid isthmus (a common site for catheter ablation).
  - The ECG characteristics of atrial flutter are:
    - Atrial rate 240–340 bpm.
    - Identical, recurring, regular sawtooth shaped flutter waves without an isoelectric baseline.
    - The flutter waves are negative in the inferior leads (II, III, and aVF) when the atrial flutter is counterclockwise (Fig. 32–8).
    - The flutter waves are positive in the inferior leads (II, III, and aVF) when the atrial flutter is clockwise.
    - The ventricular response will be variable depending on the degree of atrioventricular block.
    - Management of atrial flutter is similar to that of atrial fibrillation with the exception that catheter based ablation is a highly successful curative procedure for atrial flutter.

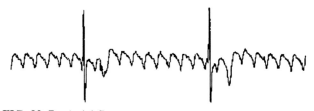

FIG. 32–7 Atrial flutter.
SOURCE: Reprinted with permission from Frank G. Yanowitz, MD
http://library.med.utah.edu/kw/ecg/

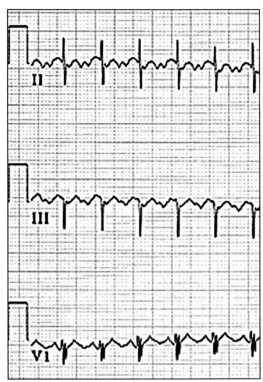

FIG. 32–8 Counterclockwise typical atrial flutter. Reprinted with permission from Frank G. Yanowitz, MD http://library.med.utah.edu/kw/ecg/

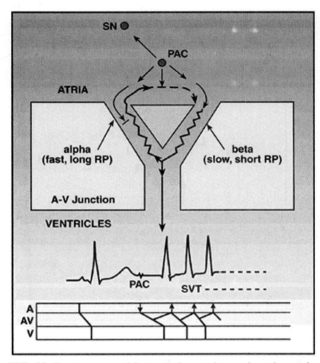

FIG. 32–9 Anatomy of fast and slow pathways in atrioventricular nodal reentry tachycardia. A-V, atrioventricular; PAC, premature atrial contraction, SN, sinus node; SVT, supraventricular tachycardia; RP, refractory period.
SOURCE: Reprinted with permission from Frank G. Yanowitz, MD http://library.med.utah.edu/kw/ecg/

- Atrioventricular nodal reentry tachycardia (AVNRT) is a paroxysmal supraventricular tachycardia often seen in structurally normal hearts.
  - The reentry circuit involves a fast and slow pathway within the atrioventricular node (Fig. 32–9).
  - The onset and termination of AVNRT is sudden.
  - AVNRT responds acutely to vagal maneuvers such as the Valsalva maneuver and cough. Adenosine or verapamil given as a rapid intravenous bolus will terminate this arrhythmia.
  - The RP interval is short in AVNRT. The P wave may not be apparent if it occurs within the QRS complex. The P wave may be visible at the end of the QRS complex or in the ST segment (Fig. 32–10).
  - Catheter based ablation of AVNRT is successful in more than 95% of cases, but it is associated with a small risk of complete AV block.

- Atrioventricular reentry tachycardia has a similar clinical presentation to AVNRT. AV reentry tachycardia is characterized by sudden onset and spontaneous termination.
  - The reentry circuit involves an accessory pathway which may be concealed (absence of a delta wave) or manifest (delta wave present).
  - As in AVNRT, AV reentry tachycardia responds acutely to vagal maneuvers as well as medications that slow conduction in the AV node such as adenosine or verapamil.
  - AV nodal blocking medications (β-blockers, verapamil) are contraindicated in patients with Wolff-Parkinson-White syndrome. These agents can precipitate cardiac arrest by enhancing the preexcited ventricular rate response by decreasing the degree of concealed retrograde conduction into the accessory pathway.

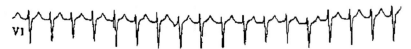

FIG. 32–10 Atrioventricular nodal reentry tachycardia.
SOURCE: Reprinted with permission from Frank G. Yanowitz, MD http://library.med.utah.edu/kw/ecg/

Lead V₁

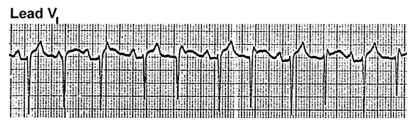

Atrial tachycardia with variable AV block

FIG. 32–11 Atrial tachycardia with variable AV block.
SOURCE: Reprinted with permission from Frank G. Yanowitz, MD http://library.med.utah.edu/kw/ecg/

- Catheter based ablation is successful in more than 95% of of AV nodal reentry tachycardias.
  - The ECG in AV reentry tachycardia is characterized by a short RP interval, 1:1 AV conduction, and a P wave in the ST segment or T wave.
  ○ Atrial tachycardias usually originate from an automatic ectopic focus that is located somewhere in the atria.
    - The ECG characteristics include a long RP interval, gradual initiation (warm up), and gradual termination (cool down) of the tachycardia, and P wave morphology and axis that is different from the normal sinus P wave axis and morphology.
    - Paroxysmal atrial tachycardia with AV block should raise the possibility of digoxin toxicity.
    - Atrioventricular nodal blocking medications and vagal maneuvers do not usually terminate atrial tachycardias. Nevertheless, these strategies may augment AV nodal block and uncover an ectopic atrial tachycardia.
    - The treatment for atrial tachycardia consists of slowing the ventricular rate with AV nodal blocking agents (see Fig. 32–11). In addition, antiarrhythmic drug therapy can be initiated with class Ia, Ic, or III drugs. Catheter based ablation is an alternative curative therapy in many patients with atrial tachycardias.
- Sinus node reentry tachycardia occurs within the sinus node cluster of cells and is conducted throughout the heart in an otherwise normal fashion.
  ○ Sinus node reentry tachycardia is characterized by a long RP interval.
  ○ Vagal maneuvers and adenosine will terminate the tachycardia.
  ○ β-adrenergic antagonists, calcium channel antagonists, and digoxin are useful medications to prevent recurrences.
  ○ The P waves will be identical in axis and morphology as the sinus P waves on ECG.
  ○ Catheter based ablation is rarely needed to treat sinus node reentry tachycardia.
- Multifocal atrial tachycardia (MAT) is associated with multiple P wave morphologies (at least three different morphologies) and variable PP and PR intervals (Fig. 32–12).
  ○ This tachycardia is commonly seen in patients with chronic obstructive pulmonary disease.
  ○ The rate of this tachyarrhythmia is generally slower than in other atrial arrhythmias and the treatment is focused on correcting the underlying pathologic process.
- Junctional ectopic tachycardia is caused by accelerated automatic discharges from a region near the His bundle.
  ○ The atria may not be activated in the retrograde fashion. Rather, the atria may remain in sinus rhythm or may be characterized by an ectopic atrial rhythm.
  ○ Atrioventricular dissociation may occur with a junctional ectopic tachycardia.
  ○ Junctional ectopic tachycardia is usually seen in patients with structural heart disease.

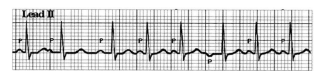

FIG. 32–12 Multifocal atrial tachycardia.

○ This rhythm is managed by treating the underlying process. Antiarrhythmic medications can be used. Catheter based ablation for cure is possible, but carries a risk of complete AV block since the focus is in close proximity to the atrioventricular node.

TACHYARRHYTHMIAS ASSOCIATED WITH ACCESSORY PATHWAYS

• Ventricular preexcitation appears on the ECG as a delta wave which slurs the upstroke of the R wave (Fig. 32–13).
• A delta wave on ECG indicates the presence of an accessory pathway or bypass tract which rapidly conducts the electrical impulse in the antegrade direction from atria to ventricles. It is associated with a short PR interval (<120 msec).
• Preexcitation is seen on the ECG in approximately 1.5 per 1000 people. Preexcitation is also seen in patients with Ebstein anomaly.
• Wolff-Parkinson-White (WPW) syndrome is a clinical syndrome characterized by preexcitation. The atrial tachyarrhythmia in WPW occurs in the presence of an antegrade conducting accessory bypass tract.
• Ventricular preexcitation is associated with an increased risk of sudden death, likely secondary to an accessory pathway that conducts impulses rapidly to the ventricle. Such a phenomenon can degenerate into ventricular tachycardia or ventricular fibrillation.
• Intermittent loss of preexcitation during normal sinus rhythm suggests a lower risk of sudden death.
• Patients who develop atrial fibrillation in the presence of a rapidly conducting accessory pathway are also at increased risk for sudden death. Risk stratification can be accomplished with electrophysiologic testing.
• Ventricular preexcitation can usually be cured via catheter based ablation techniques.
• The treatment for an acute episode of atrial fibrillation in the setting of ventricular preexcitation involves the use of procainamide or synchronized direct current cardioversion. Treatment with AV nodal blocking agents may increase conduction via the accessory pathway and accelerate the ventricular response, thus precipitating ventricular fibrillation.

VENTRICULAR TACHYARRHYTHMIAS

• Ventricular tachycardia is defined as at least three consecutive ventricular complexes with a rate greater than 100 bpm. Nonsustained ventricular tachycardia lasts less than 30 seconds.
  ○ Ventricular tachyarrhythmias are a common cause of sudden cardiac death and often accompany cardiac disease.
  ○ Patients with a wide complex tachycardia present a diagnostic dilemma eg, they may have either ventricular tachycardia or supraventricular tachycardia with aberrant conduction. The clinical and ECG characteristics that distinguish between these two types of wide complex tachycardias are as follows:
    ▪ Patients with coronary artery disease and wide complex tachycardia are much more likely to have ventricular tachycardia than supraventricular tachycardia with aberrant conduction.
    ▪ Brugada's criteria permit the clinician to distinguish ventricular tachycardia from supraventricular tachycardia with aberrant conduction:
      • Absence of RS complexes in all precordial leads is consistent with ventricular tachycardia
      • If the interval from the onset of the QRS complex to the nadir of the S wave is >100 msec in one precordial lead, the rhythm is likely ventricular tachycardia.
      • If there are more QRS complexes than P waves, the rhythm is likely ventricular tachycardia.
      • If ventricular tachycardia morphology is present in V1 and V6, the rhythm is likely ventricular tachycardia.

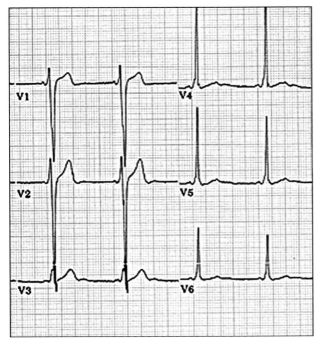

FIG. 32–13 Ventricular preexcitation.
SOURCE: Reprinted with permission from Frank G. Yanowitz, MD
http://library.med.utah.edu/kw/ecg/

- Fusion beats, capture beats, atrioventricular dissociation, QRS duration greater than 140 msec and a northwest axis are common findings on the ECG that suggest ventricular tachycardia.
  - Acute management of sustained ventricular tachycardia depends on the hemodynamic stability of the patient.
- A hemodynamically unstable patient with ventricular tachycardia receives direct current cardioversion.
- A pulseless patient with ventricular tachycardia should be defibrillated.
- Hemodynamically stable patients receive intravenous antiarrhythmic medications such as amiodarone, lidocaine, or procainamide.
- The reversible causes of ventricular tachycardia should be corrected such as hypokalemia, hypomagnesemia, hypotension, myocardial ischemia, and medications.

MISCELLANEOUS TACHYARRHYTHMIAS

- An accelerated idioventricular rhythm is usually secondary to a ventricular focus which usurps control of the ventricles by the sinoatrial node.
  - The rate is characteristically between 60 and 110 beats per minute. Atrioventricular dissociation is usually present.
  - Accelerated idioventricular rhythm is usually accompanied by severe ischemic heart disease and may occur after reperfusion of an occluded coronary artery.
  - No therapy is required unless the patient is hemodynamically unstable.
- Polymorphic ventricular tachycardia with a normal QT interval is generally only seen with myocardial ischemia.
- Polymorphic ventricular tachycardia with a prolonged QT interval is referred to as torsade de pointes. Torsade de pointes can degenerate quickly into ventricular fibrillation. Torsade de pointes is characterized by a shifting QRS axis on the ECG; the so called twisting of the pointe.
  - Torsade de pointes is associated with long QT syndromes, which may be congenital or acquired.
  - The acquired long QT syndromes are associated with many drugs and electrolyte abnormalities (hypokalemia and hypomagnesemia). The acquired long QT may also be a forme fruste of a congenital long QT syndrome.
  - Congenital long QT syndromes are inherited as specific genetic mutations.
- Bundle branch reentry ventricular tachycardia involves the right and left bundle branches as the antegrade

and retrograde conduction pathways in the reentry circuit.
  - There is usually underlying His-Purkinje conduction system disease.
  - The diagnosis is confirmed by an electrophysiologic study
- Specialized ventricular tachycardias can arise from the right or left ventricular outflow tracts.
  - Specialized tachycardias may be triggered by adrenergic stimulation. These tachycardias are usually terminated by adenosine. Catheter based ablation is frequently curative for specialized tachycardias.
- Ventricular tachycardia that arises from right ventricular dysplasia has a right ventricular origin and therefore a left bundle branch block morphology. The frequency of this arrhythmia varies according to the extent of dysplasia. Catheter based ablation is initially effective, but this rhythm disturbance may recur. Insertion of an implantable defibrillator is usually needed to prevent sudden cardiac death
- Other conditions associated with ventricular tachycardia include dilated cardiomyopathies, Brugada's syndrome, hypertrophic cardiomyopathy, infiltrative cardiomyopathies such as amyloidosis and sarcoidosis, Duchenne muscular dystrophy, tetralogy of Fallot, and myocarditis.
- Implantable cardioverter-defibrillators (ICD) are now standard of care as primary or secondary prevention for sudden cardiac death from ventricular tachycardia or fibrillation in virtually all cardiomyopathic conditions.

BIBLIOGRAPHY

Gregoratos G, Abrams J, Epstein AE, et al. ACC/AHA/NASPE 2002 guideline update for implantation of cardiac pacemakers and antiarrhythmia devices: summary article: a report of the American College of Cardiology/American Heart Association Task Force on Practice Guidelines. *Circ.* 2002;106(16):2145–2161.

Griffin BP, Topol EJ, eds. *Manual of Cardiovascular Medicine.* 2nd ed. Philadelphia : Lippincott Williams & Wilkins; 2004.

Murphy JG. *Mayo Clinic Cardiology Review.* 2nd ed. Philadelphia: Lippincott Williams & Wilkins; 2000.

Zipes DP. *Braunwald's Heart Disease: A Textbook of Cardiovascular Medicine.* 7th ed. Philadelphia: Elsevier Saunders; 2005.

Zipes DP, Camm AJ, Borggrefe M, Buxton AE, et al. ACC/AHA/ ESC 2006 guidelines for management of patients with ventricular arrhythmias and the prevention of sudden cardiac death: a report of the American College of Cardiology/American Heart Association Task Force and the European Society of Cardiology Committee for Practice Guidelines. *J Am Coll Cardiol.* 2006;48(5):e247–346.

33 ATRIAL FIBRILLATION

Frank L. Bleyer

INTRODUCTION

- Atrial fibrillation is the most common sustained arrhythmia. Atrial fibrillation is characterized by the absence of organized atrial contractions. The electrocardiogram shows the absence of P waves with rapid oscillations and irregular R-to-R intervals (Fig. 33–1).
- Atrial fibrillation is associated with multiple small wandering reentry (microreentry) circuits in the atrium. This disorganized electrical activity impairs mechanical contraction of the atria, which contributes to thrombus formation and decreased stroke volume.
- Atrial fibrillation is usually accompanied by atrial enlargement or strain and is often the consequence of heart disease.

ETIOLOGY

- Atrial fibrillation is more common in men than in women, and its incidence increases with age.
- Atrial fibrillation occurs commonly with rheumatic heart disease and mitral stenosis. It is also associated with many other clinical disorders including the following:
  - Thyroid disease
  - Coronary artery disease
  - Congestive heart failure
  - Hypertrophic cardiomyopathy
  - Mitral valve prolapse
  - Mitral regurgitation
  - Acute myocardial infarction
  - Postcardiac surgery
- Noncardiac causes include the following:
  - Hypertension
  - Acute alcohol intoxication
  - Cholinergic drugs
  - Hypoxemia
  - Noncardiac surgery

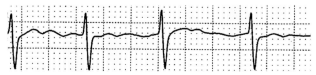

FIG. 33–1 Note irregular R-R intervals and absence of P-waves.

SYMPTOMS

- Symptoms can vary from none to significant hypotension, lightheadedness, palpitations, chest pain, and shortness of breath. The loss of atrial contraction may worsen heart failure symptoms in patients with impaired left ventricular function, diastolic heart failure, or valvular heart disease.
- Patients can exhibit minimal symptoms, regardless of the ventricular rate. However, patients who are asymptomatic usually have adequate rate control.

TREATMENT

ANTICOAGULATION

- Atrial fibrillation is associated with an increased risk of transient ischemic attacks (TIA) and stroke. There is a sixfold increased incidence of embolic events in patients with atrial fibrillation. Conditions that further increase this risk include congestive heart failure, diabetes mellitus, hypertension, age greater than 65 years, and a prior history of TIA/cerebrovascular accident.
- Anticoagulation with warfarin to achieve a international normalized ratio (INRs) of 2.0 to 3.0 has been shown to reduce the risk of ischemic stroke by 68%.
- Patients younger than 65 years of age without heart disease (ie, isolated atrial fibrillation), hypertension or diabetes mellitus are substantially less likely to develop thromboembolic complications. Importantly, the use of warfarin is not indicated in these patients. Currently, low-risk patients are treated with 325 mg of aspirin daily.
- All patients older than 60 years of age or any patient with a history of coronary artery disease, diabetes, hypertension, previous embolic event, or echocardiographic findings of left atrial enlargement, left ventricular dysfunction, or significant mitral annular calcification should be treated with warfarin. International normalized ratios should be maintained between 2.0 and 3.0.

RATE CONTROL
- The symptoms of atrial fibrillation are significantly improved with rate control. Indeed, most patients will be asymptomatic with rate control.
- β-Blockers, calcium channel blockers (diltiazem, verapamil), *Digitalis*, and amiodarone are all effective at controlling the ventricular rate. A target resting heart rate of less than 80 to 90 beats per minute is desirable.
- If a patient exhibits significant symptoms during an episode of atrial fibrillation with a rapid ventricular response, (ie, shortness of breath, chest pain) the

clinician should induce rapid rate control with intravenous drug therapy (metoprolol, diltiazem, esmolol, or verapamil). Intravenous digoxin can be effective, but its onset of action is delayed compared with the β-blockers or nondihydropyridine calcium channel blockers. Notwithstanding, digoxin is considered a first-line agent in patients who present with significantly impaired ventricular function.

DOSING REQUIRED TO ACHIEVE RATE CONTROL

- Diltiazem: 20 to 25 mg intravenously over 10 minutes followed by a 10 mg/h infusion
- Verapamil: 5 to 15 mg over 5 minutes followed by a 0.05 to 0.2 mg/min infusion
- Metoprolol: 5 mg intravenously over 5 minutes; may repeat as necessary
- Esmolol: 0.5 μg/kg intravenously over 1 minute followed by 50 μg/kg/min; titrate by 50 μg/kg/min to a maximum of 200 μg/kg/min; a repeat loading dose may be administered
- Amiodarone: 150 mg intravenously over 10 minutes followed by 1 mg/min over 6 hours then 0.5 mg/min
- In refractory cases, a combination of agents can be employed. Careful continuous monitoring for hypotension and bradycardia is required.
- Patients who present with rapid heart rates, but without significant symptoms, can be managed with oral medications:
  - Metoprolol: 25 to 50 mg by mouth every 6 hours
  - Diltiazem: 30 to 60 mg by mouth every 6 hours
  - Amiodarone: 200 to 400 mg by mouth three times a day
- Oral digoxin can control the ventricular rate quite well in the resting state; however, with increasing activity, breakthrough tachycardia is common. A second drug can be added to improve rate control. Amiodarone increases the plasma level of digoxin, necessitating a reduction in the digoxin dose.
- If life-threatening symptoms accompany atrial fibrillation (hypotension, pulmonary edema, ischemic heart disease), immediate treatment with electrical cardioversion is warranted.
- Some patients will convert to normal sinus rhythm with rate controlling drugs alone. Bradycardia (<50/min or symptomatic) is relatively common following chemical cardioversion. If such drugs are required for chronic rate control, placement of a permanent pacemaker is recommended.
- If the ventricular rate cannot be adequately controlled with pharmacologic agents, ablation of the AV node and placement of a permanent pacemaker should be considered.

RATE CONTROL VERSUS RHYTHM CONTROL

- Considerable controversy exists regarding the role of cardioversion followed by suppressive medications compared to rate control and therapeutic anticoagulation in the management of atrial fibrillation.
- Most patients who revert to sinus rhythm will have recurrent episodes of atrial fibrillation. Drugs such as amiodarone, flecainide, propafenone, sotalol, and dofetilide have been shown to decrease recurrent episodes of atrial fibrillation. Amiodarone is approximately twice as effective as other agents, but it remains a third-line agent because of its significant toxicity profile.
- The Atrial Fibrillation Follow-Up Investigation of Rhythm Management (AFFIRM) and Electrical Cardioversion for Persistent Atrial Fibrillation (RACE) trials evaluated whether rate control or rhythm control was superior. Overall the results indicate no advantage to a rhythm control strategy and underscored the importance of maintenance of long-term anticoagulation with an INR >2.0.
- Patients who present with new onset atrial fibrillation or acute atrial fibrillation in the postoperative period, acute alcohol intoxication or thyrotoxicosis, if not self-limiting, may warrant a trial of rhythm control, while maintaining the INR >2.0
- Patients who experience adverse symptoms with atrial fibrillation or are refractory to chronic heart rate control should be considered for rhythm control.
- The clinical history guides the choice of antiarrhythmia therapy used to suppress recurrent episodes of atrial fibrillation. Flecainide and propafenone are used in patients with no structural heart disease. Sotalol should be used in patients with coronary artery disease, but preserved left ventricular function. Amiodarone is the optimal choice in patients with coronary artery disease, age >75 years, and those with left ventricular dysfunction.

ACUTE CARDIOVERSION IN THE HOSPITAL

- Patients with atrial fibrillation associated with hemodynamic instability require acute cardioversion with synchronized countershock.
- If hemodynamically stable, rate control should be instituted as described above. If the duration of atrial fibrillation is <48 hours, patients can be safely cardioverted to normal sinus rhythm. If there are no clinical or echocardiographic features indicating an increased risk for cardiac emboli, patients can be discharged without warfarin anticoagulation.

- If the duration of atrial fibrillation is greater than 48 hours or unknown, patients should be anticoagulated before elective cardioversion. Two strategies have been employed:
  1. Warfarin anticoagulation (INR, 2.0 to 3.0) for 4–6 weeks followed be elective cardioversion. Typically the patient is maintained on oral anticoagulation for at least another 4 weeks.
  2. Alternatively, heparin is administered during the initial hospitalization to achieve a partial thromboplastin time of 60 to 70 seconds. A transesophageal echocardiogram is also performed to exclude a left atrial thrombus. Once excluded, the patient can be safely cardioverted. Following successful cardioversion, the patient should be maintained on warfarin anticoagulation for at least 4 weeks.
- If the patient has clinical or echocardiographic features consistent with an increased risk of cardiac embolization, long-term anticoagulation is recommended. Paroxysmal atrial fibrillation carries the same risk of cardiac emboli as persistant atrial fibrillation.

CONCLUSION

- Patients with atrial fibrillation almost always require pharmacological agents for rate control. Individuals at high risk for emboli (age >65, atrial enlargement, etc.) also require chronic anticoagulation. Some patients may benefit from an attempt at rhythm control (eg, transient or remediable causes of atrial fibrillation). The choice of rate controlling drugs, as well as drugs that suppress atrial fibrillation are ultimately determined by the clinical characteristics of the patient.

BIBLIOGRAPHY

Chugh SS, Blackshear JL, Shen WK, et al. Epidemiology and natural history of atrial fibrillation: Clinical implications. *J Am Coll Cardiol.* 2001;37:371.

Falk RH. Atrial fibrillation. *N Engl J Med.* 2001;344:1067.

Fuster, V, Ryden, LE, Cannom, DS, et al. ACC/AHA/ESC 2006 guidelines for the management of patients With atrial fibrillation: a report of the American College of Cardiology/American Heart Association Task Force on Practice Guidelines and the European Society of Cardiology Committee for Practice Guidelines (Writing committee to revise the 2001 Guidelines for the management of patients With atrial fibrillation). *J Am Coll Cardiol.* 2006;48:e149.

Wyse DG, Waldo AL, DiMarco JP, et al. A comparison of rate control and rhythm control in patients with atrial fibrillation. The atrial fibrillation follow-up investigation of rhythm management (AFFIRM) investigators. *N Engl J Med.* 2002;347:1825.

34 UNSTABLE ANGINA AND NON–ST ELEVATION MYOCARDIAL INFARCTION

Frank L. Bleyer

INTRODUCTION

- Unstable angina (UA) and non–ST elevation myocardial infarction (NSTEMI) are clinical syndromes characterized by myocardial ischemia without electrocardiographic ST elevation.
- Both syndromes are caused by plaque rupture and associated nonocclusive thrombus.
- Although UA and NSTEMI have a similar underlying pathophysiology, they differ in the degree of ischemia.
  ○ Although UA is not associated with a clinically detectable cardiac enzyme (creatine kinase myocardial band, myoglobin, or troponin) leak, there can be electrocardiographic (EKG) changes consistent with ischemia.
  ○ In contrast, NSTEMI is characterized by a gradual rise and fall in biomarkers for myocardial necrosis associated with anginal-like symptoms.

PATHOGENESIS

- The earliest changes that precede the development of atherosclerosis are believed to involve the endothelium (augmented permeability to lipids and other plasma constituents). These changes produce intramural lipid accumulation and eventually plaque formation.
- The advanced atherosclerotic plaque consists of a connective tissue fibrous cap that overlies a core of lipid *gruel* composed of lipid-laden foam cells, cholesterol, and necrotic cellular debris.
- Thinning of the protective fibrous cap is induced by a heightened local inflammatory state that is an early and characteristic feature of atherosclerosis. If sufficiently advanced, plaque rupture can occur and precipitate acute coronary and cerebrovascular syndromes.
- Plaque rupture exposes the thrombogenic inner lipid core of the plaque to circulating blood coagulation products. Platelet and coagulation system activation results in a localized thrombus.
- Thrombi in UA/NSTEMI are platelet rich and usually nonocclusive. In contrast, occluding thrombi are characteristic of acute STEMI and typically comprised of fibrin and red blood cells.
- The disrupted plaque and associated thrombus reduces myocardial blood flow and impairs oxygen

delivery to cardiac myocytes. However, microembolization of platelet aggregates also occlude small arteriolar and capillary beds, thus furthering ischemia. Indeed, microembolization is thought to be necessary to induce frank myocardial necrosis and the parallel release of biomarkers (creatine phosphokinase [CPK] and troponins).

EPIDEMIOLOGY

• In 2001 there were 5.6 million emergency department visits in the United States for chest pain. In patients with an eventual diagnosis of UA/NSTEMI, 5% to 10% died in-hospital or developed a recurrent MI.

CLINICAL PRESENTATION

• The classic symptoms of UA/NSTEMI are characterized by poorly localizing chest or arm discomfort described as pressure-like or tightening. The discomfort typically radiates to the jaw and arms. Symptoms may be precipitated by emotional or physical exertion or may occur spontaneously at rest.
• Often the clinical presentation is atypical, especially in the elderly (age >65), in women and in patients with comorbid conditions (diabetes mellitus).
• Atypical symptoms of UA/NSTEMI include the following:
  ◦ Epigastric pain
  ◦ Unexplained fatigue
  ◦ Dyspnea (at rest or with exertion)
  ◦ Confusion
  ◦ Nausea
  ◦ Diaphoresis
• Certain clinical features are considered characteristic of UA. These include:
  ◦ Rest angina (particularly if prolonged or associated with transient ST changes)
  ◦ New onset angina after minimal exertion
  ◦ Changes in the frequency of angina
• Features considered *not* characteristic, but often confused, with myocardial ischemia include the following:
  ◦ Pleuritic stabbing pain worse with respiration
  ◦ Lower or midabdominal pain
  ◦ Point tenderness, especially over the apex
  ◦ Pain reproduced with chest wall palpation
  ◦ Constant pain lasting for hours (especially in the absence of ST changes)
  ◦ Fleeting pain lasting only seconds
  ◦ Pain radiating to the lower extremities

INITIAL EVALUATION

• Patients presenting with symptoms suggestive of an acute coronary syndrome (ACS) should undergo a focused medical history and physical examination. An electrocardiogram (ECG) and biochemical marker measurements (CPK and CPK myocardial bands, troponins) should be obtained.
• After an initial evaluation, the clinician should estimate the likelihood of developing an adverse outcome. Although, risk stratification may prove useful in predicting outcome (death or recurrent MI) and designing the overall therapeutic strategy, almost all patients, regardless of risk, require coronary angiography.
• Tables 34–1 and 34–2 delineate features that classify patients into low, intermediate, or high *likelihood of ACS* and low, intermediate, or high *risk* of an adverse outcome.
• The Thrombolysis in Myocardial Infarction (TIMI) IIB and Efficacy and Safety of Subcutaneous Enoxaparin in Non-Q wave Coronary Events (ESSENCE) trials characterized seven variables that independently predicted outcomes in patients with UA and NSTEMI. Each variable is assigned a score of 1 when present and 0 when absent. By simply adding each variable, a TIMI risk score of 0 to 7 is calculated. Figure 34–1 correlates the TIMI risk score with the rate of composite endpoint of all cause mortality, new or recurrent MI, or severe recurrent ischemia requiring revascularization.
• The TIMI risk variables are as follows:
  ◦ Age older than 65 years
  ◦ Presence of at least three risk factors for coronary heart disease
  ◦ Prior coronary stenosis of ≥50%
  ◦ Presence of ST segment deviation on admission ECG

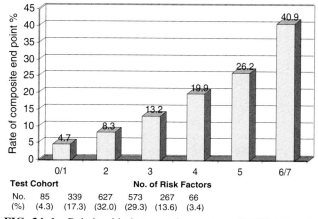

FIG. 34–1 Relationship between the number of TIMI risk variables and composite endpoint (death, new or recurrent MI, or MI requiring revascularization). (Reproduced with permission. Journal of the American Medical Assn, 2000 284;838 Copyright©2000, American Medical Association. All rights reserved)

TABLE 34–1   Likelihood That Signs and Symptoms Represent an Acute Coronary Syndrome Secondary to Coronary Artery Disease

FEATURE	HIGH LIKELIHOOD = ANY OF THE FOLLOWING:	INTERMEDIATE LIKELIHOOD = ABSENCE OF HIGH-LIKELIHOOD FEATURES AND PRESENCE OF ANY OF THE FOLLOWING:	LOW LIKELIHOOD = ABSENCE OF HIGH- OR INTERMEDIATE-LIKELIHOOD FEATURES BUT MAY HAVE:
History	Chest or left arm pain or discomfort as chief symptom reproducing prior documented angina Known history of CAD, including MI	Chest or left arm pain or discomfort as chief symptom Age > 70 years Male sex Diabetes mellitus	Probable ischemic symptoms in absence of any of the intermediate likelihood characteristics Recent cocaine use
Examination	Transient MR, hypotension, diaphoresis, pulmonary edema, or rales	Extracardiac vascular disease	Chest discomfort reproduced by palpation
ECG	New, or presumably new, transient ST-segment deviation ($\geq$0.05 mV) or T-wave inversion ($\geq$0.2 mV) with symptoms	Fixed Q waves Abnormal ST segments or T waves not documented to be new	T-wave flattening or inversion in leads with dominant R waves Normal ECG
Cardiac makers	Elevated cardiac TnI, TnT, or CK-MB	Normal	Normal

Braunwald E, Mark DB, Jones RH, et al. Unstable angina: diagnosis and management, Rockville, MD: Agency for Health Care Policy and Research and the National Heart, Lung, and Blood Institute, US Public Health Service, US Department of Health and Human Services; 1994; AHCPR Publication No. 94–0602.
CAD, coronary artery disease; CK-MB, creatine kinase myocardial band; ECG, electrocardiogram; MI, myocardial infarction; TnI, troponin I; TnT, troponin T.
SORUCE: Reproduced with permission from ACC/AHA 2002 guideline for management of patients with unstable angina and non–ST elevation myocardial infarction. American Heart Association; 2002.

TABLE 34–2   Short-Term Risk of Death or Nonfatal Myocardial Infarction in Patients with Unstable Angina

FEATURE	HIGH RISK = AT LEAST ONE OF THE FOLLOWING FEATURES MUST BE PRESENT:	INTERMEDIATE RISK = NO HIGH-RISK FEATURE BUT MUST HAVE ONE OF THE FOLLOWING:	LOW RISK = NO HIGH-OR INTERMEDIATE-RISK FEATURE BUT MAY HAVE ANY OF THE FOLLOWING FEATURES:
History	Accelerating tempo of ischemic symptoms in preceding 48 h	Prior MI, peripheral or cerebrovascular disease, or CABG, prior aspirin use	
Character of pain	Prolonged ongoing (>20 min) rest pain	Prolonged (>20 min) rest angina, now resolved, with moderate or high likelihood of CAD Rest angina (<20 min) or relieved with rest or sublingual NTG	New-onset or progressive CCS Class III or IV angina the past 2 weeks without prolonged rest pain but with moderate or high (>20 min) likelihood of CAD
Clinical findings	Pulmonary edema, most likely due to ischemia New or worsening MR murmur S$_3$ or new/worsening rates Hypotension, bradycardia, tachycardia age >75 years	Age <70 years	
ECG	Angina at rest with transient ST-segment changes > 0.05 mV Bundle-branch block, new or presumed new Sustained ventricular tachycardia	T-wave inversions >0.2 mV Pathologic Q waves	Normal or unchanged ECG during an episode of chest discomfort
Cardiac markers	Elevated (eg, TnT or Tn I >0.1 μg/mL)	Slightly elevated (eg, Tn T> 0.01 but <0.1 μg/mL)	Normal

CABG, coronary artery bypass grafting; CAD, coronary artery disease; CCS, Canadian Cardiovascular Society; ECG, electrocardiogram; IV, intravenous; NTG, nitroglycerin; TnT, troponin T.
SOURCE: Reproduced with permission from ACC/AHA 2002 guideline for management of patients with unstable angina and non–ST elevation myocardial infarction. American Heart Association; 2002 (www.acc.org).

○ Two episodes of angina in the past 24 hours
○ At least two angina episodes in the prior 24 hours
○ Elevated serum cardiac biomarkers
○ Use of aspirin in the prior 7 days
• A focused history and physical examination coupled with a surface EKG and cardiac biomarkers, allow patients to be grouped into one of the following clinical categories:
○ Noncardiac chest pain
○ Chronic stable angina
○ Possible ACS
○ Definite ACS
• The patient can also be stratified into low, intermediate, or high-risk, generally using the TIMI risk score.
• Traditional risk factors are also helpful in predicting the likelihood of coronary artery disease. Traditional risk factors for coronary artery disease include the following:
○ Family history of CAD
○ Hypertension
○ Hyperlipidemia
○ Smoking
○ Advancing age

LEVEL OF CARE

• Patients are assigned to specific treatment areas based on the initial likelihood of an ACS (ie, intensive care unit, medical floor, chest pain unit, or discharge).
• Clinical features that are consistent with noncardiac chest pain should be evaluated accordingly. Importantly, a variety of clinical conditions can elicit symptoms that mimic ACS. These include the following:
○ Musculoskeletal disease.
○ Gastrointestinal disorders (esophageal spasm, peptic ulcer disease, gallbladder disease).
○ Intrathoracic disorders including pneumonia, pleurisy, pulmonary emboli, pneumothorax, pericarditis, asthma, and chronic obstructive pulmonary disease.
○ Neuropsychiatric disorders (anxiety, hyperventilation)
○ Cutaneous disorders (shingles).
• Patients suspected of having a noncardiac etiology for their chest pain should be appropriately triaged and managed.
• Clinical features consistent with chronic stable angina may be managed with adjustments to medications, and the patient can be discharged for regular follow-up or admitted for routine observation.
• Patients classified as possible ACS must have a normal or unchanged EKG and no elevation in cardiac biomarkers. They should be pain free and their symptoms should have been mild and of short duration. These patients should have a TIMI risk score of 2 or less (Table 34–1).

• Patients who have protracted classic symptoms and/or elevation in cardiac biomarkers or EKG changes are classified as definite ACS.
• A patient classified as possible ACS with a TIMI score of 0 to 2 can be evaluated in a chest pain unit. All other patients should be admitted to a telemetry unit. Patients classified with definite ACS should be admitted to an intensive care unit (Fig. 34–2).

CHEST PAIN UNITS

• Chest pain units were developed to expedite the evaluation of patients who present with symptoms suggestive of ACS, but were otherwise low risk (TIMI score <2).
• Importantly, previous studies had indicated that patients with a chest pain syndrome secondary to an ACS, yet mistakenly discharged from the emergency department, had twice the mortality than would be expected had they been appropriately managed.
• The cost of a standard hospital admission for patients with low-risk chest pain is estimated to be $2000 to $5000. Chest pain units appear to offer similar outcomes compared to standard hospitalization but at a substantial reduction in cost and time. Indeed, several studies have suggested that the cost incurred by standard hospitalization for chest pain can be reduced by over $3000. Recent studies have questioned these early results and the precise role of the chest pain unit in the management of patients with suspected ACS is ongoing.
• Chest pain units should employ unambiguous clinical pathways (eg, preset sequence of suggested orders designed to diagnose ACS in a finite period of time, usually 6 to 12 hours). A typical patient would obtain an ECG and cardiac biomarkers in the emergency room. The chest pain unit, should deploy specially trained staff while the patient is undergoing continuous telemetry. Cardiac markers are obtained serially. If the patient exhibits recurrent symptoms, elevated biomarkers, or ECG change they are admitted to the hospital.
• Patients who remain pain free and stable with normal baseline and 6-hour cardiac biomarkers undergo risk stratification with exercise stress testing.

MEDICAL FLOOR ADMISSION

• Patients with intermediate risk can be admitted to a general medical floor with continuous telemetry. These patients should remain symptom free and without EKG changes. Trained personnel with cardiac experience should be available. Specific medical treatment should be instituted (see below).

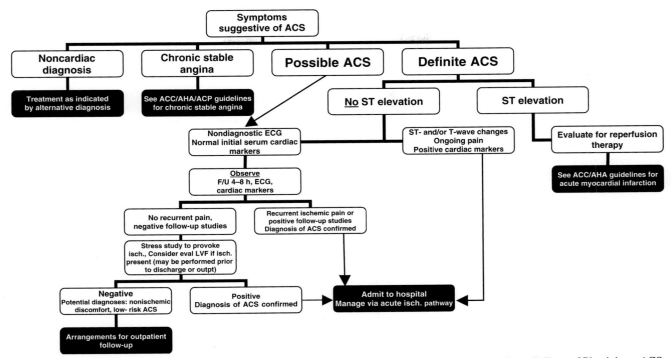

FIG. 34–2   Management algorithm for chest pain. ACC, American College of Cardiology; ACP, American College of Physicians; ACS, acute coronary syndrome; AHA, American Heat Association; ECG, electrocardiogram; F/U, following; eval, evaluation; isch; ischemic; LVF, left ventricular function.
SOURCE: Braunwald, et al. ACC/AHA practice guidelines. 2002.

INTENSIVE CARE UNIT ADMISSION

- Clinical features consistent with a high-risk of an ACS requiring admission to the intensive care unit include the following:
  - Protracted chest pain
  - EKG changes (especially changes that are evolving)
  - Elevated cardiac biomarkers
  - Malignant ventricular arrhythmias
  - Pulmonary congestion
  - Hypotension

TREATMENT

- The treatment of ACS is designed to decrease cardiac myocardial oxygen demand and increase oxygen delivery (eg, coronary flow).

OXYGEN

- Oxygen should be administered to patients with arterial saturations less than 90%.

NITROGLYCERINE

- Nitroglycerine dilates the venous bed, decreasing preload and thus myocardial oxygen demand.
- It also dilates the arterial bed (although it is much less potent) and reduces afterload (thus reducing oxygen consumption).
- Promotes collateral flow by dilating precapillary sphincters of the coronary microvasculature.
- Dilates normal and atherosclerotic epicardial coronary arteries redistributing flow to ischemic areas of the myocardium.
- Initially, 0.4 mg is administered sublingually to patients with ischemia. This dose may be repeated as needed for the symptoms and signs of ischemia.
- If pain is not relieved with sublingual nitroglycerine, intravenous (IV) nitroglycerine should be administered at a rate of 10 μg/min and increased by 5 to 10 μg/min every 3 to 5 minutes until relief of symptoms. Although 200 μg/min is commonly considered the maximal dose, higher doses can be safely administered provided that the patients blood pressure remains stable.
- The blood pressure must be monitored closely. A systolic blood pressure of >110 mm Hg should be maintained. Large abrupt decreases in blood pressure

should be avoided as they may aggravate cardiac ischemia or precipitate a cerebrovascular event.

- Tolerance to nitroglycerine develops within 24 hours and generally necessitates an increase in dosage.
- After 12 to 24 hours of symptom control, the nitroglycerine is weaned and changed to an oral preparation.

MORPHINE SULFATE

- Because morphine sulfate has analgesic, anxiolytic and vasodilatory effects, it decreases myocardial oxygen demand.
- Administered in doses of 1 to 5 mg intravenously
- Must monitor closely for hypotension and respiratory depression.
- Intravenous doses of naloxone 0.4 to 2.2 mg will antagonize morphine's effects.

β-BLOCKERS

- β-Blockers reduce blood pressure, heart rate, and contractility, decreasing myocardial oxygen demand.
- Considerable evidence supports the use of β-blockers in the management of all forms of coronary artery disease.
- Intravenous administration is recommended with protracted ischemia eg, metoprolol 5 mg intravenously every 5 minutes for three doses, then 25 to 50 mg by mouth every 6 hours.
- Bronchospasm, hypotension, and bradycardia can occur. Esmolol has a very short half-life and may prove especially useful in patients with comorbid conditions that could be worsened by β-blocker therapy (COPD).

CALCIUM CHANNEL ANTAGONISTS

- Calcium channel antagonists decrease myocardial oxygen demand and *theoretically* limit the extent and severity of myocardial necrosis.
- Calcium channel antagonists have been used to control ischemia and treat hypertension in ACS. However, the American College of Cardiology/American Heart Association (ACC/AHA) guidelines on NSTEMI (and STEMI), emphasized that no calcium channel blocker has been shown to reduce mortality in acute MI and that in certain patients they may be harmful.
- Short-acting dihydropyridine agents (nifedipine) are contraindicated in ACS in the absence of a β-blocker.
  ○ Verapamil and diltiazem are contraindicated in patients with significant left ventricular dysfunction, eg, ejections fraction <45% because of their negative inotropic effect.
  ○ In general, calcium channel blockers should only be used in patients in whom β-blockers are contraindicated.

ANGIOTENSIN-CONVERTING ENZYME INHIBITORS

- Angiotensin-converting enzyme (ACE) inhibitors have been shown to reduce mortality in patients with an acute MI with ischemic left ventricular dysfunction as well as in nonischemic cardiomyopathy.
- The HOPE and EUROPA trials demonstrated beneficial effects of ACE inhibitors in diabetic patients or patients with preexisting CAD and at least one additional risk factor but without left ventricular dysfunction. Accordingly, most patients discharged after undergoing management for UA/NSTEMI will be treated with an ACE inhibitor.
- The ACC/AHA also recommends the administration of ACE inhibitors in all postmyocardial infarct patients with left ventricular dysfunction, diabetes mellitus, and hypertension not controlled by β-blockers.

ASPIRIN

- In multiple clinical trials, aspirin has demonstrated significant benefits in patients with coronary artery disease.
- Aspirin should be administered as soon as possible in all cases of suspected ACS (eg, in the emergency department and continued daily).
- If the patient has not been receiving aspirin as an outpatient, 160 to 325 mg (chewed to maximize absorption) is recommended, followed by a dose of 81 mg daily.

UNFRACTIONATED HEPARIN AND LOW-MOLECULAR-WEIGHT HEPARIN

- Heparin accelerates the action of circulating antithrombin III, which is a proteolytic enzyme that inactivates thrombin as well as factor IXa and Xa. Heparin should be used in combination with aspirin in all patients presenting with UA or NSTEMI.
- The usual dose of unfractionated heparin is 60 to 70 U/kg (maximum 5000 U) as a bolus with an infusion of 12 to 15 U/kg/min. The partial thromboplastin time (PTT) should be maintained between 1.5 to 2.5 times control. The optimal length of treatment is not known, but most trials using unfractionated heparin (UFH) lasted 2 to 5 days.
- Low-molecular-weight heparin (LMWH) activates factor Xa. The anticoagulant effect of LMWH is more predictable than with UFH, therefore PTT monitoring is not necessary.
- In a pooled study of clinical trials comparing UFH to LMWH, patients on LMWH experienced a lower 30-day event rate without a significant increase in bleeding. This was especially evident in patients managed

conservatively (eg, not taken directly to the catheterization laboratory). Importantly, the SYNERGY trial demonstrated a statistically significant risk of bleeding in patients who were switched from UFH to LMWH and vice versa.

- Serial complete blood counts and platelet counts should be obtained daily during heparin administration. Mild to significant thrombocytopenia may occur with heparin; and autoimmune-induced thrombocytopenia (HIT) with thrombosis is a rare but catastrophic complication. If a patient has a history of heparin-induced thrombocytopenia, a direct thrombin inhibitor such as hirudin can be used. Hirudin is administered as a 0.4 mg/g IV bolus over 15 to 20 seconds followed by a continuous infusion of 0.15 mg/kg/h. The PTT should be maintained between 1.5 to 2.5 times control.

BIVALIRUDIN

- Bivalirudin is a synthetic peptide acting as a highly specific reversible inhibitor of thrombin (circulating and clot-bound). It is a reasonable alternative to heparin, although it is less well studied in the setting of acute MI.
- Its half-life is 25 minutes and it must be administered intravenously
- Bivalirudin causes a prolongation of activated partial thromboplastin time or activated coagulation time; coagulation times return to normal 1 to 2 hours following cessation.
- Predominantly cleared by the kidneys, bivalirudin requires dose reductions for dialysis patients and patients with significant (glomerular filtration rate <30 mL/min) renal impairment.

CLOPIDOGREL

- In all patients with coronary artery disease who are intolerant of aspirin (usually because of hypersensitivity), daily administration of 75 mg of clopidogrel is the alternative of choice.
- Patients with an ACS and normal EKG, and are not at high risk of bleeding or scheduled to undergo surgical revascularization, should be managed with clopidogrel (300-mg loading dose followed by 75 mg daily and continued for at least 9 months).
- In the Clopidogrel in Unstable Angina to Prevent Recurrent Events trial (CURE), Clopidogrel plus aspirin compared to aspirin alone demonstrated a 20% relative risk reduction in the primary combined endpoint of cardiovascular death, nonfatal MI, or stroke.
- Treatment with clopidogrel is beneficial whether patients undergo coronary revascularization or are treated medically.
- Bleeding is a significant problem with patients who undergo surgical coronary revascularization. If coronary artery bypass grafting (CABG) is planned, clopidogrel should be withheld at least 5 days prior to surgery.

GLYCOPROTEIN IIb/IIIa RECEPTOR INHIBITORS

- These agents inhibit the platelet IIb/IIIa receptor, which in turn impairs platelet aggregation and adhesion.
- There are three IIb/IIIa inhibitors currently available: abciximab, eptifibatide and tirofiban.
- Abciximab, is a first-generation murine monoclonal antibody that is currently reserved for use in patients undergoing percutaneous coronary intervention (PCI) in the catheterization laboratory. The GUSTO IV ACS trial evaluated the use of abciximab 24 to 48 hours before cardiac catheterization. A trend for worse outcomes was noted in the abciximab patients. Therefore, abciximab is only used in ACS when patients undergo cardiac catheterization within 6 hours.
- Studies of tirofiban and eptifibatide (nonantibody receptor inhibitors) have demonstrated an improvement in outcomes when used in ACS, especially in patients who ultimately require cardiac catheterization. These agents are especially valuable in the management of high-risk patients, that present with troponin leaks and dynamic ST changes. Tirofiban and eptifibatide should be administered as soon as possible and continued until after the PCI. In patients not requiring cardiac catheterization, a 48- to 96-hour infusion is recommended (Fig. 34–3).

STATINS

- Both primary and secondary intervention studies have shown that chronic administration of a statin reduces the incidence of ACS.
- Recently the PROVE IT TIMI 22 study provided support for the use of intense low-density lipoprotein (LDL) lowering in the setting of ACS. Patients were randomized to high-dose atorvastatin, 80 mg, every day or moderate-dose pravastatin, 40 mg, every day in the setting of an ACS and continued on the agent for 24 months. The group randomized to atorvastatin had a 16% relative risk reduction in the composite endpoint of death, MI, UA requiring rehospitalization, revascularization, and stroke.
- Therefore, aggressive cholesterol reduction with a goal of LDL <70 should begin early in the patient with ACS.

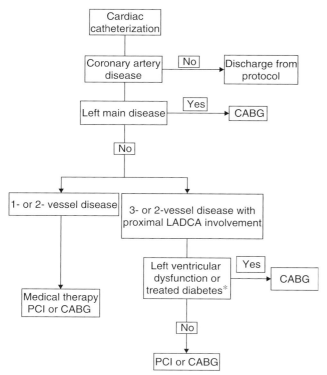

FIG. 34–3 CABG, coronary artery bypass grafting; LADG, left anterior descending coronary artery; PCI, percutaneous coronary intervention.
SOURCE: Braunwald, et al. ACC/AHA practice guidelines. 2002.

TREATMENT STRATEGIES

- The antiplatelet and antithrombotic treatment strategy is guided by an early assessment of risk and likelihood of coronary artery disease.
  - Patients who are classified as low risk can be treated with aspirin alone.
  - Patients with intermediate risk should be treated with aspirin, and LMWH or unfractionated heparin.
  - High-risk patients (positive biomarkers in the serum, dynamic EKG changes, recurrent ischemic chest pain, and a TIMI risk score ≥4) should be treated with aspirin; heparin; IIb/IIIa inhibitors; and clopidogrel (if surgical revascularization is deemed unlikely).

EARLY INVASIVE VERSUS EARLY CONSERVATIVE STRATEGIES

- Two different strategies, early conservative and early invasive, have evolved for the general management of UA and NSTEMI.
  - The early conservative approach utilizes medical management and only progresses to cardiac catheterization if recurrent ischemia develops or the patient has an abnormal noninvasive cardiac stress test.
  - The early invasive approach involves cardiac catherization within 48 hours after the onset of UA/NSTEMI and may proceed to revascularization.
- Early studies comparing these two approaches, the VAN-QUISH and TIMI IIIb, failed to reveal a difference. However, recent studies such as FRISC II, Tactics-TIMI 18, and RITA have demonstrated more favorable results with the early invasive approach. In subset analysis, it appears that higher-risk patients obtain the greatest benefit from an invasive approach. For example, patients who benefit most from the early invasive approach are those with troponin elevation, ECG ST depressions, TIMI risk scores ≥3, or high-risk clinical presentations (pulmonary edema or malignant ventricular arrhythmias). Also, patients with a previous CABG or recent (within 6 months) PCI that present with definite ACS should undergo immediate cardiac catheterization. Those with lower risk should be evaluated with a noninvasive approach, although the data are less clear in this subset.
- Each patient should be individually evaluated. Accordingly, it is essential to consider comorbidities such as age, renal function, and functional status before committing to an aggressive invasive approach (Fig. 34–4).

REVASCULARIZATION

- The indications for PCI or CABG are guided by the findings at cardiac catheterization.
- The decision to surgically or mechanically (PCI) revascularize depends on the location and number of atherosclerotic lesions as well as the left ventricular function. Clinical variables such as diabetes, age, renal function, and other comorbidities also influence the decision.
- The success rate of PCI in ACS is excellent. The use of vascular stents and IIb/IIIa inhibitors has reduced the risk of acute vessel closure and coronary restenosis to rates comparable to those observed in stable angina. The reduction in acute closure rates has decreased procedural related STEMI and the need for emergency CABG.
- CABG should be considered for patients with left main or three-vessel disease, especially with left ventricular dysfunction. Results of the Bypass Angioplasty Revascularization Investigation (BARI) trial indicates that diabetic patients with multivessel disease benefit from a CABG compared to PCI (especially when the internal mammary artery is used).
- In left main disease, surgical revascularization is the treatment of choice.
- The presence of two- or three-vessel disease with preserved left ventricular function can be treated with PCI or CABG depending on local expertise, individual preference, comorbidities, and the type and location of

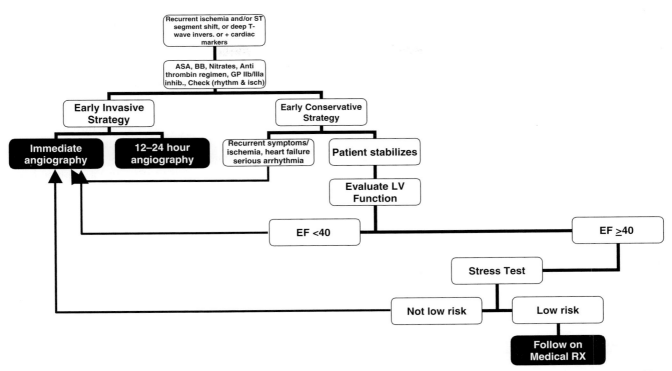

FIG. 34–4 Acute ischemia pathway. ASA, ; BB,; EF, ejection fraction; GP,; invers, inversion; isch, ischemic; LV, left ventricle; RX.

lesions. Discrete lesions favor PCI, whereas, total occlusions and multiple or long lesions favor surgery.

FOLLOW-UP

- Patients presenting with chest pain should be evaluated immediately with a focused history and physical examination, an ECG, and cardiac enzymes. These initial studies will allow an estimation of the likelihood or risk of ACS.
- The American College of Cardiology Guideline for the Management of Unstable Angina and Non–ST Segment Elevation Myocardial Infarction recommends the *mnemonic ABCDE* to guide post-hospitalization treatment:
  ○ *A*spirin and *a*ntianginals
  ○ *β*-blockers and *b*lood pressure control
  ○ *C*holesterol and *c*igarettes
  ○ *D*iet and *d*iabetes
  ○ *E*ducation and *e*xercise
  Each ABCDE is discussed with the patient and lifestyle changes and drug therapy prescribed.
- The follow up is individualized; 1- to 2-week follow-up is indicated for higher-risk patients. Low-risk patients can be followed-up by either their primary care physician or a cardiologist.

BIBLIOGRAPHY

Anderson J, Adams C, Antman E, et al. ACC/AHA 2007 guidelines for the management of patients with unstable angina/non-ST-elevation myocardial infarction: a report of the American College of Cardiology/American Heart Association Task Force on Practice Guidelines (Writing Committee to revise the 2002 Guidelines for the management of patients with unstable angina/non-ST-elevation myocardial infarction): developed in collaboration with the American College of Emergency Physicians, American College or Physicians, Society for Academic Emergency Medicine, Society for Cardiovascular Angiography and Interventions, and Society of Thoracic Surgeons. *J Am Coll Cardiol* 2007;50:e1. www.acc.org/qualityandscience/clinical/statements.htm (accessed September 18, 2007).

Antman EM, Cohen M, Bernink PJ, et al. The TIMI risk score for unstable angina/non-ST elevation MI. *JAMA.* 2000;284(7):835–842.

Bertrand ME, Simoons ML, Fox KA, et al. Management of acute coronary syndromes: acute coronary syndromes without persistent ST segment elevation. Recommendations of the Task Force of the European Society of Cardiology. *Eur Heart J.* 2000;21:1406–1432.

Cannon C, Turpie A. Unstable angina and non-ST-elevation myocardial infarction: initial antithrombotic therapy and early invasive strategy. *Circ.* 2003;107(21):2640–2645.

Gluckman TJ, Sachdev M, Schulman S, Blumenthal R. A simplified approach to the management of non-ST segment elevation acute coronary syndromes. *JAMA.* 2005;293(3):349–357.

Harrington R, Becker R, Ezekowitz M, et al. Antithrombotic therapy for coronary artery disease: The seventh ACCP conference on antithrombotic and thrombolytic therapy. *Chest.* 2004;126(3): 513S-548S.

Lee K, Lip G. Acute coronary syndromes: Virchow's triad revisited. *Blood Coagulation & Fibrinolysis.* 2003;14(7):605–625.

Ragmin F and Fast Revascularization during instability in Coronary artery disease (FRISC II) investigators. Invasive compared with noninvasive treatment in unstable coronary artery disease: FRISC II prospective randomized multicentre study. *Lancet.* 1999;354(9180):708–715.

35 ST–ELEVATION MYOCARDIAL INFARCTION

Jeffrey Ciaramita

INTRODUCTION AND DEFINITION

- The therapeutic approach to patients presenting with an ST–elevation myocardial infarction (STEMI) has advanced considerably over the past decade.
- The importance of STEMI is highlighted by the large public health burden it confers. Each year, approximately one million individuals in the United States suffer from an acute myocardial infarction (AMI), and the development of STEMI is fatal in nearly one-third of these patients.
- STEMI is a clinical syndrome that arises from coronary atherosclerosis, that is associated with plaque rupture and thrombosis. STEMI is considered an acute coronary syndrome, in which the presentation is characterized by acute ischemic chest discomfort and elevation of ST segments on the 12-lead electrocardiogram (ECG).
- Elevations of serum cardiac enzymes (creatine kinase [CK], creatine kinase myocardial band [CK-MB], or Troponin) may not be detectable for hours after the initial clinical presentation, and are thus not required for the diagnosis of STEMI. For this reason, the ECG remains the focal point in the decision pathway for diagnosis and treatment of STEMI.

PATHOLOGY

- The cardinal feature of acute coronary syndromes, including STEMI, is an abrupt coronary plaque rupture leading to thrombosis and partial or complete occlusion of the vessel. Complete occlusion of an epicardial coronary artery by a thrombus results in a STEMI.
- Plaque rupture promotes platelet activation and aggregation, and thrombin generation with thrombus formation.
- Myocardial necrosis develops when thrombus interrupts coronary blood flow resulting in impaired myocardial oxygen supply.
- Besides atherosclerosis, there are a multitude of other, less common etiologies for STEMI including restenosis, coronary spasm, arteritis, cocaine abuse, coronary emboli, and noncoronary causes of ischemia.

CLINICAL FEATURES

- Risk factors such as tobacco abuse, hypertension, hyperlipidemia, diabetes, and a family history of early heart disease increase the risk for atherosclerotic coronary artery disease.
- In many patients presenting with STEMI, a precipitating factor such as heavy exercise or emotional stress can be identified.
- Chest pain in STEMI will often be severe and prolonged, and described as crushing, constricting, squeezing, heavy, knife-like, or burning. It is substernal in location, often radiating to the left precordium, jaw, shoulder and/or arm.
- STEMI pain is usually not relieved with rest or nitroglycerin, but often improves with opiate therapy and resolves with restoration of coronary blood flow.
- Chest pain implies ongoing ischemia in STEMI, which underscores the importance of immediate therapy to relieve ischemia and limit infarction.
- Patients appear anxious or distressed, and may suffer from nausea, vomiting, profound weakness, palpitations, and diaphoresis.

INITIAL EVALUATION

- The initial evaluation of a patient presenting with symptoms suggestive of an acute coronary syndrome (ACS) includes a medical history and physical examination, 12-lead ECG, and serum cardiac enzymes.
- The presence of ST elevation on the ECG remains a prerequisite for diagnosis, therefore, all patients presenting to the emergency department with chest discomfort should have an ECG performed within 10 minutes of arrival.
- If the initial ECG is not diagnostic of STEMI, serial ECGs at 5 to 10 minute intervals may be reasonable to exclude the diagnosis of AMI in patients with a

high-index of suspicion or to differentiate AMI from other conditions that are associated with chest pain.

ROUTINE MANAGEMENT

- Treatment of STEMI is directed toward increasing or restoring myocardial oxygen supply by reestablishing coronary blood flow, while decreasing the myocardial oxygen demand.
- Initial routine measures including oxygen administration, nitroglycerin, morphine analgesia, aspirin, β-blockers, and reperfusion therapy.
- The American College of Cardiology (ACC) and American Heart Association (AHA) have established guidelines regarding therapy in STEMI patients. The following treatments have been approved as Class I or Class IIa by the ACC/AHA.

OXYGEN

- Supplemental oxygen should be administered to patients with an arterial oxygen saturation of less than 90%. It is reasonable to administer supplemental oxygen to all patients with uncomplicated STEMI during the first 6 hours.

NITROGLYCERIN

- Nitroglycerine is a arterial and venodilator that effectively decreases both afterload and preload, thus decreasing myocardial oxygen demand while increasing oxygen supply.
- Nitroglycerine is contraindicated in patients with hypotension or suspected RV infarction.
- Patients with ongoing ischemic discomfort should receive sublingual nitroglycerin. Intravenous nitroglycerin is indicated for relief of ongoing ischemic discomfort (refractory to three sublingual nitroglycerine tablets), hypertension control, or management of pulmonary congestion.

MORPHINE ANALGESIA

- Morphine is useful for analgesia and anxiety, while reducing oxygen demand through venodilation.
- Morphine sulfate, 2 to 4 mg IV at 5- to 15-minute intervals, is the analgesic of choice for management of pain associated with STEMI.

ASPIRIN

- Aspirin inhibits platelet aggregation via irreversible acetylation of cyclooxygenase which, in turn, decreases prostaglandin synthesis (eg, thromboxane A_2).
- Aspirin should be chewed by patients who have not recently consumed aspirin. The initial dose is 162 mg to 325 mg; rapid buccal absorption has been observed with nonenteric coated aspirin formulations.

β-BLOCKERS

- β-Blockers reduce heart rate and blood pressure, thus reducing myocardial oxygen demand. They also appear to reduce the extent and severity of infarction, rate of reinfarction, and frequency of ventricular arrhythmias.
- Oral β-blocker therapy should be administered promptly to all patients without a contraindication, regardless of concomitant fibrinolytic therapy or anticipated primary percutaneous coronary intervention (PCI).

REPERFUSION

- Considerable evidence exists that early and aggressive treatment aimed at restoration of coronary blood flow in an obstructed artery associated with STEMI significantly improves outcome, regardless of whether this is accomplished through PCI or fibrinolysis.
- All STEMI patients should undergo rapid evaluation for reperfusion therapy and a reperfusion strategy implemented promptly after evaluation by the medical team.

REPERFUSION THERAPY

- Timely reperfusion is the most effective therapy for restoration of myocardial oxygen balance and prevention or limitation of myocardial necrosis.
- The goal of all reperfusion strategies is to improve myocardial perfusion in the infarct zone by increasing blood flow to that area.
- Coronary blood flow is quantitatively evaluated using the TIMI (Thrombolysis in Myocardial Infarction) trial grading system. TIMI 0 is complete occlusion of the infarct artery with no flow. TIMI 1 flow is faint antegrade coronary flow beyond the occlusion, although filling of the distal coronary bed is incomplete. TIMI 2 flow is delayed or sluggish antegrade flow with complete filling of the distal territory. TIMI 3 flow is normal flow which fills the distal coronary bed completely.
- Multiple reviews of clinical data have demonstrated a linear relationship between decreasing TIMI flow and

increasing mortality rates. However, the presence of TIMI 3 flow does not assure myocardial perfusion or survival.
- Early reperfusion therapy itself is more important than the mechanism by which it is delivered. The goal time for initiating reperfusion therapy is 30 minutes door-to-administration of fibrinolytics, or 90 minutes door-to-balloon inflation for primary percutaneous intervention (PCI).

REPERFUSION THERAPY WITH FIBRINOLYSIS

- Unquestionably, fibrinolytics restore coronary blood flow, recanalize thrombotic occlusions, reduce infarct size, and improve survival rates in patients with STEMI.
- The benefits of fibrinolytic therapy appear greatest when administered early, with the *golden hour* of target therapy being treatment within one hour from the onset of symptoms.
- Absolute contraindications to fibrinolytic therapy include: any prior intracranial hemorrhage, known structural cerebral lesion, known intracranial neoplasm, ischemic stroke within the preceding 3 months (except acute ischemic stroke within 3 h), suspected aortic dissection, active bleeding or bleeding diathesis, and significant closed head or facial trauma within the last 3 months.
- The mortality benefit of fibrinolytic therapy in patients older than 75 years of age is controversial, and thrombolytic therapy in this group has generally been avoided.
- Assuming no contraindications, fibrinolysis is preferred in patients with early presentations (≤3 h), when invasive strategies are not available or when there would be an unacceptable delay before an invasive strategy can be deployed.
- Of adverse events reported with fibrinolytic use, bleeding complications are the most common. Intracranial hemorrhage is the most serious of these complications.

REPERFUSION THERAPY BY PRIMARY ANGIOPLASTY

- The methods involved in primary angioplasty have evolved from simple balloon expansion to the insertion of drug-eluting stents in combination with aggressive antiplatelet therapy.
- Primary angioplasty results in excellent reperfusion rates, with TIMI 3 flow established in greater than 90% of patients. The features which favor an invasive reperfusion strategy include cardiogenic shock, contraindications to fibrinolytics, later presentations, or when STEMI diagnosis is in doubt.

- Rescue PCI (failure of thrombolysis to restore blood flow) is recommended in STEMI patients who have developed shock within 36 hours of an AMI or have objective evidence of recurrent MI. Also, rescue PCI is reasonable for patients with hemodynamic instability and/or persistent ischemic symptoms.

INDICATIONS FOR ACUTE SURGICAL REPERFUSION IN STEMI

Indications for emergent or urgent coronary artery bypass graft (CABG) surgery include the following:
- Failed PCI with persistent pain or hemodynamic instability.
- Persistent or recurrent ischemia refractory to medical therapy with coronary anatomy suitable for surgery, yet not candidates for PCI or fibrinolytic therapy.
- Surgery is required for repair of a postinfarction ventricular septal rupture or mitral valve dysfunction.
- Cardiogenic shock within 36 hours of STEMI in patients with severe multivessel or left main disease.
- Life-threatening ventricular arrhythmias associated with severe (50%) left main stenosis and/or triple-vessel disease.

ANCILLARY THERAPIES

ANTITHROMBIN AND ANTIPLATELET AGENTS

- Antithrombin therapy with intravenous heparin has been used in the treatment of STEMI for the prevention of deep venous thrombosis (DVTs), pulmonary emboli, ventricular thrombi, and cerebral emboli. ACC/AHA guidelines strongly recommend administering weight-adjusted IV unfractionated heparin in qualified patients undergoing PCI or fibrinolytic therapy.
- Bivalirudin, a direct thrombin inhibitor, is currently an accepted alternative in patients with known heparin-induced thrombocytopenia.
- Daily aspirin is indicated in all patients without an aspirin allergy and should be administered as soon as possible in patients with STEMI, and continued indefinitely after hospital discharge.
- Thienopyridines, such as clopidogrel, exert antiplatelet activity by binding to the platelet adenosine diphosphate (ADP) receptor and inhibiting platelet aggregation. Clopidogrel is indicated for use in patients for whom PCI is planned, and in those who are unable to take aspirin due to intolerance.
- Current recommendations do not mandate clopidogrel loading prior to diagnostic coronary angiography, but several ongoing trials are addressing this.

GLYCOPROTEIN IIb/IIIa INHIBITORS

- The terminal pathway in platelet activation involves expression of the GP IIb/IIIa receptor on the platelet surface.
- Direct inhibition with agents such as abciximab, eptifibatide, and tirofiban have been used as adjunctive therapy in STEMI. Abciximab is recommended by the ACC/AHA for use before primary PCI in STEMI.

ACE INHIBITORS

- Early use of oral angiotensin-converting enzyme (ACE) inhibitors, has been widely adopted as optimal therapy for patients recently experiencing a STEMI.
- ACE inhibitors are recommended within the first 24 hours of STEMI in patients with anterior infarction, pulmonary congestion, or an ejection fraction of less than 40% in the absence of hypotension.
- Patients who are post-MI should be started on an oral ACE inhibitors within days, and if left ventricular dysfunction is present, continued indefinitely.

INSULIN

- Some trials have revealed that patients with STEMI and elevated blood glucose, benefit from strict glucose control.
- Diabetic patients who were assigned to intensive insulin therapy with IV insulin-glucose infusion for 24 hours, followed by subcutaneous insulin four times daily for 3 months demonstrated significantly lower mortality rates when compared to standard therapy.

STATINS

- Early adminstration of statins coupled with low-density population (LDL) reduction has reduced mortality and recurrent MI. Recent studies suggest that the optimal LDL after STEMI is less than 70 mg/dL.

HOSPITAL MANAGEMENT POST-STEMI

- Postreperfusion, STEMI patients should be admitted to a coronary care unit (CCU) for continuous electrical and hemodynamic monitoring.
- Supplemental oxygen may be discontinued when saturations prove stable for at least 6 hours.

- Patients should remain at bedrest for the first 12 to 24 hours, but then may slowly advance their activity level as tolerated.
- A reduced fat and cholesterol diet may be instituted immediately assuming the patient can tolerate oral feedings.
- After 12 to 24 hours of CCU observation, hemodynamically stable patients may be transferred to non-ICU hospital beds. Continued monitoring is often recommended for another 48 to 72 hours while adjusting medications and providing extensive patient counseling to maximize post-STEMI treatments and compliance.
- Cardiac rehabilatation and counseling on smoking cessation, if applicable, is essential.
- An appropriate plan for outpatient follow-up, generally within 1 to 2 weeks must be clearly articulated and discussed with the patient before hospital discharge.

BIBLIOGRPAHY

Alpert JS, Thygesen K, Antman E, Bassand JP. Myocardial infarction redefined—a consensus document of The Joint European Society of Cardiology/American College of Cardiology Committee for the redefinition of myocardial infarction. *J Am Coll Cardiol.* 2000 36:959–969.

Antman EM, Anbe DT, Armstrong PW, et al. ACC/AHA guidelines for the management of patients with ST-elevation myocardial infarction: a report of the American College of Cardiology/American Heart Association Task Force on Practice Guidelines (Committee to revise the 1999 guidelines for the management of patients with acute myocardial infarction). *Circ.* 2004;110:e82–292.

de Lemos JA, Blazing MA, Wiviott SD, et al. Early intensive vs a delayed conservative simvastatin strategy in patients with acute coronary syndromes: phase Z of the A to Z trial. *JAMA.* 2004;292:1307–1316.

Cannon CP, Braunwald E, McCabe CH, et al. Intensive versus moderate lipid lowering with statins after acute coronary syndromes. *N Engl J Med.* 2004;350:1495–1504.

Eagle KA, Guyton RA, Davidoff R, et al. ACC/AHA 2004 guideline update for coronary artery bypass graft surgery: a report of the American College of Cardiology/American Heart Association Task Force on Practice Guidelines (Committee to update the 1999 guidelines for coronary artery bypass graft Surgery). *Circ.* 2004;110:e340–437.

Keeley EC, Boura JA, Grines CL. Primary angioplasty versus intravenous thrombolytic therapy for acute myocardial infarction: a quantitative review of 23 randomised trials. *Lancet.* 2003;361:13–20.

Silber S, Albertsson P, Avilés FF, et al. Guidelines for percutaneous coronary interventions. The Task Force for Percutaneous

Coronary Interventions of the European Society of Cardiology. *Eur Heart J.* 2005;26:804–847.

Smith SC Jr, Feldman TE, Hirshfeld JW Jr, et al. ACC/AHA/ SCAI 2005 guideline update for percutaneous coronary intervention-summary article: a report of the American College of Cardiology/American Heart Association Task Force on Practice Guidelines (ACC/AHA/SCAI Writing Committee to update the 2001 guidelines for percutaneous coronary intervention). *J Am Coll Cardiol.* 2006;47:216–235.

36 CHRONIC CORONARY ARTERY DISEASE

Richard E. Stewart

OVERVIEW

- Chronic coronary artery disease spans the clinical and pathophysiologic spectrum from new onset atherosclerosis to myocardial infarction (MI).
- The clinical spectrum of atherosclerotic coronary heart disease includes eight subsets:
  1. Coronary atherosclerosis without angina or other evidence of ischemia
  2. Coronary atherosclerosis with reversible myocardial ischemia
  3. Coronary atherosclerosis with irreversible myocardial ischemia and necrosis
  4. Sudden death
  5. Syncope
  6. Cardiac arrhythmias
  7. Ischemic cardiomyopathy
  8. Atherosclerotic coronary heart disease in combination with other conditions
- This chapter deals with the stable subsets of coronary atherosclerosis with reversible myocardial ischemia. These conditions include stable angina pectoris, a positive exercise stress test, and angina equivalents.

PATHOLOGY AND PATHOPHYSIOLOGY

- Coronary atherosclerosis is the most common cause of coronary artery disease.
- This disease process is confined mainly to the intima and consists of fibrocellular proliferation intermingled with an accumulation of lipids which forms a distinctive mass called an *atheroma.*
- The atheroma is delineated from the lumen by a fibrous cap with macrophages dispersed throughout the lesion.

- In most patients, the atheroma is in an eccentric position, but concentric lesions do occur.
- As this disease process advances, lesions often display a layered appearance, suggesting different stages of plaque growth. Calcification is also seen in advanced conditions and is considered a hallmark for advanced stable coronary heart disease.
- In unstable coronary artery disease and acute coronary syndromes, thrombosis is usually present in addition to the stable atherosclerotic lesion.
- The media of the affected coronary artery is usually intact, but provides a substrate for vasospasm. Quite often, the fixed atheroma causing coronary stenosis can be aggravated by contraction of the intact muscular wall of the artery. This is common in early or premature coronary artery disease.
- Risk factors for atherosclerotic coronary artery disease include male gender, tobacco use, hypertension, diabetes mellitus, hypercholesterolemia, and various lifestyle choices including physical inactivity.
- These risk factors seem to regulate the acceleration and the time course of this disease in individuals who have a genetically determined tendency toward atherosclerosis of the coronary arteries.
- The pathophysiology of symptomatic chronic coronary artery disease is related to the oxygen delivery to the myocardial cells.
- The left ventricular myocardium in the normal heart is primarily perfused during diastole. The perfusion pressure during diastole is approximately 80 mm Hg, and the pressure within the left ventricle (which tends to oppose perfusion) is 0 to 5 mm Hg. There is less perfusion during systole because the systolic pressure in the coronary epicardial arteries is approximately equal to the systolic pressure in the left ventricle.
- The perfusion of the myocardium of the right ventricle is different from that of the left ventricle and septum because perfusion of the right ventricle occurs during both diastole and systole. This is because the pressure in the coronary arteries during the entire cardiac cycle is always higher than the pressure within the right ventricle.
- The amount of blood delivered to the myocardium must be regulated, so more blood can be delivered during exercise than during rest.
- Although, the epicardial coronary arteries can change in diameter and elicit a change in blood flow, they do not regulate coronary flow as efficiently as the small intramyocardial coronary branches, referred to as resistance arterioles.
- In the large (or epicardial) coronary arteries, coronary blood flow is not impeded until a lesion occludes approximately 50% of the luminal diameter of the artery, which is equivalent to a 75% cross-sectional obstruction.

This degree of stenosis may permit adequate myocardial perfusion at rest but not during exercise.

- Myocardial ischemia is practically envisioned as a fundamental imbalance in oxygen delivery and consumption. In chronic coronary artery disease, the atherosclerotic lesion that elicits an imbalance in supply and demand usually remains stable for a period of time. Although patients may experience symptoms of angina pectoris, the characteristics are relatively predictable.
- The supply of oxygen to the myocardium is a function of coronary artery pressure, coronary artery luminal size, and oxygen content of the blood. Oxygen demand depends on the work of the myocardium and myocardial cellular metabolism.

CLINICAL MANIFESTATIONS

- Chronic coronary artery disease can manifest as an entirely asymptomatic problem without any subjective evidence of ischemia (normal electrocardiogram, etc.). While some patients are without symptoms they will manifest a positive exercise stress test. Importantly, many patients exhibit symptoms such as shortness of breath or fatigue without classic chest pain eg, anginal equivalent. Lastly, patients with chronic coronary atherosclerotic disease can present with classic predictable exertional angina with or without other diagnostic evidence for reversible myocardial ischemia.
- The most common clinical manifestation of chronic coronary artery disease is angina pectoris caused by myocardial ischemia.
- Angina pectoris or *chest pain* is a general term used to describe chest tightness, chest pain, chest burning or aching, or simply discomfort in the chest.
- Classic angina pectoris is characterized by pain located in the retrosternal area that radiates to the left arm, the right arm, the throat, mandible, or upper back.
- The duration of the discomfort is usually 1 to 3 minutes and rarely longer than 10 minutes. If the discomfort lasts longer than 20 minutes continuously, the symptoms are more likely to reflect an acute coronary syndrome or MI.
- The typical symptoms of angina pectoris are usually precipitated by effort, emotional distress, exposure to cold, or eating.
- Classic angina pectoris caused by chronic coronary artery disease has been classified using various clinical grading systems and criteria. One common and universally accepted clinical grading system is the Canadian Cardiovascular Society System:
  - In brief, Canadian Class I angina pectoris is defined as angina not caused by ordinary physical activity but provoked by strenuous, rapid, or prolonged exertion at work or recreation. Class II angina pectoris includes symptoms of chest discomfort causing slight functional limitations brought on by ordinary activities. Class III angina pectoris is defined as angina causing marked limitations in the course of performing ordinary physical activities. Class IV angina pectoris is the inability to carry out any physical activity without symptoms of discomfort. Class IV angina pectoris also includes symptoms at rest.
- The differential diagnosis of angina pectoris caused by atherosclerotic coronary artery disease includes such disease states as esophageal reflux, esophageal spasm, esophageal rupture, peptic ulcer disease, herpes zoster, thoracic outlet syndrome, pneumothorax, mediastinal emphysema, pericarditis, aortic valve disease, and cardiomyopathy. A dissecting aortic aneurysm and pulmonary hypertensive pain is also included in this list.
- When evaluating a patient with chronic coronary artery disease, several issues must be addressed and evaluated. First, a change in the class of angina pectoris defines significant progression of disease. Accordingly, when determining this, the patient's activity level must be defined. For instance, a patient reporting stable anginal symptoms such as Class II but with a dramatic decrease in activity level requires a thorough investigation. A significant change in the symptomatic class of angina should be considered an unstable syndrome until proven otherwise.
- Anginal equivalents are symptoms caused by myocardial ischemia resulting from coronary artery disease that often are not associated with chest pain. These include dyspnea on exertion or at rest, palpitations, or fatigue.
- The pathophysiology of anginal equivalents is usually caused by transient global myocardial ischemia resulting in an elevation of left ventricular end-diastolic pressure, left atrial pressure, and pulmonary venous pressure.
- Anginal equivalents have less predictive value than typical angina pectoris, but they may be the only clues to the correct diagnosis of coronary artery disease.

PHYSICAL EXAMINATION

- The physical examination of a patient with chronic atherosclerosis is usually normal and unrevealing.
- In a stable, asymptomatic patient, physical signs that suggest coronary atherosclerosis include carotid artery bruits, abdominal bruits, or any stigmata of peripheral arterial disease.
- Physical findings in a patient with severe, chronic coronary atherosclerotic disease resulting in an ischemic cardiomyopathy may reveal an abnormal and prolonged apical impulse and atrial or ventricular

gallop sounds. The physical findings of heart failure may also be consistent with chronic and longstanding coronary artery disease.

- Physical findings in a symptomatic patient with chronic coronary artery disease (an attack of angina pectoris) include pallor and a ventricular gallop sound.

LABORATORY EVALUATION OF CHRONIC CORONARY ARTERY DISEASE

- The chest x-ray in a patient with chronic coronary artery disease is often normal. The heart may be enlarged when there is ischemic cardiomyopathy or where multiple infarcts have occurred. Radiographic evidence for heart failure may also be found in patients with ischemic cardiomyopathies. On rare occasions, calcification of the coronary arteries or the myocardium caused by old infarcts may be seen on a plain film.
- The electrocardiogram (ECG) may also be normal in patients with chronic coronary artery disease. Some patients show ST segment displacement or T-wave abnormalities. Other findings include a leftward axis deviation of the QRS complex, evidence for old MI manifested as Q waves, or a right or left bundle-branch block. The resting ECG may be normal or nondiagnostic in approximately 20% of patients with chronic coronary artery disease.
- The echocardiogram most often is normal in patients prior to the development of cardiac muscle damage. The most common abnormal findings involve left ventricular dysfunction or segmental myocardial wall motion abnormalities. Infarctions may manifest as a global left ventricular ejection fraction less than 50%. Regional wall motion abnormalities may also be observed in the presence of coronary artery disease. Advanced coronary artery disease manifesting as ischemic cardiomyopathy can present with echocardiographic findings such as left ventricular dilatation or myocardial wall thinning.
- Stress testing, either by exercise or pharmacologic infusion protocols, is indicated when the history, physical examination, and basic laboratory studies indicate that further evaluation is necessary.
- In patients with a normal baseline ECG who can exercise, treadmill exercise testing using the Bruce protocol is often diagnostic and is the preferred screening test of choice.

- Nuclear perfusion imaging using either technetium radiopharmaceuticals or thallium 201 in the form of thallous chloride is indicated in patients who have a high likelihood of false positives or negatives on routine treadmill exercise stress testing.
- Echocardiography is another imaging modality used in conjunction with exercise or pharmacologic stress. An appropriate echocardiographic window is needed to detect changes in regional myocardial wall motion and overall left ventricular function for this modality to be diagnostic.
- Coronary angiography remains the gold standard for diagnosing coronary artery disease. However, newer imaging modalities including computed tomography angiography or magnetic resonance imaging are at the forefront of cardiac diagnoses. As these newer modalities become more widespread it is likely that the evaluation of myocardial ischemia will undergo significant revision.

PREVENTION AND TREATMENT OF CORONARY ARTERY DISEASE

- There is evidence that elimination or management of risk factors may decelerate the process of atheroma formation, and atherosclerotic lesion development in the coronary arteries.
- That many individuals have significant coronary artery disease in the absence of known risk factors suggests that the etiology of this disease may be genetically determined, and that risk factors accelerate the disease process.
- Tobacco smoking should be curtailed or stopped. Hypertension should be controlled and obesity avoided. Fasting cholesterol should be determined and kept to below the current standards. Diabetes should be controlled with strict glycemic management.
- The pharmacologic treatment for chronic coronary artery disease revolves around three classes of medicines.
  - Nitrates can be used in oral or transdermal preparations. The most common form of oral nitrate is isosorbide dinitrate, which is a coronary artery dilator. Side effects can be significant, the most common being headache.
  - The second class of drugs are the β-blocking drugs. This family of pharmaceuticals is used to prevent angina pectoris by decreasing myocardial metabolic demands. In addition to preventing angina pectoris, it has been proven that β-blockers prolong the lives of selected categories of patients with chronic coronary artery disease who have

suffered a MI. These drugs also prolong life by treating and preventing various cardiac dysrhythmias.

○ The third class of medications include the calcium channel blockers. In addition to decreasing myocardial oxygen demand, these drugs also tend to prevent coronary artery spasm and are used to treat some atrial arrhythmias.

• The treatment of symptomatic chronic coronary artery disease is surgical coronary artery bypass graft surgery. Although not as popular for single- and two-vessel coronary artery disease, it may be indicated for long lesions or lesions that are not readily accessible for angioplasty.

• The mechanical treatment of symptomatic chronic coronary artery disease involves both surgical and nonsurgical procedures and techniques.

○ Surgical coronary artery bypass graft surgery has been a mainstay for the treatment of severe three-vessel coronary artery disease and two-vessel coronary artery disease associated with left ventricular dysfunction. With the advent of nonsurgical percutaneous interventions, surgical coronary artery bypass graft surgery is not as popular for single- and two-vessel coronary artery disease as it once was.

○ Percutaneous approaches include coronary angioplasty, percutaneous coronary artery stenting, and various atherectomy and plaque ablation techniques.

• With the advancement of both pharmacologic treatments and catheter-based technology along with evolving surgical techniques, the indications for specific procedures and approaches in the treatment of chronic coronary artery disease are in a constant state of flux.

BIBLIOGRAPHY

CASS Principal Investigators and Associates. Coronary Artery Surgery Study (CASS): A randomized trial of coronary artery bypass surgery survival data. *Circ.* 1983;68(5):939.

Kent KM, Rosing DR, Ewels CJ, Lipson L, Bonow R, Epstein SE. Prognosis of asymptomatic or mildly symptomatic patients with coronary artery disease. *Am J Cardiol.* 1982;49(8):1823.

Waters DD, Szlacheic J, Miller DD, Theroux P. Clinical characteristics of patients with variant death within 1 month. *Am J Cardiol.* 1982;49:658.

37 AORTIC STENOSIS

Christopher R. Longnecker

OVERVIEW

• Aortic stenosis (AS) is characterized by a stricture of the aortic valve orifice and can be secondary to congenital disease, degeneration of the valve, or rheumatic disease.

• Narrowing of the valve leaflet results in obstruction to the left ventricular outflow tract and increased work of the left ventricle (LV).

• The stenotic orifice results in turbulent blood flow which further increases the work of the LV and eventually produces left ventricular hypertrophy and heart failure.

ETIOPATHOGENESIS

• The etiology of AS can be conveniently classified into congenital valvular disease, acquired valvular disease (calcific AS), or rheumatic valve disease.

○ Congenital valvular aortic disease is associated with either a unicuspid or bicuspid aortic valve.

○ Bicuspid valves are the most common congenital cardiac anomaly, occurring in approximately 2% of the population (commissural fusion or incomplete separation during embryogenesis is believed to underlie the bicuspid anatomy). Approximately 50% of patients with a bicuspid valve will develop some degree of stenosis by the sixth decade of life.

○ It is believed that turbulence across the bicuspid valve leaflets causes fibrosis and calcium deposition.

○ Bicuspid aortic valve can also be associated with dilation of the ascending aorta, aneurysm development, aortic dissection, and aortic insufficiency (AI) suggesting a common developmental origin.

• Acquired AS is frequently secondary to degenerative changes of the valve, known as calcific AS. Age-related degenerative calcific AS is the most common cause of acquired AS in adults.

○ Risk factors associated with the development of calcific AS are similar to risk factors for coronary artery disease and include hypertension, diabetes mellitus, hypercholesterolemia, smoking, and a family history of valvular heart disease. Importantly, modification of these factors may reduce or inhibit the development of calcific AS.

• Rheumatic valve disease can also result in AS. However, rheumatic valve disease is uncommon in industrialized countries and is almost always associated with mitral valve disease.

- Other illnesses that have been associated with the development of calcific AS include:
  - Paget's disease
  - End-stage renal disease
  - Severe familial hypercholesterolemia (specifically children with homozygous type II hyperlipoproteinemia)
  - Systemic lupus erythematosus
  - Rheumatoid arthritis
  - Infection with *Chlamydophila pneumoniae*
  - Ochronosis as a result of alkaptonuria.

PATHOPHYSIOLOGY

- Narrowing of the aortic valve is usually a process which occurs over years. The LV hypertrophies in response to the increased intracavitary pressure required to eject blood across the stenotic orifice. The hypertrophied ventricle becomes less compliant, which induces diastolic dysfunction and raises left ventricular end diastolic pressure.
- Eventually, systolic dysfunction develops associated with dilation of the LV and heart failure.
- In AS the stroke volume is greatly influenced by atrial contractility. Accordingly, individuals that lose the atrial contribution to cardiac output (atrial fibrillation or atrioventricular [AV] dissociation) are quite susceptible to hemodynamic decompensation. Restoring the rhythm to normal is a priority in these settings.

CLINICAL FINDINGS

- Aortic stenosis is usually present for years before symptoms occur. Patients experience exertional dyspnea and fatigue with moderate valvular stenosis (1.0-1.5 cm^2/m^2). The classic symptoms of syncope, angina and heart failure often indicate valve area of <0.6 cm^2/m^2 (normal area 3.0-4.0 cm^2/m^2). The mortality at the symptomatic stage exceeds 90% unless the valve is replaced. (Fig. 37–1).
- Angina pectoris associated with AS may or may not be related to epicardial coronary disease. As the LV hypertrophies, coronary blood flow is reduced because the intramyocardial pressure mechanically obstructs the small penetrating arteries in the myocardium. This is particularly problematic during stress or exercise because of increased myocardial oxygen demand. Angina at rest is relatively uncommon in these patients.
- Syncope is thought to be secondary to decreased cardiac output and cerebral perfusion, usually occurring during exertion. Ventricular or supraventricular arrhythmias and transient AV block may also contribute to syncope.
- Dyspnea and congestive heart failure are the result of both systolic and diastolic dysfunction.
- Other clinical conditions that may be associated with AS include pulmonary hypertension, gastrointestinal bleeding from arteriovenous malformations, and endocarditis.

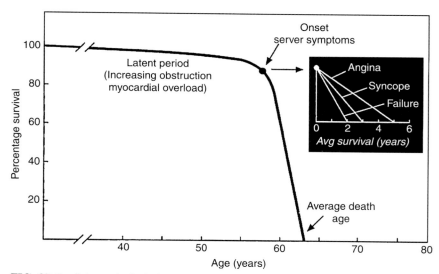

FIG. 37–1 Schematic depiction of the natural history of aortic stenosis.
SOURCE: Reproduced with permission from Aortic Stenosis JOHN ROSS, JR. and EUGENE BRAUNWALD Circulation. 1968;38:V-61-V-67

PHYSICAL EXAMINATION

- The murmur of AS is auscultated best at the right upper sternal border or base of the heart and classically radiates toward the carotid arteries. Initially, the murmur—which follows S1—peaks in early systole; but as the stenosis progresses, the murmur peaks later, becoming more intense and can be associated with a thrill at the right upper sternal border. With severe AS, the murmur may soften as left ventricular function declines.
- Most patients with AS develop parvus et tardus—a small and prolonged upstroke of the carotid arterial pulse. In patients greater than the age of 60 the cardiac upstroke may normalize or increase because of decreased compliance of the carotid arteries.
- The second heart sound may soften because of reduced movement of the aortic valve, generating a nearly inaudible S2 at the apex. In this setting, the audible S2 would only reflect closure of the pulmonic valve.

DIAGNOSTIC MODALITIES

- Calcification of the aortic valve can be visualized on the standard chest x-ray. Left ventricular hypertrophy with strain may be observed on the electrocardiogram, but this does not correlate well with the hemodynamic severity of AS.
- Echocardiography with Doppler interrogation is an excellent noninvasive tool to diagnose and evaluate AS. Echocardiography demonstrates the extent and severity of valvular thickening and calcification. The motion of the aortic valve and the severity of left ventricular hypertrophy can also be assessed by echocardiography. Aortic jet velocity, mean transvalvular gradient, and aortic valve area can also be assessed by Doppler interrogation.
- Serial echocardiography is often used to monitor disease progression; every 6 months to 1 year for severe AS (valve area <1.0 cm^2/m^2), every 1 to 2 years for moderate AS (valve area 1.0-1.5 cm^2/m^2), and every 3 to 5 years for mild disease (valve area >1.5 cm^2/m^2). Develop of new symptoms or worsening of old symptoms requires prompt evaluation.
- In patients who undergo aortic valve replacement, an echocardiogram should be performed in the early postoperative period to establish baseline function of the valve for future comparisons if problems arise.
- Cardiac catheterization can be performed when the echocardiographic images are of poor quality or there is a poor correlation between the patient's symptoms, physical findings, and the hemodynamics characterized by echocardiography. Catheterization may also be indicated in patients with suspected coronary artery disease.

If coronary artery disease is discovered, coronary artery bypass grafting can be performed in tandem with the aortic valve replacement.

AORTIC STENOSIS GRADING

- Grading of AS is accomplished by obtaining the peak aortic jet velocity, peak and mean transvalvular pressure gradient and aortic valve area after Doppler interrogation of the valve. Similar information can also be obtained during cardiac catheterization.

Grade	Valve Area (cm^2)	Peak Velocity (m/s)	Peak Grad (mm Hg)	Mean Grad (mm Hg)
Normal	3.0–4.0	1.0	<10	<10
Mild	1.5–2.5	1.0–2.0	<20	<20
Moderate	1.0–1.5	2.0–4.0	20–64	20–40
Severe/ Critical	<1.0/<0.7	>4.0	>64	>40

TREATMENT OPTIONS

- The definitive therapy for AS involves surgical replacement of the aortic valve. The surgical risk is 2% to 3%; therefore, patients should be screened carefully.
- Despite impressive advances in the surgical management of AS, medical management is the preferred initial therapy in patients with asymptomatic mild, moderate, and perhaps severe AS.
- Surgery is recommended for severe AS with symptoms, LV dysfunction, or an enlarging aortic root, and in women with severe AS who desire pregnancy.
- Surgical replacement is also indicated in patients with moderate to severe AS undergoing another cardiac surgery such as coronary artery bypass grafting.
- The choice of optimal medical therapy is of utmost importance, since several commonly used cardiac medications can precipitate complications in patients with AS. For example, diuretics may be indicated in patients with severe and symptomatic volume expansion, however their use must be monitored closely, since volume depletion can markedly impair cardiac preload (due to the stiff noncompliant ventricle) and reduce cardiac output.
- Digoxin may only be beneficial in patients with LV dysfunction or for rate control in atrial fibrillation.
- Angiotensin-converting enzyme inhibitors and other vasodilators are beneficial in patients with heart failure and mild to moderate AS. However, they should be avoided in patients with severe AS because they can cause a precipitous decrease in blood pressure by

reducing total peripheral resistance in a patient with a relatively fixed cardiac output.

- Nitrates should be used cautiously in severe AS, and are generally only used to treat angina in patients awaiting surgery. Hypotension can be a serious problem in patients receiving nitrates.
- β-Blockers are usually avoided because they tend to worsen heart failure in patients with AS.
- Prophylaxis for bacterial endocarditis should be given to patients with a murmur regardless of the severity of AS.
- Balloon valvuloplasty of a stenotic aortic valve is associated with a high complication rate and little sustained benefit. Therefore, balloon angioplasty is reserved for patients with severe AS but are poor surgical candidates.
- In patients >65 years of age there is an increase in surgical mortality and postsurgical morbidity. Nonetheless, aortic valve replacement is associated with significant benefit, since patients that tolerate the procedure achieve the expected life span of age matched controls.
- There are two main types of aortic valve replacement options: mechanical valve implantation and bioprostheses implantation. Bioprosthetic valves do not require anticoagulation but are associated with reduced durability and a smaller effective valve orifice. These valves are usually reserved for the elderly or females of child bearing age in whom warfarin therapy would be contraindicated during pregnancy. Mechanical valves have superior durability but require lifelong anticoagulation with a goal international normalized ratio of 2.5 to 3.5

PROGNOSIS

- For patients with symptomatic AS, there is a 90% mortality rate at 3 years. If a patient has isolated AS and undergoes surgical repair, their 10-year survival increases to 75%.
- For the most part, asymptomatic AS is relatively stable until complicating factors, such as congestive heart failure, ventricular enlargement, or coronary disease develop.
- Patients with coronary artery disease combined with AS fair worse than those patients with isolated AS.

BIBLIOGRAPHY

American College of Cardiology/American Heart Association. ACC/AHA guidelines for the management of patients with valvular heart disease. A report of the American College of Cardiology/American Heart Association. Task Force on Practice Guidelines (Committee on management of patients with valvular heart disease). *J Am Coll Cardiol.* 1998;32: 1486.

Carabello BA. Evaluation and management of patients with aortic stenosis. *Circ.* 2002;105:1746.

Freeman RV, Otto CM. Spectrum of calcific aortic valve disease: pathogenesis, disease progression, and treatment strategies. *Circ.* 2005;111:3316.

Palta S, Pai AM, Gill KC, Pai RG. New insights into the progression of aortic stenosis: implications for secondary prevention. *Circ.* 2000;101:2497.

38 AORTIC REGURGITATION

Joseph Polizzi

INTRODUCTION

- Aortic regurgitation (AR) is comprised of a heterogenous group of clinical disorders that injure either (1) the aortic valve leaflets or (2) the wall of the aortic root (causing dilation). The pathophysiology, clinical presentation, and management of AR vary greatly depending on whether the process is acute or chronic in nature. The symptoms of AR are primarily due to left ventricular volume and pressure overload eventuating in left ventricular dysfunction. The natural history of the disease tends to be progressive and, accordingly surgical intervention is the treatment of choice.

CONDITIONS AFFECTING THE VALVE LEAFLETS

- Rheumatic valve disease
- Calcific aortic stenosis (AR invariably accompanies this condition).
- Congenital valvular anomalies, most commonly bicuspid aortic valve.
- Iatrogenic injury: balloon valvotomy and radiofrequency catheter ablation.
- Connective tissue disorders: systemic lupus erythematosus, rheumatoid arthritis, and ankylosing spondylitis.
- Bioprosthetic valve degeneration
- Cardiac trauma
- Infective endocarditis
- Myxomatous degeneration of the valve.
- Fenfluramine-phentermine

CONDITIONS AFFECTING THE AORTIC ROOT

- Disease of the aortic root producing dilatation and aortic regurgitation are now the most common causes of isolated AR.
- Causes of aortic root dilation include
  ○ Age related aortic dilatation (altered elasticity of the root)
  ○ Systemic hypertension
  ○ Marfan syndrome
  ○ Syphilitic aortitis
  ○ Osteogenesis imperfecta
  ○ Inflammatory bowel disease
  ○ Dissecting aneurysm
  ○ Connective tissue diseases
  ○ A bicuspid aortic valve can be associated with aortic root dilation secondary to congenital anomalies of the aortic wall.

PATHOPHYSIOLOGY

- The severity of symptoms and signs associated with aortic regurgitation differ according to whether the disease is acute or chronic in onset. Nonetheless, the pathophysiology is similar regardless of the underlying process.

ACUTE AORTIC REGURGITATION

- The hallmark features of AR consist of tachycardia and increased left ventricular end-diastolic pressure (LVEDP). Because the valves do not completely efface during diastole, a portion of the stroke volume leaks back into the ventricle and raises the LVEDP. Initially, the heart may be able to compensate for the decrease in effective stroke volume by increasing total stroke volume (forward stroke volume plus regurgitant volume). However, sustained or advancing AR results in cardiac remodeling and eventually heart failure.
- When the regurgitant volume is large and acute in onset, the compensatory mechanisms (remodeling, hypertrophy and dilatation) are poorly developed, therefore the LVEDP rises rapidly (which also increases pulmonary venous pressure and congestion) and impairs effective forward flow resulting in a decline in cardiac output and cardiogenic shock.

CHRONIC AORTIC REGURGITATION

- The gradual increase in diastolic regurgitant volume permits compensatory ventricular dilatation and minimizes the increase in LVEDP. In addition, these compensatory mechanisms sustain forward stroke volume and effective cardiac output. However, as the AR progresses, the compensatory mechanisms are overwhelmed and systolic dysfunction coupled with an increase in LVEDP induces a fall in cardiac output.

CLINICAL PRESENTATION

ACUTE AORTIC REGURGITATION
- Classically patients with acute AR are ill appearing and complain of dyspnea. The physical findings reveal tachycardia, pulmonary edema, and shock.

CHRONIC AORTIC REGURGITATION
- Since compensatory mechanisms maintain cardiac output and LVEDP, these patients may remain asymptomatic for long periods of time (decades).
- Symptoms occur once left ventricular dysfunction develops. These include dyspnea with exertion, orthopnea and paroxysmal nocturnal dyspnea. If the dilatation is profound, patients may complain of pounding or a sense of throbbing in the chest. The symptoms are aggravated by emotional stress.
- Patients are exquisitely sensitive to premature ventricular contractions as the postextrasystolic beat is more forceful, thus increasing the symptom complex.
- Late in the disease course the patient may develop anginal symptoms (tends to be rare in an otherwise normal patient). Although, the coronary arteries per se are not affected by AR, if sufficiently advanced the increased LVEDP may impair subendocardial blood flow.

PHYSICAL EXAMINATION

ACUTE AORTIC REGURGITATION
- The patient will appear ill and exhibit cyanosis, tachycardic, and hypotension. The classic signs and symptoms of congestive heart failure will be present.
- Cardiac auscultation may reveal a soft or silent S_1, due to early closure of the mitral valve because of the increase in LVEDP.
- In addition, there may be an early diastolic murmur, which is much shorter than that of chronic aortic regurgitation, due to rapid equalization of pressure between the aorta and left ventricle.

CHRONIC AORTIC REGURGITATION

- On auscultation A_2 is usually soft or inaudible, an S_3 may be present.
- The diastolic murmur of AR begins immediately after A_2. It is a high-pitched decrescendo murmur heard best when the patient is leaning forward and exhaling.
- If the disease is valvular in origin the murmur is best heard at the left sternal border. However if the aortic root is involved, the murmur is often heard best at the right sternal border.
- A systolic murmur may be present because of turbulence induced by the large stroke volume.
- A severe aortic regurgitant jet may impinge on the anterior mitral valve leaflet, narrowing the mitral valve orifice. This may cause a mid-diastolic low-pitched murmur referred to as the *Austin Flint* murmur.
- Palpation of the chest may reveal a hyperdynamic and laterally displaced ventricular apex.
- A systolic thrill may be appreciated at the base of the heart, related to the augmented stroke volume.
- Peripheral signs of AR can be striking secondary to a widened pulse pressure and hyperdynamic circulation. These include:
  - *Corrigan's* pulse or *water-hammer* pulse: an abrupt rise in systolic pressure because of a large stroke volume followed by a rapid descent in diastolic pressure because of regurgitant flow.
  - *Bisferiens* pulse: two distinct impulses with each beat.
  - *Traube* sign: prominent systolic and diastolic sounds heard over the femoral arteries.
  - *Duroziez* sign: associated with a systolic murmur audible over the femoral artery when compressed proximally and a diastolic murmur when compressed distally.
  - The *Quincke* sign: characterized by visible capillary pulsation seen in the patient's lip when a glass slide is placed over the lip or when the fingernails are gently compressed.

EVALUATION

ELECTROCARDIOGRAM

- Acute AR may only present with sinus tachycardia on the 12-lead electrocardiogram (ECG).
- Chronic AR is characterized by an ECG suggestive of left ventricular enlargement/hypertrophy and left ventricular diastolic overload.
- Late in the course, as left ventricular dysfunction develops, intraventricular conduction delays may become apparent (bundle branch blocks).

CHEST X-RAY

- The left ventricle is enlarged, and the size tends to correlate with the severity and duration of AR.
- Calcification of the aortic valve may be present when there is associated AS.
- Dilation of the aortic root and the aortic arch may be visible, and if severe, may suggest aortic root disease.

ECHOCARDIOGRAPHY

- Echocardiography is essential in the evaluation of AR. Echocardiography can reveal the underlying diagnosis in some cases and determine the severity of the lesion in almost all. It also serves as a baseline that permits serial assessment of left ventricular size and function.
- 2-D echocardiography evaluates the following
  - Left ventricular systolic function
  - Left ventricular size
  - Aortic root and annulus size
  - Leaflet thickness and coaptation
  - Number of aortic valve leaflets
  - Dissection
  - Presence of other valvular abnormalities
- Doppler echocardiography provides an estimate of the severity of AR and LVEDP

CARDIAC CATHETERIZATION

- Cardiac catheterization is a valuable tool in patients whose echocardiographic data are inadequate or is discordant with the clinical findings.
- Regardless, catheterization is usually advisable to determine the presence of coronary artery disease prior to surgery. Importantly, preoperative cardiac catheterization is recommended in men older than 35 years, postmenopausal women and premenopausal women older than 35 years of age with coronary risk factors.
- Cardiac catheterization may also be used to
  - Grade the severity of AR
  - Evaluate left ventricular function
  - Evaluate end-diastolic pressures
  - Evaluate the size of the aortic root and arch
  - Exclude aortic dissection

EXERCISE TESTING

- Many patients who are asymptomatic may be so because they have gradually decreased their activity. In these settings exercise testing can determine functional capacity and elicit symptoms consistent with AR. Some studies have suggested that exercise-induced decreases in left ventricular function are associated with a poor prognosis and warrant surgical intervention.

NATURAL HISTORY

- In asymptomatic patients with severe AR and normal left ventricular systolic function, more than 45% will remain without symptoms and exhibit normal cardiac function at 10 years.
- Once symptoms develop the mortality rate exceeds 10% per year (see Table 38–1).
- Heart failure symptoms are associated with a poor prognosis. Several studies have revealed that patients with New York Heart Association (NYHA) Class III and Class IV heart failure have a four year survival rate of 30% if treated medically.

MANAGEMENT

ACUTE AORTIC REGURGITATION

- Acute AR is considered a surgical emergency and aortic valve replacement is the treatment of choice. Regardless, acute AR is associated with a high mortality and irreversible left ventricular failure.
- Before surgery the patient should ideally be stabilized with
  - Afterload reduction (intravenous vasodilators such as nitroprusside)
  - Intravenous ionotropes (dobutamine)
  - Atrial pacing, which increases the heart rate and decreases diastolic filling time, may also confer a hemodynamic benefit.
- An intra-aortic balloon pump is contraindicated because inflation of the balloon in diastole will worsen the AR.
- In acute AR due to infective endocarditis the surgery is usually delayed for 5–10 days to allow for intensive

TABLE 38–1   Natural History of Aortic Regurgitation

Asymptomatic patients with normal LV systolic function	
Progression to symptoms and/or LV dysfunction	Less than 6% per y
Progression to asymptomatic LV dysfunction	Less than 3.5% per y
Sudden death	Less than 0.2% per y
Asymptomatic patients with LV dysfunction	
Progression to cardiac symptoms	Greater than 25% per y
Symptomatic patients	
Mortality rate	Greater than 10% per y

LV, left ventricular.
SOURCE: Reproduced with permission. ACC/AHA guidelines for the management of patients with valvular heart disease. A report of the American College of Cardiology/American Heart Association. *J Am Coll Cardiol.* 1998;32(5):1486–588.

antibiotic therapy (hemodynamics permitting). This approach is preferred to reduce the postoperative risk of prosthetic valve infection

CHRONIC AORTIC REGURGITATION

- The medical treatment of chronic AR should include the following
  - All patients, no matter the severity, require endocarditis prophylaxis.
  - Patients with mild AR who are asymptomatic with normal left ventricular function require annual follow-up. If there is no change in symptoms, an echocardiogram should be performed every 2 to 3 years.
  - Patients who are asymptomatic but have echocardiographic evidence of severe AR, should undergo serial echocardiography biannually to determine cardiac size and left ventricular function.
  - Patients with severe AR should be treated with vasodilator therapy if there is evidence of left ventricular dysfunction, either by examination or by echocardiography.
    - Several agents have been studied in this setting, including angiotensin-converting enzyme (ACE) inhibitors and calcium channel blockers. Therapy with the calcium channel blocker nifedipine may delay the requirement for operative repair in patients with normal left ventricular function.
    - ACE inhibitors appear beneficial in patients with left ventricular systolic dysfunction.
- Surgical therapy is the recommended approach for patients with AR who are operative candidates. The operative mortality is estimated at approximately 4%. Candidates for surgery include:
  - All patients with symptomatic AR.
  - In asymptomatic patients with a left ventricular ejection fraction of <50% or an end-diastolic dimension on echocardiogram of >75 mm.
  - In asymptomatic patients whose ejection fraction or left ventricular end-diastolic dimension are borderline, AVR should be considered if:
    - The rate of functional decline or increase in ventricular size are relatively rapid.
    - The patient's overall functional capacity and exercise tolerance are worsening.
  - It is crucial to perform surgery prior to the development of left ventricular dysfunction, as this will significantly worsen the long term mortality after an AVR (See Fig. 38–1).
- It is generally felt that it is never too late to operate in severe AR. However, advanced cases must be evaluated thoughtfully and involve the patient, cardiologist, and cardiothoracic surgeon in the decision-making process.

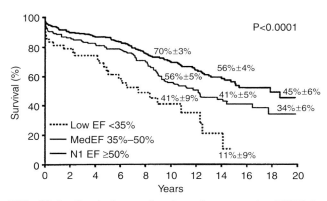

FIG. 38–1 Survival as a function of preoperative LVEF in aortic regurgitation.

EF, ejection fraction; N1, normal.

SOURCE: Reproduced with permission from Chaliki HP, Mohty D, Avierinos JF, et al. Outcomes after aortic valve replacement in patients with severe aortic regurgitation and markedly reduced left ventricular function. *Circ.* 2002;106:2687–2693.

BIBLIOGRAPHY

ACC/AHA guidelines for the management of patients with valvular heart disease. *J Am Coll Cardiol.* 32;1998:1486–1588.

Bekeredjian R, Grayburn PA. Valvular heart disease: aortic regurgitation. *Circ.* 2005;112(1):125–134.

Hemodynamic data. In: Kern MJ, ed. *The Cardiac Catheterization Handbook.* 4th ed. Philadelphia: Mosby; 2003.

Valvular heart disease. In: Zipes DP, ed. *Braunwald's Heart Disease: A Textbook of Cardiovascular Medicine.* 7th ed. Philadelphia: Elsevier Saunders; 2005.

Valvular regurgitation. In: Otto CM, ed. *Textbook of Clinical Echocardiography.* 3rd ed. Philadelphia: Elsevier Saunders; 2004.

39 MITRAL STENOSIS

Jennifer Lash

INTRODUCTION

- Mitral stenosis (MS) is an obstruction of flow from the left atrium to the left ventricle caused by narrowing of the mitral valve.
- The most common cause of MS is rheumatic valve disease; therefore, the incidence is declining in the industrialized countries.

EPIDEMIOLOGY

- Rheumatic heart disease is the precursor in 70% to 80% of cases.
- Infective endocarditis is responsible for approximately 3% of cases.
- Mitral annular calcification reportedly is responsible for 2.7% of cases.
- Rare causes of MS include systemic lupus erythematosus, rheumatoid arthritis, carcinoid heart disease, and endomyocardial fibrosis.

NATURAL HISTORY OF MITRAL STENOSIS

- In most patients with rheumatic MS, there is a 16- to 20-year latent period from the diagnosis of rheumatic fever to the onset of clinically evident MS. However, this period can be as short as 2 years in susceptible individuals (patients not receiving antibiotics for rheumatic fever or perhaps because of particularly virulent strains of streptococci).
- Once symptoms develop, the prognosis is dramatically worse and mortality increases markedly. For example the 10-year survival for patients with NYHA Class III or IV symptoms is less than 25%. Other poor prognostic factors include atrial fibrillation and the development of severe pulmonary hypertension.

PATHOLOGY

- Rheumatic heart disease is a progressive disease that is initially characterized by the formation of tiny nodules along the coapting portions of the valve leaflets. Inflammation and turbulent flow leads to the deposition of fibrin and accumulation of fibrous tissue. The commissures fuse and the cusps become rigid and calcified. This leads to a fixed, funnel shaped mitral valve morphology with a small valvular opening.

SYMPTOMS

- Symptoms may be absent in mild MS. As the stenosis progresses, symptoms appear primarily with exertion. With further narrowing of the valve orifice, symptoms are noticeable with less activity and at rest.
- Dyspnea is the most common complaint, seen in 70% of patients. It occurs when the stenotic mitral valve impedes blood flow from the left atrium to the left ventricle. This leads to an increase in left atrial pressure, which is transmitted in a retrograde fashion to the pulmonary venous system.

- Atrial fibrillation is caused by left atrial dilation secondary to the increased left atrial pressure.
- Thromboembolic manifestations (eg, stroke) are a common complication in MS, especially when atrial fibrillation accompanies the disease process.
- Hemoptysis and pulmonary edema can occur and be associated with increased cardiac output or tachycardia. Exercise, emotional stress, infection, pregnancy, or atrial fibrillation can precipitate severe symptoms in MS.
- Pulmonary hypertension is caused by long-term, chronically elevated pulmonary venous pressure, which leads to vasoconstriction, intimal hyperplasia, and medial hypertrophy of the pulmonary arterioles.

PHYSICAL EXAMINATION

- In early MS, there is a loud S1 because the increased left atrial pressure prevents the calcified leaflets from closing at the end of diastole. Systole closes the widely separated leaflets, which produces a loud first heart sound. As the disease progresses, the valve leaflets become heavily calcified and ridged and no longer open widely. Accordingly, the first sound becomes softer.
- An opening snap can be appreciated in mild to moderate MS while the leaflets are still mobile. It is heard after the S2 when listening at the apex with the diaphragm of the stethoscope.
- The murmur of MS is characterized by a low-pitched diastolic rumble best appreciated with the patient lying on the left side listening with the bell of the stethoscope positioned at the apex. The intensity of the murmur does not correlate with severity; however, the duration of the murmur directly correlates with the severity of MS.

DIAGNOSTIC TESTS

- The 12-lead electrocardiogram may reveal left atrial enlargement with large, broad P waves in lead II (>0.12 seconds), atrial fibrillation, and/or right ventricular hypertrophy.
- Echocardiography can establish the diagnosis, quantify the severity of the stenosis, and guide further therapy.
- Cardiac catheterization can provide similar information and directly measure the severity of the pressure gradient across the mitral valve.

TREATMENT

- The normal mitral valve area is 4 to 6 cm². Invasive repair of the valve is indicated when the valve area is less than 1 cm². However, intervention may also be warranted in patients with a valve area of 1.0 to 1.5 cm² accompanied by symptoms of exertional dyspnea or pulmonary hypertension.
- In mild MS, antibiotic prophylaxis is required, but no other specific medical therapy is recommended. As patients develop symptoms, medical therapy typically involves ventricular rate control with β-blockers or calcium channel blockers and careful administration of diuretics.
- Acute pulmonary congestion can occur, especially with new onset atrial fibrillation. Treatment of atrial fibrillation includes anticoagulation, diuresis, rate control, and/or cardioversion in attempt to resume sinus rhythm (See also Chap. 33, Atrial Fibrillation).
- Percutaneous balloon valvulotomy (PMV) is the preferred method of treating MS. Percutaneous balloon valvulotomy increases the mitral valve area and decreases the pressure gradient across the mitral valve. Percutaneous balloon valvulotomy is a nonsurgical approach in which a balloon is inflated across the mitral valve to mechanically open the valve at the commissures of the leaflets. It is recommended in symptomatic patients with moderate to severe MS and suitable valve morphology. It is also recommended in asymptomatic patients with moderate to severe MS associated with moderate to severe pulmonary hypertension and suitable valve morphology.
- Surgical options include open commissurotomy, where the leaflet commissures are surgically split, and mitral valve replacement with a metallic or a bioprosthetic valve. Valve replacement is indicated in patients when the valve morphology is unsuitable for PMV, moderate or severe mitral regurgitation is present, or there is a thrombus present in the left atrium despite anticoagulation.

OTHER CONSIDERATIONS

- Mitral stenosis confers an intermediate risk of endocarditis (high risk if combined with mitral regurgitation).
- Anticoagulation should be initiated in individuals with atrial fibrillation (chronic or paroxysmal), a prior embolic event, and in patients with severe MS and a large left atrium (≥5.5 cm in diameter).

BIBLIOGRAPHY

Alexander RW. *Hurst's the Heart.* New York: McGraw-Hill, 1998.

Bonow RO, Carabello BA, Chatterjee K, et al. ACC/AHA 2006 guidelines for the management of patients with valvular heart disease. A report of the American College of Cardiology/ American Heart Association Task Force on Practice Guidelines (Writing committee to revise the 1998 guidelines for the management of patients with valvular heart disease). *J Am Coll Cardiol* 2006;48:e1.

Carabello BA. Modern management of mitral stenosis. *Circ.* 2005;112:432.

Zipes DP, et al. *Braunwald's Heart Disease.* 7th ed. Philadelphia: Elsevier Saunders; 2005.

40 MITRAL REGURGITATION

Kevin Fitzgerald

INTRODUCTION

- Mitral regurgitation (MR) is characterized by backward flow of blood from the left ventricle (LV) into the left atrium (LA) during systole.
- Mitral regurgitation is caused by anatomical or functional abnormalities of the mitral valve (MV) leaflets and/or any part of the MV apparatus (chordae tendineae, papillary muscles, mitral annulus).
- It may present as a slow and indolent process such as in chronic asymptomatic MR or in a dramatic and life-threatening fashion such as with acute severe MR following an acute myocardial infarction (MI).
- The diagnosis and management of MR will predictably depend on where the patient fits in the broad spectrum of the disease process.

EPIDEMIOLOGY

- The prevalence of MR varies directly with age and inversely with severity.
- Trivial MR is often discovered during Doppler echocardiographic examination and is usually of no clinical significance.
- The Framingham investigators performed routine echocardiograms on 1696 men and 1893 women and found the prevalence of mild to severe MR to be 19% in both groups.[1]

- The Strong Heart Study studied 3486 American Indian subjects and found the prevalence of mild, moderate, and severe MR to be 19%, 1.6% and 0.2%, respectively.[2]

PATHOPHYSIOLOGY

ACUTE SEVERE MITRAL REGURGITATION

- Acute severe MR presents with severe hypotension and pulmonary edema.
- The relatively noncompliant LA is overwhelmed by regurgitant blood during systole resulting in a dramatic increase in left ventricular end-diastolic pressure (LVEDP). The LVEDP pressure is transmitted back to the pulmonary capillary bed. The pulmonary capillary hydrostatic pressure exceeds the capillary oncotic pressure and pulmonary edema ensues.
- Although the stroke volume may actually increase in acute MR (because of the decrease in total afterload), a large percentage of the stroke volume follows the path of least resistance through the defective MV which, in turn decreases effective stroke volume .
- The attendant reduction in cardiac output stimulates the expected neurohumoral compensatory mechanisms of vasoconstriction via the renin-angiotensin and sympathetic nervous systems and leads to an increase in systemic vascular resistance (systemic afterload). The increased systemic vascular resistance reduces effective stroke volume further and can precipitate cardiogenic shock. Emergent surgical intervention is usually required at this stage.

CHRONIC COMPENSATED MITRAL REGURGITATION

- Patients with chronic compensated MR may remain asymptomatic for many years.
- The left atrium dilates (associated with an increase in compliance) in response to the chronic pressure and volume overload. The increase in compliance prevents a rise in left atrial pressure and pulmonary edema.
- As the MR progresses from mild to severe, the LV compensates for the increase in LVEDP by increasing the left ventricular mass and volume. The increase in left ventricular end-diastolic volume increases contractility, increases total stroke volume, and maintains cardiac output.
- Further progression of MR induces left ventricular eccentric hypertrophy and dilatation which stretches the MV annulus and interferes with closure of the MV leaflet tips. Myocardial dysfunction ensues, impairing myocardial contractility and decreasing the total as

well as forward stroke volume. At this advanced stage, the LA pressure rises and the patient exhibits symptoms of heart failure. This is referred to as the chronic decompensated phase of MR.

ETIOLOGY

- Mitral regurgitation is caused by anatomical or functional abnormalities of the MV leaflets and/or any part of the MV apparatus. The MV apparatus includes the chordae tendineae, the papillary muscles, and mitral annulus.
- The etiology of MR can be divided into conditions primarily associated with acute or chronic MR as well as according to the specific anatomical region affected, eg, annulus versus papillary muscle.
- Acute MR may be associated with each of the following:
  - Coronary artery disease causing papillary muscle dysfunction or rupture
  - Infective endocarditis involving the mitral valve
  - Trauma
  - Connective tissue disease
  - Acute rheumatic fever
  - Dysfunction of a MV prosthesis.
- Chronic MR may be associated with each of the following:
  - Myxomatous degeneration of the MV leaflets
  - Mitral valve prolapse (MVP)
  - Connective disease diseases
  - Degenerative calcification of the MV
  - Dilated cardiomyopathy
  - Congenital heart disease
  - Rheumatic heart disease
  - Infective endocarditis

DIAGNOSIS

HISTORY

- The symptoms associated with MR depends on the following:
  - Acuteness and severity of the MR (the compliance of the LA will play a critical role in dertermining the severity of symptoms).
- Patients with mild to moderate MR are often asymptomatic for years.
- Once symptoms develop they are often nonspecific and may only include weakness and fatigue .
- Left atrial enlargement predisposes the patient to atrial fibrillation that may result in palpitations or a rapid heart rate.

- As the severity of the MR increases and the LV decompensates, patients may complain of dyspnea and exercise intolerance.
- Patients with acute severe MR present with symptoms of left-sided heart failure (respiratory distress) and sometimes right-sided heart failure (lower extremity swelling, abdominal fullness).

PHYSICAL EXAMINATION

- Mitral regurgutation is typically characterized by a holosystolic murmur at the apex of the heart, which may radiate to the axilla or the entire precordium.
- Abnormalities of the posterior MV leaflet may cause an anterior directed regurgitant jet and produce a murmur along the sternal border. This murmur can mimic the murmurs of tricuspid regurgitation or aortic stenosis.
- Abnormalities of the anterior MV leaflet may result in a MR murmur that radiates to the back.
- The intensity of the murmur does not correlate with the severity of the MR.
- The murmur may not be holosystolic. For example, the murmur associated with MVP or papillary muscle dysfunction may occur in early, mid-, or late systole.
- Severe MR may also produce a short diastolic murmur after the third heart sound that is not associated with mitral stenosis.
- Auscultation maneuvers may help to distinguish the murmur of MR from other cardiac anomalies.
  - Conditions that reduce preload (standing, early phase of the Valsalva maneuver) or afterload (amyl nitrate) reduce the intensity of the murmur.
  - Maneuvers that increase preload (squatting) or afterload (isometric exercise) increase the intensity of the murmur.
  - The late systolic murmur of MVP and hypertrophic cardiomyopathy alternatively increase with standing.
- The first heart sound may be reduced because the mitral leaflets do not close completely.
- The second heart sound may be widely split because the aortic valve closes earlier in diastole.
- If pulmonary hypertension exists, the pulmonary component of the second heart sound is prominent.
- Rapid ventricular filling may produce a third heart sound.
- Severe MR produces brisk carotid upstrokes unless there is significant LV dysfunction.
- Severe MR also produces a hyperdynamic cardiac impulse; whereas left ventricular dysfunction weakens the cardiac impulse.[3]

LABORATORY TESTING

ELECTROCARDIOGRAM

- There may be electrocardiographic (ECG) evidence of left atrial enlargement and atrial fibrillation.
- Patients with pulmonary hypertension may have ECG changes consistent with right ventricular hypertrophy.

CHEST X-RAY

- The chest film may reveal evidence of LA and left ventricular enlargement.
- Acute or decompensated MR may produce pulmonary vascular congestion on the chest film.
- Mitral annular calcification may also be evident on plain films.

ECHOCARDIOGRAPHY

- Echocardiography is the optimal tool for the diagnosis, assessment, and subsequent management of MR. Importantly, echocardiography provides an accurate assessment of the severity of MR. In particular, analysis of LA and left ventricular chamber dimensions, estimation of left ventricular systolic function (LVSF), and estimation of pulmonary artery pressure are performed.
- The indications for a transthoracic echocardiogram (TTE) published by the American College of Cardiology (ACC)/American Heart Association (AHA) include the following[4]:
  - Baseline evaluation in any patient suspected of having MR.
  - Establish the etiology of MR.
  - Periodic evaluation of left ventricular function in patients with asymptomatic moderate to severe MR.
  - Changes in signs or symptoms attributable to MR.
  - Initial evaluation after MV surgery.
  - Evaluation of pulmonary artery pressures and MR severity with exercise.
- Transthoracic echocardiography is *not* indicated for routine follow-up in asymptomatic patients with mild MR and normal left ventricular size and function.

RECOMMENDATIONS FOR FOLLOW-UP OF MITRAL REGURGITATION

- Patients with mild MR do not need routine echocardiograms. These patients require a yearly history and physical examination to screen for changes in symptoms and exercise capacity.
- In patients with moderate MR, a TTE should be done yearly or sooner if the patient develops symptoms.
- Asymptomatic patients with severe MR should undergo a TTE every 6 to 12 months.
- Indications for transesophageal echocardiography (TEE) according to ACC/AHA guidelines include the following: (1) preoperative or intraoperative assessment of patients with severe MR who are current or future candidates for MV surgery or (2) a nondiagnostic TTE. A TEE is not indicated for routine surveillance of MR.

EXERCISE STRESS TESTING

- Generally performed at the time of diagnosis and periodically thereafter to obtain an objective measure of the patient's exercise capacity. Stress testing is a valuable tool to determine the optimal timing of MV surgery.

CARDIAC CATHETERIZATION

- Angiography is indicated in patients with MR when noninvasive testing is inconclusive or when:
  - Additional hemodynamic data are required, such as pulmonary artery pressure measurements.
  - There is a discrepancy between the clinical findings and noninvasive testing.
  - Patients are at risk for coronary artery disease (especially prior to MV surgery)
  - Patients with suspected ischemic MR
- A cardiac catheterization is *not* indicated in patients with MR when MV surgery is not considered a viable option.

PROGNOSIS

- Mild to moderate MR may remain asymptomatic for 15 to 20 years after the diagnosis.
- However, severe MR not treated with MV surgery has a poor prognosis. Approximately two-thirds of these patients do not survive 8 years.[5]
- Pregnant patients with MR are at low risk for maternal/fetal complications if they have normal LVSF and New York Heart Association (NYHA) functional class I or II symptoms. High-risk patients have NYHA functional class III or IV symptoms.

TREATMENT

MEDICAL THERAPY FOR ACUTE SEVERE MITRAL REGURGITATION

- Acute severe MR requires surgical intervention. Medical therapy is considered a bridge until surgery can be carried out. Accordingly, attempts should be made to stabilize the patient until surgical correction can be accomplished. These include:
  - Nitroprusside to optimize preload and afterload.
  - In the hypotensive patient, dobutamine is utilized to increase myocardial contractility and cardiac output.

- ○ An intra-aortic balloon pump to decrease afterload and increase the mean arterial pressure.
- ○ Antibiotic therapy in the patient with MR secondary to infective endocarditis.
- ○ Prompt consultation with a cardiothoracic surgeon is required.

MEDICAL THERAPY OF CHRONIC MITRAL REGURGITATION

- Chronic MR is usually treated with vasodilator therapy, but there is little data to indicate that vasodilator therapy prolongs survival. Nonetheless, vasodilators can produce substantial symptomatic and hemodynamic improvement in patients who exhibit NYHA functional class III or IV symptoms.
- Asymptomatic patients with MR and normal LVSF do not require treatment with vasodilators unless systemic hypertension exists. Indeed, there is no rationale for utilizing vasodilator therapy in the asymptomatic patient.
- If the MR is a result of dilated cardiomyopathy, the usual therapy for heart failure (angiotensin-converting enzyme inhibitor [ACEI], β-blockers, diuretics, biventricular pacing) may reduce the severity of symptoms.
- Medical therapy for coronary ischemia can reduce the severity of ischemic MR.
- Medical therapy of atrial fibrillation with native valve MR
  - ○ Patients should be initiated on anticoagulation with warfarin to achieve a goal international normalized ratio of 2.5 (range of 2.0–3.0).
  - ○ Warfarin is generally avoided during pregnancy because of its teratogenic effects. Unfractionated heparin or low molecular weight heparin are preferred in pregnancy because neither agent crosses the placental barrier.
  - ○ Rate control can be achieved with β-blockers, nondihydropyridine calcium channel antagonists, digoxin, and amiodarone.
  - ○ Rhythm control can be achieved with antiarrhythmic drugs such as amiodarone. Electrical cardioversion can also be utilized in patients who have been anticoagulated for an appropriate period of time or have had a LA thrombus excluded with a TEE. The LA size (> 55 mm) may preclude successful cardioversion.

SURGICAL THERAPY

- Mitral valve repair is preferred over MV replacement because it is desirable to preserve as much of the MV apparatus as possible during surgical repair or replacement.

- Recommendations for MV surgery by ACC/AHA are as follows:
  - ○ Symptomatic patients with acute severe MR.
  - ○ Asymptomatic patients with chronic severe MR who fulfill the following criteria:
    - Mild to moderate LV dysfunction (left ventricular ejection fraction [LVEF] 30%–60% and/or left ventricular end-systolic dimension [LVESD] >40 mm)
    - Preserved LVSF in which MV repair is likely to be technically successful
    - Preserved LVSF with new onset atrial fibrillation
    - Preserved LVSF and pulmonary hypertension (pulmonary artery systolic pressure >50 mm Hg at rest or >60 mm Hg with exercise)
  - ○ Symptomatic patients with chronic severe MR with the following criteria:
    - Absence of severe LV dysfunction (left ventricular ejection fraction (LVEF) >30% and/or left ventricular end systolic dimension (LVESD) <55 mm)
    - New York Heart Association class III or IV symptoms and severe LV dysfunction (LVEF <30% and/or LVESD >55 mm) in whom the repair of a defective MV apparatus is highly likely to improve the clinical symptoms
  - ○ Mitral valve surgery is considered in patients with chronic severe MR secondary to LV dysfunction (LVEF <30% and/or LVESD >55 mm) who have failed optimal heart failure therapy.
- Situations in which MV surgery is not indicated include the following:
  - ○ Patients with mild to moderate MR without symptoms and normal LVSF or in whom MV repair is not feasible.
- Mitral valve surgery during pregnancy is a high-risk procedure and should only be performed when the mother is experiencing decompensated heart failure or is at high risk for death to herself or the fetus. Surgery should ideally be delayed until the fetus is viable for delivery.

PROPHYLAXIS

INFECTIVE ENDOCARDITIS

- The 2007 American Heart Association indications for infective endocarditis prophylaxis in patients with MR have changed substantially from previous recommendations.[6] The current recommendations have been designed to better reflect the prevailing evidence. Importantly, there is scant evidence that antimicrobial prophylaxis reduces the incidence of infective endocarditis except in patients at the highest risk. Patients considered at highest risk include the following:

- ○ Prosthetic mitral valves, including bioprosthetic valves
- ○ History of infective endocarditis
- ○ Acquired mitral valve disease (including mitral valve prolapse with regurgitation and those who have undergone prior valve repair) are *no* longer recommended to receive antimicrobial prophylaxis.
- Prophylaxis is also not required for pregnant patients with native MV MR who are undergoing an uncomplicated vaginal or caesarian delivery unless infection is anticipated or the patient is at high risk because of a history of endocarditis.

REFERENCES

1. Singh JP, Evans JC, Levy D, et al. Prevalence and clinical determinants of mitral, tricuspid, and aortic regurgitation (the Framingham Heart Study). *Am J Cardiol.* 1999;83(6):897–902.
2. Jones EC, Devereux RB, Roman MJ, et al. Prevalence and correlates of mitral regurgitation in a population-based sample (the Strong Heart Study). *Am J Cardiol.* 2001;87(3):298–304.
3. Zipes DP, et al. *Braunwald's Heart Disease: A Textbook of Cardiovascular Medicine.* 7th ed. Philadelphia: Elsevier Saunders; 2005.
4. Bonow RO, et al. ACC/AHA 2006 guidelines for the management of patients with valvular heart disease. *J Am Coll Cardiol.* 2006;48(3):e1–148.
5. Delahaye JP, Gare JP, Viguier E, Delahaye F, De Gevigney G, Milon H. Natural history of severe mitral regurgitation. *Eur Heart J.* 1991;12(suppl B):5–9.
6. Wilson, W, Taubert, KA, Gewitz, M, et al. Prevention of Infective Endocarditis. Guidelines From the American Heart Association. A Guideline From the American Heart Association Rheumatic Fever, Endocarditis, and Kawasaki Disease Committee. Circulation 2007; 115 published online April 19, 2007. www.circ. ahajournals. org/cgi/reprint/CIRCULATIONAHA.106.183095v1 (accessed November 11, 2007).

41 ENDOCARDITIS

Michael Forsberg

OVERVIEW

- Infective endocarditis (IE) is a microbial infection that involves the endocardial surface of the heart, principally the valves.
- Acute endocarditis is rapidly progressive with significant clinical sequelae.

- Subacute endocarditis presents over weeks to months with modest toxicity and may be associated with immunologic phenomena (glomerulonephritis).
- The development of endocarditis requires: (1) endocardial damage and (2) transient bacteremia.

EPIDEMIOLOGY

- The incidence of IE is approximately 4.2 cases per 100,000 patient years.
- Overall, the most commonly affected native valve is the mitral valve followed by the aortic valve.
- Incidence is higher among intravenous (IV) drug users.
- The tricuspid valve is the most commonly affected valve in IV drug abusers.
- Patients with underlying structural cardiac abnormalities also have a higher incidence of infection. These include patients with mitral valve prolapse, patent ductus arteriosus, ventricular septal defect, and bicuspid aortic valve.
- Prosthetic valves may be involved in up to 25% of cases of infective endocarditis.
- Mechanical prostheses have a higher risk than bioprosthetic valves during the first 3 months after implantation. Approximately 5 years after surgery the incidence equalizes between mechanical and bioprosthetic valves.

MICROBIOLOGY

- *Streptococcus* species are the most common cause of endocarditis in adult native valve endocarditis. *Staphylococcus aureus* is the second most common.
- Other causes include gram-negative bacilli, enterococci, fungi, and culture-negative endocarditis.
- In prosthetic valve endocarditis, coagulase-negative staphylococcus and *S. aureus* are the most common organisms.
- Isolation of *Streptococcus bovis* should raise the suspicion of an intra-abdominal process (ischemic colitis).
- The HACEK organisms (*Haemophilus, Actinobacillus, Cardiobacterium, Eikenella,* and *Kingella*) are associated with culture-negative endocarditis.
- Patient exposure may suggest atypical pathogens. For ecample, exposure to farm animals should suggest *Brucella* or Q fever. Exposure to birds may suggest *Chlamydia*.

CLINICAL FEATURES

- Fever is the most common symptom, present in 85% of cases.
- A murmur is present in up to 90% of cases. The quality of the murmur is determined by the valve involved.
- Embolic vascular phenomena from left sided valve lesions include splinter hemorrhages, arterial emboli to remote organs, mycotic aneurysm, conjunctival petechiae, and Janeway lesions.
- Immunologic phenomena include Osler nodes, elevated rheumatoid factor, glomerulonephritis, and Roth spots.
- Vascular and immunologic phenomena more commonly occur with subacute presentations than acute endocarditis.
- Congestive heart failure can result from valvular destruction and portends a poor prognosis.

DIAGNOSIS

- Due to the varied clinical presentations, diagnosis can be difficult.
- The diagnosis requires isolation of a typical pathogen from the blood stream and evidence of an infection (vegetation) on an endocardial surface via echocardiography.
- With subacute cases, vascular and immunologic phenomena may be prominent as compared to acute endocarditis (time course for the development of immunologic phenomena is too short).
- The Duke Criteria are a sensitive and specific set of diagnostic criteria (see Tables 88–1 and 88–2).
- Transthoracic echocardiography is the preferred initial imaging modality in suspected endocarditis with low clinical suspicion. It has been shown to have excellent specificity but lower sensitivity than transesophageal echocardiography.
- A transesophageal echocardiogram improves the sensitivity and allows evaluation of endocarditis sequelae, including valvular perforation, fistulas, and valvular abscesses.

MEDICAL TREATMENT

- The primary treatment for endocarditis is intravenous antibiotics.
- In cases of suspected endocarditis, broad spectrum antibiotics should be started after several blood cultures have been obtained.
- Once a pathogen has been isolated, specific antibiotic therapy can be tailored to the microbe based on susceptibility testing (See also Chap. 88, Cardiovascular Infections).

SURGICAL TREATMENT

- Surgical therapy in conjunction with antimicrobial therapy may be warranted in certain cases.
- Indications include moderate to severe CHF due to valvular dysfunction, unstable prosthesis, uncontrollable infection despite optimal antimicrobials, relapse after optimal therapy, *S. aureus* prosthetic valve endocarditis, or fungal infection.
- Relative indications include perivalvular extension of the infection, fistula formation, poorly responsive native valve, *S. aureus*, large (>10 mm) hypermobile vegetation, and endocarditis due to antibiotic-resistant enterococcus.

ANTIBIOTIC PROPHYLAXIS

- Antibiotic prophylaxis is recommended for patients with underlying cardiac abnormalities undergoing certain invasive procedures where transient bacteremia may occur.
- Amoxicillin given orally prior to the procedure is the treatment of choice prior to dental or upper respiratory procedures.
- Ampicillin and gentamicin are preferred prophylaxis for gastrointestinal and urinary tract procedures.

BIBLIOGRAPHY

Baddour LM, Wilson WR, Bayer AS, et al. Infective endocarditis: diagnosis, antimicrobial therapy, and management of complications: a statement for healthcare professionals from the Committee on Rheumatic Fever, Endocarditis, and Kawasaki Disease, Council on Cardiovascular Disease in the Young, and the Councils on Clinical Cardiology, Stroke, and Cardiovascular Surgery and Anesthesia, American Heart Association: endorsed by the Infectious Diseases Society of America. *Circ.* 2005;111:e394–434.

Bonow RO, Carabello BA, Chatterjee K, et al. ACC/AHA 2006 guidelines for the management of patients with valvular heart disease: a report of the American College of Cardiology/American Heart Association Task Force on Practice Guidelines (writing Committee to revise the 1998 guidelines for the management of patients with valvular heart disease) developed in collaboration with the Society of Cardiovascular Anesthesiologists endorsed by the Society for Cardiovascular Angiography and Interventions and the Society of Thoracic Surgeons. *J Am Coll Cardiol.* 2006;48(3):e1-148.

Horstkotte D, Follath F, Gutschik E, et al. Guidelines on prevention, diagnosis and treatment of infective endocarditis executive summary; the Task Force on Infective Endocarditis of the European Society of Cardiology. *Eur Heart J.* 2004;25:267–276.

42 HEART FAILURE

Stephen Kuehn

EPIDEMIOLOGY AND PROGNOSIS

- The term *heart failure* is preferred over *congestive heart failure,* because the latter term fails to encompass high-flow states.
- Approximately 5 million Americans carry a diagnosis of heart failure, with more than 550,000 new cases diagnosed per year.
- More than 1 million hospitalizations occur with a primary diagnosis of heart failure; approximately 80% of those patients are older than 65 years of age.
- The incidence of heart failure is approximately 20% in people older than the age of 60 years.
- After hospitalization, the mortality at 180 days is approximately 25%.
- The ejection fraction (EF) is an important prognostic factor but does not predict symptoms in patients with heart failure.
- Prognosis is improved significantly, especially in the short-term, if there is an identifiable, reversible cause; examples include alcoholic cardiomyopathy, severe hypertension, and primary valvular cardiomyopathy.
- Asymptomatic patients with left ventricular (LV) dysfunction have 5% or less annual mortality, whereas patients with refractory symptoms despite medical therapy have an average 6-month mortality of 50%.
- Although LV dysfunction inexorably progresses, the rate of decline of LV function in an individual patient varies considerably depending on the patients age, comorbidities, and response to therapy.
- Left ventricular dilation or right ventricular dysfunction at the time of diagnosis is a poor prognostic indicator; these patients generally do not improve symptomatically regardless of the therapeutic approach. In contrast, the mortality in these patients may improve with aggressive medical therapy.
- Additional prognostic factors include markedly reduced EF (ie, <15%), reduced maximal O_2 consumption ($\dot{V}O_2$), hyponatremia, elevated creatinine, and very poor exercise capacity (ie, inability to walk at a normal pace on level ground for more than 3 minutes).
- The most common cause of death in patients with mild to moderate (New York Heart Association [NYHA] I, II, III) heart failure is sudden cardiac death, whereas the primary cause of death in patients with severe heart failure (NYHA IV) is related to pump failure.

TABLE 42–1 New York Heart Association Functional Classification

CLASS	DESCRIPTION
I	No limitation to ordinary physical activity from cardiac disease.
II	Ordinary physical activity results in fatigue or dyspnea from cardiac disease.
III	Markedly limited from during less than ordinary activity, even ADLs; limited by dyspnea or fatigue; comfortable only at rest; caused by cardiac disease.
IV	Dyspnea or fatigue at rest or with any physical activity, caused by cardiac disease.

ADL, activities of daily living.

CLASSIFICATION AND ETIOLOGY

- The NYHA established a functional classification of heart failure (Table 42–1), whereas the ACC/AHA has developed a classification system that emphasizes the progressive nature of heart failure (Table 42–2).
- In general, heart failure can be classified as systolic (decreased myocardial contractility) or diastolic dysfunction (characterized by impaired left ventricular relaxation – either due to perturbations in active relaxation or a change in compliance). Importantly, diastolic dysfunction may occur with or without systolic dysfunction.
- The etiologic classification of heart failure is extensive (Table 42–3), the most common cause being ischemic; other common causes include valvular disease, hypertension, and inflammatory/infectious etiologies.
- Idiopathic and hypertrophic cardiomyopathies (HCM) are often familial. Hypertropic cardiomyopathy is characterized by prominent septal hypertrophy and severe diastolic dysfunction. HCM is transmitted as an autosomal dominant trait with incomplete penetrance. The molecular basis of HCM usually involves mutations in myocardial β myosin heavy chain and cardiac myosin-binding protein C genes. Many other

TABLE 42–2 American College of Cardiology and American Heart Association Classifications of Functional Stages of Heart Failure

CLASS	DESCRIPTION
A	Patient at high-risk for developing heart failure but with no structural disorder of the heart (eg, hypertension, diabetes)
B	Patient with a structural disorder of the heart but no symptoms of heart failure
C	Patient with underlying structural heart disease and past or current symptoms of heart failure
D	Patient with end-staged heart failure who may need specialized treatment, such as mechanical assist devices, continuous inotropic infusions, cardiac transplantation, or hospice care

TABLE 42–3 Etiologies of Heart Failure

Ischemic (most common)
Hypertensive
Ethanol
Viral
Infiltrative diseases (ie, amyloidosis, hemochromatosis, sarcoidosis)
Idiopathic (likely heritable)
Valvular
Postpartum cardiomyopathy
Drugs (ie, anthracyclines)

genetic disturbances have been linked to HCM, although most appear to involve myocardial contractile proteins. The vast majority of patients with idiopathic HCM are diagnosed before the age of 40.

DIAGNOSIS AND EVALUATION

- Heart failure is fundamentally defined as an imbalance in cardiac output relative to the metabolic demands of the body at normal cardiac filling pressures.
- Criteria to establish the clinical diagnosis of heart failure, such as those set forth by the Framingham group (Table 42–4), should primarily serve as a guideline.
  - The diagnosis of congestive heart failure requires the simultaneous presence of at least two major criteria or one major criterion in conjunction with two minor criteria (the minor criteria must not be caused by another condition, such as chronic lung disease).
- Etiologically, there are numerous diseases associated with the development of heart failure (see Table 42–3). Accordingly, the initial evaluation should be directed toward establishing underlying conditions, particularly those that may be reversible. In addition, the clinician should assess the patient for conditions which may unmask or exacerbate heart failure. (Table 42–5).

TABLE 42–4 Framingham Criteria for Congestive Heart Failure

MAJOR CRITERIA	MINOR CRITERIA
Paroxysmal nocturnal dyspnea	Bilateral ankle edema
Neck vein distension	Nocturnal cough
Pulmonary rales (crackles)	Dyspnea on ordinary exertion
Cardiomegaly on imaging (ie, CXR)	Hepatomegaly
Acute pulmonary edema	Pleural effusion
S3	Decrease in vital capacity by one-third from maximum recorded
Increased CVP (>16 cm H$_2$O at RA)	Tachycardia (HR >120 beats per minute)
Hepatojugular reflux	
Weight loss >4.5 kg in 5 days in response to treatment	

CVP, cardiac valve procedure; CXR, chest radiograph; HR, heart rate; RA, right atrium.

TABLE 42–5 Common Causes of Acute Exacerbation of Heart Failure

Medical noncompliance
Ischemia
Anemia
Arrhythmias (especially atrial fibrillation)
Pulmonary embolism
Uncontrolled hypertension
Acute renal failure, nephropathy
Dietary indiscretion
Fever/infection
Thyroid disease
Illicit drug use, alcohol overuse
Valvular disease (worsening, endocarditis)
Significant physical or emotional stressors
Exacerbation of other underlying disease

- Ultimately, the evaluation is intended to both seek the cause of the heart failure and to delineate the prognosis. The echocardiogram is an invaluable tool to characterize the extent and severity of heart failure. Moreover, the echocardiogram is sufficiently sensitive to permit a specific diagnosis in many patients. The echocardiogram can elucidate valvular, pericardial, or myocardial disease, provide prognostic information (EF, LV dimensions, wall thickness) and provide a baseline for future comparison. All patients should undergo a thorough evaluation for coronary artery disease, as this is the most common cause in older adults. Most patients will require an exercise stress test or possibly, cardiac catheterization. The latter is especially important in patients with several cardiac risk factors and classic symptoms of cardiac ischemia. Importantly, mechanical revascularization (ie, coronary artery bypass grafting) may reverse the LV dysfunction significantly.
- Recommended initial laboratory evaluation for patients with heart failure include a search for thyroid disease, hemochromatosis (cardiac disease is the presenting manifestation in 15%), rheumatologic conditions, and viral myocarditis. Other studies (genetic testing) may be offered depending on the clinical presentation. A plasma brain natriuretic peptide (BNP) level is useful in distinguishing heart failure (>100 pg/mL) from pulmonary causes of dyspnea. Finally, patients presenting with an acute heart failure exacerbation should undergo an evaluation for remediable causes such as medication or dietary indiscretion, acute infection, ischemia, or new arrhythmias.

PATHOPHYSIOLOGY

- Fundamentally, heart failure arises when there is decreased left ventricular stroke volume. The stroke volume depends on three interrelated factors: (1) preload or venous return, (2) myocardial contractility, and (3) afterload (impedance to forward flow). Any condition that impairs one or more of these three determinants can produce heart failure.

- For example, direct myocardial necrosis secondary to an ischemic or inflammatory process produces decreased contractility. Conversely, sustained hypertension (afterload) can injure cardiac myocytes (through remodeling and apoptosis) and reduce left ventricular function.
- Regardless of the inciting event, heart failure begets heart failure, since the systemic and local response to a decrease in LV function eventually induce cardiac remodeling (chamber dilatation) and fibrosis resulting in progression of heart failure.
- The neurohumoral response to LV dysfunction plays a critical role in the remodeling and fibrotic process. Initially, the neurohumoral response induces favorable compensatory changes that allow the heart to sustain LV stroke volume by augmenting contractility. However, sustained elevations in local and systemic neurohumoral mediators induces cardiac fibrosis. The neurohumoral systems that are particularly important in mediating this process include the sympathetic nervous system and the renin-angiotensin-aldosterone systems (RAAS).

SYMPATHETIC NERVOUS SYSTEM

- Increased sympathetic outflow is manifested by an increase in circulating catecholamines, especially norepinephrine, which augments vascular tone (afterload) resulting in myocardial stress and subsequent injury.
- β-Blockers (BBs) appear to ameliorate the deleterious effects of catecholamines and may reverse remodeling.
- Importantly, β-adrenergic receptors are downregulated in advanced failure because of chronic stimulation via catecholamines. Receptor downregulation may contribute to LV dysfunction in the advanced stages of heart failure. Importantly, BBs may induce upregulation of these receptors and augment myocardial contractility.

RENIN-ANGIOTENSIN-ALDOSTERONE SYSTEM

- Activation of the RAAS will increase sodium and water retention and heighten vascular tone. Initially, the volume expansion may facilitate LV function by augmenting preload. The increased vascular tone could augment perfusion to vital organs, including the heart. Nevertheless, sustained activation of the RAAS induces pathologic remodeling and fibrosis in the heart.

- Angiotensin-converting enzyme inhibitors (ACEIs), angiotensin receptor-blockers (ARBs), and aldosterone antagonists serve to blunt these deleterious effects, by reducing afterload (inhibiting angiotensin II), decreasing volume expansion and pulmonary congestion (by attenuating the effects of the RAAS on renal salt retention), and by decreasing the effects of these mediators on cardiac fibrosis.

MEDICAL THERAPY

- Nonpharmacologic strategies have not undergone rigorous testing. Nonetheless, it seems prudent to recommend the following to all patients with heart failure: smoking cessation, moderate consumption of alcohol (<2 drinks/d), dietary restriction of salt (2–3 g/d), 30 minutes of daily exercise, and weight reduction in obese patients.
- Pharmacologic therapy is designed to improve symptoms, retard progression of cardiac fibrosis and reduce mortality. Converting-enzyme inhibitors (or angiotensin receptor blocking agents in patients intolerant of an ACEI) are the cornerstone of pharmacologic therapy. In addition, BBs have also been shown to reduce mortality and improve symptoms in patients with heart failure. Specific BBs (carvedilol) may offer superior cardioprotection over other agents in this class. The benefits of BBs in blacks appears to be less robust. The combination of hydralazine with a long-acting nitrate is a reasonable alternative in patients intolerant of an ACEIs or ARB, as this combination also improves survival (particularly in blacks). In moderate heart failure, aldosterone antagonists (spironolactone and eplerenone) have been shown to improve survival. Diuretics are used for congestive symptoms, however there is no evidence that these agents prolong survival. Digoxin may be incorporated into the regimen when symptoms persist despite maximal therapy. Although digoxin has been shown to reduce hospitalization for heart failure, there is little evidence that mortality is improved.

ANGIOTENSIN-CONVERTING ENZYME INHIBITORS AND ANGIOTENSIN RECEPTOR BLOCKERS

- Angiotensin-converting enzyme inhibitors are the best characterized agents in the management of heart failure. They rapidly improve symptoms and significantly reduce mortality at 5 years. They are considered first-line therapy for patients with systolic dysfunction. The features of ACEIs that the clinician should be especially cognizant of include:

○ ACEIs reduce both preload and afterload, promote a natriuresis, and retard cardiac remodeling and fibrosis.

○ Drugs in this class include captopril, lisinopril, ramipril, enalapril, fosinopril, trandolapril, and quinapril. Whether specific agents within this class offer superior cardioprotection remains incompletely understood.

○ Mutliple, large randomized controlled trials have shown that ACEIs reduce mortality, decrease hospitalization rate, and improve symptoms. In addition, these studies suggest that ACEIs also reduce cardiac fibrosis and LV remodeling (Fig. 42–1).

○ Side effects associated with the ACEIs include persistent cough, angioedema, hyperkalemia, and renal insufficiency. In patients intolerant of ACEIs, the ARBs are an acceptable alternative.

○ The maximum tolerable dose should be used to gain the greatest cardioprotective benefit.

• Angiotensin receptor blockers:

○ The angiotensin receptor blockers can be used as an alternative to ACEIs in patients who are intolerant. They appear to have similar efficacy, although the data is less robust than that for the ACEIs.

○ Angiotensin receptor blockers are often used in combination with ACEIs (and the combination is likely to be superior to either agent alone), but the incidence of hyperkalemia and renal failure is increased.

○ The two ARBs that are FDA approved for heart failure include valsartan and candesartan.

β-BLOCKERS

• Like ACEIs, BBs have been shown to improve survival and symptoms in patients with LV dysfunction. The BBs are also associated with a reduction in hospitalization rate for heart failure. Several studies have indicated that combining BBs with an ACEI affords greater cardioprotection than either agent alone. BBs require several months to exert their beneficial effects.

• The BBs reduce systemic blood pressure, decrease the incidence of arrhythmias, improve cardiac remodeling, minimize myocardial ischemia, and improve cardiac symptoms.

• BBs should *not* be prescribed to patients with decompensated heart failure (pulmonary edema), as the initial negative inotropic effect can worsen heart failure. Thus, patients should be relatively stable before initiating therapy with BBs.

• Carvedilol and metoprolol succinate (XL) are the only two BBs that have been FDA approved for the treatment of heart failure.

• Adverse reactions to the BBs include fatigue, hypotension, dizziness, bradycardia, and heart block. The fatigue usually resolves if the drug is titrated slowly.

HYDRALAZINE/NITRATES

• This combination can be initiated when patients are receiving maximal heart failure therapy and continue to be symptomatic.

• This combination is also useful in patients intolerant of ACEIs and ARBs.

• Recent studies have suggested that African Americans are less responsive to ACEIs and may benefit from the hydralazine/nitrate (Hyd-NTG) combination. Interestingly, African Americans appear to liberate less nitric oxide than whites. Since hydralazine decreases nitric oxide (NO) degradation, while nitrate administration induces synthesis of nitric oxide, it is concluded that the benefit of Hyd-NTG in African-Americans is the secondary to an increase in NO. Recent studies have also demonstrated improved survival and symptoms in African Americans who received Hyd-NTG as well as ACEIs and BBs.

• Important side effects include headache and dizziness (nitrate) and drug-induced lupus (hydralazine).

DIURETICS

• Diuretics have not been shown to improve survival in heart failure and are purely administered for management of peripheral and pulmonary edema.

• Loop diuretics offer greater potency and are the preferred initial agent in the management of edema. Most patients will require daily administration of a loop diuretic to manage congestive symptoms.

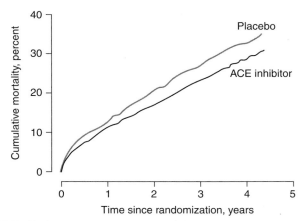

FIG. 42–1 A meta-analysis of five trials reveal that therapy with an angiotensin-converting enzyme (ACE) inhibitor significantly reduced mortality. (Flather MD, Yusuf S, Kober L, et al. *Lancet.* 2000;355:1575).

• Chronic administration of diuretics can induce significant hypokalemia and hypomagnesemia. Importantly, hypokalemia can predispose to fatal arrhythmias and aggravate digoxin toxicity. Thiazide diuretics may be used in concert with loop diuretics to augment their effect. However, these agents are *not* particularly effective in diuretic naïve heart failure patients.

• Nesiritide is a brain natriuretic peptide analogue that possesses both vasodilator and diuretic properties. It has been approved for short-term use in hospitalized patients with acute decompensated heart failure. However, recent studies suggest that neseritide may increase 6-month mortality and acutely worsen renal function. Therefore, this drug is generally reserved for use in patients who have failed a trial of intravenous loop diuretics.

ALDOSTERONE ANTAGONISTS

• Aldosterone has recently been implicated in cardiac remodeling. Moreover, the levels of aldosterone are chronically increased in heart failure. Aldosterone has also been shown to induce coronary inflammation and promote cardiac hypertrophy and fibrosis. It undoubtably also contributes to volume expansion and edema formation.

• Aldosterone antagonists (AAs) function as potassium-sparing diuretics, which may also serve to reduce the incidence of hypokalemia and attendant life-threatening arrhythmias.

• Spironolactone was associated with a 30% improvement in survival at 24 months in patients with class III to IV heart failure (Fig. 42–2).

• Eplerenone was associated with a 15 percent reduction in overall mortality at 16 months in patients who had had an MI within the preceding 2 weeks and who had an EF of 40 percent and/or diabetes mellitus.

• Spironolactone's main side effects are hyperkalemia and gynecomastia; eplerenone is less prone to produce gynecomastia.

DIGOXIN

• Digoxin is derived from the foxglove plant and has been in use for more than 200 years.

• Digoxin inhibits the sodium/potassium adenosine triphosphatase, leading to increased intracellular calcium, which is believed to augment myocardial contractility. Other important effects include an increase in parasympathetic (vagal) activity, atrioventricular nodal inhibition, and sensitization of the arterial baroreflex.

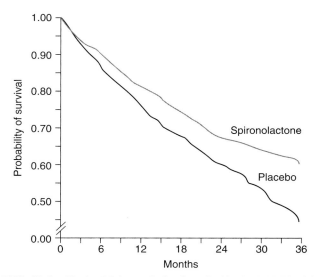

FIG. 42–2   Kaplan-Meier analysis of survival in the RALES trial shows that spironolactone reduces mortality by 30 percent. (Pitt B, Zannad F, Remme WJ, et al. *N Engl J Med.* 1999; 341:709.)

• Digoxin is associated with numerous drug interactions. Because of its narrow therapeutic index the clinician must be particularly vigilant when administering digoxin.

OTHER INOTROPES

• Intravenous inotropic therapy is used to augment cardiac output in patients hospitalized with acute decompensated heart failure. Two inotropes are currently in use, although no evidence for a survival benefit has been shown with either:

DOBUTAMINE

• Dobutamine activates β_1 receptors and increases cardiac contractility and heart rate. It also stimulates β_2 receptors, which may reduce peripheral arterial resistance and therefore afterload.

• The usual dose of dobutamine is 5 to 20 µg/kg/min.

• Adverse effects include arrhythmias and hypotension.

MILRINONE

• Milrinone inhibits phosphodiesterase, an enzyme that normally degrades cyclic adenosine monophosphate (cAMP). Cyclic AMP is a second messenger for catecholamines and, therefore inhibition of phosphodiesterase causes an increase in cardiac contractility.

• Milrinone is thought be a more potent pulmonary vasodilator than dobutamine and may be less arrhythmogenic.

• The usual dose range is 0.25 to 0.50 µg/kg/min.

DEVICE THERAPY AND TRANSPLANTATION

- Biventricular pacing with cardiac resynchronization has become an important strategy in the treatment of heart failure.
  - ○ Chronic heart failure is usually associated with myocardial conduction delays, which in turn produce dyssynchrony during myocardial contraction. Resynchronization with biventricular pacing has been shown to resynchronize the heart and improve cardiac output.
  - ○ Biventricular pacing for cardiac synchronization is indicated in patients with an EF <35%, NYHA III or ambulatory IV despite optimal medical therapy and patients who have ECG dyssynchrony defined as QRS >120 ms. A *dyssynchrony study* using echocardiography is carried out to optimize the device.
- Sudden death caused by ventricular arrhythmias is responsible for approximately half of all deaths in patients with heart failure.
  - ○ Automatic implantable cardiac defibrillators are indicated in patients resuscitated from sudden death or with symptomatic ventricular tachycardia.
  - ○ Several recent trials clearly demonstrated a survival advantage in advanced heart failure (EF <35%) treated with implantable cardiac defibrillators versus medical management.
  - ○ Therefore, defibrillators (automatic implantable cardiac defibrillators or implantable cardiac defibrillators) are indicated for patients with LV dysfunction (EF <35%) and NYHA II or III class heart failure to prevent sudden death; note that amiodarone is ineffective for this purpose.
- Ventricular assist devices:
  - ○ Ventricular assist devices are generally used as a bridge to transplantation. These invasive devices offer mechanical cardiac assistance but require surgical implantation.
- Chronic inotropic therapy:
  - ○ Chronic inotropic therapy (dobutamine, milrinone) has not been shown to improve survival; indeed it may even decrease survival. This type of support it is used solely for symptom palliation.
- Heart transplantation:
  - ○ Heart transplantation is an option for patients with end-stage heart failure refractory to medical therapy. Generally, these patients should be relatively *healthy* without significant other comorbidities. Approximately 2000 transplantations are performed each year in the United States.

BIBLIOGRAPHY

Hunt SA, Abraham WT, Chin MH, et al. ACC/AHA 2005 guideline update for the diagnosis and management of chronic heart failure in the adult: a report of the American College of Cardiology/American Heart Association Task Force on Practice Guidelines (Writing committee to update the 2001 guidelines for the evaluation and management of heart failure): developed in collaboration with the American College of Chest Physicians and the International Society for Heart and Lung Transplantation: endorsed by the Heart Rhythm Society. *Circ.* 2005;112:e154.

Maisel AS, Krishnaswamy P, Nowak RM, et al. Rapid measurement of B-type natriuretic peptide in the emergency diagnosis of heart failure. *N Engl J Med.* 2002;347:161.

Jessup M, Borenza S. Review article: heart failure. *N Engl J Med.* 2003;348(20):2007–2018.

43 AORTIC AND PERIPHERAL VESSEL DISEASE

Robert Neumayr

ARTERIAL STRUCTURE AND FUNCTION

- The arterial wall consists of three layers. The innermost layer is the tunica intima which is comprised of endothelium and connective tissue. The middle (and thickest layer) is the tunica media which is comprised of intertwining sheets of smooth muscle cells and elastic connective tissue. The tunica adventitia is the outermost layer and it is comprised of collagen and elastic tissue.
- A network of small vessels, the vasa vasorum, courses through the tunica adventitia and penetrate the tunica media to supply the arterial wall with oxygen and nutrients. The lumen of the blood vessel is enveloped by the trilaminar structure of the arerial wall.
- The main functions of blood vessels include blood transport (large conduit vessels), blood pressure regulation (small resistance arterioles), and metabolic exchange (capillaries).
- The aorta originates from the left side of the heart and is composed of three parts: (1) proximal ascending aorta, (2) arch, and (3) distal descending aorta.
- The ascending aorta courses superiorly, anteriorly, and rightward. It supports the three aortic valve leaflets and

gives rise to the three sinuses of Valsalva (the right and left coronary artery originates from the right and left sinus, respectively).

• The aortic arch courses superiorly, leftward, and then posteriorly in the mediastinum. Its branches include the brachiocephalic trunk (which continues as the right subclavian artery and the right common carotid artery), the left common carotid artery, and the left subclavian artery.

• The descending aorta is divided by the diaphragm into the thoracic aorta and the abdominal aorta; it travels inferiorly and then eventually anterior to the spine giving rise to the iliac arteries that supply the pelvis and lower extremities. While in the thorax, its branches include the bronchial, pericardial, esophageal, costal, and phrenic arteries. In the abdominal cavity, it gives rise to celiac, mesenteric, renal, gonadal, lumbar, and sacral branches.

ATHEROSCLEROSIS AND PERIPHERAL VASCULAR DISEASE

• Atherosclerosis is characterized by the deposition of lipid, inflammatory cells, cellular debris, calcium, extracellular matrix, and fibrin within the intima of the arterial wall.

• As atherosclerosis progesses, some lesions become unstable and are susceptible to rupture and ulceration which can rapidly lead to thrombosis. Rupture of the fibrous cap usually occurs at sites of thinning of the fibrous plaque that covers the advanced lesion. Thinning of the fibrous cap is thought to be secondary to influx and activation of macrophages, which release proteolytic enzymes. Thrombosis after plaque rupture as well as encroachment of plaque on luminal diameter can induce ischemia of vital organs and the extremities.

• Multiple risk factors have been associated with the development and rupture of plaque including smoking, diabetes mellitus, hypertension, hyperlipidemia, advanced age, male gender, and infiltrating inflammatory cells (clinically suspected in patients with an increase in serum inflammatory markers such as C-reactive protein, homocysteine, or fibrinogen).

• Atherosclerosis that develops in the vascular territory that supplies blood to the head and neck is referred to as cerebrovascular disease. Athersclerosis of the arteries and arterioles that perfuse the myocardium is referred to as coronary artery disease. Peripheral vascular disease refers to atherosclerosis that involves the aorta, renal, mesenteric, and lower extremity arteries and branches.

• The prevalence of peripheral vascular disease increases with age. For example, the National Health and Education Survey Database (NHANES) revealed that the prevalence of peripheral vascular disease was 0.9% between the ages of 40 and 49, 2.5% between the ages of 50 and 59, 4.7% between the ages of 60 and 69, and 14.5% after age 70.

• The clinical presentation of lower extremity peripheral vascular disease is characterized by impairment of ambulation or exercise limitation, claudication, resting limb pain, and/or nonhealing ulcers. Mesenteric ischemia is usually accompanied by postprandial abdominal pain. In general, the symptoms and signs of peripheral vascular disease reflect the distribution of the involved artery, although up to 50% of patients may experience no or mild symptoms.

• The classification of lower extremity peripheral vascular disease is based upon the severity of symptoms and signs. The Fontaine and Rutherford systems have both been used (see Table 43–1)

• Several noninvasive diagnostic modalities exist for identifying peripheral vascular disease including the ankle-brachial index (ABI), exercise treadmill test, segmental limb pressures, segmental volume plethysmography, and ultrasonography. Magnetic resonance angiography, computed tomographic angiography,

TABLE 43–1   Classification of the Severity of Peripheral Vascular Disease

FONTAINE STAGES		RUTHERFORD CATEGORIES		
STAGE	CLINICAL	GRADE	CATEGORY	CLINICAL
I	Asymptomatic	0	0	Asymptomatic
IIA	Mild claudication	I	1	Mild claudication
IIB	Moderate to severe claudication	I	2	Moderate claudication
		I	3	Severe claudication
III	Ischemic rest pain	II	4	Ischemic rest pain
IV	Ulceration or gangrene	III	5	Mild tissue loss
		III	6	Moderate tissue loss

Reprinted from Dormandy JA, Rutherford RB. Management of peripheral arterial disease (PAD). TASC Working Group. TransAtlantic Inter-Society Concensus (TASC). *J Vasc Surg.* 2000;31:S1.

and catheter-based contrast angiography are valuable, but inherently more invasive.

- Calculation of the ABI is performed by measuring the systolic blood pressure (via Doppler probe) in the brachial, posterior tibial, and dorsalis pedis arteries. The highest of the four measurements in the ankles and feet is divided by the higher of the two brachial measurements. The normal ABI is 1.0 to 1.3. Values that exceed 1.30 suggest a noncompressible calcified vessel. An ABI below 0.9 has 95% sensitivity for detecting angiogram-positive lower extremity peripheral arterial disease. An ABI of <0.90 is usually associated with claudication, while, an ABI <0.4 is consistent with severe lower extermity ischemia. ABIs and segmental pressures can be obtained before and after exercise on a treadmill in patients with a high index of suspicion for peripheral arterial disease. An MRI can determine the extent and severity of the disease in patients with an ABI <0.9, or prior to revascularization.

- General treatment options include lifestyle/risk factor modification, exercise rehabilitation programs, pharmacologic therapy, interventional procedures, surgical revascularization, and amputation:
  ○ *Risk factor modification*: smoking cessation, exercise, diet
  ○ *Exercise rehabilitation programs*: minimum of 30 minutes three times per week is useful in patients with intermittent claudication
  ○ *Pharmacologic therapy*: lipid lowering agents (β-hydroxy-methylglutaryl-coenzyme A reductase inhibitors), antihypertensives (angiotensin-converting enzyme inhibitors/angiotensin receptor blockers, diuretics, calcium-channel blockers), tight control of diabetes, antiplatelet agents (aspirin or clopidogrel), and miscellaneous agents (cilostazol or pentoxifylline)
  ○ *Interventional procedures*: angioplasty, cutting balloons, atherectomy, or endovascular stenting
  ○ *Surgical revascularization*: bypass, endarterectomy, reconstruction, or amputation

AORTIC ANEURYSMS

- An aneurysm is defined as a localized, pathologic dilatation of a blood vessel caused by disease or weakening of the vessel's wall. Generally, aortic dilatation is considered significant if the diameter is greater than 1.5 times normal or exceeds 3 cm.

- Aortic aneurysms are classified as thoracic or abdominal. Most aortic aneurysms are abdominal in location and inferior to the renal arteries. Males are affected approximately three times more commonly than women.

- Causes of thoracic aortic aneurysms include cystic medial necrosis, connective tissue disease (Marfan syndrome, Ehlers-Danlos), bicuspid aortic valve, vasculitis, infection (syphilis, tuberculosis), atherosclerosis, and trauma.

- Abdominal aortic aneurysms (AAAs) are estimated to be present in 5% to 10% of all men older than 65 years of age.

- Most AAAs are asymptomatic in nature. The clinical features may include vague abdominal or back pain, a pulsatile abdominal mass, or leg symptoms. A ruptured AAA is accompanied by severe pain and hemodynamic instability.

- The etiology of AAAs are theoretically similar to those for thoracic aneurysms but most are associated with progressive atherosclerosis and the attendant risk factors. Among these, smoking has been identified as the strongest independent risk factor.

- In patients with several risk factors and an AAA >5 cm in diameter, the annual risk of rupture is approximately 20% with an associated mortality rate as high as 75%.

- Elective surgical repair is generally recommended for aortic aneurysms ≥5.5 cm in diameter or with an expansion rate of ≥0.5 cm/y. When aortic aneurysms are <5.5 cm and asymptomatic, medical management (β-blockers, risk factor treatment) and surveillance with ultrasound (US) or computed tomography (CT) is reasonable.

- Screening with abdominal ultrasound for an AAA is usually considered in men older than 65 years of age with a history of peripheral vascular disease and risk factors (smoking, diabetes, etc.), but is not typically recommended for other patient groups.

AORTIC DISSECTION

- Aortic dissection is characterized by loss of the vessel's intimal integrity and propagation of the disruption into one or more layers of the vessel wall with subsequent intramural hematoma or false lumen formation.

- The peak incidence of aortic dissection occurs during the sixth and seventh decades of life. Men are affected 2 to 3 times more often than women. Nearly all occur in the proximal aorta (within several centimeters of the aortic valve).

- The most common presenting features of an acute dissection include severe chest, neck, or back pain (approximately 90%) characterized as sharp or tearing in nature. Syncope, dyspnea, neurologic symptoms, and anxiety may also be present. A small number of patients are asymptomatic.

- Serious sequelae of acute dissection include stroke, myocardial infarction, aortic regurgitation, heart failure, cardiac arrest, circulatory collapse, and death. The mortality exceeds 1% per hour if left untreated.
- Risk factors for aortic dissection include chronic uncontrolled hypertension, previous aneurysm, aortic coarctation, bicuspid aortic valve, arteritis, connective tissue disease, familial/genetic disease which weaken the arterial wall (Marfan syndrome), trauma, cocaine use, pregnancy, and atherosclerotic disease.
- Diagnostic modalities used to identify a dissection include the chest x-ray (which reveals mediastinal and aortic widening), echocardiography (multiplanar transesophageal approach is considerably more sensitive than transthoracic), computed tomography, magnetic resonance imaging, or angiography (considered inferior to the current noninvasive tests). The physical exam typically reveals a difference in blood pressure between arms (>20 mm Hg).
- Treatment focuses on prompt, aggressive medical therapy (β-blockers and/or vasodilators such as nitroprusside as blood pressure allows). Surgery is indicated in all proximal aortic lesions, progressive dissections, and patients who are clinical unstable or deteriorating. Uncomplicated aneurysms confined to the thoracic aorta are treated medically.

VASCULITIS AND INFECTIOUS ARTERIAL DISEASE

- Vasculitis involving the peripheral arteries is divided into noninfectious (immunologic or idiopathic) and infectious categories (See also Chap. 127, Vasculitis).
- The immunologic vasculitides are generally classified according to the size of the vessel involved. The symptoms attributed to these conditions vary from organ failure to vascular dissection depending on the site of involvement.
  - *Aorta and large arteries*: giant cell arteritis and Takayasu arteritis. May also develop large vessel vasculitis with idiopathic retroperitoneal fibrosis.
  - *Medium-sized arteries (muscular and conduit vessels)*: polyarteritis nodosa, temporal (giant cell) arteritis, Kawasaki disease.
  - *Small-sized vessels (arterioles and capillaries)*: can be associated with autoimmune disorders such as systemic lupus erythematosus; usually secondary to Wegener's granulomatosis, microscopic polyangiitis/polyarteritis, Churg-Strauss syndrome, rheumatoid arthritis, Henoch-Schönlein purpura, cryoglobulinemia, Sjögren syndrome, Behçet disease, or via a drug-induced mechanism.
- Treatment options for the vasculitides vary depending on the underlying cause but generally include antiinflammatory medications, corticosteroids, immunosuppressants, or cytotoxic agents (See also Chap. 127, Vasculitis).
- Infectious pathogens have also been associated with vessel wall inflammation. Occasionally, they produce arterial wall degeneration resulting in aneurysm formation and/or dissection. The organisms most commonly encountered include *Staphylococcus, Salmonella, Pseudomonas, Rickettsia, Treponema pallidum,* and *Mycobacterium tuberculosis.* Hepatitis B (polyarteritis nodosa) and Hepatitis C (mixed cryoglobulinemia) may also produce a systemic vasculitis, although aortic dissection and/or peripheral vascular disease would be unusual.
- Vascular infections are treated with antibiotics or antivirals as appropriate to the specific organism.

DYSPLASTIC AND THROMBOTIC ARTERIAL DISEASE

- Fibromuscular dysplasia (FMD) is an idiopathic dysplastic angiopathy of medium-size, noncoronary arterial beds (renal, carotid, mesenteric, and iliac) characterized by fibrous thickening of the arterial wall.
- Generally, FMD is identified in younger women of childbearing age. Usually, there are no clinical signs or symptoms, although refractory hypertension (renal arteries), neurologic symptoms (carotids), or limb/tissue perfusion abnormalities can arise depending on the artery involved.
- Definitive treatment for FMD generally involves surgical arterial reconstruction/bypass or endovascular interventions. These procedures can effect a cure in most patients.
- Arterial thromboembolic disease may arise from various blood coagulopathies (lupus anticoagulant or cardiolipin antibodies, mutations in prothrombin or Factor V Leiden, Factor C, S, or antithrombin III deficiencies, or systemic prothrombotic states in association with inflammatory diseases or malignancies).
- Thromboangiitis obliterans (Buerger disease) is a thrombotic/destructive process affecting the distal limb arteries of young smokers. Its appearance is similar to a vasculitis and it has been known to affect the small draining veins as well. Other than smoking cessation and limiting environmental triggers (drugs), there is no established effective therapy.

BIBLIOGRAPHY

American College of Cardiologists/American Heart Association. ACC/AHA 2005, practice guidelines for the management of patients with peripheral arterial disease (lower extremity, renal, mesenteric, and abdominal aortic). *Circ.* 2006;113(11): e463–654.

Hirsch AT, Criqui MH, Treat-Jacobson D, et al. Peripheral arterial disease detection, awareness, and treatment in primary care. *JAMA.* 2001;286:1317.

Hiatt WR. Medical treatment of peripheral arterial disease and claudication. *N Engl J Med.* 2001;344:1608.

Isselbacher EM. Thoracic and abdominal aortic aneurysms. *Circ.* 2005;111:816.

Norgren L, Hiatt WR, Dormandy JA, et al. Inter-society consensus for the management of peripheral arterial disease (TASC II). *J Vasc Surg.* 2007;45 Suppl S:S5.

Khan IA, Nair CK. Clinical, diagnostic, and management perspectives of aortic dissection. *Chest.* 2002;122(1):311–328.

Weyand CM, Goronzy JJ. Mechanisms of disease: medium- and large-vessel vasculitis. *N Engl J Med.* 2003;349:160–169.

44 DISEASES OF THE PERICARDIUM

Peter Mikolajczak and Frank Bleyer

ANATOMY AND FUNCTION

The pericardium is a fibrous sac consisting of two layers surrounding the heart. The visceral pericardium (epicardium) lines the myocardium. The parietal pericardium is a thick fibrous outer layer. These two layers are separated by a space filled with fluid ranging from 15 to 50 mL

- Although the pericardium is not essential for life it serves many subtle functions:
  - Anchors the heart in the central thorax
  - Prevents precipitous distension of cardiac chambers (because of increased venous return) that otherwise would occur with exercise
  - Anatomically restricts the spread of infection from contiguous structures (lung) to the heart
  - Secretes prostaglandins, although the functional significance of this remains incompletely understood
  - Maintains ventricular compliance and transmural cardiac pressure
  - Promotes interventricular dependence which facilitates stroke volume.
  - Allows the ventricles to generate greater isovolumic pressure at any given volume (modulates cardiac output)

CONGENITAL ABSENCE OF THE PERICARDIUM

- This is a rare condition that is characterized by partial absence of the left pericardium and is often associated with other congenital lesions such as atrial septal defect, bicuspid aortic valve, or pulmonary malformation.
- Although most patients are asymptomatic, some individuals may develop chest pain, syncope, or sudden death.
- The cardiac silhouette appears shifted and has an elongated left heart border on chest x-ray.
- Computed tomography (CT), magnetic resonance imaging (MRI), and echocardiography are usually diagnostic.

PERICARDITIS

- This is an inflammatory condition of the pericardium that is associated with the accumulation of fluid between the visceral and parietal pericardium.
- Sharp substernal chest pain is the presenting symptom. The pain typically radiates to the back and classically, to the scapula. The pain is worse with inspiration and sometimes relieved by sitting forward. At times, the pain may be difficult to differentiate from coronary ischemia or pulmonary emboli.
- A friction rub may be audible throughout the precordium. The rub is characterized by a high-pitched scratchy sound (walking on dry snow) and is classically comprised of three components (atrial systole, ventricular systole and ventricular filling).
- If a large pericardial effusion with tamponade physiology is present, the patient may be hypotensive, tachycardic, and have elevated neck veins that exhibit a prominent x descent.
- The electrocardiogram (ECG) will reveal diffuse (Fig. 44–1) ST elevation that is concave upward. PR depression can be seen in all leads except aVR. The ST elevation in pericarditis returns to baseline before the T waves invert. In contrast, in acute myocardial infarction (MI), the T wave inverts while the ST segment is still elevated (Table 44–1).
- Elevated white blood cell counts, ESR, CRP, and low grade fever may be present as well as a small troponin leak.
- 90% of the cases of pericarditis are either idiopathic or viral; however, there are a variety of important

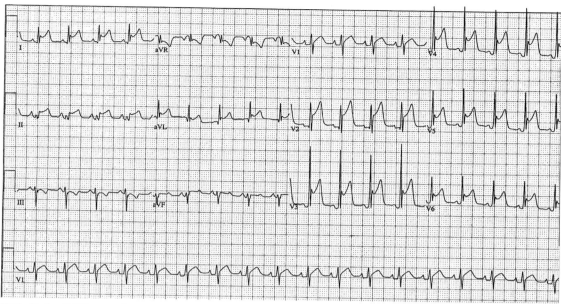

FIG. 44–1 ECG example of pericarditis. ECG, electrocardiogram.

etiologies that should be considered (tuberculosis) (Table 44–2).
• An echocardiogram may demonstrate a small to very large pericardial effusion. The size of effusion does not generally correlate with the clinical picture, albeit larger effusions are more likely to induce tamponade.
• Echocardiography is very effective in diagnosing cardiac tamponade.

TREATMENT

• Acute pericarditis of viral or idiopathic origin should be managed conservatively with nonsteroidal anti-inflammatory agents; aspirin 650 mg every 4 hours or indomethacin 25 mg three times daily. Colchicine 0.6 mg twice daily is also very effective.
• The colchicine for acute pericarditis (COPE) trial randomized patients with pericarditis to colchicine vs aspirin. Colchicine significantly improved symptoms compared to aspirin at 72 hours and decreased recurrent episodes of pericarditis at 15 months.
• Acute pericarditis will respond rapidly to corticosteroids, however, as steroids are tapered, there is a significant risk of recurrence which may evolve to steroid dependence. Therefore, steroids should be avoided, unless an underlying inflammatory disease (connective tissue disorder) is present that would require treatment with steroids.
• Uremic pericarditis responds well to intensive daily dialysis for 7-14 days.

PERICARDIAL EFFUSION AND TAMPONADE

• The inflammation of pericarditis usually promotes fluid accumulation in the pericardial sac. Moreover, blood may accumulate in the pericardial sac after myocardial rupture or aortic dissection.

TABLE 44–1   Differentiation of Pericarditis from Myocardial Infarction with ECG

MYOCARDIAL INFARCTION	PERICARDITIS
ST elevation in leads facing area of infarction with reciprocal ST depression	ST elevation all leads except aVR
No PR depression	No reciprocal changes
Convex upward ST elevation	PR depression
T waves invert before ST segment returns	Concave upward
Q wave may be present	T wave inversion after ST segment returns to baseline
	Q waves absent, may notice loss of R waves if large pericardial effusions develop

TABLE 44–2   Causes of Pericarditis

Idiopathic
Infections (viral, tuberculosis, fungal, bacteria)
Uremia
Acute myocardial infarction
Neoplasia primary or metastatic
Autoimmune disease (systemic lupus erythematosus, rheumatoid arthritis, ankylosing spondylosis)
Mediastinal radiation
Post–cardiac injury (trauma or surgery)

- As fluid accumulates, the pressure increases in the pericardial space. Pericardial pressures eventually interfere with cardiac filling resulting in cardiac tamponade.
- If fluid accumulates slowly, the pericardium can accommodate a large amount of fluid with little change in filling pressure or cardiac function. However if fluid accumulates quickly, as little as 100 mL may hinder ventricular filling and interfere with cardiac output.
- As pericardial pressure increases, atrial and diastolic ventricular pressure will compensate for the decrease in ventricular filling. However, further increases in pericardial pressure will eventually exceed the compensatory mechanisms and result in impairment of right ventricular filling. At this stage, the right and left atrial pressure and right and left ventricular diastolic pressure are equivalent to the pericardial pressure.
- System venous congestion (right heart failure) ensues and is characterized by hepatic congestion, peripheral edema, and elevation of the jugular venous pressure.
- Echocardiography is the study of choice in establishing the diagnosis of tamponade. Early diastolic collapse of the right ventricle is consistent with impairment of right ventricular filling and tamponade.
- Normally, the intrathoracic drop in pressure that occurs with inspiration is transmitted to the intracardiac chambers causing a uniform drop in cardiac pressure of 5 to 7 mm Hg. The pericardial pressure during tamponade prevents the decrease in cardiac pressure during inspiration. Rather, with inspiration, the left atrial pressure remains fixed while the pulmonary pressure decreases. This in turn decreases left heart filling, left heart stroke volume and systolic blood pressure (eg, pulsus paradoxus–the decrease in SBP exceeds 10 mm Hg).

CLINICAL FEATURES

- Patients with tamponade are usually tachycardic, hypotensive, and dyspneic. They appear anxious and may complain of chest pain.
- Jugular venous distension is present with a prominent *x* descent and no *y* descent.
- A paradoxical pulse characterized by a decrease in systolic blood pressure of >10 mm Hg on inspiration is usually present.
- An ECG may reveal low voltage or electrical alternans. Electrical alternans is characterized by beat to beat alteration in the size of the QRS complex and T wave because the heart is rotating or swinging in the fluid-filled pericardial sac.
- Echocardiography can easily identify a pericardial effusion. Importantly, right ventricular collapse in

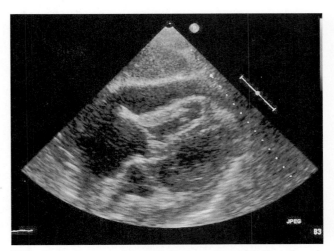

FIG. 44–2 Large pericardial effusion with early diastolic collapse of the right ventricle.

early diastole is diagnostic of tamponade. Thus, echocardiography should be promptly performed if tamponade is suspected (Fig. 44–2).

TREATMENT

- Treatment of tamponade requires emergent pericardiocentesis under fluoroscopic and echocardiographic guidance usually performed in the catheterization laboratory. Surgical drainage under direct visualization via a subxiphoid approach is also effective and may prove useful in diagnosing the etiology of an effusion (examination and culture of the fluid and pericardial biopsy).
- Routine analysis of pericardial fluid should include measurement of cell counts, specific gravity, hematocrit, and protein. A gram stain and culture for bacteria, acid-fast bacilli (AFB), cytologic examination for malignant cells, and adenosine deaminase should also be performed.

CONSTRICTIVE PERICARDITIS

ETIOLOGY

- Constrictive pericarditis is characterized by dense fibrosis, calcification, and adhesions of the parietal and visceral pericardium.
- The dense, fibrotic, calcified pericardium encases and adheres to the myocardium, restricting filling.
- Constrictive pericarditis is the culmination of months to years of chronic pericardial inflammation.

- Chronic pericardial inflammation may be due to: mediastinal irradiation, postsurgical inflammation, infection, neoplasm (breast cancer or lymphoma), autoimmune disease (systemic lupus erythematosus [SLE] or rheumatoid arthritis), uremia, sarcoidosis, methysergide therapy, or implantable defibrillator patches.
- While relatively uncommon in the industrialized world, pericardial tuberculosis remains a major cause of constrictive pericarditis in the immunocompromised host and in underdeveloped countries.

PATHOPHYSIOLOGY

- Constrictive pericarditis markedly restricts filling volumes of all cardiac chambers.
- This symmetrical restriction results in elevation and equilibration of filling pressures of all of the cardiac chambers.
- During early diastole elevated atrial pressures cause rapid ventricular filling. At mid-diastole the rigid pericardium causes ventricular filling to abruptly stop. As a result, almost all ventricular filling occurs in early diastole.
- While myocardial systolic function is preserved, the stroke volume is decreased due to impaired diastolic filling.

CLINICAL PRESENTATION

- Patients with constrictive pericarditis typically present with right heart failure symptoms.
- Early symptoms include lower extremity edema and vague abdominal complaints.
- As hepatic congestion worsens, symptoms progress to anasarca, ascites, jaundice, and cardiac cirrhosis.
- As constriction progresses patients develop exertional dyspnea, cough, and orthopnea due to elevated pulmonary venous pressures.
- End-stage constrictive pericarditis is characterized by severe fatigue, weight loss, and muscle wasting.

PHYSICAL EXAMINATION

- Physical examination reveals jugular venous distension with rapidly collapsing x and y descents. At the bedside, two prominent descents are visible with each cardiac cycle.
- Right atrial pressure paradoxically rises with inspiration; as a result jugular venous distension increases with inspiration (Kussmaul sign).

- Pulsus paradoxus (a 10 mm Hg drop is systolic blood pressure with inspiration) is present in one-third of patients with constrictive pericarditis.
- A pericardial knock, an early diastolic sound heard best at the apex and left sternal border, may be audible. The pericardial knock has a higher acoustic frequency than an S_3. The pericardial knock corresponds to early abrupt cessation of ventricular filling.
- Lower extremity edema and anasarca are often present and reflect right ventricular failure.
- Patients with hepatic congestion can develop massive hepatomegaly with palpable venous pulsations, ascites, jaundice, spider angiomata, and palmar erythema.
- A significant number of patients with constrictive pericarditis will develop atrial fibrillation and tricuspid regurgitation.
- Pleural effusions are occasionally present and may precede other symptoms or signs of constrictive pericarditis.

DIAGNOSTIC MODALITIES

- Chest x-ray may reveal right atrial enlargement and an enlarged cardiac silhouette.
- Pericardial calcification on chest x-ray should raise suspicion for tuberculous pericarditis.
- CT usually reveals pericardial calcification and thickening.
- Although the ECG is usually abnormal, it is nonspecific.
- The surface echocardiogram reveals a bright and thickened pericardium.
- Doppler flow velocity measurements reveal exaggerated respiratory variation in both mitral and tricuspid inflow velocities.

HEMODYNAMICS

- Right atrial (RA) pressure during cardiac catheterization reveals prominent x and y descents.
- The characteristic hemodynamic feature of constrictive pericarditis is the *square root sign*. At the onset of diastole there is a deep and rapid decline in right and left intraventricular pressures. During early diastole elevated atrial pressures induce rapid ventricular filling. During mid-systole the noncompliant pericardium causes an abrupt decrease in filling with a diastolic pressure plateau.
- Due to symmetrical constriction, right and left heart catheterization reveal elevation and equilibration of RA, right ventricular (RV) end-diastolic, pulmonary wedge, and left ventriclar end-diastolic pressures (~20 mm Hg).
- Normally, the RV and LV systolic pressures fall concordantly with inspiration and rise concordantly with

expiration. During constrictive pericarditis, the RV systolic pressure increases with inspiration. Due to the rigid pericardium surrounding the RV, this results in displacement of the interventricular septum into the LV. As a result, during inspiration, RV systolic pressure increases and LV systolic pressure decreases, a phenomenon known as respirophasic discordance.

TREATMENT

- Constrictive pericarditis is a progressive disease and surgical pericardiectomy is the only definitive treatment.
- In echocardiographic analysis, LV diastolic function returned to normal in 40% of patients early and in 57% of patients late after pericardiectomy.
- Medical management with diuretics and salt restriction provides symptom relief, but patients eventually become refractory.
- Sinus tachycardia is a compensatory mechanism; therefore β-blockers and calcium channel blockers should be avoided.

RESTRICTIVE CARDIOMYOPATHY

ETIOLOGY

- The hallmark of restrictive cardiomyopathy (RCM) is impaired ventricular filling with preserved systolic function.
- During RCM the ventricles require an elevated pressure to achieve a normal end-diastolic volume.

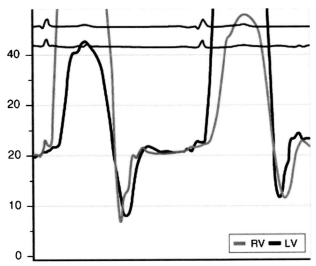

FIG. 44–3 Spontanous right ventricular and left ventricular pressure tracings in a patient with constrictive pericarditis. Tracings display equalization of diastolic pressure as well as *dip and plateau* morphology. LV, left ventricle; RV, right ventricle.

- A variety of pathologic processes may produce RCM
  - Noninfiltrative diseases: idiopathic cardiomyopathy, familial cardiomyopathy, hypertrophic cardiomyopathy, scleroderma, diabetic cardiomyopathy
  - Infiltrative diseases: amyloidosis, sarcoidosis, Gaucher disease, Hurler disease.
  - Storage disorders: hemochromatosis, Fabry's disease, and glycogen storage disease.
  - Endomyocardial disease: endomyocardial fibrosis, hypereosinophilic syndrome, carcinoid heart disease, metastatic cancer, radiation fibrosis, anthracycline, and other drug-induced fibrous endocarditis.
- Amyloidosis, especially primary (AL) amyloidosis, is a common cause of RCM.
  - Primary amyloidosis is caused by accumulation of an amyloid protein comprised of immunoglobulin light chains.
  - RCM in cardiac amyloidosis is due to replacement of normal myocardial contractile elements by infiltrative amyloidogenic deposits.
  - Cardiac amyloidosis is a common complication in primary amyloidosis and the most frequent cause of death.
- Hemochromatosis is characterized by iron accumulation in a variety of tissues.
  - Myocardial damage in hemochromatosis is thought to be due to direct tissue toxicity of the free iron moiety rather than tissue infiltration.
  - Cardiac events are responsible for death in one-third of patients with hemochromatosis.
- In sarcoidosis, a granulomatous disorder of unknown etiology, infiltration of the lungs, skin, and reticuloendothelial system dominate the clinical picture.
  - Cardiac involvement in sarcoidosis is not often recognized clinically, but is found in 20% to 30% of patients at autopsy.
  - Noncaseating granulomas infiltrate the myocardium and form fibrotic scars.
  - Sarcoid myocardial infiltration initially results in ventricular stiffening and diastolic dysfunction. Large portions of the ventricular wall may be replaced by scar leading to systolic dysfunction and aneurysm formation.

CLINICAL PRESENTATION

- Patients with RCM frequently present with exercise intolerance, dyspnea, orthopnea, fatigue, edema, and ascites.
- Exercise intolerance is due to impaired cardiac output.
- In advanced RCM hepatic congestion can result in edema, anasarca, and ascites.

- Patients with cardiac amyloidosis can present with angina and angiographically normal coronary arteries. Patients with cardiac amyloidosis may also present with conduction abnormalities, syncope, or orthostatic hypotension. Symptoms of systolic dysfunction are a common late presentation of cardiac amyloidosis.
- Sudden cardiac death is, unfortunately, a common presentation of cardiac sarcoidosis.
- Other frequent manifestations of cardiac sarcoidosis include ventricular arrhythmias, heart block, and syncope.
- One-third of patients with idiopathic RCM may present with thromboembolic complications.

PHYSICAL EXAMINATION

- Physical examination reveals jugular venous distension with rapidly collapsing *x* and *y* descents.
- Kussmaul sign may be present.
- In contrast to constrictive pericarditis, the left ventricular maximal impulse is usually prominent.
- A third heart sound may be present and, rarely, a fourth heart sound.
- Regurgitant murmurs are common.
- Peripheral edema, ascites, hepatomegaly, and a pulsatile liver are present in advanced cases.
- Patients are usually normotensive or hypotensive.

DIAGNOSTIC EVALUATION

The ECG may reveal biatrial enlargement and right ventricular hypertrophy. Sick sinus syndrome and atrial arrhythmias (especially atrial fibrillation) are common. AV and intraventricular conduction delays are common in cardiac amyloidosis and sarcoidosis.

ECHOCARDIOGRAM
- The echocardiogram characteristically reveals marked biatrial enlargement.
- Increased wall thickness and LV mass may also be seen, especially in cardiac amyloidosis.
- Patients with cardiac sarcoidosis will often have a dilated LV and regional wall motion abnormalities.

HEMODYNAMICS
- Cardiac catheterization reveals prominent *x* and *y* descents on RA pressure tracings.
- The square root sign seen in constrictive pericarditis is also present in RCM. At the onset of diastole there is a deep and rapid decline in right and left intraventricular pressures. During early diastole elevated atrial pressures cause rapid ventricular filling. During midsystole the noncompliant myocardium causes left and right ventricular filling to cease and the ventricular pressures plateau.
- Severe pulmonary hypertension and a RV systolic pressure >50 mm Hg are often present.

TREATMENT

- Excessive diuretic use in RCM may decrease ventricular filling pressures, leading to decreased cardiac output, hypotension, and hypoperfusion.
- Digoxin should be used with caution since it is potentially arrhythmogenic in patients with amyloidosis.
- The development of atrial fibrillation and the loss of atrial contraction may worsen diastolic dysfunction. It is therefore important to maintain sinus rhythm.
- Anticoagulation is recommended, especially in patients with atrial fibrillation, mitral regurgitation, and low cardiac output, due to the increased risk for atrial appendage thrombus formation.
- The median survival for cardiac amyloidosis is less than one year. Less then 5% survive more than 5 years. The prognosis remains poor despite intervention with alkylating-agent based chemotherapy.
- The course for cardiac sarcoidosis is variable with some patients progressing rapidly to death.

RESTRICTIVE VERSUS CONSTRICTIVE

- The presentation and course of constrictive pericarditis and RCM overlap in many respects and their differentiation is mandatory due to the potential for successful surgical treatment of constrictive pericarditis.
- On physical examination the LV maximal impulse is prominent in RCM and not palpable in constrictive pericarditis. A pericardial knock is consistent with constrictive pericarditis. However, the pericardial knock may be mistaken for the loud third heart sound commonly audible in RCM.
- Mitral and tricuspid regurgitation are more common in RCM.
- RCM typically is associated with increased wall thickness, while constrictive pericarditis has normal wall thickness.
- The atria are dilated more often in RCM than in constrictive pericarditis.
- On echocardiogram the pericardium can sometimes possess a thick, bright appearance in constrictive pericarditis.

- Pulmonary HTN is common in RCM and rare in constrictive pericarditis. A RV systolic pressure >60 mm Hg is indicative of RCM.
- The square root sign is seen in both constrictive pericarditis and RCM.
- Respiratory changes in LV and RV systolic pressures are concordant in RCM and discordant in constrictive pericarditis.
- Endomyocardial biopsy, CT, or MRI are useful in differentiating the two diseases by revealing myocardial scarring or infiltration (on biopsy) or pericardial thickening or calcification (on CT or MRI).

BIBLIOGRAPHY

Permanyer-Miralda G. Acute pericardial disease: approach to the aetiologic diagnosis. *Heart.* 2004;90:252–254.

Oakley C. Myocarditis, pericarditis and other pericardial diseases. *Heart.* 2000;84:449–454.

Schifferdecker B, Spodick DH. Nonsteroidal anti-inflammatory drugs in the treatment of pericarditis. *Cardiol Rev.* 2003;11: 211–217.

Little W, Freeman G. Pericardial disease. *Circ.* 2006;113: 1622–1632.

45 CONGENITAL HEART DISEASE IN THE ADULT

Abhay Laddu and Aaron Tang

ADULT CONGENITAL HEART DISEASE

GENERAL CONSIDERATIONS

- It is estimated that 85% of infants with cardiac anomalies reach adulthood.
- Approximately 750,000 American adults have congenital heart disease.
- Congenital cardiovascular malformations are generally the result of aberrant embryonic development of a normal structure, or failure of such a structure to progress beyond an early stage of embryonic or fetal development.
- Recognized chromosomal aberrations and mutations of single genes account for <10% of all cardiac malformations.

PATHOPHYSIOLOGY

- The anatomic and physiologic changes in the heart and circulation caused by congenital cardiocirculatory lesions are not static but rather progress from prenatal life to adulthood.
- Thus, malformations that are benign or escape detection in childhood may become clinically significant in the adult.

ACYANOTIC CONGENITAL HEART DISEASE WITH A LEFT-TO-RIGHT SHUNT

ATRIAL SEPTAL DEFECT

- Background
  - Atrial septal defect (ASD) is the most common congenital heart defect *seen in adults*. There is a female to male predominance.
  - ASD is usually asymptomatic in early life, but some patients appear physically underdeveloped and have a propensity for respiratory infections.
  - Cardiorespiratory symptoms occur in patients as they age.
  - The ASD can arise near the entry of the superior vena cava (*sinus venosus*; 10% of ASDs), at the atrioventricular junction (*ostium primum*; 15% of ASDs), or in the midseptum of the atria (*ostium secundum*; 75% of ASDs).
  - *Ostium primum* ASDs are often associated with trisomy 21 (Down syndrome).
  - *Patent foramen ovale* is a normal anatomical variant and not a true ASD.
- Signs and symptoms
  - Hemodynamic abnormalities correlate with the severity of the shunt.
  - Beyond the fourth decade, a significant number of patients develop atrial arrhythmias, pulmonary arterial hypertension, bidirectional shunting which advances to right-to-left shunting of blood, and cardiac failure.
  - Paradoxical emboli can occur, even with small ASDs.
  - Characteristic physical examination findings include prominent right ventricular (RV) impulse and *fixed and widely split second heart sound*. If pulmonary hypertension develops, a prominent P2 will be audible.
- Diagnostic evaluation
  - Electrocardiogram (ECG) reveals right bundle branch block in 90% of cases.
  - Chest radiograph may reveal prominent pulmonary vasculature, from increased pulmonary blood flow.

○ Surface echocardiography can identify the location of the ASD. The transesophageal echocardiography is more reliable in determining the size and location of the ASD.
• Management
○ Surgical or percutaneous closure can be performed for large, hemodynamically significant *ostium secundum* ASDs.
○ Endocarditis prophylaxis with antibiotics are not routinely recommended, because the risk of endocarditis is low.

VENTRICULAR SEPTAL DEFECTS

• Background
○ Most common congenital heart defect *in infants and children.*
○ Forty percent of ventricular septal defects (VSDs) close spontaneously by age 2 years.
○ Equally affects males and females.
○ Typical location of VSD is in the membranous septum (70% of VSDs).
○ Ventricular septal defects can also be located in the muscular septum (20% of VSDs) and near either the aortic or atrioventricular valves.
○ Hemodynamic significance depends on the size of the defect and the systemic and pulmonary vascular resistances.
○ Patients may develop pulmonary vascular obstruction, RV outflow tract obstruction, aortic regurgitation, and/or infective endocarditis.
• Signs and symptoms
○ The VSD murmur is characterized by a *loud, holosystolic sound* heard best along the left sternal border.
▪ Intensity of murmur does not correlate with the degree or severity of the VSD (ie, small, restrictive VSDs generally produce a loud murmur owing to a large intraventricular pressure gradient).
○ Adults with uncorrected VSDs and normal pulmonary pressures are generally asymptomatic.
○ *Eisenmenger complex* is characterized by a VSD with pulmonary hypertension and shunt reversal.
▪ Initially, there is left-to-right shunting with normal pulmonary vascular resistance.
▪ As blood flow increases through the pulmonary circuit, pulmonary vascular resistance increases and ultimately leads to bidirectional shunting followed by *permanent right-to-left shunting.*
▪ Patients with Eisenmenger physiology are *cyanotic* with severe pulmonary hypertension and often have *digital clubbing.*

• Diagnostic workup
○ Electrocardiographic findings vary depending on the size and significance of the defect.
▪ Small VSDs generally do not cause ECG abnormalities, whereas with large VSDs, the ECG may reveal left ventricular hypertrophy (LVH) and right ventricular hypertrophy (RVH).
○ The chest radiograph may reveal cardiomegaly and pulmonary vascular engorgement.
○ Echocardiography with color Doppler interrogation can usually define the number and location of defects in the ventricular septum as well as detect associated anomalies.
• Management
○ Surgical correction of VSDs should occur before the onset of pulmonary hypertension.
○ The severity of pulmonary hypertension is a critical determinate of prognosis.
▪ Once the pulmonary vascular resistance–to–systemic vascular resistance ratio exceeds 0.7, surgical closure is not useful.
○ These patients are at a moderate-to-high risk of developing endocarditis, and therefore require prophylactic antibiotics for selected procedures.

PATENT DUCTUS ARTERIOSUS

• Background
○ Patent ductus arteriosus (PDA) accounts for up to 10% of congenital heart disease.
○ The ductus arteriosus is a vessel leading from the bifurcation of the pulmonary artery to the aorta just distal to the left subclavian artery.
○ It is normally open in the fetus to allow right ventricular blood to bypass the high-resistance pulmonary vasculature during fetal development. This passageway usually closes within 15 hours after birth.
○ Flow across the ductus is determined by the pressure and resistance relationships between the systemic and pulmonary circulations and by the cross-sectional area and length of the ductus.
○ In most adults with a PDA, pulmonary pressures are normal and a gradient and shunt from the aorta to the pulmonary artery persist throughout the cardiac cycle, resulting in the characteristic palpable thrill and *continuous machinery murmur.*
○ Mothers of patients with a PDA may have had a history of maternal rubella infection.
• Signs and symptoms
○ There is late systolic accentuation of the classic continuous *machinery* murmur.
○ Murmur is loudest below the left clavicle.
○ Congestive heart failure usually develops at a young age.

- Patients who reach their teen years and are asymptomatic generally remain asymptomatic for the remainder of their lives.
- Rarely, adults develop exertional dyspnea, fatigue, and palpitations.
- Large left-to-right shunts through the PDA can lead to pulmonary vascular obstruction, Eisenmenger physiology with severe pulmonary hypertension, and right-to-left shunting.
- Unoxygenated blood is shunted to the descending aorta.
  - The toes, but not the fingers, develop cyanosis and clubbing, termed *differential cyanosis.*
- The leading cause of death is cardiac failure and infective endocarditis.
- Diagnostic evaluation
  - With small shunts, the ECG is normal.
  - The ECG may reveal LVH and left atrial enlargement when the shunt is large.
  - If pulmonary hypertension develops, RVH is seen on the ECG.
  - Chest radiography may reveal nonspecific pulmonary vascular engorgement.
  - Echocardiography with Doppler interrogation can reveal continuous high-velocity flow in the pulmonary trunk; The PDA can usually be visualized by two-dimensional echocardiography.
- Management
  - Surgical ligation is recommended, even for small PDAs, given their high infective endocarditis risk.
  - Patent ductus arteriosus can also be closed percutaneously with a closure device.
  - Correction of the PDA is contraindicated in patients with Eisenmenger physiology.
  - Prophylactic antibiotics are recommended for most procedures.

ACYANOTIC CONGENITAL HEART DISEASE WITHOUT A SHUNT

CONGENITAL AORTIC STENOSIS

- Background
  - Congenital aortic stenosis accounts for approximately 7% of congenital heart disease.
  - Most patients younger than age 65 years who develop aortic stenosis have a bicuspid aortic valve.
    - Commisural fusion of two of the three leaflets causes a raphe.
  - Congenital aortic stenosis is four times more common in males than females.
  - Occasionally, congenital aortic stenosis is associated with other congenital lesions.

- Over time, the bicuspid valve is exposed to increased hemodynamic stress.
- Calcium deposits on the diseased valve lead to premature valve stenosis and/or regurgitation.
- Congenital aortic stenosis is often associated with aortic root dilatation.
- Signs and symptoms
  - Carotid upstroke has diminished intensity and is delayed (*pulsus parvus et tardus*).
  - Systolic ejection murmur radiates to the carotid arteries.
    - Murmur peaks later in systole as the stenosis becomes more severe.
  - Soft aortic second sound component of the second heart sound.
  - Symptoms usually do not develop until the aortic valve area is reduced to less than 1.0 cm^2 (normal value in adults is 3.0–4.0 cm^2).
  - Symptoms are identical to those seen in patients with acquired aortic stenosis and are characterized by the classic triad:
    - *Angina*: median survival once angina develops is 5 years
    - *Exertional syncope*: median survival after syncope develops is 3 years
    - *Dyspnea/heart failure*: median survival after congestive heart failure develops is 2 years
- Diagnostic evaluation
  - The electrocardiogram may reveal LVH and left-axis deviation.
  - Aortic valve calcification can be seen on plain films of the chest.
  - Echocardiography demonstrates a bicuspid aortic valve with heavy calcification.
  - Aortic valve area can be accurately calculated by echocardiographic parameters or by hemodynamic parameters measured via cardiac catheterization.
  - A valve area of less than 0.8 cm^2 is considered severe.
- Management
  - Patients with symptomatic aortic stenosis should undergo aortic valve replacement (unrepaired symptomatic aortic stenosis carries a 5-year mortality rate of 90%).
  - Antibiotic prophylaxis prior to select procedures is recommended for patients with a bicuspid aortic valve.

COARCTATION OF THE AORTA

- Background
  - Narrowing or constriction of the lumen of the aorta.
  - The most common location is distal to the origin of the left subclavian artery near the insertion of the ligamentum arteriosum.

- Coarctation of the aorta is more frequent in males than females.
- Patients with gonadal dysgenesis (Turner syndrome) frequently present with coarctation of the aorta.
- Coarctation of the aorta is often associated with other congenital heart conditions, especially bicuspid aortic valve.
- Aneurysmal arterial dilatation of the circle of Willis produces a high risk of sudden rupture and death.
- Aortic coarctation should be considered in adults who develop hypertension in their second or third decade.
- Untreated coarctation is associated with a mean lifespan of 40 years; death is secondary to congestive heart failure, aortic dissection, ruptured intracranial aneurysm and infection of the site.
- Pregnant women with aortic coarctation are at high risk for aortic dissection.
- Signs and symptoms
  - Physical examination may reveal hypertension in the upper extremities and markedly diminished or absent femoral arterial pulses (pulse differential).
  - Late systolic murmur may be heard between the scapulae, representing blood flow through the coarctation.
  - Additional systolic and continuous murmurs over the lateral thoracic wall may reflect increased flow through dilated and tortuous collateral vessels.
  - Clinical manifestations depend on the location of the lesion and the severity of the obstruction.
  - Common clinical manifestations include headache, epistaxis, cold extremities, hypertension at a young age, and claudication with exercise.
- Diagnostic evaluation
  - The electrocardiogram is nonspecific but may reveal signs of LVH.
  - Chest films can demonstrate rib-notching, which is highly specific for coarctation.
  - Chest films may also show *the 3 sign*: indentation of the aorta at the site of coarctation, with a dilated left subclavian artery forming the upper curvature and the dilated distal aorta forming the lower curvature.
  - Echocardiography can prove difficult in visualizing the coarctation. Color Doppler assessment can aid in diagnosis and can be used to calculate a transcoarctation pressure gradient.
  - Computed tomography, magnetic resonance imaging, and aortic angiography are all helpful in diagnosing coarctation and can pinpoint the location of the lesion.
- Management
  - Surgical correction is recommended to prevent long-term complications of congestive heart failure, premature coronary artery disease, and cerebral aneurysm rupture.
  - High rates of recurrent coarctation and residual hypertension occur in patients older than 40 years who undergo surgical correction.

- Percutaneous correction is considered second line to surgical approaches.
- Prophylactic antibiotics prior to select procedures are recommended for patients with coarctation.

CYANOTIC CONGENITAL HEART DISEASE WITH INCREASED PULMONARY BLOOD FLOW

COMPLETE TRANSPOSITION OF THE GREAT VESSELS

- Background
  - In D-transposition of the great vessels, the aorta arises from the right ventricle to the right of and anterior to the pulmonary artery, which emerges from the left ventricle. This results in two separate and parallel circulations.
    - To survive, there must be mixing of oxygenated and deoxygenated blood via either a PDA, ASD, or VSD.
  - Two-thirds of infants do not have an associated shunt and rely on the ductus arteriosus or foramen ovale for communication between the parallel circulations. These infants are critically ill with severe cyanosis.
    - In these infants, an interatrial shunt is created (usually by percutaneous atrial balloon septostomy).
  - One-third of infants have some type of communication (usually an ASD or VSD) and are less symptomatic.
  - D-transposition of the great vessels occurs with a male to female predominance.
  - Without treatment, there is a 90% mortality at 1 year.
  - Prognosis depends on the severity of tissue hypoxia and the ability of the right ventricle to maintain systemic aortic pressures.
- Signs and symptoms
  - Patients with D-transposition of the great vessels present with profound cyanosis.
  - Physical examination often shows signs of other congenital cardiac lesions.
- Diagnostic evaluation
  - The electrocardiogram may reveal evidence of RVH, right-axis deviation, and right atrial enlargement.
  - Prominent pulmonary vasculature is evident on the chest radiograph.
  - Echocardiography confirms the diagnosis.
- Management
  - Surgical options
    - Atrial switch operations (Mustard or Senning)
      - Pulmonary venous return and systemic venous return are redirected at the level of the atrium via a baffle system.

- Pulmonary venous return is directed across the tricuspid valve to the morphologic right ventricle, which becomes the systemic ventricle
- Systemic venous return is directed across the mitral valve to the morphologic left ventricle
- Long-term complications: arrhythmias, ventricular failure, and baffle obstruction
  - Newer procedures aim to restore the morphologic left ventricle as the systemic ventricle, and may ultimately prove superior
- Prophylactic antibiotics are required for select procedures

CYANOTIC CONGENITAL HEART DISEASE WITH DECREASED PULMONARY BLOOD FLOW

TRICUSPID ATRESIA

- Background
  - Malformation characterized by the following:
    - Tricuspid valve atresia
    - Interatrial communication
    - Hypoplastic right ventricle and pulmonary artery
  - Tricuspid atresia is usually associated with interatrial communication.
  - Primary problem is diminished blood flow to the pulmonary circuit, causing severe cyanosis.
  - Pulmonary blood flow is often supplied by aortopulmonary collateral vessels or by a PDA.
- Signs and symptoms
  - Severe cyanosis caused by obligatory admixture of systemic and pulmonary venous blood in the left ventricle
  - Infants present with congestive heart failure
- Diagnostic evaluation
  - An ECG characteristically shows right atrial enlargement, left-axis deviation, and LVH.
  - Echocardiography delineates the anatomy.
  - Magnetic resonance imaging can also be used to visualize and characterize the defects.
- Management
  - Surgical options are aimed at increasing pulmonary blood flow and are generally palliative as opposed to curative.
  - The Fontan procedure redirects the systemic venous return directly to the pulmonary circulation.

TETRALOGY OF FALLOT

- Background
  - Most common form of cyanotic congenital heart disease
  - Accounts for 10% of all congenital cardiac abnormalities

- Four anatomic abnormalities:
  1. Large, malaligned VSD
  2. Right ventricular outflow tract (RVOT) obstruction
  3. Overriding aorta of the VSD in the right and left ventricles
  4. Right ventricular hypertrophy
  - Size of VSD and degree of RVOT obstruction determine the functional significance of this disease
    - With a large VSD, right and left ventricular pressures are generally equilibrated.
    - If RVOT obstruction is severe and systemic vascular resistance (SVR) is comparatively low, there is significant right-to-left shunting of unoxygenated blood and cyanosis (blood flow follows the path of least resistance).
    - Severe cyanosis and erythrocytosis can occur, and symptoms and sequelae of systemic hypoxemia are prominent.
  - Often associated with other congenital cardiac lesions
  - May occur in patients with DiGeorge syndrome
- Signs and symptoms
  - Cyanosis at birth
  - Digital clubbing may exist
  - Right ventricular heave, with absent pulmonic second heart sound
  - Systolic ejection murmur consistent with RVOT obstruction
  - Children develop dyspnea on exertion and learn to squat after exercise, which increases SVR, thus decreasing right-to-left shunting
  - *Tet spells* are characterized by dizziness/syncope, tachypnea, and worsening cyanosis and are caused by episodic hypoxia
    - Believed to be caused by spasm of the RVOT
    - Can be fatal
  - Patients develop reactive erythrocytosis and can develop significant problems with hyperviscosity (such as stroke)
- Diagnostic evaluation
  - The ECG shows right atrial enlargement and RVH.
  - Chest radiograph shows a boot-shaped heart (*coeur en sabot*), with prominence of the RV. Pulmonary vascular markings are diminished.
  - 2-dimensional echocardiography with color Doppler shows the large VSD, pulmonic stenosis, and severe RVH.
  - If tetralogy of Fallot was corrected during infancy or childhood, echocardiography is performed to assess the functional status of surgical baffles or shunts.
- Management
  - Without surgical correction, most patients die by their teens.
  - Avoid any medications that decrease SVR (such as vasodilators).

◦ In the past, surgical interventions were aimed at increasing pulmonary blood flow by directing venous return to the pulmonary arteries.
  ▪ Fraught with long-term complications
◦ Newer surgical techniques aim at complete surgical correction.
◦ High risk of endocarditis, so prophylactic antibiotics are required before select procedures.

BIBLIOGRAPHY

Brickner EM, Hillis LD, Lange RA. Medical progress: congenital heart disease in adults, first of two parts. *N Engl J Med.* 2000;342:256–263.

Brickner EM, Hillis LD, Lange RA. Medical progress: congenital heart disease in adults, second of two parts. *N Engl J Med.* 2000;342:334–342.

Gatzoulis MA, ed. *Adult Congenital Heart Disease: A Practical Guide.* Boston, MA: Blackwell Publishers; 2005.

Moodie DS. Adult Congenital Heart Disease. *Curr Opin Cardiol.* 1994;9:137–142.

Tede N, Foster E. *Congenital Heart Disease in Adults. Current Diagnosis and Treatment in Cardiology.* 2nd ed. Crawford M, editor. McGraw-Hill; 2003:398–443.

Thierrien J, Webb GD. *Congenital Heart Disease in Adults. Heart Disease: A Textbook of Cardiovascular Medicine.* 6th ed. Braunwald E, Zipes DP, Libby P, eds. PA: WB Saunders; 2001: 1592–1621.

Section 6
ENDOCRINOLOGY AND METABOLISM

46 DIABETES MELLITUS

Sahar Hachem and Marla Bernbaum

EPIDEMIOLOGY

- Diabetes mellitus (DM) is a chronic debilitating condition that affects more than 150 million adults worldwide, and this number is expected to double in the next 25 years.
- At present, approximately 15 to 17 million adults in the United States have diabetes, with 5 to 6 million unaware of their disease.
- The prevalence of type 2 diabetes is higher in African Americans, Asian Americans, Pacific Islanders, Hispanic Americans, and Native Americans compared with whites.[1]

PHYSIOLOGY

- In the postabsorptive state, the majority of glucose metabolism takes place in insulin-independent tissues with 50% occurring in the brain, 25% in the splanchnic area (liver plus gastrointestinal tissues), and the remaining 25% in insulin-dependent tissues (primarily muscle and to a lesser extent, adipose tissue). Approximately 85% of endogenous glucose production is derived from the liver, and the remaining 15% is produced by the kidney.
- Following glucose ingestion, the increase in plasma glucose concentration stimulates insulin release, leading to increased glucose uptake by splanchnic and peripheral tissues and suppression of endogenous glucose production (gluconeogenesis and glycogenolysis).
- Insulin inhibits lipolysis, causing a decrease in the plasma level of free fatty acid, and further enhancement of muscle glucose uptake and inhibition of hepatic glucose production.
- In the absence of insulin, gluconeogenesis and glycogenolysis proceed unchecked, and lipolysis liberates free fatty acids, which will undergo β-oxidation and produce ketone bodies.[2]

CLASSIFICATION

- Type 1 (previously designated *insulin-dependent diabetes mellitus* [IDDM])
  - An autoimmune disease in which the β-islet cells of the pancreas are destroyed, resulting in severe insulin deficiency; antibodies to insulin and β-cell components (eg, glutamic acid decarboxylase [GAD] antibodies) are often present.
  - Associated with HLA DR3, DR4 genotype; DR2 appears to be protective.
  - Patients are ketosis prone without treatment and usually younger than 35 years of age at onset.
  - Less than 50% of monozygotic twins and 10% to 15% of siblings develop type 1 diabetes.
  - Idiopathic type 1 (type 1b) diabetes has the same characteristics without the autoimmune components.[3]
- Type 2 (previously designated *noninsulin-dependent diabetes* [NIDDM])
  - A disease of insulin resistance with β-islet cell dysfunction.
  - Resistance occurs at the level of muscle and adipose tissue resulting in defective glucose disposition and increased fasting and postprandial gluconeogenesis and glycogenolysis.
  - Insulin levels can be elevated, normal, or low; 30% to 40% of patients require insulin treatment.
  - Eighty percent of patients are obese (except in Asian populations where obesity is <60%).
  - Patients are usually older than 40 years of age, but there is an increasing prevalence in young obese people.

○ Twenty-five percent of probands have an affected parent or sibling.[3]
• Gestational diabetes mellitus (GDM)
  ○ Refers to diabetes diagnosed during pregnancy.
  ○ The glucose level usually returns to normal in the postpartum period.
  ○ GDM is associated with a higher risk for DM later in life.
• Miscellaneous types
  ○ Can be caused by genetic defects in β-cell function (maturity-onset diabetes in the young [MODY] subtypes) and in insulin action, or associated with some genetic syndromes.
  ○ Can be secondary to trauma or primary disease of the pancreas (chronic pancreatitis).
  ○ Some endocrinopathies are associated with insulin resistance (ie, acromegaly, Cushing's syndrome, glucagonoma, hyperthyroidism, and pheochromocytoma).
  ○ Can be drug or chemical induced (pentamidine, glucocorticoids, phenytoin, thiazides, β-blockers, nicotinic acid) or secondary to certain infections (congenital rubella, cytomegalovirus).[3]
• Prediabetes
  ○ Impaired glucose uptake by cells but with blood glucose levels below the criteria for diabetes
  ○ Classified as either impaired glucose tolerance (IGT) or impaired fasting glucose (IFG)

DIAGNOSIS

CRITERIA FOR NONPREGNANT INDIVIDUALS

• Fasting blood glucose (FBG) greater than 126 mg/dL on two separate days, or overt symptoms of diabetes with random glucose levels elevated above 200 mg/dL, or a blood glucose level greater than 200 mg/dL following an oral glucose tolerance test (OGTT) using a 75-gram glucose challenge. (The two-hour OGTT is rarely required.)[3]

CRITERIA FOR PREDIABETES

• IGT is defined by a blood glucose greater than 140 mg/dL but less than 200 mg/dL 2 hours after a 75-gram OGTT.
• IFG is defined by a FBG greater than 100 mg/dL but less than 126 mg/dL.

CRITERIA FOR DIAGNOSIS OF GDM

• Pregnant women with a fasting plasma glucose (FPG) greater than 95 mg/dL or with a 1-hour

postprandial glucose greater than 130 mg/dL following 50 grams of oral glucose should receive a 3-hour OGTT using a 100-gram glucose bolus. The diagnosis of GDM requires any two of the four plasma glucose values at fasting, 1, 2, and 3 hours to exceed 95 mg/dL, 180 mg/dL, 155 mg/dL, and 140 mg/dL, respectively.
• Screening for GDM is recommended during the 24th through 28th week of gestation for women older than 25 years, who are overweight, have a previous history of GDM, a family history of DM, or those belonging to high-risk ethnicity groups (African American, Hispanic, Native American).
• Women with GDM should be screened 6 to 12 weeks postpartum for diabetes or prediabetes.[3]

CRITERIA FOR SCREENING ASYMPTOMATIC INDIVIDUALS

• Testing for DM should be considered in all individuals at age 45 years and older, and, if normal, it should be repeated at 3-year intervals.
• Testing should be considered at a younger age or more frequently in individuals who match the following criteria:
  ○ Obese (body mass index [BMI] >25 kg/m^2)
  ○ First-degree relative with a diagnosis of diabetes
  ○ Member of a high-risk ethnic population (African American, Hispanic, and Native American)
  ○ Delivered a baby weighing >9 lb or diagnosed with GDM
  ○ Hypertension (>140/90 mm Hg), peripheral vascular disease, acanthosis nigricans, or polycystic ovary syndrome
  ○ High-density lipoprotein (HDL) cholesterol level <35 mg/dL and/or triglyceride level >250 mg/dL
  ○ IGT or IFG on previous testing
• Although the OGTT or FPG test can be used to diagnose diabetes, the FPG test is preferred because of ease, convenience, acceptability to patients, and lower cost.[3]

SIGNS AND SYMPTOMS AT PRESENTATION

• Classic triad is polyuria, polydipsia, and polyphagia.
• Type 1 and some type 2 patients with concurrent illness can present with diabetic ketoacidosis (DKA) (10–40% of African Americans with type 2 diabetes will present with DKA); symptoms include nausea, vomiting, abdominal pain, hyperventilation (Kussmaul breathing), lethargy, and fruity breath.

- Blurred vision occurs when glucose in the lens is converted to sorbitol which produces an osmotic change and results in lens swelling.
- Type 2 diabetes can present as an incidental laboratory finding without signs or symptoms; in contrast, some patients with type 2 diabetes can *present* with long-term sequelae such as neuropathy, dermopathy, and retinal or renal pathology.

PRINCIPLES OF MANAGEMENT

Management includes insulin therapy with integration of diet, exercise, and glucose monitoring for type 1, and diet and weight loss with or without oral antiglycemic agents, insulin, insulin-enhancement agents, and glucose monitoring for type 2. For all patients, cardiac risk factors including excessive weight, dyslipidemia, and hypertension should be identified and treated.

NUTRITION THERAPY

- Patients with diabetes should receive individualized nutrition therapy.
- Use of exchanges or carbohydrate counting is recommended.
- Use of the glycemic index/glycemic load is beneficial.
- Low-carbohydrate diets (total carbohydrate <130 g/d) are not recommended.
- The 2006 nutritional recommendations for patients with diabetes are summarized in Table 46–1.
- The goal of therapy is to prevent and treat the chronic complications of diabetes by attaining and maintaining optimal metabolic control to provide adequate calories for adults, sustain normal growth and development for children and adolescents, and to meet increased metabolic needs for pregnancy, lactation, or recovery from a catabolic illness.[4]

TABLE 46–1   2006 Nutritional Recommendations for People with Diabetes

COMPONENT AND AMOUNT/DAY
Protein[a] 15–20% of the total calories
Total fat[b] <25–35% of the total calories
Saturated fat + trans fat <7% of the total calories
Carbohydrate >130 g/d
Cholesterol <200 mg/d
Sodium[c] <2300 mg/d
Fiber >14 g/1000 cal

[a]Protein for persons with nephropathy: 0.8 g/kg/d (= 10% of the total calories).
[b]Remainder of the total fat is polyunsaturated and monounsaturated fat; if high triglycerides increase the monounsaturated fat with a moderate decrease in carbohydrate (CHO).
[c]Sodium (Na) for patients with congestive heart failure (CHF): <2000 mg/d.

PHYSICAL ACTIVITY

- Regular exercise has been shown to improve blood glucose control, reduce cardiovascular risk factors, contribute to weight loss, and improve well being.
- At least 150 min/wk of moderate-intensity aerobic physical activity (50–70% of maximum heart rate) and/or at least 90 min/wk of vigorous aerobic exercise (>70% of maximum heart rate) distributed over at least 3 d/wk is recommended.
- Consider a graded exercise test with electrocardiographic (ECG) monitoring before prescribing an exercise regimen. The intensity of the regimen should exceed the demands of everyday living in previously sedentary diabetic individuals (whose 10-year risk of a coronary event is likely to be ≥10%).
- Exercise in insulin-treated patients must be coordinated with meals and insulin use.
- Exercise can exacerbate hyperglycemia or ketosis in type 1 diabetics if vigorous activity is performed when metabolic control is poor.
- In individuals taking insulin and/or insulin secretagogues, physical activity can promote hypoglycemia if the medication dose or carbohydrate consumption is not altered. To avoid hypoglycemia, consider ingestion of 15 to 30 grams of carbohydrate for each 30 minutes of exercise, or reduce the dose of rapid or short-acting insulin prior to exercise. Self-monitoring of blood glucose (SMBG) is recommended before and after vigorous exercise.[5]

PHARMACOLOGIC ANTIGLYCEMIC THERAPY

- Oral antiglycemic agents should be used in type 2 patients who have failed diet therapy alone.
- Oral agents can be used in combinations or in conjunction with insulin in type 2 patients and can also be used in combination with other available antiglycemic (insulin-enhancing) agents.
- Other insulin-enhancing agents including glucagon-like peptide-1 (GLP-1) agonists, dipeptidyl peptidase-4 inhibitors, and synthetic amylin agonists are now available.
- The comparative profile of available antiglycemic agents for treatment of type 2 diabetes is summarized in Table 46–2.

INSULIN AND INSULIN-ANALOG THERAPY

The pharmacokinetic parameters of injectable human insulin and insulin-analog preparations available in the United States are summarized in Table 46–3. Standard

TABLE 46–2   Comparative Profile of Available Oral Antiglycemic Agents[6]

ANTI GLYCEMIC AGENT	MODE OF ACTION	EXPECTED DECREASE IN HBA$_{1C}$ (%)	ADVANTAGES	DISADVANTAGES	CONTRA INDICATIONS
Biguanide (Metformin)	Decrease hepatic glucose production. Increase glucose uptake. No effect on insulin secretion.	1.5	Weight stability or modest weight loss. Inexpensive	GI side effects. Rare lactic acidosis	Renal, liver, & heart failure. Hypoxemic states with radiographic contrast procedures.
Sulfonylurea (glyburide, glipizide, glimepiride)	Enhance insulin secretion	1.5	Inexpensive	Hypoglycemia (use cautiously in frail elderly). Weight gain	Sulfonylurea allergy. Renal failure
Meglitinides (repaglinide, nateglinide)	Stimulate insulin secretion (target PPH)	1–1.5^a	Rapid onset & short duration	Three times daily dosing. Weight gain. Hypoglycemia. Expensive	Renal failure
Thiazolidinediones (rosiglitazone, pioglitazone)	Increase sensitivity to insulin	0.5–1.4	Pioglitazone causes significant improvement in TG, HDL & LDL concentration	Weight gain, fluid retention. Expensive. Occasional hepatotoxicity	Liver failure NYHA class III, IV CHF
α-Glucosidase inhibitors (acarbose, miglitol)	Reduce the absorption of carbohydrates in the proximal small intestine (target PPH)	0.5–0.8		GI side effects. Three times daily dosing. Expensive	Diarrhea. No safety data for creatinine clearance <25mL/min
GLP-1 agonists (exenatide)^b	Enhance insulin secretion (target PPH). Suppress glucagon secretion. Slow gastric motility.	0.5–1	Weight loss (2–3 kg in 6 months)	Twice daily SC injections. GI side effects (nausea and vomiting)	
DPP-4 inhibitors (sitagliptin)^c	Block degradation of GLP-1	0.6–1.4	Long-acting once daily oral tablet. Minimal GI side effects. No effect on weight.		
Amylin agonist (pramlintide)^d	Slows gastric emptying. Inhibits glucagon-induced hepatic gluconeogenesis (target PPH). Increases satiety	0.5–0.7	Weight loss (1–1.5 kg in 6 months)	Injected SC before meals. GI side effects (nausea and vomiting)	

CHF, chronic heart failure; DPP-4, dipeptidyl peptidase; GI, gastrointestinal; GLP-1, glucagon-like peptide-1;HbA$_{1c}$, glycosylated hemoglobin; HDL, high-density lipoprotein; LDL, low-density lipoprotein; NYHA, New York State Heart Association; PPH, postprandial hyperglycemia; SC, subcutaneous; TG, triglyceride.
^{a}Repaglinide is more effective at lowering HbA$_{1c}$ than Nateglinide.
^{b}Approved for use with sulfonylureas and/or metformin.
^{c}Approved for use alone and with metformin or thiazolidinediones.
^{d}Synthetic human analog of the β-cell hormone amylin that is approved as adjunctive therapy with insulin.

human insulin is synthesized using a recombinant DNA process. Structural alterations in human insulin produce insulin analogs with varying pharmacokinetic characteristics. Inhaled insulin is now also available.

INHALED INSULIN (EXUBERA)

- Efficacy comparable to subcutaneous premeal insulin.
- Faster onset of action than insulin lispro.

TABLE 46–3   Human Insulin and Insulin Analog Preparations Available in the United States[7]

INSULIN PREPARATIONS	ONSET (H)	PEAK (H)	DURATION (H)
Standard Insulin			
Short-acting			
Regular[a] Humulin R/Novolin R	0.5–1	2–3	6–8
Intermediate-acting			
NPH Humulin N/Novolin N	1.5–4	4–10	16–24
Mixtures			
70/30 Humulin/Novolin (70% NPH, 30% regular)	0.5–1	3–12	16–24
50/50 Humulin (50% NPH, 50% regular)	0.5–1	2–12	16–24
Insulin Analogs			
Rapid-acting			
Insulin lispro (Humalog)	0.2–0.5	0.5–2	3–4
Insulin aspart (NovoLog)	0.2–0.5	0.5–2	3–4
Insulin glulisine (Apidra)	0.2–0.5	0.5–2	3–4
Intermediate to long-acting			
Insulin detemir (Levemir)	1–3	No peak	14–20
Long-acting			
Insulin glargine (Lantus)	1–3	No peak	20–30
Mixtures			
75/25 Humalog (75% NPL, 25% lispro)	0.2–0.5	1–4	16–24
50/50 Humalog (50% NPL, 50% lispro)	0.2–0.5	1–4	16–24
70/30 NovoLog Neutral (70% protamine aspart, 30% aspart)	0.2–0.5	1–4	16–24

NPH, neutral protamine Hagedorn; NPL, neutral protamine lispro; NPA, neutral protamine aspart.
[a]All preparations are concentrated as U-100 (100 units/mL) with the exception of additional regular insulin available in U-500.

- Duration of action: intermediate between insulin lispro and regular insulin.
- Less than 10% of the inhaled dose is absorbed (requiring significant dosage adjustments compared with subcutaneous insulin).
- Use in conjunction with intermediate or long-acting insulin in type 1 diabetes and with oral agents, intermediate or long-acting insulin in type 2 diabetes.
- Reduces lung diffusion capacity (although this effect is not believed to be clinically significant).
- Contraindicated in lung diseases and smokers because of altered absorption and action.

INITIATION AND ADJUSTMENT OF THERAPY FOR TYPE 1 PATIENTS

- Type 1 diabetes is best treated with a combination of background basal insulin and premeal short- or rapid-acting insulin. The basal insulin is preferably initiated as insulin glargine, although twice daily neutral protamine Hagedorn (NPH) insulin or insulin detemir are alternative approaches. The rapid-acting insulin analogues are preferred for prandial coverage.
- Many patients with type 1 diabetes can benefit from continuous subcutaneous insulin infusion therapy delivered by commercially available insulin pumps.

Initiation of insulin pump therapy should be individualized, considering the patient's preferences, lifestyle, and self-care capabilities.

- There are numerous approaches to the initiation of insulin therapy, however, the treatment must be tailored to the individual needs of each patient. Two reasonable approaches are outlined below:
- *Regimen I*
  - The total insulin requirement is estimated to be 0.5 to 0.6 units/kg; lower initial doses can be used in patients with low body weight or those demonstrating high sensitivity to insulin.
  - Approximately two-thirds of the total insulin is given 30 minutes before breakfast using a combination intermediate (NPH) and short-acting (regular) insulin in a ratio of 2:1.
  - One-sixth of the total dose is given 30 minutes before supper as regular insulin and one-sixth of the total insulin dose is given as NPH at bedtime.
  - Rapid-acting insulin can be substituted for regular and given immediately before the meal.
  - Adjust dosages according to glucose response; do not adjust NPH insulin more often than every 48 hours.
- *Regimen II*
  - The total insulin requirement is estimated to be 0.5 to 0.6 units/kg.

○ Half of the total dose is administered using a basal long-acting insulin (glargine) given at bedtime.

○ Approximately one-sixth of the total dose is given as a rapid-acting insulin administered thrice daily before meals, adjusted to match the intake of dietary carbohydrate. Begin with an insulin-to-carbohydrate ratio of 1:15 (1 unit of insulin per 15 grams carbohydrate) and adjust the ratio according to glucose response.

○ A supplemental rapid-acting insulin dose (correction dose) can be added to correct for blood-glucose excursions before meals. The correction dose is calculated by dividing 1800 by the total daily insulin requirement to estimate the amount of blood glucose (mg/dL) lowered per 1 unit of insulin. (Experts disagree as to the denominator [1800 versus 1700], and 1500 is substituted if regular insulin is used).

○ Adjust glargine according to the FBG, increasing by 1 to 2 units for each 20 mg/dL of FBG over 100 mg/dL, and allowing 5 days between further increments.

○ When glucose control is stable, glargine can be shifted to any convenient consistent time each day, although, glargine injection in the morning reduces the frequency of overnight and early morning hypoglycemia.

○ Approximately one-third of type 1 patients experience a waning effect of glargine before the end of a 24-hour cycle, and require splitting the dose to twice daily.

○ Twice daily injection of detemir is an alternative to glargine.

INITIATION AND ADJUSTMENT OF THERAPY FOR TYPE 2 PATIENTS

• Lifestyle intervention is the first step in treating new-onset type 2 diabetes. However, as lifestyle intervention alone fails to achieve metabolic goals in most individuals, some diabetologists recommend the concurrent initiation of metformin, in the absence of contraindications.

• If lifestyle intervention and metformin fail to achieve glycemic goals, another medication should be added within 2 to 3 months (insulin, a sulfonylurea, or a thiazolidinedione [TZD]).

• If lifestyle, metformin, and a second medication do not result in a glycosylated hemoglobin (HbA$_{1c}$) <7%, start or intensify insulin therapy. Although three oral agents can be used, insulin therapy is preferred because of effectiveness and expense. Addition of an incretin (GLP-1 agonist or dipeptidyl peptidase-4 inhibitor) is another alternative to initiation of insulin.

• A starting dose of 10 to 15 units of intermediate or long-acting insulin given at bedtime can be added to existing oral antiglycemic agents. The dose is subsequently increased, usually by 2 units every 3 days until fasting levels are in the target range (70–130 mg/dL).

• If hypoglycemia occurs or fasting glucose levels are <70 mg/dL, the bedtime dose should be decreased by ≥4 units or 10% if the dose is higher than 60 units.

• If the HbA$_{1c}$ is still ≥7% after 2 to 3 months and the FBG is in target range, check blood glucose before lunch, dinner, and bedtime, and depending on the results, one or more insulin injections can be added.

• If prelunch blood glucose is out of range, add rapid or short-acting insulin at breakfast.

• If prebed blood glucose is out of range, add rapid or short-acting insulin at dinner.

• If predinner blood glucose is out of range, add NPH insulin at breakfast or rapid or short-acting insulin at lunch.

• The preprandial insulin dose can be prescribed according to individual sensitivities and the amount of carbohydrate to be ingested, or a regimen similar to that for type 1 diabetes can be used. In general, a dose of approximately 4 units is prescribed and then adjusted by 2 units every 3 days until the blood glucose is in range.

• Insulin should be the initial pharmacologic therapy if there are marked hyperglycemic symptoms, severe concurrent illness, contraindications to oral agents, or pregnancy.[6]

GLUCOSE MONITORING

• HbA$_{1c}$ is measured every 3 months during stabilization of therapy; once the targeted goal has been achieved, measurement can be limited to 6-month intervals.

• There is a correlation of HbA$_{1c}$ with long-term complications.

• The target HbA$_{1c}$ is <7.0% (American Diabetes Association [ADA] recommendation) or <6.5% (American Association of Clinical Endocrinologists [AACE] recommendation), eg, as close to the normal range (<6.0%) as possible without subjecting the patient to repetitive episodes of hypoglycemia.

• Self-monitoring of blood glucose (SMBG) is essential to properly adjust therapy, particularly insulin. The number of required daily SMBG measurements depends on the medications used. For patients on oral hypoglycemic regimens that are unlikely to induce hypoglycemia, routine SMBG may not be imperative but can provide feedback on meal and exercise effects. Insulin therapy requires more frequent monitoring (usually premeal as well as at bedtime).

- Additional SMBG may be necessary, for example at 2:00 AM or 1 to 2 hours after a meal to assess overnight hypoglycemia and postprandial glycemic excursions, respectively.
- The optimal glucose targets for insulin-treated non-pregnant adults are fasting and premeal levels between 90 and 130 mg/dL and bedtime levels between 110 and 150 mg/dL (ADA recommendation). If premeal glucose values are within the target range but the HbA_{1c} is not, monitoring the 1 to 2 hour post-prandial glucose to achieve a target <180 mg/dL may engender a fall in HbA_{1c}.
- For women with GDM, recommendations from the Fourth International Workshop-Conference on Gestational Diabetes suggest lowering maternal capillary blood glucose concentrations to ≤95 mg/dL fasting, ≤140 mg/dL at 1 hour, and/or ≤120 mg/dL at 2 hours after a meal.

MANAGEMENT FOR HOSPITALIZED PATIENTS

Insulin-treated patients, eating on a routine schedule, should continue home insulin regimens with adjustments according to premeal and bedtime blood glucose.

- Preparation and management for procedures or surgery
  - Insulin-treated patients who are taking nothing orally before a procedure should be scheduled for the procedure as early in the morning as possible. Start an intravenous infusion of 5% dextrose in water (D5W), or dextrose 5% in half normal saline (D51/2NS) at 125 cc/h, to run from the early morning until the procedure is completed and the patient is able to eat.
  - On the morning of the procedure, give one-half the usual dose of NPH insulin and omit the usual short- or rapid-acting insulin. If the procedure is completed by mid-morning, give the remainder of NPH with short-acting insulin, followed by a late breakfast. If the procedure is over after noon, resume the usual evening insulin schedule. An additional bolus of short-acting insulin may be required, depending on the blood glucose if a midday meal is planned.
  - Patients normally treated with basal glargine or detemir with premeal short-acting insulin can be given the full basal dose at the usual time of the evening or morning prior to the procedure, with the premeal short- or rapid-acting insulin withheld. Type 2 patients who use glargine or detemir as the sole insulin should have the dose reduced by 30% to 50%.
  - Blood glucose should be monitored before the procedure and every 4 hours until the patient is ready to eat. Treat a blood glucose over 180 mg/dL with supplements of regular insulin.

  - For insulin-treated patients undergoing long procedures (longer than 1 hour) follow the steps above with additional hourly blood glucose checks during the procedure or treat with a continuous intravenous insulin infusion, started at midnight prior to the procedure, and titrated to maintain glucose between 100 and 180 mg/dL. A separate intravenous infusion of 5% dextrose should be maintained.
  - Oral agents should be discontinued before long procedures and supplemented with subcutaneous short-acting insulin administered every 4 to 6 hours before, during, and after the procedure.
  - Metformin must be discontinued prior to surgery and all procedures requiring intravenous radiocontrast media.
- *Critically ill and postoperative patients*
  - Benefit has been established for aggressive glucose management in acute myocardial infarction (MI), postcardiac surgical patients, and possibly other critically ill patients. Intravenous insulin infusion protocols should be followed to maintain the level of blood glucose at least below 180 mg/dL, although less than 140 mg/dL appears preferable.
  - Intravenous bolus insulin should not be used in this setting as the half-life of intravenous insulin is 4 to 8 minutes.
  - All patients who are unable to eat should receive a minimum of 150 grams of daily carbohydrate to prevent ketone production (5% dextrose at 125 cc/h or 10% dextrose at 60–70 cc/h).
  - Oral antiglycemic agents are not used to treat critically ill or perioperative patients.
  - Stabile patients who are insulin-requiring and are eating normal meals should be treated with intermediate or long-acting insulin, which can be combined with premeal short- or rapid-acting insulin. Attempts should be made to establish routine doses of longer acting and premeal short- or rapid-acting insulin rather than "chasing" hyperglycemia with "sliding scale" insulin. Correction doses (supplemental short- or rapid-acting insulin) given in response to elevated glucose measurements should be used to calculate adjustments in subsequent daily insulin regimens.[8,9]

DIABETIC EMERGENCIES

- DKA and hyperglycemic hyperosmolar syndrome (HHS) are two of the most serious acute complications of diabetes.
- Hypoglycemia is another life-threatening acute complication requiring immediate treatment.

PATHOGENESIS OF DKA AND HHS

- The underlying mechanism for both disorders is secondary to a decrease in the concentration of circulating insulin associated with an increase in counter-regulatory stress hormones (glucagon, catecholamines, cortisol, and growth hormone).
- In patients with DKA, the absolute insulin deficiency results in increased activity of tissue lipase causing a breakdown of triglyceride into glycerol and free fatty acids (FFAs). FFAs are oxidized to ketone bodies causing ketoacidosis.
- Patients with HHS have a residual amount of insulin secretion that minimizes ketosis.
- When insulin is deficient, hyperglycemia results from increased gluconeogenesis, accelerated glycogenolysis, and impaired glucose use by peripheral tissues.
- Gluconeogenesis plays an important metabolic role. High levels of gluconeogenic substrates, such as amino acids (caused by accelerated proteolysis and decreased protein synthesis), lactate (caused by increased muscle glycogenolysis), and glycerol (caused by increased lipolysis) result in increased gluconeogenesis.
- In DKA and HHS, hyperglycemia causes an osmotic diuresis resulting in loss of water and electrolytes, dehydration, and decreased glomerular filtration rate (GFR), which further increase the severity of hyperglycemia. Hyperosmolarity develops in HHS patients because of prolonged osmotic diuresis coupled with poor fluid intake.[10,11]

DIABETIC KETOACIDOSIS

- Usually occurs in patients with type 1 diabetes; can occur in patients with type 2 diabetes subjected to severe stress, with increasing frequency reported among African American and Hispanic adults and children with type 2 diabetes.
- *Precipitating factors*
  - Include undiagnosed and untreated diabetes, omission of insulin or inadequate insulin treatment, trauma, severe infection, MI or cerebrovascular accident (CVA), perioperative stress and any severe physical or emotional stress.
- *Signs and symptoms*
  - Include nausea, vomiting, abdominal pain, severe dehydration, hyperventilation (Kussmaul breathing), and lethargy or coma.
- *Laboratory findings*
  - Glucose usually above 250 mg/dL but occasionally lower.
  - Acidosis with low arterial pH (<7.3), low serum bicarbonate (<18 mEq/dL), and increased anion gap.

- Positive serum and urine ketones.
- Serum potassium usually initially high, but falls precipitously with insulin and fluid infusion, and correction of acidosis. Careful monitoring of the serum potassium concentration during treatment is essential.
- Elevated serum blood urea nitrogen (BUN); elevation of creatinine may be a laboratory artifact because of ketone interference with the assay.
- Hypophosphatemia may not be apparent until after therapy is initiated.
- Elevated white blood cell (WBC) count can be caused by demargination of white blood cells in the absence of infection.
- *Treatment*
  - Consists of administration of fluids and insulin, and correction of electrolyte abnormalities.
  - Administer intravenous normal saline rapidly (1–1.5 L/h) for the first hour; after the first 1 to 2 liters, change to half normal saline to replace fluid deficit and ongoing losses (at least 4 to 6 liters) over 24 hours.
  - Initiate intravenous insulin bolus (0.15 units/kg) to saturate receptor sites, followed by insulin intravenous infusion (0.10 units/kg/h); then titrate to maintain a serum glucose of 250 mg/dL until the acidosis has resolved.
  - When glucose falls below 200 to 250 mg/dL, add 5% dextrose to the infusion to avoid starvation ketosis, protect against hypoglycemia, and reduce the risk for cerebral edema.
  - Administer bicarbonate only if the arterial pH is below 7.0 or vascular instability persists in spite of fluid management.
  - When the serum potassium is <5.3 mEq/L and the urine output is adequate, add 20 to 30 mEq potassium/L to the infusion (usually as potassium chloride), to maintain a serum potassium of 4.0 to 5.0 mEq/L.
  - Phosphate therapy is unnecessary unless serum phosphate falls below 1.0 mg/dL, or signs of severe hypophosphatemia are present. If phosphorous is required, add 20 to 30 mEq/L potassium phosphate to the infusion instead of potassium chloride.
  - Monitor every 1 to 2 hours until stable. A flow sheet should record hourly glucose, bicarbonate, venous pH, and potassium with periodic checks of BUN, creatinine, and other electrolytes.
  - Ketone levels, measured by a nitroprusside test, can fluctuate as only acetoacetate and acetone are measured and conversion from β-hydroxybutyrate to acetoacetate accelerates as serum pH increases. If available, measurements of serum β-hydroxybutyrate may prove useful. Normalization of the anion gap and increased bicarbonate levels are also reliable parameters of resolving ketoacidosis.

○ After the patient is stable for 8 to 24 hours, start subcutaneous insulin; do not discontinue the IV insulin drip during the late afternoon or overnight hours, particularly if there are insufficient available personnel to monitor patient deterioration.
○ Begin subcutaneous regular insulin at least 1 hour prior to discontinuing the IV infusion to prevent a gap in circulating insulin.[10,11]

HYPEROSMOLAR HYPERGLYCEMIC STATE

• *Precipitating factors*
  ○ Occurs in stressed type 2 non–ketone-prone diabetics often elderly patients who present with trauma, severe infection, or other catastrophic event, and are unable to replace fluid losses through oral intake.
• *Signs and symptoms*
  ○ Severe dehydration and lethargy or coma.
• *Laboratory findings*
  ○ Blood glucose in excess of 600 mg/dL, mild acidosis caused by lactic acid (pH >7.3), elevated serum osmolality (>320 mOsm/kg), marked pre-renal azotemia and variable serum sodium concentration.
• *Treatment*
  ○ Fluid replacement with normal saline followed by half normal saline with small doses of insulin (via continuous intravenous infusion) cautiously administered with blood glucose monitoring. Potassium and magnesium deficits are common and should be monitored carefully.
  ○ After glucose stabilization, subcutaneous insulin therapy can be initiated. Patients who were not treated with insulin prior to the event may not require insulin after resolution of the episode. Those discharged on insulin will require careful glucose monitoring throughout and after convalescence, as insulin requirements diminish.[10,11]

HYPOGLYCEMIA

• Occurs frequently with insulin treatment and occasionally with oral hypoglycemic agents, often as a result of unplanned exercise, inadequate intake of carbohydrate, or inappropriate dosing.
• *Symptoms*
  ○ Warning symptoms, resulting from discharge of autonomic nervous system, include nervousness, palpitations, tachycardia, diaphoresis, nausea, paresthesias of the extremities and the perioral area.
  ○ Neuroglycopenic symptoms are caused by central nervous system (CNS) glucose deprivation and include confusion, erratic emotional states, lethargy, convulsions, and coma.

○ Hypoglycemic unawareness refers to neuroglycopenia which occurs without warning symptoms. This syndrome is sometimes observed in tightly controlled insulin-treated patients, the elderly and those with longstanding diabetes who have impaired autonomic responses, and if there has been an antecedent hypoglycemic episode in the previous 24 hours.
○ Nocturnal hypoglycemia is characterized by restless sleep, nightmares, night sweats, and hypothermia.
○ The Somogyi effect refers to rebound hyperglycemia due to counter regulation that occurs several hours after a hypoglycemic episode. This may account for swings in blood glucose throughout the day, especially after overnight hypoglycemia. The treatment involves decreasing the overnight insulin or changing the timing of the intermediate-acting insulin from predinner to bedtime so that peak insulin activity occurs in the early morning hours.
• *Hypoglycemia requires immediate treatment*
  ○ In conscious patients who are able to eat, 15 to 30 grams of carbohydrate should be given (fruit juice, soda, glucose tablets, etc).
  ○ Unconscious patients who have intravenous access should receive 1 ampule of 50% dextrose IV.
  ○ Patients without IV access, who are unable to eat, should receive 1 mg glucagon by subcutaneous or intramuscular injection.
  ○ Patients on oral agents with severe hypoglycemia require hospitalization and treatment with dextrose infusion until glucose levels can be normalized and remain stable.

CHRONIC COMPLICATIONS

FACTORS CONTRIBUTING TO DEVELOPMENT OF COMPLICATIONS

• Glycemic control correlates with complications (Diabetes Control and Complications Trial {DCCT} and United Kingdom Prospective Diabetes Study {UKPDS}
• Duration of diabetes
• Genetic factors
• Coexisting medical problems: eg, hypertension, dyslipidemia, obesity

RETINOPATHY

• *Nonproliferative diabetic retinopathy (NPDR)*
  ○ Occurs eventually in all type 1 and >60% of type 2 diabetes
  ○ Staged as mild, moderate, severe, or very severe

○ Usually subclinical with microaneurysms, dot-blot hemorrhages and hard exudates.

○ Macular edema or hemorrhages near the fovea may cause severe vision impairment.

• *Proliferative diabetic retinopathy (PDR)*

○ Occurs in 25% of type 1 diabetes after 15 years, and in >70% of type 1 and 25% of type 2 diabetes over the lifetime of the patient.

○ Neovascularization with retinal tears, detachments, and scarring can lead to severe vision impairment or blindness.

○ Can be associated with neovascular glaucoma (caused by neovascularization of the iris or *rubeosis*).

• *Clinically significant macular edema*

○ Can coexist with either NPDR or PDR

○ Secondary to thickening with impaired perfusion of the central macula, threatening central vision

○ Major cause of vision loss especially in type 2 diabetes

○ Responds to early photocoagulation therapy (Early Treatment Diabetic Retinopathy Study [ETDRS])

• *Recommendations*

○ To reduce risk and progression of diabetic retinopathy both optimal glycemic control and blood pressure are essential.

○ A dilated eye examination by an ophthalmologist or optometrist should be performed within 3 to 5 years after the onset of type 1 diabetes and in patients with type 2 diabetes at diagnosis.

○ Repeat the eye examination annually or more frequently if there is evidence of progressive retinopathy.

○ Glaucoma, cataracts, cranial nerve palsies, papillopathy, and corneal trauma/infections can occur in people with diabetes and should also be evaluated.

○ Photocoagulation is delivered panretinal for all patients with high risk PDR and type 2 diabetes with severe NPDR, and is delivered locally for clinically significant macular edema; vitrectomy is reserved for patients not responsive to photocoagulation or for retinal repair.[5]

NEPHROPATHY

• Diabetic nephropathy occurs in 20% to 40% of patients with diabetes and is the leading cause of end-stage renal disease (ESRD) in industrialized nations.

• *Clinical course*

○ Hyperfiltration at the onset of diabetes.

○ Silent phase with no albuminuria, but early glomerular lesions may last for 10-15 years.

○ Microalbuminuria is the first clinical sign after 5–15 years: 30 to 300 mg/24 h (20–200 mcg/min)

○ After an additional 5-10 years, patients will develop nephrotic range proteinuria and decreasing glomerular filtration rate (GFR)

○ End-stage renal failure occurs in almost all patients with nephrotic range proteinuria.

• *Recommendations*

○ To reduce the risk and/or slow the progression of nephropathy, optimize glucose and blood pressure limit protein intake to 1.0 g/kg (if the serum creatinine exceeds 2.0-3.0 mg/dl) and initiate pharmacotherapy with an angiotensin-converting enzyme (ACE) inhibitor or an angiotensin II receptor blocker (ARBs). Dual therapy with an ACE inhibitor and ARB may further retard progressive renal injury. Published data indicates that ACE inhibitors are preferred for type 1 diabetic nephropathy whereas the ARBs are preferred in type 2 diabetic nephropathy.

○ Screen for microalbuminuria by either measuring the albumin-to-creatinine ratio in a spot early morning urine or perform a 24-hour collection. These studies should be carried out in all type 1 diabetic patients with a diabetes duration of ≥5 years and in all type 2 diabetic patients, starting at diagnosis and then yearly.[5]

MACROVASCULAR DISEASE

• Coronary artery disease (CAD) is the major cause of mortality in patients with diabetes, develops prematurely and is equally prevalent in men and women. The United Kingdom Prospective Diabetes Study (UKPDS) showed an 11% increased CAD risk for each 1% increase in HbA_{1c}.

• Diabetes is independently correlated with an increased incidence of cerebrovascular disease.

• Peripheral vascular disease, when present, is associated with an increased incidence of infection, gangrene, and amputation.

• *Recommendations*

○ Perform a diagnostic cardiac stress test for typical or atypical cardiac symptoms and/or an abnormal resting ECG.

○ Perform a screening cardiac stress test for a history of peripheral or carotid occlusive disease, a sedentary lifestyle, and age greater than 35 years prior to beginning a vigorous exercise program.

○ Screen for lipid disorders annually; the target lipid level in the diabetic is a low-density lipoprotein (LDL) cholesterol <80 mg/dL, triglycerides <150 mg/dL, and HDL cholesterol >40 mg/dL in men and >50 mg/dL in women.

○ Screen for hypertension; the goal blood pressure is <130/80 mm Hg.

○ Screen for albuminuria, and if present, begin either an ARB or ACE inhibitor.

○ Use aspirin therapy (75–162 mg/d) if other cardiovascular risk factors are present or if the patient has a history of cardiovascular disease (CVD).

○ Promote life style changes including diet/weight control, physical activity and smoking cessation.[5]

NEUROPATHY

- Can be focal or diffuse
- Usually presents as sensorimotor neuropathy and/or autonomic neuropathy
- *Sensorimotor neuropathy*
  ○ Distal symmetric polyneuropathy is the most common form of diabetic neuropathy and is characterized by paresthesias, sensory loss, and motor weakness of the distal nerves.
  ○ Focal neuropathies, including mononeuropathies and radiculopathies, can affect large mixed sensory/motor nerve trunks (eg, ulnar, median, femoral, spinal, cranial nerves III, IV, VI), usually are asymmetric and generally resolve spontaneously in 3 to 12 months. When multiple nerves are involved, the term *mononeuropathy multiplex* is applied.
  ○ Entrapment syndromes occur frequently, especially carpal tunnel syndrome, and are differentiated from mononeuropathies by electrophysiologic studies.
  ○ Diabetic amyotrophy, also known as femoral neuropathy or proximal motor neuropathy, is often bilateral, and affected patients can develop a neuropathic cachexia syndrome, which is characterized by anorexia, depression, and weight loss. Spontaneous recovery in 6 to 12 months is the rule, however, recurrences have been noted.
  ○ Treatment for pain syndromes consists of optimizing glycemic control, judicious use of analgesics, and trials of tricyclic antidepressants (amitriptyline and imipramine), anticonvulsants (gabapentin, pregabalin), 5-hydroxytryptamine and norepinephrine reuptake inhibitors (duloxetine [Cymbalta]), topical creams (capsaicin [Zostrix]), and α-lipoic acid.
- *Diabetic autonomic neuropathy*
  ○ Major clinical manifestations of diabetic autonomic neuropathy include the following:
    ▪ Cardiovascular: resting tachycardia, exercise intolerance, orthostatic hypotension, and lack of variation in heart rate during activities.
    ▪ Gastrointestinal: mild dysphagia, nausea, vomiting, early satiety, constipation, diarrhea, fecal incontinence.
    ▪ Genitourinary: urinary retention and/or incontinence; urinary tract infections; erectile dysfunction in men; and vaginal dryness, decreased perineal sensation, and dyspareunia in women.
    ▪ Sudomotor: hyperhidrosis and heat intolerance in the upper torso or anhidrosis in the lower extremities and neurovascular dysfunction.
    ▪ Treatment of autonomic neuropathy consists of symptomatic management.

- *Recommendations*
  ○ All patients with diabetes should have an annual foot examination by a healthcare professional and testing for sensation to pinprick, temperature, vibration, 10-gram monofilament pressure, and ankle reflexes.
  ○ Patients should be screened for autonomic neuropathy at the time of the diagnosis of type 2 diabetes and 5 years after onset of type 1 diabetes.[5]

FOOT COMPLICATIONS

Sensorimotor and autonomic neuropathy and peripheral arterial disease (PAD) contribute to diabetic foot complications including skin breakdown, altered foot structure, with redistribution of weight-bearing, and subsequent proclivity to ulcers, infection, and amputation.
- *Recommendations*
  ○ All individuals with diabetes should receive an annual foot examination, which includes assessment of sensory function, vascular status, and skin integrity.
  ○ Screen for PAD.
  ○ Educate patients about proper foot care and refer for special shoes/orthotics.

OTHER COMPLICATIONS

- Dermopathy
  ○ *Shin spots*, necrobiosis lipoidica diabeticorum (NLD), bullous diabeticorum, carbuncles, and folliculitis
- Connective tissue abnormalities
  ○ Reduced flexibility, Dupuytren contractures, shoulder capsulitis
- Common and unusual infections
  ○ Vaginal candidiasis, oral candidiasis, intertriginous infections
  ○ Mucormycosis
  ○ Malignant otitis externa
  ○ Emphysematous cholecystitis and pyelonephritis
  ○ Abscesses and necrotizing soft tissue infections

REFERENCES

1. Bonow RO, Gheorghiade M. The diabetes epidemic: a national and global crisis. *Am J Med.* 2004;116:2S–10S.
2. DeFronzo RA. Pathogenesis of type 2 diabetes mellitus. *Med Clin North Am.* 2004;88:787–835.
3. American Diabetes Association. Diagnosis and classification of diabetes mellitus. *Diabetes Care.* 2006;29:S43–48.
4. American Diabetes Association. Nutrition recommendations and interventions for diabetes–2006: a position statement of the American Diabetes Association. *Diabetes Care.* 2006;29:2140–2157.
5. American Diabetes Association. Standards of medical care in diabetes. *Diabetes Care.* 2006;29:S4–S42.

6. Nathan DM, Buse JB. Management of hyperglycemia in type 2 diabetes: a consensus algorithm for the initiation and adjustment of therapy. *Diabetes Care.* 2006;29:1963–1972.
7. Mooradian AD, Bernbaum M, Albert SG. Narrative review: a rational approach to starting insulin therapy. *Ann Intern Med.* 2006;145:125–134.
8. The ACE/ADA Task Force on Inpatient Diabetes. American College of Endocrinology and American Diabetes Association consensus statement on inpatient diabetes and glycemic control: a call to action. *Diabetes Care.* 2006;29:1955–1962.
9. Inzucchi SE. Management of hyperglycemia in the hospital setting. *N Engl J Med* 2006;355:1903–1911.
10. Kitabchi AE, Umpierrez GE, Murphy MB, et al. Management of hyperglycemic crisis in patients with diabetes. *Diabetes Care.* 2001;24:131–153.
11. Kitabchi AE, Umpierrez GE, Murphy MB, et al. Hyperglycemic crises in adult patients with diabetes: a consensus statement from the American Diabetes Association. *Diabetes Care.* 2006; 29:2739–2748.

BIBLIOGRAPHY

The Diabetes Control and Complications Trial Research Group. The effect of intensive treatment of diabetes on the development and progression of long-term complications in insulin-dependent diabetes mellitus. *N Engl J Med.* 1993;329: 977–986.

UK Prospective Diabetes Study (UKPDS) Group. Intensive blood-glucose control with sulphonylureas or insulin compared with conventional treatment and risk of complications in patients with type 2 diabetes (UKPDS 33). *Lancet.* 1998;352:837–853.

UK Prospective Diabetes Study (UKPDS) Group. Effect of intensive blood-glucose control with metformin on complications in overweight patients with type 2 diabetes (UKPDS 34). *Lancet.* 1998;352:854–865.

The Diabetes Control and Complications Trial/Epidemiology of Diabetes Interventions and Complications Research Group. Retinopathy and nephropathy in patients with type 1 diabetes four years after a trial of intensive therapy. *N Engl J Med.* 2000;342:381–389.

47 DISORDERS OF THE PITUITARY GLAND

Kenneth Patrick L. Ligaray

INTRODUCTION

- The pituitary gland, weighing approximately 600 mg, rests in the sella turcica. It orchestrates the coordinated secretion of other endocrine organs.

  - The anterior pituitary (adenohypophysis) is of ectodermal origin. It is connected to the median eminence of the hypothalamus by the portal vessels. These vessels allow efficient transmission of hormones from the hypothalamus to the pituitary.
  - The posterior pituitary (neurohypophysis) is of neural origin. It is derived from axons originating in the supraoptic and paraventricular nuclei of the hypothalamus.

- The anterior pituitary secretes the following hormones:
  - Growth hormone (GH)
  - Prolactin (PRL)
  - Gonadotropins
    - Follicle-stimulating hormone (FSH)
    - Leuteinizing hormone (LH)
  - Thyrotropin- or thyroid-stimulating hormone (TSH)
  - Adrenocorticotropic hormone (ACTH)
- The posterior pituitary secretes the following hormones
  - Arginine vasopressin (AVP) also known as antidiuretic hormone (ADH)
  - Oxytocin (OT)
- Various hormones modulate pituitary activity
  - Releasing factors
    - Growth hormone-releasing hormone (GHRH) for GH
    - Gonadotropin-releasing hormone (GnRH) for both LH and FSH
    - Thyrotropin-releasing hormone (TRH) for TSH and PRL (partial regulation)
    - Corticotropin-releasing hormone (CRH) for ACTH
  - Inhibitory peptides
    - Dopamine is a potent inhibitor of PRL
    - Somatostatin inhibits GH and TSH
- Other peptides may also modulate pituitary hormones
  - Vasoactive intestinal peptide (VIP) stimulates PRL.
  - Cholecystokinin (CCK) stimulates GH and inhibits TSH.
  - AVP stimulates ACTH.

DISEASES OF THE ANTERIOR PITUITARY

- Usually manifested as insufficiency or excess of one or more hormones
- Insufficiency of various hormones can be caused by tumors, infiltrative diseases, autoimmune phenomena, surgical or traumatic ablation, radiation, infarction and infections. Some are due to genetic or developmental defects.
- Excess of various hormones is usually the result of a tumor, hyperplasia, hypothalamic disease, or drug effect.

HYPOPITUITARISM

- Sudden or gradual decrease in the secretion of pituitary hormones
- Panhypopituitarism refers to generalized secretory deficiency of the anterior pituitary
- Acutely may present as adrenocortical crisis, hypoglycemia, hyponatremia, and increased sensitivity to sedative-hypnotic drugs.
- Clinical manifestations will depend on individual hormonal imbalances as described below as well as the following circumstances
  - Rapidity with which a disease affects anterior pituitary cell function
  - Severity of hormonal deficiency
  - The extent to which different anterior pituitary cells are affected

ETIOLOGY
- Isolated hormone defects are usually idiopathic or secondary to the absence of specific releasing hormones (eg, Kallmann's syndrome, deficiency of GnRH).
- Multiple hormone defects may occur secondary to a malignancy (primary or metastatic), a vascular event (eg, Sheehan syndrome), trauma, sarcoidosis, radiation, surgery, infection (eg, tuberculosis), autoimmune lymphocytic hypophysitis or be idiopathic.

DIAGNOSIS
- Clinical—suspicion based on history, signs, and symptoms should prompt appropriate diagnostic testing.
- Laboratory testing—document subnormal secretion, each hormone must be tested separately.
- Dynamic endocrine testing (stimulation tests)

DISORDERS OF GROWTH HORMONE SECRETION

- Most abundant anterior pituitary hormone. Secreted by somatotropes comprising about 50% of the anterior pituitary cells. Its growth promoting effects are mediated mostly through somatomedins or insulin-like growth factors (IGF).
- The release of growth hormone (GH) is under dual control: GHRH (stimulates) and somatostatin (inhibits). There is also negative feedback to the pituitary from GH and IGF-1.

GROWTH HORMONE DEFICIENCY
- Clinical manifestations
  - Growth retardation in children
  - In pituitary dwarfism, body proportions and primary teeth are normal, but tooth eruption is delayed.
  - In adults: increased abdominal fat, reduced muscle mass, increased LDL, decreased bone mineral density,

easy fatigability, perception of poor quality of life, increased risk of cardiovascular disease and increased inflammatory cardiovascular risk markers.
  - In diabetic patients, insulin requirements decrease.
- Diagnosis
  - Most commonly used tests
    - Insulin-induced hypoglycemia test or insulin tolerance test (best predictor). Regular insulin, 0.05 to 0.15 units/kg, is given IV. GH and glucose measurements are taken at −30, 0, 30, 60, and 120 minutes. Expected response is an increase in serum GH >5 mcg/L approximately 1 hour after the glucose has decreased to <40 mg/dL. Deficiency is confirmed by a peak GH level of <3 mcg/L.
    - Arginine/GHRH test (sufficient sensitivity and specificity to establish diagnosis)
    - Other Stimulation Tests: arginine infusion test, levodopa test, exercise
  - An inadequate increase (GH <5 mcg/L) should be confirmed with two or more stimulation tests.
  - Threshold level is 2.5 mcg/L with the use of newer, more sensitive immunoradiometric assays
  - The presence of deficiencies in three or more pituitary hormones strongly suggests the presence of GH deficiency, and in this context provocative testing may be optional.
- Management
  - Recombinant GH replacement. Start at 0.15 to 0.3 mg/d. Titration of dose is based on clinical response, side effects, and IGF-1 levels (maintain mid-normal range for age and sex).
  - Monitor at 1- to 2-month intervals during the titration phase and semiannually thereafter.
  - GH treatment is contraindicated in the presence of active malignancy, intracranial hypertension, uncontrolled diabetes, and diabetic retinopathy.
  - Use of GH as an anti aging agent or as a performance-enhancing drug for athletes is not indicated.

GROWTH HORMONE EXCESS

- Causes gigantism in *prepubertal* children and *acromegaly* in adults
- Most common cause is a somatotrope adenoma; rarely from excess GHRH, ectopic GHRH, or ectopic GH secretion
- Mixed mammosomatotrope tumors secrete both GH and PRL.
- Mortality is two to three times the expected rate, mostly from cardiovascular disease and cancer.
- Clinical manifestations of acromegaly:
  - Other features of associated hypopituitarism
  - Mass effects related to tumor expansion (visual disturbances)

- Effects of excess GH: skeletal and soft tissue overgrowth, glaucoma, exophthalmos, entrapment neuropathies, diabetes mellitus, hypercalcemia, hyperphosphatemia, hypertriglyceridemia, myopathy, hypertension, heart failure, acanthosis nigricans, fibroma, goiter, and colonic polyps
- Diagnosis
  - Document GH excess
    - Increased IGF-1 (single best test) for age and sex. IGF-1 peaks at puberty then declines thereafter.
    - Failure to suppress GH to <1 mcg/L within 1 to 2 hours after a 75 g oral glucose load
    - Fasting GH >10 mcg/L. Random levels are not recommended
    - Increased IGFPB-3 concentration is of limited utility
    - Optional tests: increase in GH response to TRH and/or L-dopa
  - Tumor localization: magnetic resonance imaging (MRI) of the pituitary is the imaging study of choice; computed tomography (CT) is less sensitive
  - Evaluate associated pituitary hormonal changes.
  - Exclude multiple endocrine neoplasms (MENs) (hyperparathyroidism, pancreatic tumors, thyroid tumors).
- Management
  - Goals of therapy
    - Lower IGF-1 to within the reference range for age and sex.
    - Lower GH levels to <1 ng/mL.
  - Treatment of choice is surgical ablation of the tumor
  - Other approaches to management
    - Medical treatment
      - Somatostatin analogues (octreotide, lanreotide)
      - Dopamine agonists (cabergoline, bromocriptine) especially if cosecreted with PRL.
      - GH receptor antagonists (pegvisomant): Importantly, with this approach GH levels may increase and, therefore, cannot be used for longitudinal monitoring.
    - Radiation therapy.

DISORDERS OF PROLACTIN SECRETION

- Unlike other pituitary hormones, PRL is predominantly under inhibitory control by dopamine. PRL is secreted by lactotropes comprising 20% of the anterior pituitary cells
- Physiologic stimulators of PRL release include TRH, VIP (vasoactive intestinal polypeptide), and estrogens. PRL provides negative feedback to the pituitary.

PROLACTIN DEFICIENCY
- Rare. May occur in panhypopituitarism or Sheehan's syndrome

- Usually manifested as failure of postpartum lactation.
- Stimulation test can be done with the use of TRH 200 to 500 mcg IV. Normal response is an increase in PRL to >2 mcg/L or an increase of >200% from baseline.

PROLACTIN EXCESS
- Most common pituitary hormone hypersecretion syndrome. Almost exclusively secondary to hypersecretion by lactotropes.
- Causes of hyperprolactinemia
  - Physiologic: pregnancy, nipple stimulation, stress
  - Pituitary tumor—most common cause is a prolactinoma; microadenoma <1 cm—female-to-male ratio 20:1; macroadenoma >1 cm
  - Pituitary stalk destruction or compression
  - Hypothalamic disease
  - Hypothyroidism
  - Renal failure—decreased PRL clearance
  - Drugs: phenothiazines, butyrophenones, reserpine, opiates, metoclopramide, tricyclic agents, estrogen
  - Chest wall disease
  - Idiopathic *functional* hypothalamic disease
- Manifestations
  - Premenopausal women: hypogonadism (infertility, oligomenorrhea, amenorrhea), galactorrhea
  - Men: hypogonadism (loss of libido, erectile dysfunction, infertility), less often galactorrhea
  - Can be associated with osteoporosis
  - Mass effects from PRL (headache and visual field deficits)
- Diagnosis
  - Serum PRL level >25 ng/mL in women, >20 ng/mL in men
  - Hook effect—an artifact in the immunoradiometric assay whereby a falsely low PRL level is reported when a large amount of PRL saturates both the capture and signal antibodies in the assay. Can be excluded by diluting the sample.
  - Macroprolactinemia—characterized by an increase in PRL that is bound to IgG. It is usually not clinically significant, since the free PRL levels are normal. Distinguished from hyperprolactinemia by gel filtration.
  - MRI (best) or CT scan of the pituitary reveals adenomas.
  - Visual field evaluation
- Management
  - Indications for treatment
    - Neurological signs and symptoms
    - Hypogonadism or other symptoms attributed to hyperprolactinemia
  - If the patient is asymptomatic one may observe
  - With symptoms (amenorrhea or infertility) dopaminergic agonists should be used

- Bromocriptine in titrated dosage. Start at 0.625 to 1.25 mg at bedtime. Preferred agent in pregnant patients.
- Cabergoline, 0.5 to 1.0 mg twice a week, is an alternative and is less likely to cause nausea.
- Reduce to lowest effective maintenance dose once the PRL level is controlled.
  - Surgery is indicated when medical therapy fails or with sudden growth of the tumor.
  - Radiation is utilized for surgical/medical failures.
  - MRI and visual field testing should be done every 6 to 12 months
  - It is preferred practice to discontinue treatment once pregnancy is diagnosed and to follow patients closely with serial PRL levels and visual field testing. Resume treatment if tumor growth occurs.

DISORDERS OF GONADOTROPIN (FSH/LH) SECRETION

- Secretion is stimulated by GnRH and is inhibited by gonadal steroids. Inhibin (a peptide produced by ovarian granulosa cells in women and Sertoli cells in men) selectively inhibits FSH, while activin (a peptide produced in various tissues, in particular, gonadal, pituitary gland, and placenta) stimulates it. Gonadotropes comprise about 10% of anterior pituitary cells.
- FSH regulates ovarian follicle development and stimulates ovarian estrogen production. It also stimulates seminiferous tubule development and regulates spermatogenesis.
- LH mediates ovulation and maintenance of the corpus luteum. It also induces testosterone synthesis and secretion by the Leydig cells.

GONADOTROPIN (FSH/LH) DEFICIENCY
- Most common clinical syndrome in the adult with panhypopituitarism.
- Either primary pituitary disease or hypothalamic disease.
- Congenital etiologies: isolated idiopathic hypogonadotropic hypogonadism (with or without associated mental retardation), Kallmann's syndrome (anosmia, red-green color blindness, midline facial abnormalities such as cleft palate, urogenital tract abnormalities, and neurosensory hearing loss), mutations in the β-subunit of FSH or LH (rare).
- Acquired etiologies: disorders that affect the hypothalamic-pituitary axis (importantly, a mass lesion in the pituitary will usually decrease secretion of the gonadotropins before ACTH or TSH).
- Excessive exercise, emotional stress, nutritional deficiencies, and critical illness can lead to hypothalamic hypogonadism

- Prolonged use of GnRH analogs, which are used to treat prostate cancer, decrease LH secretion
- Manifestations
  - Amenorrhea or menstrual irregularities, infertility, decreased vaginal secretions, decreased libido, and breast atrophy in women.
  - Sexual dysfunction (decreased libido and potency), infertility, decreased muscle mass, and reduced body hair growth in men.
- Diagnosis
  - Low baseline FSH, LH, and free testosterone levels in males; estradiol determinations in females are low, but considered optional
  - Gonadotropin reserve can be evaluated with a clomiphene stimulation test or GnRH stimulation test. However, GnRH testing adds little information unless there is isolated GnRH deficiency.
  - GnRH 100 mcg IV should increase the LH concentration by 10 international units/L and the FSH concentration by 2 international units/L, but normal responses are variable and depend on age sex, and stage of menstrual cycle.
  - A pituitary tumor should be ruled out with an MRI or CT scan.
- Treatment
  - Testosterone replacement in men. Currently available testosterone formulations include injectable, gel, and patch. Gonadotropin injections or infusions are utilized to restore fertility.
  - In women, cyclic replacement of estrogen and progesterone should be considered to maintain secondary sexual characteristics and prevent premature osteoporosis. Gonadotropin is also used to promote ovulation.

GONADOTROPIN (FSH/LH) EXCESS

- Secretory tumors are exceedingly rare; when present, 85% secrete excessive amounts of FSH rather than LH.
- Rarely tumors previously identified as nonsecretory may evolve to hypersecrete FSH/LH or their α- or β-subunits.
- FSH/LH levels are increased in gonadal failure because of the loss of negative feedback.
- Mildly elevated LH with normal FSH occurs commonly in the polycystic ovarian syndrome (PCOS)
- Management
  - For FSH/LH secretory tumors the treatment of choice is surgical ablation.
  - For gonadal failure the treatment is simply gonadal steroid replacement.
  - For PCOS, the use of oral contraceptive agents can ameliorate hirsutism and provide endometrial protection.

DISORDERS OF THYROTROPIN SECRETION

- Secretion is stimulated by TRH and is inhibited by the thyroid hormones. Thyrotropes comprise about 5% of anterior pituitary cells.
- TSH secretion is also inhibited by somatostatin, dopamine, phenytoin, and glucocorticoids.

THYROTROPIN DEFICIENCY

- Either secondary to primary pituitary disease or hypothalamic disease resulting in poorly glycosylated TSH with low biologic activity.
- Manifestations: same as primary hypothyroidism (See also Chap. 50, Disorders of the Thyroid Gland)
- Diagnosis
  - Low free T4 with normal or low TSH suggests pituitary disease
  - Low free T4 with normal or mildly elevated TSH suggests hypothalamic disease
  - The response of TSH to TRH is not useful in the evaluation of central hypothyroidism despite the underlying pathophysiology.
  - Rule out pituitary tumor (most common cause) with an MRI or CT scan
- Management
  - Levothyroxine replacement is the treatment of choice and is administered in a fashion analogous to the treatment of primary hypothyroidism. Importantly, the free T4 and not TSH must be used to monitor treatment. Pituitary-adrenal function should be evaluated before T4 therapy is initiated, because T4 accelerates cortisol metabolism and, therefore, may precipitate adrenal crisis in patients with pre-existing adrenal insufficiency
  - Central hypothryoidism often requires higher doses compared with patients with primary hypothyroidism, although the mechanism of this is poorly understood.

THYROTROPIN EXCESS

- Pituitary TSH secretory tumors are extremely rare but often large and locally invasive
- TSH hypersecretion may also occur without a tumor
- Manifestation: hyperthyroidism—unless the patient has generalized thyroid hormone resistance (which is usually familial in nature)
- Diagnosis:
  - High free T4 and high TSH
  - Disproportionate increase in the α subunit relative to TSH is strongly suggestive of a tumor.
  - MRI of the pituitary may disclose the presence of a tumor

- Management
  - Transsphenoidal resection of the tumor is effective in roughly 30%. Radiation therapy is not useful.
  - Antithyroid drugs to lower circulating thyroid hormones may benefit some but must be tempered because the decrease in thyroid hormone levels will promote an increase in TSH secretion, which, in turn, may induce expansion of a tumor
  - Somatostatin analogues (octreotide) are effective in almost all patients. Dopamine agonists are less effective but may prove particularly useful in patients with high PRL levels.

DISORDERS OF ADRENOCORTICOTROPIC HORMONE SECRETION

- Adrenocorticotropic hormone (ACTH) secretion is stimulated by CRH and inhibited by glucocorticoids. Corticotropes comprise about 20% of anterior pituitary cells.
- ACTH secretion is pulsatile, peaking at 6 AM, and achieving a nadir at midnight.

ADRENOCORTICOTROPIC HORMONE DEFICIENCY

- Any disease that involves the pituitary can lead to secondary adrenal insufficiency. In rare cases, the ACTH deficiency is isolated but more often it occurs in concert with other pituitary hormonal deficiencies (panhypopituitarism)
- Manifestations
  - Anorexia, weakness, hypotension, hyponatremia, hypoglycemia, diarrhea, and abdominal pain are usually present. Importantly, because aldosterone secretion is normal, the laboratory manifestations are quite different that those observed in primary adrenal insufficiency. In addition, hyperpigmentation is not seen since ACTH levels are low.
- Diagnosis
  - Low ACTH concentration coupled with a low cortisol level.
  - Failure of the cortisol to rise >21 mcg/dL and aldosterone >4 ng/dL 30 to 60 minutes after a dose of 0.25 mg cosyntropin IM or IV.
- Management: as in adrenal insufficiency (glucocorticoid replacement).

ADRENOCORTICOTROPIC HORMONE EXCESS

- Usually secondary to hyperplasia or an adenoma of the pituitary (Cushing disease).
- Can be secondary to adrenal failure because of the loss of negative feedback.

- Nelson's syndrome
  - Nelson's syndrome is the appearance and/or progression of ACTH-secreting pituitary macroadenomas in patients who had previously undergone bilateral adrenalectomy for Cushing's disease.
  - The tumors may be locally invasive.
  - Associated with marked hyperpigmentation because of extremely high levels of ACTH.
- Diagnosis
  - Screen with a 24-hour urine free cortisol or salivary cortisol (both of which should be elevated). If the diagnosis is in question, a 1 mg dexamethasone suppression test can be administered but false negatives are not uncommon.
  - Elevated ACTH level.
  - Differentiate from ectopic ACTH secretion by inferior petrosal sinus sampling or performing a high dose dexamethasone suppression test.
  - MRI or CT of the pituitary to rule out a tumor producing ACTH
- Management
  - The treatment of choice is transsphenoidal tumor resection
  - If surgery is unsuccessful, pituitary irradiation may be attempted. Bilateral adrenalectomy is reserved for refractory cases.

DISEASES OF THE POSTERIOR PITUITARY

DISORDERS OF ARGININE VASOPRESSIN SECRETION

- Arginine vasopressin (AVP) exerts its effects on the cortical collecting duct in the kidney, thus promoting water reabsorption and concentrating the urine. AVP is the principal hormone involved in the regulation of water homeostasis in the body.
- The major factors regulating AVP secretion include
  - Osmoreceptors: as little as a 1% rise in plasma osmolality is sufficient to stimulate AVP release.
  - Baroreceptors: decreased blood pressure stimulates AVP secretion.
  - Volume receptors
    - Decreased plasma volume stimulates AVP release.
    - Up to a 7% loss of plasma volume will not generally alter the circulating concentration of AVP.
    - A deficit in blood volume will, however, render osmoreceptors more sensitive to changes in plasma osmolality.
  - AVP is also secreted in response to stimulation of nociceptive centers (pain and stress); emetic centers (nausea and vomiting); and via chemoreceptors residing in the brainstem (hypercapnia).
  - Drugs
    - Stimulate AVP release: nicotine, clofibrate, chlorpropamide, vincristine, cyclophosphamide, barbiturates, carbamazepine, cholinergic agents, β-receptor agonists
    - Inhibit AVP release: phenytoin, ethanol, glucocorticoids, haloperidol, fluphenazine, α-receptor agonists
- Many stimuli that promote AVP release also promote thirst.
- At high plasma levels, AVP acts on vascular smooth muscle resulting in an increased tone, heightens gastrointestinal motility, induces the release of ACTH and GH, alters thermoregulation and enhances memory.

DIABETES INSIPIDUS

- Classically these patients present with polydipsia and polyuria (>2.5 L/day or >50 mL/kg/day) coupled with a dilute urine (<150 mOsm/L). Because of a slight elevation in serum sodium concentration, otherwise normal patients are extremely thirsty.
- There are two major classes of diabetes insipidus (DI):
  - Vasopressin sensitive (neurogenic or central DI)
    - Etiologies are diverse and include familial; sporadic, secondary to diseases of the hypothalamic/ pituitary unit such as head trauma or neurosurgical procedures; idiopathic forms are also recognized.
  - Vasopressin resistant (nephrogenic DI)
    - Usually familial secondary to mutations in the V2-receptor or aquaporin 2 water channels
    - Secondary causes of vasopressin resistance
      - Renal medullary disease involving the cortical collecting duct (sickle cell disease, multiple myeloma, amyloidosis, Sjögren's syndrome, medullary cystic disease).
      - Hypokalemia, hypercalcemia, protein malnutrition.
      - Drugs (lithium [up to 40%], demeclocycline, amphotericin B, gentamicin, colchicine, loop diuretics, foscarnet)
- Diagnosis
  - Primary polydipsia, which also presents with polyuria, must be distinguished from DI.
  - Importantly, a plasma osmolality exceeding 295 mOsm/kg or a serum Na concentration greater than 143 mEq/L on repeat measurements should exclude the diagnosis of primary polydipsia, which is usually associated with mild hyponatremia.
  - A water deprivation test is rarely required to establish the clinical diagnosis. If water deprivation is pursued, the patient must be hospitalized and monitored carefully for marked blood pressure or serum

sodium excursions. A water deprivation test should only be performed by a certified endocrinologist or nephrologist.

  ■ A normal urinary response to water deprivation is a rise in the serum osmolality to >300 mOsm/kg, urine specific gravity >1.010 and urine osmolality >500 mOsm/kg. In addition, there should be <5% increase in urine osmolality after vasopressin injection (DDAVP 0.03 mcg/kg IV or subQ).

  ■ In central DI, the urine osmolality will increase by 50% following vasopressin administration, whereas, there is either a small or no increase in the setting of nephrogenic DI.

  ○ An increment in urine osmolality of 150 mOsm/kg or an increase of >9% above the baseline in response to aqueous vasopressin (0.1 unit/kg subQ) will exclude nephrogenic DI.

• Essential hypernatremia is an unusual disorder, which is characterized by resetting of the central osmoreceptors (or selective destruction of osmoreceptor-mediated AVP release) without a concomitant change in AVP response to other stimuli. In other words, the AVP response profile is intact, but centered around a new, higher sodium concentration.

• Treatment
  ○ Neurogenic or central DI is treated with the AVP analogue, desamino-8-D-arginine vasopressin (DDAVP). Additional agents which appear to either promote the release of AVP or sensitize the kidney to its actions include chlorpropamide, carbamazepine, clofibrate, and thiazide diuretics (the latter agents may directly induce the expression of water channels in the apical membrane of the kidney collecting duct).
  ○ Nephrogenic DI—correct underlying electrolyte disturbances (hypokalemia and hypercalcemia), discontinuation of offending drugs (Lithium), and/or utilize thiazide diuretics with modest salt restriction; amiloride has been successful in some patients.

SYNDROME OF INAPPROPRIATE ANTIDIURETIC HORMONE SECRETION (SIADH)

• Classically presents with hyponatremia, a euvolemic clinical exam, elevated urine osmolality (>Posm) and a urine sodium concentration >40mEq/L.

• Causes
  ○ Neurohypophyseal AVP deficiency (mechanisms are poorly understood in most cases).
  ○ CNS disorders, pulmonary disease, idiopathic.
  ○ Ectopic AVP secretion: carcinoma of the lung (small cell) or pancreas, lymphomas, miscellaneous cancers, HIV infection.

• Manifestations: nausea, vomiting, muscle cramps, central nervous system manifestations seizures, coma

• Diagnosis
  ○ Hypoosmolar hyponatremia in a euvolemic patient.
  ○ Exclude hypovolemia or decreased effective intravascular volume (congestive heart failure, nephrotic syndrome, cirrhosis).
  ○ Exclude drugs that promote ADH secretion or action: chlorpropamide, vincristine, carbamazepine, phenothiazine.
  ○ Exclude endocrinopathies which present with similar biochemical features: hypopituitarism, Addison's disease, hypothyroidism.

• Treatment
  ○ Water restriction is the mainstay of therapy.
  ○ Hypertonic saline in small boluses only when the patient is severely symptomatic and only to induce a 6-8 mEq/l increase in sodium concentration (this is generally sufficient to reverse life-threatening CNS complications)
  ○ Ensure adequate solute intake to promote water loss (NaCl tablets may prove useful in this regard)
  ○ If hyponatremia is unresponsive to these measures, one may consider lithium or demeclocycline
  ○ Finally, vasopressin receptor antagonists, such as conivaptan, are available but not yet approved for use in this setting.

OXYTOCIN SECRETION

• Suckling and dilatation of the cervix stimulate secretion of oxytocin (OT).
• OT induces labor and is essential for milk ejection.
• Physiologic role of OT in men is not clear.
• Used clinically to induce labor and reduce postpartum hemorrhage.

OTHER PITUITARY DISORDERS

EMPTY SELLA SYNDROME

• The pituitary gland does not fill the sella and the remaining space is occupied by cerebrospinal fluid (CSF).
• Usually an incidental finding on imaging.
• May or may not be associated with hypopituitarism.
• Primary
  ○ Usually a normal variant
  ○ Can occur in association with other pituitary disorders
• Secondary
  ○ Following surgery, radiation, or pituitary apoplexy
  ○ Can be associated with headache and visual changes
• Management
  ○ Based on the functional status of the pituitary

- ◦ Surgery may be indicated if visual field deficits are present or CSF rhinorrhea exists.

CRANIOPHARYNGIOMA

- A slowly growing encapsulated squamous cell tumor usually occurring in children.
- These tumors may cause pituitary insufficiency, visual field defects, and hydrocephalus. A calcified area in and around the sella may be found incidentally on radiographic studies of the head.
- Treatment involves radical surgery, radiotherapy, or both. Pituitary hormone replacement is initiated if hypopituitarism exists.

PITUITARY APOPLEXY

- Potentially fatal hemorrhagic infarct of the pituitary.
- Presents as severe headache, ophthalmoplegia, visual field defects, meningismus, and acute adrenal failure.
- Patients with significant visual loss require urgent surgical decompression.
- Hypopituitarism is a likely complication.

ACKNOWLEDGMENT

This chapter is based on the original work of Dr. Arshag D. Mooradian in the *Internist's Handbook of Endocrinology and Metabolism*, 3rd ed. My most sincere gratitude for allowing me to build and learn from it.

BIBLIOGRAPHY

Henderson KE, Baranski TJ, Bickel PE, eds. *Endocrinology Subspecialty Consult*. St. Louis, MO. Department of Medicine, Washington University School of Medicine; 2005.

Melmed S and Jameson JL. Disorders of the anterior pituitary and hypothalamus. In: Jameson JL, ed. *Harrison's Endocrinology*. New York, NY: McGraw-Hill; 2006:17–56.

Mooradian AD. The hypothalamus and the pituitary gland. In: Mooradian AD, ed. *Internist's Handbook of Endocrinology and Metabolism*, 3rd ed. St. Louis, MO: Saint Louis University Health Sciences Center; 2003:83–92.

Robertson GL, Disorders of the neurohypophysis. In: Jameson JL, ed. *Harrison's Endocrinology*. New York: McGraw-Hill; 2006:57–70.

48 DISORDERS OF CALCIUM METABOLISM

Kent R. Wehmeier

NORMAL CALCIUM HOMEOSTASIS

- Maintenance of normal serum calcium is crucial to survival.
- The absorption of calcium from dietary constituents must meet or exceed losses from urine, feces, and sweat to remain in a balanced state where adequate amounts of calcium are available for physiologic functioning.
- Calcium exists in equilibrium between various ionized; complexed; or bound compartments, the relative fractions of which are determined by temperature, pH, and the concentration of binding macromolecules, such as albumin.
- A complicated signaling network has evolved to maintain calcium homeostasis in normal and during high turnover states such as pregnancy, lactation, and growth. The major regulators of calcium metabolism are parathyroid hormone (PTH), vitamin D, and calcitonin (see Table 48-1).

PARATHYROID HORMONE PHYSIOLOGY

- The calcium-sensing receptor senses the extracellular ionized calcium Ca^{2+} concentration.[1]
- Calcium-sensing receptor activation causes suppression of PTH transcription.
- Magnesium may also activate this sensor in the chief cells of the parathyroid gland but with much less affinity than calcium.
- In response to a low calcium, preproPTH is transcribed, and the resulting peptide is cleaved forming the 84 amino acid active chain of PTH.
- Pulsutile release of PTH for minute-to-minute control of Ca^{2+} (via storage granule secretion) requires magnesium.
- Low serum calcium and high serum phosphate increase PTH transcription and stabilization of PTH mRNA independent of one another and vitamin D.
- Inhibitors of PTH transcription include hypercalcemia and 1,25-dihydroxyvitamin D (1,25[OH]$_2$D).
- Furthermore, 1,25(OH)$_2$D influences transcription of the calcium-sensing receptor and the vitamin D receptor (VDR).
- PTH binds to several receptor subtypes including, (1) PTH1R (classic PTH receptor expressed in bone and kidney), (2) PTH2 (which is expressed in the CNS, GI tract and heart), and (3) novel PTH receptors referred to as C-PTHRs.

TABLE 48–1 Approximate Normal Ranges for Serum Values in Adults

MEASURE	SI UNITS	CONVENTIONAL UNITS	CONVERSION FACTOR
Ionized calcium	1.12–1.32 mmol/L	4.5–5.3 mg/dL	0.249
Total calcium	2.17–2.52 mmol/L	8.7–10.1 mg/dL	0.249
Phosphorus	0.77–1.49 mol/L	2.4–4.6 mg/dL	0.323
25(OH)D	34–91 nmol/L	14–37 ng/mL	2.5
1,25(OH)$_2$D	60–108 pmol/L	25–54 pg/mL	2.4

1,25(OH)$_2$D, 1,25-dihydroxyvitamin D; 25-hydroxyvitamin D 25(OH)D.

PARATHYROID HORMONE ACTIONS

- Of the calcium filtered by the kidney, 80% is reabsorbed in the proximal tubule (mostly via passive mechanisms).
- Parathyroid hormone triggers a conformational change and translocation of preformed voltage-dependent Ca^{2+} channels to the apical membrane of distal tubular epithelial cells causing increased Ca^{2+} reabsorption in the distal nephron.
- PTH induces the activity of 1-α hydroxylase in the proximal tubule resulting in conversion of 25-OH vitamin D to the active form (1,25-OH) of vitamin D. Parathyroid hormone also suppresses the 24-hydroxylase enzyme that inactivates vitamin D.
- Parathyroid hormone induces internalization and degradation of the sodium-dependent phosphate cotransporter in the proximal tubule, thus promoting phosphate excretion in the urine.
- PTH also decreases bicarbonate reabsorption resulting in a hyperchloremic metabolic acidosis.
- Parathyroid hormone actions on intestinal epithelial cells are thought to occur through the actions of vitamin D rather than a direct effect.
- Parathyroid hormone actions on bone cells can be divided into effects on bone-forming cells (osteoblasts) and cells involved in bone resorption (osteoclasts).
  - *Osteoblasts*: Induce bone matrix (osteoid) synthesis (type 1 collagen) and mineralization of bone.
  - *Osteoclast precursors*: Parathyroid hormone induces receptor activator of nuclear factor-κB ligand (RANKL). In the presence of macrophage colony-stimulating factor, RANKL causes differentiation of osteoclast precursors. To resorb bone, osteoclasts fuse with other osteoclasts, anchor to the bone, seal off the extracellular environment, secrete proteases to degrade the mineralized matrix, and absorb the breakdown products in small vesicles.

VITAMIN D

VITAMIN D PHYSIOLOGY

- Vitamin D$_3$ (cholecalciferol) is produced endogenously through the action of ultraviolet light, which induces photolysis of 7-dehydrocholesterol in the skin.

- Exogenous vitamin D$_3$ from animal sources (cholecalciferol) and Vitamin D$_2$ (ergocalciferol) from plant sources are absorbed and contribute to the endogenous pool of vitamin D.
- Absorption of vitamin D requires bile acids to form micelles in the small intestine and allow transport through the lymph system.
- For the purposes of simplicity, cholecalciferol (D$_3$) and ergocalciferol (D$_2$) shall be grouped under the rubric of vitamin D, but they are not equivalent therapeutically.
- Vitamin D exists in minute concentrations and is mostly bound (85%) to vitamin D–binding protein, also known as Gc globulin, with a much smaller proportion bound to albumin (15%).
- The initial step in the activation of vitamin D involves 25-hydroxylation in the liver.
- The final activation step occurs in the kidney via the action of the 1-α hydroxylase.
- This final hydroxylation step is the rate-limiting reaction and regulated negatively by 1,25[OH]$_2$D); Ca^{2+}; and phosphate.
- Positive regulators of 1-α hydroxylase include PTH, calcitonin, insulin-like growth factor 1 and γ-interferon.
- Deactivation of vitamin D occurs via the action of 24-hydroxylase.

VITAMIN D ACTIONS

- *Kidney*: 1,25(OH)$_2$D increases the expression of Ca^{2+} channels, intracellular calcium-binding proteins (calbindins-D$_{28K}$), and increases the activity of the basolateral Na$^+$/Ca^{2+} exchanger.[2] Collectively, these effects promote increased transcellular calcium transport in the kidney.
  - Phosphate reabsorption also increases as a result of vitamin D action in the kidney.
  - 1,25(OH)$_2$D suppresses the action of 1-α-hydroxylase and induces 24-hydroxylase activity, thus providing negative feedback regulation.
- *Intestine*: 1,25(OH)$_2$D increases the expression of epithelial Ca^{2+} channels, intracellular calcium-binding proteins (calbindins-D$_{9K}$), and augments Na+/Ca+ exchange, thus, promoting calcium absorption from the gastrointestinal tract.

○ To a much smaller degree, vitamin D enhances para-cellular uptake of calcium via a voltage-dependent mechanism.

- *Bone*: $1,25(OH)_2D$ induces maturation of osteoblasts resulting in the synthesis of matrix proteins and mineralization of bone.

- $1,25(OH)2D$ promotes osteoclastogenesis; mature osteoclasts are essential for bone remodeling.

CALCITONIN

CALCITONIN REGULATION

- Peptide chain synthesized by the parafollicular (or C cells) of the thyroid gland.

- Secretion is under the control of the calcium-sensing receptor. High circulating calcium levels increase calcitonin secretion.

CALCITONIN ACTION

- *Kidney*: Receptors are expressed on the proximal renal tubule. Activation of these receptors reduces calcium and phosphate reabsorption.

- *Bone*: Calcitonin induces apoptosis of osteoclasts reducing bone resorption, thus, reducing the calcium and phosphate concentration in plasma.

HYPOCALCEMIA

EPIDEMIOLOGY

- Hypocalcemia is the most common disorder of mineral metabolism in the neonatal period and is observed frequently in premature infants.

- Most common cause of hypocalcemia in adults is iatrogenic.

SYMPTOMS AND SIGNS

ACUTE

- Paresthesias, muscle cramps, tetany.
- Palpitations.
- Laryngospasm.
- Seizures.
- Chvostek sign: Elicited by tapping on the facial nerve and observing contraction of muscles in its distribution.
- Trousseau's sign: Elicited by inflating a blood pressure cuff to 20 mm Hg above the patient's systolic blood pressure. This is continued for 5 minutes or until characteristic flexion of the wrist and metacarpophalangeal joints and extension of phalangeal joints.

False-positive tests have been observed with hypomagnesemia and respiratory alkalosis.

CHRONIC

- Subcapsular cataracts.
- Basal ganglia calcification.

DIFFERENTIAL DIAGNOSIS

PARATHYROID HORMONE DEFICIENCY

- Acquired
  ○ Iatrogenic: surgery of the parathyroid or thyroid gland is the most common cause; rarely radioactive iodine ablation of the thyroid gland or external beam therapy may induce hypoparathyroidism.[1]
  ○ Magnesium deficiency or excess.
  ○ Autoimmune destruction of the parathyroid gland (polyglandular autoimmune syndrome type I).
  ○ Infiltrative diseases: iron (hemochromatosis), amyloidosis, or copper (Wilson's disease).
- Congenital
  ○ Gain-of-function mutation of the calcium-sensing receptor.
  ○ Abnormal gland development
    ▪ Multiple genetic defects have been described: X-linked and autosomal recessive hypoparathyroidism, DiGeorge's syndrome, Sanjad-Sakati syndrome and Kenney-Caffey syndrome
    ▪ Autosomal dominant mutation in the signal peptide sequence of preproPTH which impairs the conversion to active PTH
  ○ Parathyroid hormone resistance or pseudohypopara-thyroidism (target organ unresponsiveness to PTH).

VITAMIN D RELATED

- Decreased absorption of vitamin D:[3]
  ○ Poor intake.
  ○ Inflammatory bowel disease.
  ○ Intestinal resection.
  ○ Celiac disease.
  ○ Bile acid sequestrants (cholestyramine).
- Decreased synthesis of vitamin D:
  ○ Lack of sun exposure, increased skin content of melanin, excessive sunscreen use, unusual dietary practices (aversion of milk and related dairy products).
  ○ Liver failure.
  ○ Kidney failure.
  ○ Deficiency of $1-\alpha$-hydroxylase.
  ○ Oncogenic osteomalacia.
- Impaired Vitamin D metabolism:
  ○ Usually caused by medications: phenytoin, phenobarbital

- Resistance to vitamin D:
  - Mutations in the vitamin D receptor, resulting in impaired binding.

MISCELLANEOUS CAUSES

- Hungry bone syndrome after parathyroid surgery.
- Acute pancreatitis: saponification of calcium.
- Osteoblastic metastasis: breast or prostate cancer.
- Complexation: multiple transfusions—citrate, radiographic contrast—ethylenediaminetetraacetic acid.
- Hyperphosphatemia: tumor lysis syndrome, intravenous phosphate.
- Adrenal insufficiency: reduced 1-α-hydroxylation of 25(OH)D.

LABORATORY EVALUATION

- Initially obtain plasma levels of ionized Ca^{2+} (preferred over the total calcium because of the effects of albumin and other proteins on free calcium levels), phosphorus, magnesium, PTH, and vitamin D metabolites. Assessment of renal and hepatic function is essential. 25-Hydroxyvitamin D deficiency has been increasingly recognized and is readily reversible. The history should be used as a guide for obtaining additional tests.
- Electrocardiogram findings: prolonged QT interval

THERAPEUTIC APPROACH

- Acute: Indications for intravenous calcium include tetany, laryngospasm, arrhythmias, and seizures.[4]
  - Calcium gluconate 10 to 20 mL given over 10 to 15 minutes in a monitored setting will quickly resolve these life-threatening findings.
  - Continuous infusion of calcium may also be initiated: 10 ampules of calcium gluconate in 1 L of 5% dextrose in water at a rate of 50 mL/h.
  - Frequent monitoring of serum calcium is required to avoid hypercalcemia.

  - In the setting of hypomagnesemia, intravenous magnesium is necessary. Magnesium sulfate contains 48 mg/mL of elemental magnesium. Administer 2.4 mg/kg to a maximum of 180 mg over 10 minutes while following deep tendon reflexes and serial magnesium determinations.
- Chronic
  - Calcium carbonate has the highest percent of calcium by weight. Must be taken with food. Doses that exceed 500 mg of elemental calcium may be poorly absorbed since the calcium absorption is rate limited.
  - $1,25(OH)_2D$ is available orally and may be given to facilitate intestinal calcium absorption (see Table 48-2). Ergocalciferol may also prove useful (and is substantially less expensive) if the 1-α-hydroxylase (renal) and 25-hydroxylase activity (liver) is normal. In addition to monitoring serum calcium and phosphate, one should examine the 24-hour urine calcium excretion to avoid severe hypercalciuria and subsequent stone formation.

HYPERCALCEMIA

EPIDEMIOLOGY

- Most commonly secondary to primary hyperparathyroidism.
- Annual incidence of 0.1% to 0.2%.[5]

SYMPTOMS

- Mental status changes, including, fatigue, depression, lethargy, obtundation, and coma. Seizures also may occur.
- Nephrogenic diabetes insipidus, nephrolithiasis, and nephrocalcinosis have also been observed. Typically, hypercalciuria precedes hypercalcemia. Less commonly hypercalcemia is secondary to familial hypocalciuric hypercalcemia (FHH), thiazide use,

TABLE 48-2 Vitamin D Receptor Ligands for Treatment of Vitamin D Deficiency

NAME	FORMULATION	DOSE
Ergocalciferol	Oral solution 8000 IU/mL	2000 IU daily
	Capsule 50,000 IU	One capsule weekly
$1,25(OH)_2D$ (oral)	Capsule 0.25 or 0.5 μg	0.5 μg/day
$1,25(OH)_2D$ (intravenous)	1 μg/mL	0.5 μg/day

1 μg vitamin D = 40 IU; $1,25(OH)_2D$, 1,25-dihydroxyvitamin D.

and Gitelman's syndrome. Peptic ulcer disease and pancreatitis are rare presentations.
- Back pain.
- Fractures.

SIGNS

- Most are nonspecific (fatigue, weight loss, nausea), with dehydration and mental status changes being the most common.

DIFFERENTIAL DIAGNOSIS

HYPERPARATHYROIDISM
- Hypercalcemia may be quite mild and intermittent. Associated with a higher cardiovascular mortality.
- *Primary hyperparathyroidism*: three times more common in women then men.
  - Familial
    - Deactivating mutation of the calcium-sensing receptor.
    - Familial parathyroid adenomas
      - Genetic alterations may include PRAD-1/Cyclin D1 oncogene or MEN-I gene menin.
      - Jaw tumor/hyperparathyroidism
      - Multiple endocrine neoplasia I and II
      - Familial parathyroid hyperplasia
      - Familial parathyroid cancer
    - Parathyroid hyperplasia
    - Parathyroid carcinoma
- Secondary hyperparathyroidism is usually caused by chronic kidney disease.
- Tertiary hyperparathyroidism occurs when the parathyroid gland becomes autonomous.

MALIGNANCY
- Associated with increased bone resorption, increased calcium excretion, and suppression of PTH.
- Humoral hypercalcemia (increased levels of PTH-related protein) of malignancy accounts for 80% of malignancy-associated hypercalcemia's. In addition, cytokines expressed by the tumor such as interleukin-1 and 6, tumor necrosis factor-α induce local resorption of the bone and liberate calcium.
- PTH receptor P expression is observed in squamous cell cancers, renal cell carcinoma, ovarian carcinoma, and lymphomas associated with human T-lymphotropic virus 1.
- PTH receptor P binds to the PTH receptor, causing osteoclastic bone resorption, hypercalcemia, and hypophosphatemia.

- Some leukemias and lymphomas are characterized by the expression of 1-α-hydroxylase which, in turn, promotes calcitriol synthesis.
- Direct induction of osteolysis by tumor cells.
- Malignancies rarely express intact, normal PTH and, accordingly, the levels are usually low.

MISCELLANEOUS CAUSES
- Granulomatous diseases
  - Increased expression of 1-α-hydroxylase.
  - Seen in sarcoidosis, tuberculosis, silicosis, and berylliosis.
- Familial hypocalciuric hypercalcemia (FHH)
  - Inactivating mutation in the gene for the calcium-sensing receptor characterized by autosomal dominant inheritance.
  - Associated with normal or slightly elevated PTH levels.
  - A 24-hour urine calcium collection in FHH reveals less than 100 mg. In contrast, patients with primary hyperPTH usually exceed 250 mg/24h.
- Medications
  - Thiazide diuretics interfere with calcium excretion.
  - Lithium.
  - Theophylline.
- Hyperthyroidism
- Paget's disease of bone (osteitis deformans).
- Milk-alkali syndrome: associated with calcium carbonate intake that exceeds 2 g/day and milk ingestion.
- Vitamin A toxicity.
- Vitamin D toxicity.
- Immobilization.

LABORATORY EVALUATION

- Measure an ionized calcium to confirm.
- Obtain PTH levels, calcium, phosphorus, 24-hour urine calcium and creatinine, alkaline phosphatase, and complete blood count.
- With a suggestive history for malignancy or granulomatous diseases, obtain a PTH receptor P assay, thyroid-stimulating hormone, and 1,25(OH)D level.

TREATMENT

- Acute strategies:[1]
  - Symptomatic patients presenting with mental status changes or cardiovascular instability.
    - Hydration.
    - Loop diuretics ONLY when volume expanded.
    - Salmon calcitonin subcutaneously.

- Intravenous bisphosphonates: pamidronate or zoledronate.
  - Hemodialysis in patients with severe renal disease.
- Etiology specific:
  - Primary hyperparathyroidism
    - Indications for surgery include:
      - Age younger than 50.
      - Serum calcium >1 mg/dL above the upper limit of normal for the assay.
      - Nephrolithiasis.
      - Hypercalciuria >400 mg per day.
      - Osteoporosis.
      - Worsening kidney function.
        - In patients with hyperplasia, 3.5 to 4 glands are excised with forearm autotransplantation of a portion of one gland.
        - Risk of hypercalcemia after surgery is as high as 10%.
        - Reevaluation of diagnosis should be made, if the hypercalcemia is recurrent.
    - Medical therapy
      - Close follow-up of serum calcium, kidney function, and bone mineral density.
      - Oral phosphorus and estrogens have minor benefits on lowering calcium and are generally associated with significant risks.
      - No benefit to restricting dietary calcium in primary hyperparathyroidism.
      - Cinacalcet, an agonist of the calcium-sensing receptor, is approved for the treatment of hypercalcemia related to parathyroid cancer.
- Vitamin D intoxication glucocorticoids will interfere with intestinal calcium absorption.

REFERENCES

1. Pollack MR, Yu ASL. Disorders of Calcium Homeostasis. In Brenner BM, ed. *Brenner & Rector's The Kidney*. 7th ed. Philadelphia: Saunders; 2004.
2. Bouillon R. Vitamin D: from photosynthesis, metabolism, and action to clinical applications. In DeGroot LJ, Jameson LJ, Krester DD, et al, eds. *Endocrinology*. 5th ed. Boston: Elsevier; 2006:1435–1464.
3. Shoback D, Marcus R, Bikle, D. Metabolic bone disease. In Francis S, Greenspan FS, Gardner DG. *Basic and Clinical Endocrinology*. 7th ed. New York: McGraw-Hill; 2004.
4. Carpenter TO, Insogna KL. The hypocalcemic disorders: differential diagnosis and therapeutic use of vitamin D. In Feldman D, Pike JW, Glorieux, FH, eds. *Vitamin D*. 2nd ed. Boston: Elsevier; 2005:1049–1060.
5. Heath H III, Hodgson SF, Kennedy MA. Primary hyperparathyroidism: incidence, morbidity, and potential economic impact in a community. *N Engl J Med*. 1980;302:188.

49 METABOLIC BONE DISEASES

Kent R. Wehmeier

NORMAL BONE FORMATION

- Bone matrix is comprised of organic components (predominately type 1 collagen and glycosaminoglycans) and inorganic components (crystals of hydroxyapatite containing calcium, phosphorus, and other ions).
- Skeletal growth and elongation are referred to as modeling, whereas remodeling involves a tightly coupled process of bone formation and bone resorption. Imbalances in bone remodeling are associated with a variety of clinical disorders including osteoporosis, osteopetrosis, and osteomalacia.
- Mechanical forces play an important role in regulating bone modeling and remodeling.
- Bone can exist in two forms.
  - Immature or woven bone, characterized by a disordered pattern of collagen, is seen early in development, at fracture repair sites, and in some pathologic states. It is weak compared to lamellar bone.
  - Mature or lamellar bone is characterized by layers of well-organized collagen.
- Osteoblasts derived from mesenchymal stem cells initiate bone remodeling by activating adjacent osteocytes and osteoclasts which secrete collagenases and induce bone resorption. This is followed by deposition of organic matrix (osteoid) and increased local concentrations of calcium and phosphate resulting in bone mineralization. The cell biology of bone remodeling remains incompletely understood. However, some of the factors involved include, 1,25-dihydroxyvitamin D (1,25[OH]$_2$D), interleukin-1, and parathyroid hormone (PTH). For example, PTH promotes osteoclastogenesis by binding to marrow stromal cells and inducing expression of receptor activator of nuclear factor-κB ligand (RANKL). This protein binds with a receptor expressed on osteoclast precursors leading to activation of osteoclast formation.
- A dense envelope of cortical bone surrounds the spoked or honeycombed interior called trabecular or cancellous bone. Trabecular bone comprises 20% of the skeleton.
- Metabolic bone disease occurs when the opposing forces of bone formation and bone resorption (remodeling) are not in balance. For example, an increase in

bone resorption relative to bone formation results in osteoporosis. Conversely, when bone formation exceeds bone resorption, osteosclerosis or hyperostosis occurs.

OSTEOPOROSIS

- Osteoporosis is characterized by disruption of the microarchitecture of bone and loss of bone which, in turn, decreases bone strength and increases the risk of fracture. The mechanism of micoarchitectural changes in osteoporosis remains poorly understood, but is believed to be the major feature which distinguishes osteoporosis from other types of metabolic bone disease, eg, osteomalacia.
- Development of a "fragility fracture" is regarded as the hallmark e.g, hip fracture after falling from less than standing height or a vertebral fracture with activities of daily living.
- Postmenopausal osteoporosis (type 1 osteoporosis) is significantly more common when there is loss of bone in the pre- or peri-menopausal period
  - For example, reduced estrogen in the peri-menopausal period is characterized by a significant increase in osteoclastic activity that is not compensated for by new bone formation.
- Senile osteoporosis (sometimes referred to as type 2 osteoporosis) occurs in both men and women because of reduced bone formation, perhaps related to dimished production of vitamin D with advancing age.[1]

EPIDEMIOLOGY

- Age and gender are major risk factors with whites and Asian women are most commonly affected. Women older than 50 years of age have a 50% chance of suffering from an osteoporotic fracture.
- Other major factors linked to postmenopausal osteoporosis include smoking, premature menopause (onset before the age of 45 years), loss of normal menses after menarche for a prolonged period, ingestion of more than two alcoholic beverages a day, lifelong low calcium intake, family history of osteoporosis, and a body weight of less than 54.4 kg (120 lb).
- Various genetic loci (encoding collagen I, the vitamin D receptor [VDR], and the estrogen receptor) have been implicated in the development of osteoporosis, but widespread screening is not been advocated.
- Men older than 50 years of age have a 1:5 chance of an osteoporotic fracture in their lifetime. Risk factors for men include hypogonadism, ethanol use, and tobacco use. Mortality after a hip fracture has been reported as high as 37% in the first year.[2]

SECONDARY CAUSES

- Secondary osteoporosis is sometimes referred to as type 3 osteoporosis. It is almost always secondary to medications, particularly corticosteroids. A secondary cause of osteoporosis should be suspected in the following settings:
  - Fractures in patients without traditional risk factors.
  - Premenopausal women.
  - Males younger than 70 years of age.
  - Multiple fractures following low-impact trauma.
  - Bone mineral density (BMD) more than 2 standard deviations below age-matched controls.
  - Worsening BMD or fractures despite treatment.
- The causes of type 3 osteoporosis include:
  - Drugs and toxins: glucocorticoids, immunosuppressive agents, long-term progestin administration in the absence of estrogen therapy, gonadotropin hormone releasing hormone antagonists, protease inhibitors used to treat human immunodeficiency virus (HIV) infection, anticonvulsants, aluminum, excessive vitamin A adminstration, lithium, tamoxifen (premenopausal women), and anticoagulants.
  - Hypercalciuria
  - Renal tubular abnormalities caused by mutations in renal outer medullary K channels (ROMK) or the sodium-potassium-2 chloride cotransporter (NKCC2) result in decreased calcium reabsorption in the thick ascending limb of Henle. Other genetic diseases associated with hypercalciuria and metabolic bone disease include: hereditary hypophosphatemic rickets, Dent's disease, and idiopathic hypercalciuria.
  - Vitamin D deficiency has been described in a variety of clinical settings. Conceptually, vitamin D deficiency can be grouped into four clinical categories: (1) decreased intake/absorption (dietary, gastrointestinal disorders such as malabsorption, inadequate sunlight exposure), (2) decreased synthesis (liver disease, anticonvulsant therapy, kidney disease), (3) target organ resistance (hereditary vitamin D-resistant rickets), and (4) miscellaneous (diabetes mellitus, cancers, anemia, connective tissue disorders, cerebrovascular disease and chronic obstructive pulmonary disease [COPD]).[3]

HISTORY

- The history is not always helpful, since as many as 66% of vertebral fractures are asymptomatic.
- Antecedent fractures of the humerus and wrist are more common near the onset of menopause in patients who eventually develop osteoporosis.
- The onset of menarche, regularity of menses, and onset of menopause should be carefully documented.

- Premature loss of teeth is an important indicator of bone health.
- Lifestyle issues such as physical activity, calcium intake, tobacco use, and alcohol use should be recorded.

PHYSICAL EXAMINATION

- Weight and height should be assessed. It is important to quantitate the total number of teeth, since less than 20 teeth suggest a general decrease in bone health and warrant measurement of BMD. Examination of the spine should exclude the presence of kyphosis (performed with the patient standing against the wall and measuring the distance between the occipital bone and wall). Scoliosis is assessed by examining the back for curvature and prominence of the scapula as well as measurement of the distance between the ribs and pelvis. Low rib pelvis distance (less than two fingers) is associated with an increased probability of lumbar fracture.
- Also assess visual acuity, mental status, muscle strength, and balance. Various predictive tests for falls include the ability to stand on one foot, the get-up-and-go test, and standing without using arm assistance.

DIAGNOSIS

- A fracture sustained after a fall from less than standing height or with minimal trauma should suggest the diagnosis.
- Routine studies include: electrolytes, calcium, phosphorus, alkaline phosphatase, kidney and liver function, complete blood count, and thyroid-stimulating hormone.
- Depending on the history and physical examination, additional tests can include 25(OH)D and urinary calcium.
- BMD testing should be carried out in patients with a high index of suspicion or with abnormal serum chemistries.[4]
  - The World Health Organization (WHO) considers osteoporosis to be present when the patient has a BMD that falls below 2.5 standard deviations of the peak adult bone density (young adult reference mean eg, T-score) of the distal third of the radius of the nondominant forearm, femoral neck, total hip, or lumbar spine (L1–L4). A T-score of >1 and <2.5 is considered consistent with osteopenia while a score >2.5 in concert with a fragility fracture is considered consistent with severe osteoporosis. The Z-score compares BMD to that of an aged-matched population. A Z-score of >2 should prompt a thorough evaluation for secondary causes of osteoporosis.

A variety of techniques are now available to measure BMD.
  - Dual-energy x-ray absorptiometry (DXA) is the most widely used, and perhaps best studied. The accuracy and precision of DXA permits its use in monitoring therapy as well as establishing diagnosis.
  - Quantitative ultrasonography has been used to evaluate fracture risk. While reasonably good at predicting fractures in men or women, ultrasonography is not sufficiently sensitive to establish a diagnosis of osteoporosis (T-score). Based on recommendations of the International Society of Clinical Densitometry (ISCD), it should only be used when DXA is not available and should never be used to monitor therapy.[4]
  - Computed tomography of the lumbar spine overestimates the risk of osteoporosis and exposes the patient to a great deal of radiation when compared to DXA. It also provides little information regarding cortical bone density.
  - There are no universal standards that allow the information from each of these techniques to be integrated into a comprehensive diagnostic and treatment plan.
  - Osteoporosis is sometimes diagnosed on plain films when a compression fracture causes >20% reduction in vertebral body height of the lumbar or lower thoracic spine, or >30% if osteopenia is noted on plain radiographs.
- Markers of bone turnover
  - Currently available markers for bone formation include alkaline phosphatase, osteocalcin and procollagen peptides. Tissue nonspecific alkaline phosphatase is one of three transcripts produced in humans. The bone specific isozyme of this transcript can be measured clinically. However, the bone alkaline phosphatase may be normal (along with osteocalcin and the procollagen peptides) in patients with documented osteoporosis. Moreover, these assays only reflect one point in time and are influenced by many other factors such as nutrition.
  - Currently available markers of bone resorption include hydroxyproline, n-telopeptide or c-telopeptide of collagen I, pyridinium cross-links, and tartrate-resistant acid phosphatase 5b (TRAP 5b) a specific isozyme from osteoclasts, and bone sialoprotein (BSP). These are not helpful for the diagnosis of osteoporosis as they reflect only one point in time but can provide information regarding acute bone turnover.
- Bone turnover markers are sometimes used longitudinally to assess the biochemical effect of therapeutic interventions or assay the effect of PTH in hyperparathyroid patients.
- Specific guidelines on use of bone turnover markers await randomized controlled clinical trials.

TREATMENT[5]

- Nonpharmacologic
  ○ Avoidance of smoking and alcohol should be encouraged.
  ○ Counseling regarding adequate calcium intake should be offered. However, analysis of several large prospective trials has not shown a reduction in fracture incidence in otherwise normal women who consume more than 1500 mg/day of calcium (Table 49–1). In addition, vitamin D supplementation in replete individuals is not associated with a reduction in fracture incidence (Table 49–2). Accordingly, the indiscriminant use of calcium or vitamin D supplements in otherwise healthy women should be discouraged.
  ○ Variable benefits have been reported with exercise therapy for fracture prevention, however patients should be encouraged to remain active as possible as most studies suggest that aerobics and resistance training decreases the incidence of fractures (particularly in women >60 years of age) and increases BMD. Judicious use of exercise also facilitates rehabilitation from fractures.
- Pharmacologic therapy
  ○ Selection of pharmacologic therapy is based on the underlying cause of osteoporosis (see secondary causes). Thus, vitamin D deficiency, if present, must be addressed. If the patient requires glucocorticoids, they should be titrated to the lowest effective dose.
    ▪ Calcitonin was one of the first agents utilized in the management of osteoporosis. It is currently marketed in nasal form and approved only for postmenopausal osteoporosis. Calcitonin modestly reduces vertebral fractures with little effect on BMD. Side effects include rhinorrhea and epistaxis. It is not generally considered mainstay therapy.
    ▪ The bis and aminophosphonates are comprised of several oral agents approved for use in the United States: alendronate, risedronate, and ibandronate. Ibandronate is also available as an injectable that is administered four times a year. Alendronate and risedronate are also approved for male osteoporosis. In general, these analogues of pyrophosphate adhere to mineralizing surfaces and interfere with osteoclast function. For example, etidronate (a bisphosphonate) is metabolized by osteoclasts

TABLE 49–1 Optimal Calcium Intake (mg/d)

Adolescents		1300
Women	19 years of age to menopause	1000
	Postmenopause	1300
	Last trimester of pregnancy	1200
	Lactation	1000
Men	19 to 65 years of age	1000
	>65 years of age	1300

TABLE 49–2 Vitamin D Recommended Nutrient Intake (IU/D) Defined as Meeting the Nutritional Requirements of 97.5% of Apparently Healthy Individuals

Adolescents	200
19–50 years of age	200
51–65 years of age	400
>65 years of age	600
Last trimester of pregnancy	200
Lactation	200

to a compound that exchanges with the terminal pyrophosphate moiety of ATP, thus rendering it inactive. This causes a reduction in osteoclastic activity and a decrease in bone resorption. The reduction in bone resorption, increases BMD and is associated with a decrease in fracture rate. These drugs are best absorbed on an empty stomach. Side effects occur as a result of reflux into the esophagus causing irritation and rarely, ulceration. Recently, the oral bisphosphonates have been implicated in the development of osteonecrosis of the jaw.
- Serum estrogen receptor modulator (raloxifene) suppresses osteoclastic activity by binding to the estrogen receptor. Its effect on BMD is modest, but the reduction of vertebral fractures is similar to that described for alendronate. This medication is not approved for the treatment of hip fractures. Like estrogens, raloxifene increases the risk of thromboembolism, however it appears to reduce the risk of breast cancer. It is not approved for use in men.
- Parathyroid analogues are a new class of drug used in the treatment of osteoporosis, referred to as anabolic agents. PTH[1–34] when administered in a pulsatile manner induces net synthesis of bone. PTH[1–34] is approved for the treatment of osteoporosis in men and women as a daily injection (20–40 mcg/d) for 12 to 18 months. Bone density as measured by DXA are somewhat higher than those observed with the bisphosphonates, yet the fracture reduction is only somewhat better. These drugs carry a black box warning because they have been linked to the development of osteosarcoma in rodents. These agents are generally not considered first-line, although there is considerable interest in combining these drugs with the bisphosphonates, thus promoting both an increase in bone formation and a decrease in bone resorption. Side effects include dizziness, diaphoresis, hyperuricemia, hypercalcemia, and rarely, nephrolithiasis.

In summary, the bisphosphonates are the agents of choice for the management of osteoporosis. Roloxifene is a useful adjunct and is considered superior by some experts. It may offer a special advantage in patients with breast cancer. The PTH analogues can be used in both men and women, but are generally considered as third-line agents at this time.

- Adjunctive therapies should be offered to all patients and include:
  - Weight-bearing and ambulation exercises to reduce the risk of falls
  - Muscle-strengthening activities
  - Smoking cessation
  - Reducing alcohol intake
  - Vision correction
  - Household/workplace management to minimize the risk of falls
  - Identify and limit medications associated with dizziness or balance problems
  - Percutaneous vertebroplasty, kyphoplasty (use of methyl methacrylate injected into the vertebral body of a compressed vertebra to reduce pain)

OSTEOMALACIA

- Osteomalacia is characterized by decreased mineralization of bone. When identified prior to epiphysial plate closure, it is called *rickets*. Because of decreased mineralization, disorganized cartilage appears at the epiphysial plate with flaring and irregularity of the epiphysial-metaphysial junction. This can lead to shortened stature in the growing child.
- Recent reports have confirmed a resurgence of osteomalacia in the general population. Infants fed exclusively human milk without the benefit of adequate sunlight may develop rickets.[6]

EPIDEMIOLOGY

- Abnormal vitamin D metabolism is the most common cause of osteomalacia. For example, 48% of African American women aged 15 to 49 years had 25(OH)D levels of less than 15 ng/mL at the end of the winter.[7] In a study from Maine, 48% of white girls aged 9 to 11 years had 25(OH)D levels less than 20 ng/mL at the end of the winter, and 17% remained vitamin D–deficient at the end of the summer.[8]
- Other causes of osteomalacia include liver and kidney disease (impaired hydroxylation of vitamin D), gastrointestinal disease resulting in malabsorption of vitamin D, type 1 vitamin D-dependent rickets (decreased 1-α hydroxylation of vitamin D), type 2 vitamin D-dependent rickets (decreased target tissue response to 1,25(OH)2-D), osteogenesis imperfecta and fibrogenesis imperfecta (decreased matrix), and impaired renal phosphate reabsorption (X-linked hypophosphatemic rickets, hyperparathyroidism, and rare hereditary defects in renal phosphate handling).

CLINICAL MANIFESTATIONS

- Young children
  - Listless, hypotonia, poor growth, and bowing of the legs. Tetany can occur with an acute illness.
- Adults
  - Few symptoms except for chronic muscle aches or bone pain

PHYSICAL EXAMINATION

- During infancy
  - Rachitic rosary characterized by swelling at the costochondral junctions. Craniotabes or flattening of the posterior skull. Flaring of the wrist and ankles.
  - Muscular: proximal muscle weakness and waddling gait.
  - Delayed tooth eruption, dental caries, and enamel defects.
  - Short stature and limb deformities.
  - True fractures or pseudofractures.
- Postepiphysial closure (adults)
  - Signs are much more subtle and it is clinically difficult to distinguish osteomalacia from osteoporosis (many patients are asymptomatic).
  - Bone tenderness may occur.
  - Proximal muscle weakness is common.
  - True fractures and pseudofractures occur.

DIFFERENTIAL DIAGNOSIS

There are three major abnormalities responsible for most cases of osteomalacia, (1) disorders affecting vitamin D synthesis or activity, (2) diseases which alter bone matrix synthesis, and (3) conditions associated with increased renal phosphate excretion and hypophosphatemia.

- Vitamin D abnormalities
  - Decreased vitamin D intake/synthesis is secondary to either decreased dietary consumption or inadequate light exposure and malabsorption secondary to medications (bile acid sequestering agents), intestinal disease (celiac disease), hepatobiliary, or pancreatic disease. Aging is commonly associated with inadequate light exposure, therefore, 25-OH vitamin D levels should be obtained in all patients >60 years of age. The nephrotic syndrome leads to depletion of vitamin D binding protein and decreased levels of 25-OH vitamin D. Moreover, patients with chronic kidney disease may have impaired 1-α hydroxylation of 25-OH vitamin D resulting in decreased circulating levels of 1,25-OH-vitamin D. Drugs, including anticonvulsants and rifampin, impair the hydroxylation steps involved in the activation of

vitamin D. Vitamin D-dependent rickets is characterized by either reduced 1-α hydroxylation of vitamin D (Type 1, inactivating mutation in the 1-α hydroxylase gene) or resistance to the action of 1,25-OH vitamin D (Type 2 or hereditary vitamin D-resistant rickets [HVDRR], a rare autosomal recessive disorder). The vitamin D abnormalities are usually accompanied by secondary hyperparathyroidism and renal phosphate wasting.

- Decreased bone matrix
  - Diminished bone matrix synthesis is relatively uncommon but may occur with bisphosphonate therapy or when fluoride or aluminum accumulation occurs (endemic flourosis, toothpaste pica, chronic kidney disease). Osteogenesis imperfecta and fibrosing imperfecta also impair bone matrix synthesis and are associated with osteomalacia.
- Decrease serum phosphate
  - Occasionally antacid administration can impair gastrointestinal phosphate absorption, however, most clinical conditions associated with osteomalacia and hypophosphatemia are secondary to increased renal phosphate excretion. X-linked hypophosphatemic rickets (vitamin D–resistant rickets) is a rare disease caused by a mutation in the PHEX gene which encodes for an endopeptidase that degrades a phosphaturic hormone. Hereditary hypophosphatemic rickets is an autosomal recessive disorder characterized by a mutation in the renal sodium/phosphate co-transporter. Oncogenic osteomalacia (tumor-induced osteomalacia) occurs with mesenchymal tumors that produce factors such as fibroblast growth factor 23 (FGF-23) and frizzled-related protein 4 that promote renal phosphate excretion. Fanconi's syndrome is a renal tubular disorder characterized by hyperphosphaturia, glycosuria, and proximal renal tubular acidosis. It is unusual in adults, but may accompany multiple myeloma.

LABORATORY EVALUATION

- Vitamin D abnormalities are characterized by perturbations in serum calcium (usually low), serum phosphate (usually low), and elevated serum alkaline phosphatase. Secondary hyperparathyroidism is expected. The elevated PTH causes the urinary calcium level to decrease, and augments urinary phosphate excretion. A low 25 (OH)D strongly suggests impairment of gastrointestinal absorption or inadequate sunlight exposure.
- The gold standard for establishing the presence of osteomalacia is a transcortical bone biopsy with tetracycline labeling on a non-decalcified sample. Because of reduced mineralization, the osteoid seems are wide. This procedure is used infrequently for the diagnosis of osteomalacia, since the constellation of laboratory and clinical features are generally sufficient to establish the diagnosis.

IMAGING

- Radiographs in children can show radiolucent epiphyses that are widened and areas of hypomineralized bone. Pseudofractures (Looser zones or Milkman fractures) can occur on the concave side of the femoral neck, pubic rami, rib cage, and lateral aspect of the scapula.
- In adults, radiography is not helpful in distinguishing osteomalacia from osteoporosis.

TREATMENT[9]

- Must be directed at the underlying cause. Vitamin D administration (oral or intravenously) should be based on the underlying pathophysiology (see above). Indiscriminate use of vitamin D can result in hypercalciuria, hypercalcemia, nephrocalcinosis, or urolithiasis.
- Available vitamin D compounds in the United States include oral ergocalciferol (D_2) and cholecalciferol (D_3) as well as oral and parenteral 1,25(OH)$_2$D. See Table 49–3 for dosing regimens.
- Intravenous calcium may be required in some cases (see treatment of hypocalcemia).
- Correction of hypophosphatemia with potassium phosphate, although desirable, may not be required to achieve optimal bone health.

TABLE 49–3   Vitamin D Formulations and Dosing Regimens

NAME	FORMULATION	$T_{1/2}$	DOSE
Ergocalciferol	Oral solution 8000 IU/mL	<4 weeks	2000 IU daily
	Capsule 50,000 IU		One capsule/weekly
Cholecalciferol (D_3)	1000 IU capsule	<4 weeks	1000 IU daily
Calcifediol 25(OH)D_3	Tablet 20, 50 mcg	2 weeks	50–200 mcg/d
Calcitriol 1,25(OH)$_2$$D_3$	Capsule 0.25 or 0.5 mcg	6 hours	0.5 mcg/d
Calcitriol 1,25(OH)$_2$$D_3$	1 mcg/mL (intravenous)		0.5 mcg/d

PAGET'S DISEASE OF BONE

- Paget's disease is characterized by increased bone turnover ultimately producing weakened deformed woven bone. Since most patients are asymptomatic, the disease is likely grossly underestimated. Mutations (sequestrotomy 1 gene) and environmental factors such as paramyxovirus infection appear to participate in the development of Paget's disease. The abnormal bone remodeling, in rare circumstances, can lead to osteosarcoma.

EPIDEMIOLOGY[10]

- Primarily a disease of white western Europeans, New Zealanders, South Africans, Australians, and North Americans. It does not affect as many Europeans of Scandinavian decent. Men in their middle to older age are most commonly affected. As high as 1% of the population in the United States older than 40 years of age has the disease.

HISTORY

- Most are asymptomatic.
- Features suggestive of Paget's disease can include joint pain that worsens with weight bearing, increasing hat size, swelling of the proximal tibia, and loss of hearing.

EXAMINATION

- Involvement of the skull can be associated with cranial nerve deficits including hearing loss and hydrocephalus. Noticeable swelling of the mandible can be seen. The joints should be examined for associated osteoarthritis. The proximal tibia is often warm to the touch. Spinal involvement is manifested by spinal stenosis and nerve root compression syndromes.

DIAGNOSIS

- An isolated elevation of alkaline phosphatase is usually the first clue to the diagnosis of Paget's disease. Importantly, one must exclude other causes of an elevated alkaline phosphatase such as primary hyperparathyroidism and vitamin D deficiency. If a small focus is present, the alkaline phosphatase may not be increased. Bone scintigraphy is necessary to define the extent of disease. Plain films of the areas containing

TABLE 49–4 Treatment for Paget Disease

Etidronate disodium	5 mg/kg of body weight/d for 6 mo
Alendronate sodium	40 mg tablet daily for 6 mo
Tiludronate disodium	400 mg tablets daily for 3 mo
Risedronate sodium	One 30 mg tablet orally once daily for 2 mo
Pamidronate disodium	30 mg intravenously 4 h period on 3 consecutive days
Salmon calcitonin	Subcutaneous 50 to 100 units daily or three times a week for 6 mo

dense radiotracer enhancement by bone scintigraphy should be examined radiographically. Rarely, bone biopsy is needed, especially when an underlying malignancy is supected. Fortunately, osteosarcoma develops in less than 1% of cases.

TREATMENT[11]

- See Table 49–4
  - Indications
    - Symptoms resulting from active bone lesions.
    - Prophylaxis should be considered, even in asymptomatic patients, when affected sites involve weight-bearing long bones or result in nerve compression syndromes.
    - Elevation of alkaline phosphatase by itself is not an indication for treatment.
  - Bisphosphonates represent the most commonly prescribed therapy (Table 49–4).
  - Resistance to one bisphosphonate can occur. Switching to another member of this group may be effective. Bisphosphonates may cause gastric irritation after oral use; osteonecrosis of the jaw has been reported rarely.
  - Optimal markers of effective therapy have not been rigorously defined or tested.
  - Salmon calcitonin by injection can be considered in patients with hypersensitivity to the bisphosphonates. Nausea, flushing, and a shorter duration of action limits the use of calcitonin.
  - Interestingly these individuals seem more prone to develop vascular calcification.

REFERENCES

1. Green AD, Colon-Emeric C, Bastian L, et al. Does this woman have osteoporosis? *JAMA.* 2004;292:2890.
2. Seeman E, Bianchi G, Khosla S, et al. Bone fragility in men—where are we? *Osteoporos Int.* 2006;17:1577.
3. Fitzpatrick LA. Secondary causes of osteoporosis. *Mayo Clinic Proc.* 2002;77:453.

4. Official Positions of the International Society for Clinical Densitometry. http://www.iscd.org/Visitors/pdfs/ISCD_OP2005_000.pdf 2005.

5. Delaney MF. Strategies for the prevention and treatment of osteoporosis during early postmenopause. *Am J Obstet Gynecol.* 2006;194:S12.

6. Food and Agriculture Organization/World Health Organization (FAO/WHO). Human Vitamin and Mineral Requirements, 2002. www.fao.org/DOCREP/004/Y2809E/ y2809e00.htm

7. Looker AC, Dawson-Hughes B, Calvo MS, et al. Serum 25-hydroxyvitamin D status of adolescents and adults in two seasonal subpopulations from NHANES III. *Bone.* 2002;30:771–777.

8. Sullivan SS, Rosen CJ, Halteman WA, et al. Adolescent girls in Maine are at risk for vitamin D insufficiency. *J Am Diet Assoc.* 2005;105:971.

9. Whyte MP. Approach to the patient with metabolic bone disease. In Feldman D, Pike JW, Glorieux, FH, eds. *Vitamin D.* 2nd ed. Boston: Elsevier; 2005:915–929.

10. Singer FR. Paget's disease of bone. In DeGroot LJ, Jameson LJ, Krester DD, et al., eds. *Endocrinology.* 5th ed. Boston: Elsevier; 2006:1771–1782.

11. Whyte MP. Paget's disease of bone. *N Engl J Med.* 2006;355:6.

50 DISORDERS OF THE THYROID GLAND

Alan B. Silverberg

- Approximately 20 million Americans are afflicted with thyroid disease.
- 60% of the population with thyroid disorders are believed to be unaware of their abnormality.
- Women are five to eight times more likely than men to have a thyroid problem.
- Palpable thyroid nodules are found in 5% to 7% of the North American population.
- Thyroid imaging studies (radioisotope scans or ultrasounds) increase the number of nodules found in an individual and in a population. However, thyroid cancers are rare (<5% of thyroid nodules) and deaths from thyroid cancer are also very uncommon.
- Hypothyroidism (clinical and subclinical) is 10 times more prevalent than hyperthyroidism (clinical or subclinical).
- Screening for a thyroid disorder with a TSH value is controversial.
- Most thyroid diseases require lifelong follow-up and medical management.

PHYSIOLOGY

- Thyroxine (T4) is the principal product of the thyroid gland. However, T4 is sometimes considered a prohormone because it must be converted to tri-iodothyronine (T3) to exert its biological effects.
- T4 is highly protein bound, for example, 99.96% is bound to thyroxine-binding globulin (TBG), albumin, transthyretin, and lipoproteins.
- Half-life of T4 is 7 days.
- T3 is also highly protein bound (99.3%).
- Half-life of T3 is 24 hours.
- TSH controls the secretion of T4 and T3 from the thyroid gland. TSH is a glycoprotein hormone with two subunits, α (common to follicle-stimulating hormone [FSH], luteinizing hormone [LH], and human chorionic gonadotropin [HCG]) and β (unique to TSH). The half-life of TSH is 50 minutes, and its secretion is facilitated by thyrotropin-releasing hormone (TRH) secreted from the hypothalamus.
- Primary factor inhibiting TSH synthesis and secretion is T3.

PREVALENCE OF THYROID DYSFUNCTION

- Hypothyroidism is present in 2% of the adult population.
- Subclinical hypothyroidism likely accounts for an additional 5% to 17%.
- Hyperthyroidism is present in <0.2% of the adult population.
- Subclinical hyperthyroidism likely accounts for an additional 0.1% to 6.0%.

RISK OF DEVELOPING THYROID DYSFUNCTION

- Previous thyroid dysfunction
- Goiter
- Surgery or radiotherapy involving the gland or neck
- Diabetes mellitus, type 1
- Vitiligo
- Pernicious anemia
- Medications (lithium, amiodarone, interferon)
- Leukotrichia
- Family history of thyroid disease, pernicious anemia, type 1 diabetes mellitus, or primary adrenal insufficiency

ABNORMAL LABORATORY TESTS THAT ACCOMPANY HYPOTHYROIDISM

- Hypercholesterolemia
- Hyponatremia

- Anemia
- Increased creatine phosphokinase (CPK)
- Increased lactic dehydrogenase (LD)
- Hyperprolactinemia

ABNORMAL LABORATORY TESTS THAT ACCOMPANY HYPERTHYROIDISM

- Hypercalcemia
- Increased alkaline phosphatase
- Hepatocellular enzyme elevation
- Abnormal electrocardiogram (ECG) (atrial fibrillation, atrial flutter, or supraventricular tachycardia [SVT])
- Low cholesterol
- Increased ferritin
- Increased angiotensin-converting enzyme

THYROID NODULES

- Most common thyroid disorder.
- Palpable nodules are found in 5% to 7% of the North American population. Thyroid nuclear medicine scans and especially thyroid ultrasound examinations can markedly increase the detection of thyroid nodules in an individual.
- Thyroid nodules are rare in individuals younger than 20 years of age.
- Thyroid nodules increase with advancing age. It is unusual to find a multinodular thyroid gland in someone younger than 60 years of age.
- Women present with thyroid nodules six to eight times as often as men.
- Thyroid cancers are rare, occurring in less than 5% of thyroid nodules.
- Radiation exposure to the head and neck area increases the incidence of thyroid nodules and thyroid cancer. Individuals younger than 15 years of age are more likely to develop thyroid cancers secondary to radiation exposure.
- Thyroid nodules tend to cluster in families. Thyroid cancers may also be familial.
- Benign thyroid disorders that might cause nodular thyroid enlargement include Hashimoto's thyroiditis and Grave's disease.
- Medullary thyroid carcinoma (MTC) is familial 20% of the time. The familial MTCs are associated with multiple endocrine neoplasia (MEN) type 2A and 2B.

- Dysphasia, dyspnea, and dysphonia rarely occur in well-differentiated thyroid cancer but are more common with medullary and anaplastic thyroid cancers. A thyroid nodule that is increasing in size also suggests the presence of a malignancy. Pain in the thyroid gland may suggest subacute thyroiditis or hemorrhage into a thyroid nodule.
- A rock hard nodule that is fixed to surrounding structures suggests a thyroid malignancy. The incidence of thyroid cancers is the same in solitary nodular goiters and multinodular goiters. The presence of neck lymph nodes may also suggest the presence of a thyroid malignancy.

EVALUATION OF THYROID NODULES (FIG. 50–1)

- A history and careful physical examination of the thyroid gland and neck are the initial steps in evaluating nodular goiters.
- A TSH and a thyroid ultrasound are currently recommended as the first studies when evaluating the thyroid gland. If the TSH is abnormal, the likelihood of cancer is decreased but not eliminated. Ultrasound examinations of the thyroid gland can identify nodules that require further evaluation and delineate features that may suggest a thyroid malignancy.
- The fine needle aspiration biopsy (FNA Bx) of the thyroid gland or nodule is the most sensitive and specific diagnostic tool for determining whether a nodule is a malignant.

The cytopathologist will typically characterize the pathological findings in one of three ways:
1. Benign
2. Suspicious or indeterminant
3. Malignant
   - A FNA Bx that is insufficient for diagnosis should be repeated 4 to 6 weeks later.
   - All suspicious or indeterminant and malignant nodules should be surgically removed.

THYROID CANCER

- Well-differentiated, follicular cell-derived thyroid cancer consists of papillary and follicular carcinoma. Medullary thyroid cancer arises from the C cells, located in the upper two thirds of the thyroid gland. Anaplastic thyroid cancer is a poorly differentiated follicular cell derived tumor with a very poor prognosis.

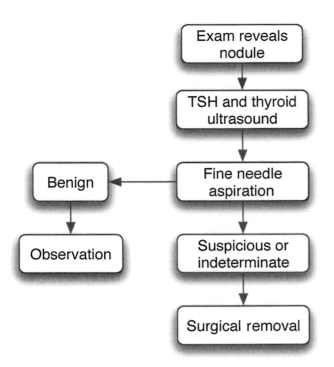

TSH: Thyroid-Stimulating Hormone.
FNA: Fine Needle Aspiration.

FIG. 50–1   Management of thyroid nodules.

- Papillary thyroid carcinoma is the most common thyroid malignancy and accounts for almost 80% of thyroid cancers. Follicular carcinoma occurs 10% to 20% of the time, and medullary thyroid cancer occurs 1% to 5% of the time. Anaplastic carcinoma is the least frequent malignancy and occurs less than 1% of the time.
- Papillary thyroid cancer is a slow-growing, well-differentiated tumor that has a very good prognosis with cancer-free survival exceeding 90% at 20 years. Distant metastases are rare at the time of presentation. This tumor spreads by local invasion and lymphatic routes to regional lymph nodes.
  ○ This is also the type of thyroid cancer associated with prior head and neck radiation exposure.
  ○ Lymph node metastases are more common in individuals younger than 20 years of age.
- Follicular carcinoma spreads by hematogenesis routes to lung and bone. Distant metastases at presentation occur less than 20% of the time.
- Medullary thyroid cancer may be sporadic (80%) or familial (20%). The serum marker for this tumor is calcitonin. The tumor arises from the thyroid C cells which produce calcitonin. It is a relatively

slow- growing tumor with a long-term survival that exceeds 80%. The familial medullary thyroid syndromes include FMTC, MEN2A, and MEN2B. The familial syndromes are associated with mutations in the RET–proto-oncogene. Metastases to regional lymph nodes, lung, bone, and liver may occur with this tumor.
- Anaplastic thyroid carcinoma usually occurs in the elderly and has a very poor prognosis.
  ○ Survival beyond year is unusual. Surgery, radiation therapy, and chemotherapy are generally not effective in prolonging survival. This is a rapidly growing tumor that presents with an enlarging neck mass and compressive symptoms, such as dyspnea, dysphonia, or dysphasia.
- Lymphomas of the thyroid are very rare and associated with prior Hashimoto's thyroiditis. They usually present as an enlarging goiter in which there is a prior history of autoimmune thyroiditis.

MANAGEMENT OF WELL DIFFERENTIATED THYROID CANCER INCLUDING PAPILLARY AND FOLLICULAR CARCINOMA (FIG. 50–2)

- Total thyroidectomy
- Radioactive iodine ablation therapy is administered 6 weeks after the total thyroidectomy when the patient is hypothyroid (TSH >50)
- Tumors <1 cm with no metastases may not require routine radioactive iodine ablation.
- After the radioactive iodine ablation, thyroid hormone is initiated and adjusted to maintain a TSH of 0.1 to 0.4 mU/L.
- Six months after surgery and radioactive iodine treatment, an I-123 whole body scan is performed after withholding thyroid hormone. Subsequent scans are performed at 6- to 12-month intervals for several years. If the studies remain negative, then the interval between studies can be lengthened.
- A serum thyroglobulin is a useful tumor marker after a total thyroidectomy. Any measurable thyroglobulin level may indicate recurrence of the tumor. The presence of anti-thyroglobulin antibodies interferes with the use of this test. The sensitivity of the thyroglobulin assay is increased if the TSH is elevated (withdrawal of thyroid hormone or after Thyrogen administration)
- Tumor recurrences have been reported as long as 20 to 30 years after the initial surgery.
  ○ Therefore, the follow-up for patients with well-differentiated thyroid cancer is lifelong.

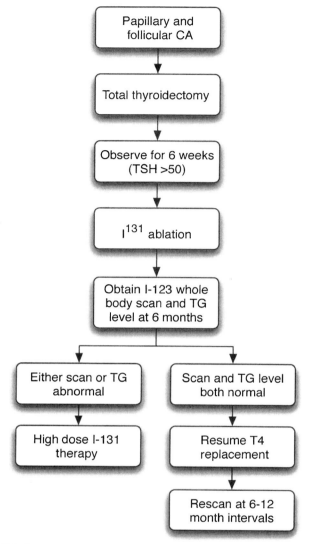

CA: Cancer.
TG: Thyroglobulin.
TSH: Thyroid-Stimulating Hormone.

FIG. 50–2 Management of well-differentiated papillary and follicular carcinomas.

THYROID FUNCTION TESTS

- TSH should be the initial test in the evaluation of hypo- or hyperthyroidism (Fig. 50–3)
- TSH is a reliable indicator of thyroid hormone status 95% of the time. The TSH is not reliable if the cause of the thyroid dysfunction is a pituitary or hypothalamic disorder.
- A normal TSH completes the workup if there is no suspicion of a pituitary or hypothalamic problem
- A decreased TSH, especially a value less than 0.1 mU/L, suggests the possibility of hyperthyroidism. If the free

T4 is elevated then the diagnosis of hyperthyroidism is established. If the free T4 is normal, a free T3 should be obtained. A normal free T3 (and a normal free T4 and decreased TSH) establishes a diagnosis of subclinical hyperthyroidism. An elevated free T3 establishes the presence of T3 toxicosis.

- An increased TSH suggests the possibility of hypothyroidism. A free T4 should be obtained to further characterize the disorder. A decreased free T4 establishes the diagnosis of hypothyroidism. A normal free T4 indicates subclinical hypothyroidism. Thyroid autoantibodies (anti-TPO and/or anti-TG) may be obtained to determine the risk of permanent hypothyroidism.
- The T3-resin uptake (T3U) is an indirect measure of the thyroid-binding globulin (TBG).
  - Thyroid hormones (both T4 and T3) are bound to TBG, albumin, and transthyretin. Thus, any change in the concentration or binding characteristics of the carrier proteins will affect the result of the measured total T4 and total T3. The TBG concentration may be increased by endogenous or exogenous estrogens, mild liver disease, or genetic factors. If the T3U result is reported as a percent, then the T3U is inversely related to the concentration of TBG. If the T3U result is reported as a ratio, then the result is directly related to the TBG concentration. TBG concentrations can be decreased by androgens, severe liver disease, acromegaly, nephrotic syndrome, and genetic factors. Reverse T3 has no biologic activity and may be useful in the evaluation of patients with euthyroid sick syndrome.
- Radioactive iodine uptake is important in the differential diagnosis of hyperthyroidism.
- Thyroid ultrasound can determine the size, shape, and consistency of the thyroid gland and/or thyroid nodule(s).
- Fine needle aspiration biopsy of the thyroid gland is important in the evaluation of thyroid nodules. It is the most sensitive and specific test for evaluation of thyroid nodules.
- Quantitative thyroglobulin is a tumor marker for papillary and follicular carcinoma of the thyroid gland. Calcitonin is a tumor marker for medullary carcinoma of the thyroid gland.

HYPOTHYROIDISM

CAUSES OF HYPOTHYROIDISM

- Primary hypothyroidism
  - Chronic autoimmune thyroiditis (Hashimoto's thyroiditis)
    - Atrophic
    - Goitrous
  - Thyroidectomy
  - Radiation

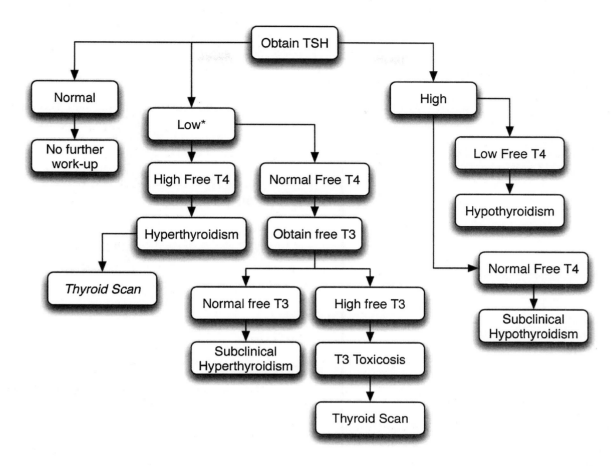

* If <0.1 suspect hyperthyroidism

TSH: Thyroid-Stimulating Hormone.

FIG. 50–3   Use of thyroid function tests (TFTs) in the evaluation of hypothyroidism and hyperthyroidism.

- ▪ Radioactive iodine therapy for hyperthyroidism
- ▪ External beam radiation to the head and neck area
  - ○ Defective thyroid hormone biosynthesis
- • Iodine deficiency
- • Enzyme abnormalities
- • Central hypothyroidism
- • Pituitary disorders
- • Hypothalamic disorders
- • Transient
- • Subacute thyroiditis
- • Silent thyroiditis
- • Postpartum thyroiditis

TREATMENT OF HYPOTHYROIDISM

- • The drug of choice is levothyroxine (L-T4)
- • In general, endocrinologists prefer branded L-T4
- • The medication should be administered on an empty stomach, 1 hour before or 2 to 3 hours after eating.

- • The medication should be administered the same time each day to promote compliance
- • The medication should not be taken with any other prescription or nonprescription medications
- • Heat, humidity, and direct sun light will degrade L-T4; therefore the medication should not be stored in a bathroom or window.
- • The approximate replacement dose is 1.4 to 1.6 mcg/kg daily
- • A general rule is to start low and titrate slowly up to the replacement dose, particularly if the patient is >65 years of age, <15 years of age, has concurrent cardiac problems, or has severe hypothyroidism.

MONITORING THYROID REPLACEMENT THERAPY

- • Primary hypothyroidism
  - ○ Monitor TSH
  - ○ Titrate the L-T4 dose to achieve a TSH value between 0.4 and 2.5

○ It takes 6 weeks to reach steady state between dose changes or when making changes between brand names or generic versions of L-T4.
• Secondary or central hypothyroidism
  ○ Monitor free T4, *not* the TSH
  ○ Titrate the L-T4 dose to achieve a free T4 level in the upper half of the normal range for the assay
• Thyroid cancer
  ○ TSH should be suppressed to 0.1 to 0.4 mU/L
  ○ If the risk of persistent or recurrent tumor is high monitor the quantitative thyroglobulin every 6 months for papillary or follicular thyroid carcinoma.
  ○ Monitor calcitonin every 6 months for medullary thyroid cancer.

MYXEDEMA COMA

• Rare, but potentially fatal disorder
• Usually occurs in the elderly
• Usually occurs in the winter months
• Usually associated with primary hypothyroidism and long-standing absence of thyroid hormone
• Treatment
  ○ Levothyroxine 300 to 500 mcg intravenously (IV) on day 1
  ○ Levothyroxine 50 to 100 mcg IV on day 2 and beyond
  ○ Dexamethasone 8 mg IV on day 1 while evaluating for the presence of adrenal insufficiency

SUBCLINICAL HYPOTHYROIDISM

• Primarily a laboratory diagnosis, characterized by a normal free T4 and a TSH that is elevated
• Few or no clinical signs or symptoms of thyroid dysfunction
• Prevalence in the United States is 4% to 8.5% and increases with age
• In women older than age 60, the prevalence is as high as 20%
• In men older than 65 years, the prevalence also rises significantly
• The prevalence in African Americans is one-third of that in the white population
• Approximately 2% to 5% per year will progress to overt hypothyroidism. The presence of thyroid autoantibodies (anti-TPO) predicts a higher risk of developing overt hypothyroidism. A TSH value >10 also predicts a higher risk of developing overt hypothyroidism
• Screening for hypothyroidism is controversial
  ○ The American Thyroid Association recommends screening for men and women beginning at age 35 and every 5 years thereafter.
  ○ The American Association of Clinical Endocrinologists recommends screening elderly women only.

○ The American College of Physicians recommends case screening in women over the age of 50.
• No clear approach to the treatment of subclinical hypothyroidism has been established
• Factors that favor the use of L-T4
  ○ Presence of anti-TPO and/or anti-TG antibodies (since the subsequent development of overt hypothyroidism is high)
  ○ Presence of a goiter
  ○ TSH >10
  ○ Perhaps older age and female sex
  ○ If no therapy with levothyroxine is started, monitor the TSH and clinical status every 6 months

THYROTOXICOSIS

DIFFERENTIAL DIAGNOSIS OF THYROTOXICOSIS

• Sustained hormone overproduction (high radioactive iodine uptake)
  ○ Graves disease
  ○ Toxic multinodular goiter
  ○ Toxic uninodular goiter or toxic adenoma
  ○ Iodine-induced (*jodbasedow*)
  ○ Trophoblastic tumor (rare)
  ○ Increased TSH secretion (rare)
• No associated hyperthyroidism (low radioactive iodine uptake)
  ○ Thyrotoxicosis factitia
  ○ Subacute thyroiditis
  ○ Painless or silent thyroiditis
  ○ Postpartum thyroiditis
  ○ Hamburger thyroiditis (rare)
  ○ Ectopic thyroid tissue (rare)
  ○ Struma ovarii

After a biochemical diagnosis of hyperthyroidism is made, a radioactive iodine uptake and scan are performed to differentiate the etiology of thyrotoxicosis. The most common causes for thyrotoxicosis are Graves disease, toxic multinodular goiter, and toxic uninodular goiter.

TREATMENT OF HYPERTHYROIDISM

• Antithyroid drugs (ATD)
  ○ Propylthiouracil (PTU)
  ○ Methimazole (Tapazole or MMI)
• Radioactive iodine
• Surgery

Which therapy is best is a matter of debate. There is no one *best* treatment. The choice of therapy largely depends on physician experience and the patient's preferences. The principal objective is to alleviate the thyrotoxicosis and its attendant symptoms.

ANTITHYROID DRUGS

- ATDs are chiefly used for long-term treatment of patients with Graves disease
  - ATDs are preferred for pregnant women, children, adolescents, before surgery, and prior to radioactive iodine therapy
  - PTU is the preferred drug during pregnancy, lactation, and for thyroid storm
  - MMI will more rapidly normalize the T4 and T3
  - PTU is supplied as a 50 mg tablet and the usual starting dose is 100 mg three times a day
  - MMI is supplied as 5 or 10 mg tablet and the usual starting dose is 30 mg daily.
  - Factors that determine the speed of recovery
    - Disease activity
    - Initial degree of hyperthyroidism
    - Intrathyroidal stores of T4 and T3, which correlates with the size of the thyroid gland
- Factors that favor a sustained remission after ATD:
  - T3-toxicosis
  - Small goiter
  - Decrease in size of the goiter during therapy
  - Normal thyroid function tests
  - Normal TSH
  - Negative tests for thyroid-stimulating immunoglobulin
  - The presence of HLA-DR4
  - Duration of antithyroid drug therapy
  - Amount of the medication needed to control the hyperthyroidism
- Clinical considerations during ATD therapy
  - Patients should be seen every 6 weeks if they are not pregnant and every 4 weeks if they are pregnant
  - Patients are usually euthyroid in 6 to 12 weeks
  - The dose of ATD should be decreased progressively as the hyperthyroidism subsides
    - A reasonable rule of thumb is to decrease the dose by 25% to 33% each visit if the free T4 and free T3 are normal.
  - The free T4 and free T3 are the best tests to monitor during ATD therapy. The TSH may remain low for months after the free T4 and free T3 are normal.
  - The dose of ATD is decreased to the lowest dose that maintains the free T4 and free T3 within the normal range.
  - ATDs are discontinued after 12 to 24 months of control of the hyperthyroidism
  - Most relapses occur within the first year off the ATDs
  - Rate of recurrent thyrotoxicosis plateaus at 50% at year 5 following discontinuation of the ATD
  - Lifelong follow-up for all patients with Graves disease is essential because hypothyroidism may occur years after successful ATD treatment.

β-ADRENERGIC ANTAGONISTS

- Ameliorate several of the clinical manifestations of hyperthyroidism.
- Also impair conversion of T4 to T3.
- Propranolol (80 mg/d), atenolol (50 mg/d), metoprolol (50 mg/d), or nadolol (40mg/d) are possible drug choices with their usual starting doses.
- The dose of β-blocker can be titrated to relieve the symptoms of hyperthyroidism (anxiety, palpitations, tremor, nervousness, and heat intolerance).
- Calcium channel blockers, such as diltiazem, can be substituted if β-blockers are contraindicated.

RADIOACTIVE IODINE THERAPY

- Most widely used treatment for adults with thyrotoxicosis in the United States.
- I-131 is the isotope of choice. It is administered orally as a capsule or a liquid. I-131 is effective as a single dose approximately 90% of the time. The typical dose range is 5 to 15 mcg. It takes 3 to 6 months for the patient to achieve a euthyroid or hypothyroid state after administering I-131.
- Contraindications
  - Pregnancy
  - Breast-feeding
- Relative Contraindications
  - Children
  - Adolescents
- It is advisable to avoid pregnancy for 6 to 12 months after I-131 therapy
  - There are no known adverse effects on the health of offspring of treated patients
- Hypothyroidism will probably occur after therapy (50% in 10 years)

SURGERY FOR HYPERTHYROIDISM

- Subtotal or total thyroidectomy is the oldest form of therapy for thyrotoxicosis.
- Very infrequently used today.
- Surgery is limited to special circumstances
  - Children
  - Adolescents
  - Middle trimester of pregnancy
  - Patients with large goiters
  - Patients with Graves ophthalmopathy
  - Patient choice
- Mortality is close to zero
- Morbidity
  - Recurrent laryngeal nerve damage
  - Hypoparathyroidism (transient or permanent) and hypocalcemia

- Preoperative preparation
  - Use ATDs to induce a euthyroid state
  - Potassium iodide (SSKI) or Lugol's solution for 10 days prior to surgery
  - β-Adrenergic antagonists are also administered

THYROID STORM

- Rare complication of poorly controlled hyperthyroidism.
- Potentially fatal.
- Pathogenesis is unknown.
- It is a clinical diagnosis—lab tests are done to confirm the clinical impression.
- Treatment
  - Large doses of ATDs: PTU 300 to 400 mg every 4 hours by mouth (PO)
  - Iodine: SSKI 3 to 5 drops every 6 hours orally
  - Dexamethasone 8 mg IV daily until adrenal insufficiency is ruled out
  - β-adrenergic antagonists either IV or PO

SUBCLINICAL HYPERTHYROIDISM

- Established when the free T4 and free T3 are normal with an undetectable TSH.
- There is an increased risk of atrial fibrillation for individuals older than 60 years of age.
- There is also an increased risk of osteopenia or osteoporosis.
- Treatment
  - Observation
  - Radioactive iodine. If the patient is older than 60 years, has osteopenia, or a cardiac problem, therapy is generally indicated

HYPERTHYROIDISM AND PREGNANCY AND LACTATION

- ATD therapy with PTU is the treatment of choice
- MMI is an acceptable alternative, but it has been associated with minor birth defects (aplasia cutis).
- ATDs are not believed to be teratogenic, however, neonatal thyroid function may be affected by transplacental passage of the ATD.
- The free T4 and free T3 are controlled to slightly above the normal range to minimize the dose of ATD.
- Thyroid function tests are monitored every 4 weeks.
- Graves disease often spontaneously improves in the later months of pregnancy.
- β-Adrenergic antagonists can be used to alleviate symptoms.

TOXIC MULTINODULAR OR SINGLE NODULE

- Toxic multinodular goiter is more common among older adults.
- Spontaneous remissions do not occur.
- Radioactive iodine or surgery is the treatment of choice.
- Surgery may be favored when the goiter or nodule is large.

EUTHYROID HYPERTHYROXINEMIA

- May be associated with increased TBG.
- Familial dysalbuminemic hyperthyroxinemia
  - Mutant albumin with low affinity and high capacity for T4, but not T3
  - Autosomal dominant inheritance

BIBLIOGRAPHY

Gharib H, Tuttle RM, Baskin HJ, et al. Subclinical thyroid dysfunction: a joint statement on management from the American Association of Clinical Endocrinologists, the American Thyroid Association, and the Endocrine Society. *Endocr Pract.* 2004;10:497–501.

Huber GH, Staub JJ, Meier C, et al. Prospective study of the spontaneous course of subclinical hypothyroidism: prognostic value of thyrotropin, thyroid reserve, and thyroid antibodies. *J Clin Endocrinol Metab.* 2002; 87:3221–3226.

Ladenson PW; Singer PA; Ain KB; et al. American Thyroid Association Guidelines for detection of thyroid dysfunction. *Arch Intern Med,* 2000;160:1573–1575.

Surks MI; Ortiz E; Daniels GH; et al. Subclinical thyroid disease: scientific review and guidelines for diagnosis and management. *JAMA.* 2004;291:228–238.

51 ADRENAL GLAND

Bahaeldeen A. Laz

INTRODUCTION

- The adrenal glands are paired organs that functionally consist of three tissues under independent control:
  - The outer cortex (zona glomerulosa) mainly controlled by the renin-angiotensin system, which regulates the release of aldosterone which, in turn, regulates sodium and potassium homeostasis.

◦ The inner cortex (zona fasciculata and zona reticularis) are primarily controlled by the corticotropin-releasing hormone (CRH)–corticotropin (ACTH) axis, which regulates the response to stress via the actions of cortisol; it also produces adrenal androgens.

◦ The medulla, which is part of the sympathetic nervous system and produces epinephrine.

GROSS STRUCTURE

• The adrenal gland in adults is a roughly pyramidal structure (2–3 cm wide, 4–6 cm long, and approximately 1 cm thick) that lies above and medial to the kidney.

• Each adrenal weighs approximately 4 g. The medulla accounts for approximately 10% of the total adrenal weight.

VASCULAR SUPPLY

• The adrenal glands are perfused by approximately 12 small arteries that originate from the aorta and the inferior phrenic, renal, and intercostal arteries. Occasionally the adrenal gland is perfused by blood originating from the left ovarian or left internal spermatic arteries.

• The right adrenal vein is short and drains into the inferior vena cava. The longer left adrenal vein usually drains into the left renal vein, either directly or after being joined by the left inferior phrenic vein.

LIGHT MICROSCOPIC STRUCTURE

• The cortex is divided into three concentric zones:

◦ The zona glomerulosa constitutes approximately 15% of the adult cortex. It consists of cells that are small and have a low cytoplasmic-to-nuclear ratio and are deficient in 17-hydroxylase activity.

◦ The zona fasciculata constitutes approximately 75% of the cortex. Its large cells have a high cytoplasmic-to-nuclear ratio and their *clear* cytoplasm is foamy and vacuolated because of abundant lipid inclusions.

◦ The innermost zona reticularis consists of irregular anastomosing cords of cells separated by thin-walled sinusoids. The cytoplasmic-to-nuclear ratio is intermediate, and the *dense* cytoplasm is lipid-poor.

◦ The cortical cuff surrounding the central vein resembles the zona glomerulosa centrally and the zona fasciculata peripherally.

ADRENAL STEROID BIOSYNTHESIS

• The major adrenal steroid hormones synthesized in the adrenal cortex include glucocorticoids (particularly cortisol), androgens, and estrogens (zona fasciculata and reticularis); and aldosterone (zona glomerulosa).

• Cholesterol is the substrate for the synthesis of all steroid hormones. The cells of the adrenal cortex can synthesize cholesterol de novo from acetate.

CORTISOL BIOSYNTHESIS

• The rate-limiting process in steroidogenesis is the transport of free cholesterol through the cytosol to the inner mitochondrial membrane. Cholesterol transport into mitochondria is mediated by the steroidogenic acute regulatory (StAR) protein.

• Pregnenolone is converted to progesterone by 3-β-hydroxysteroid dehydrogenase.

• Progesterone is converted to 17-α-hydroxyprogesterone via cytochrome P450 enzyme 17 (CYP17), which is a microsomal enzyme that catalyzes hydroxylation at the C17 position of progesterone or pregnenolone. The dual function of CYP17 allows directed steroidogenesis: 17-α-hydroxylated substrates with an intact side chain are glucocorticoid precursors, whereas generation of C19 steroids by both 17-α-hydroxylase and 17,20-hydroxylase activities directs substrate toward androgen and estrogen synthesis. In the zona glomerulosa, which lacks either isoform of CYP17 activity, pregnenolone is converted into aldosterone.

• Conversion of 17-α-hydroxyprogesterone to 11-deoxycortisol occurs via the action of CYP21A2.

• Subsequent conversion of 11-deoxycortisol to cortisol is dependent on the action of CYP11B1.

ALDOSTERONE BIOSYNTHESIS

• Progesterone is also the principal substrate for mineralocorticoid synthesis.

• In the zona glomerulosa progesterone is hydroxylated at C21 by CYP11A2 to yield deoxycorticosterone. All three terminal steps in the conversion of this intermediate to aldosterone (11-β-hydroxylation, 18-hydroxylation, and 18-methyl oxidation) are catalyzed by a single mitochondrial P450 enzyme, CYP11B2 (aldosterone synthase).

• The zona glomerulosa is well adapted for the production of aldosterone. Because it has a low concentration of 17-hydroxylase, the enzyme directs substrate along the pathways to cortisol and androgen synthesis. It is the only adrenocortical zone that has the enzyme required for the final conversion of deoxycorticosterone to aldosterone.

ADRENAL ANDROGEN BIOSYNTHESIS

- Steroids with 19 carbon atoms and androgenic activity are synthesized by the adrenals.
- Dehydroepiandrosterone (DHEA) and DHEA sulfate are the most abundant steroid hormones produced by the adrenal glands. They are generated in the zona reticularis via the conversion of 17-α-hydroxypregnenolone.
- Androstenedione, a weak androgen, is produced by side-chain cleavage of 17-α-hydroxyprogesterone via P450 C17 and is subsequently converted to testosterone by 17-ketosteroid reductase, mainly in the peripheral tissues.

CORTICOTROPIN AND CORTISOL SECRETION

- There are four patterns of pituitary ACTH and, consequently, of cortisol secretion in normal subjects:
  1. *Pulsatile*: Like other anterior pituitary hormones, ACTH is secreted in bursts, which causes a rapid increase in plasma ACTH and serum cortisol concentration. The increase in plasma cortisol induces a decrease in plasma ACTH accompanied by a slower decrement in serum cortisol, because of its delayed clearance from plasma.
  2. *Circadian rhythm*: The diurnal rhythm of cortisol secretion results from ACTH secretory episodes of greater amplitude in the morning hours.
  3. *Stress-induced secretion*: Physical stresses include severe trauma, burns, major surgery, hypoglycemia, fever, hypotension, exercise, and cold exposure.
  4. *Negative feedback inhibition by glucocorticoids*: Feedback inhibition of ACTH secretion by glucocorticoids occurs at both the pituitary and hypothalamic levels.

OTHER REGULATORY FACTORS

- Atrial natriuretic peptide (ANP) when infused into normal subjects, inhibits CRH- and vasopressin-induced ACTH secretion. In contrast, another member of the natriuretic peptide family, C-type ANP, stimulates ACTH secretion.
- Leptin activates receptors on adrenocortical cells, thus, inhibiting ACTH-stimulated aldosterone, cortisol, and dehydroepiandrosterone secretion. Leptin may also inhibit stress-induced activation of hypothalamic CRH neurons. Leptin is increased in patients with obesity, type 2 diabetes, and Cushing's syndrome.
- There is an inverse relationship between the mean daily serum cortisol concentration and body mass index.

CORTISOL

- Under basal conditions, approximately 10% is free, approximately 70% is bound to the cortisol-binding globulin, and 20% is bound to albumin.
- The major site of cortisol metabolism is the liver, where it undergoes reduction, oxidation, or hydroxylation. Subsequently conjugation with sulfate or glucuronic acid produces water soluble metabolites which are excreted in the urine.
- The kidney is the major site of extrahepatic cortisol metabolism in humans. There, cortisol is converted to cortisone by 11β-hydroxysteroid dehydrogenase type 2 (11β-HSD2).

THE PRINCIPAL ACTIONS OF GLUCOCORTICOIDS

- The glucocorticoids act as a physiological antagonist to insulin by promoting gluconeogenesis, degradation of lipids and proteins, and mobilization of extrahepatic amino acids and ketones. This leads to increased blood glucose concentrations, resulting in increased glycogen formation in the liver.
- Glucocorticoids increase blood pressure and stabilize the vascular endothelium.
- Glucocorticoids act as immunosuppressants. For example, cortisol inhibits proliferation of T-cells by inhibiting the action of interleukin-1 on T-helper cells, thus rendering them unresponsive to T-cell growth factors.
- Bone formation is impaired by interfering with bone remodeling.
- Cortisol induces a potassium shift to the extracellular compartment in exchange for sodium. This effect can produce or exacerbate hyperkalemia.
- Protracted cortisol secretion causes proteolysis (catabolism) and muscle wasting.
- Cortisol also plays a permissive role in water homeostasis by facilitating free water clearance.
- Augments appetite.
- Suppresses ACTH.
- Improves vasopressor response to various vasoactive peptides.
- Decreases the production of nitric oxide.

ALDOSTERONE

- Aldosterone is released in response to angiotensin II stimulation, and hyperkalemia.
- ACTH may acutely stimulate aldosterone synthesis and secretion.
- Aldosterone promotes reabsorption of sodium in the cortical collecting duct of the kidney and, therefore, plays an essential role in volume homeostasis.

• Aldosterone also promotes secretion of potassium and hydrogen in the distal nephron, which may induce metabolic alkalosis and hyperkalemia.

ADRENAL INSUFFICIENCY

The causes of adrenal insufficiency are typically classified into two broad categories: (1) primary (destruction of the gland) or (2) secondary (disruption of the pituitary secretion of ACTH). There are many causes of primary and secondary adrenal insufficiency, however, the most common cause of primary is autoimmune destruction of the gland, while prolonged glucocorticoid use is the most common cause of secondary adrenal insufficiency. Other causes include:

• *Primary adrenal insufficiency:* idiopathic destruction of the gland; tuberculosis (most common in underserved nations), fungal infection, infiltrative diseases, hemorrhage, metastatic cancer, and drugs such as ketoconazole, phenytoin, and rifampin.
• *Secondary adrenal insufficiency:* prolonged glucocorticoid suppression of ACTH secretion, panhypopituitarism, Sheehan's syndrome, and pituitary apoplexy.
• *Tertiary adrenal insufficiency*: said to occur when hypothalamic secretion of corticotropin-releasing factor is decreased. The most common cause of tertiary adrenal insufficiency are abrupt cessation of glucocorticoid therapy (also sometimes seen with treatment of Cushing's syndrome).

PRIMARY ADRENAL INSUFFICIENCY (ADDISON'S DISEASE)

• Bilateral adrenal destruction secondary to tuberculosis is the most common cause worldwide. In industrialized nations, tuberculosis accounts for only 7% to 20% of cases; autoimmune disease is responsible for 70% to 90%; the remainder are caused by other infectious diseases, infiltration by metastatic cancer or lymphoma, adrenal hemorrhage or infarction, or drugs.

AUTOIMMUNE ADRENALITIS
• Humoral and cell mediated process which destroys the adrenal cortex
• Autoantibodies are detectable in most (60%–70%)

Polyglandular Autoimmune Syndrome Type I and II (PGA-1/PGA-2) include autoimmune adrenalitis combined with other autoimmune endocrine disorders (thyroid autoimmune injury in type II and parathyroid injury in type 1)

• PGA-1 is a rare autosomal recessive disorder.
• Females are affected slightly more frequently than males.

• Associated with a mutation in the autoimmune regulator (AIER) a putative transcription factor localized to chromosome 21q22.3.
• Hypoparathyroidism and chronic mucocutaneous candidiasis are the classic manifestations of PGA-1.
• Adrenal insufficiency develops in the second or third decade of life.
• Malabsorption occurs in 25% of patients.
• Primary hypogonadism occurs in approximately 60% of patients.

Polyglandular Autoimmune Type II (Schmidt Syndrome, PGA-2)

• Is considerably more common than PGA-1. Importantly, primary adrenal insufficiency is virtually always seen in PGA-2.
• Autoimmune thyroid disease occurs in 20% of patients.
• Diabetes mellitus occurs in 30% of patients.
• Half of the cases are thought to be familial, and several modes of inheritance (autosomal recessive, autosomal dominant, and polygenic) have been described. Nonetheless, the precise sequence of pathogenetic events in PGA-2 are poorly understood.
• Women are affected up to three times more often than men.
• The age of onset ranges from age 20 to 40 years.
• Hypoparathyroidism does not occur in this disorder, and alopecia and pernicious anemia are much less frequent than in the type I syndrome.
• Vitiligo, myasthenia gravis, thrombocytopenic purpura, Sjögren syndrome, and rheumatoid arthritis have been described in PGA-2.

INFECTIOUS ADRENALITIS
• *Tuberculosis* can destroy the adrenal glands. Tuberculous adrenalitis results from hematogenous spread from an active infection elsewhere in the body. Extraadrenal tuberculosis is usually evident but may be clinically latent. Recovery of normal adrenal function rarely occurs after effective antituberculous therapy.
• *Disseminated fungal infections*: Several species of fungi can infiltrate the adrenal glands and cause adrenal insufficiency. Histoplasmosis and paracoccidioidomycosis (South American blastomycosis) are important causes of adrenal insufficiency in endemic areas. In contrast, adrenal insufficiency is rare in patients with cryptococcosis, coccidioidomycosis, and North American blastomycosis.
• *Human immunodeficiency virus infection*: The adrenal glands develop necrotizing adrenalitis caused by cytomegalovirus infection, but infection with *Mycobacterium avium-intracellulare* or *Cryptococcus* as well as involvement via metastatic Kaposi's sarcoma can also occur. Drugs used to treat HIV may contribute to the adrenal dysfunction in these patients.

- Some patients with acquired immune deficiency syndrome have symptoms of adrenal insufficiency but normal or high basal serum cortisol concentrations. These patients may have peripheral resistance to glucocorticoid action because of decreased affinity of type II (glucocorticoid) receptors.

ADRENAL HEMORRHAGE

- Reported in 0.3% to 1.8% of autopsy studies, although extensive bilateral adrenal hemorrhage may be present in 15% of individuals who die of shock.
- Bilateral adrenal hemorrhage is more common in males (2:1 male-to-female ratio).
- Chronic adrenal insufficiency occurs in most patients who survive bilateral adrenal hemorrhage.

Mechanisms of Nontraumatic Adrenal Hemorrhage

- The adrenal gland has a rich arterial supply but only a single drainage vein; the transition from artery to capillary plexus is so abrupt as to constitute a vascular dam.
- In stress, ACTH secretion increases, which stimulates adrenal arterial blood flow that may exceed the limited venous drainage capacity of the organ and, hence lead to vascular congestion and hemorrhage.
- Adrenal vein spasm induced by high catecholamine levels (stress/trauma) and adrenal vein thrombosis induced by coagulopathies may also lead to venous stasis and hemorrhage.

Common Causes of Adrenal Hemorrhage

- *Infectious*: sepsis, *Clostridium difficile* colitis, influenza, varicella, and malaria; Waterhouse-Friderichsen syndrome (severe hemorrhage secondary to overwhelming bacterial infection, classically meningococcemia)
- *Obstetric*: toxemia of pregnancy, spontaneous abortion, antepartum or postpartum hemorrhage
- *Hemorrhagic diatheses*: Anticoagulant use, thrombocytopenia, antiphospholipid antibody syndrome
- *Blunt trauma*
- *Complication* of granulomatous diseases, amyloidosis, and metastatic cancer
- Treatment with *ACTH* for multiple sclerosis or inflammatory bowel disease
- Right adrenal hemorrhage occurs in 2% of liver transplant recipients secondary to intraoperative ligation of the right adrenal vein

DRUGS THAT ARE ASSOCIATED WITH ADRENAL INSUFFICIENCY

- Several drugs inhibit cortisol biosynthesis: aminoglutethimide, etoposide, ketoconazole, and suramin.

- Some drugs promote the metabolism of cortisol and other synthetic glucocorticoids by inducing hepatic mixed-function oxygenase enzymes. These include phenytoin, barbiturates, and rifampin.
- Megestrol acetate is a progestin with partial glucocorticoid activity; thus, its withdrawal can occasionally cause secondary adrenal insufficiency.

CLINICAL MANIFESTATIONS OF ADRENAL INSUFFICIENCY

- The symptoms and signs of adrenal insufficiency depend on the rate and extent of loss of adrenal function, whether mineralocorticoid production is preserved, and the degree of stress. The onset of adrenal insufficiency is often very gradual, and it may go undetected until an illness or other stress precipitates adrenal crisis.

CHRONIC SYMPTOMS
- Weakness and fatigue.
- Anorexia, nausea, vomiting.
- Abdominal pain.
- Myalgias and arthralgias, postural dizziness.
- Sodium pica.
- Headache, memory impairment, and depression.
- Decreased axillary and pubic hair as well as loss of libido are common in women, in whom androgen production primarily occurs in the adrenal glands. These changes are unusual in men, in whom most androgen production occurs in the testes.

Physical Examination

- Increased pigmentation, secondary to sustained elevations in ACTH
- Hypotension, particularly when stressed
- Tachycardia
- Fever
- Decreased body hair, vitiligo

Laboratory Findings

- Hyponatremia (secondary to cortisol deficiency and the attendant decrease in free water clearance)
- Hyperkalemia (more common with a deficiency in aldosterone)
- Hypoglycemia
- Eosinophilia

ADRENAL CRISIS
- The predominant manifestation of adrenal crisis is shock; but patients often present with nonspecific symptoms such as anorexia, nausea, vomiting, abdominal pain, weakness, fatigue, lethargy, fever, confusion, or coma.

- Hyperpigmentation is not observed because of the acute nature of the insult.
- The major hormonal perturbation precipitating an adrenal crisis is a decrease in mineralocorticoid synthesis, rather than glucocorticoid deficiency. Thus, adrenal crisis can occur in patients who are receiving physiologic or even pharmacologic doses of synthetic glucocorticoid if their mineralocorticoid requirements are not met.

CORTICOSTEROID INSUFFICIENCY IN ACUTELY ILL PATIENTS

- An increase in tissue corticosteroid levels during acute illness is an important protective response.
- Many diseases and their treatments interfere with the normal corticosteroid response to illness and thus may induce tissue corticosteroid insufficiency.
- In critically ill patients, a standard corticotropin stimulation test may lack sufficient sensitivity for the diagnosis of adrenal insufficiency, because it measures adrenal reserve and not adrenal function.
- Maximally stressed patients may be secreting all the cortisol that their adrenal glands can synthesize, eg, adrenal reserve is negligible.
- Subnormal adrenal corticosteroid production during acute severe illness has been termed *functional adrenal insufficiency* to reflect the notion that hypoadrenalism can occur without obvious structural defects in the hypothalamic-pituitary-adrenal (HPA) axis.
- *Relative adrenal insufficiency* reflects an inadequate response to exogenous ACTH in which cortisol levels, although high in absolute terms, are insufficient to control the inflammatory response.
- During physiological stress the diurnal variation in cortisol secretion is lost.
- Levels of corticosteroid-binding globulin decrease rapidly in stress, causing an increase in the free cortisol level.

EFFECT OF CORTICOSTEROIDS ON THE INTEGRITY OF THE CIRCULATORY SYSTEM

- Cortisol has a vital supportive role in the maintenance of vascular tone, endothelial integrity, vascular permeability, and the distribution of total body water within the vascular compartment.
- Cortisol increases the vascular and cardiac response to the renin-angiotensin and the sympathetic nervous systems, the two most important homeostatic mechanisms in the maintenance of arterial pressure during severe sepsis.
- Cortisol is a powerful immunosuppressive hormone and modulates the inflammatory response and cytokine production. For example, cortisol potently inhibits the production of inducible nitric oxide as well as other mediators of septic shock.

DIAGNOSIS OF ADRENAL INSUFFICIENCY

- Confirmation of the clinical diagnosis of adrenal insufficiency should involve three steps:
  1. Demonstrating an inappropriately low cortisol secretion
  2. Assessing whether the cortisol deficiency is dependent on or independent of ACTH and evaluating mineralocorticoid secretion in patients without ACTH deficiency
  3. Seeking a treatable cause of the primary disorder

RANDOM CORTISOL LEVELS

- In nonstress situations, a basal cortisol level >11 μg virtually excludes ACTH-cortisol insufficiency, whereas a basal cortisol <3 μg/dl strongly suggests adrenal insufficiency.

Subnormal Response to Acute ACTH Stimulation

- A short Cosyntropin stimulation test should be performed in virtually all patients in whom the diagnosis of adrenal insufficiency is being considered, unless the diagnosis has been ruled out by a basal serum cortisol value that exceeds the normal reference range.
- Cosyntropin is an ACTH (1-24) analogue, which has the full biologic potency of native ACTH (1–39).
- A normal response to the Cosyntropin (250 μg as an intravenous bolus) stimulation test is a rise in serum cortisol concentration after 30 or 60 minutes to a peak of 18 to 20 μg/dL or more.
- Critically ill patients usually present with a high basal cortisol level and may not show a further increase after ACTH administration. Either a basal cortisol level of <20 to 25 μg/dL or an incremental response of <9 μg/dL after Cosyntropin stimulation predicts a poor outcome and identifies patients who respond favorably to glucocorticoid administration.

DIAGNOSIS OF SECONDARY ADRENAL INSUFFICIENCY

- High-dose Cosyntropin does not exclude chronic partial pituitary ACTH deficiency or deficiency of recent onset (eg, within 1 to 2 weeks after pituitary surgery).
- The adrenal glands have not yet become atrophic and are, therefore, still capable of responding to ACTH stimulation.

METYRAPONE TESTING

- Blocks cortisol synthesis by inhibiting the 11-hydroxylase enzyme.
- The overnight test is performed by administering 30 mg/kg of metyrapone orally at midnight.

- An adequate response is characterized by a plasma 11-deoxycortisol level >7 ng/dL and a plasma ACTH level >100 pg/mL.

INSULIN-INDUCED HYPOGLYCEMIA TESTING
- The stimulus of neuroglycopenia associated with hypoglycemia (blood glucose <40 mg/dL)
- In normal persons, plasma cortisol increases to >18 to 20 µg/dL and plasma ACTH response >100 pg/mL

CORTICOTROPIN-RELEASING HORMONE TESTING (1 µG/KG)
- ACTH responses are exaggerated in patients with primary adrenal failure and absent in patients with hypopituitarism. Delayed responses may occur in patients with hypothalamic disorders.

TREATMENT OF ADRENAL INSUFFICIENCY

- Adrenal insufficiency (Addison's disease) is a potentially life-threatening disorder, but some patients have few symptoms unless severely stressed.
- Patients with secondary adrenal insufficiency rarely present with symptoms or signs of glucocorticoid deficiency (such as hypoglycemia or peripheral vascular collapse during stress).
- These patients usually have symptoms of other anterior pituitary hormone deficiencies, such as infertility; impotence; fatigue; hoarseness; or constipation; or, in children, failure to grow.

TREATMENT OF ADRENAL CRISIS
- Adrenal crisis is a life-threatening emergency that requires immediate treatment.
- The initial goal of therapy in adrenal crisis is treatment of hypotension and reversal of electrolyte abnormalities and replacement of cortisol. Large volumes (2–3 L) of 0.9% saline or 5% dextrose in 0.9% saline should be infused intravenously as quickly as possible to stabilize hemodynamics.
- Glucocorticoid deficiency should be treated by immediate intravenous injection of hydrocortisone; 100 mg should be given every 6 to 8 hours.
- In contrast to glucocorticoid replacement, mineralocorticoid replacement is not acutely useful because the effects require several days to manifest.

TREATMENT OF CHRONIC PRIMARY ADRENAL INSUFFICIENCY
- Maintenance therapy with hydrocortisone: 15 to 20 mg in the morning and 5 to 10 mg at early afternoon; or a once-a-day dose of 0.75 mg for dexamethasone or 5 to 7.5 mg of prednisone.
- Maintenance therapy should also include the mineralocorticoid, fluorocortisol, at a dose of 0.05 to 0.1 mg daily.

- Patient should wear a medical tag or bracelet identifying their clinical condition.
- Triple the dose of glucocorticoid when the patient is subjected to a minor illness or injury. Consider self-injection with hydrocortisone 100 mg or dexamethasone 4 mg intramuscularly if the patient is unable to take oral medications.

CONGENITAL ADRENAL HYPERPLASIA

- Inherited as an autosomal recessive trait.
- The term *adrenal hyperplasia* derives from the tendency of the gland to undergo enlargement or hyperplasia under the sustained influence of ACTH. ACTH secretion is increased because of the decrease in cortisol biosynthesis.
- Excessive synthesis of precursor steroids with androgenic activity can cause virilization. Deoxycorticosterone, which has mineralocorticoid activity can cause hypertension.

21-HYDROXYLASE DEFICIENCY

- The most common form of congenital adrenal hyperplasia accounting for 95% of cases.
- Cortisol deficiency is the hallmark, however, severe salt wasting occurs in one-third of the patients.
- Salt wasting and hyperkalemia.
- Adrenal virilization in the female.
- In the adult form, patients have no developmental abnormalities or salt wasting but usually present with symptoms and signs of androgen excess at the time of puberty or soon thereafter.

11β-HYDROXYLASE DEFICIENCY

- Accumulation of 11-deoxycorticosterone, which has potent mineralocorticoid-like effects.
- Hypertension, metabolic alkalosis, and hypokalemia.

3-HYDROXYSTEROID DEHYDROGENASE TYPE 2 DEFICIENCY

- Inefficient or impaired cortisol synthesis with hypersecretion of DHEA.
- Severe salt wasting and hyperkalemia occur.
- Male fetus may be incompletely virilized or feminized. In the female, overproduction of DHEA may produce partial virilization.

20,22-DESMOLASE DEFICIENCY

- Extremely rare
- Global adrenocortical insufficiency and death

17α-HYDROXYLASE/17,20-LYASE DEFICIENCY

- Impaired production of glucocorticoids and sex steroids.
- 11-deoxycorticosterone production is elevated.
- Characterized by hypogonadism, hypokalemia, and hypertension.
- Female patients have primary amenorrhea and lack development of secondary sexual characteristics.
- Male patients have either ambiguous external genitalia or a female phenotype (male pseudohermaphroditism).

DIAGNOSIS OF CONGENITAL ADRENAL HYPERPLASIA

- *A CYP21A2 defect* will present will elevated serum 17-hydroxyprogesterone levels.
- *CYP11B1 deficiency* results in high 11-deoxycorticosterone and 11-deoxycortisol levels.
- *17α-hydroxylase/17,20-lyase deficiency* produces marked elevations of serum deoxycorticosterone and corticosterone.
- *3-hydroxysteroid dehydrogenase type 2 (HSD2) deficiency*: Associated with very high levels of urine DHEA and low levels of pregnanetriol and cortisol metabolites.

TREATMENT OF CONGENITAL ADRENAL HYPERPLASIA

- Daily administration of glucocorticoids to suppress ACTH.
- Treatment should be monitored with frequent measurements of serum 17-hydroxyprogesterone levels (adequate control is indicated by a level of <1000 ng/dL).
- When prenatal diagnosis has identified a female fetus affected with classic congenital adrenal hyperplasia, the mother should be treated with dexamethasone to avoid virilization of the female external genitalia.

BIBLIOGRAPHY

Allolio, B, Fassnacht, M. Clinical review: adrenocortical carcinoma—clinical update. *J Clin Endocrinol Metab.* 2006;91:2027.

Annane D. Time for a consensus definition of corticosteroid insufficiency in critically ill patients. *Crit Care Med.* 2003;31:1868–1869.

Annane D, Sebille V, Charpentier C, et al. Effect of treatment with low doses of hydrocortisone and fludrocortisone on mortality in patients with septic shock. *JAMA.* 2002;288:862–871.

Annane D, Sebille V, Troche G, et al. A 3-levelprognostic classification in septic shock based on cortisol levels and cortisol response to corticotropin. *JAMA.* 2000;283:1038–1045.

Arnaldi G, Angeli A, Atkinson AB, et al. Diagnosis and complications of Cushing's syndrome: a consensus statement. *J Clin Endocrinol Metab.* 2003;88:5593.

Bernard MH, Sidhu S, Berger N, et al. A case report in favor of a multistep adrenocortical tumorigenesis. *J Clin Endocrinol Metab.* 2003;88:998.

Castro M, Elias PC, Quidute AR, et al. Out-patient screening for Cushing's syndrome: the sensitivity of the combination of circadian rhythm and overnight dexamethasone suppression salivary cortisol tests. *J Clin Endocrinol Metab.* 1999;84:878.

Dickstein G. The assessment of the hypothalamo-pituitary-adrenal axis in pituitary disease: are there short cuts? *J Endocrinol Invest.* 2003;26:25–30.

Grumbach MM, Biller BM, Braunstein GD, et al. Management of the clinically inapparent adrenal mass. *Ann Intern Med.* 2003;138:424.

Zaloga GP, Marik P. Hypothalamic-pituitary adrenal insufficiency. *Crit Care Clin.* 2001;17:25–41.

52 FAMILIAL HYPERCHOLESTEROLEMIA
George T. Griffing

GENERAL

Familial hypercholesterolemia (FH) is a genetic disorder (autosomal dominant) that produces extreme elevations in blood levels of total cholesterol and low-density lipoprotein cholesterol (LDL). FH is associated with a high risk for premature coronary artery disease (CAD), and therefore early diagnosis and aggressive treatment is important. Furthermore, first-degree relatives should be screened so that other gene carriers can be identified and treated.

PATHOPHYSIOLOGY

Michael S. Brown and Joseph L. Goldstein received the Nobel Peace Prize in 1985 for their description of the autosomal dominant LDL receptor mutation in FH. Since then nearly 800 functional mutations of this receptor have been reported. These functional abnormalities range from 50% to completely absent receptor activity.

LOW-DENSITY LIPOPROTEIN CHOLESTEROL RECEPTOR

The LDL receptor gene is located on the short arm of chromosome 19, and the receptor protein has 860 amino acids. Two ligands on LDL bind to the receptor, apolipoprotein (apo) B-100 and apoE. Binding allows hepatic LDL uptake, which accounts for approximately 70% of circulating LDL disposal.

MUTATIONS

Several classes of mutations have been described: null alleles with complete absence of the LDL receptor; defective transport alleles, which prevent receptor insertion into the cell membrane; defective binding and internalization alleles; and defective recycling alleles that prevent dissociation of receptor and ligand.[1]

The defective hepatic LDL receptor in FH leads to elevated plasma cholesterol levels. Also, when cholesterol is not internalized by the hepatocytes, hepatic synthesis is not inhibited. This results in increased hepatic cholesterol synthesis despite high blood levels.

CIRCULATING LOW-DENSITY LIPOPROTEIN CHOLESTEROL

High circulating levels of LDL is taken up by nonreceptor scavenger pathways in nonhepatic cells. Cholesterol taken up by monocytes and macrophages lead to foam cell formation, plaque formation in the vascular endothelium, and cardiovascular disease. Cholesterol can also deposit in the skin causing xanthelasmas and xanthomas, in the eye causing corneal arcus, and in the aortic valve causing stenosis.

PREVALENCE

The prevalence of homozygous FH is 1 patient per 1 million persons, and heterozygous FH, 1 patient per 500 persons.

DEMOGRAPHICS

- Race
  - Certain countries and ethnic groups have a higher prevalence of FH including French Canadians, Christian Lebanese, South Africans, Fins, and Icelanders.
- Sex
  - There is no sex preference for FH as the gene is not on a sex chromosome. The cardiovascular manifestations of heterozygous (but not homozygous) FH appear later in women because of gender protection until the postmenopausal years.
- Age
  - The defective LDL receptor is present at birth, but the cardiovascular manifestations are related to age, as well as circulating LDL levels and other risk factors.

MORBIDITY AND MORTALITY

HOMOZYGOUS FAMILIAL HYPERCHOLESTEROLEMIA

Cholesterol deposition and diffuse atherosclerosis are the manifestations of FH. Aortic stenosis is also common. Acute myocardial infarction and sudden death can occur in very young children. Survival past childhood is unlikely without aggressive treatment. Cholesterol deposits can produce corneal arcus, tendon xanthomas, and xanthelasma.

HETEROZYGOUS FAMILIAL HYPERCHOLESTEROLEMIA

The cholesterol deposition and atherosclerosis is less severe and manifest at a later age. Men usually develop CAD by the fourth decade of life without treatment. Women lag behind by 10 or 15 years. Cholesterol deposition manifest as tendon xanthomas are most common on the Achilles tendon and the extensor tendons of the hands. Corneal arcus and xanthelasma also occur but are usually of no clinical significance.

CLINICAL

HISTORY

Children with homozygous FH can have ischemic heart disease, peripheral vascular disease, cerebrovascular disease, or aortic stenosis. Because of their young age, however, these conditions are often misdiagnosed. Symptoms of tendonitis, arthralgia, or a history of skin lesions can be present.

Homozygous patients do not survive beyond 30 years of age unless treated aggressively (see Treatment). Heterozygous FH patients, however, are asymptomatic until adulthood. Symptoms of ischemic heart disease can be present along with Achilles tendonitis and arthritic symptoms.

The family history of both homozygous and heterozygous FH is often pertinent for premature cardiovascular disease or hypercholesterolemia in one or more first-degree relatives.

PHYSICAL

Several types of xanthomas can be present:[1] planar xanthomas (on palms, fingers, elbows, buttocks, or knees), which are different from other cutaneous xanthomas because of their yellow-to-orange coloration;[2] tuberous xanthomas (around areas of trauma on hands, elbows, or knees); and[3] tendon xanthomas (on extensor tendons of hands or Achilles tendon).

Homozygous FH patients can have cutaneous xanthomas at birth and corneal arcus in early childhood. Children with heterozygous FH do not develop xanthoma or corneal arcus until a later age.

The murmur of aortic stenosis can be heard.

Xanthelasmas is a nonspecific finding that can occur in patients with normal cholesterol levels. If the diagnosis is unclear and identification of a cutaneous lesion is uncertain, a biopsy can be performed. Both xanthelasmas and the xanthomas of FH contain cholesterol, whereas, eruptive xanthomas of hypertriglyceridemia contain fat.

LABORATORY STUDIES

The defective hepatic LDL receptor in FH leads to elevated plasma cholesterol levels. Also, when cholesterol is not internalized by the hepatocytes, hepatic synthesis is not inhibited. This results in increased hepatic cholesterol synthesis despite high blood levels. The LDL levels in homozygous FH are usually higher than 600 mg/dL. In heterozygous FH with half normal and half defective receptors, the LDL levels are commonly approximately 300 mg/dL.

The finding of an isolated severely elevated LDL in the absence of secondary causes (see Differential Diagnosis) suggests the diagnosis of FH. A presumptive diagnosis of heterozygous FH can be made if the LDL level is greater than 330 mg/dL or if tendon xanthomas are present in a patient with an LDL level above the 95th percentile. Conclusive diagnosis can only be made with genetic testing.

Testing to rule out secondary hypercholesterolemia should include testing for diabetes, hypothyroidism, hepatic disease, and renal disease.

Ultracentrifugation and lipoprotein electrophoresis is usually not necessary unless significant hypertriglyceridemia is present. Genetic LDL receptor analysis is also not necessary as it will not alter therapeutic management.

IMAGING STUDIES

Echocardiography can be done to rule out aortic stenosis if a murmur is present. Radiographs of tendons to evaluate for xanthomas can be warranted in some patients.

DIFFERENTIAL DIAGNOSIS

- The following diseases are included in the differential diagnosis: dysbetahyperlipoproteinemia (type III hyperlipidemia), familial ligand defective apoB-100, familial defective apoB-100, homozygous autosomal recessive hypercholesterolemia, sitosterolemia (phytosterolemia).
- Other diseases to be considered
  ○ Familial combined hyperlipidemia
  ○ Hypothyroidism
  ○ Lipoprotein X
  ○ Nephrotic syndrome
  ○ Severe hypertriglyceridemia
  ○ Polygenic hypercholesterolemia

TREATMENT

DETERMINATION OF CARDIOVASCULAR RISK

The 2001 National Cholesterol Education Program (NCEP) Adult Treatment Panel III (ATPIII) defined target LDL levels and levels based on risk for cardiovascular disease. These guidelines were updated in 2004 to reflect accumulating evidence for lowering LDL.[2,3]

In individuals without diagnosed atherosclerotic disease, coronary heart disease (CHD) risk is determined by a number of factors:

1. Hypertension (blood pressure [BP] >140/90 mm Hg or on antihypertensive therapy).
2. Cigarette smoking.
3. High-density lipoprotein (HDL) level <40 mg/dL.
4. Male sex and age 45 years or older.
5. Female sex and age 55 years or older.
6. Family history of premature CHD: clinical CHD or sudden death in first-degree male relative younger than age 55 years or first-degree female relative younger than age 65 years.
7. An HDL level of 60 mg/dL or greater is a negative risk factor subtracted from the total.

In addition to risk-factor assessment, a 10-year risk of developing CHD can be determined by calculating the Framingham risk score, which is available through the US National Heart, Lung, and Blood Institute.

Based on the Framingham 10-year risk score and the number of risk factors, CHD risk can be stratified into low, moderate, moderate-high, high, and very-high risk categories.

1. Low-risk patients have fewer than two risk factors and a 10-year risk for a major CHD event that is less than 10%. The LDL goal is less than 160 mg/dL.
2. Moderate risk patients have two or more factors and a 10-year risk for CHD of less than 10%. The LDL goal is less than 130 mg/dL.

3. Moderate-high risk patients have two or more risk factors and a 10-year risk of 10–20%. The goal LDL is less than 130 mg/dL, and the update suggested an optional goal LDL of less than 100 mg/dL.
4. High risk includes cardiovascular disease and CHD risk equivalents. These include the following:
   a. Symptomatic carotid artery disease (transient ischemic attack or stroke of carotid origin)
   b. Peripheral artery disease
   c. Abdominal aortic aneurysm
   d. Diabetes mellitus
   e. 10-year risk less than 20%

The LDL goal for high-risk patients is less than 100 mg/dL, and the 10-year risk is greater than 20%. Besides lifestyle change, medication is recommended if the LDL level is greater than 100 mg/dL. Patients at high or very high risk have an optional LDL goal of less than 70 mg/dL.

5. Very high risk is defined as the presence of the following:
   a. Multiple other major risk factors for CHD, especially diabetes
   b. Severe, poorly controlled risk factors, especially continued cigarette smoking
   c. Multiple risk factors for the metabolic syndrome (especially triglycerides >200 mg/dL, non-HDL >130 mg/dL, and HDL <40 mg/dL)
   d. Patients with acute coronary syndromes

Patients with cardiovascular disease who are at very high risk have an optional LDL goal of less than 70 mg/dL.

LIFESTYLE CHANGES FOR FAMILIAL HYPERCHOLESTEROLEMIA

General treatment recommendations for FH include healthy diet, regular exercise, and maintaining a normal body weight.

A low-cholesterol diet in normal individuals upregulates LDL receptors and lowers circulating LDL. This does not happen in homozygous FH, however, and the impact of diet changes is negligible. Heterozygous FHLDL levels can respond to diet, however, as they can upregulate their normal complement (albeit, decreased) of LDL receptors.

The improvement in LDL levels with diet is difficult to predict because of multiple factors including the baseline diet composition, compliance with the diet, and various genetically determined biochemical factors. In general, a decrease of LDL of approximately 15% can be predicted in heterozygous patients.

As a rule, all heterozygous FH patients should be referred to a dietitian for guidance. Rather than restricting total fat, reducing the intake of saturated fat, trans fat, and cholesterol should be emphasized. Furthermore, low-fat diets are high in carbohydrates, which increase triglyceride levels and lower HDL levels. Substituting monounsaturated fats (eg, olive and canola oils, avocados, nuts) for carbohydrates, however, increases HDL levels and lowers triglyceride levels while not increasing LDL levels.

These diets should be rich in whole grains, whole fruit, and legumes and other vegetables. These foods are high in soluble fiber, which has a small (approximately 5%) cholesterol-lowering effect.

Exercise training has many cardiovascular benefits including weight loss, lowering BP, preventing diabetes mellitus, and increasing HDL. The amount of exercise should include at least moderate physical activity such as brisk walking at least 30 minutes 4 days per week.

Consideration should be given to a symptom-limited exercise stress test before undertaking a new exercise program. An exercise trainer can be useful in providing guidance implementing an appropriate program.

MEDICATION

Hydroxymethylglutaryl-coenzyme A (HMG-CoA) reductase inhibitors (statins) are the first-line medications for heterozygous FH. This is because they have the greatest LDL-lowering capability, they are well tolerated, and they have been proven in multiple clinical trials to lower CHD morbidity and mortality. The most powerful statins, rosuvastatin and atorvastatin, at their maximum approved doses, can be expected to reduce low-density lipoprotein-cholesterol (LDLC) levels 50% to 60%.[4]

Even the maximum doses of the strongest statins, however, are usually inadequate for patients with heterozygous FH, and the addition of one or more non-statin cholesterol-lowering medications is necessary.

Bile acid sequestrants (eg, cholestyramine, colestipol, colesevelam) bind to cholesterol in the gut and modestly decrease circulating LDL levels and slightly increase HDL and triglyceride levels. Care should be taken with the dose schedule as binding of other medications can interfere with their absorption.

Nicotinic acid (niacin) not only lowers LDL levels but also increases HDL and lowers triglycerides. The concern about myositis with statins is a very minor concern.

Fibric acid derivatives include gemfibrozil (Lopid) and fenofibrate (TriCor). This class of drugs is not useful in FH because they do not reliably lower LDL levels, and they substantially increase the risk of statin-induced myositis.

Ezetimibe is a cholesterol-absorption inhibitor that reduces LDL levels approximately 15%. Ezetimibe generally has minimal side effects or drug interactions. In combination with a statin, the LDL lowering is additive.

Two statin combinations are now available with either extended-release niacin (Advicor) or ezetimibe (Vytorin). These are useful medications for patients with FH.

LOW-DENSITY LIPOPROTEIN CHOLESTEROL APHARESIS

CHD patients, whose LDL level cannot be lowered below 200 mg/dL by conventional therapy, are candidates for LDL apheresis. Non-CHD patients with an LDL level >300 mg/dL are also candidates. This is expensive therapy, however, requiring treatments every 2 weeks, for the patient's lifetime.

SURGICAL CARE

Liver transplantation is an option for homozygous FH, but involves surgical risks and long-term immunosuppression. Nevertheless, a new liver provides functional LDL receptors and produces dramatic decreases in LDL levels. After transplantation, elevated LDL levels can be treated with the usual LDL-lowering medications.

Portacaval anastomosis, compared to liver transplantation, is less hazardous and requires no immunosuppression. LDL lowering is not as great, however, compared to apheresis and transplantation. Nevertheless, LDL reductions of 50% can be achieved with regression of coronary lesions, aortic lesions, and xanthomas. The mechanism for lowering LDL is unknown.

CONSULTATIONS

A child with homozygous FH should be referred immediately to a medical center that specializes in severe lipid disorders. An individual with heterozygous FH should be referred to a dietitian. If they do not reach their LDL targets, they should be referred to an endocrinologist or lipid specialist.

COMPLICATIONS AND PROGNOSIS

The complications of FH are directly related to therapy. Each of the procedures carries a small but finite risk of harm. The prognosis of untreated FH is extremely poor. Homozygous FH requires major medical intervention early in life, and heterozygous FH usually requires multidrug therapy and lifestyle intervention to correct modifiable risk factors, such as smoking, hypertension, and diabetes.[5]

REFERENCES

1. Ueda M. Familial hypercholesterolemia. *Mol Genet Metab.* Dec 2005;86(4):423–426.
2. Expert Panel on Detection, Evaluation, and Treatment of High Blood Cholesterol in Adults. Executive Summary of the Third Report of the National Cholesterol Education Program (NCEP) Expert Panel on Detection, Evaluation, and Treatment of High Blood Cholesterol in Adults (Adult Treatment Panel III). *JAMA.* May 16 2001;285(19):2486–2497.
3. Grundy SM, Cleeman JI, Merz CN, Brewer HB Jr, Clark LT, Hunninghake DB. Implications of recent clinical trials for the National Cholesterol Education Program Adult Treatment Panel III guidelines. *Circulation.* Jul 13 2004;110(2):227–239.
4. Jones PH, Davidson MH, Stein EA. Comparison of the efficacy and safety of rosuvastatin versus atorvastatin, simvastatin, and pravastatin across doses (STELLAR* Trial). *Am J Cardiol.* Jul 15 2003;92(2):152–160.
5. Marks D, Thorogood M, Neil HA, Humphries SE. A review on the diagnosis, natural history, and treatment of familial hypercholesterolaemia. *Atherosclerosis.* May 2003;168(1):1–14.

GASTROENTEROLOGY AND LIVER DISEASE

53 DISEASES OF THE ESOPHAGUS

M. Louay Omran

ANATOMY AND PHYSIOLOGY

ANATOMY

- The esophagus is a 24 cm hollow muscular tube connecting the pharynx to the stomach. It is simple in design, yet complex in function.
- The presence of a muscular sphincter at each end of the esophagus provides a seal to ensure that the esophagus remains collapsed between swallows.
- The upper esophageal sphincter (the cricopharyngeus) is a skeletal muscle that is located just below the cricoid cartilage separating the pharynx from the body of the esophagus. It remains contracted at rest to prevent swallowing of inspired air.
- The lower esophageal sphincter is located at the junction of the esophagus with the stomach. It is a 3 cm long, tonically contracted ring of circular smooth muscle fibers. The sphincter is further fortified by oblique muscle fibers known as the gastric sling as they extend from the lesser curvature to the greater curvature.
- Structurally, the esophageal wall is composed of four layers
  ○ Mucosa: squamous epithelium overlying a lamina propria and a muscularis mucosa.
  ○ Submucosa: elastic and fibrous tissue.
  ○ Muscularis propria: composed of an inner circular and an outer longitudinal muscular layer. The upper third of the esophageal musculature consists of skeletal muscle and the lower two-thirds consist of smooth muscle.

○ Adventitia: unlike the remainder of the gastrointestinal tract, the esophagus has no serosa.
- The esophageal wall derives innervation from both the parasympathetic and sympathetic nerves. The vagus nerve regulates peristalsis.
- The esophagus may be indented by adjacent structures in three locations: the aortic arch, left main bronchus, and left atrium.

PHYSIOLOGY OF SWALLOWING

Phases of swallowing are summarized in Table 53–1.

SYMPTOMS OF ESOPHAGEAL DISEASES

Since transportation of food from the mouth to the stomach is the main function of the esophagus, diseases affecting the esophagus are likely to cause disruption of this function, characterized as difficulty swallowing (dysphagia), with or without painful swallowing (odynophagia). Chest pain and globus the sensation of a lump in the throat are two symptoms potentially pointing to an esophageal disorder.

DYSPHAGIA

- Can be divided into two categories: oropharyngeal dysphagia (transfer dysphagia) and esophageal dysphagia (transport dysphagia). Table 53–2 outlines common causes and symptoms associated with each type.
- History can provide helpful clues towards a presumptive diagnosis.
  ○ Oropharyngeal dysphagia is often associated with symptoms and signs suggestive of the neurologic condition associated with it.
  ○ Dysphagia following ingestion of liquids suggests a motility disorder.

TABLE 53–1 Physiology of Swallowing

PHASES OF SWALLOWING	CONTROL	FUNCTION	DESCRIPTION
Oral	Voluntary	Preparation of food bolus	1. Food is mixed with saliva and propelled backward by the tongue as a bolus towards the pharynx
Pharyngeal	Involuntary	Transfer of food bolus into the esophagus and protection of airways	2. The larynx moves forward and the vocal folds close
			3. The upper esophageal sphincter (UES) relaxes to allow entry into esophagus
			4. The soft palate ascends to close the nasopharynx
			5. The pharyngeal constrictors contracts to push the bolus into the esophagus, breathing is inhibited
			6. The lower esophageal sphincter (LES) opens in anticipation of food delivery
Esophageal	Involuntary	Transportation of food bolus to the stomach	7. The pharyngeal contraction is propagated downwards through the esophagus as a peristalsis
			8. The bolus moves as a result of sequential relaxation of esophageal segments ahead of the contractions

○ Presence of long-standing heartburn in a patient with progressive dysphagia may suggest peptic stricture.

○ Intermittent dysphagia precipitated by solids suggests the presence of a Schatzki ring.

○ Progressive dysphagia with weight loss in an elderly patient raises the possibility of esophageal cancer.

• Diagnostic approach to dysphagia

○ If oropharyngeal dysphagia is suspected, videofluoroscopy (modified barium swallow) of oropharyngeal swallowing should be obtained.

○ If esophageal dysphagia is suspected, a barium swallow and/or upper endoscopy should be obtained to help

TABLE 53–2 Classification, Common Causes, and Symptoms of Dysphagia

TYPE OF DYSPHAGIA	TYPE OF DYSFUNCTION	COMMON CAUSES	KEY SYMPTOMS
Oropharyngeal	Structural	Zenker diverticulum Cervical osteophytes Cricopharyngeal bar Oropharyngeal tumors	Food *getting stuck* in the neck region immediately upon swallowing
	Coordination	Stroke Head trauma Cerebral palsy Multiple sclerosis Tardive dyskinesia Amyotrophic lateral sclerosis Dementia Parkinson disease	Nasal regurgitation Drooling Coughing Choking Aspiration pneumonia
Esophageal	Mechanical	Schatzki ring Esophageal web Peptic stricture Esophageal cancer Radiation injury Food impaction	Solids getting stuck in the sternal region during swallowing Chest pain
	Motility	Achalasia Diffuse esophageal spasm Nutcracker esophagus Scleroderma Eosinophilic esophagitis	Solids and liquids getting stuck in the sternal region during swallowing Chest pain

identify a mechanical cause. If a motility disorder is suspected, an esophageal manometry study is indicated.

ODYNOPHAGIA

Defined as painful swallowing, it suggests mucosal damage or sensitivity as seen in pill esophagitis and infectious esophagitis (cytomegalovirus [CMV], herpes).

CHEST PAIN

The esophagus is the most common source of atypical noncardiac chest pain. Esophageal chest pain can be due to spasm (diffuse esophageal spasm) or acid regurgitation. Some of the clues that may point to an esophageal origin of chest pain include association with meals, being position dependent, and response to antacid use.

GLOBUS SENSATION

Defined as the sensation of the presence of a lump in the throat, outside of meal time. Although it can be the result of acid reflux, it is often a sign of visceral hypersensitivity and possibly a psychological disorder.

MOTILITY DISORDERS

ACHALASIA

- Epidemiology
  - The most well-defined motor disorder of the esophagus.
  - Estimated incidence is 1:100,000; prevalence is 1:10,000.
  - Affects both genders equally.
  - Can occur at any age, but most common in the third to fifth decades.
- Pathophysiology
  - Idiopathic reduction or absence of nitric oxide-producing inhibitory neurons in the esophageal muscles, leading to heightened tone of the lower esophageal sphincter (LES) and failure of esophageal body peristalsis.
  - The failure of LES relaxation is the hallmark of achalasia and is necessary to make the diagnosis.
  - In South America, Chagas disease has similar pathologic features to achalasia. Infection with the parasite *Trypanosoma cruzi* stimulates the formation of antibodies against a parasitic antigen that carries a great resemblance to a protein on the myenteric neurons. These antibodies attach to the neurons in the myenteric plexus leading to their destruction.
- Clinical features

- Because of the absence of peristalsis and the failure of LES relaxation, dysphagia is usually present. At the time of diagnosis, all patients have dysphagia with solids, and more than half have dysphagia with liquids.
- The gradual dilatation of the esophagus and food retention in the esophageal lumen can lead to regurgitation and possible aspiration pneumonia.
- Esophageal dilatation, food fermentation, and acid production within the lumen can lead to chest pain and heartburn.
- Weight loss can be a late manifestation.
- Patients with achalasia carry approximately a 5% risk for developing squamous cell carcinoma of the esophagus.
- Diagnosis
  - Barium swallow x-ray usually reveals a dilated esophagus with air fluid levels. The lower end of the esophagus tapers down acutely giving the appearance of a bird's beak. A timed barium swallow confirms the presence of delayed esophageal emptying.
  - Manometric studies of the esophagus measuring pressure in different areas of the esophageal body and the LES during swallowing reveal the typical findings necessary for diagnosis; absence of complete LES relaxation and absence of peristalsis.
  - Upper endoscopy can only reveal indirect clues for achalasia such as the dilated food-filled esophagus in late stages and possibly absence of esophageal contraction. Endoscopy is a valuable tool to investigate the presence of pseudoachalasia, which is a tumor at the gastroesophageal junction that causes partial obstruction and mimics the clinical, radiographic, and manometric picture of achalasia. This can account for up to 5% of cases that are initially diagnosed as achalasia.
- Treatment
  - There is no curative treatment for achalasia that results in the return of normal esophageal peristalsis and sphincter relaxation during swallowing.
  - The aim is to decrease the LES pressure either chemically (medications) or mechanically (by forceful stretching) to remove the *barrier* phenomenon and allow food to be transported under the force of gravity.
  - Smooth muscle relaxants such as calcium channel blockers, nitrates, and sildenafil have been used with limited success.
  - Endoscopic treatment by forcefully dilating the LES to 3 to 4 cm with a pneumatic balloon once or twice achieves a success rate of 80% but carries a perforation risk of 3% to 5%.
  - Gastroesophageal reflux disease (GERD) can develop in approximately 10% of patients after dilatation.
  - Surgery is the most definitive treatment carrying an 85% to 90% success rate.

- Performed laparoscopically, surgery involves inducing muscular injury to the LES in a technique known as the Heller myotomy.
  - Postoperatively, 50% of patients may develop GERD.
- Patients who fail endoscopic dilatation and are considered to be a high risk for a surgical approach may benefit from endoscopically injecting botulinum toxin into the LES.[1] By attaching to and injuring the presynaptic cholinergic receptors, this toxin inhibits the release of acetylcholine from the nerve endings leading to relaxation of the LES for 3 to 12 months before new synapses develop. This technique is effective in 65% of patients, but there is always a need for repeat injection. Loss of efficacy can occur with time due to the formation of antitoxin antibodies.

SPASTIC MOTILITY DISORDERS

- Diffuse esophageal spasm
  - Possibly due to an imbalance between excitatory and inhibitory motor neurons.
  - Can present as dysphagia or chest pain. Up to 10% of patients with noncardiac chest pain may have diffuse esophageal spasm.
  - Barium esophagogram may be abnormal revealing an irregular esophageal border in a classical appearance known as *corkscrew esophagus.*
  - Definitive diagnosis is obtained by manometric studies which reveal simultaneous pressure waves suggesting simultaneous contractions.
  - Normal peristalsis and LES relaxation differentiates it from achalasia.
- Nutcracker esophagus
  - Nutcracker esophagus is a term used to define the presence of high amplitude esophageal contractions (more than 180 mm Hg) on manometry.
  - Its relationship to symptoms is debated but patients who have extremely high contraction amplitudes (>250 mm Hg) are likely to have chest pain.
  - Since not all patients who have nutcracker esophagus have chest pain, it is theorized that those who do may have increased visceral sensitivity.
- Treatment
  - The calcium channel blocker diltiazem was found to be effective in reducing both esophageal peristaltic pressure and chest pain.
  - Tricyclic antidepressants target the visceral sensitivity component.
  - Nitrates and sildenafil may be beneficial on an as-needed basis.
  - Because gastroespasophageal acid reflux can induce esophageal sm, aggressive treatment with proton pump inhibitors (PPIs) for documented reflux cases is prudent.

SCLERODERMA

- Esophageal involvement is due to the partial replacement of the esophageal smooth muscle (lower two-thirds) by collagenous tissue. This leads to a decrease or absence of peristalsis in the affected area and a significant decrease in the LES resting tone.
- Patients complain of dysphagia and are subject to acid reflux symptoms and complications.
- Diagnosis is accomplished through manometric studies that has good sensitivity. Endoscopy is indicated to investigate and treat complications of acid reflux.
- Treatment goal is to prevent acid reflux damage and to provide nutritional support as the disease progresses.

EOSINOPHILIC ESOPHAGITIS

- Suspected in young patients who present with intermittent food impaction or unexplained solid food dysphagia.
- More common in males than females.
- Probably due to eosinophil recruitment in response to environmental antigens.
- Classic endoscopic finding is a ringed or corrugated esophagus (also referred to as feline or trachea-like esophagus) in the proximal and middle sections.
- Variable, nondistinct underlying motility patterns found on manometry.
- Diagnosed by mucosal biopsy that reveals the presence of more than 20 interepithelial eosinophils per high power field.
- Topical steroids applied by swallowing of inhaled steroid formulations (metered dose inhalers without a spacer) are effective.[1]

GASTROESOPHAGEAL REFLUX DISEASE

DEFINITION

- Chronic symptoms or mucosal damage produced by the abnormal reflux of gastric contents into the esophagus.
  - Patients who have endoscopically documented mucosal damage are said to have reflux esophagitis.
  - Patients who have typical symptoms of GERD due to reflux of acid into the esophagus but do not have any mucosal damage are said to have nonerosive reflux disease (NERD).

EPIDEMIOLOGY

- No accurate data available due to the absence of a true gold standard for the diagnosis of GERD.

- U.S. population-based studies suggest that symptoms of GERD are extremely common as described below:
  - At least once a year in approximately 60% of the population.
  - At least once a month in approximately 40% of the population.
  - At least once a week in approximately 20% of the population.
- Increased incidence with aging.
- Possible protective role for *Helicobacter pylori*-induced hypochlorhydria.
- Of patients who have endoscopy for GERD symptoms
  - More than 50% have a negative endoscopy (NERD).
  - 10% have benign strictures.
  - 3% have Barrett's esophagus.
  - 1% have esophageal adenocarcinomas.

PATHOPHYSIOLOGY

- Gastroesophageal reflux occurs when the esophago-gastric barrier is compromised either transiently or permanently. Esophagitis occurs when esophageal defense mechanisms fail to protect the esophageal mucosa from the offending gastric contents.
  - Patients with severe forms of GERD (erosive esophagitis) are likely to have a mechanical disruption of the gastroesophageal junction (hiatal hernia or defective LES).
  - Patients with milder forms of GERD (NERD) are likely to have recurrent transient relaxation of a *normal* LES as the mechanism of their reflux.
  - Alcohol in moderate amounts and cigarette smoking exacerbate GERD by decreasing the LES pressure.

CLINICAL FEATURES

- Heartburn (retrosternal ascending burning sensation) and acid regurgitation (return of bitter gastric contents to the mouth) are the cardinal symptoms.
  - More frequent after meals (increased acid production) and in the supine position (loss of gravity support).
- Other symptoms include:
  - Water brash: excessive salivation in response to acid reflux.
  - Dysphagia: caused by secondary spasm and impairment of motility or by the formation of a peptic stricture.
  - Odynophagia: caused by the presence of erosive esophagitis.
  - Belching: caused by reflux of air.
  - Chest pain: caused by esophageal spasm or mucosal injury.
- Extraesophageal symptoms

- Cough: caused by reflux of acid into the respiratory tract.
- Wheezing: caused by acid irritation of the bronchi leading to bronchospasm.
- Hoarseness: caused by acid injuring the vocal cords.
- Tracheal stenosis and pulmonary fibrosis occur rarely in long-standing cases.

DIAGNOSIS

- There is no *gold standard* diagnostic tool for GERD.
- In the presence of classical symptoms, and in the absence of any signs that suggest a complicated diagnosis, a therapeutic trial with a PPI is considered to be a diagnostic tool.[2]
  - A successful trial of omeprazole twice a day has a sensitivity of 80% and a specificity of 57% for the diagnosis of GERD.
- A patient with symptoms that suggest extra-esophageal disease (chest pain, hoarseness, wheezing, etc) should undergo evaluation of the more common causes (an extraesophageal source) before GERD is pursued.
- Endoscopy is not considered a primary diagnostic tool due to its low sensitivity (50% of patients with chronic GERD symptoms have a negative endoscopy).
  - Endoscopy should be considered in select cases
    - Long-standing symptoms (more than 5–10 y)
    - Failure of empiric PPI therapy
    - Presence of alarm signs for complications: odynophagia, dysphagia, hematemesis, melena, and weight loss
- 24 to 48 hours of pH monitoring with event marking (heartburn, meals, and body position) is a useful test to document acid exposure and to correlate it with symptoms. It is not a gold standard test for GERD because it is negative in 25% of patients who have otherwise documented acid reflux (erosive esophagitis). This test can be useful to confirm diagnosis before corrective surgery, confirm diagnosis in patients with atypical or extraesophageal symptoms, and to confirm absence of acid exposure in patients who are suspected of having a *hypersensitive* esophagus.
- Barium esophagram lacks sensitivity and specificity and is only useful to evaluate a hiatus hernia, particularly preoperatively.
- Esophageal manometry has no role in the diagnosis of GERD unless motility disorders are being considered (scleredema for example).
- Impedance testing is a new diagnostic tool that allows for the detection of gas and fluid reflux through the esophagus independent of acid measurement. It can be helpful in those who have classic symptoms with negative endoscopy and pH monitoring.

TREATMENT

- Lifestyle modifications
  - Elevation of the head of the bed, avoiding heavy meals and the supine position for 3 hours after a meal, reducing intake of caffeine and chocolate, and smoking cessation are helpful logical measures to decrease the risk of acid reflux even though there is no overwhelming evidence proving their effectiveness.
- Medical therapy
  - The goal is to decrease gastric acid secretion to minimize mucosal injury in the esophagus. Accordingly, acid suppression therapy is the mainstay treatment of GERD—providing mucosal healing and symptom relief. The degree of success parallels the degree of acid suppression.
    - Acid suppressants
      - PPIs are the most potent available acid suppressants, and have an excellent success rate for the management of erosive esophagitis. See Table 53–3.
      - Both histamine H_2 receptor blockers and PPIs have modest success rates in controlling symptoms in patients with NERD (60%).
      - In a patient who is receiving a twice a day PPI and continues to have nocturnal *breakthrough* symptoms, adding a bedtime dose of an H_2 blocker can be beneficial. Unfortunately, most patients lose the benefit very quickly (days) due to tolerance.
      - When doses of equivalent potency are given, there is no significant difference in the success rates between different PPIs.
      - Despite a clinically insignificant increase in gastrin levels with long-term use of PPIs, there is no evidence that this leads to carcinoid tumors.
    - Prokinetic Agents
      - These drugs improve esophageal motility and gastric emptying and increase LES pressure.
      - These effects, if achieved, can decrease reflux and improve symptoms.
      - Metoclopramide and cisapride are prokinetic agents that fulfill this profile.

- Cisapride is no longer available in the United States because of the potential for cardiac dysrhythmias.
- Metoclopramide crosses the brain barrier and can be associated with extrapyramidal symptoms and hyperprolactinemia when used long term.
- Until newer agents are developed, there is currently no role for prokinetic drugs in the management of GERD unless associated with gastroparesis.
- Surgical treatment
  - The aim is to restore the gastroesophageal mechanical barrier to provide a *curative* solution. It is a laparoscopic, minimally invasive surgical procedure
    - Involves reconstruction of the diaphragmatic hiatus
    - Reinforcement of the LES by fundoplication
  - The ideal candidates are young patients who have documented GERD with a good response to PPIs but are concerned about taking medications long term and patients with nocturnal regurgitation and pulmonary complications.
    - Success rate is 80% to 90% when the patient is appropriately selected and the surgeon is experienced.
- Postoperative expectations
  - 5% of patients will develop persistent dysphagia.
  - Bloating (inability to belch) and diarrhea (dumping due to loss of fundus space) can occur.
  - 33% will still require long-term use of PPIs.
- Endoscopic therapy
  - Designed to improve the mechanical gastroesophageal barrier but is still an area of development with new modalities emerging and others fading away due to safety concerns.

OTHER ESOPHAGEAL DISORDERS

BARRETT ESOPHAGUS

- Acid-induced replacement of the stratified squamous epithelium that normally lines the distal esophagus by an abnormal epithelium featuring intestinal metaplasia.

TABLE 53–3   Effectiveness of Medications Used for the Treatment of Reflux Esophagitis

	H_2 HISTAMINE RECEPTOR BLOCKERS	PROTON PUMP INHIBITORS (PPI)
Mechanism of action	Block the histamine-induced stimulation of gastric parietal cells	Irreversibly bind with the proton-potassium-ATPase pump in the parietal cells
Healing of erosive esophagitis	50%	90–100%
Long-term maintenance of remission	50%	80%

- Labeled as *long segment* if extending more than 3 cm above the gastroesophageal junction.
- Predisposes to the development of adenocarcinoma of the esophagus.
- Epidemiology
  - Present in 1% of the population and in 6% to 12% of patients with symptoms of GERD.
  - Mean age at the time of diagnosis is 55 years.
  - Equal prevalence among Hispanics and whites, uncommon in blacks and Asians.
  - Male-to-female ratio is 2:1.
- Pathophysiology
  - An acquired condition resulting from severe acid-induced mucosal injury. The mechanism through which acid injury induces metaplasia is unknown.
  - Most patients with GERD do not develop Barrett's esophagus. Patients who do are likely to have had more significant acid exposure due to:
  - Hiatus hernia compromising the antireflux barriers.
  - Lower LES resting pressure than average.
- Clinical features
  - Mucosal changes do not lead to symptoms but many patients have symptoms of GERD (heartburn, regurgitation, etc).
  - There is a 0.5% annual risk for developing esophageal adenocarcinomas.
- Diagnosis
  - Corresponding to its definition, the diagnosis is made when salmon-colored mucosa (columnar) is seen endoscopically proximal to the actual gastroesophageal junction, and biopsy specimens show goblet cells suggesting intestinal metaplasia.
- Treatment
  - The goal of treatment is to minimize further mucosal injury and cellular metaplasia to ultimately prevent malignant transformation.
  - PPIs are effective in controlling reflux symptoms and decreasing acid exposure. It is not clear whether PPIs reduce the risk of malignant transformation. Similar arguments regarding antireflux surgery.
  - Because cyclooxygenase expression is increased in Barrett's esophagus and correlates positively with dysplasia and malignancy, several trials have investigated the use of aspirin or nonsteroidal antiinflammatory drugs (NSAIDs) to decrease the risk of developing adenocarcinomas.
  - Observational stud- ies revealed a potential benefit but considering that the risk of malignant transformation is low (0.5% per year), it is still not recommended to pre- scribe these agents to all patients with Barrett's esophagus.
  - Endoscopic surveillance for dysplasia is recommended on a regular basis to allow for intervention prior to malignant transformation.[3]

ESOPHAGEAL CANCER

- Epidemiology
  - The overall incidence in the United States is 3: 100,000.
  - Male-to-female ratio is 3:1.
  - Adenocarcinoma is the most common histologic type in the United States.
    - Related to acid reflux and Barrett's esophagus
    - Usually discovered in the lower esophagus
  - Squamous cell carcinoma is the most common histologic type worldwide.
  - Also related to tobacco and alcohol use.
  - Mostly in the upper and middle third.
  - Other rare histologic types include choriocarcinoma, melanoma, sarcoma, and lymphoma, and are usually found in the lower esophagus.
- Clinical features
  - Dysphagia is the typical symptom of esophageal cancer and is present in 90% of patients on presentation. It is usually progressive, involving solids then liquids. Odynophagia is a signal of advanced stage and is present in 50% of patients.
  - Other symptoms
    - Hematemesis: friable bleeding mucosa (mild) or erosion into a vessel (severe).
    - Hoarseness: involvement of the recurrent laryngeal nerve.
    - Back pain: mediastinal involvement.
- Diagnosis and staging
  - Endoscopy with biopsy.
  - Most cancers are metastatic at the time of diagnosis due to penetration of the lymphatic system near the mucosa.
  - The stage is usually expressed using the TNM system that requires knowledge of the depth of the primary tumor (T), involvement of the regional lymph nodes (N), and metastasis to distant organ (M).
    - The celiac lymph nodes are considered distant (M).
  - Endoscopic ultrasound (EUS), computed tomographic (CT) imaging, and positron emission tomography (PET) are the key tests used for staging.
    - EUS permits examination of the esophageal wall from a close proximity, and, therefore, is associated with a diagnostic accuracy of 90% for primary esophageal cancer (T), and 80% for lymph node involvement (N). EUS cannot accurately detect distant metastasis (M).
    - CT staging is important to identify distant metastasis but is less accurate than EUS for the diagnosis of primary tumor (60%) or lymph node involvement.
    - PET is a functional test that demonstrates tissue activity but not anatomical changes. It is often paired with a CT to aid in diagnostic accuracy.

- Not useful for evaluation of the primary tumor (T).
- Sensitive only for distant metastases that are >1 cm.
- Most valuable in identifying tumor involvement in a suspected lymph node.
- Very helpful in detecting residual tumor after chemotherapy and radiation therapy.
- Treatment
  - In patients with no lymph node involvement (stage I and IIA), surgery alone is recommended without the need for radiation or chemotherapy.
  - In patients with local lymph node involvement (stage IIB and IIIA), surgery alone carries a very low cure rate (10%). Adding preoperative (neoadjuvant) chemoradiation significantly increases morbidity but decreases local and regional recurrence and improves survival.[4] The decision to utilize combined therapy should be based on the patient's performance status. If surgery is not an option because of serious medical illness, combining chemotherapy (cisplatin and fluorouracil) with radiation therapy is superior to either alone.
  - In patients with significant local spread or distant metastasis (stage IIIB and IV), palliative treatment is indicated.
- Prognosis
  - Unfortunately because of the early spread of esophageal cancer, the overall 5-year survival rate remains below 15%.

REFERENCES

1. Arora AS, Perrault J, Smyrk TC. Topical corticosteroid treatment of dysphagia due to eosinophilic esophagitis in adults. *Mayo Clin Proc.* 2003;78:830–835.
2. DeVaut KR, Castell DO. American College of Gastroenterology: updated guidelines for the diagnosis and treatment of gastroesophageal reflux disease. *Am J Gastroenterol.* 2005;100: 190–200.
3. Sampliner RE, for the Practice Parameters Committee of the American College of Gastroenterology. Updated guidelines for the diagnosis, surveillance, and therapy of Barrett's esophagus. *Am J Gastroenterol.* 2002;97:1888–1895.
4. Enzinger PC, Mayer RJ. Esophageal cancer. *N Engl J Med.* 2003;349:2241–2242.

BIBLIOGRAPHY

Vaezi MF, Richter JE. American College of Gastroenterology Practice Guidelines: diagnosis and management of achalasia. *Am J Gastroenterol.* 1999;94:3406–3412.

54 DISEASES OF THE STOMACH

M. Louay Omran

GASTRIC ANATOMY AND PHYSIOLOGY

GASTRIC ANATOMY

- The stomach is divided into five anatomically defined regions that have a corresponding difference in mucosal histology:
  1. *Cardia*: a small area immediately following the gastroesophageal junction and positioned as the entrance to the stomach
  2. *Fundus*: a dome-shaped area that bulges to the left side above the cardia
  3. *Body*: a longitudinal cavity that is contiguous with the fundus and is the largest portion of the stomach
  4. *Antrum*: connects the body to the pylorus and has strong musculature
  5. *Pylorus*: a tubular structure that connects the stomach to the duodenum and contains the pyloric sphincter
- The arterial blood supply to the stomach is derived from the celiac artery through its branches (splenic, left gastric, and common hepatic), which form two arterial arcades along both curvatures of the stomach. The venous drainage accompanies the arteries and ends eventually in the portal vein. The lymphatic drainage reaches the celiac nodes. The autonomic innervation of the stomach is derived from both the sympathetic (T6–T8) and parasympathetic (vagus nerve) nervous systems.

GASTRIC HISTOLOGY

- The gastric wall is made up of four layers:
  1. The mucosa is composed of a simple layer of columnar epithelial cells.
     a. The proximal stomach contains the oxyntic glands, which are composed of parietal, chief, endocrine, mucous neck, and undifferentiated cells.
     b. The distal stomach contains the pyloric glands, which are composed of endocrine (gastrin-producing G cells) and mucous cells.
  2. The submucosa contains connective tissues, blood vessels, lymphatics, lymphocytes, and plasma cells, in addition to the submucosal plexus (Meissner).

3. The muscularis propria consists of three muscle layers: (1) inner oblique, (2) middle circular, and (3) outer longitudinal. The muscularis propria includes the myenteric (Auerbach) plexus.

4. The serosa is the outermost layer that is part of the visceral peritoneum.

GASTRIC SECRETION

- There are four major secretory products of the gastric epithelium, all of which are important either to the digestive process or to the protection of the stomach. These products are acid, proteases, intrinsic factor, mucus, and mucosal defense factors.

SECRETION OF ACID

The Parietal Cell (Oxyntic Cell)

- Responsible for gastric acid secretion from an extensive secretory network (called canaliculi) via active transport.
- Possesses five types of receptors as described below; the first three stimulate acid production and the last two inhibit acid secretion:
  1. Muscarinic cholinergic acetylcholine receptor
  2. Histamine receptor
  3. Cholecystokinin (CCK) receptor (binds gastrin)
  4. Somatostatin
  5. Prostaglandin

- Table 54–1 summarizes the chemical regulators of acid secretion in the parietal cell and their mechanism of action.

Mechanism of Acid Secretion by the Parietal Cell

- To secrete acid the resting parietal cell requires *activation,* which allows translocation of the enzyme hydrogen/potassium adenosine triphosphatase (ATPase, known as the proton pump) to the apical surface.
- Cell activation is accomplished through an increase in cytoplasmic calcium (acetylcholine mediated), or generation of cyclic adenosine monophosphate (histamine mediated). Both lead to cyclic adenosine monophosphate–dependent protein kinase activation.
- Simultaneously, a potassium-chloride cotransport transcellular pathway is activated, allowing both potassium and chloride to exit the cell through the canalicular lumen.
- Under the influence of the proton pump, the intracellular hydrogen ions (H^+) are secreted into the canalicular lumen in exchange for potassium.
- The hydrogen ion that accumulates in the canaliculus generates an osmotic gradient across the membrane that results in outward diffusion of water.
- Water, hydrogen, and chloride mixed in the canalicular lumen generate hydrochloric acid.
- The hydrogen-potassium ATPase pump is the target for the antisecretory agents known as the proton pump inhibitors (PPIs).

TABLE 54–1   Chemical Regulators of Acid Secretion in the Stomach

CHEMICAL	SOURCE	MECHANISM OF ACID SECRETION	KEY FACT
Acetylcholine	Nerve endings (response to vagus nerve stimulation)	Direct effect on M3 receptors on the PC Effect on ECLs to release histamine Effect on D cells to suppress release of somatostatin	Responsible for stress-related acid secretion
Histamine	ECL (stimulated by gastrin)	Stimulation of the H2 receptors on PC Stimulation of the H3 receptors to suppress release of somatostatin from D cells	Most important paracrine stimulator of acid secretion
Gastrin	Antral G cells (influence of mechanical stretch and protein presence in stomach)	Directly by attaching to CCK2/gastrin receptors on PC Indirectly by attaching to CCK2/gastrin receptors on the ECLs leading to histamine release	Most important trophic regulator of PC mass (hypertrophy in gastrinoma; atrophy after antrectomy, which decreases gastrin levels)
Somatostatin	D cells (influence of acid and gastrin present in stomach)	Inhibits histamine release from ECLs (major effect) Inhibits PC function Inhibits gastrin release from G cells (mild effect)	Provides negative feedback against acid secretion
PGs	Macrophages, capillary endothelial, and many other cells (influence unclear)	PGE2 has inhibitory effects on the parietal cells	PGE analogs (misoprostol) suppress acid secretion NSAIDs increase acid by inhibiting endogenous PG

CCK, cholecystokinin; ECL, enterochromaffin-like (cell); H, histamine; M, muscarinic; NSAIDs, nonsteroidal antiinflammatory drugs; PC, parietal cell; PG, prostaglandin, PGE, prostaglandin E; PGE2, prostaglandin E_2.

Regulation of Gastric Acid Secretion

- Basal acid secretion:
  - Secretion of acid is primarily dependent on the degree of basal acetylcholine production, also referred to as *vagal tone*, which varies among normal persons. Stress increases vagal tone, and men tend to have higher vagal tone than women.
- Stimulated acid secretion:
  - Three phases are involved: (1) the cephalic phase, which is predominantly cholinergic; (2) the gastric phase, which is gastrin mediated; and (3) the intestinal phase, which has a modest effect on acid secretion. Histamine plays an important role in augmenting the response in both the cephalic and gastric phases.
- Cephalic phase:
  - Thought, sight, smell or taste of food stimulates the vagus nerve:
    - Promotes acid secretion directly via the parietal cells.
    - Promotes histamine relaease from enterochromaffin-like cells.
    - Promotes gastrin release from G cells.
    - Inhibits somatostatin release from D cells.
- Gastric phase:
  - Protein degradation products (peptides) and amino acids directly stimulate the G cells to produce gastrin.
  - Distension of the stomach with food in general, leads to gastrin release mediated by gastrin-releasing peptide.
- Intestinal phase:
  - Amino acids induce a further increase in acid secretion both enterally (duodenum) through the release of gastrin and parenterally through a direct effect on the parietal cells.

SECRETION OF PROTEASES

- Pepsinogen is secreted primarily by the chief cells in the stomach under the influence of acetylcholine and peptides of the CCK/gastrin family.
- Conversion to the active protease pepsin in the stomach requires a low pH and is dependent on the presence of gastric acid.
- Pepsin is inactivated at a pH that exceeds 4. Accordingly, acid suppression facilitates ulcer healing by preventing the injurious effects of pepsin.
- Pepsin is important for the digestion of protein and results in the release of peptides and amino acids, which triggers the release of other important digestive hormones such as gastrin and CCK.

SECRETION OF INTRINSIC FACTOR

- Intrinsic factor is a glycoprotein that is secreted by the parietal cells and is necessary for the absorption of cobalamin (vitamin B_{12}).
- Secretion of intrinsic factor is stimulated via all pathways known to stimulate gastric acid secretion: histamine, gastrin, and acetylcholine.

- Cobalamin absorption:
  - Cobalamin is liberated from its dietary sources (protein and dairy products) in the stomach under the influence of acid and pepsin.
  - Cobalamin binds with R factor (present in the saliva and gastric juices).
  - When the complex reaches the duodenum, the cobalamin is released from the cobalamin-R complex under the influence of pancreatic enzymes.
  - Free cobalamin then binds to intrinsic factor (IF) to generate a new complex that is delivered to the terminal ileum.
  - In the terminal ileum, the IF-cobalamin complex binds to a specific ileal receptor, cubilin, and is actively absorbed.

SECRETION OF MUCUS AND MUCOSAL DEFENSE FACTORS

- Protection of the epithelial cells against autodigestion by acid is maintained through several defense mechanisms:
  - Mucus secreted by the gastric mucous cells (the most abundant epithelial cells), forms a continuous *blanket* covering the entire mucosa. This mucus barrier traps the bicarbonate secreted by the epithelial cells to form a mucus/bicarbonate shield that neutralizes offensive H^+ ions.
  - The epithelium itself is remarkably resistant to acid injury because of the presence of a lipid bilayer located in the apical membranes of the epithelial cells. The epithelium is also capable of rapid regeneration and repair if disrupted.
  - Back diffusion of H^+ ions into the mucosa results in a reactive increase in submucosal perfusion.
  - The submucosal blood flow buffers H^+ ions with bicarbonate and also removes excess ions.
- Any alteration in the barrier mechanism can lead to cell acidosis, necrosis, and the formation of an ulcer. This barrier alteration can occur as a result of inflammation (mucus proteolysis), exposure to nonsteroidal antiinflammatory drugs (NSAIDs), or an ischemic injury (decreased submucosal flow).

GASTRIC MOTILITY

- There are two patterns of motility depending on the presence or absence of food:
  - The fed state:
    - The gastric fundus relaxes under the influence of the vagal nerve to accommodate food as the stomach acts as a reservoir.
    - Constant and phasic contractions of the fundus ensue, creating a gradient of pressure facilitating transfer of food towards the antrum.
    - The antrum produces high-amplitude contractions that mechanically grind solids to particles <2 mm

in size before passing through the pylorus into the duodenum as a suspension designated *chyme.*

- The rate of gastric emptying depends on both the consistency and composition of the ingested material. Liquids empty quickly (20–30 min), whereas solids require 60 to 90 minutes. Fat and hypertonic fluids empty slowly because of their influence on specialized duodenal chemoreceptors leading to the release of motility-inhibiting peptides (CCK and secretin). This mechanism allows adequate time for activation of pancreatic enzymes.
- The important role of the vagus nerve in the regulation of gastric motility is highlighted in post-vagotomy patients.
  - Dumping syndrome: Loss of the accommodation reflex is responsible for accelerated emptying of liquids.
  - Gastroparesis: Decreased antral contractile activity is responsible for delayed mechanical digestion and emptying of solids.
- The fasting state:
  - High-amplitude contractile waves known as the migratory motor complex (MMC) propagate through the gastrointestinal tract every 90 minutes and serve as a *housekeeper* propelling nondigestible solid residue toward the colon.

SYMPTOMS OF GASTRIC DISEASE

DYSPEPSIA

- Defined as persistent or recurrent pain or discomfort centered in the upper abdomen. The term *discomfort* refers to symptoms such as early satiety, postprandial fullness, bloating, and nausea.
- Clinically relevant dyspepsia is defined as a relapsing or chronic condition, present for at least 12 weeks in the prior year. Gastric and nongastric causes of dyspepsia with helpful clinical clues are outlined in Table 54–2.
- Approach to dyspepsia[1]:
  - Upper endoscopy is the study of choice to diagnose peptic ulcer disease, erosive esophagitis, and gastric malignancy; and it is superior to barium radiography.
  - Upper endoscopy is indicated in all patients older than age 55 years with new-onset dyspepsia, as well as in all patients with *alarm* features such as weight loss, dysphagia, recurrent vomiting, bleeding, or anemia. In patients younger than age 55 years with uncomplicated dyspepsia, *Helicobacter pylori* should be tested for and treated if positive.
  - Abdominal imaging is performed if pancreatic or biliary tract disease is suspected.
  - Gastric emptying scan is performed in patients with recurrent vomiting.

TABLE 54–2 Gastric and Nongastric Causes of Dyspepsia with Helpful Clinical Clues

GASTRIC CAUSES	CLINICAL CLUES
Peptic ulcer disease	Presence of *Helicobacter pylori* infection on noninvasive testing, or recent NSAID use
Gastric cancer	Older age, weight loss
Gastroparesis	Postprandial fullness, early satiety, nausea, and vomiting
Helicobacter pylori	*H. pylori* infection on noninvasive testing
Infiltrative diseases	Clinical evidence of Crohn, sarcoidosis, or tuberculosis
Drug related	Use of NSAIDs, iron, potassium, digoxin, oral antibiotics (metronidazole, macrolides), bisphosphonates
Parasitic infection	History of travel abroad, diarrhea, and weight loss

NONGASTRIC CAUSES	CLINICAL CLUES
Nonerosive reflux disease	Heartburn that is relieved by antacids
Celiac disease	Caucasian, iron deficiency, anemia
Gallstones	Sudden colicky right upper quadrant pain
Chronic pancreatitis or pancreatic carcinoma	Gradual onset, postprandial pain radiating to the back
Ischemic heart disease	Exercise-related symptoms
Chronic intestinal ischemia	Fear of eating due to postprandial pain in an older smoker
Metabolic disturbances	Elevated TSH, calcium
Musculoskeletal	Pain worsened by palpation of abdominal wall, paresthesia

NSAID, nonsteroidal antiinflammatory drug; TSH, thyroid-stimulating hormone.

- Ambulatory esophageal pH testing is carried out when atypical gastroesophageal reflux disease (GERD) is suspected.
- Most patients not using NSAIDs and *H. pylori*–negative (60% of all patients with dyspepsia) have functional nonulcer dyspepsia or atypical GERD and can be treated with antisecretory agents.

NAUSEA AND VOMITING

- *Nausea* is an unpleasant sensation characterized by sickness accompanied by expectant vomiting.
- *Vomiting* is the forceful expulsion by mouth of stomach contents that is accompanied by intense contraction of the abdominal wall muscles. It should be distinguished from retching (abdominal contraction without food expulsion), regurgitation (no abdominal contraction), and rumination (regurgitation of food postprandially with subsequent chewing and swallowing).
- The vomiting center, located in the reticular formation of the medulla, receives sensory input from four major sources. When the afferent stimuli reach a certain threshold, vomiting occurs:

1. The chemoreceptor trigger zone, located in the medullary area postrema outside the blood brain barrier, functions as a *sensor* for chemical and metabolic derangements and interprets those as noxious stimuli.
2. The intraabdominal organs (gastrointestinal viscera and the peritoneum), whether affected by an infectious (food poisoning, gastroenteritis) or noninfectious (gastroparesis, biliary colic, etc.) process.
3. The vestibular system as in cases of motion sickness and vertigo.
4. The central nervous system in cases of extreme emotions, noxious smell or sights, and also in prechemotherapy anticipatory nausea.

- Depending on the source of the stimulus, a variety of receptors can be involved and eventually targeted for treatment. Identifying the cause of nausea (source of stimulus) increases the chances of success by targeting the most likely affected receptors.[2] The different nausea receptors and the medications used to target them are outlined in Table 54–3.

PEPTIC ULCER DISEASE

DEFINITION

- An ulcer is a localized mucosal breach of the stomach or duodenum that penetrates the muscularis mucosa, while erosion is a breach that does not penetrate the muscularis.
- The term *peptic* is based on the belief (now proven incorrect) that pepsin is always involved in pathogenesis.

EPIDEMIOLOGY

- The incidence of peptic ulcer disease is 0.1% (1% in *H. pylori* positive individuals).

- Lifetime prevalence is 10% but may increase to 20% if *H. pylori* is present.
- Duodenal ulcers tend to occur 2 decades earlier than gastric ulcers, but the incidence of both increases with aging.
- Men are more likely to develop a duodenal ulcer than are women.

PATHOGENESIS

- An imbalance between protective mechanisms (mucus, bicarbonate and mucosal circulation) and offensive agents (acid, pepsin, and *H. pylori*) is necessary to injure the mucosa.
- NSAIDs and/or infection with *H. pylori* are responsible for peptic ulcer disease in 90% of patients.[3]

RISK FACTORS FOR PEPTIC ULCER DISEASE
- Cigarette smokers are at an increased risk for acquiring peptic ulcer disease as well as impaired ulcer healing. These effects are proportional to the amount smoked.
- Corticosteroids augment the NSAID-related risk of peptic ulcer disease.
- Chronic anxiety may contribute to ulcer formation by heightening the cholinergic output and increasing acid production.
- Other medical comorbidities: systemic mastocytosis (increased histamine and acid production), chronic obstructive lung disease, cirrhosis, and uremia (mostly caused by metabolic acidosis and back diffusion of H^+ ions).
- There is *no* evidence that diet can cause, worsen, or treat ulcers.

ROLE OF *HELICOBACTER PYLORI*
- Only 15% of patients infected with *H. pylori* develop ulcers suggesting that both host-related factors and

TABLE 54–3   The Different Nausea Receptors and the Medications Used to Target Them

STIMULUS	REGION	RECEPTOR	PREFERRED DRUG CLASS	MEDICATION	SIDE EFFECT
Intraabdominal	MVC	5-HT-3	5-HT_3-receptor antagonists	Ondansetron, granisetron	Headache, constipation
		H_1	Antihistamines	Meclizine, dimenhydrinate	Drowsiness
Vestibular	MVC	Muscarinic	Anticholinergics	Scopolamine	Constipation, blurred vision, dry mouth
CNS	MVC	Not certain	Sedatives	Benzodiazepines	Drowsiness
Drugs		5-HT_3	5-HT_3-receptor antagonists	Ondansetron, granisetron	Headache, constipation
Metabolic	CTZ	D2	D antagonist	Chlorpromazine, haloperidol, droperidol, metoclopramide	Extrapyramidal reactions, depression, tachyarrhythmias
Toxins		NKN-1	NKN-1 receptor antagonists	Aprepitant	Fatigue, hiccups

5-HT_3, serotonin; CNS, central nervous system; CTZ, chemoreceptor trigger zone; D, dopamine; H_1, histamine zone; MVC, medullary vomiting center; NKN-1, neurokinin.

bacterial virulence factors are important. Strains producing the virulence factor, cytoxin associated gene A (CagA), are associated with increased epithelial damage.

- *H. pylori* is more likely to cause ulcers in the antrum and duodenum. Infection of the antrum damages the D cells leading to decreased somatostatin production and, hence, loss of the negative feed by somatostatin on gastrin secretion. Hypergastrinemia ensues causing an increase in acid production by the parietal cells. The increased acid load to the duodenum causes reactive *gastric metaplasia* of the duodenal mucosa, which creates new, previously absent, colonization nidus for *H. pylori*. Duodenal *H. pylori* subsequently causes inflammation in the duodenal mucosa followed by mucosal breakdown leading to ulcer formation.

ROLE OF NSAIDs

- NSAID use deprives the mucosa from cytoprotective prostaglandins required to maintain its integrity (decreased mucus and bicarbonate secretion and mucosal blood flow).
  - Erosions spontaneously occur in NSAID users.
  - Acid and pepsin secretion promotes ulcer formation.
- The risk is dose dependent. Prevalence of peptic ulcer disease is estimated to be 10% to 40% among NSAID users (most are asymptomatic).

CLINICAL PRESENTATION

- Duodenal ulcers present typically with epigastric pain, sometimes point tenderness, which tends to occur before meals and at night (hunger pain).
  - The pain is relieved by antacids and food.
  - The pain may radiate to the back if a posterior ulcer is present.
  - Nonclassic presentations include heartburn, vomiting, and weight loss.
- Gastric ulcers present with epigastric pain occurring shortly after meals.
  - Modest relief with food or antacids.
  - Anorexia, nausea and vomiting, and weight loss are more likely to be prominent compared to duodenal ulcers.
- Gastric and duodenal ulcers are frequently asymptomatic.
- Epigastric tenderness is the most frequent finding on physical examination.
- On occasion, the ulcer may present with an acute or chronic complication:
  - *Bleeding*: hematemesis, melena, or hematochezia.
  - *Perforation*: signs of an acute abdomen.
  - *Gastric outlet obstruction*: postprandial pain and distension, severe nausea and vomiting, weight loss.

DIAGNOSIS

- Upper endoscopy is the test of choice to establish the diagnosis.
  - Barium radiography is less sensitive and limited since biopsies cannot be performed.
- If a duodenal ulcer is discovered, antral biopsies to establish the presence of *H. pylori* are indicated. Biopsies of duodenal ulcers are not necessary unless Crohn's disease is suspected. The presence of multiple duodenal ulcers, especially if recurrent, should raise the question of a gastrinoma.
- If a gastric ulcer is found, biopsies from the edges of the ulcer are necessary to rule out malignancy. Antral biopsies to investigate the presence of *H. pylori* are only necessary if the ulcers are in the antrum or pyloric channel. Repeat endoscopy in 6 to 8 weeks is indicated for all gastric ulcers to confirm healing and eliminate the possibility of an unrecognized ulcerated cancer.

TREATMENT

- General principles
  - Establish acid suppression therapy to facilitate healing of the ulcer.
  - Eradicate *H. pylori* if present.
  - Remove offending agents such as NSAIDs, cigarettes, and excessive alcohol.
  - No firm dietary recommendations are needed for healing; patients should avoid foods that worsen dyspepsia.
- Acid suppression therapy:
  - PPIs are the most powerful drugs available to suppress acid production. PPIs offer >90% cure rate in 1 week, and almost 100% in 8 weeks. Histamine receptor blockers offer healing rates of 80% at 4 weeks and 90% to 95% at 8 weeks.
  - PPIs work best when the proton pump is active:
    - Best taken 30 minutes before meals.
    - Avoid coadministration with H2 blockers.
  - Table 54–4 summarizes the different medications used in the treatment of peptic ulcer disease.
- Management of *H. Pylori*-related ulcers:
  - Eradication of *H. Pylori* decreases the 1-year recurrence rate of peptic ulcer disease from 90% to 2%.
  - Detection of *H. pylori* infection can be achieved through invasive testing (requires endoscopic sampling of gastric mucosa) or noninvasive testing. Table 54–5 summarizes different detection methods for *H. pylori*.
  - A 10- to 14-day course of combination antibiotic therapy with a PPI is the treatment of choice offering a cure rate of more than 90%.[4]
  - Combine two of three antibiotics: amoxicillin, clarithromycin, metronidazole.

TABLE 54–4   Medications Used in the Treatment of Peptic Ulcer Disease

CLASS	MECHANISM	SIDE EFFECTS	KEY FACTS
Antacids (aluminum hydroxide, magnesium hydroxide, calcium carbonate)	Binding bile and pepsin Counteracting acid Promoting angiogenesis in injured mucosa	Constipation and neurotoxicity (aluminum based) Diarrhea and hypermagnesemia (magnesium based) Rebound acid stimulation and milk-alkali syndrome (calcium based)	Best used for symptomatic relief of dyspepsia
H_2 receptor antagonists (cimetidine, ranitidine, famotidine, nizatidine)	Block histamine-mediated acid secretion	Rare except cimetidine (gynecomastia, delirium in the elderly)	All have comparable effects when used at appropriate doses
PPIs (Omeprazole, lansoprazole, rabeprazole, pantoprazole, esomeprazole)	Irreversibly inactivate the proton pumps	Rare	Have a lag time to effect (should not be administered PRN)
Sucralfate	Protective barrier by binding selectively to ulcerated areas	Constipation Aluminum-related neurotoxicity	Most effective at a low pH (best taken shortly before meals)
Bismuth	Unclear (ulcer coating, binding of pepsin, stimulation of mucosal defense, suppression of *Helicobacter pylori*)	Long-term high doses may lead to neurotoxicity	Does not inhibit or neutralize gastric acid Avoid in patients with renal failure (bismuth toxicity)
PG analogs (Misoprostol)	Enhancement of mucosal defense	Diarrhea (20%) Uterine contraction and bleeding (relatively CI in women of childbearing age)	Best used for prevention of NSAID-induced gastric ulcers

CI, contraindicated; H_2, histamine; NSAID; nonsteroidal antiinflammatory drug; PG, prostaglandin; PPIs, proton pump inhibitors; PRN, on an as needed basis.

○ Urea breath test to detect *H. pylori* can be performed to confirm eradication in selected cases.
• Management of NSAID-related ulcers:
  ○ Active ulcers should be treated with PPIs; NSAIDs should be stopped whenever possible, and preferably avoided in the future.
  ○ If NSAID use is unavoidable, use the lowest possible dose and duration.
    ▪ Misoprostol or PPI combination therapy should be added in patients requiring NSAIDs.

OTHER GASTRIC DISORDERS

GASTRITIS

• Erosive and hemorrhagic gastritis:
  ○ Most commonly seen in alcoholics, NSAID users, and critically ill patients (especially ventilator dependent). Stress ulcers are most commonly seen in victims of trauma and burns.

TABLE 54–5   Diagnostic Tests for the Detection of *Helicobacter Pylori* Infection

TEST	METHOD	SENS	SPEC	LIMITATION
Invasive				
CLO test	Relies on bacterial conversion of urea to pH-raising ammonia and CO_2	95%	95%	Affected by recent use of antibiotics and PPI (within 2 wk) = false negative
Histologic examination (the gold standard test)	Relies on visually identifying bacteria	95%	99%	Interobserver variability
Noninvasive				
Serum antibodies	Relies on detection of antibodies against *H. pylori* in serum (ELISA-IgG)	90%	87%	Remains positive for a long time, so test can't be used to determine active disease or to check for cure after treatment
Stool antigen	Relies on detection of *H. pylori* in stool	90%	90%	Affected by recent use of antibiotics and PPI (within 2 wk) = false negative
Urea breath test	Relies on bacterial conversion of urea (containing a labeled carbon isotope) to ammonia and CO_2, which can be detected in breath	93%	93%	Affected by recent use of antibiotics and PPI (within 2 wk) = false negative

CLO, campylobacter-like organism; CO_2, carbon dioxide; ELISA, enzyme-linked immunoabsorbent assay; IgG, immunoglobulin G; PPI, proton pump inhibitor; sens, sensitivity; spec, specificity.

○ Epigastric pain, nausea, vomiting, hematemesis or coffee-ground emesis, and melena are the most common symptoms, but many patients remain asymptomatic.

○ In critically ill patients, prophylaxis with antisecretory therapy (H-2 receptor blockers) reduces the incidence of significant bleeding by 50%.

○ Treatment of gastritis: PPI by continuous infusion.

• Nonerosive, nonspecific gastritis:

○ Can be divided into two types: *H. pylori* gastritis (80% of cases) and autoimmune gastritis (20% of cases).

○ Table 54–6 summarizes the differences between these two types.

GASTRIC CANCER

• Higher incidence in persons who are male (2:1), older than age 60 years, and poor (low socioeconomic status).

• Risk factors: suspected dietary factors include starch as well as pickled, smoked, and nitrite-preserved foods. *H. pylori* is a strong risk factor for distal gastric cancer, whereas pernicious anemia carries an overall modest risk for gastric cancer (10%). Prior partial gastrectomy increases the risk slightly so surveillance is not justified.

• Abdominal pain, dyspepsia, and weight loss are the most common symptoms.

• A palpable mass is felt in 20% to 30% of patients. An enlarged lymph node in the left supraclavicular region is referred to as Virchow node, whereas a palpable umbilical nodule is referred to as Sister Mary Joseph nodule. Both can sometimes be found in gastric cancer.

• Diagnosis is established via endoscopy coupled with multiple biopsies (at least eight); staging requires endoscopic ultrasound and computed tomography.

TABLE 54–6   Comparison Between the Types of Chronic Nonerosive Nonspecific Gastritis

TYPE	TYPE A GASTRITIS	TYPE B GASTRITIS
Location	Fundus and body	Antrum
Histology	Gland atrophy and intestinal metaplasia	Intestinal metaplasia
Etiology	Antibodies against parietal cells (90% of patients) leading to achlorhydria and vitamin B_{12} deficiency	Infection with *Helicobacter pylori*
Gastrin	Markedly elevated gastrin	Normal or mildly elevated gastrin
Associated cancer risk	Increased risk of adenocarcinoma and carcinoid tumors	Increased risk of adenocarcinomas and low-grade B cell lymphoma (mucosa-associated lymphoid tissue lymphoma)

• Curative treatment is surgical but is only achievable with local disease. Chemotherapy for extensive disease is ineffective.

• Survival is 50% for node-negative local cancer and <10% for node-positive cancer.

GASTROPARESIS

• Chronic disorder of gastric motility that is characterized by delayed gastric emptying postprandially leading to abdominal pain, nausea, and vomiting. A clue to the diagnosis is the presence of undigested food consumed several hours before vomiting.

• In diabetics, the etiology is thought to be secondary to autonomic dysfunction, but most other cases remain poorly understood. Hypothyroidism, systemic sclerosis, amyloidosis, and prior vagotomy are the other most common known causes of gastroparesis. Any condition that causes neurogenic or myogenic dysfunction has the potential to cause gastroparesis.

• Diagnosis is achieved by performing a gastric emptying scan with radio-labeled solid low fat food. The retention of more than 60% of gastric contents at 2 hours after a meal, or more than 10% at 4 hours after a meal is diagnostic.

• There is no curative treatment unless the cause is identified and corrected (hypothyroidism for example). The goal is to improve gastric motility to reduce symptoms and maintain nutrition.[5]

• Gastric emptying can be aided by eating small meals, avoiding high residual diets (vegetables) and fat-rich food, and avoiding medications that decrease motility (anticholinergics and narcotics). Control of hyperglycemia is also important.

• Metoclopramide taken 30 minutes before meals can be useful but carries a risk of neurologic complications with long-term use. Domperidone is a peripherally acting dopamine antagonist that does not have neurological complications but carries a risk of cardiac arrhythmia and is not available in the United States. Tegaserod, a serotonin 5-HT$_4$ receptor agonist, has been used with mixed success.

• Gastric neurostimulation (gastric pacing) is an evolving modality for treatment and can be helpful in selected cases. Refractory patients may require insertion of a jejunostomy feeding tube to bypass the stomach, with or without gastric venting.

ACUTE UPPER GASTROINTESTINAL BLEEDING

• Eighty percent of all acute gastrointestinal bleedings are upper bleeds.

• Peptic ulcer disease is the most common cause of upper gastrointestinal bleeding.

- Overall mortality is 5% to 10% in patients with an upper bleed. This rate increases with advancing age.
- Usually presents as melena, possibly as hematemesis or coffee-ground emesis. Severe upper gastrointestinal bleeding may present as hematochezia and is usually associated with hemodynamic instability.
- Upper gastrointestinal bleeding is often self-limited (80%); otherwise endoscopic, angiographic, or surgical intervention may be required.
- Most rebleeding episodes occur within the first 48 hours. A visible arterial source, advanced age, active bleeding in the hospital, hemodynamic instability, and presence of comorbidities are all associated with a heightened risk of rebleeding.
- Table 54–7 summarizes different causes of gastrointestinal bleeding, their unique characteristics, and most commonly used treatment modalities.

APPROACH TO THE PATIENT WITH UPPER GASTROINTESTINAL BLEEDING

- Assess the hemodynamic status. In the first 24 to 48 hours, orthostatic measurements are more valuable than hematocrit in estimating the severity of blood loss, since hemoconcentration may result in a falsely *corrected* hematocrit.
- Obtain adequate intravenous access, initiate hydration, transfuse as needed, and correct underlying coagulopathies if present.
- Perform nasogastric lavage to confirm the diagnosis of upper gastrointestinal bleeding (bright red or coffee-ground aspirate), to rule out the diagnosis (clear aspirate with bile as evidence of negative duodenal lavage), or to identify active bleeding (continuous bright red aspirate), which carries the highest mortality risk and requires the most aggressive intervention.
- Initiate pharmacologic therapy:
  - Acid suppression therapy is required with PPIs, preferably as a continuous drip.[6] This approach has been found to decrease the risk of rebleeding from a peptic ulcer and appears to be superior to other acid suppression regimens.
  - Octreotide by continuous intravenous drip is indicated if variceal bleeding is suspected. It decreases portal hypertension by reducing splanchnic blood flow.
- Perform endoscopy to identify the source of bleeding, assess the likelihood of recurrence, and apply appropriate therapy.[7] Peptic ulcer with a visible blood vessel or adherent clot is usually treated endoscopically with injection of vasoconstrictors, with use of heat-generating therapy, or by application of a metal clip to achieve local hemostasis. Bleeding varices are treated endoscopically by band application and occasionally by sclerotherapy.
- Angiographic treatment by embolization methods (arterial bleeding), insertion of transjugular intrahepatic portosystemic shunts (variceal bleeding), or surgery may become necessary when endoscopic therapy fails or the source of bleeding is not reachable by endoscopic methods.

TABLE 54–7 Causes of Gastrointestinal Bleeding, Their Unique Features, and Most Common Treatment Modalities

CAUSE	PERCENTAGE	CHARACTERISTICS
Peptic ulcer disease	55	Often associated with *Helicobacter pylori* or NSAID use. Usually treated endoscopically. Mortality is 6–10%.
Variceal bleeding	10–20	Caused by portal hypertension. Mostly esophageal but can be gastric. Treatment is by endoscopic banding, TIPS may become necessary. Mortality is 15%.
Mallory-Weiss tears	5–15	Mostly on the gastric side of the gastroesophageal junction. Often seen in alcoholics after retching. Stops spontaneously.
Vascular anomalies	6	Hereditary hemorrhagic telangiectasia, Dieulafoy lesions, gastric antral ectasia. Treatment is endoscopic and with iron replacement.
Erosive esophagitis/ gastritis	5	Related to acid reflux (esophagitis), NSAID use, alcohol, and stress (gastritis). Treatment with antisecretory therapy.
Gastric neoplasm	1	Primary or metastatic. Effective therapy is surgical.
Aortoenteric fistula	Rare	Usually abdominal aortic graft connecting to the third part of duodenum. Proceeded by a herald bleed that stops spontaneously. Surgical exploration when suspected.
Hemobilia and hemosuccus pancreaticus	Rare	Likely trauma to liver or biliary tree (hemobilia), rupture of an aneurysm into the pancreatic duct (hemosuccus). Treatment by embolization.

NSAID, nonsteroidal antiinflammatory drug; TIPS, transjugular intrahepatic portosystemic shunt.

REFERENCES

1. Talley NJ, Vakil NB, Moayyedi P. American gastroenterological association technical review on the evaluation of dyspepsia. *Gastroenterology.* 2005;129:1756–1780.
2. Quigley EMM, Hasler WL, Parkman HP. AGA technical review on nausea and vomiting. *Gastroenterology.* 2001;120:263–286.
3. Huang JQ, Sridhar S, Hunt RH. Role of *Helicobacter pylori* infection and non-steroidal anti-inflammatory drugs in peptic-ulcer disease: a meta-analysis. *Lancet.* 2002;359:14–22.
4. Malfertheiner P, Megraud F, O'Morain C, et al. Current concepts in the management of *Helicobacter pylori* infection: the Maastricht 2–2000 Consensus Report. *Aliment Pharmacol Ther.* 2002;16:167–180.
5. Parkman HP, Hasler WL, Fisher RS. American Gastroenterological Association medical position statement: diagnosis and treatment of gastroparesis. *Gastroenterology.* 2004;127(5):1589–1591.
6. Bardou M, Touboti Y, Benhaberou-Brun D, et al. Meta-analysis: proton-pump inhibition in high-risk patients with acute peptic ulcer bleeding. *Aliment Pharmacol Ther.* 2005;21:677–686.
7. Adler DG, Leighton JA, Davila RE, et al. ASGE Guideline: the role of endoscopy in acute non-variceal upper-GI hemorrhage. *Gastrointest Endosc.* 2004;60(4):497–504.

55 DISEASES OF THE SMALL BOWEL

M. Louay Omran

ANATOMY AND PHYSIOLOGY

ANATOMY

- The small intestine is a 6 m long hollow tube that is wrapped in a serosal layer. The wall of the small bowel consists of a mucosa, submucosa, and inner circular and outer longitudinal muscular layers.
- There are two nerve cell networks: a submucosal plexus located alongside the blood and lymphatic vessels in the submucosa and a myenteric plexus located between the circular and the longitudinal muscular layers.
- The mucosa consists of the epithelium, the lamina propria (connective tissue), and the muscularis mucosa (a smooth muscle).
- The epithelium consists of a single layer of epithelial cells linked together by tight junctions.
- These cells include absorptive cells, mucus-producing cells (Goblet cells), and hormone-producing cells (endocrine cells) among others. Rapid cell turnover

allows for the entire epithelium to be replaced every 5 days. This ensures quick recovery after injurious insults such as chemotherapy.
- The intestinal mucosal surface is designed to form finger-like folds called *villi.* The surface of each epithelial cell also has finger-like projections (*microvilli*) to collectively form the "Brush Border." This *villous* pattern increases the intestinal surface area available for absorption by 600-fold compared to a nonvillous flat mucosa. The center of each intestinal villus is occupied by a capillary network that surrounds a single blind lymphatic vessel referred to as a *lacteal.* Nutrients absorbed into the capillary venous system are led to the liver via the portal vein, whereas those absorbed directly into the lacteal (mainly fat) bypass the portal vein and reach the systemic circulation directly though the lymphatic system.

PHYSIOLOGY

- The small bowel's functions include digestion, absorption, and transportation of food.
- Digestion breaks down the various components of food to their basic building blocks that can then be absorbed. The small intestine transfers the chyme (food mix) from the stomach to the colon through a complex motility pattern.
- The luminal phase of digestion depends on the function of several pancreatic enzymes and the bile acids produced by the liver. Further digestion of some nutrients is accomplished at the mucosal level by the action of the brush-border enzymes. Absorption of nutrients, minerals, and vitamins into the enterocytes occurs passively or actively via an energy-dependant mechanism.
- Absorbed nutrients and water are transported to the main circulation either indirectly via the portal vein or directly via the lymphatics. Digestion and absorption of specific nutrients are discussed in detail in the Malabsorption section.
- The motility of the small intestine displays distinct motor patterns that differ depending on its relation to a meal. The fed state is an active period characterized by intestinal segmental contractions that help mix food with digestive enzymes and allow adequate surface contact time for absorption. Phasic contractions along the length of the small bowels occur intermittently in the fed state and allow the chyme to advance slowly toward the colon. The duration of the fed state and the speed of progression of chyme are directly related to the caloric content of the meal, the higher the calories the slower the progression to allow more contact time for digestion and absorption. Between meals (the fasting state), the small intestine exhibits contractions

(migrating motor complexes) (MMCs) that are characterized by a quiescent phase that gradually progresses to propulsive movements sweeping food residue toward the colon. The MMCs are responsible for the "growling" sound heard in the fasting state and can be immediately aborted by eating.

- Although the contractions in the fed state are likely mediated by acetylcholine, motilin plays a major role in the induction of MMCs.
- In addition to digestion, absorption, and transportation of nutrients, the small intestine functions as an important barrier against invasive microorganisms, and as a "factory" producing several proteins (apolipoproteins) and hormones that mediate many of the functions of the intestine.

SYMPTOMS OF SMALL BOWEL DISEASES

DIARRHEA

- The total volume of fluids passing through the small bowel each day exceeds 8 liters which is comprised of oral intake and intestinal secretions. An average of 7 liters is absorbed in the small bowel, and 1 to 2 liters are absorbed in the colon. Conditions that lead to impaired absorption or increased intestinal secretion may result in diarrhea. Diarrhea is defined as a daily stool volume in excess of 250 mL (stool weight >250 g). Because of the difference in the composition of food residue present in the small bowel versus colon, there is a difference in the characteristics of diarrhea depending on its origin. Small bowel diarrhea is larger in volume, likely frothy and foul smelling, and is not associated with blood. Left colonic diarrhea is likely to be recurrent but has less volume, and is associated with tenesmus, mucus, and blood.
- Diarrhea can be divided into acute (less than 4 weeks) and chronic subtypes. Based on the responsible mechanism, chronic diarrhea can be further classified into four categories: osmotic, secretory, inflammatory, and functional diarrhea (Table 55–1 details the mechanisms and common causes of each category). In addition to a thorough history, the following tests help classify chronic diarrhea:
1. Serum electrolytes, albumin, and thyroid function tests
2. Complete blood count with differential

TABLE 55–1   Most Common Causes of Bacterial Infectious Diarrhea with Key Facts

Invasive	Sources	Symptoms	Treatment
Campylobacter	Poultry, water and milk, dogs and cats	Abd pain, bloody stool, Guillain-Barré, HUS, arthritis	Erythromycin or Cipro
Salmonella (non-typhi)	Poultry, eggs, milk	Fever, abd pain, no blood in stool	Supportive, Cipro if severe
Shigella	P-t-P, green onions	Fever, greenish stool, bacteremia	Amoxicillin, chloramphenicol
Escherichia coli O157:H7	Undercooked hamburger, milk, apple juice	Nausea, vomiting, headache, abd pain, HUS and TTP	No antibiotics (increased potential for complications)
Vibrio parahaemolyticus	Undercooked shellfish	Fever, bloody diarrhea	Supportive or erythromycin
Yersinia enterocolitica	Water, milk, pork	Fever, RLQ pain, nausea and vomiting, leukocytosis Ankylosing spondylitis, erythema nodosum	Aminoglycosides, trim-sulfa
Noninvasive			
Bacillus cereus	Fried rice	Early diarrhea (1–6 h) or late (12 h)	Supportive
Staphylococcus aureus	Eggs, cream, mayonnaise	No fever or vomiting or pain. Diarrhea starts in 1–6 h	Supportive
Clostridium perfringens	Rewarmed beef/turkey	Mild vomiting followed by severe diarrhea (after 12 h)	Supportive
Listeria monocytogenes	Hot dogs, cheeses	Fever, disseminated infections in ICH, extreme ages, pregnant	Ampicillin, gentamicin
E. coli (traveler diarrhea)	Water, salads	Watery diarrhea, fatigue	Supportive, Cipro or trim-sulfa
Vibrio cholerae	Water	Severe life-threatening diarrhea	Tetracycline

Abd, abdominal; Cipro, ciprofloxacin; HUS, hemolytic uremic syndrome; ICH, immune-compromised host; P-t-P, person to person; RLQ, right lower quadrant; trim-sulfa, trimethoprim-sulfamethoxazole; TTP, thrombotic thrombocytopenic purpura.

3. Stool test for lactoferrin, qualitative fat, electrolytes
4. Stool cultures, ova and parasites, *Clostridium diffi-cile* toxin, and serum C-reactive protein (CRP) when appropriate
5. Endoscopic evaluation (sigmoidoscopy or colonoscopy) unless the diagnosis is secured by the history and the above tests

• Measurement of stool electrolytes, sodium (Na) and potassium (K), are necessary to calculate the *osmolar gap*, which establishes the presence of osmotic diarrhea when it exceeds 50. The stool osmolar gap is high when a substance, other than electrolyte, is responsible for the excessive osmotic pressure, which promotes water diffusion into the intestinal lumen.
  ◦ Calculation of the stool osmolar gap = 290 − 2 (stool Na + stool K)
• Stool lactoferrin and CRP raise the suspicion of an inflammatory diarrhea. The presence of an elevated white count, positive bacterial cultures, ova and parasites, or *C. difficile* toxin identifies the presence of infectious diarrhea.
• When secretory diarrhea is identified in the absence of an infection or other obvious causes (ileal resection), intestinal secretory tumors should be considered.
• Irritable bowel syndrome is the most common cause of motility-based diarrhea, but the diagnosis relies on fulfilling the Rome diagnostic criteria and excluding other potential causes.

• Acute infectious diarrhea
  ◦ Viruses are the most common cause of gastroenteritis in the United States. Viral gastroenteritis is characterized by a brief self-limiting diarrhea (up to 5 days), mild nausea and vomiting, and absence of abdominal pain. Fever can be present but is usually low grade. Infection is acquired by contact with an infected person (Rotavirus in children, Norwalk in adults) and treatment is supportive.
  ◦ Bacterial diarrhea can be caused by enterotoxicogenic (toxin-mediated) or entero-invasive mechanisms. In entero-invasive diarrhea there is mucosal damage and ulcerations leading to intestinal bleeding and a positive stool lactoferrin assay. These abnormalities are not usually present in enterotoxicogenic diarrhea. Table 55–2 lists the most common causes of bacterial infectious diarrhea.
  ◦ Giardia is the most common diarrhea-inducing parasite in the United States, although *Entameba histolytica* is the most common in the rest of the world. *Cryptosporidium parvum* is the most common cause of parasitic diarrhea in acquired immunodeficiency syndrome (AIDS) patients.
  ◦ Giardia is acquired from contaminated water, or person-to-person spread. Acute ingestion is characterized by abdominal cramps, bloating, nausea, and watery diarrhea, although the only chronic symptom may be weight loss caused by malabsorption. Giardia is best diagnosed by detecting stool Giardia antigens and is treated with metronidazole.

TABLE 55–2   Classification of Diarrhea, Common Causes, and Important Features

TYPE	MECHANISM	COMMON CAUSES	IMPORTANT FEATURES
Osmotic	Osmotically active substances remain in the lumen attracting water by osmosis	Lactase deficiency Osmotic laxatives (lactulose, sorbitol, magnesium citrate, milk of magnesia, etc)	Osmolar gap present Stool volume is relatively low Diarrhea subsides with fasting Stops with fasting
Secretory	Abnormal secretion of electrolytes and fluids	Toxin-mediated infections *E. coli, V. cholerae, S. aureus, C. perfringens, B. cereus* Hormone-secreting tumors: VIP, gastrin, serotonin, secretin, calcitonin Nonosmotic laxatives Ileal resection (fatty acids or bile acids stimulate colonic secretion)	Leads to loss of electrolytes (hypokalemia) Stool volume is high Does not stop with fasting
Inflammatory	Mucosal damage leads to impaired absorption, excessive secretion, and increased motility	IBD, Crohn's disease, ulcerative colitis Mucosa-invasive infections: Herpes, CMV, Yersinia, *E. Coli* O157:H7, Shigella, Salmonella, Campylobacter	Stool volume is low but bloody Part of a systemic response (fever, leukocytosis, elevated CRP/ESR) Stool lactoferrin/ leucocytes present, possibly positive stool cultures Abnormal endoscopy
Motility	Slow transit leading to bacterial overgrowth or rapid transit	Diabetic neuropathy Scleroderma Hyperthyroidism IBS	Can be associated with bloating (IBS, bacterial overgrowth) Features of the underlying disease (DM, scleroderma, hyperthyroidism)

B. cereus, Bacillus cereus; C. perfringens, Clostridium perfringens; CRP, C-reactive protein; DM, diabetes mellitus; *E. coli, Escherichia coli;* ESR, sedimentation rate; IBD, inflammatory bowel diseases; IBS, irritable bowel syndrome; *S. aureus, Staphylococcus aureus; V. cholerae, Vibrio cholerae;* VIP, vasoactive intestinal peptide.

MALABSORPTION

Malabsorption is the general term used to describe impaired delivery of ingested nutrients to the blood stream. It is either the result of maldigestion, defects in the intestinal surface absorption mechanisms, or defects in transport of nutrients to the circulation. Depending on the cause, malabsorption can either be specific to a nutrient (lactose), or generalized to all nutrients when significant mucosal damage is present (celiac disease). Symptoms and signs of malabsorption include diarrhea, weight loss, and possibly abdominal pain. Increased flatulence is seen with carbohydrate malabsorption, while bulky greasy stools are seen with fat malabsorption. Complications of specific nutrient and mineral deficiency can also be seen; such as osteoporosis, iron and folate or vitamin B_{12} deficiency anemias, in addition to signs of various vitamin deficiencies.

FAT MALABSORPTION

The intestines cannot absorb dietary fat in its consumed form: long-chain triglycerides. For fat to be absorbed into the enterocyte, the following sequence must occur: emulsification, lipolysis, and micellization. Once inside the enterocyte, repackaging into chylomicrons allows transfer of lipids into the lymphatic system and then to the systemic circulation.

- Emulsification is accomplished by mastication and gastric activity leading to the formation of an aqueous lipid suspension. Formation of this suspension is necessary for the digestive enzymes to access the otherwise hydrophobic lipids. Impaired emulsification can be seen post-gastrectomy.
- Lipolysis is the break down of long-chain triglycerides to monoglycerides and free fatty acids.
- Lipolysis begins in the stomach under the influence of gastric lipase (activated by a low pH), and continues in the small intestines under the influence of pancreatic lipase and colipase (activated by a pH >7). Impaired lipolysis can be seen with pancreatic exocrine insufficiency (lipase deficiency), or in conditions leading to a lower duodenal pH (increased acid secretion resulting from a gastrinoma, or decreased pancreatic bicarbonate secretions characteristic of chronic pancreatitis). The weight loss drug, orlistat, causes intestinal fat malabsorption by inhibiting pancreatic lipase.
- Micellization occurs when bile acids (synthesized in the liver) solubilize fatty acids, monoglycerides, phospholipids, and cholesterol into water-soluble particles referred to as micelles. Because micelles are water-soluble, the contained lipids can penetrate the thin aqueous layer covering the intestinal epithelium.

While lipids enter the enterocytes, bile acids remain in the intestinal lumen until they are absorbed in the terminal ileum and recycled within the liver, (the enterohepatic cycle). Impaired micellization occurs when the concentration of duodenal bile acids is inadequate. This occurs if hepatic production or ileal absorption of bile acids is decreased as in cases of cirrhosis, Crohn's disease, or after an iliectomy. The drug, cholestyramine, is used as a cholesterol-lowering agent because it binds to bile acids and prevents their reabsorption in the ileum.

- Inside the enterocytes, the free fatty acids and the monoglycerides are reassembled into triglycerides. When phospholipids, cholesterol, and apoproteins are added, a *chylomicron* is produced. Chylomicrons exit the enterocyte through the basolateral membrane to enter the intestinal lymphatics, bypassing the portal circulation, on their way to the general circulation. Fat malabsorption is seen when the enterocytes are damaged as in the case of celiac disease, when chylomicron formation is impaired as in the case of abetalipoproteinemia (deficiency of apoprotein B), or when the intestinal lymphatics are occluded as in primary lymphangiectasia.
- The intestines are capable of absorbing 95% of the fat consumed daily. A quantitative stool fat measurement is considered positive for fat malabsorption if >6 grams of fat is found in a person consuming 100 grams of fat daily. A 72-hour stool collection optimizes the sensitivity of the assay. A less sensitive but reliable screening test is the qualitative stool fat test, which relies on identifying the presence of fat droplets in *Sudan III*-stained stool. Once steatorrhea is established, it is necessary to differentiate luminal from mucosal impairment of fat absorption. An increase in neutral fat in the stool is suggestive of lipase deficiency (pancreatic exocrine insufficiency); whereas an increase in split fat in stool is likely caused by small bowel mucosal disease. The D-xylose test, if positive, further points in the direction of mucosal dysfunction. This can be confirmed by obtaining a small bowel biopsy. If the D-xylose test is negative, pancreatic insufficiency is suspected. Further clues include the presence of a low stool elastase or pancreatic calcifications on radiographs. Confirmation of pancreatic exocrine insufficiency can be achieved through a *secretin test* that measures the bicarbonate output of the pancreas in response to secretin infusion.

CARBOHYDRATE MALABSORPTION

All ingested carbohydrates such as polysaccharides (starch) and disaccharides (sucrose, lactose) need to be broken down to monosaccharides to be absorbed. Those that cannot be broken down (cellulose) are not absorbed and result in "bulking" of the stool.

- Digestion of polysaccharides begins in the mouth (salivary amylase) and continues in the duodenum (pancreatic amylase) to produce a mixture of oligosaccharides and disaccharides.
- These are further digested to monosaccharides (glucose, galactose, fructose) under the influence of disaccharidases located in the intestinal brush border.
- Glucose and galactose are transported into the enterocytes via a sodium-dependant process mediated by the transport protein SGLT. Fructose is transported into the enterocytes by passive diffusion through the transport protein SGLT-5. Intracellular monosaccharides are eventually transported through the basolateral membrane of the enterocyte to the venous system.
- Any condition that affects one of the processes required for carbohydrate absorption (pancreas, brush border enzymes, transport proteins, intestinal mucosa) can lead to carbohydrate malabsorption. Lactose (milk) intolerance is the most common clinical example and is caused by a primary or secondary deficiency in brush border lactase activity. The drug acarbose causes intentional starch malabsorption by blocking the action of pancreatic amylase.
- Nondigested carbohydrates (cellulose) undergo a fermentation process by the colonic flora that leads to production of short-chain fatty acids that are considered the preferred energy source for the colonic epithelial cells.
- When bacteria ferment a nonabsorbed carbohydrate, hydrogen gases are produced, absorbed, and subsequently expired by the lungs. After ingestion of a particular sugar (glucose or lactulose), the presence of high amounts of hydrogen in breath reflects an increase in the sugar available to the colonic bacteria for fermentation and suggests malabsorption of that particular sugar. This observation provides the basis for the hydrogen *breath test* used for the diagnosis of carbohydrate malabsorption. False-positive results are observed if bacterial overgrowth is present.

PROTEIN MALABSORPTION

Proteins must be degraded to tripeptides, dipeptides, or amino acids to be absorbed.
- Gastric pepsins initiate proteolysis process in the stomach.
- Under the influence of bile salts, the duodenal absorptive cells release the enzyme enterokinase, which is necessary to convert pancreatic trypsinogen to trypsin, which then activates the full complement of pancreatic proteases. Pancreatic proteases convert proteins into a mixture of amino acids, dipeptides, and tripeptides. These are then absorbed via the enterocyte through highly specific sodium-dependant cotransporters.

- Any condition affecting one of the processes required for protein absorption (stomach, pancreas, intestinal enterokinase, specific amino acid transporters) can lead to protein or amino acid malabsorption. Isolated amino acid malabsorption is rare (Hartnup disease, cystinuria).
- Measurement of α_1-antitrypsin clearance allows for the diagnosis of protein-losing enteropathies.

VITAMIN AND MINERAL MALABSORPTION

Digestion of food particles liberates vitamins in a soluble form suitable for absorption as most vitamins undergo little enzymatic modification. Except for vitamin B_{12} and magnesium, which are absorbed in the ileum, most vitamins and minerals are absorbed in the proximal half of the small intestine. Conditions affecting the intestinal mucosa can lead to malabsorption of certain vitamins and minerals depending on the area affected.
- Water-soluble vitamins are absorbed by diffusion or carrier-mediated transport systems.
- Vitamin B_{12} has a unique absorption pathway that is discussed in detail in Chap. 54 (Diseases of the Stomach).
- Fat-soluble vitamins (A, D, E, and K) follow the fat absorption pathway, and are poorly absorbed when fat malabsorption is present.

CELIAC DISEASE

Celiac disease is a genetically determined immune reaction to dietary gluten that leads to damage of the proximal small bowel mucosa. In its classic full-blown form, celiac disease causes generalized malabsorption. Fortunately, most patients have a milder course, and many are asymptomatic or have subtle manifestations.

EPIDEMIOLOGY

- Common among whites of European descent. Estimated incidence in the United States may be higher than 1:250.
- Can affect up to one-third of the population because it only afflicts those with HLA-DQ2 (95% of patients) or HLA-DQ8 (5% of patients).
- Only 25% of individuals with HLA-DQ2 or HLA-DQ8 develop Celiac disease, suggesting that other environmental and immunologic factors are necessary to manifest the phenotype.

PATHOPHYSIOLOGY

- Celiac disease is secondary to a T-cell–mediated autoimmune response to glutens in the diet, affecting the intestinal submucosa of genetically susceptible individuals.
- Glutens are storage proteins that are present in wheat, barley, and rye but not in corn or rice. Glutens can be present in small amounts in oats as a contaminant.
- After ingestion of glutens, the partially digested gliadin peptides are processed by the antigen-presenting cells in the lamina propria of the small bowel. Sensitized T-cells then activate B-cells to produce immunoglobulins, and other T-cells to produce inflammatory cytokines that damage the enterocytes. One target of this autoimmune response is tissue transglutaminase (Ttg), which is also necessary for the digestion of gliadin. Inactivation of Ttg intensifies the immune response because of the accumulation of incompletely digested gliadin. The detection of immunoglobulin A (IgA) antibodies against tissue transglutaminase is now the most valuable serologic marker for the diagnosis of celiac disease.[1]
- Celiac disease causes significant changes in the villous structure in the proximal small bowel. These changes can extend to the distal small bowel in severe cases.
- Varying degrees of villous blunting and atrophy, crypt hyperplasia and elongation, and infiltration of the lamina propria with lymphocytes and plasma cells are seen. The end result is the destruction of the intestine's absorptive surface. Similar histologic findings are noted in other malabsorptive conditions such as tropical sprue, bacterial overgrowth, and Crohn's disease among others.

CLINICAL FINDINGS

- Celiac disease is one of the most commonly under-diagnosed diseases in the United States. On average,

clinical clues are present for a decade before the diagnosis is made.

- Symptoms can become evident at any age throughout adulthood, but most patients present at age 10 to 40 years. Up to 40% of people with serologic markers of celiac disease remain asymptomatic.
- Significant malabsorption of multiple nutrients is usually seen in infants. Older children and adults present with a more subtle picture (anemia or bone disease), sometimes without any gastrointestinal symptoms. As patients advance in age the more likely the disease presents in an atypical fashion. Table 55–3 summarizes the broad clinical spectrum of celiac disease.
- Dermatitis herpetiformis (DH) is a pruritic papulovesicular rash found over the extensor surfaces of the trunk and extremities and responds to a gluten-restricted diet. The suggested mechanism is autoantibodies directed against epidermal transglutaminase. Up to 10% of patients with celiac disease have DH. Conversely, more than 85% of patients with DH have celiac disease.
- Laboratory abnormalities reflect the degree of intestinal pathology. Mild cases affecting the proximal small bowel may only cause iron deficiency anemia. More extensive involvement of the small bowel can lead to other types of anemia (folate and vitamin B_{12} deficiency), prolonged prothrombin time (vitamin K deficiency), and hypoalbuminemia. Mild elevation of aminotransferases is found in up to 40% of patients.

DIAGNOSIS

- Detecting IgA Ttg antibodies carries a very high sensitivity and specificity but can be falsely negative in patients with IgA deficiency. Because IgA deficiency is prevalent in 10% of patients with celiac disease, total

TABLE 55–3   The Clinical Spectrum of Celiac Disease

TYPICAL SYMPTOMS	EXTRA INTESTINAL FEATURES	ASSOCIATED CONDITIONS	COMPLICATIONS
Chronic diarrhea	Infertility	Dermatitis herpetiformis	Refractory sprue
Bloating	Anxiety	IgA deficiency	Intestinal T-cell lymphoma
Abdominal pain	Depression	Autoimmune thyroiditis	Ulcerative jejunoileitis
Aphthous stomatitis	Fatigue	Diabetes mellitus	GI cancers
Anorexia	Arthralgia	Addison disease	
Weight loss	Osteoporosis	Microscopic colitis	
Failure to thrive	Peripheral neuropathy	Down syndrome	
	Ataxia	Rheumatoid arthritis	
	Epilepsy	Sjögren syndrome	
	Migraines	Myocarditis	
	Iron deficiency		
	Thrombocytosis		
	Elevated transaminases		
	Vitamin deficiencies		

GI, gastrointestinal; IgA, immunoglobulin A.

IgA should also be measured. IgA endomysial antibodies are highly specific, but their sensitivity depends on the expertise of the laboratory. Measurement of IgA and immunoglobulin G (IgG) antigliadin antibodies is not recommended because of poor specificity.

- Duodenal or proximal jejunal biopsy is indicated in patients who have positive serologic studies or those with a very strong clinical suspicion in spite of negative serology. A definitive diagnosis is achieved by confirming the presence of the typical histopathology and a response to a gluten-free diet.

TREATMENT

- Treatment requires complete removal of all gluten sources from the diet including medications that include gluten as a carrier. Oats can also be "contaminated" with gluten and should be eliminated. Many patients have nutritional deficiencies at the time of diagnosis requiring supplementation until intestinal recovery. Nutritional deficiencies may result in anemia (iron, B_{12}, and folate) and osteoporosis (calcium and vitamin D). Screening for and treating osteoporosis should always be done at the time of diagnosis.

COMPLICATIONS

- Lack of improvement with dietary intervention is almost always caused by incomplete removal of gluten. In a few instances, refractory celiac disease (despite a gluten-free diet) responds to treatment with steroids or immune modulators. Rarely, refractory celiac disease can be caused by the development of collagenous sprue, ulcerative jejunitis, or intestinal T-cell lymphoma, all of which carry a poor prognosis.

CROHN'S DISEASE

Crohn's disease is a chronic idiopathic segmental inflammation of the full thickness of the bowel, which can affect any area of the gastrointestinal tract from the mouth to the anus. Inflammation is mediated by an exhuberant immune reaction resulting from the interaction of bowel flora with ill-defined environmental factors in a genetically susceptible host.

EPIDEMIOLOGY

- According to the data from Olmsted County, Minnesota, the incidence of Crohn's disease is 5.8 per 100,000 and seems to be rising; the prevalence is 133 per 100,000.

- Peak incidence age is 15 to 40 years, with a second smaller peak at age 60 to 80 years. Crohn's disease is more common among people of Jewish descent, and 15% of patients with Crohn's disease have a first-degree relative with inflammatory bowel disease. Crohn's disease is more common in industrialized nations with cold climates.
- Cigarette smoking is strongly associated with the occurrence of Crohn's disease and also aggravates the course of the disease.

PATHOPHYSIOLOGY

- Several susceptibility genes have been identified, of which CARD15 is the best known. Mutations in CARD15 lead to improper handling of bacterial flora, which seems to trigger the aberrant immune response.
- The mucosa in Crohn's disease is dominated by type 1 T-helper cells capable of producing interferon-γ and interleukin-2 (IL-2) which stimulate resident macrophages to produce inflammatory cytokines including tumor necrosis factor (TNF), interleukin-1 (IL-1), interleukin-6 (IL-6), prostaglandins, and leukotrienes. This cascade is self-sustained because of the absence of programmed T-cell death (apoptosis) that signals the end of the inflammatory response. This is likely caused by loss of tolerance for bacterial antigens, which underscore the role of bacteria in the pathophysiology.
- Formation of antibodies against specific bacteria in the gut flora is used as a serologic marker of the disease. The best known antibodies are those against *Saccharomyces cerevisiae* (anti-*S. cerevisiae* antibody [ASCA]), and against *Escherichia coli*'s outer membrane protein C (anti-OmpC).

PATHOLOGY

- Inflammation in Crohn's disease is patchy and can affect any portion of the gastrointestinal tract and the perianal region. The transmural nature of the inflammation (mucosa to serosa) can lead to fibrosis, stricturing, fistulization, and abscess formation. The presence of noncaseating granulomas is highly suggestive of Crohn's disease and is seen in up to two-thirds of patients.
- Crohn's disease affects only the small bowel in 40% of cases (usually the terminal ileum), both small bowel and colon in 30% of cases, and colon only in 20% of cases. Only a small percentage of patients have oral or upper gastrointestinal involvement.
- Perianal disease affects 30% to 80% of patients with Crohn's disease. Perianal involvement includes fissuring, fistulization, and abscess formation.

CLINICAL FEATURES

- Symptom onset is usually insidious and includes right lower quadrant pain, low-grade fever, malaise, and possibly anemia. Diarrhea is seen in colonic disease. Failure to thrive and growth retardation are seen particularly in children. A palpable mass may be felt in the right lower quadrant on examination.
- Crohn's disease can also present with one of its complications. Intestinal obstruction leads to abdominal pain, distension, nausea, vomiting, and weight loss. Fistulization can occur between the small bowel and adjacent organs (enteroenteric, enterocolonic, enterovesicular and enterovaginal) or the skin. Fistulas with the mesentery can lead to abscess formation. Enterocolonic fistulas lead to small bowel bacterial overgrowth and diarrhea.
- Perianal disease causes rectal pain, discharge, and abscess formation with symptoms and signs of infection.
- The extra intestinal manifestations of Crohn's disease can be divided into those that are associated with disease activity (peripheral arthritis, ocular inflammation, and erythema nodosum) and those that are not (oral aphthous ulcers, pyoderma gangrenosum, spondyloarthropathy, and primary sclerosing cholangitis).

DIAGNOSIS

- Serum inflammatory markers such as an erythrocyte sedimentation rate (ESR) and CRP are usually elevated when Crohn's disease is active.
- Evaluation of the small bowel with barium (small bowel follow-through, enteroclysis) can reveal terminal ileum inflammation (irregular mucosa), stricturing (string sign), or fistulization. Wireless capsule endoscopy can be used to further evaluate the small bowel if necessary. Evaluation of the colon is best accomplished with a colonoscopy that reveals the typical patchy involvement; abnormal areas separated by normal mucosa (skip areas). Ulcers in Crohn's disease are deep and linear (rake ulcers) and located on an erythematous granular base with loss of the vascular pattern. Colonoscopy allows for biopsies from both the colon and terminal ileum.
- The diagnosis of Crohn's disease is based on interpretation of the clinical, laboratory, and radiographic data available. In some cases, differentiation between Crohn's disease and ulcerative colitis (UC) remains difficult, but laboratory tests can help differentiate the two conditions:
  - ASCA are positive in two-thirds of Crohn's disease patients but only 10% of patients with UC.
  - Perinuclear antineutrophil cytoplasmic antibodies (p-ANCAs) are positive in two-thirds of UC patients but only in 10% of patients with Crohn's disease.
  - Having suggestive results on both tests (+ASCA,–p-ANCA) carries a positive predictive value of 80% for Crohn's disease.

TREATMENT

- There is no cure for Crohn's disease. Thus, treatment is designed to control disease activity and minimize flare-ups. General measures include counseling for smoking cessation, nutritional support when necessary, and symptomatic management. Several medications can be used to target the disease process and are summarized in Table 55–4.[2]

TABLE 55–4 Medications Used for the Treatment of Crohn's Disease

DRUG	ROUTE	INDICATION	KEY FACTS
5-ASA	PO	Mild-moderate acute colonic dz	Efficacy questionable, no benefit in maintaining remission or preventing postoperative recurrences
Antibiotics	PO/IV	Mild-moderate acute colonic and SB dz Perianal dz	Metronidazole and ciprofloxacin have been used, beneficial in perianal disease but modest effect otherwise
Budesonide	PO	Mild-moderate SB or right colonic dz	High first-pass hepatic metabolism (90%) resulting in significantly less side effects but less effective than systemic steroids
Systemic steroids	PO/IV	Severe SB or colonic dz	Not effective in maintenance of remission, significant side effects with long-term use
Azathioprine/ 6-MP	PO	Refractory or steroid dependant dz, fistulizing dz	Response after 3–6 months, require monitoring of metabolites and signs of toxicity
Methotrexate	IM/ PO		
Infliximab	IV	Refractory or steroid dependant dz, fistulizing dz	Chimeric mouse/human or fully human monoclonal antibodies against TNF-α but have risk of infection (TB) and rare lymphomas
Adalimumab	SC		

5-ASA, 5-amino salicylic acid; dz, disease; IM, intramuscular; IV, intravenous; 6-MP, mercaptopurine; PO, oral; SB, small bowel; SC, subcutaneous; TB, tuberculosis; TNF, tumor necrosis factor.

- Acute mild-moderate Crohn's disease's is treated with 5-amino salicylic acid (5-ASA) products (Asacol, Lialda) when it affects the descending or rectosigmoid colon, and with budesonide when it affects the terminal ileum and the right colon. Antibiotics (ciprofloxacin, metronidazole) have been successful in both small bowel and colonic disease. When this approach fails, systemic steroids become necessary for short-term use, eg, they should be tapered over several weeks. Acute severe Crohn's disease requires hospitalization and administration of intravenous steroids.
- 5-ASA can be used to sustain a remission in colonic Crohn's. Immune modulators (azathioprine, mercaptopurine [6-MP]) are indicated for maintenance of remission in cases of steroid-dependence.
- Antitumor necrosis factor-α (anti-TNF-α) drugs are indicated for severe cases that are refractory to steroids; and in lieu of steroids when flare-ups occur frequently. Anti-TNF-α drugs are effective in maintaining remission and in treating fistulizing disease.
- Surgery is indicated for cases refractory to medical management particularly when complications are present (abscess, fistulas, fibrotic strictures). More than half of the patients with Crohn's disease will require surgery during their lifetime. Postsurgical recurrence is common and can occur in up to 80% of patients within 10 years after surgery. Maintenance of postoperative remission can be enhanced by the administration of oral azathioprine or 6-MP.
- Colonic Crohn's disease increases the risk of developing dysplasia leading to colon cancer. After 8 or more years of colonic Crohn's disease, patients should be screened with surveillance colonoscopies with biopsies every 1 to 2 years.

OTHER SMALL BOWEL DISORDERS

TROPICAL SPRUE

- Acute or chronic diarrhea, weight loss, and malabsorption in residents of tropical areas, particularly the Caribbean and Southeast Asia.
- Etiology remains poorly understood, but coliform bacterial infection of the small bowel seems to be an important factor. Regardless, the disease presents with mucosal injury, bowel dysmotility, and bacterial overgrowth. Folate and vitamin B_{12} deficiency are associated findings and can contribute to further mucosal damage.
- The diagnosis is strongly suspected in a person who lives or lived in a tropical area presenting with signs of malabsorption and megaloblastic anemia. A biopsy showing villous atrophy and lipid droplets adjacent to the surface epithelium supports the diagnosis. Response to treatment confirms the diagnosis.

- A combination of daily high-dose folate and antibiotics (tetracycline) for 6 months is usually adequate. Long-term folate and vitamin B_{12} supplementation are sometimes necessary.

WHIPPLE'S DISEASE

- A very rare systemic infectious disease that mainly affects white men between age 40 and 50. The disease is caused by *Tropheryma whipplei*.
- Whipple's disease typically presents as fever of unknown origin, chronic diarrhea, and joint pain. In addition to causing malabsorption, Whipple's disease can affect a variety of organs including the brain (cognitive deficit, movement disorder, seizures), heart and lungs (pleuritis, pericarditis, endocarditis), joints (migratory asymmetric arthralgia), and eyes (vitreous opacities and hemorrhage, ophthalmoplegia, and central scotoma). Untreated Whipple's disease can be fatal.
- The diagnosis is confirmed by a small intestine (or any other involved organ) biopsy, which shows periodic acid-Schiff (PAS)–positive macrophage inclusions. Polymerase chain reaction (PCR) testing for *T. whipplei* also confirms the diagnosis.
- Treatment with antibiotics should last for more than a year to prevent relapse. One regimen involves the use of doxycycline with hydroxychloroquine for 12 to 18 months.[3] Sulfonamides cross the blood-brain barrier and should be added for treatment of neurologic symptoms.

SHORT-BOWEL SYNDROME

- Short-bowel syndrome is characterized by malabsorption when less than 180 cm of functional small bowel remains. The loss of small bowel can be anatomical because of surgery (resection, bowel bypass), or functional because of small-bowel disease (Crohn's disease, ischemic injury). After bowel resection, some physiologic adaptation occurs in the remaining bowel to increase absorptive capacity. Changes can occur for up to 1 year after surgery and include slowing of motility, increase in bowel diameter, and lengthening of the villi.
- Symptoms of short-bowel syndrome include chronic diarrhea and weight loss, fatigue, abdominal pain, and edema. In addition to malabsorption, other factors contributing to the diarrhea include bacterial overgrowth if the ileocecal valve is removed, and colonic irritation if bile acid reabsorption is decreased. Symptoms and signs of vitamin and mineral deficiencies can be present including anemia, metabolic bone disease, skin changes, bleeding, and muscle cramps.
- Treatment aims at establishing adequate caloric intake, preferably orally. Medium-chain triglycerides (which

do not require digestion), high carbohydrate (except lactose), and a high fiber diet are recommended. Antidiarrheal agents and tincture of opium can be used, while cholestyramine is added to bind bile acids if colonic diarrhea is suspected. Antibiotic treatment for bacterial overgrowth is considered if the ileocecal valve is not present. Vitamins and minerals should be supplemented; and when oral intake is not adequate, total parenteral nutrition (TPN) can become necessary. Surgical solutions such as intestinal lengthening and bowel transplant are promising but not yet reliable.

ILEUS AND CHRONIC INTESTINAL PSEUDO-OBSTRUCTION

- Both conditions represent small-bowel hypomotility causing a picture of small-bowel obstruction in the absence of a mechanical cause. Symptoms are similar to those of a mechanical obstruction except for the presence of diminished or absent bowel sounds consistent with hypomotility.
- Ileus is an acute reversible syndrome seen most commonly after abdominal surgery or with infections, electrolyte abnormalities, and certain medications.
- Chronic intestinal pseudo-obstruction is chronic irreversible intestinal dysmotility that is caused by myopathies or neuropathies affecting the small intestine.[4] Common causes include diabetes mellitus, thyroid disease, systemic sclerosis, Parkinson's disease, and viral infections such as Epstein-Barr virus.
- Ileus is diagnosed by abdominal imaging, although differentiation from mechanical obstruction can be challenging and may require additional tests. Management of ileus consists of reversing the cause and providing symptomatic relief through nasogastric suction and abstaining from oral intake. Temporary support with intravenous (IV) fluids and occasionally TPN is necessary.
- The diagnosis of chronic pseudo-obstruction is suggested by the recurrent nature of the bowel obstruction in the absence of a specific reversible cause. Manometric studies are necessary to make a definitive diagnosis. Identifying the etiology of chronic intestinal pseudo-obstruction often requires full thickness biopsy of the bowel. Management is challenging and focuses on ensuring adequate nutritional intake through TPN in advanced cases. Promotility agents are not particularly effective, whereas venting gastrostomy can be useful to remove secretions.

CHRONIC INTESTINAL ISCHEMIA

- A chronic reduction in arterial perfusion of the small bowel that is caused by the presence of occlusive atherosclerotic lesions, and less frequently by vasculitis.

Considering the extensive collateral flow, ischemia can only be clinically significant if two of the three major arteries (celiac, superior mesenteric, inferior mesenteric artery) are affected.
- The most common presentation of chronic intestinal ischemia is recurrent postprandial abdominal pain (visceral angina) leading to food aversion and weight loss in the absence of any other explanation. An upper abdominal bruit can be heard in most cases. Finding of occluded arteries by angiography establishes the diagnosis. Less invasive testing such as duplex ultrasound scan and magnetic resonance angiography (MRA) can be very helpful. Treatment requires revascularization through stenting, endarterectomy, grafting, or bypass surgery. The long-term success rate is good.

ACUTE INTESTINAL ISCHEMIA

- Acute occlusion of a visceral arterial branch because of embolization, thrombosis, or arterial spasm. Occasionally, it is caused by a sudden drop in blood pressure.
- Presents with sudden onset of excruciating periumbilical pain without any significant findings on physical examination unless bowel perforation is present. Bowel infarction is suspected when lactic acidosis is found.
- Angiography is the test of choice and allows identification of the cause of ischemia, which is important for the selection of a treatment method. Emboli are treated surgically by embolectomy, thrombotic disease requires arterial bypass, whereas vasoconstriction responds to vasodilators. Any suspicion of bowel infarction requires urgent surgery and resection of the infarcted bowel.
- Despite aggressive interventions, the overall mortality is approximately 70%, which increases to 90% if bowel infarction occurs.

REFERENCES

1. National Institutes of Health. National Institutes of Health Consensus Development Conference Statement on Celiac Disease, June 28–30, 2004. *Gastroenterology.* 2005;128 (4 suppl 1):S1–9.
2. Lichtenstein GR, Abreu MT, Cohen R, et al. American Gastroenterological Association Institute technical review on corticosteroids, immunomodulators, and infliximab in inflammatory bowel disease. *Gastroenterology.* 2006;130:940–987.
3. Fenollar F, Puéchal X, Raoult D. Whipple's disease. *N Engl J Med.* 2007;356(1):55–66.
4. De Giorgio R, Sarnelli G, Corinaldesi R, et al. Advances in our understanding of the pathology of chronic intestinal pseudo-obstruction. *Gut.* 2004;53:1549–1552.

56 DISEASES OF THE COLON AND RECTUM

M. Louay Omran

ANATOMY AND PHYSIOLOGY

ANATOMY

- The colon is a 150 cm long hollow tube that is wrapped in a serosal layer. It is anatomically divided into several regions: a terminal pouch called the cecum, which is separated from the terminal ileum by the ileocecal valve; an ascending segment; a transverse segment; a descending segment; an S-shaped segment called the sigmoid colon; and the rectum.
- The wall of the colon consists of a mucosa, submucosa, and inner circular and outer longitudinal muscular layers. Except for the sigmoid colon and rectum, the circular muscle in the colon is covered with three bands of a longitudinal muscle that are known as *taeniae coli*. Because the taeniae coli do not fully surround the circular muscle, the motility of the colon is less effective and is slower than that of the small bowel. In the sigmoid colon and rectum, the longitudinal muscle completely surrounds the circular one. In the distal part of the rectum, the circular muscle thickens forming the internal anal sphincter, while striated muscle forms the external anal sphincter that, in turn, is closely connected to the pelvic floor muscles.
- There are two nerve cell networks in the colon: a submucosal plexus located adjacent to the blood and lymphatic vessels in the submucosa and a myenteric plexus located between the circular and the longitudinal muscular layers. The pudendal nerves provide input from the sacral spinal cord to the external anal sphincter and pelvic floor muscle.
- The mucosa consists of the epithelium, the lamina propria (connective tissue), and the muscularis mucosa (smooth muscle). The epithelium consists of a single layer of epithelial cells linked together by tight junctions. These cells include some absorptive cells, but are mostly mucus-producing cells (goblet cells). The colonic mucosa differs from the small intestinal mucosa by the absence of the long villi. Consequently, the absorption surface of the colon is significantly less than that of the small intestine.

PHYSIOLOGY

- The colon has a limited role in digestion but is important for stool formation and storage.

- The colon's main function is to absorb approximately 1.5 L of water daily from the stool (through a sodium transporter in exchange with potassium), to absorb chloride in exchange with bicarbonate, and to absorb vitamin K produced by the colonic flora. As a result, severe colonic diarrhea leads to significant stool losses of potassium and bicarbonate resulting in hypokalemia and metabolic acidosis. Use of antibiotics can lead to eradication of the normal colonic flora and vitamin K deficiency in those with poor nutrition.
- The colon displays two motility patterns: segmental mixing contractions with slow forward propulsion and high amplitude sweeping contractions occurring up to 10 times a day. These sweeping contractions typically occur in the morning and after meals caused by what is known as the *gastrocolic reflex* and produce the urge to defecate.
- When the rectum fills with stool and its wall stretches, a rectoanal inhibitory reflex is activated resulting in relaxation of the internal sphincter. The external sphincter remains contracted until the situation is appropriate for defecation. At that point, with abdominal straining, the rectum contracts while the external sphincter and the puborectalis muscle relax leading to a straightening of the rectoanal angle and a smooth exit of stool. On the other hand, if defecation is not desired, the brainstem sends inhibitory signals through descending nerve fibers resulting in relaxation of the rectum until the next wave of stool arrives and the contraction process is reinitiated.

SYMPTOMS OF COLORECTAL DISEASES

CONSTIPATION

- Constipation is defined as having fewer than three bowel movements a week. More complex definitions involving other markers of constipation such as the presence of hard stool, straining, and incomplete evacuation are mostly used in research settings.
- The prevalence of constipation is approximately 15% in the United States. It appears to be more prevalent with female sex, age older than 60 years, nonwhites, lower education, and a sedentary lifestyle.
- Constipation can be secondary to neurologic conditions, medications, or endocrinologic disorders (see Table 56–1), but most cases of constipation are idiopathic.
- After excluding causes of secondary constipation, the constipated patient should undergo colonoscopy or a barium enema to exclude mechanical obstruction if older than 50 years of age or if displaying warning signs for colon cancer. These signs include anemia,

TABLE 56–1   Some Causes of Secondary Constipation

NEUROLOGIC	ENDOCRINOLOGIC AND METABOLIC	DRUGS	OTHER
Autonomic dysfunction	Diabetes mellitus	Opioids	Obstruction
Parkinson disease	Hypothyroidism	Antihistamines	Pregnancy
Strokes	Hypercalcemia	Anticholinergics	Connective tissue diseases
Spinal cord injury	Hypokalemia	Antidepressants	
Multiple sclerosis		Antipsychotics	
		Antihypertensives	
		Diuretics	
		Iron/calcium/aluminum	

occult or visible rectal bleeding, unexplained weight loss, and a family history of colon cancer.

- 90% of patients with idiopathic constipation respond to simple interventions including a change in dietary habits to increase fluids and fiber, and the addition of a simple laxative. Those who do not respond are said to have *severe chronic idiopathic constipation* which can be caused by decreased colonic motility (11%), pelvic floor dysfunction (13%), both (5%), or irritable bowel syndrome (71%).
- A marker study (abdominal radiograph taken 5 days after ingestion of a marker pills) facilitates the identification of patients with decreased colonic motility. Those who are suspected of having pelvic floor dysfunction should undergo anorectal manometry with balloon expulsion testing.
- Two-thirds of patients with pelvic floor dysfunction benefit from biofeedback.
- Table 56–2 summarizes medications available for the treatment of constipation.[1]

DIARRHEA

Colonic diarrhea is discussed in Chap. 55, Small Bowel Diseases.

LOWER GASTROINTESTINAL BLEEDING

- By definition, the source of lower gastrointestinal bleeding (LGIB) must occur below the ligament of Treitz. Although only 20% of all gastrointestinal bleeding is secondary to a lower bleed, more than 90% of LGIB are from a colonic source.
- LGIB usually presents as maroon-colored stools (hematochezia). Generally speaking, the left colon is the source of bright red blood per rectum, while the right colon is the source of LGIB presenting as melena.
- Diverticulosis is the most common cause of LGIB when all ages are combined. Arteriovenous malformation (AVM) is a common cause of LGIB in older individuals while hemorrhoids are a common cause of LGIB in younger individuals. Other common causes of LGIB include neoplasms (colon polyps and cancer), inflammatory conditions (ulcerative colitis), radiation or ischemic injury of the colon, and a variety of infectious causes.
- The approach to the patient with LGIB involves hemodynamic support, correction of an underlying coagulopathy, and immediate exclusion of an upper source of bleeding which carries a higher mortality risk.[3]

TABLE 56–2   Medications Available for the Treatment of Constipation

CATEGORY	MECHANISM OF ACTION	MEDICATIONS
Bulk forming	Absorb liquids leading to swelling of fiber and increase in fecal mass	Metamucil Methylcellulose Polycarbophil
Softeners	Decrease surface tension of stool allowing water to be mixed in to soften stools	Docusate
Lubricants	Coat stool surface to decrease friction	Mineral oil
Osmotics	Attract water into the intestinal lumen following an osmotic gradient created by electrolytes or nonabsorbed sugars	Sorbitol Lactulose Polyethylene glycol Milk of magnesium Magnesium citrate
Stimulants	Irritate the walls of the intestinal to stimulate contractions/motility	Bisacodyl Senna Cascara
Promotility agents	Stimulates intestinal motility by facilitating enteric cholinergic transmission	Tegaserod Misoprostol Colchicine
Water secretors	Selectively activate chloride channels enhancing intestinal fluid secretion	Lubiprostone

- Colonoscopy is both diagnostic and therapeutic and is the most helpful test in establishing a diagnosis in LGIB. It is limited only by the need for bowel preparation which will delay its utilization. Technetium-tagged red blood cell radionuclide scanning can be used to localize the source of bleeding to a region, but is limited to bleeding at a rate exceeding 0.1 mL/min.
- Mesenteric angiography is more accurate than radionuclide scanning at localizing the source of the bleeding and can offer the option for therapeutic intervention. It is however limited by its poor sensitivity when the rate of bleeding is less than 0.5 mL/min.
- Many causes of LGIB (diverticula, AVM, hemorrhoids) are amenable to endoscopic treatment with a variety of techniques including thermal coagulation, vasoconstricting injection therapy, metallic clips, and banding.

FECAL INCONTINENCE

- Fecal incontinence is the most common symptom of rectoanal disease. Its prevalence is estimated to be 10% to 15% of the population, with a significantly higher prevalence in the elderly and nursing home residents; 50% of nursing home residents suffer from fecal incontinence.
- Fecal incontinence is defined as a continuous or recurrent uncontrolled passage of fecal material for at least one month in an individual older than 3 years of age.
- To maintain continence, a variety of anatomic structures and physiologic functions must be intact. Relevant anatomic structures include the rectum, the internal and external sphincters, and the pelvic floor. Relevant physiologic functions include stool consistency, rectal distensibility, anorectal reflexes, and cognitive function. The causes of fecal incontinence are summarized in Table 56–3.
- Patients with minor fecal incontinence do not need extensive testing and can be managed by increasing fiber intake to improve stool consistency, using antidiarrheal agents, and alleviating constipation in those with incontinence is caused by incomplete stool evacuation.[2] When this approach fails, a structured evaluation of the rectum is indicated using flexible sigmoidoscopy.

TABLE 56–3   Causes of Fecal Incontinence

MECHANISM	CAUSES
Liquid stools	Diarrheal illnesses
Stool overflow	Fecal impaction
	Rectal obstructing lesions
Central and cognitive dysfunction	Dementia, strokes, multiple sclerosis
Sphincter dysfunction	Traumatic injury (surgery, obstetric injury)
	Autonomic dysfunction (diabetes)
Pelvic floor dysfunction	Lax pelvic floor, chronic straining, rectal prolapse

- Anorectal manometry tests the physiologic interaction between the rectum, the sphincters, and the pelvic floor. Evacuation proctography can further delineate the interaction among these different areas during defecation. Anal ultrasonography and sphincter denervation measurements evaluate the sphincter anatomy and innervation. Based on the etiology of incontinence, biofeedback (if rectal sensation is maintained) and surgery are options for treatment.

ULCERATIVE COLITIS

Ulcerative colitis (UC) is a chronic idiopathic inflammation of the colonic mucosa and submucosa which begins in the rectum (proctitis) and extends proximally to the sigmoid colon (distal colitis), splenic flexure (left-sided colitis), and cecum (pancolitis). Approximately 10% of patients have inflammation in the terminal ileum known as *backwash ileitis*. Like Crohn's disease, inflammation is thought to be mediated by an immune reaction in a genetically susceptible host.

EPIDEMIOLOGY

- According to the data from Olmsted County, Minnesota, the incidence of UC is 7.3 per 100,000 and seems to be rising; the prevalence is 181 per 100,000.
- The peak incidence age is 20 to 40 years, with a second smaller peak at age 60 to 80 years. UC is more common among Jews and in urban areas. 10% to 15% of patients with UC have a first-degree relative with inflammatory bowel disease.
- Cigarette smoking appears to exert some protective effect against UC, and many patients relate the onset of symptoms to smoking cessation. Appendicitis leading to appendectomy at a young age appears to offer protection against UC.

PATHOLOGY

- Mucosal inflammation in UC is contiguous without skip areas, with clear demarcation between the affected area and the remainder of the colon. Since UC does not extend beyond the mucosa, it is not associated with fistulization, abscess formation, or perianal disease. Unlike Crohn's disease, noncaseating granulomas are absent in UC.
- Microscopically, an inflammatory infiltrate in the mucosa and submucosa forms crypt abscesses.
- In long-standing disease, crypt distortion and architectural changes are noted. Pseudopolyps represent granulation tissue within distorted glands that give the appearance of a polyp.

CLINICAL FEATURES

- The onset of symptoms is usually more sudden than Crohn's and includes crampy abdominal pain, urgency and diarrhea (nocturnal in more severe cases), and rectal bleeding.
- Fever, weight loss, and upper GI symptoms may also be seen in severe cases. The presence of decreased bowel sounds, diffuse abdominal tenderness with rebound suggests the development of toxic megacolon and possibly perforation.
- UC activity can be classified as mild, moderate, or severe. The criteria used to classify severe disease include the presence of more than six stools a day (usually bloody), significant blood loss (reflected by an increased heart rate and a drop in hematocrit), signs of systemic inflammation (fever, elevated sedimentation rate, or C-reactive protein), and malnutrition (weight loss and low albumin).
- One-third of UC patients have extra intestinal manifestations. Similar to Crohn's, extra intestinal manifestations can be divided into those associated with disease activity (peripheral arthritis, ocular inflammation, and erythema nodosum) and those that are not (oral aphthous ulcers, pyoderma gangrenosum, spondyloarthropathy, and primary sclerosing cholangitis).
- The course of UC is characterized by acute exacerbations and remissions even in the absence of therapy.

DIAGNOSIS

- Serum inflammatory markers such as the erythrocyte sedimentation rate (ESR) and C-reactive protein (CRP) are usually elevated when UC is active.
- Evaluation of the colon is best accomplished with flexible sigmoidoscopy or colonoscopy that reveals signs of inflammation including loss of the normal vascular pattern, tissue granulation, friability, and ulcer formation. Pseudopolyps may be seen in long-standing disease. Colonoscopy permits directed biopsies to confirm the diagnosis.
- Perinuclear antineutrophil cytoplasmic antibodies (p-ANCA) are positive in two-thirds of UC patients while anti–*Saccharomyces cerevisiae* antibodies (ASCA) are present in only 10% of UC patients. When both tests are obtained (+ p-ANCA, - ASCA) a positive predictive value of 64% for UC can be acheived.
- The diagnosis of UC is ultimately based on interpretation of the clinical, laboratory, and radiographic data. In some cases, differentiation between Crohn's and UC remains difficult.

TREATMENT

- Total proctocolectomy with creation of an ileostomy is curative. Clearly this is not a desirable option in most cases considering that UC is usually a disease which manifests at an early age. Alternatively, several medications are available to achieve the more practical goal of controlling disease activity and minimizing flare-ups. Medications used for the treatment of UC and their specific indications are summarized in Table 56–4.
- Acute mild to moderate UC can be treated with 5-aminosalicylic acid (5-ASA) products (Asacol, Pentasa, Colazal) given orally or rectally depending on the extent of the disease. Rectal steroids (foam or enema) are also an option. Cases that fail to respond can be treated with systemic steroids with a rapid taper over several weeks.[4]
- Acute severe UC requires hospitalization and administration of intravenous (IV) steroids.
- Cyclosporine and Infliximab are options for refractory cases.

TABLE 56–4 Medications Used for the Treatment of Ulcerative Colitis

DRUG	RT	INDICATION	KEY FACTS
5-ASA	PO	Mild-moderate dz	Effective for induction and maintenance of remission
Systemic steroids	PO/IV	Severe	Not effective in maintenance of remission, significant side effects with long term use
Azathioprine/ 6-MP	PO	Refractory or steroid-dependent dz	Response after 3–6 months, require monitoring of metabolites and signs of toxicity
Infliximab	IV	Refractory or steroid-dependent dz	Chimeric mouse/human or fully human monoclonal antibodies against TNF-α, but have risk of infection (TB) and rare lymphomas

ASA, aminosalicylic acid; dz, disease; IV, intravenous; 6-MP, 6-mercaptopurine; PO, orally; RT, route of administration

- Maintenance of a remission can be achieved with 5-ASA. Immune modulators (azathioprine, 6-mercaptopurine) and anti–tumor necrosis factor-α (anti–TNF-α) drugs are indicated for sustained remission in patients requiring frequent steroid administration or are steroid dependent.
- Surgery is indicated for cases refractory to medical management, particularly when toxic megacolon is present. Curative surgeries involve a total proctocolectomy with permanent ileostomy (Brooke ileostomy), or proctocolectomy with continent ileostomy (Kock pouch). Most patients wish to avoid having an ileostomy and opt for colectomy with the creation of an ileal pouch (with rectal or anal anastomosis). Patients with a pouch have a 50% chance of developing acute pouchitis within 1 year of surgery, and a 10% chance of developing chronic pouchitis.
- When present, pouchitis can be treated successfully with antibiotics.
- The diagnosis of UC confers an increased risk of developing dysplasia leading to colon cancer.
- The risk is estimated to be 0.5% to 1% per year or 10% to 20% after 20 years of disease.
- Screening colonoscopy with surveillance biopsies every 1 to 2 years is indicated after 8 years of pancolitis or 15 years of left-sided colitis.

COLORECTAL CANCER

- Colorectal cancer (CRC) is the 4th most common cause of cancer and 2nd most common cause of cancer mortality in the United States. The incidence and mortality are higher in men and in African Americans.
- The lifetime risk of developing CRC is 6%.
- The factors associated with an increased risk of CRC include:
  ○ Aging, particularly, in patients older than 50 years of age
  ○ A personal history of colorectal adenoma or CRC is associated with a three- to six-fold increase in the incidence of a future adenoma or CRC
  ○ Having a first-degree relative with CRC doubles the risk of CRC
  ○ Chronic UC and colonic Crohn's disease are associated with an increased risk of CRC (25% after 25 years). The risk is higher with pancolitis and in patients who have primary sclerosing cholangitis.
  ○ Genetic predisposition (familial polyposis)
  ○ Consumption of diets high in fat and red meat and low in fiber increase the risk of CRC
  ○ Alcohol consumption is associated with a modest increase in risk of CRC
  ○ Smoking for more than 20 years confers a higher risk of CRC
  ○ Sedentary lifestyle

PATHOPHYSIOLOGY

- 98% of CRCs are adenocarcinomas
  ○ Almost all CRCs arise from a preexisting adenoma although only 1% of adenomatous polyps progress to CRC
  ○ Characteristics of polyps that carry a high risk of progression to CRC
    - Larger than 1 cm
    - Have villous or tubovillous histology
    - Presence of three or more polyps
- The progression from adenoma to adenocarcinomas is mediated by a variety of mutations or through chromosomal and microsatellite instability. An overlap between these mechanisms is common.
- Genetic mutations thought to play an important role in the development of CRC include
  ○ Aberrant tumor suppressor genes
    - *APC* mutations (*gatekeeper gene*) are found in early adenomas
    - *P53* mutations are usually found in advanced carcinomas
  ○ Cancer-suppressing genes
    - *DCC* mutations are found in adenomas with severe dysplasia
  ○ Cancer promoting genes *oncogenes*
    - K-*ras* is present in 50% of large adenomas
  ○ DNA mismatch repair gene abnormalities
    - Are responsible for microsatellite instability and include: *hMLH1, hMLH2, hMLH3, hMLH6, hPMS1, and hPMS2*
- 60% to 70% of CRCs are sporadic noninherited cancers.
- 20% to 30% of CRCs are familial, but have an unknown genetic basis.
- Up to 10% of CRCs are caused by defined inherited syndromes
  ○ Familial adenomatous polyposis (FAP): caused by mutations in the APC tumor suppressor gene. FAP is manifested by the presence of hundreds of polyps by the second decade of life and is associated with a 100% chance of developing CRC. Gardner's syndrome is FAP with extraintestinal manifestations such as desmoid tumors and osteomas; Turcot's syndrome is characterized by FAP and brain tumors.
  ○ Hereditary nonpolyposis colon cancer (HNPCC): caused by a mutation in a DNA mismatch repair gene, is manifested by early-onset CRC (fourth decade) and is most likely to occur proximal to the splenic flexure. Patients with HNPCC have an increased risk of noncolonic cancer both gastrointestinal (stomach, small bowel) and nongastrointestinal (biliary tree, ovaries, endometrium). The Muir-Torre syndrome is characterized by HNPCC associated with sebaceous gland tumors.

CLINICAL FEATURES

- Symptoms and signs associated with CRC often arise late in the disease and depend on the location:
  - Right-sided colon cancer presents with iron deficiency anemia caused by slow blood loss, weight loss, abdominal pain, and possibly a palpable cecal mass.
  - Left-sided colon cancer presents with constipation caused by obstruction, rectal bleeding, and abdominal pain.
- The presence of bacteremia with *Streptococcus bovis* should suggest CRC and prompt a colonoscopy.

DIAGNOSIS AND STAGING

- Colonoscopy is the diagnostic test of choice in patients suspected of having CRC. Flexible sigmoidoscopy and barium enema are inferior alternatives.
- Once the diagnosis is made, preoperative staging is important and requires an abdominal and pelvic computed tomography (CT) scan and a chest radiograph. Endoscopic ultrasound is indicated for accurate staging of rectal cancers.
- CRC stage is the most important factor in predicting survival. The prognosis of CRC is superior than rectal cancer of an equivalent stage.
- CRC staging is accomplished using the TNM classification or the Duke staging system. Using the TNM classification, tumors that are not associated with lymph node or distant metastasis (N0M0) are considered early stage (I or II depending on whether the serosa is involved). These tumors have the best prognosis with survival exceeding 75% in 5 years. Tumors involving the lymph nodes without distant organ involvement are considered stage III and carry a 5-year survival of 40% to 70%. Tumors involving distant metastasis (stage IV) have a dismal 5-year survival rate of 5%.

TREATMENT

- Surgery alone is curative for early stage colon cancer (I and II) and rectal cancer (I).
- Adjuvant chemotherapy with 5-fluoruracil (5-FU), leucovorin, and oxaliplatin is indicated for stage III colon cancer, while chemotherapy in addition to radiation are indicated for stage II and III rectal cancer.
- Palliative surgery, chemotherapy, and possibly radiation therapy are indicated for stage IV CRC.

PREVENTION

- Screening for CRC
  - In average risk patients >50 years of age (those without a history of CRC, adenomatous polyps, inflammatory bowel disease, or colon cancer in a family member). The following tests are options
    - Annual fecal occult blood or sigmoidoscopy every 5 years
    - Double contrast barium enema every 5 years
    - Colonoscopy every 10 years
    - CT colography and stool DNA analysis are novel techniques that are not yet approved for screening
  - High-risk patients (history of CRC, polyps, inflammatory bowel disease or familial)
    - First-degree relatives with CRC should undergo colonoscopy at age 40 or 10 years before the onset of CRC (whichever sooner). Repeat colonoscopy every 5 to 10 years (depending on age of onset).
    - Patients with genetic syndromes should undergo aggressive screening with flexible sigmoidoscopy or colonoscopy at an early age and repeat every 1 to 2 years depending on the syndrome.
    - Patients with inflammatory bowel disease should undergo colonoscopy every 1 to 2 years with surveillance biopsies performed in patients with extensive disease for more than 9 years.
- Surveillance
  - History of adenomatous polyps
    - Colonoscopy every 5 years for low-risk persons
    - Colonoscopy every 3 years for high-risk persons (a polyp larger than 1 cm, 3 or more polyps, villous histology)
  - History of curative surgery for CRC
    - Colonoscopy 1 year after surgery, repeat after 3 years then every 5 years if no polyps are found.[5]

IRRITABLE BOWEL SYNDROME

DEFINITION

- Irritable bowel syndrome (IBS) is a gastrointestinal disorder characterized by chronic recurrent abdominal pain, altered bowel habits and disordered defecation associated with bloating, in the absence of an identifiable organic etiology.

DEMOGRAPHICS

- IBS is the most commonly diagnosed gastrointestinal condition and the second most common cause for absenteeism from work in the United States.
- IBS affects 10% to 15% of the population in the United States and Europe.
- IBS affects all ages but is more common in young women (2:1).

PATHOPHYSIOLOGY

- Remains uncertain.
- Several observations suggest that visceral hypersensitivity plays a critical role. This is underscored by demonstrating a heightened pain response and cerebral activity after rectal distention with a balloon when compared to controls. This is also the basis for using neuromodulators such as tricyclic antidepressants in the treatment of IBS.
- Altered intestinal and colonic motility is also believed to play an important role, particularly in constipation-predominant IBS. Altered motility may be secondary to perturbations in serotonin synthesis and secretion. This observation provides the basis for using tegaserod in the management of IBS.
- Inflammation may participate in a subgroup of patient especially those with diarrhea-predominant IBS. This was suggested by studies which revealed the presence of an inflammatory infiltrate in the intestinal wall of patients with IBS.
- The role of stress and psychologic factors have long been considered since stress is associated with worsening symptoms, and IBS patients have a higher prevalence of physical and sexual abuse in their background compared to controls. Corticotrophin-releasing factor is a mediator of stress that also causes abdominal pain and alters colonic motility.
- Small intestinal bacterial overgrowth has been recently implicated in a large subgroup of patients with IBS.

CLINICAL MANIFESTATIONS

- Recurrent severe crampy abdominal pain that is not associated with signs of organic disease (bleeding, nocturnal symptoms, or weight loss in the absence of depression). This pain typically improves with defecation and worsens with eating. Stress can aggravate pain frequency or intensity.
- Change in bowel habits manifested as constipation, diarrhea, or alternating bouts of both is a very common clinical presentation. Constipation is associated with straining and incomplete evacuation. Diarrhea is preceded by urgency and can be associated with mucus.
- Bloating is common and can lead to frequent belching. Upper gastrointestinal symptoms and dyspepsia are also prevalent in patients with IBS.
- Conditions such as fibromyalgia, back pain, headaches, dyspareunia, dysuria, and sleep disturbances are more common among IBS patients.

DIAGNOSIS

- There is no gold standard or diagnostic marker for IBS.
- The Rome Criteria were created by an international working group in Rome, Italy, to unify the definition of IBS in research protocols.[6] The Rome Criteria require the presence of abdominal pain or discomfort for at least 3 days per month in the previous 3 months associated with two of the following: improvement with defecation, onset associated with a change in stool frequency, or a change in the form of stool.
- The American Gastroenterological Association recommends the diagnosis of IBS to be based on the presence of suggestive symptoms (Rome Criteria) coupled with exclusion of other gastrointestinal conditions that mimic IBS. The presence of warning symptoms and signs that may suggest an organic disease (bleeding, anemia, severe diarrhea, significant weight loss, fever, or nocturnal symptoms), or a family history of colon cancer or inflammatory bowel disease should be noted as they clearly change the diagnostic approach.
  - In the absence of these warning factors, a simple work up including a complete blood count, basic chemistries, screening for celiac disease (particularly in white patients with diarrhea), and screening for thyroid disease is usually adequate. There is only a 5% chance of missing another condition that is responsible for IBS symptoms when employing such an approach.
  - The presence of warning signs mandates a more extensive workup including stool studies to exclude infection and malabsorption, blood tests to include liver function tests, C-reactive protein and ferritin, and an endoscopic examination (sigmoidoscopy or colonoscopy) to investigate colon cancer in older patients, and to exclude inflammatory bowel diseases in younger patients with diarrhea. Mucosal colonic biopsies are indicated for patients with persistent diarrhea to exclude microscopic colitis.

TREATMENT

- There is no curative approach. Once the diagnosis is established, treatment should focus on patient education, reassurance, psychological support, and modification of dietary factors that may worsen symptoms (caffeine use, poor fiber intake, lactose intolerance). Pharmacologic intervention is indicated for patients with symptoms that are affecting their quality of life.
- Using neuromodulating agents (such as tricyclic antidepressants) was found to be beneficial in decreasing pain and improving global symptoms of IBS. Tricyclic antidepressants should be used in doses smaller than those used for depression and should be titrated slowly. Selective serotonin reuptake inhibitors can also be used when patients have concomitant depression.

- The efficacy of antispasmodics (anticholinergics) in treating pain has been questioned in several meta-analyses. It is reasonable to use them on an as-needed basis, especially when pain is anticipated , eg, recurrent postprandial pain.
- Patients with diarrhea-predominant IBS may benefit from selective use of antidiarrheal agents such as loperamide. 5-hydroxytryptamine-3 (5-HT3) receptor antagonists are available for those refractory patients with severe diarrhea but only after informing the patient that these drugs can be associated with ischemic colitis.
- Women with constipation-predominant IBS may particularly benefit from the use of 5-hydroxytryptamine-4 (5-HT4) receptor agonists which stimulate colonic motility and decrease bowel sensitivity. IBS patients on tegaserod (Zelnorm) experience improvement in abdominal pain, bloating, and stool frequency. Unfortunately, tegaserod was recently removed from the market by the manufacturer because of concerns of cardiovascular complications related to its use.
- A few recent reports suggested that patients with bacterial overgrowth can benefit from the use of antibiotics. The main improvement noted was with bloating.
- The use of probiotics is gaining popularity as an adjunctive treatment method but large well designed studies proving their efficacy are lacking.

OTHER COLONIC AND RECTAL DISEASES

DIVERTICULAR DISEASE

- Diverticulosis
  - Diverticuli represent protrusions of the colonic mucosa through areas weakened by the penetration of the vasa recta into the colonic wall.
  - The prevalence of diverticulosis increases with age, rising from 30% at age 60 years, to 70% by 80 years of age.
  - Diverticulosis is usually asymptomatic but complications include infection (diverticulitis) in 20% of patients, and bleeding in 5% of patients. Segmental inflammation of the sigmoid colon with resulting fibrosis and stricturing may occur.
- Diverticulitis
  - When stool obstructs the lumen of a diverticulum, an increase in the diverticular pressure ensues leading to decreased blood supply and necrosis. Diverticulitis is a contained perforation of a diverticulum with the formation of a pericolonic abscess. When the perforation is large it can lead to peritonitis and a life-threatening presentation.
  - The typical presentation includes left lower quadrant pain, fever, and leukocytosis. Physical examination reveals left lower quadrant tenderness and occasionally a palpable mass. Peritoneal signs can be seen in severe cases.
  - The diagnosis of diverticulitis is based on clinical evidence without the need for imaging. If the diagnosis is in doubt or there is a need to rule out complicated presentations, CT can be performed and is more than 80% sensitive. Flexible sigmoidoscopy should be avoided.
  - Treatment of acute diverticulitis is achieved by hydration and a 10-day course of antibiotics. The route of administration can either be oral or intravenous depending on the severity of the presentation. Antibiotics should target both gram-negative bacilli and anaerobes. Large abscesses should be drained percutaneously, while surgery is indicated in cases of overt perforation and peritonitis.
  - Contrary to common belief, dietary modifications such as avoiding seeds have no proven benefit in the prevention of diverticulitis.
- Diverticular bleeding
  - 5% of patients with diverticulosis suffer a significant gastrointestinal bleeding.
  - Up to 50% of patients hospitalized for lower gastrointestinal bleeding have a bleeding diverticulum.
  - Diverticular bleeding is typically painless and self-limited.
  - Since the risk of recurrent diverticular bleeding is approximately 25% after the first episode and 50% after a second episode, surgery to remove the affected segment of the colon should be entertained after a second bleed from the same segment. The use of endoscopy to pinpoint the bleeding source is complicated by the fact that diverticular bleeding often stops spontaneously before colonoscopy is done. Therefore, early colonoscopy after a quick bowel purge is preferred.

ISCHEMIC COLITIS

- Ischemic colitis is characterized by segmental inflammation and ulceration of the colonic mucosa as a result of a decrease in blood flow. In most cases the decreased blood flow is caused by a transient drop in blood pressure. Ischemic colitis usually afflicts older individuals with atherosclerotic disease.
- Ischemic colitis presents as bloody diarrhea with mild crampy abdominal pain.
- Plain abdominal radiographs may reveal submucosal edema described as *thumb printing*. Colon wall thickening can be seen on computed tomography. Endoscopy reveals segmental patchy erythema with ulceration of the affected area, but endoscopy is only indicated to exclude other possible causes of colitis.
- Treatment is usually supportive by ensuring adequate hydration, adequate perfusion pressure, and broad spectrum antibiotics.

CLOSTRIDIUM DIFFICILE COLITIS

- *C. difficile* colonizes the gut of 3% of community-dwelling individuals and 20% of patients hospitalized for more than 1 week. Most, but not all cases of *C. difficile* colitis, are associated with antibiotic use. Patients at an increased risk include older individuals, those weakened by severe illnesses such as intensive care unit patients, burn unit patients, and patients with cancer.
- *C. difficile* produces two types of toxins. Toxin A causes cytotoxicity and apoptosis allowing toxin B to penetrate and cause cellular necrosis. The disruption of the intestinal epithelium leads to diarrhea and the formation of pseudomembranes. If the inflammation penetrates into the deeper layers of the colon wall it may cause toxic dilatation of the colon (toxic megacolon).
- Diarrhea is the main feature of *C. difficile*-associated disease. It typically starts after 1 to 2 weeks of antibiotic use but can occur after only one dose. Although Clindamycin is the antibiotic most frequently linked to *C. difficile* colitis in the literature, any antibiotic can cause it.
- Mortality is less than 5% in the normal host but rises to 20% in the elderly or the immune suppressed host. Toxic megacolon significantly raises mortality.
- Enzyme-linked immunosorbent assay (ELISA) for the detection of toxin A or B in stool is the most common test used for the diagnosis because of its sensitivity and ease of use.
- Treatment consists of discontinuation of the offending antibiotic (if possible) and supportive care (IV hydration, gentle use of antidiarrheals). This approach is usually adequate for mild disease but more severe cases require the use of an antibiotic against *C. difficile*, and possibly hospitalization. Metronidazole and vancomycin given orally are equally effective against *C. difficile* and are usually administered for 7 to 14 days. Metronidazole is less expensive than vancomycin and should be the first line choice. Patients who fail to respond to metronidazole may benefit from the addition of a toxin-binding resin (cholestyramine), or can be switched to vancomycin.
- Despite adequate treatment, 25% of patients suffer a recurrence. Recurrent cases are treated with a repeat course of the antibiotic used to achieve response during the first episode. A prolonged treatment course with or without a tapering regimen may be used in recurrent disease.

COLONIC PSEUDOOBSTRUCTION (OGILVIE SYNDROME)

- Colonic pseudo-obstruction is characterized by severe adynamic dilatation of the colon (usually cecum, ascending, and transverse) in the absence of a mechanical obstruction.
- It usually occurs in hospitalized patients who are post-operative, critically ill, or using high-dose narcotics.
- After exclusion of mechanical obstruction, appropriate treatment includes intravenous hydration and discontinuation of the offending agents (narcotics).
- Severe resistant cases can be treated with careful endoscopic decompression of the colon or with the use of intravenous neostigmine with close patient monitoring.

HEMORRHOIDS

- Hemorrhoids are dilated vessels in the submucosa of the lower rectum arising from the superior and inferior hemorrhoidal veins. Vessels above the dentate line are referred to as *internal*, while those below the dentate line are referred to as *external*.
- Hemorrhoids occur as a result of conditions that increase the intrapelvic pressure such as pregnancy, pelvic tumors, prolonged standing or sitting, and chronic straining as a result of constipation.
- Symptoms of hemorrhoids include rectal bleeding (bright red blood coating the stool or noted while wiping), skin and anal irritation, and pain.
- Internal hemorrhoids are classified into four grades
  - Grade I: hemorrhoids remain above the dentate line
  - Grade II: hemorrhoids prolapse out of the anal canal but reduce spontaneously
  - Grade III: hemorrhoids prolapse out of the anal canal but require manual reduction
  - Grade IV: hemorrhoids are irreducible
- Grades I and II are treated conservatively with a high-fiber diet, analgesic creams, steroid suppositories, and sitz baths. Resistant hemorrhoids require more aggressive intervention such as endoscopic banding or hemorrhoidectomy.[7] Hemorrhoidectomy is the more definitive treatment but carries a higher risk of complications (pain, hemorrhage, constipation, and urinary tract infection).
- Grades III and IV are usually treated with surgical hemorrhoidectomy.
- Thrombosed external hemorrhoids are treated with clot excision if presenting within 72 hours of occurrence, otherwise with conservative symptomatic management.

ANAL FISSURE

- A traumatic tear in the lining of the anal canal, mostly occurring in the posterior midline and caused by straining and chronic constipation. While usually self-healing, many fissures progress to chronic fissuring because the associated internal sphincter spasm causes further widening of the fissure and a decrease in blood supply resulting in ulceration.

- Patients usually complain of severe pain associated with defecation and during rectal examination, and occasionally note blood on tissue paper.
- The diagnosis is made by observing a fresh tear in the anal mucosa. Chronic fissures may expose the internal sphincter and be associated with a skin tag.
- Treatment is straightforward and involves topical analgesics and sitz baths. The use of topical nitroglycerin or calcium channel blockers may help decrease the anal sphincter pressure and allow the fissure to heal. Refractory cases can be treated with Botox injection and ultimately surgically by lateral internal sphincterotomy. The surgical approach is associated with a risk of fecal incontinence.

REFERENCES

1. American College of Gastroenterology Chronic Constipation Task Force. Evidence-based approach to the management of chronic constipation in North America. *Am J Gastroenterol.* 2005;100(suppl 1):S1-S21.
2. Cheetham M, Brazzelli M, Norton C, et al. Drug treatment of fecal incontinence in adults. *Cochrane Database System Rev.* 2003;CD002116.
3. Zuccaro G. Management of the adult patient with acute lower gastrointestinal bleeding. *Am J Gastroenterol.* 1998;93:1202–1208.
4. Kornbluth, A, Sachar, DB. Ulcerative colitis practice guidelines in adults (update): American College of Gastroenterology, Practice Parameters Committee. *Am J Gastroenterol.* 2004;99:1371–1385.
5. Winawer S, Fletcher R, Rex D, et al. Colorectal cancer screening and surveillance: clinical guidelines and rationale-Update based on new evidence. *Gastroenterology.* 2003;124:544–560.
6. Longstreth GF, Thompson G, Chey WD, et al. Functional bowel disorders. *Gastroenterology.* 2006;130:1480–1491.
7. American Gastroenterological Association medical position statement: diagnosis and treatment of hemorrhoids. *Gastroenterology.* 2004;126:1461–1462.

57 LIVER AND BILIARY DISEASES

Adrian M. Di Bisceglie

ANATOMY AND PHYSIOLOGY

- The liver has a dual afferent blood supply, from the hepatic artery and the portal vein—the liver derives approximately 60% of its oxygen supply from the portal vein. Blood entering the liver passes through portal triads into hepatic sinusoids lined with fenestrated endothelium and the space of Disse, which contains cells of the reticuloendothelial system (Kupffer cells) and hepatic stellate cells (myofibroblasts). When activated, these myofibroblasts produce collagen, an important element in development of cirrhosis.
- Bile is produced by hepatocytes and excreted into bile canaliculi, which merge to form bile ductules lined by biliary epithelium. Bile drains from the left and right hepatic ducts into the common hepatic duct. Bile is stored in the gallbladder, which contracts after meals and empties its contents into the duodenum via the common bile duct.

SYMPTOMS AND SIGNS OF LIVER DISEASE

- Symptoms and signs of liver disease depend on the type of liver disease and correlate with the mechanism of liver injury as described below (Table 57–1)

TABLE 57–1 Signs and Symptoms of Liver Disease

		SYMPTOMS	PHYSICAL SIGNS
Acute liver injury		Fatigue, nausea, vomiting	Jaundice
Chronic hepatitis		Fatigue, right upper quadrant pain	Hepatomegaly
Cirrhosis	Portal hypertension	Increasing abdominal girth, hematemesis, hematochezia	Ascites, bleeding varices, splenomegaly
	Hepatic encephalopathy	Confusion, difficulty concentrating	Asterixis, loss of consciousness, coma
	Decreased hepatic synthetic function	Easy bruising, ankle swelling	Ecchymoses, ankle edema, jaundice
	Miscellaneous		Loss of muscle bulk, gynecomastia, spider angiomas, palmar erythema
Cholestasis		Pruritus, dark urine, pale stools	Jaundice, hyperpigmentation, skin changes from scratching
Liver tumors		Weight loss, pain in right upper quadrant	Irregular hepatomegaly, vascular bruit, friction rub

LIVER FAILURE AND LIVER TRANSPLANTATION

- The manifestations of liver injury can be grouped into four categories:
  1. *Loss of hepatic synthetic function*: Direct injury to the hepatocyte resulting in decreased synthetic function primarily manifest by hypoalbuminemia, hyperbilirubinemia, and hypoprothrombinemia.
  2. *Portal hypertension*: Hepatic fibrosis and remodeling (cirrhosis) reduce the flow of blood through the low pressure portal venous system. This results in the development of venous collaterals which bypass the liver; these collaterals occur at the sites of portosystemic anastomosis and cause gastroesophageal and rectal varices and prominent veins in the abdominal wall. Portal hypertension also results in the accumulation of fluid in the abdomen (ascites) and hypersplenism (splenomegaly and pancytopenia).
     - Treatment of variceal bleeding is a medical emergency and requires resuscitation with intravenous fluids and blood. Pharmacotherapy with intravenous octreotide reduces the portal pressure. This is usually followed by endoscopic therapy with band ligation or sclerosing injection of varices. The use of noncardioselective β-blockers such as propranolol and nadolol significantly reduce the risk of subsequent bleeds.
     - β-Blockers also have an important role in the prophylaxis of variceal bleeding—preventing the primary bleeding episode in individuals known to have cirrhosis and large gastroesophageal varices. Refractory bleeding may be controlled by transjugular intrahepatic portosystemic shunt (TIPS).
     - Ascites is generally managed with salt restriction (<2g/day) and diuretics (spironolactone and furosemide). Refractory ascites may be controlled by TIPS.
  3. *Hepatic encephalopathy*: This ranges in severity from mild confusion and difficulty sleeping to unresponsive coma. Hepatic encephalopathy is associated with hyperammonemia. In association with chronic liver disease, encephalopathy is purely functional and reversible. However, when encephalopathy arises in the setting of acute liver failure it may be secondary to cerebral edema, which if severe may be complicated by uncal herniation and death.
     - Hepatic encephalopathy is treated with lactulose, a nonabsorbed sugar that causes osmotic diarrhea and acidifies the lumen of the colon, thus reducing the absorption of ammonia.
     - Nonabsorbable antibiotics also decrease the bacterial load in the colon and hence the production of ammonia.
  4. Vascular changes including systemic vasodilatation and a hyperdynamic circulation may precipitate hepatopulmonary syndrome and hepatorenal syndrome, both serious and potentially life-threatening complications of cirrhosis that reverse promptly after liver transplantation.
     - Liver transplantation is now commonly performed for patients with end-stage liver disease (more than 5000 cases each year in the United States).[1] Organ allocation for adults in the United States is based on the MELD system (Model for End-Stage Liver Disease). The MELD score is calculated based on serum bilirubin, prothrombin time, and serum creatinine levels. Organs are allocated first to those individuals with the highest MELD scores.
       - Liver transplantation is associated with 5-year survival rates of 80% to 85%. Liver conditions with the best survival after liver transplantation are primary sclerosing cholangitis (PSC), primary biliary cirrhosis (PBC), autoimmune hepatitis, and hepatitis B; liver tumors tend to have the worst prognosis.
       - Hepatitis C, the most common indication for liver transplantation is associated with universal recurrence of hepatitis C virus (HCV) infection and some graft loss caused by recurrent cirrhosis beginning approximately 5 years after a successful transplant.
       - The use of long-term immunosuppressive therapy is critical for preventing rejection of the liver graft. The mainstays of immunosuppressive therapy are cyclosporine and tacrolimus.
       - Corticosteroids are used early in the posttransplant period and to treat episodes of rejection.
       - Other more recent agents used to immunosuppress the liver transpant recipient include mycophenolate mofetil and rapamycin.

VIRAL HEPATITIS

- Viral hepatitis represents a major cause of acute and chronic liver disease. Chronic hepatitis accounts for 40% to 50% of liver transplants performed in the developed western world.
  - There are five known viral agents that cause hepatitis. They are usually grouped into those that cause only acute hepatitis: hepatitis A virus (HAV) and hepatitis E virus (HEV) versus those that are associated with both acute and chronic liver injury (hepatitis B, C, and D).
  - Interestingly, those organisms associated with acute liver injury are transmitted by the enteral route, whereas the three viral agents that are associated with both acute and chronic hepatic injury (hepatitis B virus [HBV]), HCV and hepatitis D virus (HDV), are all parenterally transmitted by contact with contaminated blood or blood products.[2,3] HDV infection only occurs in patients with HBV infection.

TABLE 57–2   Serologic Testing for Hepatitis B

CLINICAL STATES	TESTS HBsAg	ANTI-HBs	TOTAL ANTI-HBc	IgM ANTI-HBc	HBeAg	ANTI-HBe	HBV DNA	ALT
Acute hepatitis B	+	–	+	+	+	–	+	elevated
HBeAg positive chronic hepatitis B	+	–	+	–	+	–	$>10^{5*}$	elevated
HBeAg negative chronic hepatitis B	+	–	+	–	–	+	$>10^{4*}$	elevated
Immune tolerant	+	–	+	–	+	–	$>10^{5*}$	normal
Inactive carrier	+	–	+	–	–	+	$<10^{4*}$	normal
Recovered	–	+	+	–	–	+	–	normal
Vaccinated	–	+	–	–	–	–	–	normal

ALT, alanine aminotransferase; anti-HBc, antibody to hepatitis B core antigen; anti-HBs, antibody to hepatitis B surface antigen; HBeAg, hepatitis Be antigen; HBsAg, hepatitis B surface antigen; HBV DNA, hepatitis B viral DNA.
*HBV DNA in copies/mL

○ The forms of viral hepatitis cannot be reliably distinguished on clinical grounds alone and, therefore, require the use of sensitive and specific serologic assays to distinguish them. For patients with acute viral hepatitis, tests for hepatitis B surface antigen (HBsAg), immunoglobulin M (IgM) antibody to hepatitis B core antigen (IgM anti-HBc), antibody to hepatitis C virus (anti-HCV), hepatitis C viral RNA and IgM antibody to the hepatitis A virus (IgM anti-HAV) should be ordered. For those with chronic hepatitis (>6 mo), HBsAg and anti-HCV usually suffice as an initial screen.

• Serologic testing for HBV infection is particularly complex and is summarized in Table 57–2.
  ○ Chronic viral hepatitis may result in chronic liver injury with inflammation and fibrosis.
  ○ Progressive fibrosis may lead to cirrhosis and liver failure or be complicated by hepat\ocellular carcinoma (HCC).
  ○ A liver biopsy is an important modality of determining the severity of chronic viral hepatitis.
  ○ Several systems have emerged for grading and staging of hepatitis. The one most commonly used applies four grades to the severity of necrosis and inflammation and four grades to the severity and degree of fibrosis, with stage 4 being synonymous with cirrhosis.
  ○ Treatments of viral hepatitis have become much more successful and effective over the last decade (see Table 57-3). Therapy with pegylated interferon and ribavirin can eliminate HCV infection in approximately 50% of treated patients, whereas treatment with nucleoside and nucleotide analogues is able to control and suppress HBV infection in almost all treated patients.

AUTOIMMUNE LIVER DISEASES (SEE TABLE 57-4)

• Autoimmune hepatitis is a chronic liver disease associated with hepatic inflammation, which may progress to hepatic fibrosis, cirrhosis and liver failure. Although the mechanism of autoimmune hepatitis remains obscure, 2 types have been described: (1) Classic (type 1) autoimmune hepatitis occurs in women of all ages and (2) ALKM-1 (type 2) autoimmune hepatitis is only seen in young women.

TABLE 57–3   Treatment of Chronic Viral Hepatitis

	CHRONIC HEPATITIS B	CHRONIC HEPATITIS C	CHRONIC HEPATITIS D
Indications	HBeAg positive or negative chronic hepatitis B	Active liver disease based on liver biopsy or elevated ALT	Active liver disease based on liver biopsy or elevated ALT
Agents used	Evolving but likely interferon or lamivudine	Pegylated interferon plus ribavirin	Pegylated interferon monotherapy
Endpoints of therapy	Suppression of HBV DNA, loss of HBeAg, loss of HBsAg	Loss of hepatitis C virus RNA from serum	Suppression of HDV RNA and normalization of ALT
Duration of therapy	Interferon 12 mo; nucleos(t)ides 12 mo to indefinite	6 to 12 mo	12 mo to indefinite

ALT, alanine aminotransferase; HBeAg, hepatitis Be antigen; HBsAg, hepatitis B surface antigen; HBV DNA, hepatitis B viral DNA.

TABLE 57–4   Autoimmune Liver Diseases

	AUTOIMMUNE HEPATITIS	PRIMARY BILIARY CIRRHOSIS	PRIMARY SCLEROSING CHOLANGITIS
Gender preponderance	Female	Female	Male
Ages	All	Mean age = 55	Mean age = 40
Disease associations	Thyroid disease, idiopathic pulmonary fibrosis	Thyroid disease; Sjögren's syndrome	Inflammatory bowel disease
Diagnostic test	ANA, hyperglobulinemia, liver biopsy	AMA, liver biopsy	ERCP or MRCP
Treatment	Immunosuppressives (corticosteroids, azathioprine)	Ursodeoxycholic acid	None
Benefit from liver transplantation when advanced	Yes	Yes	Yes

AMA, antimitochondrial antibody; ANA, antinuclear antibody; ERCP, endoscopic retrograde cholangiopancreatogram; MRCP, magnetic resonance cholangiopancreatography.

○ Characteristic features include elevated serum aminotransferases, hyperglobulinemia, circulating autoantibodies directed toward smooth muscle, actin, nuclear antigens, and liver kidney microsomes, and chronic inflammation with prominence of plasma cells on liver biopsy.
○ Autoimmune hepatitis responds to immunosuppressive agents, particularly corticosteroids.
○ Therapy is typically initiated with corticosteroids in patients with severe disease, eg, 5–10 fold increase in aminotransferases, bridging necrosis, 2 fold increase in circulating gamma globulins.
○ Azathioprine may be added to enhance the response to corticosteroids or to provide a steroid sparing effect. Mycophenolate mofetil has been successfully administered to patients refractory to standard immunosuppressive therapy. Controversy exists regarding the optimal duration of therapy, however, patients may require life-long therapy to avoid relapses of hepatitis, which occur in more than 50% when immunosuppression is withdrawn.
• Primary biliary cirrhosis is a liver disease characterized by inflammation of and injury to the bile ductules, eventually resulting in their complete disappearance.[4] Hence, PBC has features of cholestatic liver disease, with elevations of serum alkaline phosphatase, pruritus, and jaundice.
○ Primary biliary cirrhosis occurs with a female preponderance (90%) and tends to present after middle age. The diagnosis can be established with certainty in patients presenting with features of cholestatic liver disease and seropositivity for antimitochondrial antibody. The liver biopsy reveals characteristic features of bile duct injury, sometimes associated with granulomatous inflammation and bile duct loss.
○ Treatment of PBC is with ursodeoxycholic, a nontoxic bile acid that replaces other toxic bile acids

accumulating in the presence of cholestasis. Ursodeoxycholic acid is associated with significant improvement in serum biochemistries and even in histologic features of PBC, but controversy remains as to whether ursodeoxycholic acid significantly affects the long-term progression of PBC to cirrhosis and liver failure.
• Primary sclerosing cholangitis has features of an autoimmune disease, but its pathogenesis remains uncertain.[5] Primary sclerosing cholangitis is characterized by injury to intrahepatic and extrahepatic bile ducts, associated with fibrosis and stricturing, resulting in clinical and biochemical features of cholestasis similar to PBC.
○ In contrast to PBC, PSC is a male-predominant condition (70%) and the mean age at diagnosis is 40 years of age. It often occurs (perhaps as often as 90%) in association with inflammatory bowel disease such as ulcerative colitis or Crohn's disease.
○ Primary sclerosing cholangitis is diagnosed by the characteristic clinical and serum biochemical picture with appropriate imaging confirmating bile duct strictures and dilatation (such as magnetic resonance cholangiopancreatography [MRCP] or endoscopic retrograde cholangiopancreatogram [ERCP]). Although liver biopsy is not essential for the diagnosis, it may reveal characteristic features of onion-skin fibrosis around bile ductules with loss of intrahepatic bile ducts.
○ There is no effective treatment for PSC, but patients with advanced liver disease caused by PSC benefit from liver transplantation.

OTHER LIVER DISEASES

• Fatty liver diseases include those caused by alcohol (alcoholic hepatitis) and a miscellaneous group of diseases referred to as nonalcoholic fatty liver disease (NAFLD).

○ Sustained alcohol ingestion (>40 g/day for women and >80 g/day for men) may result in alcoholic hepatitis and cirrhosis.

○ Alcoholic hepatitis is a condition characterized by an acute onset of jaundice, painful hepatomegaly, fever, and leucocytosis. Liver biopsy shows characteristic features of Mallory hyaline, fatty change, and polymorphonuclear leucocyte infiltration. Alcoholic hepatitis has a poor prognosis, despite treatment with corticosteroids and pentoxifylline. Cirrhosis may follow or be associated with alcoholic hepatitis. There is no specific treatment except for liver transplantation, which is typically done only after a period of abstinence from alcohol (typically at least 6 months).

○ Nonalcoholic fatty liver disease (NAFLD) is associated with obesity, diabetes, insulin resistance, and the metabolic syndrome.[6] There is a range of severity from simple steatosis to nonalcoholic steatohepatitis to cirrhosis. Although there is no specific therapy for NAFLD, attempts at treatment are aimed at control of diabetes and weight loss.

• Inherited metabolic diseases may also affect the liver, including hemochromatosis, Wilson disease and α_1-antitrypsin deficiency.

PRIMARY LIVER CANCER

• Two main primary liver cancers may occur: hepatocellular carcinoma (HCC) and cholangiocellular carcinoma (CCC).[7]

○ HCC is the more common of the two and is almost always associated with chronic viral hepatitis or an underlying liver disease. It often occurs against a background of cirrhosis. The diagnosis of HCC is based on dynamic imaging studies that reveal the characteristic arterial hypervascularity of this tumor (multiphasic computed tomography or magnetic resonance imaging), sometimes confirmed with a liver biopsy. Serum α-fetoprotein levels are elevated to more than 400 ng/mL in 60% to 80% of patients with HCC, particularly with large and more advanced tumors.

○ Potentially curative treatments of HCC may be applied when the tumor is relatively small (single tumor, <5 cm in diameter), using surgical resection, liver transplantation, or local ablation with radiofrequency or ethanol injection.

○ Chemoembolization has been shown to prolong survival in patients with more advanced tumors.

○ Often the prognosis of patients with HCC is determined by the presence and severity of associated cirrhosis and liver failure.

○ Two major forms of CCC are recognized: peripheral and central. Typically, the peripheral form is not associated with underlying liver disease, whereas the central type often occurs with primary sclerosing cholangitis. Cholangiocellular carcinoma has a poor prognosis. The most effective form of therapy is surgical resection, but even that has limited benefit in most cases.

DISEASES OF THE GALLBLADDER

• The most common conditions afflicting the gallbladder are related to the presence of gallstones (cholelithiasis).[8] There are two main types of stones: cholesterol stones and pigment stones.

○ Cholesterol stones arise when bile is supersaturated with cholesterol but require nucleation with mucin or other glycoproteins to manifest. Pigment stones are comprised largely of bilirubin and arise predominantly in patients with chronic hemolytic states, cirrhosis, Gilbert's syndrome, or cystic fibrosis.

○ Gallstones are usually clinically silent unless they become impacted in the cystic duct or Hartman's pouch where they obstruct the outflow of bile. This may occur transiently, in which case they cause episodes of right upper quadrant pain (biliary colic), or if sufficiently prolonged, acute cholecystitis.

○ Acute cholecystitis is characterized by right upper quadrant pain, tenderness to palpation (including a positive Murphy's sign), low-grade fever, and leucocytosis. The diagnosis can be confirmed by ultrasonography or other imaging study showing the presence of gallstones and thickening of the gallbladder wall. Radionuclide scanning with technetium 99m–labeled *N*-substituted iminodiacetic acids (hepatoiminodiacetic, dimethyl iminodi- acetic, diisopropyl iminodiacetic acid) show nonvisualization of the gallbladder.

○ Treatment of acute cholecystitis is initially with intravenous antibiotics, but cholecystectomy is usually required to prevent further episodes of acute cholecystitis.

○ Cholecystectomy is generally performed through the laparoscopic route, but may sometimes need to be done by open laparotomy.

○ Additional complications of gallstones include chronic cholecystitis, biliary obstruction with cholangitis and pancreatitis. (See also Chap. 58, Diseases of the Pancreas.)

REFERENCES

1. Said A, Lucey MR. Liver transplantation: an update. *Curr Opin Gastroenterol.* 2006;22:272–278.

2. Lok ASF, McMahon BJ. AASLD Practice Guidelines: chronic hepatitis B. *Hepatology.* 2007;45:507–539.

3. Strader DB, Wright T, Thomas DL, Seeff LB. AASLD Practice Guidelines: diagnosis, management and treatment of hepatitis C. *Hepatology*. 2004;1147–1171.
4. Heathcote EJ. AASLD Practice Guidelines: management of primary biliary cirrhosis. *Hepatology*. 2000;31:1005–1013.
5. MacFaul GR. Chapman RW. Sclerosing cholangitis. *Curr Opin Gastroenterol*. 2006;22:288–293.
6. Brunt EM, Janney CG, Di Biscegllie AM, et al. Nonalcoholic steatohepatitis: a proposal for grading and staging the histological lesions. *Am J Gastroenterol*. 1999;94:2467–2474.
7. Hayashi PH, Di Bisceglie AM. The progression of hepatitis B- and C-infections to chronic liver disease and hepatocellular carcinoma: presentation, diagnosis, screening, prevention, and treatment of hepatocellular carcinoma. *Infect Dis Clin North Am*. 2006;20:1–25.
8. Greenberger N, Paumgartner G. In Kasper DL, Braunwald E, Fauci AS, eds. *Harrison's On-Line*. 16th ed. 2007 www.harrisononline.com.

58 DISEASES OF THE PANCREAS

Adrian M. Di Bisceglie

ANATOMY AND PHYSIOLOGY

- The pancreas is a retroperitoneal parenchymal organ with exocrine glands that produce secretions into the pancreatic duct which drains into the duodenum via the sphincter of Oddi. Embryologically, there are two pancreatic ducts, the ventral and dorsal, which usually fuse and drain into a common duct. Occasionally, however, they remain separate and a small accessory duct (of Santorini) may drain separately into the duodenum (pancreas divisum).
- In addition to the exocrine function of the pancreas, which secrete digestive enzymes in an alkaline solution, the pancreas has a significant endocrine function as hormones are produced by pancreatic islets (insulin, glucagon, somatostatin, gastrin).
- The anatomy of the biliary and pancreatic ducts can be imaged by endoscopic retrograde cholangiopancreatogram (ERCP). In this procedure, the biliary ampulla is cannulated at the time of upper gastrointestinal endoscopy, water-soluble contrast is injected and a radiograph is obtained. A more recent noninvasive alternative is magnetic resonance cholangiopancreatography (MRCP), which captures images by magnetic resonance imaging with three-dimensional computerized reconstruction of the biliary tree and pancreatic ducts.

- A functional assay of pancreatic exocrine function can be obtained following the administration of secretin (secretin stimulation test). In this assay, secretin is administered intravenously, and pancreatic secretions are collected through a catheter placed in the distal duodenum. The secretions are then assayed for bicarbonate concentration, lipase and trypsin activity.

SYMPTOMS OF PANCREATIC DISEASE

- A characteristic feature of pancreatic disease is abdominal pain, which can be severe in acute and chronic pancreatitis or with pancreatic cancer. The pain is typically epigastric, continuous, and radiates to the back.
- Pancreatic exocrine dysfunction can cause steatorrhea and malabsorption. (See also Chap. 55, Diseases of the Small Bowels.) Patients complain of producing large, bulky, offensive-smelling stools and develop features of fat malabsorption, including deficiency of fat-soluble vitamins.
- Pancreatic endocrine dysfunction results in insulin deficiency and diabetes mellitus.

ACUTE PANCREATITIS

- Pancreatitis is defined as an inflammation of the pancreas and has been described in association with a variety of causes. In general, pancreas should be divided into acute pancreatitis and chronic pancreatitis, the acute condition being further characterized by full reversibility after the episode.
- There are two pathologically distinct forms of pancreatitis, interstitial and hemorrhagic, the latter being more severe. The causes of acute pancreatitis are shown in Table 58–1.
- Patients with acute pancreatitis (Table 58–2) develop upper abdominal pain, typically with vomiting. Physical examination reveals tenderness in the epigastrium without rebound. An ileus can occur and be associated with abdominal distension.
- The features of severe pancreatitis include hypotension and shock, subcutaneous fat necrosis, and retroperitoneal hemorrhage characterized by a Gray-Turner sign (large ecchymoses in the flanks) or Cullen's sign (ecchymoses around the umbilicus).
- It is important to recognize that hyperamylasemia is not synonymous with pancreatitis. For example, several other conditions can cause upper abdominal pain, vomiting and hyperamylasemia including perforated viscus, bowel obstruction, mesenteric ischemia, and cholecystitis. Thus, the diagnosis of acute pancreatitis is based on a constellation of clinical and

TABLE 58–1   Etiology of Acute Pancreatitis

Alcohol
Gallstones
Pancreatic obstruction
Sphincter of Oddi dysfunction
Pancreas divisum
Carcinoma of the pancreas
Metabolic
Hypertriglyceridemia
Hypercalcemia
Genetic disorders
Hereditary pancreatitis (associated with mutations in the trypsinogen
    gene and CFTR, the transporter which is defective in cystic fibrosis)
Drugs and toxins
Poisons (insecticides, methanol, scorpion venom)
Immunosuppressants (azathioprine, 6-MP, cyclosporine, tacrolimus,
    corticosteroids)
Antivirals and antibiotics (ddI, pentamidine, trimethoprim-
    sulfamethoxazole) others (furosemide, thiazide diuretics, ACE
    inhibitors)

ACE, angiotensin-converting enzyme; CFTR, cystic fibrosis
transmembrane conductance regulator; ddI, didanosine; 6-MP,
mercaptopurine.

laboratory findings with radiologic evidence of pancreatic inflammation.

- Approximately 20% of patients with acute pancreatitis have a severe course, associated with prolonged morbidity and even mortality. There are several systems for grading the severity of pancreatitis, including Ranson's criteria and the Simplified Glasgow criteria.
- According to Ranson's scheme, the presence of three or more of the following clinical features predict a severe outcome: On admission,
  - Age >55 years
  - Leukocytosis
    - White cell count >16,000/mm^3
    - Serum aspartate aminotransferase (AST) >250 U/L

TABLE 58–2   Diagnostic Tests in Acute Pancreatitis

CHARACTERISTIC BLOOD TESTS

Serum amylase	Elevated (>2 ULN)
Serum lipase	Elevated
Ancillary blood tests	
Blood count	Leukocytosis
Liver tests	Increased bilirubin and transaminases
Serum calcium	Decreased
Imaging studies	
CT of the abdomen	Pancreatic enlargement, inhomogeneity, surrounding fluid
Chest x-ray	Pleural effusion, atelectasis, features of ARDS
Ultrasound	Can show gallstones in gallbladder or bile duct

ARDS, acute respiratory distress syndrome; CT, computed tomography;
ULN, upper limits of normal.

TABLE 58–3   Complications of Acute Pancreatitis

Local complications
Pancreatic phlegmon
Infected pancreatic phlegmon
Pseudocyst formation
Pancreatic ascites
Hemosuccus pancreaticus
Systemic complications
Renal failure
Respiratory failure

  - Lactate dehydrogenase (LDH) >350 U/L
  - Serum glucose >200 mg/dL
  - After 48 hours
    - Hematocrit decrease by >10%
    - Blood urea nitrogen (BUN) increased by >5mg/dL
    - Serum calcium <8 mg/dL
    - Partial pressure of alveolar oxygen (P$_a$O$_2$) <60 mm Hg
    - Base deficit >4 mEq/L
    - Fluid sequestration >6 L
- There is no proven therapy for acute pancreatitis. Treatment is aimed at supportive care (minimizing pancreatic secretions by fasting and by maintaining optimal fluid balance) and early recognition of complications such as an infected phlegmon. ERCP is indicated after gallstone pancreatitis to remove any stones remaining in the common bile duct and perform a sphincterotomy of the sphincter of Oddi, prior to cholecystectomy.
- There are many possible complications of acute pancreatitis, which can occur in the hours, days, or weeks after the onset of the illness. They are generally classified into local and systemic complications (Table 58–3).
- Pancreatic phlegmon refers to a large area of pancreatic necrosis with edema, generally detectable by computed tomography (CT) scan. This can become infected resulting in pancreatic abscess.
- Pancreatic pseudocyst, a fluid-filled area within the pancreas with no epithelial lining, generally takes several weeks to develop from a phlegmon. A pseudocyst can also become infected.
- If the pancreatic duct is disrupted by pancreatitis (as well as other causes), pancreatic secretions can leak into the abdomen and cause peritoneal inflammation, resulting in pancreatic ascites, characterized by a high concentration of peritoneal amylase.
- Any large blood vessel within the pancreas can be disrupted by localized inflammation in the wall of a pseudocyst, resulting in hemorrhage through the pancreatic duct (hemosuccus pancreaticus).
- Renal failure occurs initially as a result of intravascular volume depletion. Acute respiratory distress syndrome (ARDS) is a dreaded and often lethal complication of acute pancreatitis associated with capillary leaking, resulting in hypoxemia and respiratory failure.

CHRONIC PANCREATITIS

- Chronic pancreatitis is a persistent inflammatory disease of the pancreas associated with morphologic or functional damage to the pancreas.
- The causes of chronic pancreatitis include alcohol, malnutrition (*tropical pancreatitis*), and genetic causes (hereditary pancreatitis and cystic fibrosis). Approximately 20% of cases of chronic pancreatitis have no obvious etiology.
- Clinical features of chronic pancreatitis include abdominal pain, weight loss, malabsorption, and diabetes mellitus. Weight loss is complex, however in part, since eating certain foods may exacerbate the pain, and patients avoid eating. Malabsorption caused by pancreatic exocrine insufficiency can also contribute to weight loss. Pancreatic endocrine insufficiency is caused by loss of pancreatic islet cells and results in glucose intolerance.
- The diagnosis of chronic pancreatitis can be established with functional or structural studies. Functional studies assess pancreatic exocrine function by testing for the presence of malabsorption. Classically, this involves quantitation of fat in a 72-hour stool collection while on a 100g fat diet (>7 g/day of fat is considered abnormal). A random test for fecal fat is a simple screening procedure as is a test for the presence of fecal elastase (sensitivity and specificity of 95%). Serum concentrations of amylase and lipase are often normal in patients with chronic pancreatitis because of the patchy nature of the injury. Structural studies (CT or ERCP) are aimed at demonstrating either the characteristic pancreatic calcification of chronic pancreatitis or dilatation of the pancreatic duct.
- The management of chronic pancreatitis is typically focused on control of pain, which can be chronic and severe. It is important to eliminate precipitating factors such as alcohol and a high-fat diet. If simple analgesics are not effective or if significant fat malabsorption exists, administration of pancreatic enzyme supplements should be offered. Pancreatic enzymes require an alkaline environment to promote activation and, therefore, are usually given with an acid suppressant in the form of an H_2-blocker or a proton pump inhibitor.
- Celiac plexus block by injection of alcohol or steroids has had limited success in relieving pancreatic pain and should be considered experimental.
- Pain that persists despite the use of narcotic analgesics merits evaluation with an ERCP for the presence of a pancreatic duct stricture (which can be dilated or even stented) or stones in the pancreatic duct, which can be removed.
- Surgery is reserved for severe and refractory cases. Pancreaticojejunostomy has been used to drain a dilated pancreatic duct although a pancreatic resection is occasionally performed in an attempt to relieve severe pain.
- Pancreatic exocrine insufficiency is treated with purified extracts of pancreas containing active pancreatic enzymes. The extract is sprinkled over food.

TUMORS OF THE PANCREAS

- Tumors of the pancreas include ductal adenocarcinoma, endocrine neoplasms, carcinoid tumors, lymphomas, and other rare tumors.
- Adenocarcinoma is by far the most common tumor of the pancreas, accounting for approximately 90% of tumors. There are more than 30,000 new cases of pancreatic carcinoma each year in the United States. This is a highly lethal cancer, and the mortality rate approximates the incidence rate.
- Common risk factors for pancreatic cancer include smoking and chronic pancreatitis.
- The clinical presentation of pancreatic cancer depends on its location. Thus tumors in the head of the pancreas can cause obstruction of the common bile duct or pancreatic duct, whereas tumors in the body or tail of the pancreas tend to present at a more advanced stage with abdominal pain, weight loss, and diabetes. Acute pancreatitis can be the initial presenting syndrome.
- Obstruction of the common bile duct by pancreatic cancer can cause biliary obstruction and jaundice (typically painless jaundice, as opposed to biliary obstruction by gallstones which is painful).
- The diagnosis of pancreatic cancer is suggested by the presence of a mass in the pancreas seen on imaging studies such as CT, magnetic resonance imaging (MRI), ultrasound, or ERCP. Preoperative diagnosis can be difficult as the pancreas is difficult to access for biopsy. Cytologic examination obtained by endoscopic brushings of the epithelium or fine needle aspiration combined with endoscopic ultrasound examination can be misleading, and pancreatic cancer can readily be confused with chronic pancreatitis. Serum levels of the tumor marker CA19–9 are sometimes elevated in patients with pancreatic cancer.
- The optimal treatment of pancreatic cancer is surgery. Pancreaticoduodenectomy (the Whipple procedure) is recommended provided there has been minimal local spread of the tumor (particularly vascular invasion) or distant metastases. Adjuvant chemotherapy is used after surgery. In general pancreatic cancer is chemoresistant, thus extensive or recurrent pancreatic cancer after surgery does not respond well to systemic chemotherapy.

TABLE 58–4   Pancreatic Endocrine Tumors

TUMOR	HORMONE PRODUCED	RESULTING SYNDROME
Gastrinoma	Gastrin	Zollinger-Ellison syndrome
Insulinoma	Insulin	Hypoglycemia
Glucagonoma	Glucagon	Glucagonoma syndrome
VIPoma	VIP	Watery diarrhea, hypokalemic alkalosis
Somatostatinoma	Somatostatin	Somatostatinoma syndrome
GRFoma	growth hormone RF	acromegaly
ACTHoma	ACTH	Cushing syndrome
Nonfunctioning	None	Mass effects

ACTH, corticotropin; GRF, gonadotropin-releasing factor; RF, releasing factor; VIP, vasoactive intestinal peptide.

PANCREATIC ENDOCRINE TUMORS

- These are tumors that are presumed to originate from the islet cells of the pancreas or related cells in the wall of the duodenum. They are often functional and produce the hormones from their cell of origin. Excess production of these hormones lead to characteristic clinical syndromes (Table 58–4).
- These tumors have neuroendocrine features and can be benign or malignant. Malignancy can be difficult to establish purely based on histologic appearance and can sometimes only be established after metastases have occurred. Wherever possible, if the tumor can be identified, it should be surgically removed.
- Zollinger-Ellison syndrome is caused by production of gastrin by neuroendocrine tumors, resulting in extreme overproduction of gastric acid and refractory peptic ulceration. The diagnosis is suggested by fasting hypergastrinemia. Therapy is directed at controlling acid hypersecretion with proton pump inhibitors.
- Glucagonomas produce glucagon, which causes a characteristic syndrome of rash (necrolytic migratory erythema), diabetes mellitus, and weight loss. The diagnosis is suggested by finding elevated serum levels of glucagon. The syndrome can be controlled by the administration of the long-acting somatostatin analogue, octreotide. Zinc therapy can diminish the rash.
- Tumors that secrete vasoactive intestinal peptide (VIP) can cause a syndrome of watery diarrhea and hypokalemic alkalosis. The diarrhea is profuse and cholera-like. The diagnosis of a VIPoma is suggested by diarrhea that exceeds 3 L/day even while fasting. The use of octreotide can alleviate symptoms.
- Insulinomas are usually benign tumors that cause hypoglycemia associated with hyperinsulinemia.

An insulinoma must be distinguished from factitious hypoglycemia caused by surreptitious administration of insulin by the patient via measurement of C-peptide levels—if these are raised, with hypoglycemia and hyperinsulinemia, this suggests the insulin is of endogenous origin, likely from an insulinoma.
- Other pancreatic endocrine tumors are summarized in Table 58–4.

BIBLIOGRAPHY

American Gastroenterological Association. American Gastroenterological Association medical position statement: treatment of pain in chronic pancreatitis. *Gastroenterology.* 1998; 115(3):765–776.

American Gastroenterological Association. American Gastroenterological Association medical position statement: epidemiology, diagnosis, and treatment of pancreatic ductal adenocarcinoma. *Gastroenterology.* 1999;117(6):1464–1484.

Banks PA, Freeman ML. Practice guidelines in acute pancreatitis. *Am J Gastroenterol.* 2006;101:2379–2400.

Gomez-Rivera F, Stewart AE, Arnoletti JP, et al. Surgical treatment of pancreatic endocrine neoplasms. *Am J Surg.* 2007;193:460–465.

Larson SD, Nealon WH, Evers BM. Management of gallstone pancreatitis. *Adv Surg.* 2006;40:265–284.

Owyang, C. Pancreatitis. In Goldman L, Ausiello D, eds. *Cecil Textbook of Medicine.* 22nd ed. Philadelphia, PA: Saunders; 2004:879–885.

Yadav D, Lowenfels AB. Trends in the epidemiology of the first attack of acute pancreatitis: a systematic review. *Pancreas.* 2006;33:323–330.

Section 8
HEMATOLOGY

59 BONE MARROW AND BONE MARROW FAILURE

Catherine Iasiello

The hematopoietic system is comprised of three cellular components:
- Red cells which transport oxygen from the lungs to the tissues
- White cells which protect against infection
- Platelets which are involved in hemostasis

Abnormalities of the production or function of these cells result in hematological disease.

BONE MARROW STRUCTURE AND FUNCTION

The cellular components of blood are derived from a pool of stem cells. In the embryo, the yolk sac, liver and spleen, produce blood cells. However by 5 months gestation, hematopoietic cell production is fully established in the bone marrow. At birth, all bones contain hematopoietic marrow, but in the adult active marrow is restricted to the axial skeleton, upper humeri, and proximal femora. The bone marrow accounts for 5% of an adult's weight and is responsible for the generation of over a trillion cells every day, including 70 billion neutrophils and 200 billion red cells. Normal marrow contains a lineage of immature precursors and a storage pool of mature cells for release at times of increased demand. Up to 10 times the circulating number of neutrophils are stored in the marrow, whereas red cell storage pools and circulating pools are equal in size. In normal marrow, 50% to 60% of cells are dedicated to myeloid cell production.

Anatomically, the bone marrow occupies the intertrabecular spaces in trabecular bone. Hematopoietic cells reside in a framework of reticular cells and collagen in intimate contact with stromal cells, adipocytes, and macrophages, which provide the necessary microenvironment for cell growth. Normal marrow has a characteristic ultrastructural organization. Nests of red cell precursors cluster around a central macrophage, which provides iron and serves to phagocytically extract nuclei. Megakaryocytes are large cells which produce and release platelets into vascular sinuses. White cell precursors are clustered around the bone trabeculae with maturing cells migrating toward the vascular sinuses. Plasma cells normally comprise less than 5% of the marrow cells and are scattered throughout the intertrabecular spaces.

HEMATOPOIETIC STEM CELLS

Cells produced by the bone marrow are derived from a finite number of pluripotent stem cells that are capable of differentiating into any type of mature hematopoietic cell. A total population of 1 to 2×10^6 pluripotent stem cells produces more than 10^{11} cells each day. Injury to stem cells by drugs or irradiation results in bone marrow failure. Pluripotent stem cells differentiate into lineage-committed stem cells which produce myeloid cells, erythroid cells, and megakaryocytes. Stem cells can be recognized by their surface expression of the CD 34 antigen; only 0.1% to 0.3% of the marrow cells are stem cells. The proliferation and differentiation of stem cells is under the control of a variety of growth factors produced by stromal cells, fibroblasts, and macrophages. Some, such as granulocyte macrophage colony stimulating factor (GM-CSF), interleukin-3 (IL-3), and stem cell factor, act on several lineages at both early and late time points. Others, such as erythropoietin, granulocyte colony stimulating factor and thrombopoietin, are lineage-specific.

MATURE BLOOD CELLS

RED CELLS

- Structure and function
  - The mature red cell is a 7.5 μm biconcave disc, which delivers oxygen to the tissues from the lungs and carbon dioxide in reverse direction. The red cell does not have a nucleus and has no mitochondria. The normal red cell lifespan is approximately 120 days. The red cell must pass through the smallest capillaries in the circulation and, therefore is distensible. The membrane is comprised of a lipid bilayer to which a skeleton of filamentous proteins is attached via special link proteins. Inherited abnormalities of these proteins result in derangements in membrane structure resulting in the formation of abnormally shaped cells called spherocytes and elliptocytes as the cells pass through the microvasculature of the spleen. Red cells are subjected to osmotic stress in the pulmonary and renal circulation. However, cell volume is maintained by active ion pumps that control intracellular concentrations of sodium, potassium, chloride, and bicarbonate. Membrane proteins inserted into the lipid bilayer also form the antigens recognized by blood grouping.
- Development
  - The earliest red cell precursors in the bone marrow are nucleated. These cells divide rapidly and produce progressively smaller daughter cells which undergo hemoglobinization. Maturation is complete when the nucleus is extruded but ribosomal proteins are still present in the cytoplasm. Reticulocytes lose this remnant material over several days, resulting in the production of a mature red cell. These cells are eventually released into the systemic circulation. Red cell production is controlled by erythropoietin, a hormone produced by renal tubular interstitial cells in response to hypoxia. Erythropoietin stimulates committed erythroid stem cells to proliferate and decreases the maturation time for red cells.

WHITE CELLS

- Structure and function
  - Five major types of white cell are present in normal blood: neutrophils, eosinophils, basophils, monocytes, and lymphocytes. In children up to the age of seven, lymphocytes are the predominant cell, but after age 7, neutrophils are the most abundant cell type. Neutrophils, eosinophils, and basophils are classified as granulocytes, because they contain prominent cytoplasmic granules.

- Neutrophils
  - Mature neutrophils are 10 to 14 μm in diameter, with a multilobular nucleus containing two to five segments. Their main function is to recognize and ingest foreign substances and microorganisms, which are then degraded intracellulary. Two types of granules are present in neutrophils: primary granules and the more abundant secondary granules. Primary granules contain myeloperoxidase and other proteins that are important for microbial elimination. They are released intracellularly. Secondary granules contain a number of membrane proteins such as adhesion molecules and components of the oxidase enzyme. Upon degranulation the contents of secondary granules are released extracellulary.
  - The earliest precursor of the neutrophil is the myeloblast, which differentiates into the promyelocyte which contains primary granules. Promyelocytes become myelocytes, which contain both primary and secondary granules. The final steps in maturation involve the conversion of the metamyelocyte to the mature segmented neutrophil. The entire process takes from 17 to 25 days. Importantly, a large storage pool exists in the bone marrow. Neutrophils in the circulation may be freely circulating or attached to the endothelium (marginated). These two pools are equal in size. Exercise or catecholamines demarginate the cells and increase the number of neutrophils in the circulation. Myelocytes or metamyelocytes are normally only found in the marrow but may appear in the circulation in infectious or toxic states. A variety of clinical conditions increase the appearance of immature myeloid precursors in the blood as well as immature (nucleated) red cells; this is referred to as a leukoerythroblastic reaction.
- Eosinophils
  - Eosinophils are similar in size to neutrophils but usually only comprise 1% to 6% of the circulating white cells. They possess bilobed nuclei and display prominent orange granules on staining. They are phagocytic and their granules contain a peroxidase capable of generating reactive oxygen species and proteins involved in the intracellular destruction of helminths and protozoa.
- Basophils
  - Basophils are the same size as neutrophils but comprise only 1% of the circulating white cells. They contain dense black granules. Basophils bind IgE antibody on their surface, and exposure to the appropriate antigen elicits degranulation resulting in the release of histamine, leukotrienes, and heparin. These cells are involved in hypersensitivity reactions.
- Monocytes
  - Monocytes are the largest of the white cells, with a diameter of 12 to 20 μm and an irregular nucleus

surrounded by an abundant pale blue cytoplasm containing occasional cytoplasmic vacuoles. These cells can migrate to the tissue compartment and transform into macrophages, Kupffer cells, or antigen-presenting dendritic cells. Macrophages phagocytose debris, apoptotic cells, and microorganisms. When activated, they produce a variety of cytokines, such as IL-1, tumor necrosis factor (TNF), and GM-CSF. Monocytes remain in the circulation for 8–70 hours, while macrophages have a maximum lifespan of several months.

- Lymphocytes
  - Lymphocytes are heterogeneous in size, with the smaller cells being the same size as red cells and the largest similar to neutrophils. Small lymphocytes are circular with scanty cytoplasm, but the larger cells are more irregular with abundant blue cytoplasm. The majority of lymphocytes in the circulation are T cells (80%), which can be recognized by their expression of CD antigens. They mediate cellular immunity and two major subtypes have been characterized: CD4+ helper cells and CD8+ suppressor cells. The B cells mediate humoral immunity and can be recognized by their expression of immunoglobulin light chains (2:1 ratio of kappa and lambda). Their lifespan can vary from several days to many years.

BONE MARROW FAILURE

The bone marrow failure syndromes are a group of disorders than can be either inherited or acquired. These diseases reflect disorders of the hematopoietic stem cell that can involve either one cell line or all of the cell lines (erythroid, myeloid or megakaryocytic). The lymphocytes, which are involved in lymphoproliferative disorders, are usually spared. The pathophysiology of marrow failure involves the following mechanisms: (1) a decrease in or damage to the hematopoietic stem cells or their microenvironment, resulting in hypoplastic or aplastic bone marrow; (2) maturation defects (eg, Vitamin B12 or folate deficiency); and (3) differentiation defects (eg, myelodysplasia).

The prevalence of bone marrow failure secondary to hypoplastic or aplastic anemia is low in the United States and Europe (2 to 6 cases per million persons) compared to the prevalence of bone marrow failure secondary to acute myelogenous leukemia and multiple myeloma (27 to 35 cases per million persons). The frequency of myelodysplasia, on the other hand, has increased from 143 cases reported in 1973 to approximately 15,000 cases annually in the United States. This is likely an underestimation of the actual prevalence,

which is believed to be closer to 35,000 to 55,000 new cases a year.

Pancytopenia occurs when red blood cells, white blood cells, and platelets are all affected.

The specific causes of marrow failure include:
- Aplastic anemia (initially all 3 cell lines may not be affected) is either:
  - Congenital; for example, Fanconi anemia.
  - Acquired: injury from viruses (hepatitis B virus, Epstein-Barr virus, parvovirus), autoimmune, ionizing radiation, antineoplastic agents, poisons (eg, benzene) and drugs (eg, chloramphenicol).
- Single-cell line deficiencies are less common, and include:
  - Myelodysplasia: caused by a defect in the differentiation of precursor cells
  - Acute myeloid or lymphoblastic leukemia
  - Infiltration of the marrow (eg, lymphoma, multiple myeloma, carcinoma, hairy cell leukemia)
  - Megaloblastic anemia (vitamin B12 or folate deficiency)
  - Myelofibrosis: fibrosis of the bone marrow associated with radiotherapy, Hodgkin disease, polycythemia vera, and malignant transformation
- The history can help distinguish inherited causes from acquired causes. Inherited bone marrow failure is usually diagnosed in young adults but may remain undiagnosed until the fifth or sixth decades of life. These diseases should be considered if any of the following are present: subtle but characteristic physical anomalies, hematologic cytopenias, unexplained macrocytosis, myelodysplastic syndrome, acute myelogenous leukemia, or squamous cell cancer (even in the absence of pancytopenia). Siblings of a patient with Fanconi anemia who develop abnormal blood counts should also be investigated.
- Exposure to toxins, drugs, environmental hazards, and recent viral infections (eg, hepatitis) should be noted.

The manifestations of bone marrow failure are secondary to the clinical effects of cytopenia. Patients with severe anemia may present with pallor and/or signs of congestive heart failure, such as shortness of breath. Bruising (ecchymoses, petechiae), gum bleeding, or nosebleeds suggest thrombocytopenia. Fever, cellulitis, pneumonia, or sepsis suggest neutropenia. The presence of hepatomegaly, splenomegaly, or lymphadenopathy suggests a diagnosis of leukemia or lymphoma.

BIBLIOGRAPHY

Benayahu D, Akavia UD, Shur I. Differentiation of bone marrow stroma-derived mesenchymal cells. *Curr Med Chem.* 2007; 14(2):173–179.

Bone marrow. Encyclopædia Britannica. 2007. *Encyclopædia Britannica Online.* 17 April 2007. http://www.britannica.com/eb/article-9080586.

Dawon J. Congenital pancytopenia associated with multiple congenital anomalies. *Pediatrics.* 1955;15:325.

Ho AD, Punzel M. Hematopoietic stem cells: Can old cells learn new tricks? *J Leukoc Biol.* 2003;73:547–555.

Rolink AG, Massa S, Balciunaite G, Ceredig R. Early lymphocyte development in bone marrow and thymus. *Swiss Med Wkly.* 2006;28;136(43–44):679–683.

Salacz ME, Lankiewicz, MW, Weissman DE. Management of thrombocytopenia in bone marrow failure: A review. *J Palliat Med.* 2007;10(1):236–244.

Schatteman GC, Dunnwald M, Jiao C. Biology of bone marrow-derived endothelial cell precursors. *Am J Physiol Heart Circ Physiol.* 2007;292(1):H1–18.

Travlos GS. Normal structure, function, and histology of the bone marrow. *Toxicol Pathol.* 2006;34(5):548–565.

Young NS. Acquired bone marrow failure. In: Handin RI, Stossel TP, Lux SE, eds. *Blood: Principles and Practice of Hematology.* Philadelphia, PA: JB Lippincott; 1995:293–365.

60 RED BLOOD CELL DISORDERS

Krishnamohan R. Basarakodu, Stephen L. Graziano, Scott W. McGee, Rajesh R. Nair, Michael C. Perry, Arun Rajan, Huda Salman, and Allison P. Wall

THE WORKUP OF ANEMIA
Allison P. Wall

CLINICAL EVALUATION

- Anemia is a common diagnosis and is detected in 20% to 40% of hospitalized patients. An initial history and physical provide important clues to the etiology of the anemia. Important details of the history include ethnicity/family history (congenital causes), social history including habits, dietary history (nutritional deficiencies), previous medical history (renal function, malignancies), and surgical history.
- Common presenting clinical symptoms include weakness, fatigue, dyspnea on exertion, and dizziness. Physical examination findings include pallor (skin, mucous membranes, and conjunctivae), hypotension, tachycardia, and a systolic ejection murmur.

PATHOPHYSIOLOGY

- Anemia is defined as a hemoglobin (Hb) concentration and hematocrit (HCT; packed cell volume of red blood cells [RBCs]) below the lower limit of normal based on the patient's age, sex, and geographic location (altitude of residence); generally a Hb of 12 g/dL in women and 14 g/dL in men is considered normal. The average life span of a RBC is 120 days. One percent of the body's red cells are replaced each day to compensate for normal losses. The mechanisms responsible for anemia include decreased production of red cells, accelerated destruction of red cells, or blood loss. These mechanisms can occur simultaneously and collectively contribute to the develop of anemia.

LABORATORY EVALUATION

- The initial laboratory evaluation should include a complete blood cell count (CBC), reticulocyte count, erythropoietin (EPO) level, and evaluation of the peripheral smear. Special attention should be directed toward analyzing the red cell indices to aid in formulating a differential diagnosis. The RBC indices group anemias according to size (microcytic, normocytic, macrocytic) and Hb concentration (hypochromic, normochromic, hyperchromic) (Table 60–1).
- Common red cell indices reported by the blood bank include the following (Table 60–2):
  - Mean corpuscular volume (MCV); approximates the mean size of red cells.
  - Mean corpuscular hemoglobin (MCH); approximates the absolute Hb content.
  - Mean corpuscular hemoglobin concentration (MCHC); approximates the concentration of Hb relative to the size of the red cell.
  - Red cell distribution width (RDW) is a measurement of the coefficient of variation of red cell volume.

TABLE 60–1 Categories of Anemias Based on Mean Corpuscular Volume

MICROCYTIC (<80)	NORMOCYTIC (80–100)	MACROCYTIC (>100)
Iron deficiency	Blood loss (acute)	B_{12} deficiency
Blood loss (chronic)	Anemia of chronic disease	Folate deficiency
Thalassemia	Aplastic anemia	Drug-induced megaloblastic anemia
Lead poisoning	Uremia	Liver disease
Sideroblastic anemia	Mixed nutritional deficiencies	Hypothyroidism

TABLE 60–2   Red Cell Indices and Reticulocyte Count (RC)

HIGH RDW	LOW RC	HIGH RC
Low MCV	Iron deficiency	β-Thalassemia, sickle cell disease
Normal MCV	MDS, early iron, B$_{12}$, and folate deficiency	Sickle cell disease
High MCV	MDS, B$_{12}$, and folate deficiency	Chronic liver disease, hemolysis
NORMAL RDW		
Low MCV	Anemia of chronic disease	
Normal MCV	Anemia of chronic disease	
High MCV	Aplastic anemia, chemotherapy, EtOH	Chronic liver disease

EtOH, ethyl alcohol; MCV, mean corpuscular volume; MDS, myelodysplastic syndromes; RDW, red cell distribution width.

- The reticulocyte count indicates whether the bone marrow's response to the anemia is appropriate and aids in the classification of anemia (Table 60-3). There are two methods employed to determine whether the bone marrow's response to the anemia is appropriat:

$$\text{Absolute reticulocyte count (ARC)}$$
$$= \text{reticulocytes (\%)} \times \text{RBC count/mm}^3$$

  ○ An ARC <100,000 indicates a hypoproliferative bone marrow.

$$\text{Reticulocyte index (RI)}$$
$$= \text{reticulocytes (\%)} \times \text{(patient HCT/normal HCT)}$$

  ○ RI >3 indicates an appropriate marrow response.
- Erythropoietin (EPO) is a protein produced by the kidney in response to hypoxia. Erythropoietin stimulates red cell precursors in the marrow and promotes an erythrocytosis. The EPO level assesses whether adequate EPO is available for hematopoiesis. IF the

TABLE 60–3   Classification of Anemia on the Basis of ARC or RI

HYPERPROLIFERATIVE ANEMIAS	HYPOPROLIFERATIVE ANEMIAS
RI >3 or ARC >100,000	*RI <3 or ARC <100,000*
Bone marrow damage, marrow aplasia	Blood loss
Renal disease	Hemolysis
Inflammation, chronic infections	Hemoglobinopathies
Iron deficiency	Red cell membrane abnormality
Thalassemia	Therapeutic response to treatment of iron/B$_{12}$/folate deficiency
Sideroblastic anemia	
B$_{12}$ deficiency	
Folate deficiency	
Refractory anemia	
Drug toxicity	

ARC, absolute reticulocyte count; RI, reticulocyte index.

level is appropriate then a presumptive diagnosis of EPO resistance is considered. Patients with anemia caused by decreased EPO production (eg, renal insufficiency) respond well to EPO administration. Similarly, patients with anemia of chronic disease also respond to EPO administration (albeit, the response is less robust).

PERIPHERAL BLOOD SMEAR

- The peripheral smear is a useful tool in the evaluation of anemia (Table 60–4). Review of the peripheral smear may reveal red cell fragments (hemolytic anemia), rouleaux formation (myeloma), and nucleated red cells (marrow infiltration). Commonly encountered red cell morphologies such as microcytic hypochromic red cells suggest iron deficiency or thalassemia. Macrocytic red cells suggest an underlying megaloblastic anemia.

BONE MARROW EXAMINATION

- In some patients, a bone marrow examination is necessary to establish the diagnosis (eg, patients with refractory anemia). Using local anesthesia and sterile technique, the posterior superior iliac spine is accessed and a bone marrow biopsy and aspirate obtained. The aspirate provides a rich source of hematopoietic cells that are subjected to morphologic analysis. The biopsy specimen is also a useful

TABLE 60–4   Significance of Findings in a Peripheral Smear

PERIPHERAL SMEAR	CLINICAL DISORDERS
Schistocytes, fragmented red cells	DIC, TTP, HUS, HELLP, severe burns
Nucleated red cells	Reticulocytosis
Rouleaux formation	Multiple myeloma, MGUS
Basophilic stippling	Lead poisoning, thalassemia, hemolysis
Sickle cells	Hemoglobin SS or SC disease, S-β thalassemia
Howell-Jolly bodies	Splenectomy, functional asplenia
Burr cells	Uremia
Spherocytes	Hereditary spherocytosis, autoimmune hemolytic anemia
Hypersegmented neutrophils	Pernicious anemia, B$_{12}$ deficiency, folate deficiency
Teardrop cells	Myelofibrosis, myelodysplasia, thalassemia
Target cells	Liver disease, hemoglobinopathies (ie, thalassemia)
Spur cells	Liver disease
Ovalocytes	Megaloblastic anemia
Bite cells	Unstable hemoglobin, glucose-6-phosphate dehydrogenase deficiency, and other oxidant-induced hemolysis
Intraerythrocytic inclusions	Malaria, babesiosis

DIC, disseminated intravascular coagulation; HELLP, hemolysis, elevated liver enzymes, and low platelet (count); HUS, hemolytic uremic syndrome; MGUS, monoclonal gammopathy of undetermined significance; TTP, thrombotic thrombocytopenic purpura.

tool to assess the overall cellularity of the bone marrow. Complications such as bleeding, infection, or pain can occur (although, uncommonly) at the biopsy site.

IRON-DEFICIENCY ANEMIA
Krishnamohan R. Basarakodu

EPIDEMIOLOGY

- Iron-deficiency anemia is the most common cause of anemia throughout the world and is the most common nutritional deficiency worldwide. In the United States, approximately 10% of women of child-bearing age and children <5 years of age are deficient in iron. Iron deficiency is also common in the patients greater than 60 years of age. The prevalence of iron-deficiency anemia in the United States varies widely by age, sex, and race. It is estimated that 2% of adult men, 9% to 12% of non-Hispanic women, and 20% of African American and Mexican American women are iron deficient. Iron deficiency is by far the most common hematologic disorder encountered in general practice.

ETIOLOGY AND RISK FACTORS

- Iron-deficiency anemia results from one or more of the following conditions:
  - Nutritional deficiency of iron
    - Vegetarian/vegan diet (which is low in iron)
    - Cow's milk rather than breast milk during infancy (cow's milk has a similar amount of iron as breast milk but the bioavailability is less)
  - Defects in iron absorption
    - Gastric bypass surgery
    - Gastric atrophy
    - Irritable bowel disease
    - Achlorhydria
    - Celiac disease
    - Medications that interfere with iron absorption (antacids, calcium and pancreatic enzyme supplements, tetracyclines)
    - Dairy products (phosphates)
    - Tea (tannins)
    - Phytates and phosphonates in vegetables
  - Increased demand for iron
    - Premature birth
    - Postnatal and adolescent growth spurt
    - Pregnancy
    - Lactation
  - Increased loss of iron
    - Gastrointestinal blood loss

- Genitourinary blood loss
- Child birth
- Trauma
- Surgery
- Blood donation
- Excessive phlebotomy
- Scaling skin disorders (psoriasis)
- Intravascular hemolysis
- Pulmonary hemosiderosis and Goodpasture syndrome
- Parasitic infestation (hook worm, amebiasis, *Helicobacter pylori*)

BIOLOGY OF IRON HOMEOSTASIS

- Dietary iron exists in two states: heme and nonheme. Ninety percent of iron consumed in the diet exists in the nonheme form, while 10% is derived from heme. Heme iron, found in animal protein, is better absorbed than nonheme iron. Nonheme iron is found in vegetables and some animal protein. Its absorption is enhanced by ascorbic acid while heme iron absorption is inhibited by dairy products, phosphates, phytates, and tannins in tea.
- Dietary nonheme iron exists in the ferric state, whereas, iron is absorbed in the ferrous state. Gastric acidity is essential for the conversion of ferric iron to ferrous iron prior to absorption. Ferrous iron is absorbed in the duodenum and upper jejunum by the divalent metal transporter 1. Heme iron is internalized by a heme carrier protein in the presence of an alkaline pH. Inside the enterocyte iron is released from heme by heme oxygenase-1. Iron is delivered to the basolateral membrane where it is transported to the interstitial space by ferroportin-1. Ferrous iron is then converted to ferric iron by hephaestin. Ferric iron binds to transferrin, a serum iron-transport protein and is transported into the circulation. Ferroportin is negatively regulated by hepcidin, an iron regulatory hormone. When iron is in excess, hepcidin binds to ferroportin, and the complex is internalized and degraded, which in turn prevents iron absorption.
- Transferrin transports iron to erythroid precursors that express transferrin receptors (TfR). Iron-bound transferrin binds to the transferrin receptor and is internalized. Iron is released and exported from the endosomal vesicle to the mitochondria by divalent metal transporter-1, where it is coupled with protoporphyrin to form the heme molecule. Heme then combines with globin protein, forming Hb. Transferrin receptors and transferrin are then recycled to the cell surface and circulation, respectively. Any remaining iron in the cell combines with the protein apoferritin to generate

ferritin. If the amount of apoferritin is insufficient, the remaining iron will be deposited and stored in tissues as hemosiderin. Iron can be mobilized from these storage deposits and transported back to erythroid precursors when needed.

- An additional source of iron is derived from senescent erythrocytes. Every day approximately 1% of senescent erythrocytes are phagocytosed by reticuloendothelial cells, mostly in the spleen. Approximately 20 mg of iron is released from the reticuloendothelial system (RES) into plasma each day where it binds to transferrin and is transferred to erythroid precursors for heme synthesis. Hepcidin also plays an important role in the release of iron from reticuloendothelial cells.

- Normal adult males have a total body iron content of 4 to 4.5 g and adult females have approximately 3.5 to 4 g. Two-thirds of the iron in the body is present as Hb in erythrocytes. Each milliliter of red cells (packed red blood cells) contain 1 mg of iron while 1 mL of whole blood has 0.5 mg. In males, 1000 mg of iron and in women 500 mg exist as storage iron, mostly as ferritin. Hemosiderin is primarily located within macrophages in the marrow, liver, and spleen. A small quantity of iron is present in myoglobin and cytochrome enzymes. Approximately 3 mg of iron is bound to circulating transferrin, which recycles approximately 10 times per day.

- Iron metabolism in humans is controlled by absorption rather than excretion. Iron is regularly lost from the body through exfoliation of intestinal epithelium, skin, bile, and through urinary excretion. There are no physiologic mechanisms that regulate iron excretion, therefore losses must be compensated for by an increased intake or absorption. Adult males and postmenopausal females lose approximately 1 mg of iron per day. Menstruating women lose twice this amount. During pregnancy, lactation, and growth, iron intake and absorption must increase. The normal diet is comprised of 10 to 20 mg of iron and approximately 5% to 10% is absorbed.

- When iron is required for erythrocyotis, the storage sites (mononuclear phagocyte system) provide the first-line of defense. Initially ferritin levels decrease and tissue and bone marrow iron is depleted. This is followed by a decrease in serum iron levels, and then total iron binding capacity increases. The density of transferrin receptors on erythroid precursors increases and the extracellular component of the transferrin receptor is shed into the circulation where its serum concentration increases two- to fourfold. With severe iron deficiency, red cells become microcytic and hypochromic and eventually pencil- or cigar-shaped cells are noted on the peripheral smear.

CLINICAL FEATURES

SYMPTOMS
- Often asymptomatic
- Fatigue
- Exercise intolerance
- Difficulty swallowing
- Headache
- Learning and behavioral problems in children

SIGNS
- Pallor
- Glossitis
- Esophageal webs
- Koilonychia
- Papilledema in infants
- Tachycardia with or without flow murmurs
- Cardiac decompensation (high output failure)
- Splenomegaly (rare)

LABORATORY FINDINGS

- Low ferritin level
- Low iron level
- High total iron-binding capacity (TIBC)
- Low transferrin percentage saturation
- Increased erythrocyte zinc protoporphyrin levels
- Low MCV, MCH, and MCHC
- Decreased bone marrow stainable iron
- Increased soluble transferrin receptor (sTf-R) levels
- Ratio of sTf-R to ferritin is usually >2.5
- Thrombocytosis (reactive)
- Elevated RDW

PERIPHERAL SMEAR FINDINGS

- Microcytosis
- Hypochromia
- Anisocytosis
- Poikilocytosis
- Cigar- or pencil-shaped cells and, rarely, target cells

CAVEATS AND CAUTIONS IN INTERPRETING LABORATORY RESULTS

- Ferritin is an acute phase reactant and its level increases in the presence of infection, inflammatory disorders, cancer, or liver injury. Serum ferritin levels greater than 100 μg/L are rare in iron deficiency and a level less than 12 μg/L is a highly specific indicator of iron deficiency.

- Serum iron, TIBC, and transferrin percentage saturation levels may be normal in early iron deficiency.
- Low MCV, MCH, and MCHC are seen only when iron-deficiency anemia is severe and has been present for weeks or months.
- Increased erythrocyte zinc protoporphyrin levels are found in both iron deficiency and lead poisoning.
- Increased serum transferrin receptor levels are not specific for iron deficiency and is also seen with erythroid hyperplasia (effective or ineffective erythropoiesis), myelodysplasia, myeloproliferative, and lymphoproliferative disorders.
- A bone marrow biopsy to establish the diagnosis of iron deficiency is rarely needed.

DIAGNOSIS

- Iron-deficiency anemia is characterized by three stages: (1) iron-store depletion, (2) iron-deficient erythropoiesis, and (3) iron-deficiency anemia.
- With iron-store depletion, ferritin levels decrease to less than 40 μg/L and sTf-R levels begin to increase. Bone marrow stainable iron decreases to near undetectable levels. Serum iron, TIBC, and Hb levels remain normal.
- With iron-deficient erythropoiesis, ferritin levels decline further to less than 20 μg/L, serum iron levels decrease, TIBC increases, and transferrin saturation is less than 15%. Stainable iron stores are absent and sideroblasts are reduced. Hemoglobin levels decrease slightly, but there is no change in red cell morphology.
- With the onset of iron-deficiency anemia, serum ferritin levels decrease to less than 12 μg/L. Serum iron decreases, TIBC increases and sTf-R levels are markedly elevated, and transferrin saturation decreases to less than 10%. Stainable iron and sideroblasts are absent. Hemoglobin levels decrease to less than 10 g/dL and red cell morphology changes. Microcytic, hypochromic cells appear in the circulation with severe iron deficiency; bizarre-shaped cells including pencil cells and target cells appear at this stage.

DIFFERENTIAL DIAGNOSIS

ANEMIA OF CHRONIC DISEASE

- In anemia of chronic disease, ferritin levels are generally increased, serum iron and TIBC are low, and the transferrin saturation usually exceeds 10%. The sTf-R levels are normal and the sTf-R/ferritin ratio is <2.5 (it

is >2.5 in iron-deficiency anemia). Stainable bone marrow iron is present.

THALASSEMIA

- In thalassemia, serum iron and TIBC are normal and the transferrin saturation is >20%. Stainable iron stores are strongly positive. A hemoglobin electrophoresis should establish the diagnosis.

SIDEROBLASTIC ANEMIA

- In sideroblastic anemia, the serum iron and TIBC are increased and bone marrow iron staining reveals characteristic ringed sideroblasts.

LEAD POISONING

- In lead poisoning, the blood lead levels are usually high, and on peripheral smear, basophilic stipling and target cells may be observed.

TREATMENT

- Packed red blood cell transfusions should be administered to severely anemic patients with symptoms of dyspnea, exercise intolerance, or cardiac decompensation or if they require surgery.
- The cause of iron deficiency should always be investigated and treated appropriately. It is preferable to treat iron deficiency with oral iron. There are several oral iron preparations available. Oral medicinal iron is always in the ferrous form. Ferrous sulfate is the least expensive preparation, and a 325 mg tablet contains 66 mg of elemental iron. Ferrous gluconate, ferrous fumarate, and polysaccharide iron complex are similar preparations with somewhat different iron composition. Enteric-coated or slow-release preparations may be better tolerated but are not absorbed as efficiently and are expensive. Iron should ideally be administered on an empty stomach to promote optimal absorption. The side effects of oral iron include epigastric distress, constipation, or diarrhea. Lowering the dose or consuming it with food decreases epigastric distress but retards the absorption. Constipation or diarrhea should be treated supportively. Ascorbic acid enhances iron absorption, accordingly, it is common practice to add 250 mg of ascorbic acid at the time of iron administration. One tablet of ferrous sulfate iron 3 to 4 times a day results in the absorption of approximately 50 mg of elemental iron.
- The reticulocyte count increases within 7 days of oral iron supplementation and Hb levels begin increasing by 1 to 2 weeks. If there is no increase in Hb after 2 weeks of treatment, suspect poor compliance, continued iron loss (bleeding), malabsorption, or an erroneous diagnosis.

As the Hb level increases the absorption of iron decreases. This tends to be associated with a relative flattening of the Hb dose-response relationship. Once the anemia is corrected, iron supplementation should continue for 4 to 6 months to fully replenish the stores. Iron supplementation is always provided during pregnancy.

- Patients with intolerable side effects to oral iron, impaired iron absorption or compliance, or those with ongoing blood loss may benefit from parenteral iron. There are three parenteral iron formulations available in the United States: iron dextran, iron sucrose, and sodium ferric gluconate. After parenteral administration, the iron-carbohydrate complex is metabolized by the RES and iron is released into circulation. Transferrin transports the liberated iron to the liver, spleen, and bone marrow.

Iron Dextran

- Iron dextran is the only preparation that can be given intravenously or intramuscularly. Iron dextran can, theoretically, be administered as a single dose to restore the patient's iron status to normal (total dose infusion). However, the disadvantages to this preparation include a 2% to 3% incidence of serious adverse effects including anaphylactic reactions and delayed hypersensitivity reactions (after 24 to 48 hours). The delayed reaction is characterized by myalgia, arthralgia, headache, and malaise. The allergic reactions are believed to be dependent on the dextran component. A test dose is required before administering iron dextran. Moreover, the release of iron is modest and requires weeks to elicit a biological response. Intramuscular injection produces pain and staining of skin at the injection site and is associated with erratic delivery and absorption.

Sodium Ferric Gluconate

- Sodium ferric gluconate is given intravenously, and up to 80% of the iron is available for transport by transferrin within 24 hours. Anaphylactic or delayed reactions are negligible and a test dose is not required. A maximum of 125 mg of iron can be administered at one time. Therefore, it is usually given as 8 weekly doses.

Iron Sucrose

- Iron sucrose is given intravenously. Anaphylactic reactions are negligible and a test dose is not required. A maximum of 100 mg of iron can be given at one time and can also be repeated weekly as required. The iron deficit is calculated based on the fact that 1 gm of hemoglobin contains 3.3 mg of elemental iron. The manufacturers package insert should be consulted prior to administering iron parenterally.

ANEMIA OF CHRONIC DISEASE
Rajesh R. Nair

INTRODUCTION

- Anemia of chronic disease is also termed *anemia of chronic inflammation.* It is associated with infectious diseases, neoplasia, connective tissue diseases, heart disease, trauma, and diabetes and is characterized by hypoproliferative, normocytic, and normochromic RBC indices (Table 60–5).
- It is the second most prevalent cause of anemia after iron-deficiency anemia.
- The pathogenesis of anemia of chronic disease is characterized by perturbations in iron transport and cellular uptake. For example, iron is diverted from the circulation into storage sites (rather than RBC precursors) leading to iron-restricted erythropoiesis.

PATHOPHYSIOLOGY

- The underlying inflammatory medical condition induces the release of cytokines including interleukins and tumor necrosis factor (TNF). Overall these mediators alter iron disposition, interfere with the synthesis or action of erythropoietin, and attenuate the life span of red cells, resulting in anemia.
- The proliferation and differentiation of erythroid precursors, erythroid burst-forming units, and erythroid colony-forming units are impaired, which, in turn, is related to the deleterious effects of interferon (IFN)-α, IFN-β, IFN-γ, TNF-α, and interleukin-1. Interferon-γ appears to be the most potent inhibitor of erythropoiesis.
- Tumor cells that secrete proinflammatory cytokines damage erythroid progenitor cells. In addition, tumors may aggravate anemia by promoting blood loss, inducing malnutrition/malabsorption (vitamin deficiencies), inducing hypersplenism, stimulating autoantibody production (autoimmune hemolysis in chronic lymphocytic

TABLE 60–5   Causes of Anemia of Chronic Disease

Infection
Viral infection, human immunodeficiency virus
Bacterial
Parasitic
Fungal
Cancer
Hematologic
Solid tumor
Autoimmune
Rheumatoid arthritis
Systemic lupus erythematosus
Sarcoidosis
Vasculitis
Chronic kidney disease

leukemia), interfering with renal function, and producing marrow suppression via the intrinsic effects of chemotherapy and radiation.

- Erythropoietin synthesis is inversely proportional to tissue oxygenation and Hb levels. Although the erythropoietin level may be increased in anemia of chronic disease, it is insufficient to sustain normal erythropoiesis. Importantly, several cytokines appear to down-regulate the erythropoietin receptor resulting in a blunted erythropoietin response.
- Iron is acquired by the macrophage by erythrophagocytosis and the transmembrane uptake of ferrous iron by the protein divalent metal transporter 1 (DMT1). In contrast, ferroportin is a transmembrane exporter of iron. Interferon γ, lipopolysaccharide, and TNF-α up-regulate the expression of divalent metal transporter 1, and down-regulate the expression of ferroportin causing iron to be effectively trapped in the macrophage. Iron trapped in the macrophage leads to a *de facto* state of iron deficiency.
- Cytokines also exert direct toxic effects on progenitor cells by inducing the formation of labile free radicals such as superoxide anion.
- Infiltration and growth of tumor cells or microorganisms wthin the bone marrow, (human immunodeficiency virus infection, hepatitis C, and malaria) may also produce anemia.
- Anemia associated with chronic kidney disease is chiefly secondary to decreased synthesis of erythropoietin. However, the uremic state itself may also impair erythropoiesis.

THE ROLE OF HEPCIDIN

- Hepcidin is an acute phase protein composed of 25 amino acids, which is directly involved in iron homeostasis (see Biology of Iron Homeostasis).
- Hepcidin decreases iron absorption in the small intestine, and mobilization from the placenta and macrophage. Hepcidin binds to ferroportin and induces internalization and degradation of the complex, thus preventing iron absorption or mobilization. Interleukin-6 appears to play an important role in regulating hepcidin and by extension is likely involved in the pathogenesis of the anemia associated with chronic inflammation
- Interestingly, hepcidin knockout mice develop severe iron overload (hemosiderosis).

LABORATORY EVALUATION

- In both anemia of chronic disease and iron-deficiency anemia, the serum concentration of iron and transferrin saturation are reduced, reflecting absolute iron deficiency or hypoferremia (accumulation of iron in the RES) in iron deficiency anemia or the anemia of chronic disease, repectively.
- In chronic disease, the decrease in transferrin saturation primarily reflects a decrease in serum iron. In iron-deficiency anemia, transferrin saturation also reflects an increase in transferrin. Transferrin levels are usually decreased in anemia of chronic disease.
- The search for an underlying cause of iron deficiency should include a detailed history to rule out a dietary cause. Frequently, iron deficiency indicates pathological blood loss such as dysfunctional uterine bleeding in women or chronic gastrointestinal bleeding from peptic ulcer disease, duodenal ulcer, inflammatory bowel disease, angiodysplasia, intestinal adenomas, gastrointestinal cancer, or parasitic infections.
- The evaluation of anemia of chronic disease must also include a determination of the status of whole-body iron to rule out iron-deficiency anemia.
- Ferritin is used as a marker of iron storage, and a level <15 ng/mL is generally assumed to reflect absent iron stores.
- A ferritin level of >30 ng/mL provides a positive predictive value of (92%–98%) in the evaluation of iron deficiency anemia.
- Patients with anemia of chronic disease, typically exhibit normal or increased ferritin levels, reflecting increased storage and retention of iron within the RES.
- The serum ferritin concentration, must be interpreted cautiously in chronic inflammatory diseases because ferritin is also an acute phase reactant.
- Examination of the bone marrow for iron content and distribution of iron may prove useful. In the ACD, bone marrow macrophages contain normal or increased quantities of storage iron, whereas erythroid precursors reveal decreased or absent iron staining.
- The soluble transferrin receptor is a truncated fragment of the membrane receptor that is shed into the circulation in iron deficiency. In contrast, levels of soluble transferrin receptors in ACD are not usually increased, in part, because transferrin-receptor expression is decreased by pro-inflammatory cytokines.
- A determination of soluble transferrin receptor levels by means of commercially available assays can distinguish patients with anemia of chronic disease from patients iron deficiency (characterized by reduced ferritin levels and high levels of soluble transferrin receptors).

TABLE 60–6   Iron Studies in the Evaluation of Anemia of Chronic Disease Versus Iron Deficiency Anemia

VARIABLE	ANEMIA OF CHRONIC DISEASE	IRON DEFICIENCY	COMBINED DEFICIENCY
Iron	Decreased	Decreased	Decreased
Transferrin	Decreased	Increased	Variable
Transferrin sat	Low	Very low	Low
Ferritin	Increased	Decreased	Variable
Soluble transferrin receptor	Normal	Increased	Variable
Ratio of soluble transferrin receptor to log ferritin	<1	>2	>2

- The ratio of the concentration of soluble transferrin receptor to the log of the ferritin level may also be helpful. A ratio of less than 1 suggests anemia of chronic disease, whereas a ratio of greater than 2 suggests absolute iron deficiency coexisting with anemia of chronic disease (Table 60–6).
- Anemia of chronic disease is characterized by a normochromic, normocytic anemia; and a low reticulocyte count.
- Measurement of erythropoietin levels is useful only for anemic patients with Hb levels of less than 10 g/dL, because erythropoietin levels at higher Hb concentrations remain well within the normal range.
- The ACD is usually accompanied by an elevation in acute phase reactants such as fibrinogen and C-reactive protein.

TREATMENT

RATIONALE FOR TREATMENT

- Anemia of chronic disease remains underrecognized and undertreated.
- ACD causes a compensatory increase in cardiac output to maintain systemic oxygen delivery. ACD is associated with a poor prognosis in a variety of conditions including coronary artery disease, pulmonary disease, and chronic kidney disease.
- In patients with renal failure who are receiving dialysis and in patients with cancer who are undergoing chemotherapy, correction of the anemia to a Hb level of 11-12 g/dL is associated with an improvement in the quality of life.
- Anemia has been associated with a relatively poor prognosis among patients with chronic kidney disease.
  - For example, dialysis patients with a Hb level of <8 g/dL are associated with a doubling of the odds

of death, as compared with a Hb level of 10 to 11 g/dL.
  - Hematocrit levels that are maintained between 33% and 36% are associated with the lowest risk of death among patients undergoing dialysis.

GENERAL ASPECTS IN TREATMENT

- Guidelines recommend that the target Hb be approximately 11 to 12 g/dL in patients with cancer or chronic kidney disease (somewhat higher in kidney disease).
  - Importantly, recent studies suggest that attempts to normalize the hematocrit in these settings are associated with a poor prognosis. One prospective, multicenter trial involving patients who underwent dialysis designed to achieve normal HCT levels (more than 42%), as compared with lower levels (more than 30%), with the use of a combination of erythropoietin therapy and intravenous iron dextran was halted because of increased mortality in the high-HCT cohort.
  - Intravenous iron should be administered in ACD if the response to erythropoietin is suboptimal.

TREATMENT OPTIONS

- Transfusion:
  - Blood transfusions are widely used as a rapid and effective therapeutic intervention. Transfusions are particularly helpful in patients with severe anemia (in which the Hb is less than 8.0 g/dL) or life-threatening anemia (in which the Hb is less than 6.5 g/dL), particularly when the condition is aggravated by complications such as bleeding.
  - Blood-transfusion therapy has been associated with increased survival rates in anemic patients with myocardial infarction, but transfusion itself has also been linked to increased mortality in patients who are critically ill. The exact role of erythropoiesis stimulating agents in this setting remains controversial.
  - It is important to recognize that the latest guidelines for the management of ACD in patients with cancer or chronic kidney disease do not recommend regular blood transfusion therapy in their management algorithms because of the risks associated with transfusion therapy, such as iron overload and sensitization to human leukocyte antigens.
  - The preferred therapy for ACD is directed toward correction of the underlying disorder, rather than replacement therapy with red cell transfusions.
- Iron therapy:
  - Oral iron is poorly absorbed in ACD because of down-regulation of ferroportin in the duodenum. In addition, iron therapy for ACD is controversial.

○ For example, iron is an essential nutrient for proliferating microorganisms, and the sequestration of iron into the RES is believed to represent a defense strategy to inhibit the growth of pathogens.

○ Nonetheless iron supplementation should be considered for patients who are unresponsive to therapy with erythropoietic agents because of functional iron deficiency.

○ In addition to absolute iron deficiency accompanying ACD, functional iron deficiency develops under conditions of intense erythropoiesis.

○ Parenteral iron has been shown to augment the erythropoietic response to erythropoiesis stimulating agents in patients with cancer who are undergoing chemotherapy and in patients undergoing dialysis even when iron stores appear adequate (normal ferritin and transferrin saturation). In particular, it is advisable to administer parenteral iron to dialysis patients with a ferritin of <200 ng/mL and a transferrin saturation of <25%.

○ Iron therapy is currently not recommended for patients with anemia of chronic disease who have a high or normal ferritin level (greater than 100 ng/mL), owing to possible adverse outcomes in this setting (see chronic kidney disease exception above).

• Erythropoietic agents:

○ Erythropoietic agents are currently approved for use in the ACD that accompanies chemotherapy, chronic kidney disease, and infection with human immunodeficiency virus (HIV) undergoing myelosuppressive therapy.

○ The percentage of patients with anemia of chronic disease who respond to therapy with erythropoietic agents is 25% in the myelodysplastic syndromes, 80% in multiple myeloma, and up to 95% in rheumatoid arthritis and chronic kidney disease.

○ Three erythropoietic agents are currently available— epoetin-α, epoetin-β, and darbepoetin-α, which differ in terms of their pharmacokinetic and pharmacodynamic properties eg, receptor-binding affinity, and serum half-life (Table 60–7).

○ Erythropoietin can exert additional biologic effects. It exerts an antiinflammatory effect in rheumatoid arthritis, resulting in a reduction of disease activity (mechanism unknown).

○ Additionally, the erythropoietic agents inhibit apoptosis and may promote cell growth and proliferation. These effects may inhibit cell death after organ injury (spinal cord injury, kidney damage, or liver disease). Conversely, these progrowth effects may prove undesirable. For example, a recent study

TABLE 60–7   Package Insert Dosing Schedule Erythropoietic Agents and Titration

STARTING DOSE	DOSING ADJUSTMENTS
Epoetin-α 150 U/kg subcutaneously three times weekly	Increase dose to 300 U/kg subcutaneously three times weekly
Epoetin-α 40,000 U/kg subcutaneously every week	Increase epoetin alfa to 60,000 U/kg subcutaneously weekly
Darbepoetin 2.25 µg/kg subcutaneously every week or darbepoetin 500 µg subcutaneously every 3 weeks	Increase dose to 4.5 µg subcutaneously weekly

If hemoglobin increases by 1 g/dL in 2-week period, dose should be reduced by 25%.
If hemoglobin exceeds 13 g/dL, hold therapy, reinitiate therapy when hemoglobin decreases to less than 12 g/dL at 25% dose reduction.

investigating the effect of therapy with epoetin on the clinical course of patients with metastatic breast carcinoma was discontinued because of a trend toward higher mortality among patients receiving the drug.

○ A double-blind prospective study investigating whether target Hb levels greater than 13 g/dL for women and greater than 14 g/dL for men improved regional tumor control among patients undergoing radiation therapy for squamous-cell carcinoma of the head or neck showed a recurrence rate among patients who were treated with epoetin that was higher than that among patients treated with placebo.

○ Thus, these agents should be used with caution in patients with these tumors. The FDA currently recommends a target Hb level of 11 to 12 g/dL in patients with an underlying malignancy.

MONITORING THERAPY

• Before initiation of therapy with an erythropoietic agent, iron deficiency should be treated.

• The Hgb response to administration of an erythropoietic agent, should be determined after 4 weeks of therapy and at intervals of 2 to 4 weeks thereafter.

• If the Hb level increases by less than 1 g/dL, the iron status should be reevaluated and iron supplementation considered. If iron-restricted erythropoiesis is not present, a 50% escalation in the dose of the erythropoietic agent is reasonable (Table 60–7).

• The dose of the erythropoietic agent will require adjustment once the Hb concentration reaches 12 g/dL.

• If no response is achieved after 8 weeks of optimal dosage in the absence of iron deficiency, a patient is

TABLE 60–8 Adverse Effects of Erythropoietic Therapy

Hypertension
- Blood pressure should be controlled prior to initiating therapy.
- Seizures have been reported in chronic renal failure patients.

Thrombosis
- High target hemoglobin (42 ± 3%) is associated with increased mortality and an increased incidence of vascular events.
- The hemoglobin target should be <12 g/dL to decrease the risk of thrombosis.

Pure red cell aplasia
- Between 1998 and 2004, almost 200 cases of PRCA were reported in patients treated with erythropoietin. More than 90% of cases occurred with Eprex, an epoetin α product used outside the United States.
- Patients who develop resistance to erythropoietic drugs should be evaluate for PRCA.

PRCA, pure red cell aplasia.

considered unresponsive to erythropoietic agents. Other conditions that may contribute to a poor response should be reviewed and managed aggressively (inflammatory disorders, uremia).
- The complications of erythropoiesis stimulating agents are summarized in Table 60–8.

MEGALOBLASTIC ANEMIA
Scott W. McGee

- The term *megaloblastic* describes the characteristic appearance of the red cell precursors in the bone marrow. Megaloblastic anemias are caused by impaired DNA synthesis. Because the MCV is elevated (>100 fL), megaloblastic anemias are classified as macrocytic anemias. Because of perturbed DNA synthesis, the nucleus and cytoplasm mature at different rates, giving rise to cells with large, immature-appearing nuclei and a normal cytoplasm. This is referred to as *nuclear-cytoplasmic asynchrony.*
- There are numerous causes of megaloblastic anemia, but by far the most common are folate deficiency, cobalamin (vitamin B_{12}) deficiency, and certain drugs. Any disorder or condition leading to a deficiency of one or both of these nutrients, or that interferes with DNA synthesis, can precipitate a megaloblastic anemia.

PATHOGENESIS

- Folate is a cofactor for the enzyme that converts deoxyuridine monophosphate to deoxythymidine monophosphate. The products undergo additional phosphorylation reactions, producing the deoxytriphosphate compounds (deoxythymidine triphosphate [dTTP], deoxyuridine triphosphate [dUTP]). When dTTP is deficient, dUTP is incorporated into DNA. The cell attempts to correct the base substitution, however, in the absence of dTTP, DNA fragmentation and cell death ensue.
- Cobalamin is a required cofactor for the enzymes involved in producing bioactive folate. Therefore, it is believed that cobalamin deficiency leads to megaloblastic anemia by engendering a deficiency of usable folate (the methylfolate trap hypothesis).

PHYSIOLOGY

- For normal adults, the daily requirement of folate is 50 μg. Foods rich in folate include green vegetables and fruits. The average daily American diet contains 400 to 600 μg of folate. Because some of the dietary folate may not be readily absorbed, the recommended daily allowance of folate is 0.4 mg. The total folate content in the average adult is approximately 5 mg. Therefore, when folate intake is deficient, megaloblastic anemia develops over a period of many months (>4 months). Folate requirements are increased when cell turnover or cell synthetic rates rise eg, hemolytic anemias, alcoholism, pregnancy, and lactation (6-fold increase). Folate is absorbed mostly in the proximal jejunum, therefore, clinical conditions that induce injury at this site may impair folate absorption (sprue).
- Cobalamin is synthesized from specific microorganisms. The dietary sources of cobalamin include meat, liver, seafood, and dairy products. Individuals not consuming these products must receive a cobalamin supplement to prevent deficiency. The average Western diet contains up to 30 μg of cobalamin per day, but only between 1 to 5 μg is absorbed. The average adult's total body cobalamin content is 2 to 5 mg. Because the average daily losses of cobalamin amount to less than 0.1% of the body pool, it may take years to develop cobalamin deficiency even with complete abstinence. The recommended daily allowance of cobalamin for adults is 5 μg.
- The absorption of cobalamin requires intrinsic factor, a glycoprotein synthesized and secreted by the parietal cells of the stomach. Additionally, gastric secretions contain R proteins, which bind cobalamin. Cobalamin in the diet is released via digestive enzymes in the stomach. Once free, the cobalamin is bound by R proteins in the stomach, and the cobalamin-R complexes are then degraded by pancreatic enzymes in the duodenum. The free cobalamin is then bound by intrinsic factor, and the intrinsic factor-cobalamin complex interacts with the intrinsic factor receptor, cubilin, and is subsequently absorbed. The terminal ileum has the highest density of cubilin.

GENERAL CLINICAL FEATURES OF MEGALOBLASTIC ANEMIA

- The symptoms of megaloblastic anemia parallel those of anemia in general: weakness, fatigue, dyspnea, and light-headedness. Pallor and jaundice combine to produce the classic lemon-yellow skin of megaloblastic anemia. Additionally, patients may develop a beefy, red smooth tongue, weight loss, thrombocytopenia, and neutropenia. Classically, the neutrophils have hypersegmented nuclei (>5 lobes).

COBALAMIN (VITAMIN B₁₂) DEFICIENCY

- In addition to the general features listed above, cobalamin deficiency can produce a neurologic syndrome that may precede the development of megaloblastic anemia. Importantly, the neurological manifestations require immediate treatment to prevent irreversible deficits. The initial symptoms are usually characterized by paresthesias of the fingers and feet along with a decrease in proprioception and vibratory sense. If left untreated, the syndrome can progress to spastic ataxia. The syndrome is caused by demyelination of the dorsal and lateral columns of the spinal cord. Dementia mimicking Alzheimer disease may also develop. *Megaloblastic madness* describes patients with cobalamin deficiency who develop psychosis.
- Diagnosis:
  - Serum B_{12} levels are almost always low. In borderline cases, serum methylmalonic acid and homocysteine levels can be measured; both are elevated in B_{12} deficiency. Once the diagnosis is established, the underlying cause must be determined. Anti-intrinsic factor and antiparietal cell antibodies should be quantitated to establish the diagnosis of pernicious anemia. Upper endoscopy may reveal an intestinal cause (malabsorption). The three-part Shilling test is largely of historical significance and is rarely used today.
- Treatment:
  - Treatment consists of vitamin B_{12} 1000 μg intramuscularly daily for 7 days, then weekly for 1 month, then monthly for life unless the underlying etiology is correctable. B_{12} administration produces a reticulocytosis within 5 to 7 days, followed by resolution of hematologic abnormalities in 2 to 3 months. The neurologic symptoms may not resolve, particularly if they have been present for a significant period of time.

FOLATE DEFICIENCY

- Unlike cobalamin, there is are no neurological abnormalities associated with folate deficiency. However, administration of folate to a cobalamin-deficient patient can correct the anemia but will have no effect on the neurologic features. Therefore, it is imperative to distinguish B_{12} deficiency from folate deficiency.
- Diagnosis:
  - Both serum and RBC folate levels should be measured. The serum folate reflects recent folate intake (preceding few days) and, therefore can be falsely normal after a single folate-rich meal. The RBC folate levels, which reflect folate turnover during the preceding 2 to 3 months, are a better indicator of tissue stores.
- Treatment:
  - Folate deficiency is treated with oral folate 1 mg/day. To prevent a relapse, treatment should be continued for at least 2 years.

DRUG-INDUCED MEGALOBLASTIC ANEMIA

- A variety of drugs have been associated with the development of a megaloblastic anemia (Table 60–9). Some drugs, such as zidovudine, may induce a macrocytosis without concomitant anemia. Offending drugs should be discontinued, if possible.

HEMOGLOBINOPATHIES
Huda Salman

INTRODUCTION

- Hemoglobinopathies are characterized by production of structurally defective Hb caused by abnormalities in formation of the globin portion of Hb.
- Structural Hb variants typically are based on a point mutation in a globin gene that produces a single amino acid substitution in a globin chain. Although most are of limited clinical significance, a few important subtypes have been identified.
- Homozygotes for HbC and HbS (sickle cell disease) will most likely have significant clinical manifestations, whereas HbE and HbD homozygotes may be mildly symptomatic or not at all. Diagnosis of heterozygotes may be important for genetic counseling.

TABLE 60–9   Drugs that Cause Megaloblastic Anemia

5-Fluorouracil	Methotrexate
6-Mercaptopurine	Neomycin
Acyclovir	Omeprazole
Arsenic	Pemetrexed
Azathioprine	Phenobarbital
Carbamazepine	Phenytoin
Colchicine	Pyrimethamine
Cytarabine	Sulfasalazine
Hydroxyurea	Triamterene
Lansoprazole	Trimethoprim
Metformin	Zidovudine (AZT)

- Thalassemia results from quantitative reductions in globin chain synthesis. Diminished β-globin chain synthesis produces β-thalassemias, whereas decreased α-chain production produces α-thalassemias.
- The severity of clinical manifestations in these disorders relates to the amount of globin chain produced and the stability of residual chains present in excess. The thalassemia minor syndromes are characterized clinically by mild anemia with persistent microcytosis. Thalassemia intermedia (ie, HbH disease), is characterized by a moderate, usually compensated hemolytic anemia that may present with clinical symptoms during a period of physiologic stress such as infection, pregnancy, or surgery. The thalassemia major syndromes produce severe, life-threatening anemia. α-Thalassemia major usually is incompatible with life; β-thalassemia major presents in infancy and requires lifelong transfusion therapy and/or bone marrow transplantation for successful control of the disease. Double heterozygosity for certain structural variants and/or thalassemia syndromes may also lead to severe clinical disease.

NORMAL HEMOGLOBIN STRUCTURE

- Hemoglobin is a tetrameric protein with four peptide chains: two α or α-like chains and two β or β-like chains. The amino acids in the globin polypeptide chain are assembled in a long convoluted knot within which lies the heme moiety, which carries a molecule of O_2. Heme iron is in the Fe^{++} (ferrous) form, and does not change its valence with release of O_2. Abnormalities that result in a change to the ferric (Fe^{+++}) form, results in a Hb molecule that has impaired O_2 carrying capacity (methemoglobin, HbM). The α_1/β_2 interface is an important region for the unique O_2-carrying function of Hb, and abnormalities in this area will alter Hb O_2 affinity. The areas of the molecule where the globin chains are in contact with each other or with the heme molecules are functionally important and have been highly conserved throughout evolution.

HEMOGLOBIN SYNTHESIS

Hemoglobin synthesis is directed by controlling genes that are switched on and off at certain stages of life, resulting in different globin chain synthesis at different stages. The genes controlling α-like globin chains are located on chromosome 16, whereas genes for β-like chains are located on chromosome 11. The switch from γ chain to β chain production starts at approximately the ninth gestational week, when Hb A becomes detectable. Fetal Hb synthesis declines but persists until 9 months of age, at which time the switch is complete. Accordingly, β chain abnormalities do not manifest at birth. A small amount of fetal Hb (1% or less) persists in adults in a small clone of cells referred to as F cells.

A third minor normal Hb seen in adults is HbA_2 (α_2/δ_2). Normal A_2 levels are 1% to 3%. The clinical importance of HbA_2 is that it is elevated in the beta thalassemias. To summarize, normal hemoglobins are comprised of HbA = 96%, HbF = 1%, HbA_2 = 3%.

CLASSIFICATION OF ABNORMAL Hb SYNTHESIS
1. Production of structurally normal, but decreased amounts of globin chains (the thalassemias)
2. Production of structurally abnormal globin chains (eg, HbS, HbC, HbE)
3. Failure to switch globin chain synthesis (hereditary persistence of fetal Hb, a condition that influences the severity of clinical manifestations of other hemoglobinopathies)

- Inheritance of all of the aforementioned disorders is autosomal codominant. Codominant is the most accurate terminology, because heterozygosity produces discernible but minor clinical findings.

THALASSEMIAS

DEFINITION
- Genetically decreased globin chain synthesis results in thalassemia. Theoretically, there are as many types of thalassemias as there are types of globin chains. The most clinically relevant are the α- and β-thalassemias.

GENETICS
- The thalassemias are all caused by mutations in the globin gene cluster. The defects are numerous (more than 250 different mutations have been described), and include deletional or nondeletional mutations. These genetic mutations are best known for their geographic and ethnic clustering.

α-Thalassemias
- α-Thalassemias are characterized by decreased α chain synthesis. Deletion defects are most common, but nondeletional defects have been described. There are two α-globin genes per haploid genome; thus the abnormality can result from one to four gene deletions. No α-globin is produced by the gene in α0, and α+ is characterized by reduced globin gene product. Silent carrier state is characterized by a single gene deletion coupled with three intact genes; there is no clinical abnormality. The two-gene deletion produces a minor clinical condition with a mild hypochromic,

microcytic anemia, similar to iron deficiency. Deletion of three genes, or HbH disease results in moderate anemia that is hypochromic and microcytic; there is hepatosplenomegaly caused by extramedullary hematopoiesis. Deletion of all four genes is incompatible with life and results in hydrops fatalities or intrauterine death.

Diagnosis

- Analysis of the complete blood count reveals hypochromia, microcytosis, and mild anemia with two or three gene deletions. Confirmation of decreased α-chain synthesis is determined by globin chain synthesis measured in reticulocytes. Restriction fragment polymorphism is used for prenatal diagnosis. Decreased synthesis of α-chain results in an excess of non–α-chains, which are insoluble and form tetramers. These abnormal Hb tetramers can be demonstrated by the presence of red cell inclusions on cresyl blue stain and by Hb electrophoresis. Bart Hb (γ_4-tetramers) is found in the first few weeks of life and Hb (Fig. 60–1) H (β_4-tetramers) can be found in older patients.
- Because the genes for α- and β-thalassemia reside on separate chromosomes, they can be coinherited. Coinheritance of α-thalassemia can exert beneficial effects on the phenotype (clinical severity) of β-thalassemia as well as the structural hemoglobinopathies, for example sickle cell disease.

β-Thalassemia

- B-Thalassemia is associated with more than 200 point mutations and, rarely, by deletions. It is clinically heterogeneous because various genetic lesions impair globin-chain synthesis to differing degrees. However, genotypic variability at known loci is often insufficient to explain the disparate phenotypes of individual patients with the same genotype, and other genetic modifiers may exist.
- One β-globin gene carrying a thalassemia mutation manifests as thalassemia trait.
- Two β-globin genes carrying a thalassemia mutation, at least one of which is mild; one β-globin thalassemia mutation in combination with excess α-globin genes (less common) defines thalassemia intermedia. Thalassemia major is characterized by two β-globin genes carrying a severe thalassemia mutation.

PATHOPHYSIOLOGY

- Decreased β-chain synthesis leads to an excess of α chains, some of which are incorporated into hemoglobins that do not have β-chains, such as HbF ($\alpha_2\gamma_2$) or HbA$_2$ ($\alpha_2\delta_2$). Residual free α-chains form tetramers, which are quite insoluble. They accumulate and precipitate within red cells, leading to increased fragility and death. The RBC life span is thus shortened. The cells may also be destroyed within the marrow leading to ineffective erythropoiesis. The reduction in β-chains leads to decreased Hb content per cell, hypochromia, and microcytosis.

CLINICAL MANIFESTATIONS AND MANAGEMENT

- Children with thalassemia major present at approximately 6 months of age with anemia that can be severe and symptomatic.
- The anemia that is associated with thalassemia may be accompanied by ineffective erythropoiesis, with marrow expansion and extramedullary hematopoiesis in the liver, spleen, and other sites, such as bone (paravertebral masses). Transfusion therapy, which is the mainstay of treatment, allows for normal growth and development and suppresses ineffective erythropoiesis (Fig. 60–2).
- Transfusion-transmitted infections (primarily hepatitis B and C) are an important cause of death in countries where proper testing is unavailable.
- Iron overload results from transfusional hemosiderosis and excess gastrointestinal iron absorption. Iron deposits in the heart, liver, and multiple endocrine glands produce severe injury to these organs, with variable organ failure.
- The endocrinopathies can be treated with hormone replacement. However, the most serious result of iron overload is cardiotoxicity, for which chelation therapy is required. Individualization of doses of deferoxamine lead to fewer untoward effects (hearing loss, bone dysplasia); and development of oral chelators and combined chelation therapy has improved compliance and efficacy.

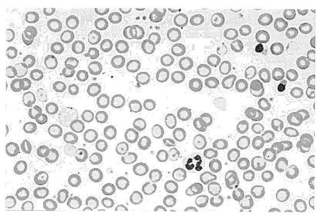

FIG. 60–1 Thalassemia peripheral smear.

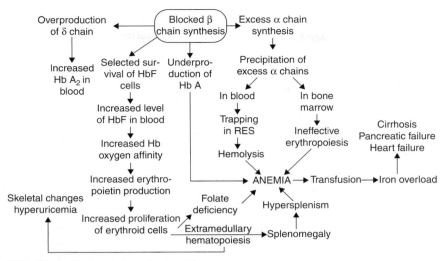

FIG. 60–2 Thalassemia pathophysiology.
Hb, hemoglobin; HbA$_2$, minor fraction of adult hemoglobin; RES, reticuloendothelial system.

- Thalassemia can be cured by bone marrow transplantation. Hematopoietic stem-cell transplantation with the use of related or unrelated donors is a viable alternative that generally results in an excellent outcome for low-risk patients. If transplantation is successful, transfusions, and usually chelation therapy, are no longer necessary. There is a small risk of serious complications (death, graft failure or rejection, and graft versus host disease). Furthermore, growth failure and endocrinopathies, particularly gonadal dysfunction, can still occur.
- All of the above factors, in addition to the availability of adequate support in various geographical regions, must be considered when deciding whether to perform transplantation in a particular patient.
- Experimental therapies to ameliorate the anemia that have been or are currently under investigation include fetal Hb modifiers and antioxidants. In the future, gene therapy or other molecular methods may be feasible.

STRUCTURAL HEMOGLOBINOPATHIES
- These defects usually result from a point mutation in the α- or β-globin gene, which produces an amino acid substitution in the polypeptide chain of the Hb molecule. This results in a functional abnormality whose effects depend on the location of the missense mutation. The mutation could produce the following:
  ○ No physiological abnormality or symptoms
  ○ An increased tendency to aggregate (HbS, HbC)
  ○ Instability of the Hb molecule resulting in hemolysis
  ○ Altered O$_2$ affinity (increased or decreased)
  ○ Decreased O$_2$ carrying capacity (HbM)
- There are more than 400 different abnormal hemoglobins described to date. Fortunately, most are rare and

cause no clinical disease. Sickle cell disease is a frequent and clinically relevant hemoglobinopathy.

SICKLING DISORDERS
- SS disease: homozygosity for the mutant HbS (no normal β-alleles, no HbA, also referred to as *sickle cell anemia*).
- SC disease: double heterozygosity for two β-chain mutants, HbS and HbC (no normal β-alleles, no HbA).
- Sickle β-thalassemia: double heterozygosity for HbS and β-thalassemia. One β-gene directs the synthesis of HbS, the other is either completely suppressed and the patient has no HbA (S β–thal) or incompletely suppressed and the patient produces a small amount of HbA (S β+ thal). HbA$_2$ is elevated in these conditions.
- SO Arab and SD disease: double heterozygosity for HbS and HbO or HbD, respectively.
- Hereditary persistence of fetal Hb with HbS, where there is a failure to switch from γ- to a β-chain synthesis coinherited with HbS. Patients have high levels of HbF and very mild clinical symptoms because of the protective effects of HbF.

Pathophysiology of Sickling
- In its deoxygenated state, HbS is extremely insoluble. Polymer formation within the RBC causes a shape change to the sickled form that gives the disease its name. Sickling is accompanied by increased rigidity, loss of deformability, increased adhesiveness to endothelial cells, and red cell membrane damage, all of which adversely affect the flow properties of the red cells through the microvasculature. This produces

vasoocclusion, which promotes a vicious cycle of stasis, tissue hypoxia, tissue acidosis, increased viscosity, further polymer formation, and further vasoocclusion which perpetuates the cycle. Membrane damage reduces the red cell life span to 15 days instead of 120 days, resulting in a hemolytic component.

Clinical Features

- All the sickling disorders previously mentioned are associated with similar clinical features; the double heterozygous states generally have a milder clinical course.
  - Hemolytic anemia results in pallor, jaundice, increased fatigue, gallstones, and growth retardation.
  - Aplastic crises may occur following viral infections, where there is transient marrow suppression resulting in a life-threatening fall in Hb synthesis.
  - Vascular obstruction from intravascular sickling results in episodic musculoskeletal pain, which is variable and unpredictable but can be disabling if frequent and severe. Although called *pain crises,* pain attacks are usually uncomplicated and not life threatening. Specific complications of obstruction include
    - Acute bone pain or infarction at all ages
    - Dactylitis, a swelling of the hands and feet, is a classic early childhood symptom.
    - Osteonecrosis of the spine and femoral heads is often seen in adults and commonly causes chronic pain.
    - Splenic sequestration crisis, a sudden pooling of blood in the spleen with hypovolemic shock, is a life-threatening and recurrent syndrome of early childhood.
    - Strokes are uncommon, but are often recurrent and associated with high morbidity. Ischemic and hemorrhagic catastrophes can occur in the brain.
    - Acute chest syndrome, pulmonary infarction, and/or pneumonia are common and indistinguishable from another.
    - Beginning in early childhood there is a lifelong risk of bacterial infections, which can be fatal. This is secondary to splenic infarction (autosplenectomy) from vasoocclusion and fibrosis.
    - Renal manifestations: There is often loss of urine-concentrating capacity caused by sickling in vessels around the loop of Henle; large volumes of dilute urine are produced even in young children, underscoring the need for copious fluid intake at all times to avoid dehydration. Other renal problems include hematuria and glomerular disease (nephrotic syndrome).

- Other manifestations of vasoocclusion include priapism, trophic leg ulcers, and blindness.
- The disease is extremely variable in its severity. Factors that affect disease severity have not been clearly defined and are the subject of considerable debate, but likely include:
  - Presence of genetic markers such as the β-gene haplotype
  - Coinheritance of α-thalassemia (beneficial)
  - Amount and distribution of HbF (higher levels are beneficial)

Sickle Cell Trait

- This is a benign, carrier state; and most individuals have no clinical symptoms. The incidence of the trait in African Americans is 10%. In certain tribal areas of India the incidence approaches 30%. Sickle cell trait can cause hematuria and loss of urine-concentrating capacity. Symptoms from intravascular sickling have been reported with strenuous exercise at high altitudes and flying at high altitudes in unpressurized aircraft.

Diagnosis

- The patient's clinical history and physical findings are extremely helpful.
- The presence of HbS is easily detected by the inexpensive and highly sensitive solubility test, even in the carrier state. Hemoglobin electrophoresis confirms the exact phenotype.
- The presence of hemolytic anemia (low Hb, high reticulocyte counts, bilirubin, and lactate dehydrogenase and morphologic sickling on peripheral blood smear).

Management Strategies

- Symptomatic and supportive care of complications such as pain episodes with analgesics, (often narcotics), local heat packs, adequate hydration, acid-base balance, avoiding hypoxia and exposure to cold, and treatment of febrile episodes early and aggressively with antibiotics.
- Judicious use of blood transfusions to prevent strokes in children, to treat pneumonia if there is respiratory distress, for severe anemia (Hb <5, usually with aplastic crisis or splenic sequestration), or during high-risk pregnancies.
- Early diagnosis can be established by screening newborns, and routine daily prophylactic penicillin and pneumococcal vaccine are used to prevent the high childhood mortality associated with infections.
- Psychosocial support and self-help groups are important for improved disease adjustment, especially for adults. Pain attacks are often capricious, severe, and frequent and can be an important barrier to self-determination and independent living.

- Recent advances in bench research have been applied to the management of sickle disease:
  - Agents that stimulate fetal Hb production such as hydroxyurea decrease sickling.
  - Bone marrow or cord blood stem cell transplantation from an HLA-identical sibling is a high-risk procedure that can be curative. It is used for certain high-risk individuals, such as those developing a stroke in childhood.
  - Antisickling agents such as membrane-active drugs are being tested in phase 2 and 3 clinical trials.
  - Gene therapy is being intensely pursued.

RARER STRUCTURAL HEMOGLOBINOPATHIES

The Unstable Hemoglobins

- These usually occur from amino acid substitutions near the heme pocket resulting in a Hb which is unstable. A prototype is Hb Zurich. The instability causes the heme moiety to separate from the globin chain after the slightest oxidative stress. The denatured Hb precipitates in the red cell and forms Heinz bodies, which promote splenic sequestration of the cells resulting in a hemolytic anemia.
- The diagnosis is established by demonstration of a hemolytic anemia, detection of Heinz bodies (by staining), and via the heat precipitation test. Hemoglobin electrophoresis is not always useful because of the tendency of the Hb to rapidly denature.
- One should avoid oxidant drugs, transfuse as clinically indicated, and splenectomize if the anemia is severe.

Hemoglobins With High O_2 Affinity

- The prototype is Hb Bethesda. The amino-acid substitution is near the $\alpha_1\beta_2$ interface, resulting in tight binding of O_2. Release of O_2 to tissues is delayed, producing tissue hypoxia. The hypoxia induces Hb synthesis because of increased erythropoietin levels.
- The diagnosis is established by the presence of familial erythrocytosis (polycythemia), exclusion of other causes of erythrocytosis (polycythemia vera, cyanotic heart disease), high red cell mass, high arterial O_2 saturation, and a markedly *left*-shifted O_2 dissociation curve.
- One should maintain the HCT <70% by phlebotomy to prevent hyperviscosity syndromes.

Hemoglobins With Low O_2 Affinity

- The prototype is Hb Kansas. The amino-acid substitution is also near the $\alpha_1\beta_2$ interface, but this results in decreased O_2 affinity. The Hb extracts O_2 poorly from the lungs, and deoxyhemoglobin levels increase, producing cyanosis.

- The diagnosis is established by examining the O_2 dissociation curve, which is *right* shifted. The Hb level and red cell mass are normal.
- No specific management is necessary or effective. The cyanosis is relatively well tolerated if strenuous activities are avoided.

Hemoglobins M

- The prototype is HbM Boston. The amino acid substitution is near the heme pocket, close to the site of the iron molecule. The mutant Hb cannot maintain iron in its ferrous state, and the resulting Hb is persistently detected as methemoglobin with impaired O_2 carrying capacity. This results in a chronic cyanotic state.
- The diagnosis is established by documenting a history of cyanosis since birth, with a normal O_2 saturation, brown discoloration of freshly drawn blood, and spectrophotometry to confirm the presence of methemoglobin. Electrophoresis also demonstrates the abnormal Hb. No management is required, because the quantity of HbM is insufficient to cause physiologic derangements.

Hemoglobins C, D, E

- These structural variants are synthesized at a lower rate than normal β-chains and comprise less than half the total Hb in heterozygotes. Heterozygous HbC (AC) produces target cells but no anemia. Homozygous C (CC) produces a mild hemolytic anemia, significant red cell morphologic changes (target cells, Hb crystals and microspherocytes), and mild splenomegaly. Heterozygous E (AE) causes a mild thalassemia phenotype with microcytosis and hypochromia. Homozygous E (EE) results in a moderate thalassemic phenotype, with significant hypochromia, microcytosis and a mild anemia. HbE migrates as HbC and HbA$_2$, close to HbO Arab on Hb electrophoresis (Fig. 60–3). A combined E–β-thalassemia inheritance results in a transfusion dependent thalassemic phenotype. Hemoglobin E is common in Southeast Asia and in certain areas of the Indian subcontinent.

PREVENTION OF HEMOGLOBINOPATHIES

- Premarital screening and genetic counseling is easy and inexpensive. It should involve nondirective genetic counseling for couples at risk and target populations with a high prevalence of the hemoglobinopathy traits.
- Prenatal diagnosis can be performed by chorionic villus sampling (CVS). Challenges include technical difficulties of the various methods used, as well as the expense. Furthermore, for safety and effectiveness, at risk pregnancies should be analyzed in the first trimester (8 to 14 weeks gestation). This requires

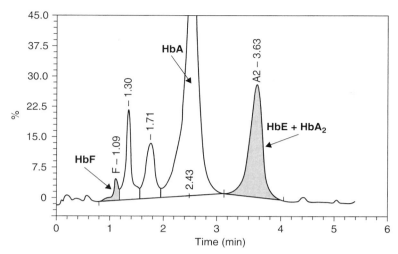

FIG. 60–3 HbE on Hb electrophoresis. Hb, hemoglobin; HbA$_2$, minor fraction of adult hemoglobin.

awareness-raising programs in communities with a high prevalence of the genetic defect. The choice of a therapeutic abortion for affected pregnancies can be difficult due to cultural and religious beliefs. Recent studies report a higher acceptance of prenatal diagnosis with a previously affected child. The costs of transfusion and chelation are prohibitive for families in developing countries. A useful strategy is universal screening for hemoglobinopathies among all pregnant women in high-risk areas of the country, initiated by midwives, who could also be trained to provide genetic counseling. Carrier women who are pregnant can then be referred for CVS to a local facility, and the sample sent to a tertiary laboratory for testing. Funding for this type of program, while expensive, can be cost-saving compared to the costs of treating the hemoglobinopathy.

• Preconceptional diagnosis and implantation of normal embryos after *in vitro* fertilization is an alternative that is currently available in the West. It is extremely expensive and cannot be recommended routinely.

• In-utero therapy using stem cell transplantation is an interesting and potentially exciting technology that could aid couples at risk not opting for termination. It allows for the relative non-immunocompetent fetus to more easily accept the stem cell transplant without graft versus host disease.

TRANSFUSION SAFETY IMPROVEMENTS

• The mainstay of care of patients with hemoglobinopathies continues to be blood transfusion support. Thus, transfusion safety is an important consideration,

particularly the avoidance of transfusion transmitted infections. Donor screening has long been in place in developing countries. The Indian Drug and Cosmetics Act of 1992 requires that blood collected for transfusions be tested negative for hepatitis B, HIV, syphilis, and malaria. However, using a less sensitive test like reverse passive hemagglutination is permitted; and the more sensitive enzyme-linked immunosorbent assay techniques are infrequently used. Thus, donor screening may be ineffective in some areas of the country. Other pitfalls are the use of expired kits and reagents and improper standard operation procedures. Numerous studies from India have indicated the risks of transfusion-transmitted infections.

• Simply changing from paid or *replacement* donors to voluntary donors can greatly reduce the prevalence of transfusion-transmitted infections. Such a change reported in the Japanese literature resulted in a reduction of transfusion-transmitted hepatitis from 51% to less than 15%. Other strategies recommended include reducing the use of inappropriate blood transfusions; increased use of self-donated units that are stored and auto-transfused for elective surgical procedures; use of intraoperative blood salvage techniques for surgical procedures; and effective, inexpensive testing of donors for infectious diseases. The development of central packaging of equipment, consumables, and data handling processes is important in controlling quality of procedures, thus making blood transfusions safer. An independent national monitoring body should perform monitoring of blood safety. Training of personnel who handle blood banking facilities is also important, particularly for the storage and transport of blood. Recent published studies from India have shown a slight decrease in the seropositive rate of blood donors for HIV and hepatitis B virus in the past 6 to 7 years. Seropositivity is consistently higher for *replacement* versus volunteer donors in these studies, suggesting the importance of encouraging a volunteer donor system.

STEM CELL TRANSPLANTATION

An improved technique of stem cell transplantation using HLA-matched sibling donors is now a curative procedure for the hemoglobinopathies. There is recent interest in nonmyeloablative stem cell transplantation, which has less morbidity and leads to chimerism in the recipient. This is still investigational in most countries.

HEMOLYTIC ANEMIA
Arun Rajan, Stephen L. Graziano

INTRODUCTION

- Hemolytic anemias results from premature destruction of RBCs and the inability of the bone marrow to compensate for the fall in RBC mass.
- Hemolysis can result from a wide variety of causes and RBC destruction can occur either within or outside of the vasculature (Table 60–10).
- Patients may present with nonspecific symptoms such as fatigue, dyspnea or palpitations, or with indirect hyperbilirubinemia or hemoglobinuria.
- A detailed history and physical examination is helpful in establishing the etiology of hemolysis. This includes a history of recent infections, exposure to drugs and toxins, as well as a detailed family history.
- Physical findings can vary considerably. In addition to pale mucosae, the patients may present with jaundice, splenomegaly, or peripheral edema.
- Laboratory studies include a panel of biochemical tests performed on peripheral blood and examination of the peripheral blood smear for characteristic morphological changes seen in RBCs. Flow cytometry can also be used to diagnose specific conditions such as paroxysmal nocturnal hemoglobinuria and underlying myeloproliferative or lymphoproliferative disorders.
- General principles of management include observation during mild hemolysis and transfusion support and consideration of splenectomy with significant hemolysis causing symptomatic disease. Specific maneuvers include steroid therapy in immune hemolysis and plasmapheresis for thrombotic thrombocytopenic purpura.

TABLE 60–10   Causes of Hemolytic Anemia

Hereditary hemolytic anemia

Red blood cell membrane disorders
 Cytoskeletal abnormalities
  Hereditary spherocytosis
  Hereditary elliptocytosis
  Hereditary pyropoikilocytosis
 Lipid disorders
  Hereditary stomatocytosis
  Hereditary abetalipoproteinemia
 Abnormalities of membrane antigens
  McLeod syndrome
 Abnormalities of membrane transport
  Hereditary xerocytosis
Red blood cell enzyme deficiencies
 Pyruvate kinase deficiency
 Glucose-6-phosphate deficiency
 Other enzyme deficiencies
Defects in the hemoglobin molecule
 Sickle cell disease
 Unstable hemoglobins

Acquired hemolytic anemia

Immune hemolytic anemia
 Warm-antibody hemolytic anemia
 Transfusion reactions
 Cryopathic syndromes
  Cold agglutinin disease
  Paroxysmal cold hemoglobinuria
  Cryoglobulinemia
Mechanical damage to red blood cells
 Macroangiopathic hemolytic anemia
  March hemoglobinuria
  Hemolysis caused by artificial heart valves
 Microangiopathic hemolytic anemia
  Hemolytic-uremic syndrome
  Thrombotic thrombocytopenic purpura
  Disseminated intravascular coagulation
  Vasculitis syndromes
 Mechanical damage caused by infectious agents:
  Malaria, Babesiosis
Red cell membrane disorders
 Spur cell anemia
Hypersplenism
Chemical and toxin-mediated damage
 Arsenic, copper, snake and spider venoms
Physical injury to red blood cells
 Radiation-induced damage
 Heat-induced damage
Paroxysmal nocturnal hemoglobinuria

CLASSIFICATION OF HEMOLYTIC ANEMIA

- Hemolytic anemias have been classified using a variety of clinical and biochemical features:
  ○ Hemolysis caused by intracorpuscular defects (abnormalities intrinsic to the RBC) versus extracorpuscular mechamisms (not caused by a RBC defect per se)
  ○ Hereditary versus acquired hemolytic anemia
  ○ Immune versus nonimmune mediated hemolytic anemia

PATHOPHYSIOLOGY OF SPECIFIC TYPES OF HEMOLYTIC ANEMIA

- Red blood cell enzyme defects:
  - Because the mature RBC has no nucleus, it depends on glycolysis for the generation of energy. Therefore, defects in the glycolytic pathway can compromise generation of adenosine triphosphate within the RBC and shorten its lifespan. The various enzyme deficiencies that have been described are pyruvate kinase (approximately 95%), glucose phosphate isomerase (approximately 4%), phosphoglycerate kinase, triose phosphate isomerase, and phospho-fructokinase (all very rare). These disorders are all inherited and most are inherited in an autosomal recessive pattern. However, phosphoglycerate kinase deficiency is a sex-linked disorder and affected males have severe hemolytic anemia. Most other enzyme deficiencies present as congenital non-spherocytic hemolytic anemia.
  - Glucose-6-phosphate dehydrogenase (G6PD) deficiency: This is the most common enzyme defect affecting the hexose-monophosphate shunt. Because of the absence of reduced glutathione, red cells in these patients are prone to oxidative damage. Hemoglobin within these RBCs precipitates when exposed to oxidative stress and forms Heinz bodies (hence the term *Heinz body hemolytic anemia*). Because the G6PD gene is located on the X chromosome, G6PD deficiency is also sex linked. Most patients with the disorder have a single or two base substitutions that alters the properties of G6PD, thereby affecting enzyme activity. Patients develop nonspherocytic hemolytic anemia, especially when exposed to drugs, toxins, or infectious agents.
  - Other enzyme defects include members of the hexose-monophosphate shunt such as glutathione peroxidase and 6-phosphogluconate dehydrogenase and enzymes of nucleotide metabolism such as pyrimidine 5′-nucleotidase.
- Defects in the Hb molecule (hemoglobinopathies): A wide variety of defects can involve the Hb molecule itself leading to a decrease in the RBC lifespan and premature destruction. These disorders include sickle cell disease, thalassemias, and hemoglobinopathies caused by unstable hemoglobins.
  - Sickle cell disease arises as a result of a point mutation resulting in the substitution of valine for glutamic acid at the sixth position of the β-globin polypeptide. The disease is inherited in an autosomal recessive fashion. In the deoxygenated state, the sickle Hb molecule forms intracellular polymers and alters the shape of the red cell. Because of aberrant expression of adhesion molecules on these red cells,

they also have an increased propensity to adhere to vascular endothelium.

  - Hemoglobin C disease occurs because of substitution of lysine for glutamic acid at the sixth position of the β-globin polypeptide. Red cells containing HbC are less deformable and hence more susceptible to fragmentation. As the red cell loses its cell membrane, it forms microspherocytes. Red cell lifespan is shortened and splenomegaly is often seen in these patients.
  - Unstable hemoglobins arise as a result of mutations that change the amino acid sequence of the globin chains. This compromises the structural integrity of the Hb molecule, resulting in its denaturation and precipitation within the red cell. When Hb precipitates, it forms inclusion bodies that can damage the cell membrane. These inclusion bodies appear as Heinz bodies on staining the red cell with specific dyes.
- Red blood cell membrane defects:
  - Hereditary spherocytosis: In approximately 80% of the cases the disorder is inherited in an autosomal dominant fashion and affects cytoskeletal proteins, primarily spectrin and ankyrin. Loss of the cell membrane results in the cell assuming a spherical shape. This makes it much less flexible and prone to splenic sequestration.
  - Hereditary elliptocytosis is an autosomal dominant disorder caused by defects in spectrin and erythrocyte membrane protein 4.1.
  - Hereditary pyropoikilocytosis is related to defects in the cytoskeletal protein spectrin. Red blood cells undergo lysis at approximately 45°C.
  - Hereditary stomatocytosis is an autosomal dominant condition with abnormal permeability of the red cell membrane to sodium and potassium. Some patients lack the erythrocyte membrane protein 7.2. Others may lack the Rh proteins.
- Paroxysmal nocturnal hemoglobinuria (PNH) is a clonal disorder acquired at the level of the stem cell. The affected stem cell has an inactivating mutation affecting the pig-A gene on the X chromosome. This gene is needed for the synthesis of a glycophosphatidylinositol anchor to which a number of proteins bind on the cell surface. Among these proteins are the decay-accelerating factor (CD55) and the membrane inhibitor of reactive lysis (CD59). Lack of these proteins results in increased sensitivity of the RBC to lysis by members of the complement cascade. Patients with PNH are more prone to venous thrombosis and may actually exhibit pancytopenia due to deficient hematopoiesis.
- Spur cell anemia: In patients with advanced liver disease, the RBC membrane consists of excess cholesterol

without an excess in the concentration of total membrane phospholipids. These conditions lead to the formation of spur cells and target cells, respectively. Spur cell membranes are less deformable than normal. Therefore, an increased proportion of these cells are destroyed in the spleen, leading to the development of hemolytic anemia.

- Immune hemolytic anemia: A large number of conditions can lead to the development of antibodies that damage RBCs resulting in immune hemolysis. The two key features of immune hemolysis are a shortened red cell lifespan and the presence of circulating antibodies directed against red cells.
  - Warm antibody hemolytic anemia is most often caused by immunoglobulin G (IgG) antibodies that develop in response to protein antigens. The antibody-coated red cells adhere to phagocytes and are destroyed. Complement activation can also lead to hemolysis. The various causes of warm-antibody hemolytic anemia include lymphoproliferative disorders (chronic lymphocytic leukemia, non-Hodgkin lymphoma), lupus and other collagen vascular disorders, infections, and drugs (described later). The degree of hemolysis in these patients varies considerably.
  - Cold-reactive antibodies usually develop against polysaccharide antigens and are of the immunoglobulin M (IgM) type. Polyclonal cold agglutinins can develop as a result of infections, most commonly infectious mononucleosis and *Mycoplasma pneumoniae.* Monoclonal cold agglutinins are associated with an underlying neoplasm such as lymphoma.
  - Paroxysmal cold hemoglobinuria is caused by the Donath-Landsteiner antibody that is directed against the P antigen and induces complement-mediated hemolysis. Unlike most cold-reactive agglutinins, the Donath-Landsteiner antibody is of the IgG type. Paroxysmal cold hemoglobinuria is associated with viral infections or may be autoimmune, although in the past it was associated with tertiary syphilis.
- Traumatic hemolysis: As the name suggests, it is caused by physical damage to the RBCs as they course through the vasculature.
  - Macrovascular hemolysis is most commonly associated with artificial heart valves. It may also be seen in individuals with severe aortic stenosis and those who have undergone an aortofemoral bypass.
  - Microangiopathic hemolysis is caused by RBCs that are damaged by fibrin strands or platelet aggregates in the microcirculation. Hemolytic uremic syndrome (HUS), thrombotic thrombocytopenic purpura (TTP), eclampsia, and disseminated intravascular

coagulopathy are among the conditions that are associated with microangiopathic hemolysis. Adenocarcinomas of the stomach, breast, and lung can also lead to microangiopathic hemolysis.

- Most cases of idiopathic TTP occur as a result of autoantibody formation against the metalloprotease ADAMTS13, which normally cleaves von Willebrand factor. Presence of large multimers of Willebrand factor leads to microvascular thrombosis, microangiopathic hemolysis, and thrombocytopenia. The classic pentad of TTP includes microangiopathic hemolytic anemia, thrombocytopenia, fever, renal and neurologic abnormalities. The peripheral blood smear demonstrates the presence of schistocytes. The reticulocyte count and lactate dehydrogenase levels are elevated and haptoglobin levels diminished. Coagulation parameters including the prothrombin time and activated partial thromboplastin time are usually normal.
- Hemolytic uremic syndrome is a thrombotic microangiopathy seen in children that is usually associated with a preceding diarrheal illness caused by a Shiga-toxin producing gram-negative microorganism. It leads to oliguric or anuric renal failure.
- Disseminated intravascular coagulopathy results from widespread generation of microthrombi within the vasculature when natural anticoagulant mechanisms are overwhelmed. Most commonly it occurs because of exposure of blood to tissue factor. Disseminated intravascular coagulopathy results in thrombocytopenia, reduced fibrinogen levels, elevated D-dimer and fibrinogen degradation products, and an abnormal coagulation profile with an elevation in prothrombin time and partial thromboplastin time.
- Drug-induced hemolysis occurs by three distinct mechanisms:
  1. Drugs such as α-methyldopa induce hemolysis by a mechanism similar to warm antibody hemolytic anemia. The drug induces formation of IgG antibodies directed against red cell antigens. However, there are no antibodies directed against the drug itself. The antibody-coated red cells are destroyed as a result of splenic sequestration, usually leading to mild to moderate hemolysis.
  2. Drugs such as penicillin act as haptens and form a complex with RBC surface proteins against which antibodies are formed. Immunoglobulin G antibodies predominate and red cells are destroyed as a result of splenic sequestration. Hemolysis is usually mild to moderate.
  3. Drugs such as quinidine incite antibody formation and form ternary complexes with the antibody and RBC membrane constituents. Either IgG or IgM antibodies may predominate and hemolysis occurs as a result of direct complement-mediated injury or

splenic and hepatic clearance of complement-coated red cells. Hemolysis is often sudden and severe resulting in hemoglobinuria.

- Toxin-induced hemolysis: Red cell damage can occur as a result of infections (malaria), heavy metal exposure (arsenic, lead, copper), and other environmental toxins (spider venom, bee and wasp stings). Physical agents such as 100% oxygen and heat can also result in hemolysis.

DIAGNOSIS

- A thorough history and physical examination can prove useful in defining the underlying etiology of hemolysis.
- Symptoms of anemia itself are nonspecific and include weakness, fatigue, progressive shortness of breath, dizziness, and extremity swelling.
- Some patients may develop jaundice or pass blood in urine.
- Patients may demonstrate splenomegaly on examination.
- Laboratory studies aid in diagnosing the underlying etiology:
  - Hematology panel: The degree of hemolysis determines the severity of anemia. Ongoing hemolysis is associated with a compensatory bone marrow response that is manifest as an increased reticulocyte index. However, if the bone marrow is hypoproliferative (eg, caused by marrow infiltration by cancer cells or during aplastic crises), the reticulocyte count maybe normal or decreased.
  - Biochemical tests: Hemolysis is associated with indirect hyperbilirubinemia, low or absent haptoglobin, and an elevated level of lactate dehydrogenase. With intravascular hemolysis, urine analysis reveals hemoglobinuria and hemosiderinuria.
  - Examination of the peripheral smear: Characteristic morphologic changes of the RBCs may prove invaluable in establishing a diagnosis (Table 60–11). In addition, the presence of atypical myeloid cells may suggest the presence of an underlying myeloproliferative disorder.
  - Other specific laboratory studies include the following:
    - Antiglobulin test: Helps establish a diagnosis of immune hemolytic anemia. The test is designed to detect the presence of immunoglobulin or complement-coated RBCs (direct antiglobulin test) or the presence of antibodies in the patients' serum that react with RBC antigens (indirect antiglobulin test). For the direct antiglobulin test (Coomb's test), the patient's RBCs are mixed with rabbit or mouse antibodies directed against human IgG or

TABLE 60–11 Morphological Changes in Red Blood Cells that Aid in Diagnosis of Hemolytic Anemia

RED CELL MORPHOLOGY	HEMOLYTIC SYNDROME (AND OTHER CONDITIONS)
Acanthocyte (Spur cell)	Spur cell anemia Abetalipoproteinemia Postsplenectomy Severe liver disease
Spherocyte	Hereditary spherocytosis Immune hemolytic anemia Hemoglobin C disease Posttransfusion Infection-associated hemolysis
Elliptocyte (Ovalocyte)	Hereditary elliptocytosis Myelodysplastic syndrome Thalassemia Iron-deficiency anemia
Schistocyte	Microangiopathic hemolytic anemia Hemolysis caused by prosthetic heart valves March hemoglobinuria
Target cell	Cholestasis and liver disease Hemoglobin C disease and Hemoglobin C trait Iron deficiency Thalassemia
Dacryocyte (Tear-drop cell)	Myelofibrosis Myelodysplastic syndrome Hereditary pyropoikilocytosis Hereditary elliptocytosis Severe iron deficiency Megaloblastic anemia Thalassemia
Echinocyte (Burr cell)	Renal disease Malnutrition Gastric cancer
Stomatocyte	Hereditary stomatocytosis Hereditary spherocytosis Alcoholic liver disease
Leptocyte	Thalassemia Obstructive liver disease
Sickle red cells	Sickle cell syndromes
Heinz bodies	Unstable hemoglobin variants Oxidant stress

complement. The presence of IgG or complement on the RBCs results in agglutination of the red cells, which constitutes a positive Coomb's test (Fig. 60–4). Antibodies in the serum can be detected by incubating the patient's serum with normal RBCs and then running the direct antiglobulin test on the sample. This is known as the indirect Coombs test.

- Flow cytometry: In addition to aiding in the diagnosis of an underlying myeloproliferative disorder, flow cytometric analysis is used for the diagnosis of PNH. A clonal population of cells deficient in CD55 and CD59 expression can be detected in this disorder.

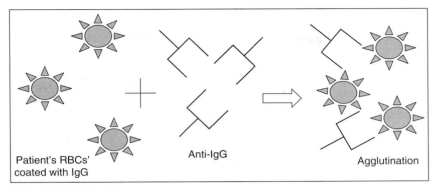

FIG. 60–4 Mechanism of direct antiglobulin (Coomb's) test.

- Enzyme assays: Specific enzymatic assays can help diagnose red cell enzyme deficiencies. Of note the test may be false-negative during an acute hemolytic episode if older red cells that contain the defective enzyme have already undergone lysis.
- Hemoglobin electrophoresis: Structurally abnormal Hb molecules such as HbS and HbC display a characteristic migration pattern on gel electrophoresis. Hence, this technique helps in the diagnosis of sickle cell syndromes.
- Heinz body preparation: Heinz bodies represent denatured globin that arises as a result of oxidative damage to Hb. They can be detected when peripheral blood is incubated with supravital stains such as brilliant cresyl blue and then examined under the microscope. They appear as stained inclusions close to the red cell membrane. The Heinz body preparation is useful in detecting the presence of unstable Hb variants, because they may not display an abnormal pattern on gel electrophoresis. Other tests used to diagnose the presence of unstable hemoglobins include the isopropanol stability test or the heat stability test.

MANAGEMENT (FIGURE 60–5)

- General principles of management:
  - Mild cases of hemolytic anemia do not need any specific therapy. If the patient is asymptomatic, blood counts could be followed closely to ensure hematological stability. If the patient is symptomatic, blood transfusion might be indicated.
  - Splenectomy could benefit many patients with symptomatic anemia, because the pathogenesis of many subtypes of hemolytic anemia involves splenic sequestration of red cells, leading to decreased RBC survival.

  - If a drug-induced etiology is suspected, the offending agent should be withdrawn and supportive therapy offered.
  - Autoimmune hemolytic anemia usually needs upfront treatment with steroids.
  - Certain subtypes of hemolytic anemia warrant specific treatment measures. An important example is TTP, which is a potentially fatal disorder unless it is rapidly diagnosed and treatment with plasmapheresis instituted.
- Treatment of specific subtypes of hemolytic anemia:
  - Red blood cell enzyme defects
    - Most patients do not need any specific therapy.
    - Blood transfusions can be considered in patients with severe anemia or bone marrow hypoplasia.
    - Folic acid supplementation at a dose of 1 mg/day is recommended in patients with severe hemolysis
    - Patients with pyruvate kinase deficiency may benefit from splenectomy. However, splenectomy is not as beneficial in other red cell enzyme deficiencies.
    - Because G6PD-deficient patients usually have self-limited hemolysis, offending drugs (oxidizing agents) should be avoided in these patients (Table 60–12).
  - Sickle cell disease
    - Management of acute pain crises: Patients should be well hydrated and often need opioid analgesics for optimal pain control.
    - Acute chest syndrome is a medical emergency needing aggressive therapy. If an underlying lung infection is suspected, empiric antibiotic therapy is reasonable considering the serious nature of this complication. Patients should be transfused to keep the HCT level greater than 30%. If the patient remains hypoxic, exchange transfusion can be considered.
    - For patients experiencing frequent complications, including repeated episodes of acute chest

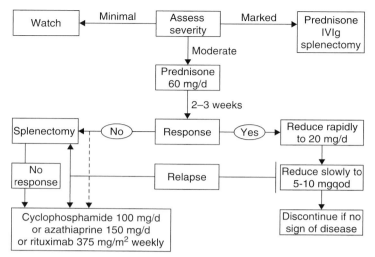

Source: Kasper DL, Braunwald E, Fauci AS, Hauser SL, Longo DL, Jameson JL, Isselbacher KJ: *Harrison's principles of Internal Medicine*, 16th Edition; http://www.accessmedicine.com

FIG. 60–5 Algorithm used to guide the treatment of immune hemolytic anemia.

syndrome, attempts can be made to increase the level of fetal Hb. This helps slow down the sickling process. The most extensively used drug for this purpose is hydroxyurea.

- Red blood cell transfusion is indicated in patients who develop symptomatic anemia, splenic sequestration, multiorgan dysfunction, or stroke. Chronic RBC transfusion might be beneficial in patients at a high risk for stroke.

○ Red cell membrane disorders
  - Hereditary spherocytosis: In symptomatic individuals, splenectomy leads to correction of anemia. Patients with symptomatic gall bladder disease should undergo cholecystectomy and splenectomy

TABLE 60–12 Drugs to Avoid in Patients With Glucose-6-Phosphate Dehydrogenase Deficiency

Acetanilid
Dapsone
Doxorubicin
Furazolidone
Glibenclamide
Isobutyl nitrite
Methylene blue
Nalidixic acid
Niridazole
Nitrofurantoin
Phenazopyridine
Phenylhydrazine
Primaquine
Sulfacetamide
Sulfamethoxazole
Sulfanilamide
Sulfapyridine
Thiazolsulfone
Toluidine blue
Urate oxidase

to prevent formation of intrahepatic gallstones. Individuals with chronic hemolysis and pregnant women should receive folic acid supplementation.
○ Paroxysmal nocturnal hemoglobinuria
  - Treatment of anemia: Prednisone can be used at a dose of 0.25 to 1 mg/kg/day to decrease the severity of acute hemolytic exacerbations. Androgens have also been used to treat anemia of PNH either alone or with steroids. Blood transfusion should be considered in the setting of severe anemia.
  - Folate supplementation is recommended in view of increased erythropoiesis in these patients. Iron replacement should also be considered if an iron panel suggests iron deficiency.
  - Eculizumab is a humanized monoclonal antibody against complement C5 that has been shown to dramatically reduce the degree of hemolysis in patients with PNH. It has also been shown to decrease the risk of venous thrombosis.
  - Paroxysmal nocturnal hemoglobinuria patients who develop venous thrombosis should receive lifelong anticoagulation. Selected patients considered to be at high risk for venous thrombosis could be considered for primary prophylaxis with warfarin.
  - The only curative modality for these patients is allogenic stem cell transplantation.
○ Immune hemolytic anemia
  - Patients with mild hemolysis can be observed.
  - If the degree of hemolysis is significant, corticosteroids are the cornerstone of therapy. For severe hemolysis, splenectomy should be considered (Figure 60–5). Of note, splenectomy has no role in the treatment of paroxysmal cold hemoglobinuria, because hemolysis is not extravascular.

- In cases requiring high doses of steroids to maintain stable Hb levels, or in those who are unresponsive to or relapse after splenectomy, treatment with intravenous immunoglobulin (IVIG), danazol, mycophenolate mofetil, or rituximab can be considered.
  - ○ Thrombotic thrombocytopenic purpura
    - ▪ Therapeutic plasma exchange should be instituted as soon as a diagnosis of TTP is made. For idiopathic TTP, corticosteroids are also usually started along with plasma exchange. Once the platelet count has increased to >150,000/μL for two consecutive days, plasma exchange can be discontinued and a steroid taper begun.
    - ▪ The anti-CD20 antibody rituximab seems to be beneficial in relapsed or refractory cases of TTP and autoimmune hemolytic anemia.

ERYTHROCYTOSIS
Michael C. Perry

- *Erythrocytosis* refers to any elevation in the number of RBCs, whereas the term *polycythemia* should be reserved for the myeloproliferative disorder polycythemia rubra vera (PRV) characterized by the expansion of neoplastic hematopoietic stem cells. The diagnosis should be considered when the HCT is >48% in a woman or >52% in a man, or when the Hb is >16.5 g/dL in women or >18.5 g/dL in men.
- Red blood cell production in humans is controlled by the trophic hormone erythropoietin (EPO); 90% of EPO is synthesized by the kidneys in response to hypoxia. In the kidney EPO-producing cells sense hypoxia through reductions in Hb concentration (anemia), reduced oxygen saturation (hypoxemia), decreased oxygen saturation from Hb (high O_2 affinity hemoglobins), or reduced oxygen delivery to the kidney (renal vascular occlusion). A negative feedback inhibition system reduces EPO levels with increased oxygen delivery. Therefore, EPO-independent production, as in PRV, suppresses EPO levels and EPO-driven erythropoiesis, characteristic of secondary erythrocytosis, is associated with normal or high EPO levels.
- Erythrocytosis may also be described as *primary* erythrocytosis (PRV) or *secondary* (all other causes) (Table 60–13). Secondary erythrocytosis can be appropriate, that is, a response by the body to hypoxia (such as that encountered at high altitudes), or inappropriate (no hypoxic drive exists). Finally, the number of RBCs may seem to be increased because of a decrease in plasma volume, creating a relative erythrocytosis.
- Relative erythrocytosis (Table 60–14) is usually caused by a decreased plasma volume with sparing of

TABLE 60–13 Classification of Erythrocytosis

Primary
Polycythemia rubra vera
Secondary
Appropriate
High altitude
Cardiopulmonary disease
Hemoglobinopathy
Inappropriate
Tumors
Renal vascular disease
Endocrine disorders
Familial or hereditary disorders
Relative
Plasma shift
Spurious

the RBC mass. This may occur through excessive sweating, hyperemesis, burns, diabetic ketoacidosis, diarrhea, fluid deprivation, or diuretics. Correction of the fluid loss corrects the Hb/HCT to normal values.
- Physical examination should concentrate on the presence or absence of cyanosis, clubbing, and pulmonary or cardiac disease, looking for possible secondary causes of erythrocytosis. Splenomegaly should raise the concern for PRV.

TABLE 60–14 Relative Erythrocytosis

Secondary to decreased plasma volume:
Sweating
Hyperemesis
Burns
Diabetic ketoacidosis
Diarrhea
Fluid deprivation
Diuretic
Spurious erythrocytosis
Clinical Features
Middle-aged males
Stocky
Tense
Symptoms
Headache
Dizziness
Increased sweating
Physical examination
Plethora
Hypertension
Blood
Increased Hct (rarely >60)
Normal WBC
Platelets
Other lab
Hyperlipidemia
Hyperuricemia
Cause
High normal red cell mass plus low normal plasma volume
Treatment
None (for the increased Hct)

Hct, hematocrit; WBC, white blood cell.

- So-called *spurious erythrocytosis* is seen in stocky, tense middle-aged men (35 to 55 years of age) who may complain of headache, dizziness, or increased sweating. On examination they are found to be plethoric and hypertensive. Their HCTs are increased, but rarely greater than 60; and white blood cell and platelet counts are normal. They may also have hyperuricemia and hyperlipidemia. The cause is a high normal red cell mass with a low normal plasma volume. No therapy is required for the increased HCT.

- Erythrocytosis is considered appropriate when it is the result of compensation to minimize tissue hypoxia (Table 60–15). This might result from exposure to high altitudes, cardiac disease (such as cyanotic congenital heart disease), pulmonary disease, or high-affinity Hb (abnormal Hb that does not release oxygen appropriately in response to tissue needs). Mutant hemoglobins with high oxygen affinity are often discovered by eliciting a family history and then performing the appropriate Hb electrophoresis. This compensatory erythrocytosis follows a benign course.

- The misnomer *smoker polycythemia* is an elevation in HCT in a chronic smoker. Smoking causes increased levels of carbon monoxide which bind irreversibly to the Hb molecule, inhibiting the release of oxygen to the tissues. This leads to hypoxemia and the resultant compensatory erythrocytosis. The diagnosis is established by confirming an increased red cell mass with decreased plasma volume, an elevated blood carboxyhemoglobin, and a left-shifted O_2 disassociation curve (Fig. 60–6). Cessation of smoking will correct the problem, if it can be accomplished.

- Secondary erythrocytosis is considered inappropriate in the absence of tissue hypoxia (see Table 60–15).

TABLE 60–15   Absolute Polycythemia

Appropriate secondary polycythemia

The result of compensation to minimize tissue hypoxia:
Altitude
Cardiac disease
Pulmonary disease
Abnormal Hb

Inappropriate secondary polycythemia

Renal lesions
Hypernephroma
Hydronephrosis
Cystic disease
Renal artery stenosis
Transplantation rejection
Bartter syndrome
Tumors
Hepatoma
Uterine leiomyoma
Cerebellar hemangioblastoma
Pheochromocytoma

Hb, hemoglobin.

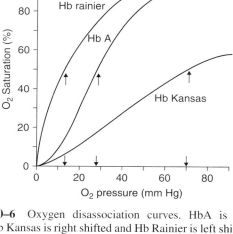

FIG. 60–6 Oxygen disassociation curves. HbA is normal, while Hb Kansas is right shifted and Hb Rainier is left shifted and less likely to release hemoglobin in the tissues. Hb, hemoglobin.

The mechanisms are usually renal in origin such as tumor, cyst, or obstruction, which leads to increased erythropoietin production. Additionally, extrarenal erythropoietin production by tumors such as hepatomas, uterine leiomyomas, cerebellar hemangioblastomas, and pheochromocytomas can produce erythrocytosis. Correction of the renal problem or resection of the tumor usually resolves the situation. Androgens and anabolic steroids can also produce an erythrocytosis.

- The key distinction to make in the patient with an elevated Hb is to separate primary polycythemia (PRV) from the myriad other causes (see Chap. 65, Myeloproliferative Disorders) (Fig. 60–7). It is advisable to first repeat the blood counts before initiating an extensive diagnostic evaluation. Historically, the evaluation of an elevated Hb/HCT began with the measurement of red cell mass and plasma volume via nuclear medicine techniques. This procedure is less commonly performed today. Investigation usually begins when the HCT is 56 or higher in a patient with normal plasma volume. An arterial blood gas and a serum erythropoietin level will help determine whether hypoxemia is contributing to the situation and may classify the process into primary and secondary causes. Although PRV is associated with low levels of erythropoietin (EPO) in greater than 90% of cases, secondary causes typically are characterized by elevated EPO values. An abdominal computed tomography scan can evaluate the liver, kidneys, and uterus, looking for tumors and renal abnormalities; if the issue is still unresolved, evaluation of the partial pressure of oxygen necessary for 50% binding aids in the diagnose of mutant hemoglobins.

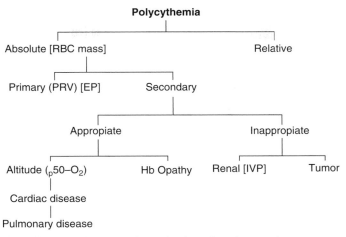

FIG. 60–7   Decision tree for evaluation of erythrocytosis. EP,; IVP,; PRV, polycythemia rubra vera; RBC, red blood cell.

- Recently, it has been shown that greater than 95% of patients with PRV harbor a mutation in the JAK2 gene. Several reference labs are now able to assay for the V617F mutation, and its presence in a patient with erythrocytosis is diagnostic of PRV.
- For treatment of PRV, please see Chap. 65, Myeloproliferative Disorders. For secondary causes of erythrocytosis, treatment is aimed at controlling the underlying cause (smoking cessation, resection of EPO-secreting tumors), and using phlebotomy for symptom management. It must be remembered when using phlebotomy in these patients that symptoms can be worsened if the HCT is reduced to the normal range. Conversely, significant improvement in symptoms can be achieved by small reductions in HCT. Therefore, the target reduction in HCT is usually modest and the target HCT for each patient is determined individually based on symptoms.

BIBLIOGRAPHY

Allen RH, Seetharam B, Podell ER, et al. Effect of proteolytic enzymes on the binding of cobalamin to R protein and intrinsic factor: In vitro evidence that a failure to partially degrade R protein is responsible for cobalamin malabsorption in pancreatic insufficiency. *J Clin Invest.* 1978;61:47.

Alperin JB, Hutchinson HT, Levin WC. Studies of folic acid requirements in megaloblastic anemia of pregnancy. *Arch Intern Med.* 1966;117:681.

Babior BM. Folate, cobalamin, and megaloblastic anemias. In: Lichtman MA, Beutler E, Kipps TJ, et al, eds. *Williams Hematology.* 7th ed. New York, NY: McGraw-Hill; 2006:497.

Berlin NI, Wasserman LR. Polycythemia vera: A retrospective and reprise [review]. *J Lab Clin Med.* 1997;130:365.

Beutler E, Hoffbrand AV, Cook JD. Hematology. *Am Soc Hematol Educ Program.* 2003;40–61.

Birgegard G, Wide L. Serum erythropoietin in the diagnosis of polycythaemia and after phlebotomy treatment. *Br Haematol J.* 1992;81:603.

Bolton-Maggs PH. Hereditary spherocytosis: New guidelines. *Arch Dis Child.* 2004;89:809.

Brown SM, Gilbert HS, Krauss S, Wasserman LR. Spurious (relative) polycythemia: A nonexistent disease. *Am J Med.* 1971;50:200.

Bunn HF, Rosse W. Hemolytic anemias and acute blood loss. In: Kasper DL, Braunwald E, Fauci AS, Hauser SL, Longo DL, Jameson JL, eds. *Harrison's Principles of Internal Medicine.* 16th ed. New York, NY: McGraw-Hill, 2005:607.

Butterworth CE Jr, Santini R Jr, Frommeyer WB Jr. The pteroylglutamate components of American diets as determined by chromatographic fractionation. *J Clin Invest.* 1963;42:1929.

Copelan EA, Balcerzac SP. Secondary polycythemia. Wasserman LR, Berk PD, Berlin NI, eds. *Polycythemia Vera and the Myeloproliferative Disorders.* Philadelphia, PA: WB Saunders; 1995:195.

Coyer SM. Anemia: Diagnosis and management. *J Pediatr Health Care.* 2005;19(6):380–385.

DiLazzaro V, Restuccia D, Foglia D, et al. Central sensory and motor conduction in vitamin B_{12} deficiency. *Electroencephalogr Clin Neurophysiol.* 1992;84:433.

Dunn LL, Rahmanto YS, Richardson DR. Iron uptake and metabolism in the new millennium. *Trends Cell Biol.* 2007;17(2):93–100.

Fairbanks VF, Klee GG, Wiseman GA, et al. Measurement of blood volume and red cell mass re-examination of Cr-51 and I-125 methods (corrected version of Vc666). *Blood Cells Mol Dis.* 1996;22:169.

Food and Nutrition Board. *National Research Council: Recommended Dietary Allowances.* Washington, DC: National Research Council; 1968.

Fraser TN. Cerebral manifestations of Addisonian pernicious anemia. *Lancet.* 1960;2:258.

Frenette PS, Atweh GF. Sickle cell disease: Old discoveries, new concepts, and future promise. *J Clin Invest.* 2007;117:850.

Gaziev D, Galimberti M, Lucarelli G, et al. Bone marrow transplant from alternative donors for thalassemia: hLA-phenotypically identical relative and HLA-nonidentical sibling or parent transplant. *Bone Marrow Transplant.* 2000;25: 815–821.

George JN. Thrombotic thrombocytopenic purpura. *N Engl J Med.* 2006;354:1927.

Gräsbeck R. Calculations on vitamin B_{12} turnover in man. *Scand J Clin Lab Invest.* 1959;11:250.

Hagedorn CH, Alpers DH. Distribution of intrinsic factor-vitamin B_{12} receptors in human intestine. *Gastroenterology.* 1977;73:1019.

Halstead CH. Folate deficiency in alcoholism. *Am J Clin Nutr.* 1980;33:2736.

Hedlund B. Hemoglobins of human embryos, fetuses, and neonates. In: Fairbanks VF, ed. *Hemoglobinopathies and Thalassemias.* New York, NY: Brian C. Decker; 1980:14–17.

Heidel F, Lipka DB, von Auer C, et al. Addition of rituximab to standard therapy improves response rate and progression-free survival in relapsed or refractory thrombotic thrombocytopenic purpura and autoimmune haemolytic anaemia. *J Thromb Haemost.* 2007;97:228.

Herbert V, Zalusky R. Interrelations of vitamin B_{12} and folic acid metabolism: Folic acid clearance studies. *J Clin Invest.* 1962; 41:1263.

Herbert V. Biology of disease: Megaloblastic anemias. *Lab Invest.* 1985;52:3.

Herbert V. Experimental nutritional folate deficiency in man. *Trans Assoc Am Physicians.* 1962;75:307.

Herbert V. Minimal daily adult folate requirement. *Arch Intern Med.* 1962;110:649.

Heyssel RM, Bozian RC, Darby WC, et al. Vitamin B_{12} turnover in man: The assimilation of vitamin B_{12} from natural foodstuff by man and estimates of minimal daily requirements. *Am J Clin Nutr.* 1966;18:176.

Higgs DR, Sharpe JA, Wood WG. Understanding alpha globin gene expression: A step towards effective gene therapy. *Semin Hematol.* 1998;35:93–104.

Higgs DR, Vickers MA, Wilkie AO, et al. A review of the molecular genetics of the human [alpha]-globin gene cluster. *Blood.* 1989;73:1081–1104.

Hill A, Richards SJ, Hillmen P. Recent developments in the understanding and management of paroxysmal nocturnal hemoglobinuria. *Br Haematol J.* 2007;137:181.

Hillman RS, Adamson J, Burka E. Characteristics of vitamin B_{12} correction of the abnormal erythropoiesis of pernicious anemia. *Blood.* 1968;31:419.

Hillman RS, Ault KA, Rinder HM. Iron deficiency anemia. *Hematology in Clinical Practice.* 4th ed. New York, NY: McGraw-Hill; 2005;12:53–64.

Hoffbrand AV, Newcombe BFA, Molin DL. Method of assay of red cell folate activity and the value of the assay as a test for folate deficiency. *J Clin Pathol.* 1999;19:17.

Hoffman PC. Immune Hemolytic Anemia-Selected Topics. *Hematology Am Soc Hematol Educ Program.* 2006;13.

Horne MC. *Iron Deficiency: Bethesda Handbook of Clinical Hematology.* Philadelphia, PA: Lippincott Williams & Wilkins, 2005;1–10.

Josephson CD, Su LL, Hillyer KL, et al. Transfusion in the patient with sickle cell disease: A critical review of the literature and transfusion guidelines. *Transfus Med Rev.* 2007;21:118.

Kahn MJ, Leissinger C. Underproduction anemias. *Am Soc Hematol Self-Assessment Program.* 2005;71–85.

Killip S, Bennett JM, Chambers MD. Iron deficiency anemia. *Am Fam Physician.* 2007;75(5):671–678.

Lawrence JN, Berlin NI. Relative polycythemia; the polycythemia of stress. *Yale J Biol Med.* 1952;24:498.

Lindenbaum J, Savage DG, Stabler SP, et al. Diagnosis of cobalamin deficiency: II. Relative sensitivities of serum cobalamin, methylmalonic acid and total homocysteine concentrations. *Am J Hematol.* 1990;34:99.

McMullin MF, Bareford D, Campbell P, et al. Guidelines for the diagnosis, investigation and management of polycythaemia/erythrocytosis. *Br Haematol J.* 2005;130:174.

Motulsky AG. Frequency of sickling disorders in blacks US. *N Engl J Med.* 1973;288:31–33.

Muirhead H, Cox JM, Mazzarella L, Perutz MF. Structure and function of haemoglobin. 3. A three-dimensional Fourier synthesis of human deoxyhaemoglobin at 5.5 Angstrom resolution. *J Mol Biol.* 1967;28:117–156.

Olivieri NF. The [beta]-thalassemias. *N Engl J Med.* 1999;341: 99–109.

Parker C, Omine M, Richards S, et al. Diagnosis and management of paroxysmal nocturnal hemoglobinuria. *Blood.* 2005; 106:3699.

Pauling L, Itano HA, Singer SJ, et al. Sickle cell anemia: A molecular disease. *Science.* 1949;110:543–548.

Pearson TC, Messinezy M. Investigation of patients with polycythaemia [review]. *J Postgrad Med.* 1996;72:519.

Rasmussen K, Vyberg B, Pedersen KO, et al. Methylmalonic acid in renal insufficiency: Evidence of accumulation and implications for diagnosis of cobalamin deficiency. *Clin Chem.* 1990; 36:1523.

Richman DD, Fischl MA, the AZT Collaborative Group, et al. The toxicity of azidothymidine (AZT) in the treatment of patients with AIDS and AIDS-related complex: A double-blind, placebo-controlled trial. *N Engl J Med.* 1987;317:192.

Ronquist G, Theodorsson E. Inherited non-spherocytic haemolysis due to deficiency of glucose-6-phosphate dehydrogenase. *Scand J Clin Lab Invest.* 2007;67:105.

Scott LM, Tong W, Levine RL, et al. *JAK2* Exon 12 mutations in polycythemia vera and idiopathic erythrocytosis. *N Engl J Med.* 2007;356:459–468.

Silverstein SB, Rodgers GM. Parenteral iron therapy options. *Am J Hematol.* 2004;76(1):74–78.

Smith ADM. Megaloblastic madness. *Br Med J.* 1960;2:1840.

Smith JR, Landaw SA. Smokers' polycythemia. *N Engl J Med.* 1978;298:6.

Spivak JL. Polycythemia vera: Myths, mechanisms, and management. *Blood.* 2002;100:4272.

Titenko-Holland N, Jacob RA, Shang N, et al. Micronuclei in lymphocytes and exfoliated buccal cells of postmenopausal women with dietary changes in folate. *Mutat Res.* 1998; 417:101.

Turgeon ML. Hypochromic anemias and disorders of iron metabolism. In: *Clinical Hematology Theory and Procedures.* 4th ed. Philadelphia, PA: Lippincott Williams & Wilkins; 2005:131–144.

Victor M, Lear A. Subacute combined degeneration of the spinal cord: current concepts of the disease: Value of serum vitamin B$_{12}$ determinations in clarifying some of the common clinical problems. *Am J Med.* 1956;20:896.

Vilter CF, Vilter RW, Spies TD. The treatment of pernicious and related anemias with synthetic folic acid: I. Observations on the maintenance of a normal hematologic status and on the occurrence of combined system disease at the end of one year. *J Lab Clin Med.* 1947;32:262.

Weinreb NJ. Relative polycythemia. In: Wasserman LR, Berk PD, Berlin NI, eds. *Polycythemia Vera and the Myeloproliferative Disorders.* Philadelphia, PA: WB Saunders WB. 1995:226.

Wians FH, Urban JE, Keffer JH, Kroft SH. Discriminating between iron: Deficiency anemia and anemia of chronic disease using traditional indices of iron status vs transferrin receptor concentration. *Am J Clin Pathol.* 2001;115(1): 112–118.

Zumberg M, Kahn MJ. Iron metabolism, iron overload and the porphyrias. *Am Soc Hem Self-Assessment Program.* 2005;54–70.

61 WHITE CELL DISORDERS

C. Daniel Kingsley

The white blood cell (WBC) count from a complete blood count (CBC) is comprised of five main cell lines. Normally the count in adults will vary between 4500 and 11,000 cells/mm^3. Although abnormalities in the total WBC count are easily recognized, abnormalities in the absolute count of the various subtypes can be challenging. The formula used to calculate the absolute count of a particular white cell line is shown below using lymphocytes as an example:

Absolute lymphocyte count

= (Total WBC × Percent lymphocytes) ÷ 100.

For the cell lines that normally are present in small numbers (eg, basophils), accuracy is assured by using a direct count rather than a calculated one. Each time a white cell disorder is suspected, a careful history, physical examination, and inspection of the peripheral blood smear is mandatory. All three of these evaluations are inexpensive, yet indispensable.

Although early WBC precursors (eg, myelocytes or metamyelocytes) can be seen in the peripheral smear during pregnancy or during a leukemoid reaction, blasts are never normally seen and therefore, suggest a serious hematologic disorder. Other important findings on the peripheral smear include Auer rods or lymphoid cells with cleaved nuclei, cerebriform nuclei, hyperlobulated nuclei, or hairy cytoplasm. The above findings suggest an underlying leukemia or lymphoma. A leukoerythroblastic peripheral smear (early WBC precursors and nucleated RBCs) often accompanies marrow replacement with metastatic cancer or marrow fibrosis (myelofibrosis). Accordingly, the findings noted above require further evaluation including a bone marrow biopsy and aspirate.

Microorganisms, fungi, and helminthes can occasionally be identified within WBCs. For example, *Histoplasma*, *Ehrlichia*, *Plasmodium*, *Babesia*, and yeast can sometimes be diagnosed from examination of the peripheral blood smear or a bone marrow aspirate.

NEUTROPHILS

Neutrophils comprise the primary white blood cell line and are referred to as *granulocytes* (neutrophils, basophils, and eosinophils). The neutrophil granules contain myeloperoxidase, lactoferrin, gelatinase, and alkaline phosphatase, all of which are important in host defense. Bands (immature neutrophils) and mature neutrophils (polymorphonuclear neutrophil [PMN]) are normal in the standard peripheral blood smear. During periods of stress, the storage WBC pool (marginated WBCs) can liberate up to 10 times the usual number of cells; moreover new neutrophils can be generated in less than 2 days. Neutrophils circulate for 6 hours, but may last up to 5 days in tissues. The normal absolute neutrophil count (ANC) is 1500 to 8000 cells/mm^3. However, racial differences exist and African Americans may normally have an ANC as low as 1000 cells/mm^3. There is an increased risk of infection when the ANC is below 1000/mm^3 and a high risk of infection when below 200/mm^3.

While clinicians tend to focus on the number of neutrophils, the function and appearance of neutrophils may also herald a clinical disturbance. Patients with the Pelger-Huët anomaly (both inherited and acquired as a result of myelodysplasia) have bilobed mature neutrophils with no noted dysfunction. The neutrophils' granules are abnormal in both the Alder-Reilly anomaly (resembling toxic granules) and the May-Hegglin anomaly (resembling Döhle bodies), but both do not confer an increased risk of infection. Megaloblastic anemia and uremia are causes of hypersegmentation of the nuclei of neutrophils.

NEUTROPHILIA

Neutrophilia is defined as an ANC above 8000 cells/mm^3. Spurious leukocytosis can be caused by platelet clumping and precipitated cryoglobulin particles, both of which are misinterpreted as white cells. Spurious neutrophilia can be readily excluded by examination of the peripheral smear. Often the history and physical examination reveals the cause of an elevated count. Infections will raise the count and produce toxic granulation, Döhle body formation, and cytoplasmic granulation. Leukemoid reactions are associated with a normal leukocyte alkaline phosphatase (LAP) score, minimal left shift, no basophilia, no eosinophilia, and usually are characterized by counts between 50,000 and 100,000 cells/mm³. Glucocorticoid use causes demargination of the PMNs and decreased egress into the body tissues. Administration of lithium, catecholamines, all-trans retinoic acid, or granulocyte-colony stimulating factor also produce neutrophilia. Any inflammatory or stressful state can generate neutrophilia, including vasculitis, malignancy, myeloproliferative disorders, recent vigorous exercise, eclampsia, labor, seizures, thyroid storm, depression, posttraumatic stress disorder, recent vaccination, snake bites, poisoning, recent surgery, electric shock, or thermal burns. Cigarette smoking is likely the most common cause of mild neutrophilia, with a doubling of the ANC in a two pack per day smoker. The ANC will normalize in 1 to 2 years, but can take up to 5 years after smoking cessation. Splenectomy is an often overlooked but common medical cause of persistent neutrophilia. Acute leukemia and a leukoerythroblastic peripheral smear can both be associated with neutrophilia and are discussed elsewhere. Persistent mild neutrophilia is a normal variant in approximately 2% of the population. These patients are asymptomatic

The evaluation of neutrophilia involves a careful history, physical examination, and inspection of the peripheral smear. A sedimentation rate or C-reactive protein may be helpful to rule out inflammatory disorders. Selected patients may require a bone marrow biopsy and further laboratory testing and imaging if an underlying malignancy is suspected.

NEUTROPENIA

Neutropenia is defined as an ANC below 1500 cells/mm³. Mild neutropenia (1000–1500 cells/mm³) confers no increased risk of infection, moderate neutropenia (500–1000 cells/mm³) conferes a significant risk, and severe neutropenia (<500 cells/mm³) has a very high risk of infection. This abnormality can be further divided into the acquired and congenital neutropenias.

Congenital neutropenias are very rare, usually associated with recurrent, severe infections since childhood, a positive family history, and include infantile agranulocytosis, congenital dysgranulopoietic neutropenia, reticular dysgenesis, dyskeratosis congenita, Fanconi anemia, and Shwachman-Diamond-Oski syndrome.

Cyclic neutropenia is usually a familial syndrome that presents in childhood with fatigue, malaise, anorexia, mouth ulcers, and neutropenia occurring roughly every 3 weeks. As opposed to other congenital neutropenias, cyclic neutropenia tends to be mild and benign.

Acquired neutropenias are by far the more common and more varied subgroup of the two. Post infectious neutropenia is the most common acquired isolated neutropenia, and usually is mild, self-limited, and virally related. Epstein-Barr, human immunodeficiency virus (HIV), and infectious hepatitis cause more severe and prolonged neutropenia. Occasionally overwhelming infections cause neutropenia as the bone marrow, and its reserves are unable to compensate for the ongoing requirements. Drug-induced neutropenia is the second most common acquired neutropenia and is caused either by induction of antibodies or direct toxicity to the marrow. Chemotherapy, clozapine, quinidine, gold, phenothiazine, sulfonamides, semisynthetic penicillins, ticlopidine, chloramphenicol, ethanol, rifampin, and H_2-blockers are the most commonly implicated medications. Megaloblastic anemias can be associated with neutropenia. There is a direct correlation between spleen size and the degree of neutropenia. Autoimmune neutropenia can be caused by thymomas, transfusions, suppressor T cells, and rheumatologic disorders such as Felty syndrome, systemic lupus erythematosus, and rheumatoid arthritis. Patients on hemodialysis can experience complement-activated leukopenia. Leukemias, myelophthisis, myelodysplasia, and aplastic anemia can also be associated with neutropenia but these conditions will typically present with other hematologic abnormalities.

As always, a history, including the patient's extended family, physical examination, and peripheral smear examination are invaluable. If thrombocytopenia or anemia are also discovered, a bone marrow biopsy should almost always be performed in the absence of a clear etiology. If the patient is asymptomatic with mild neutropenia and has evidence of a recent viral infection or new medication, they may be observed. Any new or suspicious medication should be discontinued, if possible, and the CBC repeated in 1 to 2 weeks. More frequent CBCs should be performed if cyclic neutropenia is suspected. Patients who are symptomatic with moderate to severe neutropenia should undergo bone marrow aspiration. If the etiology is not obvious, testing including serum vitamin B_{12}, folate, HIV, antinuclear antibodies, antineutrophil antibodies, Coomb's test, and serum protein electrophoresis should be performed. Most patients with neutropenia can be safely managed at home, however, depending on the severity of neutropenia, they should avoid fresh fruit, vegetables, flowers, black pepper, humidifiers, and acutely ill individuals.

NEUTROPHIL DYSFUNCTION

For the immune system to work effectively, a patient needs both quantitatively and qualitatively adequate neutrophils. Neutrophil dysfunction should be suspected if a patient with chronic recurrent bacterial infections has a normal number of neutrophils. In these individuals one must exclude disorders of complement, immunoglobulins, and T cells. Chédiak-Higashi anomaly is the best known syndrome of neutrophil dysfunction. Pathognomonic large granules in both PMNs and lymphocytes should prompt an evaluation for this syndrome. Drugs, such as corticosteroids, salicylates, ethanol, epinephrine, doxorubicin, and colchicine, are known to impair neutrophil function. Myelodysplastic syndromes and myeloproliferative disorders can cause both quantitative and qualitative perturbations in neutrophils. Patients with Kartagener syndrome and Job syndrome are prone to infections because of neutrophil dysfunction. Complement deficiency syndromes will present in a fashion similar to neutrophil dysfunction and must be excluded. Patients with diabetes, sickle cell anemia, graft-versus-host disease, and malnutrition all are prone to recurrent infections because of impaired neutrophil function.

LYMPHOCYTES

Lymphocytes are the second most common WBC, comprising 15% to 40% of the circulating white cells. The absolute lymphocyte count usually ranges between 1000 and 5000 cells/mm^3. Lymphocytes consist of T cells (CD4$^+$ and CD8$^+$), B cells, and natural killer cells and are important for modulating humoral and cellular immunity. The peripheral smear usually reveals two types of lymphocytes—a small lymphocyte with clumped chromatin and a thin rim of deep blue cytoplasm, and a large granular lymphocyte with abundant cytoplasm and azurophilic granules. Atypical lymphocytes are frequently seen after viral infections and can be confused with malignant lymphocytes.

LYMPHOCYTOSIS

An absolute lymphocyte count above 5000 cells/mm^3 is the hallmark of lymphocytosis. Viral infections are the usual cause of a reactive lymphocytosis. Many viral infections are lumped under the term infectious lymphocytosis, which is virtually always benign. Infectious mononucleosis is associated with atypical lymphocytes that peak 3 weeks into the illness and can persist for up to 2 months. It is also associated with pharyngitis,

lymphadenopathy, and splenomegaly. Epstein-Barr virus and cytomegalovirus are the main causes of infectious mononucleosis. The principal bacterial infection associated with lymphocytosis is *Bordetella pertussis*, whereas most other bacterial infections do not cause a lymphocytosis. Typhoid fever, toxoplasmosis, measles, infectious hepatitis, and HIV are all associated with a lymphocytosis. Splenectomy will increase all blood counts. Allergic and hypersensitivity reactions are common causes of noninfectious lymphocytosis. Thyrotoxicosis, ulcerative colitis, Crohn disease, serum sickness, and vasculitis have all been reported to cause a lymphocytosis. Malignant causes of lymphocytosis include chronic lymphocytic leukemia, acute lymphocytic leukemia, mycosis fungoides, Sézary syndrome, hairy cell leukemia, Waldenström macroglobulinemia, and large granular leukemia.

LYMPHOPENIA

Lymphopenia is defined as an absolute count of less than 1000 cells/mm^3 and is considered severe when the counts are less than 700 cells/mm^3. Many inherited immunoglobulin diseases cause lymphopenia; these include Wiskott-Aldrich syndrome, ataxia-telangiectasia, X-linked agammaglobulinemia, severe combined immunodeficiency, and DiGeorge syndrome. Chemotherapy, radiation therapy, aplastic anemia, and advanced malignancies are also causes of lymphopenia. Whipple disease, intestinal lymphectasia, severe right-sided heart failure, and thoracic duct drainage are all causes of lymphopenia induced by gastrointestinal loss of the lymphocytes. HIV causes destruction of the CD4$^+$ T-cell lymphocyte, which can induce lymphopenia. Tuberculosis is associated with lymphopenia that resolves several weeks after initiation of effective therapy. Systemic illnesses associated with lymphopenia include myasthenia gravis, sarcoidosis, and systemic lupus erythematosus. Low lymphocyte counts are also associated with renal failure and elevated corticosteroid levels. Viral infections causing postinfectious lymphopenia include measles, mumps, chickenpox, and infectious hepatitis.

LYMPHOCYTE DYSFUNCTION

Lymphocytes play a key role in the immune system, contributing to both cellular and humoral defenses. Lymphocyte dysfunction, either because of decreased production of immunoglobulins, decreased production of cytokines, or impaired proliferative response to antigen, is associated with serious complications. The most common causes of decreased immune function associated with lymphocyte dysfunction are common variable immunodeficiency syndrome (which is characterized by low levels of IgG and reduced IgA or IgM), serum immunoglobulin A (IgA), and immunoglobulin G (IgG) subclass deficiency.

MONOCYTES

Monocytes are the largest circulating WBC. They have a distinctive folded nucleus, grayish-blue cytoplasm, and vacuoles. They normally comprise less than 10% of the total WBC, and should not exceed 800 cells/mm^3. After circulating for approximately a day, monocytes egress into tissues where they transform into macrophages

MONOCYTOSIS

A monocytosis can be seen in many inflammatory conditions including tuberculosis, collagen vascular disease, and bacterial endocarditis. Monocytosis has been reported in patients with depression, and those that are pregnant. Splenectomy has also been associated with a monocytosis. Malignancies and myeloproliferative disorders are commonly associated with a monocytosis. Monocytes also tend to increase during neutropenia and recovery from agranulocytosis, which can be misleading in patients with leukemia as well as those recovering from chemotherapy.

MONOCYTOPENIA

Monocytopenia does not occur in isolation but may be seen in conditions characterized by pancytopenia. Hairy cell leukemia and aplastic anemia are two disorders that are associated with a severe monocytopenia and serious infections. Glucocorticoid use has also been described in conjunction with a monocytopenia.

BASOPHILS

Basophils are bilobed granulocytes that stain dark blue-black with Wright stain. In tissues they are known as mast cells. They circulate for 6 to 12 hours. The granules contain histamine, heparin, and glycosaminoglycans. A normal basophil count is relatively low, comprising only 2% of the total white count or roughly 80 cells/mm^3. Nonetheless, the total count is abnormal in basophilic leukemia and the myeloproliferative disorders. Mast cells possess the characteristic staining of basophils and originate from CD34$^+$ cells.

BASOPHILIA

Basophilia is defined as an absolute basophil count greater than 80 cells/mm^3 and is seen in a variety of inflammatory conditions and hypersensitivity reactions. Patients with myeloproliferative disorders will often present with basophilia. As previously mentioned, splenectomy will cause an elevation in all blood counts. Hyperlipidemia has been associated with basophilia. Both smallpox and chickenpox have been associated with an elevation in the basophil count. Cutaneous mastocytosis and urticaria pigmentosa tend to be benign diseases of childhood that are associated with basophilia, but systemic mastocytosis tends to be progressive with end-organ damage and short survival times.

BASOPENIA

Basopenia is uncommon but has been associated with glucocorticoid use, ovulation, and hyperthyroidism. Hypersensitivity reactions have been associated with basopenia, but the mechanism remains obscure and may simply represent a laboratory artifact.

EOSINOPHILS

Eosinophils are bilobed granulocytes that stain orange or red with Wright's stain. Eosinophils circulate for 6 to 12 hours prior to egressing into the target tissue. Eosinophilic granules contain major basic protein, eosinophil-derived neurotoxin, peroxidase, and eosinophil cationic protein. There is a diurnal variation in eosinophil counts with a twofold increase in the evening in relation to the plasma cortisol levels. A normal eosinophil count will comprise up to 8% of the total white count or 500 cells/mm^3. Eosinophils are an important defense against parasitic infections.

EOSINOPHILIA

Eosinophilia is commonly observed in neoplastic, infectious, or allergic diseases. Acute leukemias (especially acute myelomonocytic [M_4] with inversion of chromosome 16) and chronic myelogenous leukemia are associated with a clonal expansion of eosinophils. Lymphomas (Hodgkin, non-Hodgkin, and cutaneous T cell), metastatic cancers, and myeloproliferative disorders can be associated with nonclonal eosinophilia. Infections are a cause of eosinophilia with helminthic infestations the most common. Allergic disorders are the most common cause of eosinophilia seen in developed countries. Atopic conditions such as asthma and allergic rhinitis commonly present with increased tissue eosinophils and less commonly blood eosinophilia. Drug reactions are another well-known cause of eosinophilia. Medical conditions associated with eosinophilia include vasculitis, rheumatoid arthritis, systemic lupus erythematous, cholestatic hepatitis, Addison disease, Churg-Strauss syndrome, Wiskott-Aldrich syndrome, Job syndrome, Well syndrome, and chronic kidney disease. Splenectomy will raise the total WBC and total eosinophil count. Radiotherapy is also associated with eosinophilia. Hypereosinophilic syndromes are associated with sustained, massive eosinophilia, involvement of multiple organs, and can lead to end-organ dysfunction. Systemic mastocytosis is associated with serum eosinophilia in one-fifth of the cases.

EOSINOPENIA

Eosinopenia is very uncommon and has been associated with glucocorticoid use, acute infections, and epinephrine. Drug-induced agranulocytosis as a cause of eosinopenia has been described.

BIBLIOGRAPHY

Ascensao JL, Oken MM, Ewing SL, et al. Leukocytosis and large cell lung cancer. A frequent association. *Cancer.* 1987;60:903.

Beutler E, Lichtman MA, Coller BS, Kipps TJ, Seligsohn U, eds. *Williams Hematology.* 6th ed. New York, NY: McGraw-Hill; 2001.

Boggs DR, Joyce RA. The hematopoietic effects of lithium. *Semin Hematol.* 1983;20:129.

Butterfield JH. The eosinophil and eosinophilia. In Tefferi A, ed. *Primary Hematology.* Totowa, NJ: Humana Press; 2001:161.

Christensen RD, Hill HR. Exercise-induced changes in the blood concentration leukocyte populations in teenage athletes. *Am J Pediatr Hematol Oncol.* 1987;9:140.

Constantinou CL. Differential diagnosis of neutropenia. In Tefferi A, ed. *Primary Hematology.* Totowa, NJ: Humana Press; 2001:93.

Dale DC, Fauci AS, et al. Comparison of agents producing a neutrophilic leukocytosis in man. Hydrocortisone, prednisone, endotoxin, and etiocholanolone. *J Clin Invest.* 1975;56:808.

Darko DF, Rose J, Gillin JC, et al. Neutrophilia and lymphopenia in major mood disorders. *Psychiatry Res.* 1988;25:243.

Downey H, McKinlay CA. Acute lymphadenosis compared with acute lymphatic leukemia. *Arch Intern Med.* 1923;32:82.

Freidenberg WR. Disorders of granulocytes: Qualitative and quantitative. In Mazza JJ, ed. *Manual of Clinical Hematology.* 3rd ed. Philadelphia, PA: Lippincott Williams & Wilkins; 1995:155.

Hillman RS, Ault KA, Rinder HM. *Hematology in Clinical Practice.* 4th ed. New York, NY: McGraw-Hill; 2002.

Jakobsen BW, Pedersen J, Egeberg BB. Postoperative lymphocytopenia and leucocytosis after epidural and general anaesthesia. *Acta Anaesthesiol Scand.* 1986;30:668.

Kay NE. Benign lymphocyte disorders. In: Mazza JJ, ed. *Manual of Clinical Hematology.* 3rd ed. Philadelphia, PA: Lippincott Williams & Wilkins; 1995:274.

Mason BA, Lessin L, Schechter GP. Marrow granulocyte reserves in black Americans. Hydrocortisone-induced granulocytosis in the "benign" neutropenia of the black. *Am J Med.* 1979;67:201.

McBride JA, Dacie JV, Shapley R. The effect of splenectomy on the leucocyte count. *Br J Haematol.* 1968;14:225.

Parry H, Cohen S, Schlarb JE, et al. Smoking, alcohol consumption, and leukocyte counts. *Am J Clin Pathol.* 1997;107:64.

Patel KJ, Hughes CG, Parapia LA. Pseudoleucocytosis and pseudothrombocytosis due to cryoglobulinemia. *J Clin Pathol.* 1987;40:120.

Savage RA. Pseudoleukocytosis due to EDTA-induced platelet clumping. *Am J Clin Pathol.* 1984;81:317.

Shoenfeld Y, Tal A, Berliner S, et al. Leukocytosis in non hematological malignancies—A possible tumor-associated marker. *J Cancer Res Clin Oncol.* 1986;111:54.

Solanki DL, Blackburn BC. Spurious leukocytosis and thrombocytopenia. A dual phenomenon caused by clumping of platelets in vitro. *JAMA.* 1983;250:2514.

Tefferi A. Blood eosinophilia: A new paradigm in disease classification, diagnosis, and treatment. *Mayo Clin Proc.* 2005;80:75.

Tefferi A. Leukocytosis and the chronic leukemias. In Tefferi A, ed. *Primary Hematology.* Totowa, NJ: Humana Press; 2001:175.

Telerman A, Amson RB, Delforge A, et al. A case of chronic aneosinocytosis. *Am J Hematol.* 1987;12:187.

Turgeon ML, ed. *Clinical Hematology Theory and Procedures.* 4th ed. Philadelphia, PA: Lippincott Williams & Wilkins; 2005.

Van Tiel E, Peeters PH, Smit HA, et al. Quitting smoking may restore hematological characteristics within five years. *Ann Epidemiol.* 2002;12:378.

Waterbury L. *Hematology.* 4th ed. Baltimore, MD: Williams & Wilkins; 1996.

Yam LT, Yam CF, Li CY. Eosinophilia in systemic mastocytosis. *Am J Clin Pathol.* 1980;73:48.

62 NORMAL HEMOSTASIS AND BLEEDING DISORDERS

Hans-Joachim Reimers

PHYSIOLOGY OF HEMOSTASIS

Following injury to a blood vessel, blood platelets adhere to exposed subendothelial structures such as collagen. This process is aided by adhesive proteins such as von Willebrand factor (vWF). Collagen binding sites on blood platelets have been well characterized. The platelet membrane glycoprotein integrin α_2 β_1 is a high affinity binding site, while platelet glycoprotein VI binds to collagen with a lower affinity. Similarly, collagen- and platelet-binding sites for vWF have been identified. Upon binding of platelets to collagen, signals are generated that induce platelet shape change, the platelet release reaction, and ultimately platelet aggregation. As part of the platelet activation processes, conformational changes occur in the platelet membrane including assembly of the glycoprotein IIb/IIIa complex which serves as the fibrinogen receptor. Fibrinogen molecules link activated platelets, thus leading to platelet aggregation.

Platelets contain α granules (which store a variety of adhesive proteins and coagulation factors) as well as dense or δ granules which store small molecules (eg, adenine nucleotides, serotonin and divalent cations). During the platelet release reaction the contents of these granules are extruded into the surrounding fluid. Adenine diphosphate (ADP) serves to recruit more platelets into the aggregate since platelets also have receptors for ADP. Another substance that helps to recruit more platelets into the growing platelet aggregate is thromboxane A2 (TXA2) which is formed during platelet activation from platelet arachidonate.

During platelet activation, the platelet plasma membrane undergoes further important changes. Serine phosphatidyl residues which are on the inside of the platelet membrane in the resting platelet, become exposed on the outside (*flip-flop*), and serve as a phospholipid binding site for the assembly of the coagulation enzymes. Binding of the coagulation enzymes to the platelet surface (as well as other cell surfaces) ensures localization of clot formation to the site of injury, rather than causing disseminated intravascular coagulation (DIC).

Thrombin formed on the platelet surface cleaves fibrinopeptides A and B from the fibrinogen molecule and thereby allows fibrin monomer polymerization and stabilization of the platelet aggregate by fibrin formation. Thrombin is also a very powerful platelet-aggregation inducing agent, and thus serves to amplify the hemostatic process.

Platelet aggregation and fibrin formation is fine tuned by an elaborate system of positive and negative feedback loops and inhibitors. Disorders of platelet adhesion and aggregation can be referred to as disorders of primary hemostasis, while the coagulopathies may be summarized as disorders of secondary hemostasis.

APPROACH TO THE BLEEDING PATIENT

A quantitative or qualitative deficiency of platelets (thrombocytopenia, thrombocytopathy), von Willebrand

TABLE 62–1   Bleeding History: Goals

Establish

- Likelihood of abnormal bleeding
- Congenital/inherited or acquired bleeding disorder
- Mode of inheritance
- Association with underlying illness (comorbidity)
- Association with medication/drugs/transfusions
- Site of bleeding
  - Mucocutaneous
  - Joints
  - Retroperitoneal
  - Soft tissues
- Type of bleeding
  - Spontaneous
  - Provoked
  - Prolonged initial bleeding (abnormal primary hemostasis)
  - Delayed bleeding (abnormal secondary hemostasis)

factor (von Willebrand disease [vWD]), or coagulation factors (hemophilia), as well as vessel wall disorders and rarely a deficiency of inhibitors of fibrinolysis may underlie abnormal bleeding. Bleeding disorders may be inherited, congenital or acquired. Bleeding can occur spontaneously or be provoked by injury or surgery. Bleeding disorders may present themselves with different physical signs depending on the underlying defect.

Much valuable information in regard to the presence and categorization of a possible bleeding disorder can be obtained by a *thorough history* (Table 62–1). Some relevant questions are summarized in Table 62–2.

The *first goal* in taking the personal history is to establish the likelihood of abnormal bleeding. A significant bleeding disorder will reveal itself most likely by either evidence of spontaneous bleeding or by excessive bleeding after challenge by trauma or surgery, and in women by excessive menstrual bleeding. Abnormal surgery-related bleeding includes more than anticipated need for blood transfusions or blood transfusions after minor surgery such as tonsillectomies or tooth extractions.

TABLE 62–2   Bleeding History: Questionnaire

- Have you ever experienced a serious bleeding complication during or after a surgical procedure?
- Have you ever experienced excessive vaginal bleeding immediately after childbirth or perineal bleeding from an episiotomy?
- Have you experienced persistent menorrhagia in the absence of fibroids or other uterine abnormalities?
- Do you experience brisk or prolonged bleeding after minor cuts or exaggerated bruising after minor trauma?
- Have you ever developed a joint bleed, or retroperitoneal hematoma in the absence of major trauma?
- Have you ever experienced spontaneous bleeding?
- Has any member of your family experienced severe bleeding complications, perhaps requiring transfusions of red blood cells?
- Do you have any known medical problems?
- Do you take any prescription medications, over-the-counter medications, or homeopathic remedies on a regular basis?
- Have you noticed any unusual rashes or easy bruisability?

TABLE 62–3   Selected Drugs That May Cause Thrombocytopenia

- Antiarrhythmics
- Procainamide
- Quinidine
- Glycoprotein IIIb/IIIa antagonists
  - Abciximab
  - Eptifibatide
  - Tirofiban
- Antimicrobial agents
  - Amphotericin B
  - Linezolid
  - Rifampin
  - Trimethoprim-sulfamethoxazole
  - Vancomycin
- Histamine H_2 blockers
  - Cimetidine
  - Ranitidine
- Carbamazepine
- Heparin
- Hydrochlorothiazide
- NSAIDS
- Quinine

TABLE 62–4   Selected Drugs That Affect Platelet Function

- Cyclooxygenase inhibitors
  - Aspirin
  - Nonsteroidal antiinflammatory drugs (NSAIDS)
- Adenosine diphosphate (ADP) receptor antagonists
  - Ticlopidine
  - Clopidogrel
- Glycoprotein IIb-IIIa receptor antagonists
  - Abciximab
  - Tirofiban
  - Eptifibatide
- Drugs that increase cyclic adenosine monophosphate (AMP)
  - Adenyl cyclase activators
    - PGE_1, PGD_2; PGI_2; analogs
  - Phosphodiesterase inhibitors
    - Dipyridamole
    - Cilostazol
    - Methylxanthines
    - Caffeine
    - Aminophylline
- Nitric oxide, nitric oxide donors
- Antimicrobials
  - Penicillins
  - Cephalosporins
  - Hydroxychloroquine
- Cardiovascular drugs
  - β-Adrenergic blockers
  - Vasodilators
  - Diuretics (furosemide)
  - Calcium channel blockers
  - Quinidine
  - ACE-inhibitors
- Psychotropic drugs
  - Tricyclic antidepressants
  - Serotonin-reuptake inhibitors
  - Phenothiazines
- Dextran
- Vitamin E
- Garlic, ginger, other *alternative medications*

PGD, prostaglandin D: PGE, prostaglandin E; PGI, prostaglandin I

Excessive spontaneous bleeding includes frequent nose-bleeds requiring packing or other interventions.

The *second goal* is to establish whether the bleeding disorder is inherited, congenital or acquired. A family history and the age of onset of the bleeding disorder will help to answer this question. If the bleeding disorder appears to be acquired later in life, association with other medical problems or medication needs to be explored. Tables 62–3 and 62–4 list some medications that can cause thrombocytopenia or platelet dysfunction and associated increased risk of bleeding.

Thirdly, the type of bleeding and the site of bleeding may help to distinguish between a defect of primary hemostasis (platelet plug formation) and secondary hemostasis (fibrin stabilization of hemostatic clot). If bleeding is arrested initially after injury, but delayed bleeding occurs, a coagulopathy is more likely than a platelet disorder or vWD. In contrast, if initial arrest of bleeding is prolonged, a platelet disorder, vWD or a vascular problem is more likely. Mucocutaneous bleeding is characteristic for defects in primary hemostasis (platelet-related or vWF-related). Retroperitoneal bleeding is more likely associated with coagulopathies. Joint bleeding is typical for the classical hemophilias A (factor [F] VIII deficiency) and B (F IX deficiency). Spontaneous bleeding usually signifies a more pronounced bleeding disorder (eg, severe hemophilia A with F VIII level <1%) than provoked bleeding with surgery (eg, mild hemophilia A with F VIII level of 5%–30%).

The physical examination may provide further evidence of abnormal bleeding. Table 62–5 summarizes signs that may provide immediate evidence of active or prior bleeding.

Some signs found on physical examination (Table 62–6) may give clues to vascular conditions that are associated with abnormal bleeding in the absence of platelet disorders, vWD, or coagulopathies.

These conditions include Ehlers-Danlos syndrome, Osler-Weber-Rendu syndrome, scurvy, and nonthrombocytopenic purpura in amyloidosis. In contrast, the morphological appearance of senile purpura, purpura simplex, or psychogenic purpura may be suggestive of a hemorrhagic diathesis. However, these conditions are *not* associated with abnormal bleeding (Table 62–7).

TABLE 62–5   Evidence of Bleeding

- Petechiae (<3 mm)
- Purpura (>3 mm)
- Ecchymosis
- Sites of previous or active bleeding
- Hemarthrosis
- Hematomas

TABLE 62–6 Signs of Conditions Associated with Abnormal Bleeding but Normal Hemostatic Screening Tests

SIGN	CONDITION
Joint laxity	Ehlers-Danlos syndrome
Skin hyperelasticity	
Paper-thin scars	
Mucosal and visceral telangiectasias	Osler-Weber-Rendu syndrome
AV malformation	
Aneurysms	
Diffuse petechiae	Vitamin C deficiency
Perifollicular purpura	Scurvy
Corkscrew hairs	
Purpura (nonthrombocytopenic)	Amyloidosis

AV, arteriovenous

LABORATORY EVALUATION

A detailed personal and family history of the patient suggests whether or not a patient has a clinically significant bleeding disorder. Laboratory testing, in contrast, is useful to delineate the exact cause of the bleeding disorder. However, a routine platelet count, activated partial thromboplastin time (aPTT), and prothrombin time (PT) may be normal in a patient with a bleeding disorder (eg, some forms of von Willebrand disease, mild hemophilia, thrombocytopathies, factor XIII deficiency, antiplasmin deficiency, vascular disorders) whereas a patient with prolonged aPTT may have a thrombotic problem but no bleeding disorder (eg, lupus anticoagulant). Thus, additional laboratory testing is usually required either to determine the cause of an abnormal screening test or the cause of a bleeding disorder in a patient with normal platelet count, aPTT and PT.

Thrombocytopenia is usually recognized immediately because almost all patients have an automated blood count (CBC) performed as initial laboratory evaluation. Common causes of thrombocytopenia are summarized in Table 62–8.

However, the platelet count may be falsely low as a result of platelet clumping. This occurs in about one of

TABLE 62–7 Signs of Conditions Suggestive of but not Associated with Abnormal Bleeding

SIGN	CONDITION
Reddish purplish ecchymoses on extensor surfaces of upper extremities; loose fitting skin; loss of subcutaneous fat	Senile purpura
Bruising in relation to menses	Purpura simplex
Bruises with bizarre distribution pattern (areas accessible to patient)	Psychogenic purpura
Skin fragility, purplish striae, flexor and extensor surfaces of upper and lower extremities and torso	Cushing syndrome

TABLE 62–8 Pathophysiology of Thrombocytopenias

- Hereditary/Congenital
- Acquired
  - Immune thrombocytopenia
    - acute (viral infection)
    - chronic (adult)
    - drug-induced (heparin, quinidine, etc.)
  - Nonimmune
  - Diminished production (bone marrow infiltration, aplasia, toxic)
  - Increased destruction/consumption (infection; surgery, DIC; extracorporeal circulation; thrombotic thrombocytopenic purpura)
  - Sequestration (enlarged spleen)

DIC, disseminated intravascular coagulation

every one thousand specimens. Therefore, all specimens with thrombocytopenia must be reviewed under the microscope. In some patients, the clumping is caused by calcium ion binding to ethylenediaminetetraacetic acid (EDTA) in the CBC specimen. Repeat testing must be carried out in these patients using Na-citrate, heparin or no anticoagulant. Inspection of the blood smear may also provide important clues in other patients with thrombocytopenia (Table 62–9).

Giant platelets may be found in Bernard-Soulier syndrome as well as in the May-Hegglin anomaly. The latter inherited disorder also shows typical leukocyte inclusions. Giant platelets, by definition, are as large or larger than the size of a red blood cell. *Large platelets* are

TABLE 62–9 Review of Peripheral Blood Smear

MORPHOLOGY	PLATELET NUMBER	CONDITION
Normal platelets	Increased	Inflammation
Normal platelets	Increased	Cancer
Normal platelets (RBC: microcytosis, hypochromia)	(Increased)	Iron deficiency
Giant platelets	Increased	Essential thrombocytosis
Giant Platelets (Deficient ristocetin-induced platelet aggregation)	Decreased	Bernard-Soulier syndrome
Giant platelets (Leukocyte inclusions)	Decreased	May-Hegglin anomaly
Large platelets (Pelger-Huet cells, leukocyte hypogranulation)	Decreased	Myelodysplastic syndrome.
Small platelets	Decreased	X-linked thrombocytopenia (defective Wiscott-Aldrich syndrome protein)
No platelet granules	Decreased	Gray platelet syndrome (α-granule deficiency)
Schistocytes	Decreased	TTP/HUS DIC Malignant hypertension

DIC, disseminated intravascular coagulation; RBC, red blood cells; HUS, hemolytic uremic syndrome; TTP, thrombotic thrombocytopenic purpura.

TABLE 62–10   Acquired Disorders of Platelet Function

- Drugs
- Uremia
- Severe liver disease
- Monoclonal gammopathies
- Mechanical platelet damage (extracorporeal circulation; hemodialysis)
- Myeloproliferative disorders
- Myelodysplastic disorders

somewhat smaller and can be seen in patients with myelodysplastic syndrome in addition to the characteristic bilobed hypogranulated leukocytes (Pelger-Huet cells) as well as in pseudo–vWD (platelet-type vWD). *Small platelets* are typical for X-linked thrombocytopenia characterized by a defective Wiskott-Aldrich syndrome protein. *Platelets devoid of granules* by light microscopy are characteristic of the gray platelet syndrome in which the platelet α-granules are absent. The presence of *schistocytes* in a thrombocytopenic smear is a hallmark of thrombotic thrombocytopenic purpura and hemolytic uremic syndrome but can also be observed in patients with DIC and malignant hypertension.

Abnormal platelet function as a cause of petechial or purpuric bleeding may be observed in patients with normal, high or low platelet counts. Abnormal platelet function can be acquired or inherited (Tables 62–10 and 62–11).

The underlying biochemical and pathological aberrations have been elucidated only partially. There is no

TABLE 62–11   Selected Congenital Disorders of Platelet Function

- Glycoprotein (GP) abnormalities
  - Glanzmann thrombasthenia   GP IIb/IIIa
  - Bernard-Soulier syndrome   GP Ib/IX/V
  - Pseudo-vWD   GP Ib
  - Defect in collagen binding   GP Ia/IIa, GP VI, GP IV
- Defects of platelet secretion and signal transduction
  - Storage pool defects
    - Dense δ-granule deficiency
    - Gray platelet syndrome (α-granule deficiency)
    - Combined α- and δ-granule deficiency
  - Release or secretion defects (signal transduction defects)
    - Defects in receptors for agonists (ADP, thrombin, epinephrine)
    - Defects in calcium mobilization
    - Defects in G-protein activation
    - Defects in phosphatidyl inositol metabolism
    - Defects in protein phosphorylation
  - Abnormalities of the prostaglandin pathway
    - Defect in arachidonic acid production: phospholipase A₂ defect
    - Cyclooxygenase deficiency
    - Thromboxane synthetase deficiency
    - Lack of response to thromboxane A₂
- Disorders of platelet coagulant activity
  - Scott Syndrome: defective Factor Va-Xa binding to platelet surface
  - Defects in platelet–coagulation protein interaction
- Disorders of plasma proteins that interfere with platelet function
  - Von Willebrand disease (vWD)
  - Congenital afibrinogenemia

TABLE 62–12   Laboratory Assessment of Primary Hemostasis

- Review of blood smear
- Bleeding time
- Platelet function analyzer (PFA-100)
- Platelet aggregation studies
- Platelet granule contents and release products
- von Willebrand factor
  - Antigen
  - Ristocetin cofactor activity
  - Collagen binding activity
  - F VIII binding activity
  - Multimeric composition

single routine laboratory test which recognizes abnormal platelet function with high sensitivity and specificity. Methods available in specialized laboratories are summarized in Table 62–12.

The *bleeding time* depends on platelet number and function, platelet adhesion molecules such as vWF, vascular factors (eg, Ehlers-Danlos syndrome, vitamin C deficiency, vasculitis) as well as the structure of skin and subcutaneous tissue (eg, actinic changes, senile purpura), and on the experience of the technician performing the test. Therefore, the bleeding time should only be used in conjunction with other tests of platelet function (eg, PFA-100 analyzer, platelet aggregation and release studies, vWF analysis) by specialized hemostasis laboratories and hemostaseologists.

The *PFA-100 tes*t is sometimes referred to as an *in vitro bleeding time*. It measures the *closure time* of a capillary coated with either epinephrine/collagen or with ADP (adenosine diphosphate)/collagen under standardized high flow conditions. It is sensitive to adhesive proteins (such as vWF) and platelet number and function as well as to the hematocrit. It excludes the vessel wall as a determinant.

Platelet aggregation studies can be carried out in a small number of specialized laboratories. Platelet aggregometry, using ADP, collagen, arachidonate or ristocetin as agonists, is able to identify platelet dysfunction secondary to receptor abnormalities, defects in signal transduction or release of granule constituents.

Von Willebrand factor is a multimeric plasma glycoprotein composed mostly of identical subunits of about 250 kDa in size. High molecular weight (HMW)-vWF multimers mediate platelet adhesion at sites of vascular injury by binding to connective tissue and to platelets. VWF also binds and stabilizes blood clotting factor VIII. Therefore, defects in vWF can cause bleeding with features typical of platelet dysfunction, or of mild to moderately severe hemophilia A, or of both. Quantitative deficiencies are measured with an antigen assay, structural abnormalities are measured by determining the multimeric composition, and platelet binding

TABLE 62–13   Laboratory Assessment of Secondary Hemostasis

Prothrombin time
Activated partial thromboplastin time
Thrombin time
Coagulation factor assays
Mixing studies

of vWF is measured with the ristocetin cofactor activity assay. Tests are also available to determine the collagen binding activity and the factor VIII binding activity of vWF (Table 62–13).

The initial screening tests to look for a defect in *secondary hemostasis (coagulopathy)* are an activated partial thromboplastin time (aPTT), a prothrombin time (PT), and a thrombin time. To perform a prothrombin time, tissue factor, phospholipids, and calcium are added to citrated patient plasma. A normal *prothrombin time* will depend on the presence of sufficient factor VII (*extrinsic pathway*), factor X, factor V, factor II, and fibrinogen (*common pathway*). Synthesis of factor II, VII, and X are vitamin K dependent; factor V synthesis is Vitamin K independent. All of these factors are synthesized in the liver. A *normal aPTT* will depend on the presence of sufficient amounts of contact activation factors (HMW-kininogen, prekallikrein, Hageman factor [F XII]) as well as F XI, F IX, F VIII (*intrinsic pathway*). and the factors of the *common pathway*. An aPTT test is performed by adding a *foreign surface* such as kaolin, a phospholipid and calcium to citrated patient plasma. It is noteworthy that prolongation of the aPTT caused by deficiency of contact activation factors is not associated with a bleeding disorder. This indicates that this pathway of activation of the coagulation cascade is not important in vivo. In contrast, a prolonged aPTT caused by F VIII, IX, or XI deficiency is associated with a clinical bleeding disorder (hemophilia A, B, and C). It is also noteworthy that the common pathway is more sensitive to the PT than the aPTT. This means that the prothrombin time becomes prolonged first when the concentration of the common pathway factors are reduced. Therefore, the aPTT test is very useful to measure deficiencies of F VIII, IX, and XI, whereas the PT is very good in reflecting deficiencies of F II, V, VII, and X. The *thrombin time* is performed by adding thrombin to citrated patient plasma, and the time until blood clotting occurs is recorded. The thrombin time is dependent on the fibrinogen concentration and any inhibitors of thrombin (such as heparin) or inhibitors of fibrin polymerization (such as fibrin degradation products or paraproteins). If one of the screening tests is abnormal (prolonged), the next step is to determine whether this is caused by a coagulation factor deficiency or the presence

of an inhibitor. A *mixing study (50:50 mix)* serves this purpose. An abnormal screening test will normalize upon mixing with normal pool plasma if there is a factor deficiency (because the deficient factor will be at least 50% in the mixed sample. This is generally sufficient to normalize the coagulation time.) Conversely, the clotting time will remain prolonged if there is an inhibitor in the patient specimen since it will also inactivate the coagulation factor in the normal pool plasma (lupus anticoagulant; inhibitors of specific coagulation factors).

If a factor deficiency is suspected based on the mixing study, the concentration of the specific factor in the patient sample can be determined (factor assay).

THROMBOCYTOPENIAS

A normal platelet count is between 150,000 and 350,000/μL. Thrombocytopenia is defined as a platelet count less than 100,000/μL. The bleeding time starts to increase when the platelet count falls below 100,000/μL, and injury or surgery may provoke excessive bleeding. Spontaneous bleeding usually occurs only at platelet counts below 20,000/μL, while serious hemorrhage is usually only observed at platelet counts less than 10,000/μL.

The cause of a low platelet count can be secondary to *diminished production* caused by marrow injury due to drugs (eg, chemotherapeutic agents, ethanol), irradiation, or marrow failure as a consequence of other disorders (such as aplastic anemia). The marrow can be infiltrated by solid tumors or leukemia or replaced by fibrosis. There are also a number of rare inherited thrombocytopenias associated with diminished platelet production (Table 62–14).

Table 62–15 outlines factors that suggest a hereditary thrombocytopenia.

Sequestration of platelets may be responsible for thrombocytopenia if an enlarged spleen can be demonstrated.

Accelerated platelet destruction may occur as the result of an *immune mechanism* such as in neonatal thrombocytopenia, alloimmune thrombocytopenia, viral illness-related thrombocytopenia in children, human immunodeficiency virus (HIV), hepatitis C related thrombocytopenia, drug-related thrombocytopenia (eg, heparin, quinine, quinidine), thrombocytopenia in association with lupus erythematosis, lymphoma, and chronic lymphocytic leukemia. Chronic autoimmune thrombocytopenia can also occur in adults without any recognizable cause. Patients with classic thrombotic thrombocytopenic purpura have been found to possess an antibody against the enzyme ADAMTS 13 which is responsible for the degradation of the very high molecular weight multimer of

TABLE 62–14 Inherited Thrombocytopenias

SYNDROME	GENE MUTATION	INHERITANCE
• Mediterranean	GP Ib α	autosomal dominant
○ Macrothrombocytopenia		
• Di George/velocardiofacial syndrome	GP Ib β	autosomal dominant
• MYHS-related thrombocytopenia	MYH 9, fibrillin-I	autosomal dominant
○ May-Hegglin anomaly Fechtner, Epstein and Sebastian Syndromes		
• Thrombocytopenia with predisposition for leukemia	RUNX 1 (CBF A2, AML 1)	autosomal dominant
• Paris-Trousseau/Jacobsen syndromes	FL 11	autosomal dominant
• Congenital amegakaryocytic thrombocytopenia	C-Mp1	autosomal recessive
• Chromosome 10/THC2	FLJ1 4813	autosomal dominant
• Thrombocytopenia with radioulnar synostosis	HOXA 11	autosomal dominant
• Thrombocytopenia and absent radii (TAR)	Unknown	autosomal recessive
• GATA 1-related thrombocytopenia with dyserythropoiesis	GATA 1	X-linked
• Wiskott-Aldrich syndrome	WASP	X-linked

vWF. In the absence of this enzyme, there is an increased risk of platelet aggregation in the microcirculation with end organ damage.

Increased platelet destruction or consumption caused by nonimmune mechanism occurs in extracorporeal circulation, surgery, infection and DIC. DIC can be diagnosed if there is evidence of platelet consumption (low platelet count), prothrombin consumption (prolonged prothrombin time), evidence of an effect of thrombin on the fibrinogen molecule (presence of fibrin monomer, fibrin degradation products, hypofibrinogenemia) in the setting of appropriate clinical circumstances (source of endotoxin or tissue factor such as bacteremia, extensive burns, trauma, heat stroke, metastatic carcinoma, giant hemangioma, retained dead fetus, mismatched blood transfusion, or acute promyelocytic leukemia).

The thrombocytopenia of pregnancy is probably caused by dilution (intravascular volume expansion).

THROMBOCYTOPATHIES

Acquired disorders of platelet function are quite common, especially those caused by medications and

TABLE 62–15 Reasons to Suspect Hereditary Thrombocytopenia

- Family history of thrombocytopenia (parent-child; maternal uncle-nephew)
- Lack of response to treatment for autoimmune thrombocytopenia
- Persistence of stable thrombocytopenia for years
- Bleeding out of proportion to the platelet count (associated platelet dysfunction)
- Onset at birth
- Diagnostic features on blood smear (giant platelets; Döhle bodies; microcytosis)
- Associated features (absent radii; mental retardation, renal failure; impaired hearing, cataracts)

drugs. Disorders associated with impaired platelet function are listed in Table 62–10. In contrast, inherited thrombocytopathies are rare. Table 62–11 outlines some of the known molecular defects.

VON WILLEBRAND DISEASE (VWD)

VWD is a bleeding disorder caused by inherited defects in the concentration, structure or function of von Willebrand factor (vWF). VWD is classified into three primary categories.

Type 1 includes partial quantitative deficiency; type 2 includes qualitative defects; and type 3 includes complete deficiency of vWF. Type 2 is divided into 4 subcategories (Table 62–16).

Acquired disorders that mimic vWD are referred to as acquired von Willebrand syndrome.

Patients with type 1 vWD have a high probability of responding to DDVAP (desmopressin), whereas those with type 2 and type 3 usually do not. Therefore, the

TABLE 62–16 Classification of Von Willebrand Disease

TYPE	DESCRIPTION
1	Partial quantitative deficiency of vWF
2	Qualitative vWF defects
2A	Decreased vWF-dependent platelet adhesion and a selective deficiency of high-molecular-weight vWF multimer
2B	Increased affinity for platelet glycoprotein Ib
2M	Decreased vWF-dependent platelet adhesion without a selective deficiency of high-molecular-weight vWF multimer
2N	Markedly decreased binding affinity for factor VIII
3	Virtually complete deficiency of vWF

vWF, von Willebrand factor.

latter need to be treated with vWF replacement for bleeding complications or during surgery.

COAGULOPATHIES

Congenital bleeding disorders are rare in comparison to the acquired bleeding disorders (Table 62–17).

The most common, hemophilia A, is an X-linked disorder with a frequency of approximately 1:10,000. In its severe form (<1% factor VIII), it is usually diagnosed during the first year of life. Preferred treatment is early prophylaxis with factor replacement 2 to 3 times per week to avoid recurrent joint bleeds and disabling hemophilic arthropathy.

Factor VIII, IX, and XI deficiency are usually recognized by a prolonged aPTT in patients with a bleeding problem. However, mild forms may have a normal aPTT, and the diagnosis will only be made if the physician pursues the workup of a patient with a bleeding disorder vigorously.

Patients with afibrinogenemia or dysfibrinogenemia will be recognized by a prolonged thrombin time (and normal PT and aPTT).

Factor II, V, VII, and X deficiency will cause a prolonged prothrombin time. In severe factor II, V, and X deficiency, the aPTT will *also* be prolonged (factor II, V, X are common pathway factors). In contrast, even severe factor VII deficiency will cause only a prolongation in the PT (FVII is an extrinsic pathway factor).

In contrast to the congenital bleeding disorders, acquired coagulopathies are common. Liver disease is the most common cause of an acquired coagulopathy (other than intentional anticoagulation), since all coagulation factors other than factor VIII are synthesized in the liver (note that F VIII is usually increased in patients with liver disease). In liver disease, it is common to find initially a prolonged PT, and in more advanced disease a prolonged aPTT and PT. In contrast to the congenital coagulopathies, further workup of a prolonged PT and aPTT by single factor assays reveals low levels of all factors synthesized in the liver, rather than a single low factor.

It is important to distinguish the coagulopathy of liver disease from vitamin K deficiency (which is a frequent problem in intensive care unit patients). In vitamin K deficiency, F II, VII, IX, and X will be low; factor V is normal because F V synthesis does not require vitamin K. In clinical practice, it is therefore helpful to measure F VII and F V simultaneously to distinguish liver disease from vitamin K deficiency.

Antibodies to coagulation factors are a rare but very serious clinical problem. The most common is an antibody to factor VIII in hemophilic patients who are on prophylaxis; an *autoantibody* to factor VIII develops in approximately 1 of one million people per year (acquired hemophilia). Treatment should always occur in specialized centers.

DIC with consumption coagulopathy has been addressed above. DIC screening (platelet count, prothrombin time, fibrin monomer, D-dimer, fibrinogen) should be performed in patients in the appropriate clinical setting. Treatment addresses the underlying disease, and substitution of components that have been consumed and are responsible for bleeding complications (platelets, fibrinogen).

Anticoagulation can be associated with serious bleeding complications when outside the therapeutic range. Fast reversal may have to be initiated with use of oral or intravenous vitamin K in combination with fresh frozen plasma.

VASCULAR DISORDERS

Table 62–18 summarizes hemostatic disorders caused by blood vessel wall defects. *Senile* (*atrophic* or *actinic*) *purpura* is common in older and debilitated patients, but can also be seen in patients after excessive solar exposure. UV light increases the breakdown of collagen. Characteristic location is the extensor surface of the forearms. Slight trauma or stretching of the skin can cause physical rupture with subcutaneous bleeding.

TABLE 62–17 Coagulopathies

- Congenital bleeding disorders
  - Hemophilia A   (factor VIII deficiency)
  - Hemophilia B   (factor IX deficiency)
  - Hemophilia C   (factor XI deficiency)
  - Rare bleeding disorders
    - Afibrinogenemia/Dysfibrinogenemia
    - Factor VII deficiency
    - Factor V deficiency
    - Factor X deficiency
    - Factor II deficiency
- Acquired coagulopathies
  - Liver disease
  - Vitamin K deficiency
  - Antibody to coagulation factor
  - Disseminated intravascular coagulation
  - Anticoagulation

TABLE 62–18 Hemostatic Disorders Caused by Blood Vessel Wall Defects

- Aging/Actinic changes
- Chronic therapy with glucocorticosteroids
- Vitamin C deficiency
- Amyloidosis
- Heritable disorders of connective tissue
- Hereditary hemorrhagic telangiectasia
  - (Osler-Weber-Rendu disease)

Cortisol is known to decrease collagen synthesis, while collagen catabolism is not affected. Thus, collagen becomes scarce, resulting in capillary fragility. The glucocorticoid-related purpura also occurs primarily on the extensor surfaces of the forearms. The skin is thin, and extravasated blood therefore accumulates superficially. The perifollicular hemorrhage characteristic of scurvy (*vitamin C deficiency*) has become a rare condition. Vitamin C is necessary to convert proline into hydroxyproline. This reaction is needed to crosslink collagen fibers. Weakened collagen compromises microvascular strength.

Purpuric bleeding can be found in about 15% of patients with *amyloidosis*. Amyloid material is deposited between the endothelium and the basement membrane. Therefore it increases capillary fragility, but it can also impair the ability of arterioles to constrict, thereby causing prolonged bleeding.

Subcutaneous hemorrhages may be encountered in *inherited metabolic disorders of the connective tissue* such as the Ehlers-Danlos syndrome, pseudoxanthoma elasticum, osteogenesis imperfecta, and Marfan syndrome. Bleeding in these disorders is usually a result of tearing of fragile subcutaneous tissues and skin rather than spontaneous purpuric lesions. Postsurgical wound healing is impaired. Clinically these conditions are recognized by extreme joint laxity and skin stretching.

The Osler-Weber-Rendu syndrome is an autosomal dominant inherited disorder characterized by telangiectasias (small arteriolar-venous malformation). The huge capillary dilatations are caused by lack of or alterations of a structural protein called endoglin. Several subtypes have been described with unique alterations of the endoglin gene. Bleeding occurs because of rupture of the lesions. Telangiectasias occur most often on hands, fingernail beds, lips, tongue, and surface of the face. They become more apparent with age. Most of the clinically relevant bleeding comes from the nose. However, the most troublesome bleeding is chronic gastrointestinal bleeding. Nose bleeding is best handled by cauterization or laser ablation. Gastrointestinal bleeding is initially best treated by iron substitution. Estrogen therapy may be helpful in some patients.

TREATMENT PRINCIPLES

THROMBOCYTOPENIA

The first task is to determine the cause of the thrombocytopenia. More specifically, one needs to determine whether the thrombocytopenia is an isolated, independent problem (eg, inherited nonimmune thrombocytopenia, immune thrombocytopenia) or secondary to another condition (eg, infection, surgery, drug-related, immune thrombocytopenia in the context of HIV, lupus erythematosus, hepatitis C; splenic sequestration, bone marrow disorder).

Acute immune thrombocytopenia with a platelet count of less than 10,000/μL may be responsive to glucocorticoids, intravenous gamma globulin, anti-Rhesus factor (anti-D) antibodies (in Rh positive patients), CD-20 antibody (Rituximab), or splenectomy. Thrombocytopenia in the context of thrombotic thrombocytopenic purpura requires immediate treatment with plasmapheresis. Inherited nonimmune thrombocytopenias will only require platelet transfusion support with significant bleeding or with scheduled surgery. Secondary thrombocytopenias require treatment of the underlying problem, if possible, and platelet support only for bleeding complications.

THROMBOCYTOPATHY

Inherited thrombocytopathies need to be characterized and classified in order to direct treatment of bleeding complications (platelet transfusion; DDVAP).

Acquired thrombocytopathies need to be classified with regard to *drug-related* thrombocytopathy, *transient* thrombocytopathies (eg, extracorporeal circulation), or production of abnormal platelets (myelodysplastic syndrome [MDS]) or comorbidity-related thrombocytopathy (eg, uremia). Treatment, therefore, may involve omission of the offending drug, platelet replacement for acute bleeding in MDS, and adjunctive measures such as DDVAP and optimization of hematocrit in patients with renal function impairment.

VON WILLEBRAND DISEASE

The treatment of von Willebrand disease depends on the type and clinical severity. Type 1 vWD may be treated with DDVAP for bleeding and minor surgery. However, support with vWF-concentrate (vWF rich-FVIII concentrate) may be needed for prolonged perioperative support. Type 2 vWD (qualitative deficiency) usually requires replacement for major bleeding and perioperative support until wound healing has occurred. Type 3 vWD always requires vWF replacement. In patients with frequent bleeding as well as joint bleeding, prophylaxis is to be considered.

COAGULOPATHIES

The prophylactic treatment of patients with severe hemophilia A and B has been proven to be very effective in avoiding hemophilic arthropathies. *All* hemophilia patients, whether severe, moderate or mild by laboratory and clinical criteria, need factor support perioperatively. This treatment needs to be guided by physicians experienced in the care of these patients. Known hemophilic patients with acute injuries, especially skull trauma, need to receive factor replacement *prior to* any diagnostic procedures and laboratory assessment. The dose, frequency, and duration of factor treatment for acute bleeds depends on the site of bleeding (2 weeks for brain bleed, factor level 80–100 units/dL; 1–2 days for *ordinary* joint bleed; factor level 40–60 units/dL).

Coagulopathy caused by vitamin K deficiency will be corrected within several hours by administration of vitamin K. Coagulopathy caused by liver disease can only be treated by replacement of coagulation factors synthesized in the liver. Commonly, fresh frozen plasma is utilized. When determining the necessary quantity, one needs to remember that the factor concentration in pooled plasma is close to 100 units/dL; and in general factor levels of >30 units/dL are needed for effective hemostasis.

Hemostatic support is needed for patients with DIC/consumption coagulopathy who bleed and are thrombocytopenic and/or hypofibrinogenemic. Patients with DIC frequently have platelets with abnormal function and, therefore, need platelet support at higher platelet concentrations than patients with immune thrombocytopenias. Fibrinogen replacement is needed for patients with fibrinogen levels below 100 to 150 mg/dL. Cryoprecipitate, which is rich in fibrinogen, is used for this purpose.

BIBLIOGRAPHY

Cattaneo M. Inherited platelet-based bleeding disorders. *J Thromb Haemost.* 2003;1:1628–1636.

Rao AK. Inherited defects in platelet signaling mechanisms. *J Thromb Haemost.* 2003;1:671–681.

Nurden AT. Qualitative disorders of platelet and megakaryocytes. *J Thromb Haemost.* 2005;3:1773–1782.

Balduini C, Cattaneo M, Fabris F, et al. Italian Gruppo di Studio delle Piastrine. Inherited thrombocytopenias. A proposed diagnostic algorithm from the Italian Gruppo di Studio delle Piastrine. *Haematologica.* 2003;88:582–592.

Sadler JE, et al. Update on the pathophysiology and classification of von Willebrand disease: A report of the Subcommittee on von Willebrand Factor. *J Thromb Haemost.* 2006;4:2103–2114.

63 THROMBOPHILIA
Ganesh C. Kudva

EPIDEMIOLOGY

- Deep vein thrombosis (DVT) and/or pulmonary embolism are collectively referred to as venous thromboembolic (VTE) disease.
- Pulmonary embolism almost always follows deep vein thrombosis of the lower extremities; rarely of the upper extremities, or the right heart.
- In the absence of treatment, pulmonary embolism occurs in 50% of cases of DVT over 3 months.
- If untreated pulmonary embolism carries a 10% to 25% mortality. With treatment, mortality is reduced to 1.5% for pulmonary embolism and 0.4% for DVT.
- Long-term morbidity includes pulmonary hypertension (3%–4%) and postthrombotic syndrome (30%).
- In the United States 2 million cases of DVT and 600,000 cases of pulmonary embolism are estimated to occur annually.
- Between 60,000 to 200,000 deaths likely occur annually in the United States because of pulmonary embolism.
- Although thrombophilia was originally used to describe an inherited tendency (demonstrable by a laboratory test) toward recurrent venous thromboembolism, of late it has been applied to acquired conditions and arterial thrombosis. This discussion is confined to hypercoagulable states causing VTE (Tables 63–1 to 63–3).

PATHOPHYSIOLOGY

- Normally, blood is maintained in the fluid state by an equilibrium between coagulation factors and natural anticoagulants such as antithrombin III and proteins C and S. The negatively charged endothelium prevents contact with tissue factor, a potent initiator of coagulation and collagen that binds to platelets and enables formation of a platelet plug.
- The Virchow triad, consisting of stasis, vessel wall injury, and hypercoagulability, is still helpful in broadly understanding the pathogenesis of VTE.

TABLE 63–1 Inherited Thrombophilia

Antithrombin III deficiency
Protein C deficiency
Protein S deficiency
Factor V Leiden mutation
Prothrombin G20210A mutation
Dysfibrinogenemia

TABLE 63–2 Risk Factors for Thrombosis/Acquired Thrombophilia

AGE	CANCER
Major surgery	Heart failure
Trauma	Antiphospholipid syndrome
Immobilization (cast or bed)	Myeloproliferative disorders
Long-distance travel	PNH
Pregnancy and puerperium	Heparin-induced thrombocytopenia
Hormone therapy (estrogens, progestins)	Obesity
Drugs (L-asparaginase)	Venous catheters
Smoking	Previous VTE

- Venous thromboembolism may be unprovoked (idiopathic) in approximately 40% to 50% of cases or provoked by a number of identifiable risk factors, which may upset the delicate procoagulant-anticoagulant balance, in 50% to 60% of patients.
- Fifty percent of patients with inherited thrombophilia that develop a first episode of VTE are provoked. In addition, many thrombophilic patients suffer their first event later in life. These observations have led to a two-hit theory to explain the pathogenesis: (1) an underlying (likely genetic) predisposition to thrombosis (thrombophilia) and (2) an acquired risk factor which precipitates thrombus formation.

HEREDITARY THROMBOPHILIA

ANTITHROMBIN III DEFICIENCY

- Characterized by Egeberg in 1965 in a Norwegian family with thrombophilia.
- Antithrombin III is a potent natural anticoagulant that inhibits thrombin activity.
- In the absence of antithrombin III, thrombin remains persistently active leading to VTE.
- Incidence: whites 0.02%, patients with the first episode of DVT 1%, antithrombin III deficiency is present in 4% of thrombophilic families.
- Autosomal dominant mode of inheritance.
- Heterozygous state leads to VTE.
- Homozygous state is incompatible with life.
- Likely to cause heparin resistance as heparin acts by potentiating antithrombin activity.

TABLE 63–3 Complex Thrombophilia

Hyperhomocysteinemia
Hyperfibrinogenemia
Elevated factor VIII
Elevated factor IX
Elevated factor XI

- Antithrombin III infusions are especially helpful in these patients.

PROTEIN C DEFICIENCY

- Discovered by Griffin and coworkers in 1981.
- Protein C is a natural anticoagulant.
- In the presence of cofactor protein S, it inactivates activated factors V and VIII.
- Incidence: whites 0.2%, patients with the first episode of VTE 3%, thrombophilic families 6%.
- Autosomal dominant mode of inheritance.
- Heterozygous state leads to VTE.
- Homozygous state leads to neonatal purpura fulminans.

PROTEIN S DEFICIENCY

- Discovered by Comp, Schwartz, and coworkers in 1984.
- Protein S is a natural anticoagulant.
- It acts as a cofactor in the inactivation of activated factors V and VIII by protein C.
- Incidence: whites 0.2%; first episode of VTE 1% to 2%, thrombophilic families 6%.
- Autosomal dominant mode of inheritance.
- Heterozygous state leads to VTE.
- Homozygous state leads to neonatal purpura fulminans.

FACTOR V LEIDEN MUTATION

- Discovered by Dahlbeck and coworkers in 1993.
- Mutation was further characterized by Bertina and colleagues from Leiden in 1994.
- G1691A mutation results in an amino acid substitution (R516Q) in factor V that promotes resistance to the action of activated protein C.
- Persistantly activated factor V leads to thrombosis.
- Incidence: whites 4% to 7%, first VTE 20%, thrombophilic families 40%.
- Founder mutation believed to have evolved approximately 30,000 years ago.
- Autosomal dominant mode of inheritance.
- Heterozygous state leads to a fourfold rise in the risk of VTE.
- Homozygous state leads to a 40- to 80-fold rise in thrombotic risk.

PROTHROMBIN MUTATION G20210A

- Discovered by Poort and colleagues in 1996.
- Characterized by a mutation in 3' untranslated region of the prothrombin gene resulting in higher levels of

prothrombin (by an ill-defined mechanism) leading to increased thrombin formation.

- Incidence: whites 2%, first DVT 6%, thrombophilic families 18%.
- Autosomal dominant mode of inheritance.
- Heterozygous state leads to threefold rise in risk of VTE.
- Risk of thrombosis in the homozygous state is unknown.

DYSFIBRINOGENEMIA

- Extremely rare disorder characterized by a dysfunctional fibrinogen molecule.
- May be silent or associated with bleeding or arterial or venous thrombosis.
- Autosomal dominant mode of inheritance.

ACQUIRED THROMBOPHILIA

AGE, OBESITY, AND SMOKING

- The risk of a first VTE increases exponentially after 55 years of age.
- The risk in patients younger than age 15 years is <1/100,000/y; at 55 the risk is 62/100,000/y, and at age 80 the risk is 600/100,000/y.
- Interplay of other risk factors is believed to underlie the increased risk with advancing age.
- Obesity and smoking are independent risk factors that double the thrombotic risk.

SURGERY AND TRAUMA

- Certain types of surgery confer especially high risk: orthopedic procedures such as knee and hip replacements are the most common. It is also particularly prevalent after abdominal surgery.
- The mechanism leading to thrombosis is thought to be secondary to release of tissue factor coupled with prolonged immobilization.
- Thromboprophylaxis was first established as effective in these surgical settings.

IMMOBILIZATION (INCLUDING CASTS) AND LONG-DISTANCE TRAVEL

- Mechanism of thrombosis is believed to be secondary to stasis caused by inactivity of the calf or any other muscle that acts as a venous pump.
- Thromboprophylaxis has been established in patients with medical illness.

PREGNANCY AND HORMONAL (ESTROGEN AND PROGESTIN) THERAPY

- Thrombotic risk is increased fourfold.
- Greatest risk is in the puerperium.
- Several mechanisms are operative: reduced protein S, increased coagulation factor levels, reduced venous tone caused by estrogens, compression of the left iliac vein (enlarging uterus) resulting in stasis, and release of tissue factor at delivery.
- The absolute risk is not high enough to justify routine thromboprophylaxis in pregnancy.

CANCER AND CHEMOTHERAPY

- Cancer increases the risk of VTE fourfold or more.
- Multiple mechanisms play a role: release of tissue factor from the tumor, compression of veins leading to venous stasis, surgery and immobilization, frequent use of venous catheters, and drugs such as L-asparaginase and tamoxifen.
- L-Asparaginase may reduce synthesis of the natural anticoagulants antithrombin III, protein C and S.
- Low-molecular weight heparin has greater efficacy than warfarin in treating VTE in cancer patients.

VENOUS CATHETERS

- Because catheters are placed in upper extremity veins, they are the main cause of upper extremity venous thrombosis.
- Catheter-induced thrombosis is caused by mechanical venous trauma induced by the catheter.
- Catheters are the major cause of venous thrombosis in younger individuals.
- Only 10% of idiopathic deep venous thrombosis occurs in the upper extremities.
- Idiopathic upper extremity thrombosis is rarely caused by thrombophilia alone.

ANTIPHOSPHOLIPID SYNDROME

- Characterized by an antiphospholipid antibody directed against complexes of phospholipid and proteins such as β_2-glycoprotein I or prothrombin.
- The antibody may be detected by a coagulation test (lupus anticoagulant) or serological assays (anticardiolipin or anti-β_2-glycoprotein I immunoglobulin G or immunoglobulin M antibodies).
- Clinically, these patients present with either venous or arterial thrombosis or recurrent miscarriage.

MYELOPROLIFERATIVE DISORDERS

- Polycythemia vera and essential thrombocythemia, among others are associated with an increased risk of thrombosis partly caused by erythrocytosis and thrombocytosis.
- A complete blood count usually reveals the diagnosis.
- Thrombosis of visceral veins such as the portal vein and superior mesenteric vein may occur before the phenotypic manifestation of myeloproliferative disorders (and may be identified by the JAK2 mutation).
- Correction of blood counts significantly reduces thrombotic risk.

PAROXYSMAL NOCTURNAL HEMOGLOBINURIA

- Rare, acquired clonal disorder caused by a mutation in the PIG-A gene, which encodes for an enzyme involved in the terminal step of the synthesis of the glycosylphosphatidylinositol anchor; a molecular anchor for many membrane proteins on hematopoietic cells.
- Red cells lack a membrane protein (CD59 or Membrane Inhibitor of Reactive Lysis) that confers protection against complement-mediated lysis. Thus patients with this disorder develop intravascular hemolysis.
- Patients with this disorder may develop pancytopenia or aplastic anemia.
- The mechanism of thrombosis is unclear but occurs only in patients who are anemic.

HEPARIN-INDUCED THROMBOCYTOPENIA

- Heparin-induced thrombocytopenia is a well-known but potentially fatal complication of heparin and low molecular weight heparin (LMWH) therapy.
- It is caused by an antibody against complexes of platelet factor 4 and heparin or LMWH.
- Usually, thrombocytopenia occurs 5 to 14 days after starting heparin/LMWH therapy; earlier if previously exposed.
- Thirty percent of patients develop arterial or venous thrombosis.
- The diagnosis is confirmed by heparin antibody detection via enzyme-linked immunosorbent assay or serotonin release assay methods.
- Treatment includes immediate discontinuation of heparin/LMWH and anticoagulation with a direct thrombin inhibitor such as argatroban or lepirudin.
- Warfarin may be substituted after the platelet count exceeds 100,000/μL.

- Continue anticoagulation for at least 1 month even in the absence of thrombosis.
- In the event of thrombosis, anticoagulation is continued for 3 to 6 months.
- Avoid heparin use in the future.

COMPLEX THROMBOPHILIA

HYPERHOMOCYSTEINEMIA

- Associated with an fourfold increased risk of initial and recurrent VTE.
- Hyperhomocysteinemia may be inherited as well as acquired.
- Deficiencies of vitamins B_{12} and B_6 and folic acid, renal failure, and hypothyroidism may be associated with hyperhomocysteinemia.
- However, recent studies suggest that hyperhomocysteinemia is only a marker of and is not involved in mediating thrombosis because correction of hyperhomocysteinemia with supplemental folic acid, B_{12} and B_6 does not reduce the incidence or recurrence of VTE.[1]

ELEVATED FACTOR LEVELS

- Elevated levels of factor VIII, XI, IX, and fibrinogen may be inherited or acquired.
- Levels higher than 150% of normal increase thrombotic risk by two- to fourfold.

TREATMENT OF VENOUS THROMBOEMBOLISM

- Anticoagulation with heparin followed by warfarin for at least 3 to 6 months. Less than 3 months is inadequate. For patients whose VTE is provoked, a short course (<3 months) of warfarin may be adequate if the inciting factor is eliminated. Extended anticoagulation has been demonstrated to be beneficial for up to 2 years after an initial unprovoked event.[2] For those with recurrent VTE (three or more events) indefinite anticoagulation is recommended.

SCREENING PATIENTS FOR THROMBOPHILIA

- Obtain a thorough history, careful physical examination, and systematic laboratory evaluation together with a chest x-ray. These studies may establish the diagnosis of VTE and reveal most inciting factors. The chance of finding one or more thrombophilic conditions in patients with idiopathic VTE has increased from <10% to >50% in the last decade following the

TABLE 63–4 Screening for Thrombophilia in Venous Thromboembolism

Unprovoked VTE, especially younger than age 55
Multiple VTE
VTE in unusual sites: visceral veins, cerebral veins, and so forth
Family history, especially of unprovoked VTE
Recurrent (three or more) miscarriages

VTE, venous thromboembolism.

discovery of factor V Leiden and prothrombin G20210A mutation. A comprehensive hypercoagulable work-up must be undertaken when hypercoagulability is suspected (Table 63–4).

• The diagnosis of thrombosis after provocation does not usually warrant a workup for inherited thrombophilia if the offending factor can be eliminated, because elimination of the risk factor reduces the risk of recurrent VTE to that of individuals without thrombophilia.[3] In the event of unprovoked VTE, workup for inherited thrombophilia is worth pursuing, especially if the patient is a candidate for extended anticoagulation (Table 63–5).

FAMILY SCREENING FOR THROMBOPHILIA

• First-degree relatives of individuals with inherited thrombophilia have a 50% chance of inheriting these autosomal dominant traits. However, screening for inherited thrombophilia in healthy individuals with a family history of VTE must be carefully considered, weighing the benefits of such knowledge against potential problems with insurability, particularly because the absolute lifetime risk of thrombosis is still quite low despite a high relative risk (Table 63–6). Besides patient preference, other considerations for testing include, the use of intensive antithromboprophylaxis in high-risk situations such as during pregnancy and the puerperium and counseling patients regarding oral contraceptive therapy. At present there is no clear benefit to thrombophilia testing in asymptomatic children.

TABLE 63–5 Indications for Extended Anticoagulation in Unprovoked Venous Thromboembolism

Homozygous factor V Leiden
Compound heterozygosity for factor V Leiden and prothrombin G20210A
Antithrombin III deficiency
Protein C deficiency
Protein S deficiency
Dysfibrinogenemia
Antiphospholipid syndrome
Cancer

TABLE 63–6 Relative and Absolute Risk of Thrombosis

HETEROZYGOUS THROMBOPHILIA	RELATIVE RISK	ABSOLUTE RISK
Antithrombin III deficiency	fivefold	1/1000
Protein C deficiency	sevenfold	1/700
Protein S deficiency	sixfold	1/800
Factor V Leiden	sevenfold	1/700
Prothrombin G20210A	threefold	1/1600

REFERENCES

1. Ray JG, Kearon C, Yi Q, et al. Homocysteine-lowering therapy and risk for venous thromboembolism-a randomized trial. *Ann Intern Med.* 2007;146:761.
2. Kearon C, Ginsberg JS, Kovacs MJ, et al. Comparison of low-intensity warfarin therapy with conventional-intensity warfarin therapy for long-term prevention of recurrent venous thromboembolism. *N Engl J Med.* 2003;349:631.
3. De Stefano V, Martinelli I, Mannucci PM, et al. The risk of recurrent deep venous thrombosis among heterozygous carriers of both factor V Leiden and the G20210A prothrombin mutation. *N Engl J Med.* 1999;341:801.

BIBLIOGRAPHY

Colman RW, Hirsh J, Marder VJ, et al. *Hemostasis and Thrombosis: Basic Principles and Practice.* Philadelphia, PA: Lippincott Williams & Wilkins; 2001.
Cushman M. Epidemiology and risk factors for venous thrombosis. *Semin Hematol.* 2007;44:62.

64 MYELODYSPLASIA

Scott McGee

DEFINITION AND CLASSIFICATION

Myelodysplastic syndrome (MDS) is comprised of malignant stem-cell disorders characterized by dysplasia and ineffective erythropoiesis.[1] The French-American-British (FAB) classification originally relied on peripheral blood and bone-marrow findings to determine the

TABLE 64–1   FAB Classification of MDS

TYPE	BONE MARROW BLASTS (%)	PERIPHERAL BLOOD BLASTS (%)	AUER RODS	MONOCYTES (>1000 μ/L)	RINGED SIDEROBLASTS
RA	<5	≤1	No	No	No
RARS	<5	≤1	No	No	Yes
RAEB	5–20	<5	No	No	±
CMML	≤20	<5	No	Yes	±
RAEB-T[a]	21–30	OR ≥5	±	±	±

CMML, chronic myelomonocytic leukemia; FAB, French-American-British; MDS, myelodysplastic syndrome; RA, refractory anemia; RAEB, refractory anemia with excess blasts; RAEB-T, refractory anemia with excess of blasts in transformation; RARS, refractory anemia with ring sideroblasts; WHO, World Health Organization.
[a]The WHO classification considers ≥20% blasts to be acute leukemia.

type of MDS[2] (Table 64–1). The World Health Organization (WHO) recently revised this system to include cytogenetics[3] (Table 64–2).

- MDS can occur de novo or as a result of damage sustained from exposure to mutagens such as chemotherapy or radiation (therapy-related MDS [T-MDS]).[4]
- T-MDS responds less well to therapy and has a worse prognosis than de nova MDS.
- Among the conditions classified as MDS, there is a variable risk of transformation to acute leukemia, which is highest for refractory anemia with excess blasts-2 (RAEB-2) (40%) and lowest for refractory anemia with ring sideroblasts (RARS) (5%).[5]

EPIDEMIOLOGY

- The exact incidence of MDS is unknown but is thought to exceed that of acute leukemia, which has an incidence of 2.1 cases per 100,000.[6]
- The risk for acquiring MDS increases with advancing age such that it is rare in patients younger than 50 years of age. However, it has been described in children.

CLINICAL PRESENTATION

- The clinical presentation is variable. Some patients can present with fatigue or dyspnea related to anemia.

TABLE 64–2   WHO Classification of MDS

Refractory anemia (RA)
Refractory anemia with ringed sideroblasts (RARS)
Refractory cytopenia with multilineage dysplasia
Refractory cytopenia with multilineage dysplasia and ringed sideroblasts
Refractory anemia with excess blasts-1 (RAEB-1)
Refractory anemia with excess blasts-2 (RAEB-2)
MDS unclassified
MDS with isolated del(5q)

MDS, myelodysplastic syndrome; WHO, World Health Organization.

Less commonly, patients can present with recurrent infections from neutropenia or bleeding related to thrombocytopenia.[7] Others can be completely asymptomatic and come to the clinicians attention because of incidental laboratory abnormalities.

LABORATORY FINDINGS

- Patients are almost always anemic and have a low reticulocyte count. Anemia can be the only abnormality, or it can be accompanied by leukopenia and/or thrombocytopenia.
- Approximately 50% of patients present with pancytopenia (anemia, leukopenia, and thrombocytopenia).
- Paradoxically, the bone marrow will be hypercellular in 90% of cases.
- On the peripheral blood smear ovalomacrocytosis (large, oval-shaped red cells) is a classic finding. Elliptocytes and tear drop forms may also be identified.
- Ringed sideroblasts are red-cell precursors in the bone marrow that have five or more iron granules around the nucleus when the marrow is stained for iron.[8] They are characteristic of RARS but can be seen in any of the MDS subtypes.
- Granulocytes often display decreased segmentation of the nucleus. A special abnormality known as the *pseudo–Pelger-Huet* anomaly occurs when the neutrophils are bilobed.[9]
- Platelets are often large and can be hypogranular. Platelets that are as large as the red cells are termed *giant platelets*.

DIAGNOSIS

- MDS should be considered in patients with unexplained cytopenias or monocytosis.[10]
- Examination of the blood smear and bone marrow is required to demonstrate the required dysplastic features.[11]

- Other conditions that may contribute to the blood and bone marrow findings must be excluded (see Differential Diagnosis below).

PROGNOSIS

Although the WHO and FAB classifications facilitate the diagnosis, they do not provide information on prognosis.[12] An international workshop on MDS developed the International Prognostic Scoring System (IPSS) for MDS (Table 64–3).[13] The IPSS uses the percentage of bone marrow blasts, karyotype, and number of cytopenias to provide an overall score which classifies patients into one of four prognostic groups with significantly different median survivals (Table 64–4).

- The time to progression to acute leukemia was also significantly different in each of the four risk groups:
  ○ Low: 9.4 years
  ○ Intermediate 1: 3.3 years
  ○ Intermediate 2: 1.1 years
  ○ High: 0.4 years
- Other prognostic factors that are associated with a poor prognosis include transfusion dependence,[14] p53 mutations or loss of heterozygosity,[15] CD34 positivity of bone marrow nucleated cells, increased serum β_2-microglobulin,[16] and mutations in the FLT3 gene.[17]

DIFFERENTIAL DIAGNOSIS

Several diseases can present with clinical features that overlap with MDS (Table 64–4). Because treatments for these conditions and MDS are significantly different, it is critical to establish the correct diagnosis.

TREATMENT

- Goals of treatment for MDS include the following:
  1. Control of symptoms related to cytopenias
  2. Improvement in quality of life
  3. Improvement in survival
  4. Prevention of progression to acute leukemia
- The only curative treatment for MDS is allogeneic hematopoietic cell transplant. Unfortunately, lack of suitable donors, advanced patient age, and concomitant medical comorbidities render the large majority of patients ineligible for transplant. It is important to realize that transplant-related mortality and relapse rate at 5 years can be as high as 40%.
- Treatments have been divided into either *high* or *low* intensity as follows:[18]
  ○ *High-intensity* treatment usually requires hospitalization and carries a significant risk of treatment-related mortality. Combination chemotherapy and hematopoietic cell transplantation are included under this category
  ○ *Low-intensity* treatment is outpatient-based and includes growth factors, differentiation-inducing agents, biologic response modifiers, and low-intensity chemotherapy
- Supportive care entails treating infections with antibiotics and administering red-cell and platelet transfusions for symptomatic anemia and thrombocytopenia, respectively.

TABLE 64–3   IPSS for MDS

VARIABLE	SCORE				
	0	0.5	1.0	1.5	2.0
Bone marrow blasts (%)	<5%	5–10%		11–20%	21–30%
Karyotype[a]	Good	Intermediate	Poor		
Cytopenias[b]	0 or 1	2 or 3			

RISK GROUP	IPSS SCORE	MEDIAN OS
Low	0	5.7 y
Intermediate-1	0.5–1.0	3.5 y
Intermediate-2	1.5–2.0	1.2 y
High	2.5–3.5	0.4 y

IPSS, International Prognostic Scoring System; MDS, myelodysplastic syndrome; OS, overall survival.
[a]Karyotype definitions:
Good: normal; -Y; del(5q); del(20q)
Poor: complex (≥3 abnormalities); abnormal chromosome 7
Intermediate: all others
[b]Cytopenia definitions:
Red blood cells (RBCs): hemoglobin (HGB) <10 g/dL
White blood cells (WBC): absolute neutrophil count <1800 μ/L
Platelets: platelet count <100,000 μ/L

TABLE 64–4   Differential Diagnosis of MDS

Aplastic anemia
Megaloblastic anemia
Myelofibrosis
Atypical CML
HIV infection
Drugs:
    Valproic acid
    Mycophenolate
    Ganciclovir

CML, chronic myelogenous leukemia; HIV, (human immunodeficiency virus); MDS, myelodysplastic syndrome.

- Chronic red-cell transfusions can lead to iron overload, which will require chelation therapy.
- The response of patients with MDS to hematopoietic growth factors (granulocyte-macrophage colony-stimulating factor [GMCSF], granulocyte colony-stimulating factor [GCSF], and erythropoietin [EPO]) has been disappointing. Interestingly, the combination of EPO and GCSF has been shown to decrease transfusion requirements in patients with low-serum EPO and IPSS low or intermediate-1 risk.[19]
- The biologic response modifiers, thalidomide and its derivative, lenalidomide (Revimid) can function as anticytokines in MDS.
- Thalidomide has produced responses in some low-risk MDS patients, but side effects (neuropathy, fatigue, constipation) generally outweigh the benefit.[20]
- Lenalidomide, which does not cause significant neuropathy, has been effective in low-risk MDS patients, particularly those with deletion 5q.[21] Indeed, this agent is Food and Drug Administration (FDA)-approved for patients with transfusion-dependent anemia caused by low or intermediate-1 risk MDS with a deletion 5q cytogenetic abnormality.
- Low intensity chemotherapy is an option for patients with intermediate or high IPSS risk MDS.
- Cytarabine is the most widely studied agent. It has not, however, proven to be very effective with complete response rates below 20%.[22]
- Azacytidine (Vidaza), a pyrimidine nucleoside analog, functions as both a direct cytotoxic agent as well as a DNA hypomethylating agent (methylation of promoter regions silences gene expression while reversing the methylation can permit expression of genes).[23] It has been shown to delay time to death and leukemic transformation, improve quality of life, and increase survival in MDS patients in a recent phase III trial.[24] Azacytidine is FDA-approved for use in refractory anemia (RA) or RARS (if accompanied by neutropenia, thrombocytopenia, or transfusion dependency), refractory anemia with excess blasts (RAEB), refractory anemia with excess blasts in transition (RAEB-T), and chronic myelomacrocytic leukemia (CMML).

- Decitabine (Dacogen) is also a pyrimidine nucleoside analog with potent DNA hypomethylating properties. In a phase II trial, it improved survival of IPSS high risk patients to 1.2 years (expected survival for this group is only 0.4 years).[25] Decitabine has been FDA-approved for use in patients with treated, untreated, de novo, and secondary MDS of all FAB subtypes and intermediate-1, -2, and high-risk IPSS groups.
- High-intensity chemotherapy employs regimens similar to those used for the treatment of acute myelogenous leukemia. Response rates for MDS are not as good as they are for acute leukemia, likely because of patient factors (older age, poor cytogenetics).[26] MDS patients with intermediate-2 or high-risk IPSS scores and good performance status should be considered for high-intensity therapy followed by hematopoietic cell transplantation.[27]

RECOMMENDATIONS

- The National Comprehensive Cancer Network (NCCN) recommendations for MDS include the following:[18]
  - Patients ≤60 years of age with good or excellent performance status and in the IPSS low or intermediate-1 category should be considered for low-intensity therapy or supportive care.
  - Patients ≤60 years of age with good or excellent performance status and in the IPSS intermediate-2 or high-risk category should be considered for high-intensity therapies.
  - Patients >60 years of age with good performance status and in the IPSS intermediate-2 or high-risk categories should be considered for low-intensity therapies, although selected patients can be considered for high-intensity treatments.
  - Patients >60 years of age with good performance status and in the IPSS low or intermediate-1 categories should be considered for supportive care or low-intensity therapies.
  - Patients with poor performance status, regardless of age, should be offered supportive care, although selected patients may be candidates for low-intensity therapies.

REFERENCES

1. Doll, DC, List, AF. Myelodysplastic syndromes. *West J Med.*1989;151:161.
2. Bennett, JM, Catovsky, D, Daniel, MT, et al. FAB Cooperative Group: proposal for the classification of the myelodysplastic syndromes. *Br J Haematol.* 1982;51:189.

3. Brunning, RD, et al. Myelodysplastic syndromes: Introduction. In: Jaffe, ES, Harris, NL, Stein, H, Vardiman, JW, eds. *World Health Organization Classification of Tumours. Pathology and Genetics of Tumours of Haematopoietic and Lymphoid Tissues.* Lyon: IARC Press; 2001.

4. Levine, EG, Bloomfield, CD. Leukemias and myelodysplastic syndromes secondary to drug, radiation, and environmental exposure. *Semin Oncol.* 1992;19:47.

5. Sanz, GF, Sanz, MA, Vallespi, T, et al. Two regression models and a scoring system for predicting survival and planning treatment in myelodysplastic syndromes: A multivariate analysis of prognostic factors in 370 patients. *Blood.* 1989;74:395.

6. Aul, C, Gattermann, N, Schneider, W. Age-related incidence and other epidemiological aspects of myelodysplastic syndromes. *Br J Haematol.* 1992;82:358.

7. Foucar, K, Langdon RM, 2d, Armitage, JO, et al. Myelodysplastic syndromes. A clinical and pathologic analysis of 109 cases. *Cancer.* 1985;56:553.

8. Hast, R. Sideroblasts in myelodysplasia: Their nature and clinical significance. *Scand J Haematol Suppl.* 1986;45:53.

9. Kuriyama, K, Tomonaga, M, Matsuo, T, et al. Diagnostic significance of detecting pseudo–Pelger-Huet anomalies and micro-megakaryocytes in myelodysplastic syndrome. *Br J Haematol.* 1986;63:665.

10. Steensma, DP, Bennett, JM. The myelodysplastic syndromes: Diagnosis and treatment. *Mayo Clin Proc.* 2006;81:104.

11. Bowen, D, Culligan, D, Jowitt, S, et al. Guidelines for the diagnosis and therapy of adult myelodysplastic syndromes. *Br J Haematol.* 2003;120:187.

12. Greenberg, PL, Sanz, GF, Sanz, MA. Prognostic scoring systems for risk assessment in myelodysplastic syndromes. *Forum (Genova).* 1999;2: 917-944.

13. Greenberg, P, Cox, C, Le Beau, MM, et al. International scoring system for evaluating prognosis in myelodysplastic syndromes. *Blood.* 1997;89:2079.

14. Balducci, L. Transfusion independence in patients with myelodysplastic syndromes: Impact on outcomes and quality of life. *Cancer.* 2006;106:2087.

15. Christiansen, DH, Andersen, MK, Pedersen-Bjergaard, J. Mutations with loss of heterozygosity of p53 are common in therapy-related myelodysplasia and acute myeloid leukemia after exposure to alkylating agents and significantly associated with deletion or loss of 5q, a complex karyotype, and a poor prognosis. *J Clin Oncol.* 2001;19:1405.

16. Gatto, S, Ball, G, Onida, F, Kantarjian, HM. Contribution of β-2 microglobulin levels to the prognostic stratification of survival in patients with myelodysplastic syndrome (MDS). *Blood.* 2003;102:1622.

17. Georgiou, G, Karali, V, Zouvelou, C, et al. Serial determination of FLT3 mutations in myelodysplastic syndrome patients at diagnosis, follow up or acute myeloid leukaemia transformation: Incidence and their prognostic significance. *Br J Haematol.* 2006;134:302.

18. National Comprehensive Cancer Network (NCCN). NCCN practice guidelines for the myelodysplastic syndromes. *J Nat Compr Canc Netw.* 2003;1456. www.nccn.org/professionals/physician_gls/default.asp. Accessed March 8, 2005.

19. Negrin, RS, Stein, R, Doherty, K, et al. Maintenance treatment of the anemia of myelodysplastic syndromes with recombinant human G-CSF plus erythropoietin: Evidence for in vivo synergy. *Blood.* 1996;87:4076.

20. Moreno-Aspitia, A, Colon-Otero, G, Hoering, A, et al. Thalidomide therapy in adult patients with myelodysplastic syndrome. *Cancer.* 2006;107:767.

21. List, A, Kurtin, S, Roe, DJ, et al. Efficacy of lenalidomide in myelodysplastic syndromes. *N Engl J Med.* 2005;352:549.

22. Miller, KB, Kim, K, Morrison, FS, et al. The evaluation of low-dose cytarabine in the treatment of myelodysplastic syndromes: A phase-III intergroup study [erratum *Ann Hematol* 1993;66:3164]. *Ann Hematol.* 1992;65:162.

23. Cheson, BD. Standard and low-dose chemotherapy for the treatment of myelodysplastic syndromes. *Leuk Res.* 1998;22 (suppl 1):S17.

24. Silverman, LR, Demakos, EP, Peterson, BL, et al. Randomized controlled trial of azacitidine in patients with the myelodysplastic syndrome: A study of the cancer and leukemia group B. *J Clin Oncol.* 2002;20:2429.

25. Wijermans, P, Lubbert, M, Verhoef, G, et al. Low-dose 5-aza-2′-deoxycytidine, a DNA hypomethylating agent, for the treatment of high-risk myelodysplastic syndrome: A multicenter phase II study in elderly patients. *J Clin Oncol.* 2000;18:956.

26. Tricot, G, Boogaerts, MA. The role of aggressive chemotherapy in the treatment of the myelodysplastic syndromes. *Br J Haematol.* 1986;63:477.

27. de Witte, T, Suciu, S, Verhoef, G, et al. Intensive chemotherapy followed by allogeneic or autologous stem cell transplantation for patients with myelodysplastic syndromes (MDSs) and acute myeloid leukemia following MDS. *Blood.* 2001;98:2326.

65 MYELOPROLIFERATIVE DISORDERS

Sri Laxmi Valasareddi

The myeloproliferative disorders are a group of clonal hematopoietic stem cell diseases characterized by overproduction of one or more hematologic cell lines.

WHO Classification:
1. Polycythemia vera
2. Essential thrombocythemia
3. Chronic idiopathic myelofibrosis
4. Chronic myelogenous leukemia
5. Chronic neutrophilic leukemia
6. Chronic eosinophilic leukemia/hypereosinophilic syndrome
7. Chronic myeloproliferative disorders, unclassifiable

POLYCYTHEMIA VERA

Polycythemia vera (PV) is a clonal disorder arising in the multipotent hematopoietic progenitor cell that is responsible for the accumulation of morphologically normal red cells, white cells, and platelets. A definable stimulus and nonclonal hematopoiesis must be excluded. It is distinguished from other myeloproliferative disorders by the presence of elevated RBC mass. It was first described by Vasquez in 1892 and in 1951 classified as a myeloproliferative disorder by Dameshek.

EPIDEMIOLOGY

- Incidence is 2.3 per 100,000
- Median age at diagnosis is 60 years
- Male to female ratio is 1.2:1

PATHOGENESIS

PV is caused by one or more genetic events in a single hematopoietic progenitor cell that leads to an increase in red cell production and a variable increase of platelets and myeloid cells. A possible explanation for the hypersensitivity of hematopoietic progenitor cells to growth factors and other cytokines has been provided by a study of the cytoplasmic tyrosine kinase Janus kinase 2 (JAK2), a gene located on the short arm of chromosome 9 (9p). JAK2V617F is an acquired somatic mutation with replacement of valine by phenylalanine at position 617 in the Janus Kinase 2 protein. JAK-2 phosphorylates itself and adjacent receptors which leads to a cascade of erythroid-specific signaling which inhibits erythroid apoptosis and promotes proliferation and differentiation. JAK-2 inhibits itself, down-regulating the erythropoietin signal. JAK2 mutations are present in up to 95% of patients. The presence of the mutation distinguishes PV from secondary polycythemia. The mutation is not specific and is present in 50% to 60% of patients with essential thrombocytosis and 40% to 50% with agnogenic myeloid metaplasia (AMM). Seventy percent of patients are heterozygous and 30% are homozygous. Homozygosity is associated with a higher Hb level, more severe pruritus and a higher risk of myelofibrosis, but similar disease duration and incidence of thrombosis/bleeding.

CLINICAL FEATURES

- Headache, weakness, dizziness, and excessive sweating
- Pruritus (after a warm bath)
- Erythromelalgia or burning pain in the hands and feet associated with erythema, pallor, or cyanosis
- Transient visual disturbances
- Thrombosis: Venous in the lower extremities, pulmonary, mesenteric, splenic, portal vessels and hepatic vessels causing the Budd-Chiari syndrome and arterial thrombi in the coronary or cerebrovascular circulation
- Hemorrhage as a result of thrombocytosis or an acquired von Willebrand syndrome
- Gastrointestinal symptoms such as epigastric distress with gastroduodenal erosions and peptic ulcer disease.

PHYSICAL FINDINGS

- Splenomegaly in 70%
- Facial plethora in 65%
- Hepatomegaly in 40%
- Engorgement of the optic fundus veins
- Excoriation of the skin due to pruritus
- Stigmata of a prior thrombotic event such as stroke, deep venous thrombosis, or superficial thrombophlebitis
- Gouty arthritis

LABORATORY FINDINGS

- Red cell mass (RCM) >36 mL/Kg in men and >32 mL/Kg in women using isotope dilution
- Hb >16.5 g/dL, HCT >50% in women
- Hb >18.5 g/dL, HCT >56% in men
- Thrombocytosis: Platelets >400,000
- Leukocytosis: white blood cell (WBC) >12,000 (mostly neutrophils)
- Elevated leukocyte alkaline phosphatase (LAP) in 70% (non specific)
- Elevated serum B12 level
- Low serum erythropoietin (EPO)
- Bone marrow is hypercellular with erythroid hyperplasia and increased megakaryocytes. There is absence of stainable iron in 94% of patients.

DIAGNOSIS

WHO criteria to establish the diagnosis
- Basic criteria
  1. Demonstration of an increased RCM or increased hemoglobin concentration, or an elevated hematocrit.
  2. Disorders causing secondary erythrocytosis are absent, including hypoxia, familial polycythemic

disorders, high-affinity hemoglobins, truncated EPO receptor, and ectopic EPO production by a tumor.

In addition to the two basic criteria listed above, one of the following should also be present: splenomegaly or a clonal genetic abnormality other than the Philadelphia chromosome (or BCR-ABL fusion gene), or spontaneous endogenous erythroid colony formation *in vitro*.

If these are not present, the diagnosis can be established in the presence of the two basic criteria plus two (or more) of the following:

• Platelet count >400,000/µL
• White blood cell count >12,000/µL
• Low serum EPO levels
• Bone marrow examination which reveals panmyelosis with prominent erythroid and megakaryocytic proliferation

DIFFERENTIAL DIAGNOSIS

• Secondary polycythemia is characterized by elevated red cell mass, elevated erythropoietin levels (because of tissue hypoxia) and increased leukocyte alkaline phosphatase. These patients do not develop thrombocytosis, leukocytosis, or splenomegaly.
• Relative polycythemia, also called Gaisböck disease or apparent polycythemia. These individuals have a contraction erythrocytosis because of a decrease in plasma volume.

TREATMENT

The goals of treatment are to minimize symptoms and the long term complications of the disease (thrombosis, bleeding, myelofibrosis, acute leukemia, or other malignancies).

1. Phlebotomy is the treatment of choice. The goal is to maintain the hematocrit below 45% in men and 42% in women. Phlebotomy does not control thrombocytosis and, indeed, may aggravate it.
2. Hydroxyurea is an antimetabolite that inhibits DNA synthesis. It is used in concert with phlebotomy in patients who are at high-risk for thrombosis (age over 70, prior thrombosis, platelet count >1,500,000/µL, presence of additional cardiovascular risk factors). Its main side effects are gastrointestinal irritation, leukopenia, stomatitis, and oral and leg ulcers.
3. Anagrelide interferes with maturation of megakaryocytes and is used mainly in patients who are refractory to other treatments and have persistent thrombocytosis. Side effects include palpitations, tachycardia, dizziness, nausea, diarrhea, and fluid retention. It is contraindicated in patients with cardiac, liver or kidney disease, and in pregnancy.
4. Interferon α is a biological myelo- and immunomodulatory agent. It is used in pregnancy to reduce the platelet count. Side effects include fever, arthralgias, myalgias, headache, anorexia, and depression. It is contraindicated in patients with advanced cardiac, liver, or kidney disease.
5. Radioisotope phosphorous-32 and chlorambucil were the first clinically useful cytoreductive agents, but they are rarely used today. They are effective in reducing platelet count, phlebotomy requirements, and leukocyte counts, but the risk of leukemia is 10% to 15% over 15 years. They can be considered for refractory disease and in patients with contraindications to the use of other agents.

PROGNOSIS

If left untreated, the median survival is 6 to 18 months. With treatment the median survival exceeds 10 years. The most common cause of mortality is thrombosis or transformation into acute myelogenous leukemia or a *spent* phase.

ESSENTIAL THROMBOCYTHEMIA

Essential thrombocythemia (ET) was first recognized in the 1930s. It is the most common MPD.

EPIDEMIOLOGY

• Incidence is 2.5:100,000/yr
• Median age at diagnosis is 60 years
• It is 1.5 to 2.0 times more common in women

PATHOBIOLOGY

• Thrombocytosis in ET results from an intrinsic proliferative abnormality of megakaryocyte progenitor cells
• The JAK2 gene mutation leads to constitutive tyrosine kinase phosphorylation activity that promotes hypersensitivity to local or circulating cytokines
• JAK2 mutations have been identified in 50% to 60% of patients with ET

CLINICAL FEATURES

- 50% are asymptomatic
- Vasomotor symptoms are observed in 40%
  - Headache
  - Lightheadedness
  - Atypical chest pain
  - Acral paresthesias and cyanosis
  - Cutaneous ulcers
  - Erythromelalgia
  - Transient visual disturbances
- Thrombosis occurs in 10% to 50%
  - Arterial: cerebral (transient ischemic attack [TIA], cerebrovascular accident [CVA]), coronary, ophthalmic, and distal extremities
  - Venous: deep extremities, pelvic, mesenteric, hepatic, portal
- Hemorrhage: GI, mucosal, epistaxis, urogenital, deep-seated hematomas
- Obstetric: First trimester abortion
- Splenomegaly may be present in 25% to 50%

LABORATORY FINDINGS

- Platelet count >600,000/μL
- Large or giant platelets in the circulation
- Leukocytosis in ~50%
- Occasional eosinophil and megakaryocyte fragments in the peripheral blood
- Nucleated red cells and immature myeloid cells ~25% in the peripheral blood
- Leukocyte alkaline phosphatase (LAP) score is typically elevated
- Bone marrow is usually hypercellular. There are increased numbers and clusters of large megakaryocytes with hyperploid nuclei

DIAGNOSIS

ET is diagnosed in patients with sustained elevations of the platelet count >600,000/μL after exclusion of reactive thrombocytosis and other myeloproliferative disorders.

DIFFERENTIAL DIAGNOSIS

The most common cause of an elevated platelet count is reactive thrombocytosis. Causes include:
- Chronic infections such as tuberculosis or pneumonitis
- Inflammatory bowel disease
- Connective tissue disorders
- Anemia due to iron deficiency or hemolysis
- Drugs such as vincristine or growth factors
- Malignancy

Transient elevation in platelet number can occur with blood loss, acute infections, inflammation, and recovery from thrombocytopenia.

RISK STRATIFICATION

- Low risk (all of the following)
  - Age younger than 60 years
  - No history of thromboembolism
  - Platelet count <1,500,000/μL (without a bleeding history or acquired vWD)
  - No cardiovascular risk factors (smoking, hypercholesterolemia, hypertension, obesity)
- Intermediate risk
  - Neither low- nor high-risk features
- High risk (one or both)
  - Age ≥60 years
  - History of thromboembolism

TREATMENT

- Treatment is based on risk stratification
- The low-risk group does not require platelet reduction therapy. Low-dose aspirin may be administered if there is no history of bleeding
- Intermediate-risk group
  - Low-dose aspirin to reduce cardiovascular events; monitor for bleeding/bruising
  - Platelet-lowering agents should be employed in patients with platelet counts >1,500,000/μl and/or with bleeding symptoms
- High-risk groups are treated with platelet lowering therapy as well as low-dose aspirin
- Aspirin is also helpful in treating vasomotor symptoms
- In the event of acute thrombosis or hemorrhage, platelet pheresis to reduce the count to <600,000/μL should be considered
- Platelet-lowering agents
  - Hydroxyurea is an antimetabolite that can reduce the thrombosis rate and normalize the platelet count
  - Anagrelide is a prostaglandin synthetase inhibitor. It selectively inhibits platelet production without suppressing other lineages and also inhibits platelet aggregation at high doses. It is preferred over hydroxyurea for younger patients but should be used with caution in cardiac disease due to its vasodilatory effects. It is tenfold as expensive as hydroxyurea
  - Interferon α is the agent of choice for symptomatic or otherwise high-risk women with ET who desire

pregnancy, as the above agents are contraindicated in pregnancy

PROGNOSIS

Most patients will have a normal life expectancy if major bleeding or thrombotic complications can be avoided. Rare patients develop extensive myelofibrosis with myeloid metaplasia or AML (≤1%).

AGNOGENIC MYELOID METAPLASIA

Agnogenic myeloid metaplasia (AMM), also known as idiopathic myelofibrosis or primary myelofibrosis, was first described in 1879 by Hueck. It was included in the myeloproliferative disorders in 1951 by Dameshek, because of the similarity in clinical picture and bone marrow pathology with PV, ET, and CML.

EPIDEMIOLOGY

- Annual incidence rate of AMM is 0.5 to 1.5 cases per 100,000 persons
- Median age at diagnosis is 60 years
- Male-to-female ratio is approximately 1:1
- There is a link between radiation exposure, exposure to industrial solvents such as benzene and toluene, and exposure to radioactive contrast material (Thorotrast)
- There is some evidence of genetic transmission with a higher incidence noted in Ashkenazi Jews

PATHOGENESIS

- The mechanism of the disease process is not well understood but is believed to arise from a somatic mutation of a pluripotent hematopoietic progenitor cell which results in chronic myeloproliferation and atypical megakaryocytic hyperplasia.
- Megakaryocyte-derived growth factors resulting in fibroblastic proliferation have been shown to promote reactive fibrosis and also regulate hematopoiesis by selectively acting on early progenitor cell growth.
- Ineffective hematopoiesis and extramedullary hematopoiesis are chief characteristics of this disease.

CLINICAL FEATURES

There is a heterogeneous presentation with 20% of patients having no symptoms at the time of diagnosis.

When symptoms occur, they include
- Fever, night sweats, weight loss
- Weakness, fatigue, dyspnea on exertion (as a consequence of anemia)
- Petechiae, ecchymoses, or GI hemorrhage (caused by thrombocytopenia and abnormal platelet function)
- Bone pain
- Thromboembolic events such as pulmonary emboli and portal vein thrombosis
- Gouty arthritis

PHYSICAL FINDINGS

- Splenomegaly is present in 90% of patients
- Hepatomegaly in 70%
- Portal hypertension (10%–20%) with increased splanchnic flow (because of splenomegaly and/or intrahepatic obstruction) is associated with extramedullary hematopoiesis
- Pulmonary hypertension secondary to extramedullary hematopoiesis in the lungs and the development of pulmonary fibrosis
- Skin involvement is rare but may present with surface ulcers, bullae, nodules, or erythematous plaques
- Osteosclerosis with diffuse or patchy increase in bone density producing a mottled appearance on radiologic studies is seen in 25% to 66% of patients with AMM

LABORATORY FINDINGS

- Anemia is usually normocytic, normochromic secondary to ineffective RBC production and shortened RBC survival. Hemolytic anemia is common (15%)
- Leukopenia (13%–25%)
- Leukocytosis (30%)
- Thrombocytosis (>500,000)
- Thrombocytopenia (<100,000) in a third of patients in the myelofibrotic phase
- Defective platelet aggregation
- Disseminated intravascular coagulation (15%) (characterized by thrombocytopenia, decreased factor V and VII, increased fibrin split products)
- Elevated lactate dehydrogenase
- Increased serum vitamin B12 levels
- Hyperuricemia (60%)
- Alkaline phosphatase and γ-glutamyltransferase (GGT) enzyme elevations (50%)
- The JAK2 V617F gene mutation is seen in 50% of patients with AMM
- The peripheral blood smear reveals leukoerythroblastosis with nucleated red blood cells and immature myeloid elements. Teardrop erythrocytes, giant platelets, and megakaryocytic fragments are also seen

- Bone marrow examination: Bone marrow aspiration usually yields a dry tap.
- Bone marrow biopsy reveals fibrosis and is generally associated with atypical megakaryocytic hyperplasia and thickening and distortion of the bony trabeculae.

DIFFERENTIAL DIAGNOSIS

AMM is a diagnosis of exclusion, and therefore other causes of myelofibrosis must be ruled out. These include
- Other myeloproliferative disorders: polycythemia vera, essential thrombocythemia, and CML (BCR/ABL)
- Lymphoid disorders such as lymphomas, hairy cell leukemia, and multiple myeloma
- Nonhematologic disorders such as infections, metastatic cancers, gray platelet syndrome, pulmonary hypertension
- Connective tissue disorders such as systemic lupus erythematosus (SLE)
- Secondary hyperparathyroidism from renal osteodystrophy or vitamin D deficiency
- Myelodysplastic syndrome with fibrosis
- Acute myelofibrosis is seen with acute megakaryocytic leukemia (M7)

TREATMENT

Asymptomatic patients without adverse prognostic factors such as hemoglobin <10 g/dL, platelets <100,000/L, white blood cell count <4 or >30 $\times$ 10^9/L, and absence of constitutional symptoms, can be observed without treatment.

Allogeneic stem cell transplantation is the only curative treatment for AMM. This is limited to patients who are younger than 60 years of age with high-risk AMM and who have an HLA-matched donor.

Palliative treatment options include:
- Hydroxyurea for splenomegaly, thrombocytosis, and leucocytosis
- Alkylating agents such as melphalan for splenomegaly, thrombocytosis, and leucocytosis
- Steroids and/or cyclosporine for immune-mediated complications such as autoimmune hemolytic anemia
- Danazol and other androgens have been used to treat the anemia
- Thalidomide, an antiangiogenesis drug, has been used successfully to treat anemia and thrombocytopenia
- Lenalidomide which has a similar mechanism of action as thalidomide, is more potent, with fewer adverse effects, and is undergoing investigation for the treatment of AMM

- Etanercept, which is a tumor necrosis factor-α inhibitor, exerts a beneficial effect on the constitutional symptoms
- Blood transfusions as needed for anemia
- Erythropoietin if the serum level is inappropriately low
- Splenectomy for painful splenomegaly, refractory cytopenias or portal hypertension
- Splenic irradiation for painful splenomegaly, if patients are not surgical candidates.
- Radiation therapy to the liver for symptomatic hepatomegaly. Radiation is also used in areas of extramedullary hematopoiesis to control local symptoms or complications

PROGNOSIS

- Mean survival is approximately 5 years (1–30 years)
- The incidence of leukemic transformation ranges from 5%–30% in the first 10 years
- Primary causes of death are infection, leukemic transformation, and heart failure

CHRONIC MYELOID LEUKEMIA

Chronic myeloid leukemia (CML) is a clonal disorder arising in the hematopoietic stem cell, characterized by dysregulated production of a particular lineage of mature myeloid cells with fairly normal differentiation. The Philadelphia chromosome is invariably associated with this disorder.

EPIDEMIOLOGY

- The incidence is 1 to 2 cases per 100,000 population
- Median age at diagnosis is 65 years
- Male-to-female ratio is 1.3 to 2.2:1

PATHOGENESIS

The Philadelphia chromosome (Ph) is a balanced translocation between the long arms of chromosome 9 and 22, t (9, 22). This translocation juxtaposes c-abl, a protooncogene from chromosome 9 to the break point cluster region (BCR) on chromosome 22 giving rise to a fusion gene. The fusion protein (BCR-ABL), with increased tyrosine kinase activity, causes aberrant activation of multiple signaling pathways implicated in the pathogenesis of this disease. The Philadelphia chromosome is detectable in 90% to 95% of patients. About half the patients without detectable Ph chromosome by cytogenetic analysis will express the BCR-ABL fusion gene by FISH analysis. The remaining patients are considered true Ph chromosome negative or atypical CML and have a poor prognosis. The pathobiology of atypical CML is not known.

CLINICAL FEATURES

- Asymptomatic disease is discovered on routine blood work in up to 50% of the patients
- Fatigue, anorexia, weight loss, and night sweats are observed in the remainder
- Petechiae and bleeding episodes are common due to platelet dysfunction
- Splenomegaly causing abdominal discomfort and early satiety
- Gouty arthritis
- Bone pain
- Symptoms of leukostasis such as headache, priapism, and focal neurological deficits

LABORATORY FINDINGS

- Leukocytosis with counts >100,000/µL in up to 70%
- Anemia which is normocytic, normochromic
- Platelets are >600,000 to 700,000 in up to 30%
- Leukocyte alkaline phosphatase score is low
- Vitamin B12 levels are elevated
- Peripheral blood smear reveals a left shift with myeloid cells in various stages of maturation. There is almost always an increase in basophils and eosinophils
- Bone marrow aspiration and biopsy in the chronic phase shows hypercellularity with increased myeloid-to-erythroid ratio and megakaryocytes. Myelofibrosis may also be seen
- The Ph chromosome or BCR-ABL rearrangement is detected in 97% of patients

DIAGNOSIS

The diagnosis is established by confirming the presence of leukocytosis in the absence of infection. The presence of peripheral blood basophilia is almost universal. A definitive diagnosis requires the detection of the Ph chromosome or BCR-ABL fusion gene in typical CML.

DIFFERENTIAL DIAGNOSIS

1. Infections
2. Leukemoid reaction
3. Chronic myelomonocytic leukemia
4. Polycythemia vera
5. Essential thrombocythemia
6. Ph chromosome positive acute myeloid or lymphoblastic leukemia

CLINICAL COURSE

There are three phases that comprise the clinical course of this disease.
1. Chronic phase: Most patients are diagnosed in the chronic phase. The duration between the onset of the chronic phase and development of the acute phase is approximately five years. It is believed to be significantly longer with the advent of improved therapies.
2. Accelerated phase: This phase is ill defined. It is characterized by increasing leukocytosis, basophilia, thrombocytopenia or thrombocytosis, increasing numbers of blasts in the peripheral blood, and worsening splenomegaly.
3. Acute or blast phase: The blastic phase is characterized by 30% or more blasts in the peripheral blood and signs and symptoms of acute leukemia.

TREATMENT

- Allogeneic stem cell transplantation is curative and is the preferred option in younger patients with a suitable donor
- Imatinib mesylate is an oral Bcr- Abl tyrosine kinase protein inhibitor. The goals of treatment of CML are to achieve a hematologic remission (normal complete blood count [CBC]) and no evidence of organomegaly), a cytogenetic remission (0% Ph-positive cells), and a molecular remission (negative polymerase chain reaction (PCR) for the mutated BCR/ABL m-RNA). The main side effects of imatinib are nausea, diarrhea, fluid retention, rash, and myelosuppression. Nilotinib and Dasatinib are newer tyrosine kinase inhibitors which have been used in patients intolerant to imatinib or unresponsive to imatinib
- Hydroxyurea was the most commonly used myelosuppressive agent before the advent of imatinib
- Interferon α was the treatment of choice in older patients who were not candidates for bone marrow transplantation
- Busulfan is an alkylating agent that was used to treat CML in the past. While not curative, the initial clinical response to busulfan is similar to that observed with hydroxyurea.

BIBLIOGRAPHY

Blacklock HA, Royle GA. Idiopathic erythrocytosis—a declining entity. *Br J Haematol.* 2001;115:774–781.

Campbell PJ, Green AR. The myeloproliferative disorders. *N Engl J Med.* 2006;355(23):2452–2466.

Cervantes F. Modern management of myelofibrosis. *Br J Haematol.* 2005;128:583–590.

Cortelazzo S, Finazzi G, Ruggeri M, et al. Hydroxyurea for patients with essential thrombocythemia and a high risk of thrombosis. *N Engl J Med.* 1995;332:1132–1136.

Cortes JE, Talpaz M, Kantarjian H. Chronic myelogenous leukemia: A review. *Am J Med.* 1996;100:555–570.

Deininger MW, Goldman JM, Melo JV. The molecular biology of chronic myelogenous leukemia. *Blood.* 2000;96:3343–3356.

Faderl S, Talpaz M, Estrov Z, Kantarjian HM. Chronic myelogenous leukemia: Biology and therapy. *Ann Intern Med.* 1999;131:207–219.

Garcia-Manero G, Faderl S, O'Brien S, et al. Chronic myelogenous leukemia: A review & update of therapeutic strategies. *Cancer.* 2003;98:437–457.

Geary CG. The story of chronic myeloid leukaemia. *Br J Haematol.* 2000;110:2–11.

Harrison CN, Campbell PJ, Buck G, et al. Hydroxyurea compared with anagrelide in high-risk essential thrombocythemia. *N Engl J Med.* 2005;353(1):33–45.

Harrison C. Pregnancy and its management in the Philadelphia negative myeloproliferative diseases. *Br J Haematol.* 2005;129:293–306.

Lee SJ. Chronic myelogenous leukaemia. *Br J Haematol.* 2000;111:993–1001.

Mesa RA, Li CY, Ketterling RP, et al. Leukemic transformation in myelofibrosis with myeloid metaplasis: A single-institution experience with 91 cases. *Blood.* 2005;105:973–987.

Michiels JJ, Abels J, Steketee J, et al. Erythromelalgia caused by platelet-mediated arteriolar inflammation and thrombosis in thrombocythemia. *Ann Intern Med.* 1985;102:466–471.

Michiels JJ, Koudstaal PJ, Mulder AH, et al. Transient neurologic and ocular manifestations in primary thrombocythemia. *Neurology.* 1993;43:1107–1109.

Michiels JJ. Erythromelalgia and vascular complications in polycythemia vera. *Semin Thromb Hemost.* 1997;23:441–445.

Passamonti F, Rumi E, Pungolino E, et al. Life expectancy and prognostic factors for survival in patients with polycythemia vera and essential thrombocythemia. *Am J Med.* 2004;117:755–766.

Peggs K, Mackinnon S. Imatinib mesylate—the new gold standard for treatment of chronic myeloid leukemia. *N Engl J Med.* 2003;348:1048–1050.

Savage DG, Szydlo RM, Goldman JM. Clinical features at diagnosis in 430 patients with chronic myeloid leukaemia seen at a referral centre over a 16-year period. *Br J Haematol.* 1997;96:111–114.

Schafer AI. Molecular basis of the diagnosis and treatment of polycythemia vera and essential thrombocythemia. *Blood.* 2006;107:4214–4218.

Smith RE, Chelmowski MK, Szabo EJ. Myelofibrosis: A review of clinical & pathologic features & treatment. *Crit Rev Oncol Hematol.* 1990;10:305–312.

Steurer M, Gastl G, Jedrzejczak WW, et al. Anagrelide for thrombocytosis in myeloproliferative disorders. *Cancer.* 2004;101:2239–2245.

Tefferi A, Silverstein MN, Noel P. Agnogenic myeloid metaplasia. *Semin Oncol.* 1995;22:327–340.

Tefferi A. Myelofibrosis with myeloid metaplasia. *N Engl J Med.* 2000;342:1255.

Tefferi A, Lasho TL, Schwager SM, et al. The clinical phenotype of wild-type, heterozygous, and homozygous JAK2V617F in polycythemia vera. *Cancer.* 2006;106:631–639.

Tefferi A, Spivak JL. Polycythemia vera: Scientific advances and current practice. *Semin Hematol.* 2005;42:206–222.

Tefferi A. Risk-based management in essential thrombocythemia. *American Society of Hematology Education Program Book. Hematology.* 1999;172–177.

66 ACUTE LEUKEMIAS

Krishnamohan R. Basarakodu

ACUTE LYMPHOBLASTIC LEUKEMIA

DEFINITION

- Acute lymphoblastic leukemia (ALL) is a heterogeneous group of lymphoid disorders that result from a clonal expansion of immature lymphoid cells in the marrow, blood, and other organs.

EPIDEMIOLOGY

- In the United States, 5000 new cases are diagnosed each year
- It is the most common leukemia in children, representing 80% of acute leukemias
- It accounts for less than 20% of acute leukemias in the adult
- ALL is characterized by a bimodal age distribution with an early peak at 4 to 5 years of age and a second peak around age 50

ETIOLOGY/RISK FACTORS

- Trisomy 21 (Down syndrome)
- Immunodeficiency/human immunodeficiency virus infection

- Klinefelter syndrome
- Excessive chromosomal fragility
  - Fanconi anemia
  - Bloom syndrome
  - Ataxia-telangiectasia
- Viral infections
  - Epstein-Barr virus is associated with mature B-cell ALL
  - Human T-cell lymphotropic virus-1 associated with adult T-cell leukemia/lymphoma

FRENCH-AMERICAN-BRITISH AND WORLD HEALTH ORGANIZATION CLASSIFICATIONS

FRENCH-AMERICAN-BRITISH CLASSIFICATION
- The FAB scheme is an older classification that uses morphological criteria including cell size, cytoplasm, nucleoli, basophilia, and vacuolization. This system classifies ALL into three categories, L1 (small uniform cells), L2 (large varied cells), and L3 (large varied cells with vacuoles). L3 is associated with mature B-cell ALL (Burkitt's lymphoma). The French-American-British classification scheme has largely been abandoned since it has no clinical or prognostic significance.

WORLD HEALTH ORGANIZATION CLASSIFICATION
- The WHO classification relies on morphology as well as immunogenetics (immunophenotyping). This system reflects the prognosis of the disease and provides a rationale for optimal therapy. The WHO system recognized two main subtypes: (1) precursor-B cell, and (2) precursor-T cell. These subtypes are further subdivided on the basis of cytogenetic abnormalities.
- Precursor B-cell ALL/lymphoblastic lymphoma (70%–75%)
  - Cytogenetic subgroups and associated genes
    - t(9;22)(q34;q11.2) or Philadelphia chromosome subtype is seen in 20% of adults and 5% of children with ALL (3-year survival of 75%)
    - t(v;11q23); mixed lineage leukemia gene (3-year survival of 25%)
    - t(1;19)(q23;p13); abnormal PBX1/E2A genes (3-year survival of 20%)
    - t(12;21)(p13;q22); abnormal TEL/AML1 genes (3-year survival of 20%)
  - Chromosome number also influences prognosis. For example, hypodiploidy is associated with a 3-year event free survival of 10%, whereas hyperdiploidy >50 is associated with 3-year event free survival of 30%–50%.
- Mature B-cell ALL (L3) or Burkitt's lymphoma accounts for <5% of all ALLs.

- Precursor T-cell ALL/lymphoblastic lymphoma accounts for 20%–25%

CLINICAL FEATURES

RELATED TO MARROW INFILTRATION
- Bone pain
- Dyspnea and fatigue (anemia)
- Infections (neutropenia)
- Bleeding (thrombocytopenia)

RELATED TO TISSUE INFILTRATION
- CNS involvement (common with Mature B-cell ALL)
- Abdominal masses and ileocecal intussusception (common with mature B-cell ALL)
- Bulky lymphadenopathy and hepatosplenomegaly (common with T-cell and mature B-cell ALL)
- Lytic bone lesions and hypercalcemia (common with adult T-cell ALL)

RELATED TO INCREASED BLASTS IN THE CIRCULATION
- Headache, confusion, and retinal hemorrhages from hyperviscosity (rare)

LABORATORY FINDINGS

- Leukocytosis with lymphocytosis
- Blasts (>20%) on the peripheral smear and bone marrow
- Anemia
- Neutropenia
- Thrombocytopenia
- Hyperviscosity (rare)
- Tumor lysis syndrome with hypocalcemia, hyperphosphatemia, hyperkalemia, and acute renal failure

DIAGNOSTIC WORKUP

- Complete blood count with differential
- Peripheral smear review
- Comprehensive metabolic panel
- Lactate dehydrogenase
- Bone marrow aspirate and biopsy for morphology, immunocytochemistry, flow cytometry, cytogenetics (fluorescence in situ hybridization [FISH] and polymerase chain reaction [PCR] if necessary)
- Chest radiograph
- Multigated angiogram scan or two-dimensional echo (before anthracycline use)
- Lumbar puncture

- Human leukocyte antigen (HLA) typing if transplant is a consideration
- Directed imaging as necessary based on signs and symptoms

ADVERSE PROGNOSTIC FACTORS

- Advanced age (>60 years)
- Adverse cytogenetics
  ○ t(9;22)
  ○ t(4;11)
  ○ Trisomy 8
  ○ Hypodiploidy
- White blood cell count >50,000/μL
- Prolonged time to complete remission (CR) (>4–6 wk)

TREATMENT

- Treatment of ALL is complex and is divided into induction, consolidation-intensification, central nervous system (CNS) sterilization (during induction and consolidation), and maintenance.
- The backbone of all induction regimens include a combination of vincristine, anthracyclines, and corticosteroids.
- Improved outcomes have been obtained by intensifying the induction with cytarabine and cyclophosphamide in T-cell ALL and with fractionated doses of cyclophosphamide and high dose methotrexate in mature B-cell ALL.
- Consolidation therapy involves repeated application of modified induction regimens.
- Central nervous system sterilization consists of intrathecal chemotherapy with high-dose methotrexate, cytarabine, steroids, and high-dose systemic chemotherapy with agents that cross the blood-brain barrier (methotrexate, L-asparaginase, and cytarabine), and CNS irradiation.
- Central nervous system sterilization can be achieved with a combination of intrathecal chemotherapy and high-dose systemic chemotherapy without CNS irradiation.
- Maintenance therapy includes daily 6-mercaptopurine, weekly methotrexate, and monthly pulses of vincristine and prednisone for 3 years.
- Rituximab (anti-CD20 monoclonal antibody) is being used with increasing frequency to treat patients who express CD20.
- Imatinib mesylate is used to treat Philadelphia chromosome–positive ALL.

- Maintenance therapy is not given to patients with mature B-cell ALL because they respond well to short–term, dose-intensive regimens and relapses are rare after the first year of remission.
- Radiation to both testis is recommended for testicular leukemia.
- Allogeneic stem cell transplant is considered in CR1 for high-risk patients with HLA-matched siblings.

TREATMENT OF RELAPSED ACUTE LYMPHOBLASTIC LEUKEMIA
- Patients with relapsed ALL have a poor prognosis
- Response rates are lower and are shorter with a median survival of 6 months
- Allogeneic stem cell transplant should be considered in second complete remission

LATE COMPLICATIONS OF THERAPY

- Acute myelogenous leukemia (AML) (especially with alkylating agents and topoisomerase II inhibitors)
- Cardiomyopathy
- Thyroid dysfunction
- Infertility
- Growth retardation
- Osteoporosis
- Avascular necrosis of bone
- Learning disabilities
- Central nervous system tumors

ACUTE MYELOGENOUS LEUKEMIA

DEFINITION

- Acute myelogenous leukemia (AML) is a malignant disease of hematopoietic progenitor cells characterized by maturational arrest and uncontrolled proliferation with concomitant inhibition of normal hematopoiesis by malignant cells.

EPIDEMIOLOGY

- Accounts for 10,000 deaths annually in the United States
- Median age at diagnosis is 70 years, however it increases in incidence with each decade
- Slightly more common in males (3:2)
- Most common malignant myeloid disorder in adults
- Accounts for approximately 80% of acute leukemias in adults

ETIOLOGY/RISK FACTORS

GENETIC DISORDERS ASSOCIATED WITH AML
- Down's syndrome, Bloom syndrome, Klinefelter syndrome, Fanconi anemia, Kostmann syndrome, ataxia-telangiectasia, and Wiskott-Aldrich syndrome

ENVIRONMENTAL RISK FACTORS
- Benzene, herbicide and pesticide exposure, ionizing radiation

TREATMENT-ASSOCIATED RISK FACTORS
- Alkylating agents or topoisomerase II inhibitors

PREEXISTING HEMATOLOGIC DISORDERS
- Myelodysplasia, myeloproliferative disorders, and paroxysmal nocturnal hemoglobinuria

PATHOPHYSIOLOGY

- The prevailing hypothesis is that normal blasts require at least two genetic "hits" to induce blast transformation. The first hit is thought to inhibit normal differentiation and the second hit induces uncontrolled cellular proliferation.

CLASSIFICATION

FRENCH-AMERICAN-BRITISH AND WORLD HEALTH ORGANIZATION CLASSIFICATIONS
- The French-American-British (FAB) classification is an older classification but is still in common use. It is based on cytomorphology and cytochemistry. It divides AML into eight subtypes (M0 to M7) as follows:
  - M0: minimally differentiated AML
  - M1: AML without maturation
  - M2: AML with maturation
  - M3: Acute promyelocytic leukemia (APL)
  - M4: Acute myelomonocytic leukemia
  - M5: Acute monocytic leukemia
  - M6: Acute erythroleukemia
  - M7: Acute megakaryocytic leukemia
- The WHO classification system incorporates cytogenetics, molecular genetics, therapy-related AML, and acute biphenotypic leukemias into the existing FAB formulation. This classification groups patients into favorable, intermediate and unfavorable categories. Nevertheless, most patients will receive similar induction therapy. The WHO classification scheme is outlined below (four major categories are included):

- Acute myelogenous leukemia with recurrent cytogenetic translocations:
  - Acute myelogenous leukemia with t(8;21)(q22;q22)
  - Acute myelogenous leukemia with abnormal bone marrow eosinophils and chromosomal inversion (inv)(16)(p13q;q22) or t(16;16)(p13;q11)
  - Acute promyelocytic leukemia with (15;17) (q22;q11) and variants, promyelocytic leukemia/ retinoic acid receptor-α
  - Acute myelogenous leukemia with 11q23 (mixed lineage leukemia gene) abnormalities
- Acute myelogenous leukemia with multilineage dysplasia
  - With prior myelodysplastic syndromes (MDS)
  - Without prior MDS
- Acute myelogenous leukemia and MDS, therapy related
  - Alkylating agent related
  - Topoisomerase II inhibitor related
  - Other types
- Acute myelogenous leukemia, not otherwise categorized
  - Acute myelogenous leukemia, minimally differentiated
  - Acute myelogenous leukemia, with maturation
  - Acute myelogenous leukemia, without maturation
  - Acute myelomonocytic leukemia
  - Acute monocytic leukemia
  - Acute erythroid leukemia
  - Acute megakaryocytic leukemia
  - Acute panmyelosis with myelofibrosis
  - Acute biphenotypic leukemias

CLINICAL FEATURES

RELATED TO BONE MARROW FAILURE
- Dyspnea and fatigue (anemia)
- Infections (neutropenia)
- Bleeding (thrombocytopenia)

RELATED TO TISSUE INFILTRATION
- Gum hypertrophy
- Skin involvement (Sweet's syndrome)
- Central nervous system dysfunction and cranial nerve palsies
- Chloromas (tumors of myeloid blasts)

RELATED TO INCREASED NUMBER OF BLASTS IN THE CIRCULATION
- Headache, confusion, and retinal hemorrhages from hyperviscosity secondary to leukostasis

RELATED TO RELEASE OF GRANULES FROM BLASTS

Bleeding from disseminated intravascular coagulation (DIC) (mostly in acute promyelocytic leukemia [APL])

LABORATORY FINDINGS

- Leukocytosis
- Blasts on peripheral smear and bone marrow (≥20%)
- Anemia
- Thrombocytopenia
- Hyperuricemia with high tumor burden
- Hyperviscosity
- Tumor lysis syndrome with hypocalcemia, hyperphosphatemia, hyperkalemia, and acute renal failure
- Disseminated intravascular coagulation picture mostly with APL

DIAGNOSTIC WORKUP

- Complete blood count with differential
- Peripheral smear review
- Comprehensive metabolic panel
- Disseminated intravascular coagulation panel
- Lactate dehydrogenase level
- Bone marrow aspirate and biopsy for morphology, immunocytochemistry, flow cytometry, cytogenetics (FISH and PCR if necessary)
- Chest radiograph
- Multigated angiogram scan or two-dimensional echo (before anthracycline use)
- Lumbar puncture in select patients after clearance of blasts from the circulation
- Human leukocyte antigen typing of patient and siblings if the patient is a transplant candidate
- Human immunodeficiency virus, herpes simplex virus, Cytomegalovirus, varicella, and hepatitis B and C serologies
- Directed imaging as necessary based on signs and symptoms

PROGNOSTIC FACTORS

UNFAVORABLE

- Age older than 60 years
- Cytogenetics: –5, –7, 11q23, or complex karyotype
- Therapy-related AML is associated with a much worse prognosis
- Acute myelogenous leukemia arising from a preexisting hematologic disorder
- Presence of FMS-like tyrosine kinase 3 internal tandem repeats

- Multidrug-resistance phenotypic expression
- Poor performance status
- Leukocytosis >50,000/µL

FAVORABLE

- Cytogenetics: t(8;21), inv(16), t(16;16),
- t(15;17)

TREATMENT

TREATMENT OF ACUTE MYELOGENOUS LEUKEMIA (EXCEPT ACUTE PROMYELOCYTIC LEUKEMIA)

- Divided into two phases: induction and consolidation
- Goal of induction is to achieve a CR
- Goal of consolidation is to prevent relapse and confer long-term survival

INDUCTION

- The most common chemotherapy regimen for induction is referred to as 7 + 3: 7 days of continuous intravenous cytarabine plus 3 days of bolus intravenous anthracycline (daunorubicin or idarubicin).

CONSOLIDATION

- Used for patients with favorable cytogenetics by employing high-dose cytarabine (ARA-C).
- For younger patients with intermediate- and high-risk cytogenetics without HLA-matched sibling donors, three to four cycles of high-dose chemotherapy with ARA-C is administered

HEMATOPOIETIC STEM CELL TRANSPLANTATION

- For younger patients with intermediate- (normal karyotype) or high-risk cytogenetics, allogeneic-matched sibling stem cell transplant should be considered in the first remission.

TREATMENT OF ACUTE MYELOGENOUS LEUKEMIA IN OLDER PATIENTS

- Older patients have a poor prognosis because of comorbidities, unfavorable cytogenetics, and poor performance status
- Patients without significant comorbidities may receive standard induction with 7 + 3.
- Low-dose cytarabine may be used for consolidation because high dose therapy is not associated with an improved outcome.

TREATMENT OF RELAPSED ACUTE MYELOGENOUS LEUKEMIA

- Human leukocyte antigen–matched stem cell transplant may be performed if a donor is available.

- For patients without a suitable donor, repeat the initial regimen or administer a high-dose cytarabine-containing regimen if the initial complete remission (CR) was longer than one year.
- Patients with an initial CR less than one year in duration should be considered for a clinical trial.

TREATMENT OF ACUTE PROMYELOCYTIC LEUKEMIA

- Acute promyelocytic leukemia is the most curable subtype of AML.
- All-trans-retinoic acid (ATRA) restores normal myeloid maturation by overriding the t(15;17) protein-induced blockade of the retinoic acid receptor.
- Most commonly, ATRA plus anthracycline-based chemotherapy is used for induction, anthracycline-based regimen for consolidation, and ATRA plus low-dose mercaptopurine and methotrexate for maintenance.
- With use of aforementioned therapy, 80% to 90% achieve CR and 70% to 75% are cured.
- APL is associated with high incidence of consumptive coagulopathy, however the use of ATRA has decreased its incidence.
- Treatment of APL with ATRA is associated with Retinoic acid syndrome, which is characterized by pleural and pericardial effusions, edema, weight gain, hypotension, and pulmonary infiltrates.
- Retinoic acid syndrome is effectively treated with early administration of dexamethasone.
- Arsenic trioxide is used for relapsed and refractory APL.

ACUTE MYELOGENOUS LEUKEMIA IN PREGNANCY

- During pregnancy, 40% of AMLs occur in the first trimester, 40% in the second trimester, and 20% in the third trimester
- Induction chemotherapy can be safely given beyond the first trimester.
- Delaying chemotherapy until delivery is not considered safe.

BIBLIOGRAPHY

Annino L, Vegna ML, Camera A, et al. Treatment of adults with acute lymphoblastic leukemia (ALL): Long-term followup of the GIMEME ALL 0288 randomized study. *Blood.* 2002;99: 863–871.

Berman E, Heller G, Santorsa J, et al. Results of a randomized trial comparing idarubicin and cytosine arabinoside with daunorubicin and cytosine arabinoside in adult patients with newly diagnosed acute myelogenous leukemia. *Blood.* 1991; 77:1666–1674.

Bishop JF, Matthews JP, Young GA. A randomized trial of high-dose cytarabine in induction in acute myeloid leukemia. *Blood.* 1996;87:1710–1717.

Cassileth PA, Harrington DP, Appelbaum FR, et al. Chemotherapy compared with autologous or allogeneic bone marrow transplantation in the management of acute myeloid leukemia in first remission. *N Engl J Med.* 1998;339: 1649–1656.

Densmore JJ, Camitta BM, Williams ME. Acute lymphoblastic leukemia and lymphoblastic lymphoma. *Am Soc Hematol Self-Assessment Program.* 2005:228–235.

Durrant IJ, Prentice HG, Richards SM. Intensification of treatment of adults with acute lymphoblastic leukemia: results of U.K. Medical Research Council randomized trial UKALL XA. *Br J Haematol.* 1997;99:84–92.

Faderl S, Jeha S, Kantarjian HM. The biology and therapy of adult acute lymphoblastic leukemia. *Cancer.* 2003;98: 1337–1354.

Giles FJ, Keating A, Goldstone AH, et al. Acute myeloid leukemia. *Hematology (Am Soc Hematol Educ Program).* 2002;73–110.

Gokbuget N, Hoelzer D. Recent approaches in acute lymphoblastic leukemia in adults. *Rev Clin Exp Hematol.* 2002;6: 114–141.

Kantarjian HM, O'Brien S, Smith TL, et al. Results of treatment with hyper-CVAD, a dose-intensive regimen, in adult acute lymphocytic leukemia. *J Clin Oncol.* 2000;18:547–561.

Larson RA, Dodge RK, Burns CP, et al. A five-drug induction regimen with intensive consolidation for adults with acute lymphoblastic leukemia: Cancer and Leukemia Group B Study 8811. *Blood.* 1995;84:2025–2037.

Mayer RJ, Davis RB, Schiffer CA, et al. Intensive postremission chemotherapy in adults with acute myeloid leukemia. Cancer and Leukemia Group B. *N Engl J Med.* 1994;331: 896–903.

Pui C-H, Rellins MV, Downing JR. Acute lymphoblastic leukemias. *N Engl J Med.* 2004;350:1535–1548.

Solomon S, Malkovska V. Acute myelogenous leukemia. *Bethesda Handbook of Clinical Hematology.* 2005:135–150.

Tallman MS, Nabhan C, Camitta BM. Acute Myeloid Leukemia. *Am Soc Hemol Self-Assessment Program.* 2005:211–227.

Thomas DA, Cortes J, O'Brien S, et al. Hyper-CVAD program in Burkitt's type adult acute lymphocytic leukemia. *J Clin Oncol.* 1999;17:2461–2470.

Vogler WR, Velez-Garcia E, Weiner RS, et al. Phase III trial comparing idarubicin & daunorubicin in combination with cytarabine in acute myelogenous leukemia: A Southeastern Cancer Study Group Study. *J Clin Oncol.* 1992;10:1103–1111.

Wiernik PH, Banks PL, Case DC, et al. Cytarabine plus idarubicin or daunorubicin as induction and consolidation therapy for previously untreated adult patients with acute myeloid leukemia. *Blood.* 1992;79:313–319.

Yates J, Glidewell O, Wiernik P, et al. Cytosine arabinoside with daunorubicin or Adriamycin for therapy of acute myelocytic leukemia: a CALGB study. *Blood.* 1982;60:454–462.

Zittoun RA, Mandelli F, Willemze R, et al. Autologous or allogeneic bone marrow transplantation compared with intensive chemotherapy in acute myelogenous leukemia. European

Organization for Research and Treatment of Cancer (EORTC) and the Gruppo Italiano Malattie Ematologiche Malignedell' Adulto (GIMEME) leukemia Cooperative Groups. *N Engl J Med.* 1995;332:217–223.

67 CHRONIC LYMPHOCYTIC LEUKEMIA

Krishnamohan R. Basarakodu

DEFINITION

• Chronic lymphocytic leukemia (CLL) is a chronic lymphoproliferative disorder with clonal expansion of mature, functionally incompetent lymphocytes. B-cell CLL is identical to small lymphocytic lymphoma (SLL) but is believed to represent a different stage characterized by nodal enlargement.

EPIDEMIOLOGY

• CLL is the most common leukemia in the United States, accounting for 31% of all leukemias.
• The median age at diagnosis is 70 years and the male to female ratio is 1.7:1.
• It is rare in people younger than 30 years of age and almost never seen in children. It is extremely uncommon in Asian countries for ill-defined reasons.
• It is the only leukemia not associated with radiation exposure. For example, a cohort of patients studied after exposure to ionizing radiation from the atomic bomb (study period from 1950–1987) revealed a significantly increased incidence of leukemias except CLL.
• Ninety-five percent of CLLs in the United States are B-cell CLLs.
• There is a high incidence of lung, gastrointestinal (GI), and skin cancers in patients with CLL.

ETIOLOGY AND RISK FACTORS

• These are largely unknown. Rarely, environmental and occupational risk factors have been implicated but they have not been proven. Family history (first-degree relatives) and Agent Orange exposure have been implicated in some studies.

PATHOPHYSIOLOGY

• The lymphocytes in CLL resemble mature circulating lymphocytes but they are clonal B-cells arrested in the final stages of development.
• Although the lymphocytes proliferate relatively slowly, they are long-lived secondary to abnormalities in apoptosis.

CHROMOSOMAL ABNORMALITIES

• Cytogenetic abnormalities are present in 80% of cases and have prognostic implications. The most common abnormality is trisomy 12 (15%) and the most common structural abnormality involves the long arm of chromosome 13 (13q). Other cytogenetic abnormalities include: 11q deletion, 17p deletion, 6q deletion, and t(11;14). The cytogenetic abnormalities can occur at any time during the disease process. Changes tend to be associated with a poor prognosis and progressive disease.

CLINICAL FEATURES

Many patients are asymptomatic (20% to 25%). Approximately 10% to 15% present with the classic B-symptoms of lymphoma (fever, weight loss, night sweats, and extreme fatigue). More than 50% will present with one or more of the following findings:
• Lymphadenopathy (predominantly peripheral; the nodes tend to be round, firm and nontender, seen in 90%)
• Infections (bacterial and viral)
• Anemia, thrombocytopenia, or a marked elevation in WBC count (20% to 30%)
• Splenomegaly (60%)
• Hepatomegaly (15%)

LABORATORY FINDINGS

• Leukocytosis with an absolute lymphocytosis >5000 μ/L is considered essential for the diagnosis. Many patients present with extreme elevations in lymphocyte counts (often exceeding 100,000 to 200,000/microL). Hyperviscosity may rarely occur with counts that exceed 200,000/μL

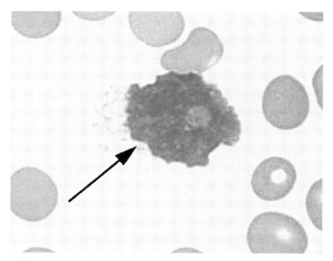

FIG. 67–1 Characteristic smudge cell in CLL.

- *Smudge cells* are flattened cells noted on the peripheral smear (Fig. 67–1). These cells represent damaged small lymphocytes during preparation of the slide. The fragility of small lymphocytes is characteristic of CLL.
- Anemia (secondary to bone marrow failure, autoimmune hemolysis, splenic sequestration, and/or pure red-cell aplasia)
- Thrombocytopenia (bone marrow failure, autoimmune destruction, and splenic sequestration)
- Hypogammaglobulinemia is present in 50% of patients
- Elevated lactate dehydrogenase (LDH) (especially in patients with Richter's transformation eg, aggressive large cell lymphoma developing in a patient with CLL)
- Elevated serum-β_2-microglobulin
- Elevated serum uric acid level is common but nonspecific.

DIAGNOSIS

- An absolute, and sustained (usually 3-6 months) lymphocytosis of >5000 µ/L is required for the diagnosis.
- The lymphocytosis cannot be explained by other causes (viral infections, some leukemias).
- The monoclonal lymphocytes must express B-cell markers (CD19, CD20, CD21, CD23, and CD24). The cells should also express the T-cell antigen, CD5 and either kappa or lambda light chains. Flow cytometry is invaluable in establishing the diagnosis of CLL.
- A bone marrow biopsy is not necessary for the diagnosis.

- Clinical data, morphology, and flow cytometry differentiate CLL from other leukemias and lymphomas (see below).

DIFFERENTIAL DIAGNOSIS

- Prolymphocytic leukemia (morphology of the cells is quite different)
- Leukemic phase of mantle cell lymphoma or follicular lymphoma (these cells do not express CD23)
- Hairy cell leukemia (bone marrow biopsy and peripheral smear will show characteristic cells)
- Waldenström macroglobulinemia
- Splenic lymphoma with villous lymphocytes

STAGING

- Two staging systems have been employed: Rai and Binet.
  - The Rai system groups CLL into five stages (0–IV) based on the presence or absence of lymphadenopathy, hepatosplenomegaly, anemia (hemoglobin [Hb] <11 g/dL), and thrombocytopenia (platelet count <100,000 µ/L).
  - The five stages of the Rai system are stratified as follows: low risk (stage 0), intermediate risk (stage I–II), and high risk (stage III–IV).
  - The Binet system groups CLL patients into three stages (A–C) based on the number of clinical areas exhibiting lymphadenopathy and the presence or absence of anemia (Hb <11 g/dL in men, <10 g/dL in women) and thrombocytopenia (platelet count <100,000 µ/L).
- Both systems do not employ recently identified genetic or molecular markers for prognostication.

PROGNOSTIC FACTORS

- All of the following have been associated with an unfavorable prognosis:
  - 17p deletion, 11q deletion, ZAP 70 expression, or CD38 expression
  - Absence of immunoglobulin VH (IGVH) somatic hypermutation
  - Advanced Rai or Binet stage
  - Rapid lymphocyte doubling time (<12 months)
  - Initial lymphocyte count >50,000 µ/L
  - Elevated LDH or serum-β_2-microglobulin
  - Increased expression of serum-soluble CD25 receptors.

- The following are associated with a favorable prognosis:
  ○ Isolated 13q deletion or ZAP 70 negativity
  ○ Presence of IGVH somatic hypermutation

INDICATIONS FOR TREATMENT

- The diagnosis of CLL itself is not an indication for treatment. Indeed, most patients are discovered incidentally and are asymptomatic. Moreover, these patients may have very slow progression and the risks of chemotherapy must be weighed against the indolent nature of this disorder. Factors which may favor early treatment include:
  ○ Rapid lymphocyte doubling time.
  ○ Progressive cytopenias secondary to bone marrow involvement.
  ○ Autoimmune anemia and thrombocytopenia.
  ○ Bulky or progressive lymphadenopathy.
  ○ Massive or progressive splenomegaly.
  ○ Symptoms related to the disease (weight loss, fever, chills and night sweats).
  ○ Recurrent infections.

TREATMENT

- Chlorambucil was the agent of choice for many decades. The principal goal of therapy was palliation, however newer agents have been associated with complete remissions, sometimes of long duration. Accordingly, the treatment of CLL is undergoing revision. A complete remission is defined by the National Cancer Institute Working Group (NCI/WG) as follows: absence of symptoms attributable to CLL, normal physical examination, absolute lymphocyte count <4000/µL, absolute neutrophil count >1500/µL, platelet count >100,000/µL, hemoglobin concentration >11 g/dL, bone marrow lymphocytosis <30 percent, and no lymphoid nodules on bone marrow biopsy.
- Fludarabine is the most effective single agent in CLL, but has not been shown to prolong survival.
- The addition of Rituximab (anti-CD20 monoclonal antibody) induces a more complete response rate but is associated with greater toxicity.
- Concurrent fludarabine-based chemotherapy with rituximab produces better response rates than sequential therapy.
- Fludarabine alone or combined with rituximab with or without cyclophosphamide is now considered the first-line treatment for most patients.
- Alemtuzumab (anti-CD52 monoclonal antibody) can be used in patients who do not respond to fludarabine.

- Patients who relapse after 1 year of a disease-free interval can be treated with the initial regimen again.
- Allogenic stem-cell transplant should be considered for young patients with high-risk features and relapsed disease, but it is associated with high treatment-related morbidity and mortality.

COMPLICATIONS

- Autoimmune cytopenia is usually treated with steroids (other treatments include intravenous immunoglobulin [IVIG], splenectomy, cyclosporine, or rituximab).
- Recurrent infections in patients with hypogammaglobulinemia are managed with monthly IVIG.
- Richter's transformation may occur in 10% of CLL patients.
- Transformation to acute prolymphocytic leukemia occurs in 2% to 5% of CLL patients.
- Second malignancies of the skin, GI tract, and lung are common in CLL patients.

BIBLIOGRAPHY

Abbasi S, Cheson B. Chronic lymphocytic leukemia. *Bethesda Handbook Clin Hematol.* 2005;177–185.

Borthakur G, Bueso-Ramos CE, O'Brien S. Chronic lymphocytic leukemia and associated disorders. *MD Anderson Manual Med Oncol.* 2006;39–55.

Byrd JC, Peterson BL, Morrison VA, et al. Randomized phase 2 study of fludarabine with concurrent versus sequential treatment with rituximab in symptomatic, untreated patients with B-cell chronic lymphocytic leukemia: results from Cancer and Leukemia Group B 9712 (CALGB 9712). *Blood.* 2003;101:6–14.

Crespo M, Bosch F, Villamor N, et al. ZAP-70 expression as a surrogate for immunoglobulin-variable-region mutations in chronic lymphocytic leukemia. *N Engl J Med.* 2003;348:1764–1775.

Densmore JJ, Williams ME. Lymphoproliferative diseases. *Am Soc Hematol Self-Assessment Program.* 2005;236–272.

Hamblin TJ, Davis Z, Gardiner A, et al. Unmutated IgV(H) genes are associated with a more aggressive form of chronic lymphocytic leukemia. *Blood.* 1999;94:1848–1854.

Hegde UP, Wilson WH, White T, et al. Rituximab treatment of refractory fludarabine-associated immune thrombocytopenia in chronic lymphocytic leukemia. *Blood.* 2002;100:2260–2262.

Kay NE, Hamblin TJ, Jelinek DF, et al. Chronic lymphocytic leukemia. *Hematology Am Soc Hematol Educ Program.* 2002;193–213.

Keating MJ, Flinn I, Jain V, et al. Therapeutic role of alemtuzumab (Campath-1H) in patients who have failed fludarabine: Results of a large international study. *Blood.* 2002;99:3554–3561.

O'Brien SM, Kantarjian HM, Cortes J, et al. Results of the fludarabine and cyclophosphamide combination regimen in chronic lymphocytic leukemia. *J Clin Oncol.* 2001;19:1414–1420.

Rai KR, Freter CE, Mercier RJ, et al. Alemtuzumab in previously treated chronic lymphocytic leukemia patients who also had received fludarabine. *J Clin Oncol.* 2002;20:3891–3897.

Yee KW, O'Brien SM. Chronic lymphocytic leukemia: Diagnosis and treatment. *Mayo Clin Proc.* 2006;81:1105–1129.

68 HODGKIN LYMPHOMA

Rami Owera

DEFINITION

- Hodgkin lymphoma (formerly called Hodgkin's disease) is a clonal hematopoietic malignancy that arises within the lymph node.
- Classically, the involved tissue is comprised of a small number of large multinucleated cells referred to as Hodgkin/Reed-Sternberg (HRS) cells.
- The remainder of the involved tissue contains a background of nonneoplastic inflammatory cells.

CLASSIFICATION

The WHO classification system divides the Hodgkin lymphomas into two categories: (1) Classic Hodgkin lymphoma (HL), and (2) Nodular lymphocyte predominant Hodgkin lymphoma (NLPHL). Classic HL is further subdivided as follows:
- Nodular sclerosis: NSHL
- Mixed cellularity: MCHL
- Lymphocyte depleted: LDHL
- Lymphocyte rich: LRHL

EPIDEMIOLOGY

- 7800 new cases are diagnosed each year and approximately 1500 deaths secondary to HL occur in the United States each year.
- There is a bimodal age distribution. The first peak occurs in the third decade; the second peak occurs in the sixth and seventh decades

- It is common in males than females
- The nodular sclerosis subtype is more common in patients from a higher socioeconomic class
- Mixed cellularity and lymphocyte depletion subtypes are more common in lower socioeconomic classes
- Chronic Epstein-Barr virus (EBV) infection increases the risk of developing HL. EBV DNA can be detected in HL specimens and is also localized to the malignant cells using in situ hybridization.

PATHOPHYSIOLOGY

- HRS cells are CD30 positive in 95% and CD15 (granulocyte antigen) positive in 85% of all cases.
- B-Cell specific activation protein (BSAP) is present in 90% of HRS cells
- HRS cells contain monoclonal immunoglobulin (Ig) gene rearrangements in almost all cases, which suggest a B-cell origin

CLINICAL PRESENTATION

- Asymptomatic lymphadenopathy is the presenting feature in more than two-thirds of all cases
- Cervical, mediastinal, axillary, and inguinal areas are the most commonly involved sites
- B-symptoms are common (25% to 30%) and include fever, night sweats, and weight loss. Other constitutional symptoms include fatigue, pruritus, and alcohol-induced pain
- Mediastinal bulky disease may produce chest pain, shortness of breath, cough, and rarely superior vena cava (SVC) syndrome
- Retroperitoneal lymphadenopathy may cause back pain and ureteral obstruction
- Nephrotic syndrome has been described in HL. The glomerular lesion is usually characterized by changes consistent with nil lesion (minimal change disease) or focal glomerulosclerosis.
- Urticaria, erythema nodosum, erythema multiforme, and skin necrotizing lesions are rare
- Anemia of chronic disease and hemolytic anemia have also been characterized

DIAGNOSTIC STUDIES

- Excisional biopsy of an enlarged lymph node is required to establish the diagnosis

- Routine laboratory tests including a complete blood count (CBC) with differential, comprehensive metabolic panel, erythrocyte sedimentation rate (ESR), lactate dehydrogenase (LDH), albumin, and uric acid are necessary. These tests are primarily useful to exclude other organ involvement.
- Imaging studies, including a standard chest x-ray and computed tomography (CT) scan of the chest, abdomen, and pelvis are performed to define the extent of the disease.
- Bone marrow aspiration and biopsy should be considered for patients with advanced disease, B symptoms, or markedly abnormal CBC to exclude other malignant processes and infection.
- Laparotomy and splenectomy are no longer routinely performed.

DIFFERENTIAL DIAGNOSIS

- Non-Hodgkin lymphoma
- Metastatic cancer
- Infectious mononucleosis
- Sarcoidosis
- Fungal infection
- Tuberculosis
- Drug toxicity (phenytoin)

STAGING

- The Cotswolds revision of the Ann Arbor staging system is used to stage the disease
  ○ Stage I: Involvement of a single lymph node region or lymphoid structure.
  ○ Stage II: Involvement of two or more lymph node regions on the same side of the diaphragm.
  ○ Stage III: Involvement of lymph node regions or structures on both sides of the diaphragm
  ○ Stage IV: Involvement of extranodal sites
- All classes are subclassified to indicate the presence (B) or absence (A) of systemic (B) symptoms (fever, drenching night sweats, or weight loss >10% of normal weight). In addition, the involvement of a single extranodal site is classified as IE, while extension to a contiguous site is classified as E, as in Stage IIIE. Involvement of the spleen is designated by the letter S, as in stage IIIs. And finally, the presence of "bulky disease," referring to larger masses of cancerous tissue, is indicated by the letter X.

PROGNOSTIC FACTORS

- The following factors are associated with a worse prognosis
  ○ Sex: male>female
  ○ Age: older than 50 years
  ○ Stage IV disease
  ○ Anemia: hemoglobin (Hb) <10.5
  ○ Leukocytosis: white blood cell (WBC) >15,000
  ○ Lymphopenia: lymphocyte count <600 or 8% of the total WBC
  ○ Hypoalbuminemia: albumin <4.0
- For patients with early stages I and II, the following factors are associated with an unfavorable prognosis
  ○ Bulky mediastinal lymphadenopathy
  ○ Age older than 50 years
  ○ B symptoms and an ESR greater than 30 mm/h
  ○ An ESR greater than 50 mm/h without B symptoms
  ○ Involvement of four or more lymph node regions

TREATMENT

- For early stage I, II disease
  ○ Chemotherapy consists of four cycles of ABVD (doxorubicin, bleomycin, vinblastine, dacarbazine) followed by radiation therapy to the involved sites (5-year survival exceeds 90% in children)
- For advanced stage III, IV disease
  ○ Six to eight cycles of ABVD chemotherapy (5-year survival is 87%–95%). Involved field radiation therapy only for patients with bulky mediastinal disease
- For relapsed disease
  ○ Salvage chemotherapy with six to eight cycles of chemotherapy that was not used previously (for example, consider MOPP [mechlorethamine, vincristine, procarbazine, and prednisone]).
  ○ High-dose chemotherapy followed by autologous stem cell transplantation should be considered in patients that relapse early (within 12 months) or have relapsed for the second time.

TREATMENT RELATED SIDE EFFECTS

- From chemotherapy
  ○ Bone marrow suppression
  ○ Myelodysplasia
  ○ Cardiomyopathy (doxorubicin)
  ○ Pulmonary fibrosis (bleomycin)
  ○ Sterility (MOPP)
  ○ Peripheral neuropathy

○ Secondary malignancy
○ Aseptic necrosis
• From radiation therapy
  ○ Bone marrow suppression
  ○ Hypothyroidism
  ○ Cardiomyopathy
  ○ Pericarditis
  ○ Pneumonitis
  ○ Coronary artery disease
  ○ Spinal cord injury

SECONDARY MALIGNANCY

• The estimated risk of a second tumor is 15% to 20% at 15 years (breast, thyroid, and sarcomas are the most common)
• The breast cancer relative risk is significantly higher in younger patients treated with radiation therapy
• Routine screening mammography should begin 8 to 10 years after completing radiation therapy
• Smoking cessation to reduce the risk of lung and head and neck cancers is advisable

SURVIVAL SUMMARY

• Cause specific survival with treatment
  ○ Early stage (IA and IIA) with a favorable prognosis
  ○ 85% to 90% at 10 years
• Early stage with unfavorable prognosis
  ○ 70% to 80% at 10 years
• Advanced stage III and IV
  ○ 50% to 60% at 10 years

BIBLIOGRAPHY

Cavalli F. Rare syndromes in Hodgkin's disease. *Ann Oncol.* 1998;9 Suppl 5:S109.

Harris NL. Hodgkin's disease: Classification and differential diagnosis. *Mod Pathol.* 1999;12:159–176.

Healey EA, Tarbell NJ, Kalish LA, et al. Prognostic factors for patients with Hodgkin's disease in first relapse. *Cancer.* 1993; 71:2613–2620.

Henry-Amar M. Second cancers after radiotherapy and chemotherapy for early stages of Hodgkin's disease. *J Natl Cancer Inst.* 1983;71:911–923.

Howell SJ, Grey M, Chang J, et al. The value of bone marrow examination in the staging of Hodgkin's lymphoma: A review of 955 cases seen in a regional cancer centre. *Br J Haematol.* 2002;119:408–411.

Jaffe ES, Harris NL, Stein H, Vardiman JW, eds. World Health Organization Classification of Tumours. *Pathology and Genetics of Tumours of Hematopoietic and Lymphoid Tissues.* Lyon: IARC Press; 2001.

Kuppers R, Klein U, Schwering I, et al. Identification of Hodgkin and Reed-Sternberg cell-specific genes by gene expression profiling. *J Clin Invest.* 2003;111:529–537.

Lister TA, Crowther D, Sutcliffe SB, et al. Report of a committee convened to discuss the evaluation and staging of patients with Hodgkin's disease: Cotswolds meeting. *J Clin Oncol.* 1989;7: 1630–1639.

Mauch PM, Kalish LA, Kadin M, et al. Patterns of presentation of Hodgkin disease. Implications for etiology and pathogenesis [see comments]. *Cancer.* 1993;71:2062–2066.

Mauch PM. Controversies in the management of early stage Hodgkin's disease [see comments]. *Blood.* 1994;83:318.

Mendenhall NP, Cantor AB, Barre DM, et al. The role of prognostic factors in treatment selection for early-stage Hodgkin's disease. *Am J Clin Oncol.* 1994;17:189–199.

Mueller N, Evans A, Harris NL, et al. Hodgkin's disease and Epstein-Barr virus. Altered antibody pattern before diagnosis. *N Engl J Med.* 1989;320:689–695.

Oza AM, Ganesan TS, Leahy M, et al. Patterns of survival in patients with Hodgkin's disease: Long follow up in a single centre. *Ann Oncol.* 1993;4:385–396.

Tucker MA, Coleman CN, Cox RS, et al. Risk of second cancers after treatment for Hodgkin's disease. *N Engl J Med.* 1988;318:76–88.

van Leeuwen FE, Klokman WJ, Hagenbeek A, et al. Second cancer risk following Hodgkin's disease: A 20-year follow-up study. *J Clin Oncol.* 1994;12:312–319.

69 NON-HODGKIN LYMPHOMA

Osama Qubaiah and Paul Petruska

• The non-Hodgkin lymphomas (NHLs) are a heterogeneous group of disorders featuring malignant proliferation of B or T lymphocytes that may invade any organ, but usually involve lymph nodes, spleen, peripheral blood, and bone marrow. They can range from indolent to aggressive malignancies. Therefore, treatment must be individualized according to each patient's disease behavior. Although our understanding of the pathobiology of the NHLs has improved, it is still difficult to predict the course of the disease regardless of the classification scheme employed. For example, it is common for patients with aggressive NHLs to undergo cure, whereas patients with indolent forms may respond poorly to therapy (although their 5-year survival may still be quite good).

EPIDEMIOLOGY

• Non-Hodgkin lymphomas have increased in frequency in the United States between 1950 and the late 1990s for reasons that are poorly understood.

- The incidence has been steadily rising in North America, Europe, and Australia at a rate of approximately 2% to 3% per year for the past 30 years.
- In 2007, approximately 63,190 new cases of NHL will be diagnosed, whereas approximately 18,660 will die, making it the fifth most common cancer in both men and women.
- Non-Hodgkin lymphomas are more frequent in patients older than 65 years of age and in men, with a male to female ratio of 1.1:1
- The median age at diagnosis occurs in the sixth decade of life, but Burkitt's lymphoma and lymphoblastic lymphoma typically occur in younger patients.
- T-cell lymphomas are more common in Asia, whereas follicular lymphoma is more common in western countries. Extranodal nasal-type natural killer (NK)/ T-cell lymphoma has a characteristic geographic distribution in Southeast Asia and South America.
- Adult T-cell leukemia/lymphoma, which is associated with human T-cell lymphotropic virus (HTLV) I, is more common in southern Japan and the Caribbean.

ETIOLOGY

- Immunosuppression related to human immunodeficiency virus (HIV) infection or the delayed effects of immunomodulation for solid organ transplantation, are associated with an increased incidence of NHL. These settings can promote B-cell proliferation and susceptibility to tumor-associated viruses such as Epstein Barr. Other immunoregulatory disorders such as Hashimoto's thyroiditis, rheumatoid arthritis, and sicca syndromes are also associated with an increased risk of developing NHL.
- Primary immunosuppression syndromes in children can also increase the risk of developing NHLs such as:
  ○ Ataxia telangiectasia
  ○ Wiskott-Aldrich syndrome
  ○ Common variable immunodeficiency
  ○ Severe combined immunodeficiency
  ○ X-linked lymphoproliferative disorder
- Occupational exposure to certain pesticides and herbicides has been associated with an increased risk for developing NHL. Agricultural workers with cutaneous exposure to these agents have a two- to sixfold increased incidence of NHL.
- Some infectious agents have also been implicated in the pathogenesis of NHLs:
  ○ *Helicobacter pylori* infection can induce mucosa-associated lymphoid tissue (MALT) lymphoma. This lymphoma is dependent on sustained antigenic stimulation by *H. pylori*.

○ Epstein Barr virus is clearly associated with Burkitt's lymphoma, HIV-related B-cell lymphoma, as well as extranodal nasal-type NK/T-cell lymphoma.
○ Human herpesvirus 8 is associated with the development of Kaposi's sarcoma and primary effusion lymphoma, seen most commonly in acquired immune deficiency syndrome.
○ HTLV-I is associated with adult T-cell leukemia/lymphoma.
○ Chronic hepatitis C virus infection has been linked to the occurrence of lymphoplasmacytoid lymphoma and immunocytoma.
○ Simian virus 40 (SV40) sequences were found to be a contaminant of polio vaccines administered in the late 1950s and early 1960s. It has been postulated that this exposure may be a contributing factor to the increasing incidence of NHLs.
- See Table 69–1 for a list of etiologic risk factors for the development of NHLs.

CLASSIFICATION

- Over the past three decades several classification systems have been used for NHL. The current standard classification is the World Health Organization (WHO) Classification of Hematological Malignancies

TABLE 69–1   Etiologic Risk Factors for the Development of Non-Hodgkin Lymphomas

Infectious:

Epstein-Barr virus
Human T-cell lymphotropic virus 1
Human immunodeficiency virus
Hepatitis C virus
Helicobacter pylori
Human herpesvirus 8

Inherited Immunodeficiency Syndromes:

Klinefelter syndrome
Chédiak-Higashi syndrome
Ataxia telangiectasia syndrome
Wiskott-Aldrich syndrome
Common variable immunodeficiency disease

Acquired Immunodeficiency Diseases:

Iatrogenic immunosuppression
HIV-1 infection
Acquired hypogammaglobulinemia

Autoimmune Disease:

Sjögren syndrome
Celiac sprue
Rheumatoid arthritis
Systemic lupus erythematosus

Chemical or Drug Exposure:

Phenytoin
Digoxin
Radiation
Prior chemotherapy and radiation therapy

TABLE 69–2 World Health Organization Classification of Non-Hodgkin Lymphoma

B CELL	T CELL
Precursor B-Cell Neoplasm	**Precursor T-Cell Neoplasm**
Precursor B lymphoblastic leukemia/lymphoma (precursor B-cell acute lymphoblastic leukemia)	Precursor T lymphoblastic leukemia/lymphoma (precursor T-cell acute lymphoblastic leukemia)
Mature (Peripheral) B-Cell Neoplasms	**Mature (Peripheral) B-Cell Neoplasms**
B-cell chronic lymphocytic leukemia/small lymphocytic lymphoma	T-cell prolymphocytic leukemia
B-cell prolymphocytic leukemia	T-cell granular lymphocytic leukemia
Lymphoplasmacytic lymphoma	Aggressive NK-cell leukemia
Splenic marginal zone B-cell lymphoma (+/− villous lymphocytes)	Adult T-cell lymphoma/leukemia (HTLV-I +)
Hairy cell leukemia	Extranodal NK-/T-cell lymphoma, nasal type
Plasma cell myeloma/plasmacytoma	Enteropathy-type T-cell lymphoma
Extranodal marginal zone B-cell lymphoma of MALT type	Hepatosplenic γδ T-cell lymphoma
Mantle cell lymphoma	Subcutaneous panniculitis-like T-cell lymphoma
Follicular lymphoma	Mycosis fungoides/Sézary syndrome
Nodal marginal zone B-cell lymphoma (+/− monocytoid B cells)	Anaplastic large-cell lymphoma, primary cutaneous type
Diffuse large B-cell lymphoma	Peripheral T-cell lymphoma, not otherwise specified
Burkitt lymphoma/Burkitt cell leukemia	Angioimmunoblastic T-cell lymphoma
	Anaplastic large-cell lymphoma, primary systemic type

HTLV, human T-cell lymphotropic virus; MALT, mucosa-associated lymphoid tissue; NK, natural killer.

(Table 69–2), which categorizes lymphoid neoplasms into the following categories:
○ B-cell neoplasms
○ T- and NK-cell neoplasms
○ Hodgkin lymphoma
• Further subcategorization of these tumors employs morphology, immunophenotype, genetic features, and clinical symptoms. Within the B and T-/NK-cell categories, two major subcategories are recognized:
1. Precursor neoplasms, corresponding to the earliest stages of differentiation
2. Peripheral or mature neoplasms, corresponding to more differentiated stages
• NHLs can also be classified according to whether they are indolent or aggressive (Table 69–3).

TABLE 69–3 Classification of Non-Hodgkin Lymphomas Into Indolent Versus Aggressive Types

INDOLENT LYMPHOMAS	AGGRESSIVE LYMPHOMAS
B Cell:	**B Cell:**
Follicular grades I, II, IIIa	Mantle cell
Marginal zone	Follicular grade IIIb
Mucosa associated lymphoid tissue	Diffuse large B cell
Nodal	Mediastinal large B cell
Chronic lymphocytic leukemia/small lymphocytic lymphoma	Burkitt and Burkitt-like
	Precursor B lymphoblastic
T Cell:	**T Cell:**
Mycosis fungoides/Sézary syndrome	Systemic anaplastic large cell
Primary cutaneous anaplastic large cell	Peripheral T cell
	Precursor T lymphoblastic
	Adult T-cell leukemia/lymphoma

GENETIC ABNORMALITIES

• Non-Hodgkin lymphomas are associated with genetic abnormalities. Specific and sometimes diagnostic abnormalities are well established.
○ Some NHLs have no known associated genotype (It is often assumed that genetic abnormalities exist but have yet to be identified in these patients).
○ Most genetic abnormalities likely involve immunoglobulin gene rearrangement resulting in fusion of immunoglobulin promoter and enhancer regions with various oncogenes, thus inducing their expression.
• See Table 69–4 for a list of the most common genetic abnormalities.

STAGING

• Complete staging of NHLs requires the following:
○ Complete history
○ Physical examination
○ Computed tomography (CT) of neck, chest, abdomen, and pelvis
○ Bone marrow biopsy
• Currently, positron emission tomography (PET) is considered a critical imaging study to accurately stage NHLs.

TABLE 69–4   Common Genetic Abnormalities in Non-Hodgkin Lymphomas

GENETIC ABNORMALITY	ASSOCIATED DISEASE	ONCOGENE INVOLVED	FUNCTION
t(14;18)	Follicular lymphoma	BCL-2	Antiapoptosis
t(11;14)	Mantle cell lymphoma	Cyclin D1	Cell cycle regulator
t(8;14), t(2;8), t(8;22)	Burkitt lymphoma	c-myc	Transcription factor
t(3;14)	Large B-cell lymphoma	BCL-6	Transcription factor
t(2;5)	Anaplastic large-cell lymphoma	ALK	Transcription factor
t(11;18)	MALT	BCL-10	Antiapoptosis

MALT, mucosa-associated lymphoid tissue.

- Brain imaging with CT or magnetic resonance imaging (MRI) is necessary in patients with the following:
  ○ Burkitt's or lymphoblastic lymphoma
  ○ Aggressive histology lymphoma involving the bone marrow, sinonasal region, or testis.
- PET scanning is extremely valuable to determine the response to therapy, since CT scans often show shadowing that represents scarring rather than tumor burden. Such patients would incorrectly be classified as partial responders.
- The Ann Arbor staging system was implemented to define the stage of NHLs according to tumor burden, eg, localized disease (stage I) versus extensive disease (stage IV) as well as clinical symptoms, eg, fever, night sweats, and weight loss.
- See Table 69–5 for detailed Ann Arbor staging definitions for NHLs.

PROGNOSTIC FACTORS

- The International Prognostic Index (IPI) was developed to predict outcome in patients with aggressive NHLs based on pretreatment clinical characteristics (Table 69–6).
- Each risk factor in Table 69–6 is assigned 1 point. The total score determines the risk group in which the patient falls. Table 69–7 summarizes the risk groups and their corresponding 5-year overall survival.
- Age-adjusted IPI risk features were also defined for patients younger than 60 years of age. Table 69–8 and Table 69–9 summarizes risk groups and their 5-year overall survival according to age-adjusted IPIs.
- Other poor prognostic features for NHLs include the following:
  ○ β_2-Microglobulin level >1.5 times normal.
  ○ Expression of bcl-2 in large B-cell lymphoma (BCL).
  ○ High anti-Ki 67/MIB-1, indicating a high proliferative potential
- Expression of BCL-6 in large BCL was found to confer a good prognosis.

EVALUATION AND WORKUP AT PRESENTATION

- The initial patient evaluation should include the following:
  ○ Complete history with particular emphasis on eliciting B-symptoms (fever and chills, drenching night sweats, fatigue, pruritus, weight loss)
  ○ Physical examination
  ○ Complete blood count
  ○ Serum lactate dehydrogenase (LDH)
  ○ Liver function tests and kidney function tests
  ○ Uric acid level
  ○ Chemistry profile including serum calcium
  ○ Serum protein electrophoresis
  ○ Serum β_2-microglobulin
  ○ Computed tomography scan of chest, abdomen, and pelvis with contrast (if possible)
  ○ Whole body PET scan
  ○ Bone marrow aspiration and biopsy
  ○ Cerebrospinal fluid examination, when indicated

TABLE 69–5   Ann Arbor Staging System

Stage I	Single lymph node region (I) or single extranodal organ or site (IE)
Stage II	Two or more nodal regions, same side of diaphragm (II), or localized extranodal extension plus one or more nodal regions (IIE)
Stage III	Nodal involvement on both sides of the diaphragm (III) which may be accompanied by localized extralymphatic extension (IIIE) or splenic involvement (IIIS)
Stage IV	Dissemination to one or more extranodal tissues or organs (bone marrow, liver), with or without nodal involvement
A	Asymptomatic
B	Unexplained fever >38°C
	Night sweats
	Unexplained weight loss >10% baseline within 6 months of staging
E	Extranodal disease
X	Bulky disease (>10 cm maximum diameter, or mediastinal mass > one-third maximal chest diameter)

TABLE 69–6   International Prognostic Index

Age >60 years
Lactate dehydrogenase > normal
Performance status 2–4
Stage III or IV
>1 Extranodal site of disease

TABLE 69–7   Risk Groups According to the International Prognostic Index

RISK GROUP	RISK SCORE	5-YEAR OVERALL SURVIVAL (%)
Low	0–1	73
Low-intermediate	2	51
High-intermediate	3	43
High	4–5	26

TABLE 69–9   Risk Groups According to Age-Adjusted International Prognostic Index for Patients Younger Than 60 Years

RISK GROUP	RISK SCORE	5-YEAR OVERALL SURVIVAL (%)
Low	0	83
Low-intermediate	1	69
High-intermediate	2	46
High	3	32

LOW-GRADE NON-HODGKIN B-CELL LYMPHOMAS

B-CELL SMALL LYMPHOCYTIC LYMPHOMA

- B-cell small lymphocytic lymphoma (SLL) accounts for approximately 7% of all NHLs. Importantly, it commonly presents as a chronic leukemia.
- Patients usually present with lymphadenopathy.
- The diagnosis is easily made when mature B lymphocytes express CD5.
- Approximately three-quarters of these patients also have evidence of bone marrow involvement.
- The diagnosis can be morphologically confused with lymphoplasmacytic lymphoma, mantle cell lymphoma, and nodal marginal zone B-cell lymphoma; but only mantle cell lymphoma and SLL are CD5$^+$ (Fig. 69–1).
- The International Prognostic Index should be calculated in all patients:
  - If low, no treatment is necessary and the patient can be observed until there is evidence of disease progression.
  - If high, treatment with a multiagent chemotherapy regimen is indicated.
- Some of the commonly used regimens are as follows:
  - Cyclophosphamide, doxorubicin (Adriamycin), vincristine, prednisone, and rituximab (CHOP-R).
  - If anthracyclines are contraindicated because of cardiac disease, then CVP-R can be used, which omits doxorubicin (Adriamycin)from CHOP-R.
  - Alemtuzumab is a monoclonal antibody with good activity. It eliminates both B and T cells, so patients must be treated with prophylactic antibiotics, antifungals, and antivirals.

TABLE 69–8   Age-Adjusted International Prognostic Index Risk Factors for Patients Younger Than 60 Years.

LDH > normal
Performance status 2–4
Stage III–IV

LDH, lactate dehydrogenase.

- Allogeneic bone marrow transplantation is the only curative treatment modality and should be considered in young patients in otherwise good health.

EXTRANODAL MARGINAL ZONE B-CELL LYMPHOMA OF MALT

- Most MALT lymphomas occur in gastric mucosal sites, but the intestinal mucosa can also be involved.
- It can also occur in extranodal nonmucosal sites including the lungs, periorbital soft tissue, salivary glands, and thyroid.
- Most patients present with an isolated mass in these extranodal sites or a gastric ulcer.
- Most cases of gastric MALT lymphoma are associated with *H. pylori* infection where it is believed to arise from chronic stimulation of the B and T lymphocytes in the stomach by *H. pylori*.
- If the stomach is involved, the most common presentation is that of peptic ulcer disease but occasionally the lymphoma can present as a gastric mass and result in mechanical obstruction.
- At presentation, the tumor is usually confined to the stomach but can involve the draining lymph nodes.

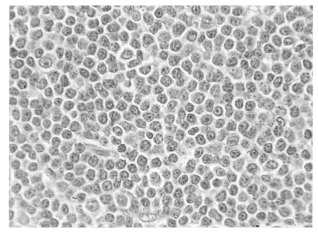

FIG. 69–1 Small lymphocytic lymphoma. Notice the presence of mature lymphocytes.

- Characteristic karyotypic abnormalities include the following:
  - t(11;18)(q21;q21)
  - Less commonly t(1;14)(p22;q32)
  - Rarely, trisomies of chromosomes 3, 7, 12, and 18
- More than two-thirds of gastric MALT lymphomas regress with successful eradication of *H. pylori* infection; this is less well documented in the presence of a large mass. Failure to respond to effective antibiotic treatment indicates either large cell transformation or t(11;18) positivity. In that case a local treatment modality such as gastric radiotherapy is usually effective, but single agent chemotherapy can still be viable.

NODAL MARGINAL ZONE LYMPHOMA

- This condition was previously called *monocytoid B-cell lymphoma.*
- Approximately one-third of patients who carry this diagnosis have an extranodal MALT lymphoma, hence a search for an extranodal lymphoma should always be carried out in such patients.
- No characteristic karyotypic abnormalities have been defined.
- Treatment usually focuses on palliation of symptoms, but chemotherapy can be used to treat progressive disease.
- Median survival is approximately 10 years.

FOLLICULAR LYMPHOMA

- Follicular lymphoma comprises approximately 30% of all NHLs. Usually, the diagnosis can be established with an adequate biopsy specimen. Morphologically, a follicular pattern of growth is virtually diagnostic (Fig. 69–2). The tumor is composed of small and large

cells in varying proportions. The grade of the tumor is dependent on the relative distribution of these cells in a microscopic field, and can be either composed of predominantly small cells, predominantly large cells, or a mixture. Patients who have predominantly large-cells have poor prognosis and may only respond to salvage therapies.

  - The presence of t(14;18) and expression of BCL-2 are confirmatory.
  - Reactive follicular hyperplasia (infections) can create diagnostic dilemmas.
  - The presentation of follicular lymphoma is classically characterized by painless lymphadenopathy.
  - Extranodal involvement is rare and patients usually have a low IPI, but 10% will have a high index.
  - The Follicular Lymphoma International Prognostic Index (FLIPI) is used to predict outcome in these tumors. Table 69–10 details variables used in calculating a FLIPI score.
- Each of the variables in Table 69–10 is assigned a score of 1 and summed. Patients are then classified into risk groups as follows:
  - Low risk (FLIPI 0–1)
  - Intermediate risk (FLIPI 2)
  - High risk (FLIPI ≥3)
- Table 69–11 details the 5- and 10-year survival based on FLIPI score.
- Follicular lymphoma is very responsive to chemotherapy and radiation therapy. It is estimated that approximately 25% of patients experience a spontaneous regression. There is controversy regarding initial treatment of asymptomatic patients, and some experts believe that treatment with rituximab is better than a watch and wait approach.
  - Involved-field radiation therapy is an option in localized disease.
  - When chemotherapy is indicated, use of single-agent chemotherapy, like chlorambucil or cyclophosphamide, or the use of combination chemotherapy, like CVP or CHOP, is appropriate.
  - Presently, chemotherapy treatment almost always involves rituximab. This agent induces a complete remission in 50% to 75% of patients and as many as 20% of remain free of disease for longer than 10 years.

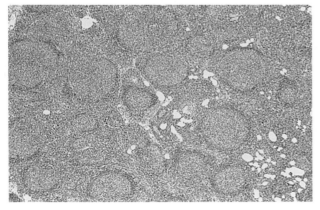

FIG. 69–2 Follicular lymphoma. Nodular growth pattern of tumor with effacement of nodular architecture.

TABLE 69–10   Follicular Lymphoma International Prognostic Index

Age ≥60 years
Ann Arbor stage III–IV
Hemoglobin <12 g/dL
Serum LDH level > upper limit of normal
Number of nodal sites >4

LDH, lactate dehydrogenase.

TABLE 69–11   Risk Groups According to Follicular Lymphoma International Prognostic Index and Their Overall Survival

RISK GROUP	RISK SCORE	5-YEAR OVERALL SURVIVAL (%)	10-YEAR OVERALL SURVIVAL (%)
Low	0–1	90.6	70.7
Intermediate	2	77.6	50.9
High	≥3	52.5	35.5

○ Multiple newer agents have recently been shown to be active in the treatment of follicular lymphoma, including radiolabeled antibodies such as Y 90 ibritumomab tiuxetan (Zevalin) and I 131 tositumomab (Bexxar). Both of these are indicated for relapses.

○ Interferon-α also has shown benefit in trials originating from Europe.

○ Autologous and allogeneic bone marrow transplantation are used in patients with relapses and can lead to long disease-free survival in carefully selected patients.

○ Follicular lymphoma with predominance of large cells should be treated more aggressively using anthracycline-based combination chemotherapy regimens, which can result in an overall survival comparable to patients who have other follicular lymphoma subtypes.

LYMPHOPLASMACYTIC LYMPHOMA

• Lymphoplasmacytic lymphoma is the WHO designation for Waldenström macroglobulinemia. The tumor is composed of plasmacytoid lymphocytes which produce monoclonal immunoglobulin M.

○ It is a disease of the elderly (>65 years of age).

○ Lymphoplasmacytic lymphoma usually presents with lymphadenopathy, splenomegaly, anemia, and less frequently with symptoms of hyperviscosity.

○ Bone marrow infiltration is universal.

○ Patients can also develop cryoglobulinemia or cold autoimmune hemolytic anemia.

○ Patients are treated expectantly and there is no indication for treatment of an asymptomatic patient. Effective first-line chemotherapeutic agents include fludarabine and cladribine, which are also effective for relapsing disease. Rituximab is also effective as both initial therapy and for relapsing disease. Autologous and allogeneic stem cell transplantation are other modalities of treatment that can be employed in selected patients.

• Patients with symptomatic hyperviscosity should undergo the following:

○ Urgent plasmapheresis to lower the concentration of the circulating monoclonal immunoglobulin M

○ Immediate treatment with chemotherapy to control the malignant plasma cell proliferation.

HIGH-GRADE NON-HODGKIN B-CELL LYMPHOMAS

DIFFUSE LARGE B-CELL LYMPHOMA

• These tumors are the most common type of NHLs constituting approximately 33% of the cases.

• Patients can present with lymph node involvement and/or extranodal involvement, with the latter seen in approximately 50% of patients at the time of diagnosis.

• Bone marrow involvement is seen at presentation in approximately 20% of patients.

• The gastrointestinal tract is a common site of extranodal involvement, accordingly gastrointestinal symptoms are frequently reported by patients.

• The diagnosis can be established by morphologic examination of a lymph node biopsy (Fig. 69–3).

• BCL-6 and CD10 expression confer a better prognosis, whereas BCL-2 expression confers a poorer prognosis.

• The IPI score is predictive of survival. An IPI score of 0 to 1 is associated with a 5-year survival > 70%. In contrast, a score of 4 to 5 is associated with a 5-year

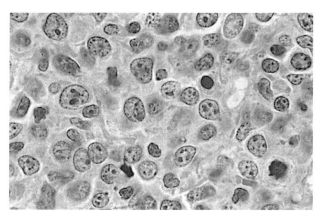

FIG. 69–3   Diffuse large B cell lymphoma. Cells are large with vesicular chromatin and prominent nucleoli.

survival of 20%. In a recent study, the expression of several genetic markers proved useful in predicting overall survival, while adding to the predictive power of the IPI.

- Cure rates of 80% to 90% are expected with stage I disease or nonbulky stage II disease after 3 to 4 cycles of cyclophosphamide, doxorubicin, Oncovin (vincristine), and prednisone (CHOP) plus rituximab and involved field radiation therapy.
- In the remaining patients who have more advanced disease, the recommended treatment is 6 to 8 cycles of combination chemotherapy, such as CHOP and rituximab. Approximately 70% of these patients are expected to achieve a complete remission, and more than half of those will be cured.
- Accumulating evidence suggests that patients who have an IPI score ≥3 have a better event-free and overall survival with autologous stem cell transplantation than with combination chemotherapy with CHOP. However, no comparison to CHOP plus rituximab has been studied.
- Patients who relapse should receive salvage chemotherapy followed by high-dose chemotherapy and autologous stem cell transplantation if the lymphoma is chemosensitive.

MANTLE CELL LYMPHOMA

- This aggressive lymphoma comprises approximately 6% of all NHLs. It was recognized as a separate entity only in the past decade. Mantle cell lymphoma (MCL) can be confused with other small cell B-cell lymphomas like small cell lymphocytic lymphoma. They both have aberrant expression of CD5 in malignant B cells. However, cyclin D1 and t(11;14) positivity are diagnostic of MCL.
  - Usually MCL presents with palpable lymphadenopathy and systemic symptoms (fever, weight loss).
  - Approximately two-thirds of the patients have stage IV disease at presentation, with frequent bone marrow and peripheral blood involvement.
  - Gastrointestinal involvement is characteristic of MCL, and patients can develop lymphomatosis polyposis.
  - Approximately 25% of patients survive more than 5 years, but almost all of these have low IPIs at presentation.
- Treatment of MCL is generally unsatisfactory.
  - The occasional patient with localized disease can be treated with chemotherapy followed by radiation therapy.
  - In patients who present with wide-spread disease, aggressive combination chemotherapy regimens should be employed.

- One of the most commonly used combination regimens is HyperC-VAD alternating with high-dose methotrexate and cytarabine, in combination with rituximab. Collectively, this regimen consists of cyclophosphamide, vincristine, doxorubicin, dexamethasone, cytarabine, high-dose methotrexate, and rituximab.
- If the patient is a good candidate, hematopoietic stem cell transplantation should be offered.
- Both autologous and allogeneic transplantation have been used successfully.
- In general, the results of treatment with chemotherapy alone are discouraging; but recent data indicate improving results when patients are treated with HyperC-VAD (see above) followed by autologous stem cell transplantation.

MEDIASTINAL LARGE B-CELL LYMPHOMA

- Mediastinal large B-cell lymphoma is most commonly seen in young females.
- It usually presents with a bulky anterior mediastinal mass.
- Because of the location, such tumors commonly cause superior vena cava syndrome.
- Patients usually have a high LDH and low serum β_2-microglobulin.
- Clinically, mediastinal large B-cell lymphoma resembles Hodgkin lymphoma.
- Frequently, mediastinal large B-cell lymphoma can progress to involve extranodal sites.
- Treatment should include an anthracycline-containing regimen.

BURKITT'S LYMPHOMA

- Burkitt's lymphoma is the most rapidly growing human tumor.
- It is a rare disease in adults constituting less than 1% of NHLs, but is more commonly seen in children (approximately 30% of NHLs).
- Burkitt's lymphoma is classified into three categories:
  1. Endemic: seen in African children and usually presents with a jaw or facial mass
  2. Sporadic: seen in Western countries
  3. HIV-related
- It usually presents with bulky abdominal lymphadenopathy and involvement of the gastrointestinal and genitourinary tracts.
- In both endemic and sporadic cases, most of the tumors are Epstein Barr virus positive.
- The diagnosis can be established morphologically, but cytogenetic analysis can aid in confirming the diagnosis.

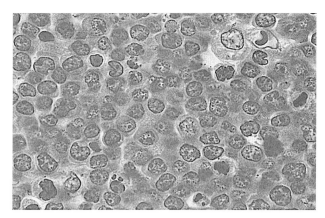

FIG. 69–4 Burkitt lymphoma. Cells are uniform in size and shape with multiple nucloeli. Notice starry sky histiocyte in the upper right.

- The cells are medium in size and homogeneous (Fig. 69–4).
- The demonstration of a malignant B-cell clone with the characteristic cytogenetic abnormalities t(8;14), t(2;8), or t(8;22) is confirmatory. All characterized translocations lead to deregulated expression of the c-myc protooncogene, which promotes cellular proliferation.
- Because central nervous system (CNS) involvement is common, lumbar puncture should be performed at the time of diagnosis and intrathecal chemoprophylaxis administered as part of the routine treatment regimen.
- Once the diagnosis is established, treatment should begin as soon as possible to prevent rapid growth of the tumor.
  - It is crucial to aggressively hydrate and administer allopurinol to all patients before chemotherapy to prevent tumor lysis syndrome.
  - Intensive chemotherapy combination regimens that employ high doses of cyclophosphamide are commonly employed.
  - With aggressive chemotherapy, cure rate approach 70% to 80%.
  - Unfortunately, treating relapses is commonly doomed to failure, and chemotherapy is usually ineffective.

LOW-GRADE NON-HODGKIN T-CELL LYMPHOMAS

MYCOSIS FUNGOIDES/SÉZARY SYNDROME

- Mycosis fungoides is a disease of older patients (usually 60 years of age or older).
- Males are more commonly affected.

- The diagnosis of mycosis fungoides is often delayed for years, as it is commonly confused as a chronic skin condition.
- It progresses from patchy involvement of the skin to plaques then to nodular skin involvement.
- A skin biopsy in the early stages of the disease may not disclose the diagnosis, however a characteristic biopsy finding is the so-called *Pautrier microabscesses* located in the epidermis (Fig. 69–5).
- Sézary syndrome represents the advanced stage of mycosis fungoides. It is characterized by progression to nodal disease and organ infiltration with circulating monoclonal T cells along with erythroderma.
- Treatment of localized skin disease includes:
  - Topical nitrogen mustard
  - Electron beam radiotherapy
  - Photochemotherapy using oral psoralen and ultraviolet irradiation
- In patients with systemic dissemination, palliation is the primary goal.
  - Responses to methotrexate and steroids are generally poor, as is the response to multiagent chemotherapy regimens.
  - Targeting the interleukin-2 receptor or the retinoid pathway has been investigated and holds promise.

HIGH-GRADE NON-HODGKIN T-CELL LYMPHOMAS

ANAPLASTIC LARGE T-CELL LYMPHOMA

- Anaplastic large T-cell lymphoma (ALCL) affects younger individuals.
- Males are affected more often than females.
- Before the discovery of current immunohistochemical and cytogenetic techniques, this lymphoma was referred to as undifferentiated carcinoma.
- Approximately half of the patients present at an early stage disease (ie, stage I or II).
- Patients commonly have systemic symptoms and elevated LDH, but bone marrow involvement is rare.
- Skin involvement is frequent and patients can have a less aggressive disorder referred to as cutaneous ALCL, which is believed to be related to lymphomatoid papulosis.
- ALCL cells typically express several T-cell markers including the following:
  - CD30.
  - Expression of anaplastic lymphoma kinase (ALK) protein (ALK-positive patients are usually younger and have a better prognosis)
  - Cytogenetics reveal translocation t(2;5).

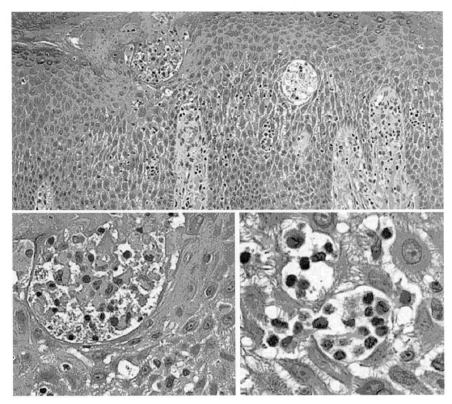

FIG. 69–5 Mycosis fungoides. Pautrier microabscesses in the epidermis.

- IPI predicts prognosis.
  - Treatment should include an anthracycline-based combination chemotherapy regimen.
  - Cure rates approaching 70% have been reported even with advanced stage disease.

ADULT T-CELL LYMPHOMA/LEUKEMIA

- This lymphoma is related to HTLV-I infection, which is a blood-borne virus. It can be acquired by blood product transfusion, sexually, or transmitted transplacentally.
- The highest risk of development of lymphoma is observed in patients who acquire the infection through breast milk (2.5%).
- Latency period is long and averages 55 years.
- Patients usually have an aggressive course marked by the following:
  - Wide-spread lymphadenopathy
  - Hepatosplenomegaly
  - Lytic bone lesions
  - Hypercalcemia
  - Skin infiltration
- Typically, bone marrow involvement is limited and anemia and thrombocytopenia are uncommon.

- The diagnosis is established when the malignant cells express T-cell immunohistochemical markers along with the presence of HTLV-I antibodies.
- The cells themselves are called flower cells because of the characteristic indentation of the nuclei (Fig. 69–6).
- Treatment should include multiagent chemotherapy regimens, but complete remissions are rare.

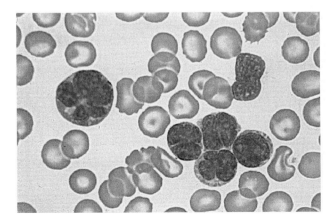

FIG. 69–6 Peripheral smear from a patient with adult T cell lymphoma/leukemia showing characteristic multiple nuclear lobules of malignant cells known as "flower cells".

PERIPHERAL T-CELL LYMPHOMA

- Several clinical syndromes are included in this category and summarized in Table 69–12.
- Peripheral T-cell lymphoma represents approximately 7% of all NHLs.
- Hemophagocytic syndrome can be associated with any of these clinical syndromes and is characterized by the following:
  ○ Severe anemia secondary to the ingestion of red blood cells by monocytes and macrophages.
  ○ This syndrome is associated with a high case fatality rate.
- Patients usually present with a high IPI.
- The 5-year survival is approximately 25%.
- The diagnosis rests on revealing the expression of CD4, a T-cell marker.
- Malignant cells can also express CD8, but less commonly.
- Translocations involving the T-cell antigen receptor genes on chromosomes 7 or 14 may be present, but no diagnostic cytogenetic abnormality has been identified.
- Identifying a monoclonal T-cell population with a T-cell receptor gene rearrangement also confirms the diagnosis.
- Treatment regimens are similar to those used for diffuse large B-cell lymphoma (DLBCL), but the response is worse.
- Hematopoietic stem cell transplantation should always be considered in such patients.

OTHER NON-HODGKIN LYMPHOMAS

PRECURSOR T-OR B-LYMPHOBLASTIC LYMPHOMA

- Lymphoblastic lymphoma overlaps with acute lymphoblastic leukemia to a great extent. These lymphomas are rapidly fatal without aggressive treatment and are mostly of T-cell origin. They are much more common in children. More than 80% of patients present with stage III or IV disease present with an elevated LDH. More than 50% have B-symptoms .
  ○ Precursor B-cell lymphoblastic lymphoma mostly presents in children and young adults with lymphadenopathy or bone involvement. The bone marrow is frequently involved and its involvement correlates with CNS infiltration.
  ○ Precursor T-cell lymphoblastic lymphoma generally presents in young males with a large mediastinal mass that is frequently associated with pleural effusions, superior vena caval obstruction, tracheal obstruction, or a pericardial effusion.
  ○ The initial treatment should be with a systemic intensive multiagent chemotherapy regimen along with intrathecal chemotherapy.
  ○ Patients should be aggressively prophylaxed against tumor lysis syndrome.
  ○ If an optimal chemotherapy regimen is used, it is unclear if autologous stem cell transplantation will lead to additional benefit.

IMMUNODEFICIENCY-ASSOCIATED LYMPHOPROLIFERATIVE DISORDERS

- Immunodeficiency, whether congenital or acquired, can be associated with the development of lymphoproliferative disorders. These can be NHLs or less commonly Hodgkin lymphomas. NHL's are usually of B-cell origin, but rarely can be of T-cell origin. They are associated with a poor prognosis, and treatment is rarely curative. Sometimes, reducing immunosuppression in patients with solid organ or stem cell transplantation can be helpful. Also, there is recent data to suggest that rituximab is particularly beneficial in this lymphoma.

PRIMARY CENTRAL NERVOUS SYSTEM LYMPHOMA

- Primary CNS lymphoma is a rare disorder.
- Primary CNS lymphoma may occur de novo or in association with immunosuppression secondary to HIV infection or solid or stem cell transplantation.
- Most of these lymphomas are of B-cell origin and usually are of the DLBCL subtype.
- The mainstay of treatment is methotrexate combined with corticosteroids.
- Radiation therapy is an option, but radiation-related neurological toxicity can be problematic.
- Primary CNS lymphoma usually carries a poor prognosis.

TABLE 69–12 Peripheral T-Cell Lymphoma Clinical Syndromes

Angioimmunoblastic T-cell lymphoma
Extranodal T-/NK-cell lymphoma of nasal type
Enteropathy-type intestinal T-cell lymphoma
Hepatosplenic γδ T-cell lymphoma
Subcutaneous panniculitis-like T-cell lymphoma

NK, natural killer.

BIBLIOGRAPHY

American Cancer Society. Cancer facts and figures 2007. http://www.cancer.org. Accessed September, 2007.

American Society of Hematology Self Assessment Program, 2nd ed. 2005.

Cheson BD, Pfistner B, Juweid ME, et al. Revised response criteria for malignant lymphoma. *J Clin Oncol.* 2007;25(5): 579–586.

Armitage JO, Fargo DL. Malignancies of lymphoid cells. In: Harrison's *Principles of Internal Medicine.* 16th ed. 641–655.

International non-hodgkin's lymphoma prognostic factors project. A predictive model for aggressive non-Hodgkin's lymphoma. *N Engl J Med.* 1993;329(14):987–994.

Jaffe ES, Harris NL, Stein H, Vardiman JW. *World Health Organization Classification of Tumours. Pathology and Genetics of Tumours of Haematopoietic and Lymphoid Tissues.* Lyon: IARC Press; 2001.

Juweid ME, Stroobants S, Hoekstra OS, et al. Use of positron emission tomography for response assessment of lymphoma: consensus of the Imaging Subcommittee of International Harmonization Project in Lymphoma. *J Clin Oncol,* 2007; 25(5):571–578.

Lossos IS, Czerwinski DK, Alizadeh AA, et al. Prediction of survival in diffuse large B-cell lymphoma based on the expression of six genes. *N Engl J Med.* 2004;350:1828–1837.

Milpied N, Deconinck E, Gaillard F, et al. Initial treatment of aggressive lymphoma with high-dose chemotherapy and autologous stem-cell support. *N Engl J Med.* 2004;350:1287–1295.

Solal-Céligny P, Roy P, Colombat P, et al. Follicular lymphoma international prognostic index. *Blood.* 2004;104(5):1258–1265.

70   MULTIPLE MYELOMA AND RELATED DISORDERS

Christopher N. Hueser

MULTIPLE MYELOMA

BACKGROUND

- Multiple myeloma (MM) is a disease that is characterized by the neoplastic proliferation of a single clone of plasma cells engaged in the production of monoclonal immunoglobulins (M proteins). Such clones proliferate in the bone marrow and frequently invade boney structures thereby producing characteristic symptoms. For the diagnosis of MM, there must be evidence of related organ or tissue impairment such as elevated blood **C**alcium, **R**enal insufficiency, **A**nemia and/or **B**one lesions, easily remembered by the mnemonic **CRAB**.

EPIDEMIOLOGY

- Multiple myeloma is the common plasma cell malignancy
  - One percent of all malignancies
  - Thirteen percent of all hematologic malignancies
  - In the United States 14,000 cases are diagnosed, resulting in 13,000 deaths
  - Incidence: males > females; African Americans > whites
  - Mean age at the time of diagnosis is 69 years of age.

CLINICAL FEATURES

- Immunosuppression.
  - Hypogammaglobulinemia as well as a decrease in the function of circulating immunoglobulins is common. The decrease in immunoglobulin function is caused by the myeloma-associated paraprotein.
  - Generalized marrow failure occurs because of proliferation of myeloma cells in the marrow cavity.
- Renal Failure: There are two major causes of renal insufficiency.
  - Myeloma kidney
    - Urine studies reveal large, waxy casts. The extent of cast formation correlates directly with the concentration of free urinary light-chains and the severity of renal insufficiency. Myeloma kidney is more often encountered with λ–light-chains.
  - Hypercalcemia
    - It is the initial presentation in 15% to 30% of patients. Increased serum levels of calcium can lead to lethargy, constipation, nausea, and vomiting. Furthermore, hypercalcemia can result in hypercalciuria promoting an osmotic diuresis, polydipsia, and polyuria, ultimately leading to dehydration and prerenal azotemia. Hypercalcemia appears to directly impair renal perfusion, contributing to prerenal azotemia. Calcium levels should be analyzed by obtaining an ionized calcium level as the total calcium is influenced by the serum proteins (particularly albumin).
- Neurologic Complications
  - Radiculopathy is the most common neurologic complication. This complication can be secondary to a vertebral mass lesion or pathologic fracture.
  - Spinal cord compression is an oncologic emergency and warrants immediate intervention by radiation oncologists and neurosurgeons.
  - Polyneuropathy occurs secondary to the neuropathic effect of the paraprotein on peripheral nerves. Although, not common in MM, when it occurs, polyneuropathy is usually associated with amyloid deposition.

- Skeletal system
  - Bone pain results from osteolytic lesions leading to pathologic fractures. The pain occurs particularly in the back or chest and is usually worse with movement.
  - Overall there is impaired osteoblastic activity and increased osteoclastic activity leading to bone resorption.
  - Pathognomonic "punched out" lesions can be observed on skull films.
- Hematologic
  - Anemia can be secondary to marrow infiltration, decreased erythropoietin levels, and increased levels of proinflammatory cytokines such as interleukin 6 (IL-6) and tumor necrosis factor-α (TNF-α). The anemia is usually normocytic and normochromic.

DIAGNOSTIC WORKUP

- History and physical examination
- Complete blood count with differential
- Complete metabolic panel
- Serum protein electrophoresis (SPEP)
- Urine protein electrophoresis (UPEP)
- Skeletal survey
- Peripheral blood smear (rouleaux formation)
- β_2-Microglobulin levels
- Bone marrow biopsy and aspirate (malignant plasma cells)
- Quantitative serum immunofixation studies
- Lactate dehydrogenase (LDH)
- Alkaline phosphatase
- C-reactive protein (CRP)
- Magnetic resonance imaging (MRI) of the head, spine, and pelvis to determine extent of disease (especially with solitary plasmacytoma)
- MRI of the spine to evaluate for cord compression

LABORATORY FINDINGS

- The hallmark of myeloma is increased monoclonal antibodies, the M-protein, in the serum and urine. If the monoclonal protein is readily filtered across the glomerular basement membrane, a serum M-spike may not be seen, although depression of other antibodies occurs regardless.
- A normocytic, normochromic anemia is commonly seen.
- Hypercalcemia is present at diagnosis 20% of the time.

RADIOLOGIC FINDINGS

- Characteristic "punched out" lesions seen on skull x-rays is pathognomic. Osteoporosis may also occur. Fractures occur in more than 80% of cases.

DIAGNOSTIC CRITERIA AND DIFFERENTIAL DIAGNOSIS

- For diagnostic criteria and differential diagnosis of multiple myeloma, see Tables 70–1, 70–2, and 70–3.

TREATMENT

- Multiple chemotherapeutic regimens have been successfully used in the treatment of MM. Therapy is generally withheld in patients with asymptomatic disease who have no evidence of progression. Smoldering MM (see below) is not treated unless the patient develops a marked rise in M-protein, lytic bone lesions, a solitary plasmacytoma, renal disease or hypercalcemia. Importantly, the presence of cytogenetic abnormalities (chromosome 13q deletion), increased β_2-microglobulin, and an elevated plasma cell labeling index are poor prognostic features. Most chemotherapy-based regimens produce a response in > 50% of the patients (MPT regimens; melphalan, prednisone, and thalidomide). Newer agents that may prove useful include proteasome inhibitors (bortezomib) and antiangiogenesis agents.
- Autologous peripheral stem cell transplantation (AST) is the only option for cure. Typically, patients must be <65 years of age and be early Durie-Salmon

TABLE 70–1   Diagnostic Criteria for Multiple Myeloma[a]

MAJOR CRITERIA

Plasmacytoma
Plasmacytosis of the bone marrow >30% plasma cells
Monoclonal protein
  IgG >3 g/dL
  IgA >2 g/dL
  Urine-κ or light chains >1 g/dL

MINOR CRITERIA

Lytic bone lesion
Plasmacytosis of the bone marrow 10%–30% plasma cells
Monoclonal protein less than major criteria
Hypogammaglobulinemia

[a]Diagnosis established by presence of one major and one minor criteria or three minor criteria.

TABLE 70–2   Durie and Salmon Classification of Multiple Myeloma

STAGE I

Hemoglobin >10 g/dL
Calcium <12 mg/dL
0–1 Lytic bone lesions or solitary plasmacytoma only
IgG <50 mg/dL, IgA <30 mg/dL
Urine light chain M-component on protein electrophoresis 4 g/24 h

STAGE II

Neither stage I nor III

STAGE III

Hemoglobin <8.5 g/dL
Calcium >12 mg/dL
>5 Lytic bone lesions
IgG >7 0 mg/dL, IgA >50 mg/dL
Urine light chain M-component on protein electrophoresis >12 g/24 h

SUBCLASSIFICATION

A	Creatinine <2 mg/dL
B	Creatinine >2 mg/dL

SOURCE: Adapted from Durie BG, Salman SE. A clinical staging system for multiple myeloma. *Cancer.* 1975;36:842–854.

stage (II to III) to be considered for myeloablative therapies.

COURSE AND PROGNOSIS

- The median survival of patients with symptomatic MM is 30 to 36 months. Unfortunately, chemotherapy has had little impact on overall survival. Indeed, survival is influenced to a greater extent by time to progression than by initial response to chemotherapy. Clearly, AST can result in long-term survival in some patients.

- Patients will eventually succumb to marrow failure, develop myelodysplasia or infection.

MM VARIANTS (TABLE 70–3)

SMOLDERING MULTIPLE MYELOMA (SMM)

- SMM is characterized by an M-protein >3 g/dL and greater than 10% bone marrow plasma cells.
- Importantly, SMM is characterized by the *absence* of bone lytic lesions, anemia, renal insufficiency, or hypercalcemia. These patients should *not* be treated.
- The median time to progression to overt MM is 26 months.

PLASMA CELL LEUKEMIA

- Monoclonal plasma cells can be detected in the blood of patients with active MM (but are usually not found in patients with SMM or MGUS). Plasma cell leukemia is a rare complication of late-stage MM. It has also been described as a primary or de novo disease (60% of cases). It is characterized by abundant (20%) plasma cells in the peripheral blood (flow cytometry). The prognosis of plasma cell leukemia is very poor.

SOLITARY PLASMACYTOMA

- Solitary plasmacytomas are comprised of plasma cells. They can involve the bone (solitary plasmacytoma of the bone) or soft tissue (extramedullary plasmacytoma). Most involve the bone and generally present with bone pain.
- The diagnosis is based on a biopsy revealing a monoclonal plasma cell population with no other lesions (lytic) on the skeletal survey. In addition, the bone

TABLE 70–3   Differential Diagnosis of Myeloma and Related Disorders

	MM	MGUS	NSMM	SMM	AMYLOIDOSIS	WM
M-protein(g/dL)	>3	<3	None	>3	<3	>3
Bone marrow Plasma cells	>10%	<10%	>10%	>10%	<10%	>10%
Lytic lesions	often	absent	often	absent	absent	absent
Symptoms	often	absent	absent	absent	often	often
Abnormal renal Function	± present	absent	± present	absent	± present	
Hypercalcemia	± present	absent	± present	absent	absent	absent
Anemia	often	absent	often	absent	absent	often

MM, multiple myeloma; MGUS, monoclonal gammopathy of unknown significance; NSMM, nonsecretory multiple myeloma; SMM, smoldering multiple myeloma; WM, Waldenström macroglobulinemia.

marrow must be normal and there is no evidence of an M-protein in the serum or urine. Fifty to sixty percent of patients with solitary plasmacytomas progress to overt MM in 3 to 10 years. Tumoricidal radiation is the treatment of choice for bony or extramedullary plasmacytomas.

NONSECRETORY MYELOMA (NSMM)

- Nonsecretory myeloma is characterized by the absence of detectable monoclonal M-protein in both serum and urine. It accounts for 1% to 5% of all patients with MM. Patients are treated in the same fashion as those with secretory MM.
- The response of NSMM to therapy is based on improvement in constitutional symptoms, improvement in end-organ function (renal disease), and reduction of plasmacytosis in the bone marrow.

MONOCLONAL GAMMOPATHY OF UNDETERMINED SIGNIFICANCE (MGUS)

BACKGROUND

- MGUS is defined by the presence of a monoclonal protein in patients with no other features of multiple myeloma (lytic lesions, anemia, hypercalcemia) or other neoplastic condition (B-cell lymphoproliferative disorder). The M-protein must be <3g/dL and the bone marrow must have <10% plasma cells. Importantly, a variety of nonmalignant disorders including connective tissue diseases (lupus, rheumatoid arthritis), HIV infection, hepatitis C infection, and urticaria have been described in association with MGUS.

EPIDEMIOLOGY

- The prevalence of MGUS is 3.2% in persons older than 50 years of age and 5.3% in those older than 70 years of age. The incidence of MM is approximately 1% per year in these patients.
- The median age of diagnosis is 70 years.
- There is a higher incidence in African Americans than in whites.

SYMPTOMS

- Patients are usually asymptomatic, and the MGUS is typically discovered incidentally.

DIAGNOSTIC WORKUP

- The workup is designed to exclude overt MM, other neoplastic disorders (leukemias and lymphomas) and nonmalignant disease (HIV and hepatitis C). A careful history and physical examination is essential. Otherwise, the patient should undergo routine laboratory testing including a CBC, metabolic profile, SPEP and UPEP.
- A skeletal survey and bone marrow aspirate (only if the serum monoclonal concentration is greater than 1.5 g/dL) is also usually performed.

LABORATORY FINDINGS

- Elevated total serum protein concentration with an M-component of <3 g/dl.
- Less than 10% bone marrow plasma cells.
- Absence of bone lytic lesions.
- Absence of end-organ damage.

AMYLOIDOSIS

- Primary amyloidosis is characterized by deposition of β-amyloid in tissues and organs. The amyloidogenic protein can be derived from either (1) light chains (AL) or (2) inflammatory proteins (AA). Rarely, the amyloidogenic protein is related to a genetic disorder such as the heredofamilial fever syndromes. There are no specific diagnostic blood, serum, or radiologic tests for amyloidosis. The diagnosis can only be confirmed by Congo red staining of affected tissue. The specific type of amyloid can also be characterized histologically.

EPIDEMIOLOGY

- Median age of diagnosis is 65 years.
- Two-thirds of the patients are male.
- The incidence is approximately 3000 cases per year.

CLINICAL MANIFESTATIONS

- Commonly patients present with weakness, fatigue, and/or weight loss. Another common finding is purpura that usually occurs in the face, neck, and upper eyelids.
- In patients with congestive heart failure, pedal edema and dyspnea are characteristic.
- Hoarseness or a change in voice can also be a presenting symptom. Macroglossia occurs in approximately 10% of patients.

- In patients with autonomic neuropathy, paresthesias and syncope are seen.

LABORATORY FINDINGS

- Proteinuria is present in 70% of patients at the time of diagnosis, one-third of whom have proteinuria in the nephrotic range. An M-protein is found in 90% of patients.

ORGAN INVOLVEMENT

- Cardiac
  - The clinical outcome and the likelihood of patients responding to treatment is, in large part, determined by the extent of cardiac involvement at the time of diagnosis.
  - Heart failure is the cause of death in >50% of patients.
- Renal
  - Progressive glomerular injury leading to renal failure is also common and confers a very poor prognosis.
- Liver
  - Hepatomegaly without imaging abnormalities on computed tomography (CT) or MRI occurs in one-sixth of patients. The liver can become engorged to the extent that patients experience early satiety and weight loss.
- Nervous system
  - Autonomic dysfunction can manifest as severe diarrhea alternating with constipation.
  - Orthostatic hypotension can be severe and limit therapy options aimed at reducing nephritic edema.
  - Peripheral neuropathy is common and primarily affects the sensory neurons. It occurs most often in the lower extremities. Of those patients who do experience upper extremity neuropathy, one-half have carpal tunnel syndrome. Gabapentin and amitriptyline often fail to provide benefit in these patients.

DIAGNOSIS

- If the level of circulating monoclonal protein and plasma cell percentage in the bone marrow are consistent with MGUS and there is nephrotic syndrome, chronic heart failure (CHF), peripheral neuropathy, carpal tunnel syndrome, or massive hepatomegaly, the most likely diagnosis is primary amyloidosis.
- Ultimately amyloid deposits must be demonstrated in tissue. Clearly, a biopsy of an affected site (kidney) is preferable to random tissue sampling. Nonetheless, a random transcutaneous fat biopsy is positive 80% of the time. If an abdominal fat biopsy fails to provide a diagnosis, a bone marrow biopsy and aspiration can be performed. If both the abdominal fat pad and bone marrow biopsies are negative then a rectal biopsy is indicated. The rectal biopsy is positive 75% of the time.
- A positive biopsy specimen produces an apple-green birefringence under polarized light with Congo red staining.

TREATMENT

- Amyloid cardiomyopathy is best treated with supportive care. Salt restriction and loop diuretics can be used. Caution should be used when attempting to reduce afterload with angiotensin-converting enzyme inhibitors as postural hypotension is commonly associated with amyloidosis.
- Amyloidosis responds to MM-based therapy (see above).
- Peripheral blood stem cell transplantation (PBSCT) has been rarely utilized, but may offer a cure.

WALDENSTRÖM MACROGLOBULEMIA

BACKGROUND

- Waldenström's macroglobulinemia (WM) is a clonal disorder of small lymphocytes producing a malignant clone of plasma cells which synthesize immunoglobulin M (IgM). The bone marrow shows a pathognomonic lymphoplasmacytic infiltrate.

EPIDEMIOLOGY

- The incidence of WM range between 3.4 per million person-years among men and 1.7 per million person-years among women, and increases with age.
- WM accounts for approximately 2% of all hematologic malignancies.
- It is more common among whites than African Americans.
- The median age at diagnosis is 63 years.

CLINICAL MANIFESTATIONS

- Presenting symptoms are usually nonspecific and include fatigue, weight loss, anorexia, and weakness.

- Symptoms caused by monoclonal IgM include Raynaud's phenomenon, amyloidosis, cold agglutinin hemolytic anemia, and peripheral neuropathy.
- Hepatosplenomegaly and lymphadenopathy are present in 15% to 25% of patients.
- Hyperviscosity symptoms, such as epistaxis, blurred vision, dyspnea, or headache can occur.
- If hyperviscosity is suspected, a funduscopic examination should be performed, and blood viscosity should be measured.
- Increased plasma volume and anemia can worsen heart failure.

LABORATORY FINDINGS

- The erythrocyte sedimentation rate is almost always markedly elevated in WM (>100) and the thrombin time is frequently prolonged.
- Anemia (usually normochromic, normocytic) is the most common laboratory finding in symptomatic patients. The peripheral smear typically reveals prominent rouleaux formation.
- Hepatosplenomegaly and/or lymphadenopathy is seen in approximately 50% of patients. Computed tomography of the chest, abdomen, and pelvis should be performed as part of the staging workup.
- A lymphoplasmacytic infiltrate with mast cells is seen on bone marrow biopsy.

TREATMENT

- Initiation of therapy should be based on the presence of constitutional symptoms, progressive symptoms, complications such as hyperviscosity syndrome, renal insufficiency, peripheral neuropathy, or cryoglobulinemia.
- No defined treatment algorithm exists for WM as there are few clinical trials.
- Agents that have been employed with success for WM include alkylating agents (chlorambucil), nucleoside analogs (fludarabine), and the monoclonal antibody, rituximab.

BIBLIOGRAPHY

Bladé J, Kyle RA. Nonsecretory myeloma, immunoglobulin D myeloma, and plasma cell leukemia. *Hematol Oncol Clin North Am.* 1999;13:1259–1272.

Channan-Khan A, Miller KC. Supportive care in multiple myeloma. *Clin Lymphoma Myeloma.* July 2006;42–50.

Comenzo RL. Amyloidosis. *Curr Treat Options Oncol.* 2006;7: 225–236.

Durie BG, Salman SE. A clinical staging system for multiple myeloma. *Cancer.* 36:842–54. 1975.

Kyle RA. Clinical aspects of multiple myeloma and related disorders including amyloidosis. *Pathol Biol.* 1999;47:148–157.

71 TRANSFUSION MEDICINE

Marian Petrides and Allison Lisle

BLOOD COMPONENT COLLECTION AND PROCESSING

Most of the blood processed in the United States is collected as whole blood, anticoagulated with citrate which is rapidly metabolized by the recipient after transfusion. The collected whole blood is processed by centrifugation into packed red blood cells (RBCs), fresh frozen plasma (FFP), and platelets.[1] Whole blood (WB) derived platelet units are typically pooled into four-unit to six-unit unit batches immediately prior to release from the transfusion service.

Cryoprecipitate is obtained by thawing a unit of FFP in the refrigerator overnight, then centrifuging the FFP in a refrigerated centrifuge and harvesting the precipitate.[1] The remaining plasma can be refrozen and substituted for whole FFP in the treatment of patients with thrombotic thrombocytopenic purpura.

Platelets, RBCs, and FFP can also be collected by apheresis, which offers the advantage of leukocyte reduction of cellular products (RBCs and platelets) during processing.[1] A single apheresis platelet unit is the therapeutic equivalent of four to six units of WB-derived platelets. Thus, use of an apheresis platelet unit will reduce the recipient's exposure to donor proteins by threefold to fivefold when compared with a pool of WB-derived platelets.

CONTENTS

- A unit of RBCs contains approximately 180 mL of RBCs in 30 to 70 mL of plasma. 100 mL of a preservative solution may be added to extend shelf life. The hematocrit of a typical unit without an additive is 70% to 80%, whereas additive solution RBC units have a hematocrit of 55% to 60%. The RBCs in a unit must be compatible with ABO antibodies present in the recipient, but the small amount of plasma that accompanies the RBCs is of little concern in adults because it is diluted in a much larger plasma volume (approximately 3 L in a 70 kg patient).

- A WB-derived platelet unit contains platelets in approximately 50 mL of plasma, so a six-unit pool (sometimes referred to as a *six pack*) has a volume of approximately 300 mL. A six-unit pool of WB-derived platelets contains approximately the same number of platelets as are found in a single apheresis platelet unit, which has a comparable volume (300 mL). Platelets should be plasma-compatible with the recipient's RBCs if at all possible. If ABO incompatible platelets must be given, transfusion of O platelets into an A, B, or AB patient should be avoided if possible.
- FFP contains on average 1 international unit per mL of each of the coagulation factors (proteins C and S and antithrombin), along with 2 to 4 mg/mL of fibrinogen. The typical volume of an FFP unit is 200 to 250 mL. FFP must be thawed for 20 to 30 minutes in a 37°C water bath prior to use. The ABO antibodies present in the unit must be compatible with the antigens present on the recipient's RBCs.
- Each unit of cryoprecipitate contains approximately 200 mg fibrinogen and no less than 80 international units of factor VIII in 5 to 15 mL of plasma. Cryoprecipitate must be thawed prior to use and is pooled by the transfusion service (typical pool size of 10 units) prior to issue. As with platelets, plasma compatibility with recipient RBCs is preferred.

INDICATIONS FOR TRANSFUSION

When discussing common transfusion indications, it must be recalled that not every patient who fulfills the standard criteria for transfusion must receive a transfusion. Likewise, some patients who do not fulfill criteria can still benefit from prophylactic transfusion in the appropriate clinical setting. Symptomatic patients may require therapeutic transfusion at any measured laboratory value.

RED BLOOD CELLS

RBCs are transfused to increase oxygen-carrying capacity.[1,6] In patients with sickle cell anemia, RBC transfusions are also used to reduce the percentage of hemoglobin S in an effort to reduce viscosity and improve transit through the microvasculature.[2]

A recent study in medical and surgical critical care patients revealed that patients whose hemoglobin was maintained between 7 and 9 g/dL showed no statistically significant difference in survival or multiorgan dysfunction when compared with those maintained between 10 and 12 g/dL.[3] This supports a transfusion *trigger* of 7 g/dL in asymptomatic young patients with acute-onset anemia. Patients with known ischemic cardiovascular

disease, significant respiratory dysfunction, and diabetics at risk for silent ischemia may require transfusion therapy to maintain the hemoglobin at higher levels (9–10 g/dL)—at least until clear data emerge regarding risks in this subset of patients. Patients with symptomatic anemia unresponsive to fluid replacement require RBC transfusion regardless of the measured hemoglobin level.[4]

PLATELETS

Several studies conducted in thrombocytopenic patients with acute myelogenous leukemia (except M3) have documented the importance of maintaining a platelet count ≥10,000/μL in the absence of bleeding, fever, hypersplenism, coincident coagulopathy (including heparin) or anatomic lesions at risk of bleeding (esophageal varices). In patients with these comorbidities, ≥20,000/μL should suffice as prophylactix. Patients with active hemorrhage benefit from a platelet count exceeding 50,000/μL and those at risk of critical space bleed (central nervous system, spinal cord; eye; lung) may benefit from prophylactic transfusion to maintain the platelet count above 100,000/μL. Patients with congenital platelet dysfunction may require therapeutic transfusion in the setting of active bleeding, regardless of the platelet count.[4]

FRESH FROZEN PLASMA

Numerous studies have shown that prothrombin time (PT) and partial thromboplastin time (PTT) are poor indicators of the risk of bleeding after invasive procedures unless the values are greater than 1.5 times the midnormal value. Thus, prophylactic FFP need only be given when deficiency of coagulation factors results in marked (more than 1.5 times midnormal) prolongation of the PT or PTT.[4] It is important to recall in this context that 1.5 times the midnormal PT corresponds to an international normalized ratio (INR) of 2.0. Indeed, a recent study revealed that less than 1% of patients with mildly prolonged INRs (1.1–1.85) who received FFP transfusion showed complete correction, and only 15% showed correction halfway to normal.[5] As with RBCs and platelets, therapeutic use is a different matter and should be initiated when bleeding is felt to be related to an underlying coagulopathy.

CYROPRECIPITATE

Cryoprecipitate is transfused primarily to restore fibrinogen in patients who are profoundly hypofibrinogenemic (fibrinogen less than 100 mg/dL).[4,6] In patients bleeding profusely, it is advisable to initiate thawing and pooling of cryoprecipitate at a slightly higher fibrinogen level (125 mg/dL). Although cryoprecipitate also contains factor VIII and von Willebrand factor, there are alternative (specific) blood products used to replace these deficiencies.[2] Cryoprecipitate has been used successfully to treat bleeding in patients with uremic platelet dysfunction unresponsive to DDAVP. In addition, cryoprecipitate is used to replace factor XIII in the rare patient who is factor XIII deficient.[6]

PRETRANSFUSION COMPATIBILITY TESTING

ABO AND Rh TYPE

Prior to transfusion, a sample from the patient must be tested to determine the recipient's ABO group and Rh status (presence or absence of the D antigen). This is done by testing red cells from the patient with reagent antibody (anti-A, anti-B, and anti-D).

Since anti-A and anti-B are *naturally occurring* antibodies that are reliably present whenever the respective antigens are lacking on the patient's red cells, ABO grouping consists of testing the recipient's red cells as above (*forward type*), then confirming the presence of the expected antibodies in his/her plasma (*reverse type*). If the ABO group determined on forward typing does not match that found on reverse typing, the patient may receive group O RBCs and group AB plasma but should not receive ABO type-specific blood until the discrepancy is resolved (Table 71–1).[2]

Reverse typing is not used for Rh testing because anti-D is always an immune antibody, that is, it does not appear in patients who have never been transfused. Patients who are D-negative (Rh negative) should receive D-negative RBCs, except in an emergency. When the need for blood is emergent and no ABO-compatible Rh negative units are available, it is safe to transfuse Rh positive RBCs so long as the patient is not known to have produced anti-D. The risk associated with transfusing Rh positive RBCs to an Rh negative

patient without anti-D is the development of anti-D (40%–80% of the time) weeks to months later. Conversely, Rh negative patients who have produced anti-D must receive Rh negative blood for the remainder of their lives.[2]

ANTIBODY SCREEN: INDIRECT COOMBS TEST

There are 29 identified blood group antigen systems, many with multiple allelic pairs.[7] Thus, establishing that patients receive ABO and Rh compatible blood is insufficient. Accordingly, the recipient must be screened for clinically significant antibodies directed against these minor blood group antigens.

The usual screening test examines the reactivity (non-ABO antibodies) of recipient plasma against two or three reagent group O red blood cells of known antigenic specificity. Because the technique used in antibody screening and antibody identification involves pre-incubating recipient plasma with reagent red cells before addition of the Coomb's reagent (rabbit antibody against human IgG), the technique is referred to as the indirect antiglobulin test (IAT), more commonly known as the *indirect Coombs test*.

The plasma from patients with a positive antibody screen is then tested against a panel of 12 to 16 group O RBCs of known antigenic composition to determine the antigenic specificity of the detected antibody. When a putative specificity is determined, the final step involves antigen phenotyping the recipient's own RBCs to ensure that they are antigen negative, and thus incapable of generating the antibodies identified with the IAT.[2]

CROSSMATCH

Once the specificity of the antibody is defined, ABO compatible units are tested and those that are antigen-negative are selected. The final step, the crossmatch, involves testing the recipient's plasma against these antigen-negative units.[2] An incompatible crossmatch suggests the presence of an additional, unsuspected antibody and requires further evaluation.

DIRECT ANTIGLOBULIN TEST

Unlike the indirect Coomb's test, which detects circulating antibody in the recipient's plasma, the direct antiglobulin test (DAT), also known as the direct Coomb's test, screens for antibody that is bound to the recipient's circulating red cells in vivo. The DAT involves mixing recipient red cells with Coomb's

TABLE 71–1 Expected Antibodies Based on ABO Group

ABO GROUP	EXPECTED ANTIBODY IN PLASMA
A	Anti-B
B	Anti-A
O	Both anti-A and anti-B
AB	No antibody

TABLE 71–2 Summary of Safe Transfusion Practice

PATIENT ABO GROUP	RBCs TO TRANSFUSE	FFP, PLATELETS, CRYO TO TRANSFUSE[a]
A	A, O	A, AB (has no antibody
B	B, O	B, AB (has no antibody)
O	O	A, B, AB, O
AB	A, B, AB, O	AB

[a]Mandatory for FFP, preferred for platelets and cryoprecipitate.
Cryo, cryoprecipitate; FFP, fresh frozen plasma; RBCs, red blood cells

reagent, and examining the cells for agglutination or hemolysis.

The DAT has two major uses: evaluation of autoantibodies (these antibodies are bound to the recipient's RBCs as well as transfused RBCs) and the evaluation of possible hemolytic transfusion reactions (in which case the alloantibody would be bound only to transfused red cells and not to the patient's own RBCs).[2] See Table 71–2 for a summary of safe transfusion practices.

TRANSFUSION REACTIONS

Transfusion reactions can be innocuous or life-threatening, depending on the underlying mechanism(s). Thus, whenever a transfusion reaction is considered, the transfusion should be discontinued, the transfusion service notified immediately, and a posttransfusion blood sample (ethylenediaminetetraacetic acid (EDTA)-anticoagulated tube preferred) sent to the blood bank as soon as possible. In most cases, the blood product should be returned promptly to the blood bank along with all attached tubing (needle removed).

ACUTE HEMOLYTIC TRANSFUSION REACTION

ETIOLOGY
• Preformed antibody (usually anti-A or anti-B) in the recipient binds to antigens on the red blood cells in the transfused unit, causing activation of complement and the membrane attack complex. This is accompanied by cell lysis and the liberation of cellular contents (*cytokine storm)* resulting in hypotension and activation of the coagulation system.[2]

CLINICAL PRESENTATION
• Acute onset hemoglobinemia/hemoglobinuria, hypotension, disseminated intravascular coagulation (DIC), flank pain, pain at the infusion site, chest pain/sense of impending doom, fever, rash, and dyspnea may all be

seen. Sometimes fever or rash may be the initial presenting symptoms. Onset usually occurs within 4 hours of transfusion.

TREATMENT
• Discontinue the transfusion and release a posttransfusion blood sample to the blood bank immediately. Hemodynamic support with intravenous (IV) fluids and vasopressors is usually required. Ventilatory support may also be required. Once the causative antibody is identified, antigen-negative units can be transfused, if needed.[2]

PREVENTION
• By employing rigorous protocols involving the recipient, sample, and blood product, these reactions are rare.

DELAYED HEMOLYTIC TRANSFUSION REACTION

ETIOLOGY
• Occurs when preformed antibody is absent (or present in an amount insufficient for detection) in the recipient's pretransfusion sample, although the recipient has previously been sensitized. Occasionally may be caused by brisk production of new antibody.

CLINICAL PRESENTATION
• Unexplained drop in hemoglobin or rise in indirect bilirubin 2 days to 2 weeks following transfusion. May also be detected by the blood bank as a newly identified antibody in a recently transfused patient.

TREATMENT
• Identify antibody specificity. All future transfusions must be antigen-negative, even if antibody is no longer detectable in the laboratory.

PREVENTION
• Once the antibody is identified, use only antigen-negative RBC units.

FEBRILE NONHEMOLYTIC TRANSFUSION REACTION (FNHTR)

ETIOLOGY
• Cytokines and other biological response modifiers are liberated from blood products during storage. Alternatively, white blood cells (WBCs), WBC stroma, or platelets in the blood product react with preformed antibody (often human leukocyte antigen [HLA] antibody) in the recipient resulting in pyrogen release.

CLINICAL PRESENTATION

- Rigors, fever (unexplained increase in temperature of at least 1°C), possibly hypertension and tachycardia. Hypotension is not a feature.

TREATMENT

- Discontinue the transfusion, and release the posttransfusion blood sample and the remainder of the unit to the blood bank immediately. The blood bank will test for hemolysis and obtain a Gram stain and bag culture on the implicated unit to exclude sepsis. If the clinical suspicion of sepsis (see below) and the Gram stain are negative, the patient is treated for the fever and rigors with antipyretics and meperidine, respectively.

PREVENTION

- Leukocyte reduction of cellular blood products reduces the incidence of FNHTR.[2]

SEPTIC TRANSFUSION REACTION

ETIOLOGY

- Bacterial contamination of transfused unit.

CLINICAL PRESENTATION

- Fever, hypotension, possibly septic shock

TREATMENT

- Discontinue the transfusion and immediately send a posttransfusion blood sample and the remainder of unit to the blood bank for analysis and culture. Maintain IV access, administer fluids intravenously and vasopressors as required, initiate broad-spectrum antibiotic coverage.

PREVENTION

- Careful visual inspection of blood products at the time of issue for discoloration, clots, bubbles, or hemolysis. Platelet units are routinely tested for bacterial contamination following collection, although the final culture results may not be available until after issue. Infuse all blood components within 4 hours of issue from the blood bank.[2]

ALLERGIC (URTICARIAL) REACTION

ETIOLOGY

- Soluble allergens present in the transfused unit

CLINICAL PRESENTATION

- Urticaria in the absence of respiratory distress or angioedema.

TREATMENT

- Antihistamines

PREVENTION

- Unlikely to recur. Reaction is flow rate dependent, so transfuse cellular products as slowly as possible. Premedicate with antihistamines. If recurrent reactions, consider a different antihistamine and/or corticosteroid premedication. Rarely, patients with multiple allergic reactions to RBCs may benefit from washed RBCs.[2]
- If there is an extensive rash, swelling of the mouth or tongue (angioedema), or respiratory distress, observe anaphylaxis precautions with subsequent transfusions.

ANAPHYLACTIC/ANAPHYLACTOID REACTION

ETIOLOGY

- Classically these reactions are secondary to anti-IgA antibodies in IgA deficient recipients. The antibody interacts with IgA in the transfused unit.[2] Miscellaneous allergens (drugs or diluents added to the blood product) may also trigger the response, as may passive infusion of IgE antibody from donor to recipient.[4]

CLINICAL PRESENTATION

- Anaphylaxis is characterized by severe dyspnea, laryngospasm (stridor), and hypotension.

TREATMENT

- Discontinue the transfusion and treat the anaphylactic reaction with epinephrine, antihistamines and IV corticosteroids. The recipient should be tested for antibody directed against IgA.

PREVENTION

- If anti-IgA antibody is identified, the patient must receive blood products from IgA-deficient donors (frozen, deglycerolized RBCs or RBCs washed in 3 L saline are also acceptable).[4] If the patient is not IgA deficient and is anti-IgA antibody negative, then the clinician should obtain a thorough history to identify potential allergens.

TRANSFUSION-RELATED ACUTE LUNG INJURY (TRALI)

ETIOLOGY

- TRALI is characterized by neutrophil sequestration and degranulation in the pulmonary capillary bed, releasing pro-inflammatory cytokines that result in pulmonary capillary leak. Two theories have evolved to explain this reaction: (1) Donor anti-granulocyte or anti-HLA antibodies bind to antigens on the recipient's granulocytes in the pulmonary microvasculature, and (2) Lipid and cytokine mediators contained within blood products activate (prime) neutrophils in the pulmonary microvasculature of susceptible individuals. A composite theory that invokes components of both mechanisms may be involved in the pathogenesis of this complication.

CLINICAL PRESENTATION

- An acute respiratory distress syndrome (ARDS)-like picture, during the transfusion or within 6 hours (usually within 2 hours) after the end of the transfusion in patients with no previous history of acute lung injury and in the absence of an alternate explanation for acute lung injury. The chest x-ray reveals pulmonary edema without cardiomegaly. The central venous pressure (CVP) and pulmonary capillary wedge pressure (PCWP) are not elevated (eg, noncardiogenic pulmonary edema).

TREATMENT

Supportive care is all that can be offered eg, oxygen and ventilatory support. Uncomplicated TRALI usually resolves within 1 week, however, 5% to 10% of cases are fatal.

PREVENTION

- No special precautions are required as recurrent TRALI is rare, although the recipient should not receive blood products from the original donor. The blood bank will initiate an investigation of the donor for anti-HLA or anti-human neutrophil antigen (anti-HNA) antibodies. If these antibodies are detected, the donor should be excluded from further donation of plasma-containing products.[2]

REFERENCES

1. *Circular of Information for the Use of Human Blood and Blood Components.* AABB; July 2002.
2. Petrides M, Stack G. *Practical Guide to Transfusion Medicine.* Bethesda, MD: AABB Press; 2001.
3. Herbert PC, Wells G, Blajchman MA, et al. A multicenter, randomized, controlled clinical trial of transfusion requirements in critical care. *New Engl J Med.* 1999;340(6):409–417.
4. Petrides M, AuBuchon J. To transfuse or not to transfuse: An assessment of risks and benefits. In: Mintz PD, ed. *Transfusion Therapy: Clinical Principles and Practice.* 2nd ed. Bethesda, MD: AABB Press; 2005.
5. Abdel OI, Healy B, Dzik WH. Effect of fresh-frozen plasma transfusion on prothrombin time and bleeding in patients with mild coagulation abnormalities. *Transfusion.* 2006;46: 1279–1285.
6. Becker J, Blackall D, Evans C, et al. *Guidelines for Blood Utilization Review.* Bethesda, MD: AABB; 2001.
7. Brecher ME, ed. *AABB Technical Manual.* 15th ed. Bethesda, MD: AABB; 2005.

72 ONCOLOGIC SCREENING AND DETECTION

Syed Huq

BACKGROUND

- Oncologic screening has received considerable attention over the past few decades with the aim of reducing the burden of neoplastic diseases, given the possibility of cure in the early stages of many neoplasms.
- In recent years, the incidence of cancer has risen. In 2006, approximately 1.4 million people were diagnosed with cancer and up to 560,000 people succumbed to cancer. It is estimated that 3% to 35% of these deaths could have been averted through the adoption of screening methods.[1]
- Adherence to current screening recommendations is still imperfect, with the Institute of Medicine estimating that up to 20% of new cancers and up to 30% of cancer-related deaths may be averted through the routine adoption of proven screening methods.[2]

SCREENING: GENERAL PRINCIPLES

- A screening test refers to a test that is carried out in asymptomatic populations with the aim of detecting early disease. These tests are usually not diagnostic but identify patients who warrant further workup using specific confirmatory testing such as a tissue biopsy with histopathologic examination (eg, breast mass).
- Several examination methods, laboratory tests, and imaging modalities have been used for screening; but all must meet certain criteria before routine use can be advocated.
  - The screening test must detect cancers before the onset of symptoms.
  - Treatment initiated on the basis of a positive screening test must improve outcome as compared to standard treatment of symptomatic patients.
  - The outcome should reflect a reduction in cause-specific mortality, but in certain settings, reduction of all-cause mortality may be reasonable (eg, in the elderly).
  - The test or examination should ideally be noninvasive and cost-effective.
- The accuracy of screening tests is usually expressed in terms of sensitivity and specificity. *Sensitivity* refers to the diagnostic power of a test to detect disease in people who truly have the disease, whereas *specificity* refers to the ability of a test to identify people without the disease. Screening tests ideally have a high specificity and sensitivity.
- Screening studies, intrinsically, are biased, which may amplify the potential benefits of the study. The common biases encountered include the following:
  - *Lead-time bias*: This occurs when a screening test can identify a disease early, but early treatment does not result in improved survival.
  - *Overdiagnosis or length-time bias*: Sensitive screening methods can sometimes identify indolent diseases that progress slowly or at all, thus, having minimal impact on survival. Screening in this setting can result in harm to the patient, as a result of the side effects of unnecessary therapy. Some authors cite this bias in their criticism of the routine use of prostate-specific antigen (PSA) screening for prostate cancer.
  - *Selection bias*: This bias reflects randomization and sample size, eg, study subjects may differ significantly from the population at large. For example, volunteers in screening studies may have greater health awareness and other lifestyle factors that produce better outcomes, regardless of the screening test. This may overestimate the benefit of the screening test in question.
- To minimize the occurrence of bias, recommendations for screening must be generated from well-designed prospective randomized controlled trials,

which measure cause-specific mortality. These studies provide the best estimates of the benefits or harms of a screening modality.

- It is not always possible to conduct such large-scale population studies, because of cost and logistics. Hence, observational case-control and cohort studies are sometimes used to develop clinical practice guidelines in settings where the disease burden is significant and randomized clinical trials are unavailable.
- Widely accepted cancer screening guidelines include those published by the United States Preventive Services Task Force (USPSTF), American Cancer Society (ACS), National Cancer Institute (NCI), and medical specialty societies. Some of these are summarized in Table 72–1.

BREAST CANCER SCREENING

- Breast cancer accounts for greater than 200,000 new cases each year, and results in approximately 40,000 deaths per year. The average lifetime risk for breast cancer is approximately 8%.[1]
- Three different modalities are commonly employed for screening average risk women for breast cancer:
  1. *Self-breast examination*: Although a monthly self-breast examination has been recommended for all women older than age 20 years, there has been no randomized trial showing a mortality benefit. However, a large proportion of cancers are usually first identified by the patient, hence, most authorities recommend counseling women on proper self-breast examination.
  2. *Clinical breast examination*: Both the USPSTF and ACS recommend a regular clinical breast

examination, but the frequency and demographics (age range) differ, as shown in Table 72–1. Randomized trials have shown some benefit of a high-quality clinical breast examination, and the mortality benefit of screening mammography is enhanced by 5% to 20% when combined with clinical breast examinations.[3]
  3. *Mammography*: Based on a large number of randomized trials and subsequent meta-analysis, regular screening mammography has been shown to decrease breast cancer mortality. It is estimated that in women between 40 and 70 years, regular screening mammography offers a 15% relative risk reduction in breast cancer mortality.[3]

- The age at which breast cancer screening should start has been the subject of considerable debate. The current consensus opinion of the ACS and the NCI is to begin yearly mammography for all women older than 40 years of age. Thus, a comprehensive breast cancer screening strategy would include regular self-breast examinations every month, a clinical breast examination yearly, and an annual mammogram starting at age 40 years.
- Magnetic resonance imaging (MRI) of the breast appears to be particularly useful in younger women as well as in women with dense breast tissue, in whom mammography is less sensitive. This technique has not yet been formally evaluated in a screening scenario, and thus cannot be recommended routinely to all patients.
- Genetic testing for BRCA1 and 2 mutations is reserved for patients with a high-risk family history, which includes two or more first-degree relatives with breast or ovarian cancer. These mutations have incomplete penetrance, hence referral for genetic counseling for a full discussion of prevention options, including chemo-prevention, is useful.[4]

TABLE 72–1 Current Screening Recommendations for Selected Cancers

CANCER	AMERICAN CANCER SOCIETY	USPSTF GUIDELINES
Breast cancer	*All females*	*All females*
• Monthly SBE	>20 y	Not recommended
• Clinical breast examination	>40 yearly, 20–40 every 3 y	>50 y, yearly
• Mammogram	>40 yearly	0–75 every 1–2 y
Cervical cancer	*All females*	*All females*
Pap cytology	Begin 3 y after intercourse, or at 21 y, repeat yearly	18–65 every 1–3 y
Colon cancer	*All patients*	*All patients*
• FOBT	>50 y, every y	>50 y, every y
• Sigmoidoscopy	>50 every 3–5 y	>50 (intervals not specified)
Prostate cancer	*All males*	
• PSA	>50 every y	No recommendation
• DRE	>40 every y	No recommendation
Skin cancer	Skin examination 20–40 y every 3 y	No recommendation, except for high-risk subgroups

DRE, digital rectal examination; FOBT, fecal occult blood test; Pap, Papanicolaou; PSA, prostate-specific antigen; SBE, self-breast examination; USPSTF, United States Preventive Services Task Force.

CERVICAL CANCER SCREENING

- Although its incidence in the United States has been steadily decreasing, cervical cancer is the second most common cancer worldwide. The Papanicolaou (Pap) cytology test represents one of the triumphs of oncologic screening with an estimated 70% decline in cervical cancer related mortality.[3]
- Interestingly, there have never been any randomized trials done to establish efficacy, but numerous population and cohort studies have confirmed the extraordinary mortality reduction of regular Pap screening.
- Screening appears to be effective when started within 3 years of intercourse, or at age 21 years. Pap screening should be continued yearly, until age 30 when women who have had three or more consecutive normal tests may be tested every 2 to 3 years.
- High-risk individuals, which include those with a history of sexually transmitted disease, multiple sexual partners, or those with a history of an abnormal Pap, should continue yearly testing.
- Women who have had a hysterectomy and cervix removal for a benign illness do not appear to benefit from continued yearly screening. Similarly, women older than the age of 70 years, with a normal Pap in the last 10 years, also may choose to stop screening.
- The etiologic agent associated with virtually all cervical cancers is the human papillomavirus (HPV). The use of reflex HPV DNA testing in patients who demonstrate atypical squamous cells of undetermined significance on Pap cytology appears to enhance the sensitivity of cytological testing in identifying both invasive cervical cancer as well as carcinoma in situ.
- A wide array of assays are available for cytological testing: Liquid based cytology and DNA testing appear to be superior to conventional cytology, but definitive data are lacking, and the choice should be based on local expertise and availability.
- The recent introduction of a quadrivalent HPV vaccine marks a new step in the prevention of cervical cancer. This appears to be effective in preventing up to 80% of HPV infections and subsequent cervical neoplasia and is now recommended for girls aged 13 years and older. However, this vaccination has not yet eliminated the requirement for regular Pap cytological examinations.

COLORECTAL CANCER SCREENING

- Colorectal cancers account for almost 150,000 cases every year, with approximately 58,000 deaths. Although mortality has been decreasing, the incidence has remained stable.
- Screening remains underutilized in colon cancer, with only approximately 30% of the target population (all patients older than age 50 years) undergoing regular screening. Importantly, most colorectal cancers occur within premalignant lesions such as adenomas, which could be detected and removed prior to the development of invasive cancer.
- There are four modalities recommended for colorectal screening. Not all are available in all settings. Colorectal screening is recommended in adults older than the age of 50 years.
  1. *Fecal occult blood testing (FOBT)*: Annual or biannual testing of consecutive stool specimens for the presence of occult blood has been shown to reduce mortality by up to 30%. Earlier trials appeared to show an increase in sensitivity by rehydrating specimens; but specificity drops, leading to unneccesary secondary procedures (endoscopy). All patients with a positive FOBT should undergo an endoscopic examination of the colon and rectum. Adherence to this screening modality occurs in less than 50% of unselected patients.
  2. *Flexible sigmoidoscopy*: This has been studied alone and in combination with FOBT. Most studies have evaluated the 60 cm flexible sigmoidoscopic examination. This allows adequate examination of the distal colon. Adenomas identified in this region should prompt a full colonoscopic examination to exclude additional proximal lesions. The optimal frequency for such examinations is unclear, but most authorities recommend a 5-year interval. Adding annual FOBT to regular sigmoidoscopic examination increases the sensitivity by 5% to 8% to over 76% in patients with an advanced adenoma or invasive cancer.
  3. *Colonoscopy*: The mortality benefits of full colonoscopy have not yet been fully evaluated, but it is estimated that this modality can identify neoplastic lesions in 25% of patients with a normal sigmoidoscopy and single FOBT. This technique is especially useful for high-risk patients with a family history of colon cancer or with ulcerative colitis. Most specialty societies recommend a full colonoscopy once every 10 years starting at age 50 years. The interval should be shortened for those who have polyps and those who have lesions >10 mm, tubular adenomas, or sessile polyps, which are considered advanced lesions.[3]
  4. *Double contrast barium enema*: A single trial that compared double contrast barium enema to colonoscopy found that the barium study only identified half as many polypoid lesions as colonoscopy. Given the decreased sensitivity of double contrast barium studies, most societies recommend the use of endoscopic evaluation.

- High-risk patients include those with a family history of colon cancer, in whom screening should begin at least 10 years prior to the age of the affected family member at diagnosis. Patients with a history of breast and ovarian cancer should be considered at increased risk, given the possibility of hereditary nonpolyposis colon cancer syndrome in these populations. Finally, patients with inflammatory bowel disease, particularly ulcerative colitis, should undergo regular surveillance colonoscopies given the increased incidence of invasive cancer in this population.
- Newer techniques include the evaluation of stool for DNA mutations in exfoliated neoplastic cells. A trial comparing this modality to FOBT found the sensitivity improved from 20% to approximately 50%. This test is still not widely available but these initial results are promising.
- Virtual colonoscopy or computed tomography (CT) colonography requires a similar bowel preparation to a colonoscopy. Following colonic insufflation with air via a rectal tube, abdominal computed tomographic images are obtained, and a three-dimensional reconstruction of the colon is generated. Studies have compared this to conventional colonoscopy with similar results for polyps greater than 6 mm. The reproducibility of this test is still unproven, and no mortality data exist about the benefits of this procedure.

PROSTATE CANCER SCREENING

- Prostate cancer is the most common cancer in males and remains the second most common cause of cancer-related deaths in men, with approximately 230,000 cases and 28,900 deaths yearly.
- Screening for prostate cancer is accomplished through a combination of an annual digital rectal examination (DRE) and an annual PSA test.
- The PSA is a serological test that has a sensitivity of 80% to 85% but a rather low specificity, since levels are often elevated in benign prostatic hyperplasia.[3]
- The DRE has a sensitivity of approximately 60% but also suffers from a lack of specificity. Patients with a positive DRE should undergo both PSA measurement and a transrectal ultrasound.
- There is a high proportion of indolent prostate cancers in males > 60 years of age, and mathematical models have estimated that routine screening may yield a false-positive diagnosis of prostate cancer in up to 50% of males between the ages of 55 and 67 years. Such studies have ignited controversy regarding the role of prostate cancer screening. The USPSTF does not support or refute prostate screening, whereas the ACS and the American Urological Association recommend that

men older than age 50 years be offered screening after a discussion of the potential benefits and risks.[5]
- Data from two large ongoing trials assessing the mortality benefits of prostate screening for patients between the ages of 50 to 75 years are pending. Older studies have not suggested a benefit when screening patients above the age of 75 years, and consensus statements do not recommend screening males with a life expectancy less than 10 years.

SKIN CANCER SCREENING

- Skin cancer has steadily increased over the last few decades, thought to be primarily a result of increased recognition and reporting rather than a true increase in prevalence. There were 800,000 nonmelanoma skin cancers, with approximately 54,000 cases of melanoma, in 2006.[1]
- Interventions, including regular screening examinations, have reduced the incidence of melanomas internationally; but in the United States progress has been less impressive.
- There is no clear consensus about optimal screening for skin cancer. The USPSTF does not recommend screening average risk patients but does recommend yearly skin examinations for patients with a history of premalignant lesions or a family history. The ACS recommends a thorough skin examination by a clinician every 3 years for patients between the ages of 20 and 40 years.[3]
- There have been no trials that have examined the benefits of clinician screening.
- A single study showed some mortality benefit of regular skin self-examination, but this has not been reproduced. Nonetheless, the promotion of regular skin self-examination may prove a useful adjunct to other public health awareness programs.

LUNG CANCER SCREENING

- Lung cancer is the largest cause of cancer mortality accounting for approximately 174,000 new cases and 162,000 deaths.[1]
- Previous efforts at screening using chest radiographs have shown no mortality benefit. In addition, false positives ranged from 4% to 15% leading to unnecessary additional procedures with attendant patient risks.
- Sputum cytology has been studied in conjunction with the chest radiograph. Although this combination may detect lung cancers earlier, there does not appear to be a significant mortality benefit.

- Currently, there are no screening recommendations from any of the clinical guideline development organizations for asymptomatic individuals.
- Helical CT of the chest has received increasing attention since it can detect lesions smaller than 1 cm. Both false-positive results and overdiagnosis remain enormous concerns with helical CT. The invasive nature of a percutaneous biopsy or thoracotomy and the attendant risks preclude the routine use of these procedures except in unusual or compelling settings. A recent large, uncontrolled study evaluating the use of annual CT scanning of middle-aged smokers suggested significant mortality benefits; but the lack of a control group renders this study largely inadequate. The results of the ongoing National Lung Screening Trial, comparing the use of helical CT to chest x-ray, is anxiously awaited to clarify the role of helical CT.[3]

SCREENING: FUTURE DIRECTIONS

- The emergence of new techniques in molecular biology, particularly proteomics, may help identify the expression of unique surface proteins associated with asymptomatic cancers. High throughput laser desorption machines can identify many such proteins, and these assays may ultimately characterize specific patterns associated with different types of cancer. Although this technique is promising, it is still in its infancy and has not been used for routine cancer screening.
- Results from other studies, including a large study evaluating the use of serum cancer antigen 125 measurements and transvaginal ultrasound for the screening of ovarian cancer, may help identify new screening paradigms.
- One of the great challenges of screening has been adherence to current screening recommendations. Overall, it is estimated from patient interviews, that although 70% of women had had a mammogram and Pap smear recently, only 35% to 40% of men and women had an FOBT or colonoscopy. Continued education and patient counseling by physicians and physician extenders have been found to double or triple response rates. Disadvantaged populations, including ethnic minorities and patients without health insurance, may be particularly important targets for education and screening.

REFERENCES

1. American Cancer Society. *Cancer Facts and Figures, 2006.* Atlanta, GA: American Cancer Society; 2006.
2. National Cancer Policy Board and IOM. *Fulfilling the Potential of Cancer Prevention and Early Detection.* Washington, DC: National Research Council, Institute of Medicine; 2003.
3. National Cancer Institute. *PDQ Cancer Screening/Prevention Summary.* Bethesda, MD: National Cancer Institute. http://www.cancer.gov/cancertopics/pdq. Accessed February 2007).
4. US Preventive Services Task Force. *Guide to Clinical Preventive Services.* International Medical Publishing, 1996.
5. Babaian RJ, Mettlin C, Kane R, et al. The relationship of prostate-specific antigen to digital rectal examination and transrectal ultrasonography: findings of the American Cancer Society National Prostate Cancer Detection Project. *Cancer.* 1992;69:1195.

73 CANCER TREATMENT OVERVIEW

Michael C. Perry

INTRODUCTION

The mention of the words "cancer" or "leukemia" is enough to paralyze thoughts in most individuals, and it is best to plan for several visits to discuss the diagnosis and its implications. Having family members or friends in the room also provides another set of ears to recall what was said (and not said). If the clinician is sure of the diagnosis then the patient must be told in clear, unmistakable language of the presence of the malignancy, the plans for further evaluation, and a brief explanation of possible therapies. It is best not to engage in a detailed discussion of therapy until all necessary information has been collected to avoid confusion.

DIAGNOSIS

It is seldom, if ever, appropriate to treat a patient without histologic confirmation of malignancy. This can come in the form of a cytologic diagnosis as from a Papanicolaou (Pap) smear in cervical cancer, of sputum cytology in lung cancer, or examination of ascitic or pleural fluid. Needle biopsies can also confirm a cancer, although larger biopsies, such as excision of an involved lymph node, can provide larger amounts of tissue needed for special stains, cytogenetics, molecular biology studies, and so forth. Careful communication with the surgeon and pathologist in advance of the procedure can be extremely helpful in assuring that adequate tissue, appropriately handled, is available for analysis. If a lymphoma is suspected, for example, flow cytometry will be uniformly requested, as well as cytogenetics in addition to the routine stains. For breast cancer, the tissue should be sent for hormone and HER2-neu receptors. If there is doubt about the exact classification of the tumor (common in sarcomas and lymphomas), then the slides should be sent to a reference pathologist prior to the initiation of therapy. For non-Hodgkin lymphomas repeat biopsy after a recurrence can reveal transformation of the disease to a more aggressive type, which would alter therapy.

STAGING

Staging is used to determine the extent of the disease and to make comparison of treatments at different centers meaningful. Clinical staging is done by the clinician, whereas pathologic staging is performed by the pathologist who has tissue available for analysis. The tests used for clinical staging vary from cancer to cancer. In general, chest x-rays, computed tomography (CT), and radionuclide scans are used for solid tumors, and bone marrow aspiration and biopsy are added for hematologic malignancies. Positron emission tomography (PET) scans are rapidly becoming part of routine staging because of their ability to identify metastases that might have otherwise gone undetected. Hematologic and chemistry function tests are routinely done but do not influence staging. For most tumors, the **TNM** system is used, with differing **T** stages, for example, assigned for increasing size or invasion of the primary tumor. **N** designations indicate the extent of lymph node involvement, and **M** designations indicate the presence or absence of metastases. These are combined into stages, typically four stages, indicated by Roman numbers I through IV for least to most involved. Lymphomas and other hematologic malignancies have separate staging systems, and the reader is referred to the appropriate chapters. Once staging is complete then discussions of treatment and prognosis can proceed.

• Treatment options typically consist of surgery, radiation therapy (RT), or chemotherapy, or a combination of modalities. Historically, surgery was usually attempted first and if the cancer proved to be unresectable, then RT was used for local control, with chemotherapy used only after failure of both local therapies. Currently, the treatment sequence may be reversed with chemotherapy, with or without RT, then surgery. This *neoadjuvant* approach may permit preservation of vital functions such as maintaining the function of the larynx with laryngeal cancer or preserving rectal function with anal cancer. This *organ-sparing* approach is gaining momentum for several tumor types.

SURGERY

Complete removal of the cancer and involved lymph nodes is the goal of most oncologic surgery, but surgery can also provide tissue for a diagnosis and staging, debulk a tumor, bypass an obstruction, or establish venous access.

For some cancers, such as lung or pancreatic primaries, complete resection is virtually the only chance for cure, but all too often this is not possible, and most patients with these cancers will require additional modalities, although, the likelihood of long-term survival is low.

Surgical procedures can range from simple biopsies to complex operations. Importantly, the general medical condition of patients plays a key role in determining whether an extensive surgery is indicated. A young, healthy 55-year-old might be a candidate for a radical prostatectomy, wheres a 90-year-old man with multiple comorbid illnesses would not likely be. In addition to knowledge of coexisting medical conditions, simple questions about the presence or absence of weight loss and a determination of the patient's performance score or a geriatric assessment can assist in the choice of procedure or therapy.

RADIATION THERAPY

Ionizing radiation can be used in cancer treatment for cure or for palliation. It can be used alone or in combination with chemotherapy with the latter sensitizing the cancer cells to radiation, or providing an adjuvant effect. RT can be part of primary therapy, adjuvant therapy, or multimodality therapy. Radiation can be provided through a distant source, such as a linear accelerator (teletherapy), or locally (brachytherapy) through application of a radioactive source. Bone-seeking intravenous radioisotopes, such as strontium or samarium, are often very helpful in relieving pain from bone metastases from breast or prostate cancer, and radioactive iodine is an effective therapy for some forms of thyroid cancer. Several types of cancer, such as early cervical cancer, lymphomas, head and neck cancer, can be cured with radiation therapy alone, whereas others such as lung and esophageal cancer are often candidates for combined chemoradiation therapy. The goal of concurrent chemotherapy/RT is to sterilize the primary tumor with the radio sensitizing properties of chemotherapy added to RT, while the chemotherapy eradicates distant metastases. Unfortunately, both local control and the eradication of distant metastases often remain unachieved goals.

When the goal of RT is palliation for painful bone metastases, bronchial obstruction, or to treat brain metastases, the course of therapy is typically short.

Because both surgery and radiation therapy are local therapies one must be cautious to avoid injuring adjacent normal structures. Normal tissue tolerance, which varies among different organs and tissues, often prevents the use of radiation doses that could otherwise eradicate cancers. Radiation therapy is also limited by tumor hypoxia: large, bulky tumors are frequently relatively radioresistant, whereas well-oxygenated tumors can be more effectively treated at lower doses.

CHEMOTHERAPY

Chemotherapy, or more accurately systemic therapy, includes traditional chemotherapy, hormonal therapy, adminstration of biologic response modifiers, and targeted therapies. Chemotherapy can be used in the neoadjuvant setting, as an adjuvant after surgery or radiation therapy, as part of planned multimodality therapy, for palliation, and less commonly, alone. The list of metastatic cancers cured by chemotherapy alone is short and includes Hodgkin and non-Hodgkin lymphomas, acute leukemias, testicular cancer, and a few rare tumors. The addition of chemotherapy to surgery and radiation therapy as part of planned multimodality therapy can cure several malignancies, mostly in the pediatric setting.

Hormonal therapy is used to treat breast and prostate cancers. Most prostate cancers are androgen sensitive, and androgen depletion through orchiectomy, estrogens, or antiandrogens will, at least temporarily, produce responses in metastatic disease. Approximately one-third of premenopausal women and three-quarters of postmenopausal women with breast cancer will have tumors that bear estrogen and/or progesterone receptors. In premenopausal women, oophorectomy or the antiestrogen tamoxifen can produce responses. In postmenopausal women, tamoxifen, or one of a group of aromatase inhibitors that inhibit the conversion of hormones in fat or muscles into estrogen, will produce an excellent response.

Classical chemotherapy consists of a variety of agents from several chemical classes including, alkylating agents, antimetabolites, topoisomerase inhibitors, antitumor antibiotics, and enzymes. Unfortunately, these drugs are nonspecific and also injure other rapidly reproducing tissues, such as bone marrow, gut, and hair follicles. Expected side effects thus include bone marrow suppression with neutropenia, thrombocytopenia and anemia, mucositis, diarrhea, and hair loss. For many malignancies combinations of chemotherapeutic agents from different classes are used to produce greater cell kill and reduce the likelihood of resistance. Few metastatic cancers are cured by chemotherapy, and chemotherapy is most effective when the tumor burden is lowest, that is, in the adjuvant setting after surgery for early stage breast cancer. Specific chemotherapy programs are listed under individual tumor types elsewhere in the text.

Targeted agents are drugs directed at a specific molecular point or target, such as a protein tyrosine kinase, or the presence of a specific antigen on a tumor cell. Tyrosine kinase inhibitors include imatinib, erlotinib, and gefitinib. Perhaps the best example of the success of tyrosine kinase inhibitor therapy is the dramatic response of chronic myelogenous leukemia to imatinib (Gleevec). Imatinib also has activity against gastrointestinal stromal cell tumors.

Erlotinib, directed against the epidermal growth factor receptor (EGFR), has antitumor effects in patients whose non–small-cell lung cancers have a specific EGFR mutation. The vascular endothelial growth factor receptor (VEGFR) inhibits the formation of new blood vessels that are critical for tumor growth. Anti-VEGFR agents, such as bevacizumab, prevent vascular endothelial growth factor (VEGF) from inducing its signal in endothelial cells, thereby preventing their division. Bevacizumab has antitumor effects in metastatic colorectal cancer, non–small-cell lung cancer, and breast cancer. Thalidomide inhibits angiogenesis through an unknown pathway and is effective against multiple myeloma.

Bortezomib (Velcade), a unique drug, is a reversible inhibitor of the proteasome pathway that normally regulates the intracellular concentration of many proteins. It has been effective in the treatment of refractory multiple myeloma and non-Hodgkin lymphomas.

The development of monoclonal antibodies directed against an antigen found on cancer cells represents an additional treatment modality, often complementary to conventional chemotherapy. Examples include alemtuzumab, cetuximab, rituximab, and trastuzumab. Trastuzumab has recently been shown to add significantly to disease-free survival in HER2-neu–positive patients who receive adjuvant therapy for early stage breast cancer. These monoclonal antibodies can be used alone (naked), or, in some cases, labeled with a radioactive molecule to enhance cell killing. This radioimmunoconjugate approach has been most effective in the treatment of hematologic malignancies.

BIBLIOGRAPHY

Perry, MC. Principles of cancer treatment. In: *Cecil Medicine*. Philadelphia, PA: Elsevier; 2007:Chapter 192, 1193–1201.

74 CENTRAL NERVOUS SYSTEM TUMORS

Nancy F. McKinney

GENERAL

- Central nervous system (CNS) tumors include tumors of the brain parenchyma, the meninges, and the cranial nerves.
- These may be benign or malignant, but because of their location, and the fact there is often little room for growth, all CNS tumors are potentially life threatening.

- CNS tumors may be primary or metastatic from other sites. Metastatic brain tumors (eg, from cancers of the breast or lung) outnumber primary CNS tumors tenfold.
- The annual incidence of primary CNS tumors is about 14 cases per 100,000 people, and this number is increasing. These tumors comprise a heterogeneous group of malignancies.
- Glial tumors account for the majority of primary CNS neoplasms (approximately 50%–60%), with meningiomas accounting for about 25%, schwannomas for about 10%, and other CNS tumors accounting for the remainder.

ETIOLOGY AND EPIDEMIOLOGY

- The etiology of primary CNS tumors is poorly understood. Most cases are sporadic. There are some known environmental factors such as radiation exposure, prior cranial irradiation, exposure to petrochemicals, and electromagnetic field exposure. Despite media coverage, there is no evidence linking cellular phone use, diet soda consumption, or smoking with primary brain tumors. There is an increased incidence of primary CNS lymphoma caused by human immunodeficiency virus (HIV) infection.
- A very small proportion of primary CNS tumors are inherited. These tend to arise in childhood and are part of the following familial brain tumor syndromes:
  ◦ Turcot syndrome (DNA mismatch repair genes).
  ◦ Li-Fraumeni syndrome (germ line mutations of p53).
  ◦ Tuberous sclerosis (the classic CNS tumor is characterized by a subependymal giant cell astrocytoma in 5% to 10% of patients with tuberous sclerosis).
  ◦ Neurofibromatosis type 1 (increases the likelihood of optic pathway glioma and brainstem glioma).
- The incidence of primary CNS neoplasms increases with age and peaks at approximately 75 to 85 years of age. The peak incidence of gliomas is approximately 60 to 65 years of age. Gliomas have a 2:1 male predominance; while meningiomas have a 2:1 female predominance.
- The incidence of primary CNS lymphoma has increased dramatically since the 1970s. This is partly a result of the emergence of HIV/AIDS. However, the incidence has also increased in non–HIV-infected individuals.

SIGNS AND SYMPTOMS

- The symptoms of CNS tumors may be nonspecific such as headache, seizures, nausea and vomiting, loss of consciousness, cognitive dysfunction, memory problems, and mood or personality change, or they may reflect neurologic dysfunction specific to the area of the tumor, such as weakness, spasticity, aphasia, and/or visual-spatial dysfunction. High-grade tumors typically present with symptoms of increased intracranial pressure, such as headache or focal neurological signs. Low-grade or benign tumors often present with seizures or are incidentally found on imaging studies.

EVALUATION

- Basic laboratory testing is generally normal in patients with primary CNS neoplasms. However, if a brain lesion is identified, it is important to search for a primary systemic cancer, as this is far more common than a primary CNS tumor.
- Lumbar puncture may induce brain herniation in patients with mass lesions and increased intracranial pressure, and therefore should only be performed in patients with suspected meningitis or leptomeningeal involvement of tumor.
- If a brain lesion is suspected, computed tomography (CT) scanning is an excellent and convenient imaging study to rule out hemorrhage. In addition, CT scanning can identify mass effects with contrast enhancement. Nonetheless, magnetic resonance imaging (MRI) is the imaging study of choice for brain tumors, as it has the highest sensitivity and specificity. MR spectroscopy may differentiate brain tumors from other types of intracranial lesions and can distinguish between infiltrative malignancies (glioma and lymphoma) and circumscribed tumors (metastasis, meningioma, and germinoma).
- Once a brain lesion is identified, the workup should include CT scanning of the chest and abdomen to evaluate for a primary malignancy. The remainder of the workup should include a focused evaluation to exclude other malignancies including a breast examination for women, colonoscopy for patients with bowel symptoms, rectal examination, and bone scan for patients with bony pain.
- If the brain is found to be the only site of disease, the patient should be referred to a neurosurgeon for resection or biopsy of the affected site.

SYMPTOMATIC TREATMENT OF CNS NEOPLASMS

- Glucocorticoids such as dexamethasone (10 mg bolus followed by 4 mg IV or PO every 6 h) are important in decreasing the edema in the brain surrounding the tumor and improving neurologic function. Steroids should be initiated when there is a high index of suspicion of CNS tumor causing mass effect.
- Anticonvulsants such as phenytoin or valproic acid, or newer agents such as levetiracetam, are indicated if the patient presents with seizure activity. There is some debate as to whether anticonvulsants should be

administered prophylactically if the patient has a tumor in an area with great potential for producing seizures (eg, cerebral cortex). Most experts do not recommend the prophylactic use of anticonvulsants, because of the risk of adverse effects.

- Patients should also be aggressively treated for nausea, headache, depression, and anxiety. As part of a comprehensive management strategy, patients should also receive speech, physical, and occupational therapy to promote an independent lifestyle.

GLIOMAS

- Gliomas account for over 60% of primary CNS malignancies. They are derived from glial cells and include astrocytomas, oligodendrogliomas, and ependymomas.
- Glial tumors are classified based on their histopathologic features. Importantly, in 2000, the World Health Organization revised their classification of gliomas based on histologic grade. The factors that are used to determine grade include degree of cellular atypia, mitotic activity, cellularity, vascular proliferation, and degree of necrosis. Generally speaking, the higher the grade, the more aggressive the tumor, and the poorer the prognosis.
- Glial tumors are histologically heterogenous with aberrant proliferation and varying degrees of apoptosis. The tumor cells quickly develop resistance to therapy. They tend to infiltrate the surrounding tissues, and they are highly vascular with aggressive and disorganized angiogenesis. As a general rule, they do not metastasize.
  - Grade I Histologies
    - Pilocytic astrocytoma
    - Giant cell astrocytoma
    - Ganglioglioma
    - Myxopapillary ependymoma
    - Dysembryoplastic neuroepithelial tumor
  - Grade II Histologies
    - Well-differentiated low-grade astrocytoma (diffuse, infiltrative, fibrillary)
    - Oligodendroglioma
    - Ependymoma
    - Mixed oligodendroglioma/astrocytoma
  - Grade III Histologies
    - Anaplastic astrocytoma
    - Anaplastic oligodendroglioma
    - Anaplastic ependymoma
    - Mixed anaplastic oligodendroglioma/anaplastic astrocytoma
  - Grade IV
    - Glioblastoma multiforme (GBM)

MOLECULAR GENETICS

Activation of oncogenes, inactivation of tumor suppressor genes, and deregulating DNA repair genes have all been characterized in gliomas. Different genetic abnormalities are associated with specific types of gliomas, different grades of tumors, and different sensitivities to therapies.

Genetic profiling determines prognosis more accurately than by histologic subtype or grade. This is an area of extensive investigation.

Some examples of key genetic alterations that appear to be important in the development of gliomas are described below:

Epidermal growth factor receptor (EGFR) gene amplification: this may arise de novo or develop in a preexisting lower grade glioma. It is seen in about 30% of primary GBM, and 8% of secondary GBM.

Disruption of p53: the p53 tumor suppressor protein is involved in cell cycle arrest, cell repair or involution after DNA damage, and apoptosis. Inactivation of p53 is common in gliomas, either due to a direct mutation or loss, *p14*ARF mutation, or human double-minute 2 (HDM2) amplification.

CDKN2A/p16 deletion: this factor is an upstream mediator of pRB function. The result of deletion of CDKN2A/p16 is loss of cell cycle control and uncontrolled proliferation.

Inactivation of PTEN/MMAC1 tumor suppressor gene on chromosome 10: this disturbance is associated with malignant progression to glioblastoma, and is seen in 30% to 50% of GBM.

Platelet-derived growth factor receptor (PDGFR): This gene product is amplified or overexpressed in many malignant gliomas.

Loss of chromosome 19q: This is unique to glial tumors and is not a feature of other human cancers. This is the only genetic alteration shared by all three histologic subtypes of malignant glioma. It is of unclear significance in astrocytomas. In oligodendrogliomas, the combined loss of chromosome 1p and 19q is associated with improved prognosis and may predict increased chemosensitivity as well as longer recurrence free survival.

Loss of the distal region of chromosome 10q: This is the most common genetic abnormality in newly diagnosed GBM. It occurs equally in primary and secondary GBM. It is the only genetic abnormality that has been found to confer a negative prognosis independent of clinical factors.

PROGNOSIS AND SURVIVAL

Despite the fact that primary CNS tumors rarely metastasize, they are still very difficult to treat secondary to their location and the presence of the blood brain barrier.

The prognosis for patients with high-grade gliomas is dismal: a 2004 population based study found an overall survival of glioblastoma to be 42.4% at 6 months, 17.7% at 1 year, and 3.3% at 2 years.

Prognostic factors include pathologic grade (lower is better), the patient's age (younger is better), performance status (higher is better), the size of tumor (smaller is better), the extent of surgery (complete resection is better), and as noted above molecular genetics; with loss of chromosome 10q being a negative prognostic factor, and combined loss of chromosome 1p and 19q associated with improved survival in oligodendrogliomas.

In general, the median survival for low-grade gliomas (grade II) is between 5 and 10 years, for anaplastic gliomas (grade III) is between 2 and 3 years, and for GBM (grade IV) is 12 to 15 months. However, with the addition of temozolomide in combination with radiation therapy, these figures appear to be improving.

ASTROCYTOMAS

- Astrocytomas are the most common form of primary CNS neoplasms, and include low-grade astrocytomas, anaplastic astrocytomas (AA), and GBM

LOW-GRADE ASTROCYTOMAS
- There are rare forms of grade I astrocytoma, including juvenile pilocytic astrocytoma, subependymal giant cell astrocytoma, ganglioglioma, and pleomorphic xanthoastrocytoma that are common in children and have a very good prognosis after definitive surgical excision alone.
- Low-grade diffuse astrocytomas tend to occur in young adults, and the mean age of presentation is 30 to 35 years. They are found mainly in the cerebral hemispheres. Even though these tumors are slow growing and of low malignant potential, they are diffusely infiltrating, difficult to cure with surgery and radiation, and are still generally lethal. They have a median 5-year survival of 36% to 55%, and a 10-year survival of 26% to 43%. Low-grade astrocytomas may also progress to higher grade gliomas with time.
- Therapy for diffuse low-grade astrocytoma is initially surgery, with the maximal resection possible without causing significant neurologic morbidity. Gross total resection (GTR) is not possible in the majority of the patients, given the diffuse histologic nature of the tumors.
- Following surgery, radiation therapy is standard of care, as it has been shown to provide a survival advantage and improve quality of life in patients with low-grade diffuse astrocytomas.

- There is currently no clear role for chemotherapy in low-grade astrocytomas; however, temozolomide has been shown in several phase II trials to be active in these tumors, and is an area of clinical study.

HIGH-GRADE ASTROCYTOMAS
- High-grade astrocytomas include anaplastic astrocytomas and glioblastoma multiforme; these tumors are quite aggressive and are generally fatal within years despite aggressive multimodality therapy.
- Anaplastic astrocytomas (AA) are characterized histologically by diffusely infiltrating cells and increased nuclear atypia and mitotic activity. GBM exhibits high mitotic activity and either endothelial proliferation or necrosis.
- The peak incidence of AA is in the fourth decade; the peak incidence of GBM is in the fifth decade.
- The optimal therapy of high-grade astrocytoma includes surgery with the goal of maximal resection (>98% of the tumor). This has the benefit of providing adequate tissue for diagnosis, improving neurological function, as well improving progression-free and overall survival.
- Following surgery, limited-field radiation therapy (RT) of 60 Gy in 30 fractions is standard of care as this has shown a palliative survival benefit. Higher RT doses do not appear to improve outcome. Radiosensitizers, stereotactic radiosurgery, and interstitial brachytherapy have been studied, but have yet to show a clear clinical benefit.
- Until 1999, there was only a very small benefit to systemic chemotherapy above surgery and radiation in high-grade astrocytomas (approximately 8%–10% absolute benefit). There are several obstacles to chemotherapy delivery in high-grade gliomas, including the blood-brain barrier (BBB) (the BBB efflux proteins transport chemotherapy drugs out of the CNS), and dysfunctional tumor vasculature that reduces drug delivery to the tumor. In addition, the histologic and genetic heterogeneity characteristic of high-grade gliomas acts as a defense mechanism, because the tumor soon develops resistance to both conventional and targeted chemotherapeutic agents.
- Chemotherapy regimens that have been traditionally used include PCV (procarbazine, lomustine, and vincristine) and BCNU (carmustine). These appear to have greater activity in AA than in GBM.
- In 1999, temozolomide, an oral alkylating agent was shown to be active in patients with recurrent AA and GBM, with few adverse effects, leading to improvement in progression-free survival. This has since been studied in GBM in the adjuvant setting in combination with radiation therapy, followed by 6 months of maintenance temozolomide. Overall survival at 24 months

was 26.5% in the RT plus temozolomide group compared to 10.5% with radiation alone. Progression-free survival at one year was 26.9% in the combination arm compared to 9.1% in the RT alone arm, and at two years was 10.7% compared to 1.5%. These figures were statistically significant and led to the current recommendations of radiotherapy plus temozolomide followed by maintenance temozolomide as the new standard of care following maximal surgical resection in GBM. Concurrent RT with temozolomide is being studied in AA; however, as the drug is highly active in AA, many clinicians are using the same regimen as with GBM.

- Patients with recurrent high-grade gliomas tend to do very poorly. Symptom management with steroids, antiseizure medications, antiemetics, and social support is very important. If the patient chooses active treatment, neurosurgery and excision of the majority of the recurrent tumor may palliate symptoms. Gliadel wafers (CCNU impregnated wafers) may be placed in the tumor bed at the time of surgery. Radiation therapy may be an option with a lower dose; the major complication being radiation necrosis. Stereotactic radiotherapy, photodynamic therapy, and GliaSite balloon are all modalities that are being studied in the recurrent setting. If the patient has not been treated with temozolomide, this should be administered for recurrent disease. However, following failure of temozolomide, there is no consensus on second or third line chemotherapeutic agents that may be used, and none have very high efficacy. Carmustine (BCNU), lomustine (CCNU), carboplatin, etoposide, irinotecan, and oxaliplatin have all been used with modest success.

OLIGODENDROGLIOMAS

- Oligodendrogliomas are rare, comprising about 15% of gliomas and about 5% of primary CNS neoplasms. The peak incidence is 55 to 64 years of age, and this incidence is increasing. In general, these tumors have a better prognosis than astrocytomas of equal grade, and overall they have a median survival of 10 years.
- These tumors are diffuse and histologically are often characterized by an admixture of astrocytic and oligodendroglial cells. They contain calcified areas in about one-third of cases. On light microscopy, the cells are round with perinuclear halos (*fried eggs*) with an acutely branching (chicken wire) capillary pattern. Anaplastic oligodendrogliomas have increased cellularity, high mitotic rate, and pleomorphism (grade III). If they exhibit endothelial proliferation or necrosis, they are considered GBM.
- The molecular genetics of oligodendrogliomas have prognostic implications. The most frequent molecular alteration is allelic loss of 1p and 19q, with loss of 1p in 83%, and loss of 19q in 66%, and combined loss in 66%. The combined loss of chromosome 1p and 19q has been associated with improved prognosis and improved responsiveness to chemotherapy. Methylguanine-methyltransferase (MGMT) is down regulated in the majority of oligodendrogliomas, especially those with loss of 1p and 19q.

- Treatment for oligodendrogliomas involves GTR, if possible. However, subtotal resection is usually done, regardless. Radiation therapy is performed in the adjuvant setting following resection with up to a cumulative dose of 50 to 54 Gy for low-grade tumors, and 60 to 65 Gy for anaplastic tumors.
- Oligodendrogliomas are more chemosensitive than astrocytomas. Traditional first-line adjuvant therapy is PCV (procarbazine, lomustine [CCNU], and vincristine). However, recent trials examining temozolomide monotherapy suggest that this may be equally effective, with less toxicity.
- For recurrent oligodendrogliomas, temozolomide has been shown to be effective in patients who progress while on PCV. Interestingly, PCV has been shown to be effective in patients who progress on temozolomide. Carboplatin also appears to have modest activity in the recurrent setting.

EPENDYMOMA

- Ependymomas are an uncommon group of glial tumors that account for <10% of brain tumors, and 25% of spinal cord tumors. About 75% are low grade. There is equal male-to-female ratio, and this tends to be a disease of childhood, with a median age of diagnosis of 5 years of age. In children they tend to behave as aggressive intraventricular tumors; in adults they tend to be benign spinal cord tumors.
- The overall survival at 10 years is 45% to 55%. Unlike other gliomas, ependymomas may metastasize through the CSF, so-called drop metastasis.
- They are believed to arise from ependymal cells lining the ventricular system. Histologically they appear low grade; well demarcated; with areas of calcification, hemorrhage, and cysts. The classic finding is of pseudorosettes of spindle shaped cells arranged around blood vessels. If they exhibit high cellularity or mitoses, they are designated anaplastic ependymoma (grade III).
- The standard treatment for ependymomas includes resection followed by adjuvant radiotherapy. There is no proven benefit for chemotherapy in adults. As with other gliomas, GTR is associated with a better outcome than partial resection.
- GTR alone may be sufficient for low-grade ependymomas (grade I).

- Adjuvant radiation therapy is standard of care for grade II and III ependymomas. Craniospinal irradiation is recommended with CSF seeding or for patients with anaplastic ependymoma, because of the high risk of drop metastasis.
- Patients with recurrent ependymomas do poorly and generally die within a few months. Palliation may include aggressive surgical resection, re-irradiation, or stereotactic radiosurgery. Chemotherapy may have a role in palliation but remains investigational.

MENINGIOMA

- Meningiomas are common primary CNS neoplasms that arise from the dural cover of the brain, 90% are benign. They account for 13% to 26% of primary CNS neoplasms. They usually are attached to the dura, may invade the skull, but only occasionally invade the brain. There is a 2:1 female-to-male predominance, and the average age at diagnosis is between 40 and 70 years of age.
- Most meningiomas are sporadic, however, there are causative events that have been identified, including prior cranial irradiation, a personal history of breast cancer, and neurofibromatosis type 2.
- Meningiomas tend to be slow growing and form well-circumscribed masses that can be easily *shelled out* by the surgeon. They do not tend to infiltrate into surrounding brain tissue. Histologically, they are divided into histologic grades I, II, and III based on their nuclear atypia, mitotic rate, cellularity, vascular proliferation, and degree of necrosis. Approximately 90% of meningiomas are grade I and follow a benign clinical course. Grade II meningiomas have a higher rate of recurrence (30%–40%) than grade I tumors (7%–20%). Grade III meningiomas, or anaplastic meningiomas have malignant cytology and/or a high mitotic rate. These often invade the brain, they commonly recur, and they may metastasize.
- There are several genetic mutations that have been characterized in the meningiomas
  - Monosomy 22, with mutation of the NF2 gene on 22q12 is an early event in the development of the tumor.
  - Losses of 1p, 9p, 3p, 6q, 14q, 10q are commonly seen as the disease progresses, and are associated with increasing histological grade.
  - Overexpression of p53 protein is common and may predict the potential for malignant behavior.
- Meningiomas are usually asymptomatic, and are incidentally found on imaging studies. It is estimated that 2% to 3% of the population have asymptomatic meningiomas. In these cases, it is recommended to follow the patient with repeat CT or MRI of the brain.

- When symptomatic, meningiomas most commonly present with seizures, but may present with symptoms of increased intracranial pressure, nausea, headache, or focal neurological signs.
- If a meningioma presents with neurological symptoms, it should be surgically resected if possible. Complete resection should be attempted, as meningiomas commonly recur if they are not entirely removed, including the dura and overlying bone. However, the location in relationship with vital neural or vascular structures often precludes this, and partial excision in combination with adjuvant radiotherapy increases the time to recurrence.
- Stereotactic radiosurgery uses multiple beams of radiation aimed from many directions to converge at the tumor while minimizing radiation dose to the rest of the brain. This is an option for patients with small tumors that are in locations difficult to access by traditional neurosurgical techniques or in patients who are not surgical candidates.
- Meningiomas tend to be chemoresistant, and the use of chemotherapy in this disease remains investigational.

PRIMARY CNS LYMPHOMA

- Primary CNS lymphomas (PCNSL) are non-Hodgkin lymphomas that present in the CNS. These are rare and may occur in the brain, meninges, spinal cord, or eyes. The incidence is increasing, and this is believed to be secondary to its association with immunosuppression and human immunodeficiency virus (HIV). Patients with HIV have a 3600-fold increased risk of developing PCNSL over immunocompetent people. Immunosuppression from organ transplantation, autoimmune disease, and congenital immunodeficiencies also increases the incidence of PCNSL.
- The prognosis of PCNSL is poor compared to histologically similar extranodal lymphoma occurring outside the CNS. It is common to have a dramatic clinical and radiographic response to therapy; however, recurrent disease is common, and much more difficult to treat.
- The most common histology of PCNSL is diffuse large B-cell lymphoma, comprising nearly 90% of cases.
- Clinically, patients often present with signs of increased intracranial pressure, headaches, and neurological signs. Multifocal disease and leptomeningeal seeding is common.
- Diagnosis should include contrast-enhanced MRI, and evaluation of cerebrospinal fluid (CSF) with lumbar puncture, cell count, cytology, flow cytometry, and immunoglobulin heavy-chain rearrangement studies. Classic findings on the CSF are elevated white count, and high protein concentration, as well as low glucose level compared to serum level. CSF cytology may be

abnormal; however, in most cases it is normal, and serial samples may be necessary if leptomeningeal disease is suspected. Stereotactic biopsy of the brain lesion is usually required for the diagnosis. Ophthalmologic evaluation should be part of the evaluation, as well as a complete history and physical examination and chest films and CT scans to rule out metastatic lymphoma.

- Lymphomas tend to be steroid sensitive; therefore glucocorticoids should be withheld if possible until a tissue diagnosis has been obtained.

- Unlike other CNS neoplasms, the only therapeutic role of surgery is for diagnosis, and chemotherapy and radiation therapy are the mainstays of treatment. Concurrent chemotherapy with high dose systemic methotrexate (doses of 2–8 g/m^2) and whole-brain radiation therapy (WBRT) is associated with complete responses in over 50% of patients, and 2-year survival of 43% to 73%, with tolerable toxicity. These responses have been improved with the use of a methotrexate-based combination chemotherapy regimens in addition to WBRT.

- One of the complications of combined chemotherapy and WBRT is late neurotoxicity, and this risk increases significantly with increasing age and poor performance status.

- Chemotherapy alone is an option for patients with PCNSL who are older than 60 years of age and those with poor performance status. High-dose methotrexate either as a single agent, or in combination with other agents produces impressive complete radiographic response rates of 30% to 90%. While cure is possible, the vast majority of patients will relapse.

- Radiation therapy alone has good overall response rates (80%–90%), but these responses are not durable, and the associated late toxicities are high, making this a poor choice for a single modality of treatment.

- Salvage therapy for PCNSL is an area of considerable study. Most patients will relapse or progress following initial therapy. Accepted second-line therapies include repeat high-dose methotrexate, temozolomide, temozolomide plus rituximab, and high-dose chemotherapy with autologous stem cell transplant. Repeat whole brain irradiation may be performed; however, the neurotoxicity associated with this is often unacceptable. These patients tend to do dismally following relapse.

BRAIN METASTASIS

- Metastatic disease to the CNS from systemic malignancy is the most common cause of CNS neoplasm— nearly tenfold more common than primary CNS neoplasms. The majority of brain metastases occur by hematogenous spread. The most common origin of brain metastasis is the lung, followed by breast, renal, melanoma, and colon cancers; however, nearly any type of cancer can metastasize to the brain, including lymphomas.

- Once a malignancy metastasizes to the brain it is generally incurable, and, on average, the patient has only months to live. There is a role for surgery in select cases of metastatic disease, including certain cancers such as melanoma or renal cell cancer where the brain is the only site of metastatic disease, or where the extracranial disease is stable. Otherwise, if there are multiple brain lesions, surgery is reserved for large or symptomatic lesions.

- Radiation therapy is the primary treatment modality for brain metastasis, and has been shown to increase survival and to palliate symptoms. In patients who have already undergone whole brain irradiation, stereotactic radiosurgery is an option for small lesions if they are few in number (generally fewer than 4).

- Chemotherapy may be used to treat CNS metastasis in certain cases, especially in tumors such as small cell lung cancer and germ cell tumor, which are highly chemosensitive. This has the advantage of treating the systemic disease as well.

BIBLIOGRAPHY

Athanassiou H, Synodinou M, Maragoudakis E, et al. Randomized phase II study of temozolomide and radiotherapy compared with radiotherapy alone in newly diagnosed glioblastoma multiforme. *J Clin Oncol.* 2005; 23(10): 2372–2377.

Batchelor T, Loeffler J. Primary CNS lymphoma. *J Clin Oncol.* 2006;24:1281–1288.

Baehring JM. An update on oligodendroglial neoplasms. *Curr Opin Neurol.* 2005;18:639–644.

Butowski NA, Sneed PK, Chang SM, et al. Diagnosis and treatment of recurrent high-grade astrocytoma. *J Clin Oncol,* 2006; 24(8):1273–1280.

Gonzalez J, Gilbert M. Treatment of astrocytomas. *Curr Opin Neurol.* 2005;18:632–638.

Hegi ME, Diserens AC, Gorlia T, et al. MGMT gene silencing and benefit from temozolomide in glioblastoma. *N Engl J Med.* 352:2005;10:997–1003.

Henson JW. Treatment of glioblastoma multiforme. *Arch Neurol.* 2006;63:337–341.

Lang F, Gilbert M. Diffusely infiltrative low grade gliomas in adults. *J Clin Oncol.* 2006;24(8):1236–1245.

Ohgaki H, Dessen P, Jourde B, et al. Genetic pathways to glioblastoma: A population-based study, *Cancer Res.* 2004;64: 6892–6899.

Pan E, Prados M. Primary neoplasms of the central nervous system, In: Kufe DW, Pollock RE, Bast RC, et al. eds. *Cancer Medicine 6*. Hamilton, ON: BC Decker; 2003:1195–1226.

Reardon DA, Rich JN, Friedman HS, et al. Recent advancement in the treatment of malignant astrocytoma. *J Clin Oncol.* 2006;24(8):1253–1265.

Soffietti R, Nobile M, Ruda R, et al. Second-line treatment with carboplatin for recurrent or progressive oligodendroglial tumors after PCV chemotherapy: A phase II study. *Cancer.* 2004;100:807–813.

Stupp R., Dietrion PY, Kraljevic O, et al. Promising survival for patients with newly diagnosed glioblastoma multiforme treated with concomitant radiation plus temozolomide followed by adjuvant temozolomide. *J Clin Oncol.* 2002;20(5):1375–1382.

Stupp R, Mason WP, van den Bent MJ, et al. Radiotherapy plus concomitant and adjuvant temozolomide for glioblastoma. *N Engl J Med.* 2005;352(10):987–996.

Whittle IR, Smith C, Navoo P, et al. Meningiomas. *Lancet.* 2004;363:1535–1543.

75 HEAD AND NECK TUMORS

Huda Salman

INTRODUCTION

- Cancer of the head and neck refers to a collection of cancers, predominantly squamous cell carcinoma (SCC), arising from a variety of regions. The head and neck region consists of five anatomically distinct regions:
  1. The oral cavity, which includes the lips, buccal mucosa, anterior tongue, floor of the mouth, hard palate, upper gingiva, lower gingiva, and retromolar trigone.
  2. The pharynx, which is divided into the oropharynx, nasopharynx, and hypopharynx. The oropharynx includes the tonsillar area, tongue base, soft palate, and posterior pharyngeal wall. The hypopharynx includes the pyriform sinuses, posterior surface of the larynx (postcricoid area) and inferoposterior, inferolateral pharyngeal walls.
  3. The larynx, which is divided into three anatomic regions: (1) supraglottic larynx, (2) glottic larynx (true vocal cords and the mucosa of the anterior and posterior commissures), and (3) the subglottic larynx (extends to the inferior border of the cricoid cartilage).
  4. The nasal cavity and the paranasal sinuses, which include the maxillary, ethmoid, sphenoid, and frontal sinuses.
  5. The major salivary glands which include the paired parotids, submandibular and sublingual glands, and the minor salivary glands.

PATHOLOGY

SQUAMOUS CELL CARCINOMA

- More than 90% of all head and neck cancers are SCCs.

HISTOLOGIC GRADE

- There are three histologic grades based on the extent of keratinization: A well-differentiated tumor is characterized by >75% keratinization; a moderately differentiated tumor, by 25% to 50%; and a poorly differentiated tumor, by <25%.
- In general, the more poorly differentiated a lesion, the higher the incidence of regional metastases and the poorer the prognosis. Histologic grade has been an inconsistent predictor of clinical behavior, however. Features that predict aggressive behavior include perineural spread, lymphatic invasion, and tumor spread beyond the lymph node capsule.

OTHER TUMOR TYPES

- Other less common head and neck cancers include mucoepidermoid carcinoma, adenoid cystic carcinoma, and adenocarcinoma, all of which may arise in the salivary glands. Head and neck cancers with neuroendocrine features include small-cell undifferentiated cancer and esthesioneuroblastoma (olfactory neuroblastoma). Both Hodgkin disease and non-Hodgkin lymphoma may also be diagnosed as head and neck tumors, often involving the lymph nodes of the neck or Waldeyer ring.

EPIDEMIOLOGY AND MOLECULAR EPIDEMIOLOGY

- Head and neck cancer is a major global health issue, with a half million new cases diagnosed per year.
- There is a concern that the incidence is increasing, particularly in young adults and in women. The male/female ratio is less than 2:1, and is closing steadily. This shift in gender distribution appears to depend on adult smoking prevalence, where the proportion of men who smoke has decreased and the proportion of young females who smoke has increased. More than 20% of patients diagnosed with head and neck cancer develop a second or third primary tumor, most often within the oral cavity, caused by susceptibility of the mucosa to carcinomatous change.
- Tobacco smoking and alcohol consumption are the two most strongly implicated risk factors for the development of head and neck cancer.

- Certain viruses and chronic irritation appear to be involved as well, but the association is not as clear as with smoking and alcohol consumption.
- Attempts have been made to link variations in head and neck cancer prevalence to the ethnic composition of the population. Such variations in occurrence have been demonstrated to exist for certain tumor types, such as undifferentiated nasopharyngeal carcinoma and lymphoepithelioma-like tumors.
- Evidence of this type of relationship in SCC of the head and neck has been scarce, however.
- Therefore, regional variations in the development of head and neck cancer may be strongly related to habitual and cultural risk factors, which are prevalent in these areas. These factors include chewing tobacco, chewing areca nut either alone or with the addition of tobacco, chewing Khat leaves, smoking marijuana, and drinking Maté.
- Neoplasms arise clonally from transformed cells that have undergone specific genetic alterations in protooncogenes or tumor-suppressor genes. Tabulation of the critical genetic changes in each step of the progression of head and neck cancer from preneoplastic lesions to invasive cancer has allowed the delineation of a model of molecular progression.
- Loss of chromosomal region 9p21 is the most common of all genetic changes and occurs early in the progression of these tumors. The main effect of this loss is the inactivation of the *p16* gene, an inhibitor of cyclin-dependent kinase that is important in regulating the cell cycle.
- Approximately half of all head and neck cancers contain a mutation of the *p53* gene located at 17p. The loss of *p53* function caused by various mutations results in a progression from preinvasive to invasive lesions and increases the likelihood of further genetic progression.
- Amplification of the oncogene cyclin D1, which constitutively activates cell-cycle progression, is seen in approximately one-third of all tumors and is usually associated with invasive disease.
- Tumor-suppressor genes have not been isolated or characterized for most of the chromosomal regions that are commonly lost in these tumors.

CLINICAL PRESENTATION

- Early signs and symptoms are often vague but may point to a site of origin in the head and neck.
  - Paranasal sinus cancers and cancers of the nasal cavity may present with a nonhealing ulcer, epistaxis, or nasal obstruction.
  - Nasopharyngeal cancer presents with a mass in the neck in up to 90% of patients. Serous otitis media may occur because of eustachian tube obstruction.

Headache and cranial nerve abnormalities may be present at diagnosis.
  - Cancer of the oral cavity is associated with ulcers or masses that do not heal, dental changes or poorly fitting dentures, and in some cases referred otalgia. Tongue and lip cancers present as exophytic or ulcerative lesions often associated with pain. Patients with primary tongue lesions often have cervical nodal disease, whereas the incidence is substantially lower in patients with hard palate and lip cancers.
  - Cancer of the glottis is often manifested by persistent hoarseness. Later symptoms may include dysphagia, referred otalgia, chronic cough, hemoptysis, and stridor.
  - Cancers of the oropharynx and supraglottic larynx usually do not present with specific early warning signs and are often not clinically apparent until the development of cervical adenopathy, pain (which may be referred to the ear), dysphagia, or a fixed tongue.

DIAGNOSIS

HISTORY

- Risk factors as previously outlined, including a history of tobacco and alcohol use and environmental exposures, should be reviewed. Any adult patient with symptoms referable to the upper aerodigestive tract that have lasted longer than 2 weeks or with an asymptomatic neck mass should undergo a thorough examination with a high index of suspicion for carcinoma.

PHYSICAL EXAMINATION

- The physical examination is the best means for detecting lesions of the upper aerodigestive tract. Frequently, the initial assessment also will indicate the severity and chronicity of the disease. Because of the frequent occurrence of multiple primary tumors in patients with a head and neck tumor, careful evaluation of the entire upper aerodigestive tract is necessary at the time of diagnosis. The examination should always follow a systematic approach.

SKIN AND SCALP

- A search should be made for ulcers, nodules, and pigmented or other suspicious lesions. This part of the evaluation is frequently overlooked.

CRANIAL NERVES

- A cranial nerve evaluation is essential for any patient with a head and neck tumor or neck mass (which may be a manifestation of occult cancer). This evaluation should include assessing eye motion (cranial nerves [CNs] III, IV, and VI); testing sensation of the face (CN V); examining the muscles of facial expression by having the patient grin, grimace, raise eyebrows, close eyes tightly, show teeth, and puff out the cheeks (CN VII); testing of hearing (CN VIII); assessing gag reflex (CN IX); evaluating vocal cord mobility (CN X); and having the patient fully abduct the shoulder (CN XI) and protrude the tongue (CN XII). Even the slightest abnormality may be helpful in identifying a primary tumor.

EYES/EARS/NOSE

- The eyes, ears, and nose should be evaluated for any sign of mass effect, abnormal drainage/discharge, bleeding, or effusion.

ORAL CAVITY

- Halitosis may be the first indication of a lesion in the upper aerodigestive tract. The teeth, gingivae, and entire mucosal surface should be inspected.
- The lymphoid tissue of the tonsillar pillars should be inspected and any asymmetry noted. Tongue mobility also should be evaluated.
- The floor of the mouth, tongue, and cheeks should be palpated using a bimanual technique (one gloved finger inside the mouth and the second hand under the mandible). Palpation should be the last step of the examination because of stimulation of the gag reflex. Worrisome lesions should be biopsied.

NECK

- Examination of the neck is invaluable in identifying a mass. Palpation is the cornerstone of the examination. It is performed by grasping the tissue and feeling the nodes between the thumb and index and long fingers. The relationship of a mass to major structures, such as the salivary gland, thyroid, and carotid sheath, should be considered. Important qualities of a mass include location, character, tenderness, size, mobility, and associated thrill or bruit. The thyroid should be palpated.

INDIRECT LARYNGOSCOPY

- The nasopharynx, hypopharynx, and larynx should all be examined with care. The vocal cords should be visualized and their mobility evaluated. Mirror examination provides an overall impression of mobility and asymmetry, which may point to a hidden tumor.

DIRECT LARYNGOSCOPY

- Nasopharyngoscopes permit a thorough inspection of the upper aerodigestive tract in the office setting. Attention should be focused individually on the piriform sinuses, tongue base, pharyngeal walls, epiglottis, arytenoids, and true and false vocal cords. Also, any pooling of secretions should be noted.

ENDOSCOPY

- Approximately 5% of patients with head and neck cancer have a synchronous primary squamous cell cancer of the head and neck, esophagus, or lungs. Examination with the patient under anesthesia with endoscopy (which may include direct laryngoscopy, esophagoscopy, and bronchoscopy) and directed biopsy should be performed in all patients with an occult primary squamous cell cancer and in many patients with a known head and neck primary. Examination with the patient under anesthesia also can provide information regarding the extent of the tumor. The most common sites of silent primary tumors are the tonsils, base of the tongue, and piriform sinuses. Tumors of the nasopharynx have become easier to identify with the increased use of flexible nasopharyngoscopy. Biopsies should be performed in common areas of silent primaries in addition to the primary anatomic sites associated with lymphatic drainage of any neck mass.

LABORATORY EVALUATION

- There are no specific screening laboratory tests other than preoperative studies performed in the diagnostic evaluation of most head and neck carcinomas. Epstein-Barr virus, anticapsid antibodies, and serum immunoglobulin G are tumor markers for nasopharyngeal carcinomas.

DIAGNOSTIC IMAGING

PLAIN X-RAYS
- Posteroanterior and lateral chest x-rays should be obtained in all adult patients to eliminate the possibility

of occult lung metastasis or a second primary. A Panorex film may help delineating bony involvement in some cases of oral cavity lesions.

COMPUTED TOMOGRAPHY

- The computed tomography (CT) scan is probably the single most informative test in the assessment of a head and neck tumor. It may delineate the extent of disease and the presence and extent of lymphatic involvement and will distinguish cystic from solid lesions. Computed tomography scans of the chest, abdomen, and pelvis sometimes may identify the site of an occult primary tumor presenting with a node low in the neck. Computed tomography offers high spatial resolution and discriminates among fat, muscle, bone, and other soft tissues and surpasses magnetic resonance imaging (MRI) in the detection of bony erosion.

MAGNETIC RESONANCE IMAGING

- Magnetic resonance imaging may provide accurate information regarding the size, location, and soft-tissue extent of tumor. It provides limited information regarding bony involvement, unless there is gross involvement of the marrow space. Relatively greater sensitivity of MRI in relation to CT is offset by its decreased specificity. The main disadvantage of MRI is movement artifact, which is a particular problem in the larynx and hypopharynx. Gadolinium-enhanced MRI is probably superior to CT for imaging tumors of the nasopharynx and oropharynx.

POSITRON EMISSION TOMOGRAPHY

- Positron emission tomography (PET) has been evaluated in both primary and recurrent SCC of the head and neck. 18-Fluorodeoxyglucose (18-FDG) is the most commonly used PET radiotracer. It enters the cell and undergoes the first step in glycolysis to produce 18-FDG-6-phosphate, which reflects the metabolic rate of the tissue. The metabolic rate of malignancies is higher than that of most benign tumors or normal tissues. 18-FDG imaging therefore has the potential to distinguish between benign and malignant processes, grade tumors, identify metastases, and diagnose tumor recurrence. In head and neck cancer, 18-FDG imaging has been useful in detecting clinically occult recurrences, but it has proved less useful in identifying an occult primary site for metastatic cervical disease.

BIOPSY

- Biopsies of the primary tumor often can be performed in an outpatient setting.
- Punch or cup forceps biopsy is important in the diagnosis of mucosal lesions. The biopsy should be obtained at the border of the lesion away from areas of obvious necrosis.
- Fine-needle aspiration is a useful diagnostic modality. Multiple passes are made through the lesion with a fine-gauge (22-gauge) needle while suction is applied. Suction should be released before withdrawing the needle through surrounding soft tissue of the neck. Fine-needle aspiration has an associated false-negative rate as low as 7%. The diagnostic accuracy depends on the physician's skill and the cytopathologist's experience. Cytology is particularly useful in distinguishing a metastatic SCC from other malignant histologies. However, a negative result should not be interpreted as absence of malignancy.

CORE BIOPSY

- Core biopsy is not preferred except if the expected diagnosis is lymphoma.

OPEN BIOPSY

- Open biopsy should be performed only when a diagnosis has not been made after extensive clinical evaluation and fine-needle aspiration is nondiagnostic. The operation should be performed only by a surgeon prepared to conduct immediate definitive surgical treatment at that time (which may entail radical neck dissection).

STAGING

- In the tumor, node, metastasis (TNM) staging system for head and neck cancer (HNC) established by the American Joint Committee on Cancer (AJCC), the criteria for primary tumor (T) classification are site-specific.
- In general, T1 to T3 tumors are characterized by increasing size of the primary, whereas T4 describes invasion of muscle, bone, cartilage, or vessels; T4a designates surgically resectable disease, whereas T4b generally indicates locally unresectable disease. The classifications for lymph node involvement (N stage) are the same for all sites except nasopharyngeal cancer (Table 75–1).
- The combined T, N, and M classifications are used to assign an overall stage (I–IV, called the stage grouping) to the tumor. The AJCC stage groupings are common for all primary sites except nasopharynx (Table 75–2).
- Detection of nodal metastasis is an important determinant of prognosis. Prior to the development of CT scanning, detection of cervical metastases was based upon physical examination. However, physical examination is associated with a false-negative rate of 15% to 30% and a false-positive rate of 30% to 40%.

TABLE 75–1   American Joint Committee on Cancer Primary Tumor (T) Classification for Cancers of the Oral Cavity, Hypopharynx, and Oropharynx

Lip and oral cavity

TX	Minimum requirements to assess the primary tumor cannot be met
T0	No evidence of primary tumor
Tis	Carcinoma in situ
T1	Tumor 2 cm or less in greatest diameter
T2	Tumor more than 2 cm but not more than 4 cm in greatest dimension
T3	Tumor more than 4 cm in greatest dimension
T4	Lip: tumor invades through cortical bone, inferior alveolar nerve, floor of mouth, or skin of face (ie, chin or nose)
T4	Oral cavity
T4a	Tumor invades adjacent structures (eg, through cortical bone, into deep [extrinsic] muscles of tongue [genioglossus, hypoglossus, palatoglossus, and styloglossus], maxillary sinus, skin of face)
T4b	Tumor invades masticator space, pterygoid plates, or skull base and/or encases internal carotid artery

Hypopharynx

TX	Primary tumor cannot be assessed
T0	No evidence of primary tumor
Tis	Carcinoma in situ
T1	Tumor limited to one subsite of the hypopharynx and 2 cm or less in greatest dimension
T2	Tumor involves more than one subsite of the hypopharynx or an adjacent site, or measures more than 2 cm but not more than 4 cm in greatest diameter without fixation of hemilarynx
T3	Tumor measures more than 4 cm in greatest dimension or with fixation of hemilarynx
T4a	Tumor invades thyroid/cricoid cartilage, hyoid bone, thyroid gland, esophagus, or central compartment soft tissue
T4b	Tumor invades prevertebral fascia, encases carotid artery, or involves mediastinal structures

Oropharynx

TX	Primary tumor cannot be assessed
T0	No evidence of primary tumor
Tis	Carcinoma in situ
T1	Tumor 2 cm or less in greatest dimension
T2	Tumor more than 2 cm but not more than 4 cm in greatest dimension
T3	Tumor more than 4 cm in greatest dimension
T4a	Tumor invades the larynx, deep/extrinsic muscle of tongue, medial pterygoid, hard palate, or mandible
T4b	Tumor invades lateral pterygoid muscle, pterygoid plates, lateral nasopharynx, or skull base, or encases the carotid artery

Salivary gland

TX	Primary tumor cannot be assessed
T0	No evidence of primary tumor
T1	Tumor 2 cm or less in greatest dimension without extraparenchymal extension
T2	Tumor more than 2 cm but not more than 4 cm in greatest dimension without extraparenchymal extension
T3	Tumor more than 4 cm and/or having extraparenchymal extension
T4a	Tumor invades skin, mandible, ear canal, and/or facial nerve
T4b	Tumor invades skull base and/or pterygoid plates and/or encases carotid artery

TABLE 75–2   Staging System for Head and Neck Cancers

Stage 0	Stage IVB
Tis, N0, M0	T4b, any N, M0
Stage I	Any T, N3, MO
T1, N0, M0	Stage IVC
Stage II	Any T, any N, M1
T2, N0, M0	T1–3, N1, M0
Stage III	
T3, N0, M0	
Stage IVA	
T4a, N0 or N1, M0	
T1–4a, N2, M0	

• A mandatory component of the initial staging evaluation is a search for distant metastases, which are usually asymptomatic. The most common sites are the lungs, followed by the liver and bone. In the past chest CT was usually recommended to screen for pulmonary metastases in all patients, whereas evaluation by bone scan was only carried out if there were symptoms or signs (such as an elevated serum level of alkaline phosphatase) that suggested the presence of bone metastases. PET scans may soon replace or supplement CT and bone scans.

TREATMENT AND PROGNOSIS

• Treatment for HNC is highly complex, not only because of the variety of tumor subsites, but also because of the anatomic constraints of the head and neck region, and the importance of maintaining organ function. Following therapy for HNC, rehabilitation and restoration of speech and swallowing are critical to quality of life.

EARLY STAGE HNC

• In Stage I and II, there is no apparent lymph node involvement. Approximately 30% to 40% of patients with HNC present with early disease. These patients are generally managed with either surgery or radiation therapy (RT). The overall cure rate ranges from 60% to 98%, depending on the stage, disease site, and biologic factors (eg, overexpression of certain gene markers such as Bcl-2).

LOCOREGIONALLY ADVANCED, POTENTIALLY RESECTABLE HNC

• Locoregionally advanced disease which includes cancer metastatic to cervical lymph nodes and locally advanced primary tumors (stages III, IVa, IVb) is present in more than 50% of patients at diagnosis. These patients are generally managed with some combination of RT, surgery, and chemotherapy; and 5-year survival rates of approximately 40% to 50% can be achieved.

- Most deaths are related to locoregionally persistent or recurrent disease. Nonoperative approaches using concomitant chemotherapy and RT do not appreciably improve long-term survival rates over those achieved by surgery and RT, but an important benefit is that preservation of organ function is possible in approximately 50% of patients with larynx or hypopharyngeal primary tumors. Whenever possible, patients should be treated, at least initially, with intent to preserve the larynx.

LOCOREGIONALLY ADVANCED, UNRESECTABLE HNC

- These patients generally have a poor prognosis, with 5-year survival rates of only 10% to 30% using RT alone. Concomitant chemoradiation therapy (CRT) produces a distinct survival advantage over either RT alone or chemotherapy alone in these patients, particularly multiagent chemotherapy protocols given concomitantly with hyperfractionated radiotherapy protocols. Survival rates of up to 40% to 60% at 4 years are now being reported. However, the improved overall clinical outcomes in the CRT plus hyperfractionated radiotherapy studies comes at the cost of significant treatment-induced acute morbidity; thus, they are best utilized in patients with good performance status.

DISTANT METASTATIC AND RECURRENT ADVANCED, UNRESECTABLE HNC

- Chemotherapy is of major palliative benefit in patients with symptomatic metastatic or incurable recurrent HNC. However, whether any regimen prolongs survival is uncertain. The average survival for patients who receive chemotherapy for advanced disease is 6 to 8 months; it is only slightly less with supportive care.
- In contrast, a subset of patients who present with locally recurrent but nonmetastatic HNC may be successfully salvaged with further local treatment. For previously irradiated patients who have a potentially resectable recurrence and who are surgical candidates, 5-year survival rates after salvage surgery range from 16% to 36%, depending on the location and volume of recurrent disease.
- Increasing amounts of data support a potentially curative role for reirradiation in patients with previously irradiated recurrent unresectable HNC. Long-term survival rates of 10% to 20% can be achieved, and some studies report 5-year survival rates as high as 35% with concomitant chemotherapy and reirradiation. However, these approaches are all complicated by significant treatment-related toxicity.

BIBLIOGRAPHY

Greene, FL, Page, DL, Fleming, ID, et al, eds. *AJCC Cancer Staging Manual.* 6th ed. New York, NY: Springer-Verlag; 2002.

Berenson JR, Yang J, Mickel RA. Frequent amplification of the Bcl-1 locus in head and neck squamous cell carcinomas. *Oncogene.* 1989;4:1111–1116.

Boyle JO, Hakim J, Koch W, et al. The incidence of p53 mutations increases with progression of head and neck cancer. *Cancer Res.* 1993;53:4477–4480.

Cairns P, Polascik TJ, Eby Y, et al. Frequency of homozygous deletion at p16/CDKN2 in primary human tumours. *Nat Genet.* 1995;11:210–212.

Califano J, van der Riet P, Westra W, et al. Genetic progression model for head and neck cancer: Implications for field cancerization. *Cancer Res.* 1996;56:2488–2492.

Callender T, el-Naggar AK, Lee MS, Frankenthaler R, Luna MA, Batsakis JG. PRAD-1 (CCND1)/cyclin D1 oncogene amplification in primary head and neck squamous cell carcinoma. *Cancer.* 1994;74:152–158.

Department of Health, Social Services and Public Health (DHSSPS). *A Five-year Tobacco Action Plan 2003–2008.* Belfast, Northern, Ireland: DHSSPS; 2003.

Eakin R. Head and neck cancer. In: Spence RAJ, Johnston PG, eds. *Oncology.* Oxford, UK: Oxford University Press; 2001:191–208.

Fearon ER, Vogelstein B. A genetic model of colorectal tumorigenesis. *Cell.* 1990;61:759–767.

Forastiere AA, Goepfert H, Maor M, Pajak TF. Concurrent chemotherapy and radiotherapy for organ preservation in advanced laryngeal cancer. *N Engl J Med.* 2003;349:2091.

Hartwell LH, Kastan MB. Cell cycle control and cancer. *Science.* 1994;266:1821–1828.

Hollstein M, Sidransky D, Vogelstein B, Harris CC. p53 Mutation in human cancers. *Science.* 1991;253:49–53.

Jares P, Fernandez PL, Campo E, et al. PRAD-1/cyclin D1 gene amplification correlates with messenger RNA overexpression and tumor progression in human laryngeal carcinomas. *Cancer Res.* 1994;54:4813–4817.

Johnson NW, Warnakulasuriy S, Tavassoli M. Hereditary and environmental risk factors: Clinical and laboratory risk matters for head and neck, especially oral, cancer and precancer. *Eur J Cancer Prev.* 1996;5:5–17.

Kamb A, Gruis NA, Weaver-Feldhaus J, et al. A cell cycle regulator potentially involved in genesis of many tumor types. *Science.* 1994;264:436–440.

Koch WM, Brennan JA, Zahurak M, et al. p53 Mutation and locoregional treatment failure in head and neck squamous cell carcinoma. *J Natl Cancer Inst.* 1996;88:1580–1586.

Kotsianti A, Costopoulos J, Morgello S, et al. Undifferentiated carcinoma of the parotid gland in a white patient: Detection of Epstein-Barr virus by in situ hybridization. *Hum Pathol.* 1996;27:87–90.

Nawroz H, van der Riet P, Hruban RH, Koch WM, Ruppert JM, Sidransky D. Allelotype of head and neck squamous cell carcinoma. *Cancer Res.* 1994;54:1152–1155.

Pande P, Soni S, Kaur J, et al. Prognostic factors in betel and tobacco related oral cancer. *Oral Oncol.* 2002;38:491–499.

Pfister, DG, Laurie, SA, Weinstein, GS, et al. American Society of Clinical Oncology clinical practice guideline for the use of larynx-preservation strategies in the treatment of laryngeal cancer. *J Clin Oncol.* 2006;24:3693.

Reed A, Califano J, Cairns P, et al. High frequency of p16 (CDKN2/MTS-1/INK4A) inactivation in head and neck squamous cell carcinoma. *Cancer Res.* 1996;56:3630–3633.

Schantz SP, Yu G. Head and neck cancer incidence trends in young Americans, 1973–1997 with a special analysis for tongue cancer. *Arch Otolaryngol Head Neck Surg.* 2002;128:268–274.

Somers K, Merrick MA, Lopez ME, Incognito LS, Schechter GL, Casey G. Frequent p53 mutations in head and neck cancer. *Cancer Res.* 1992;52:5997–6000.

Soo, KC, Tan, EH, Wee, J, et al. Surgery and adjuvant radiotherapy vs concurrent chemoradiotherapy in stage III/IV non-metastatic squamous cell head and neck cancer: A randomised comparison. *Br J Cancer.* 2005;93:279.

van der Riet P, Nawroz H, Hruban RH, et al. Frequent loss of chromosome 9p21–22 early in head and neck cancer progression. *Cancer Res.* 1994;54:1156–1158.

76 BREAST CANCER

Joanne E. Mortimer

EPIDEMIOLOGY

- Breast cancer is the most common malignancy in women in the United States with an annual incidence of 182,000 cases.
- One in eight women in the United States will be diagnosed with breast cancer. This incidence is based on the assumption that the average woman will live to 80 years of age.
- The median age at diagnosis is 63 years.
- One in 200 breast cancers is diagnosed in men.
- Estrogen receptors (ERs), progesterone receptors (PRs), and HER2-neu are prognostic factors.
- African American women are less likely to develop breast cancer. However, cancers in this population tend to be high grade and triple negative (ER, PR, and HER2 negative), conferring a poor prognosis.
- Women whose breast cancers have been diagnosed on screening mammography may have a more indolent disease process.[1]
- Although 46,000 women die of breast cancer annually, the mortality rate has decreased 25% since 1990.
  - The most significant decline is in young women and women with ER positive tumors.[2]
  - Recent changes in the use of hormone replacement therapy (HRT) have also resulted in a decreased incidence in older women.

- The decline in breast cancer deaths has been attributed to improved detection and multimodality treatment of early stage disease.
- Breast cancers develop over 10 to 20 years as the ductal epithelium transforms from hyperplasia to dysplasia to ductal carcinoma in situ to an invasive ductal carcinoma.
- Breast cancer metastasizes from the primary lesion to the regional lymphatics (axillary and internal mammary lymph nodes) or hematogenously to other organs.

RISK FACTORS

- Risk factors for the development of breast cancer include: female sex, age, prolonged menstrual life, genetic predisposition, radiation, HRT.
  - Prolonged menstrual life risk factors include: menarche before age 11 years, menopause after age 55 years, nulliparity, first child after age 30 years.
  - Combined estrogen and progesterone as HRT is associated with an increased risk of developing breast cancer, whereas the risk associated with single-agent estrogen is less clear.[3,4]
  - Women with heritable predispositions for breast cancer tend to be younger at diagnosis (<40 years of age) and are more likely to develop bilateral breast cancer.
    - Breast cancer gene 1 (BRCA1) mutation carriers are at an increased risk for developing breast and ovarian cancers.
    - Breast cancer gene 2 (BRCA2) mutation carriers have an increased risk for the development of both male and female breast cancers and a higher incidence of prostate cancer.
    - Women with Cowden syndrome have a higher risk of breast cancer.
- A history of mantle-field radiation therapy to treat Hodgkin disease is associated with more than a ten-fold increased risk for breast cancer.
  - Therefore, these women are considered high risk and should be monitored closely with physical examinations and mammography.

DIAGNOSIS

- Most (75%) breast cancers are identified clinically as a mass in the breast, which is generally painless.
- A bloody nipple discharge can be indicative of an underlying malignancy; more often it is associated with a benign process such as a papilloma.
- Bilateral diagnostic mammograms are performed to clarify the abnormality and to ensure that there are no other lesions.

- In women with a newly diagnosed breast cancer, bilateral magnetic resonance imaging (MRI) of the breast can be of value in identifying a contralateral breast cancer. MRI can detect cancers in 3% of women that were not appreciated on mammography. The incidence of false-positive findings requiring biopsy is three times the rate of positive biopsies for cancer.[5]
- Confirmation of a cancer diagnosis requires tissue obtained by core biopsy or excision of the mass.
- At initial presentation, 15% of women will already have evidence of metastatic disease.
  - Inflammatory breast cancer is a clinical diagnosis characterized by erythema over two-thirds of the breast wall or evidence of peau d'orange changes.
    - Biopsy of the skin will confirm a tumor within the dermal lymphatics.
    - Patients with this presentation are treated initially with systemic therapy. Following response to systemic therapy, surgery, radiation therapy, and possibly hormonal therapy (if ER and/or PR positive) are indicated.

PATHOLOGY

- The majority (80%) of primary breast cancers present as infiltrating ductal carcinomas, with 10% to 15% presenting as invasive lobular carcinomas; the remaining histologies include colloidal, medullary, and tubular.
- Accepted prognostic factors include: tumor size, grade, nodal status, estrogen receptor/progesterone receptor status, and HER2 status.
  - Estrogen receptor and progesterone receptor status are generally determined by immunohistochemistry. Tumors that are ER and/or PR positive are considered hormonally sensitive.
  - The tumor is considered to be HER2 positive if it stains 3+ or greater by immunohistochemical assessment, or if gene amplifications of more than 2 are demonstrated using fluorescence in situ hybridization (FISH) techniques.
- Determination of hormone receptor and HER2 status are crucial to define optimal systemic therapy for early stage disease as well as recurrent/metastatic disease and, accordingly, must be performed on all new breast cancers.

SURGERY

- Surgery is important in establishing the diagnosis of breast cancer, controlling the local cancer, and staging the axilla.
  - The entire breast is treated either by mastectomy or lumpectomy and radiation therapy.

- A number of controlled trials have established that lumpectomy plus breast irradiation is equivalent to mastectomy. [6,7]
- In breast-conserving surgery, the primary breast tumor is removed in its entirety with a 1 cm margin.
- Sentinel-node mapping with technetium-99m (^{99m}Tc) and/or isosulfan blue (Lymphazurin) can accurately assess axillary nodal involvement by the cancer.[8]
  - If the sentinel node is free of tumor, the possibility of involvement in other nodes is <15%, and a full axillary dissection is generally not performed.
  - The current practice for those women who have evidence of tumor spread to the sentinel node is to perform a complete axillary dissection. Level I data to support this approach, however, is not yet available.[9]
- Radiation therapy is indicated in all women undergoing breast conservation therapy and can be indicated in women with involvement of multiple axillary nodes and in those with lymphovascular invasion by cancer.
  - Women undergoing lumpectomy (breast conservation therapy) receive postoperative radiation therapy to the breast, which has been shown to decrease the likelihood of an in-breast recurrence.
  - With cancer involvement of four or more axillary nodes, additional radiation to the chest wall and axilla has been shown to improve both local control and survival.[10,11]

SYSTEMIC ADJUVANT THERAPY

- After removal of the primary cancer, recommendations for systemic therapy to treat micrometastatic disease (adjuvant therapy) are based on the patient's stage, hormone receptor status, and HER2 status.
- Adjuvant chemotherapy has been shown to improve both recurrence-free and overall survival in women with early stage breast cancer. Specific recommendations are based on known prognostic factors. The National Cancer Institute (NCI) consensus panel recommendations for adjuvant therapy are summarized in Tables 76–1 through 76–3.
- The online program, www.http://Adjuvantonline.com is designed to aid in the decision making for adjuvant therapy recommendations. Patient information (age, tumor size, grade, ER, nodal status, and comorbid medical conditions) is input, and the 10-year relapse free and overall survivals are calculated for specific chemotherapy and hormonal therapy regimens and based on data from controlled trials.
- The addition of trastuzumab to adjuvant chemotherapy has been shown to improve both disease-free and

TABLE 76–1   Risk Categories for Women with Node-Negative Breast Cancer

	LOW RISK (HAS ALL LISTED FACTORS)	INTERMEDIATE (RISK CLASSIFIED BETWEEN LOW AND HIGH RISK)	HIGH RISK (HAS AT LEAST ONE LISTED FACTOR)
Tumor size	≤1 cm	1–2 cm	>2 cm
ER or PR status	Positive	Positive	Negative
Tumor grade	Grade 1	Grade 1–2	Grade 2–3

ER, estrogen receptor; PR, progesterone receptors.

overall survival in women with HER2 positive tumors with negative nodes and a primary tumor ≥1 cm that is ER– (or >2 cm and ER+) as well as women with axillary nodal involvement.[12,13]

- Premenopausal women with ER- and/or PR-positive tumors should receive hormonal therapy as a component of their adjuvant therapy.
  ○ Women with low-grade, ER positive/PR positive tumors, and negative axillary lymph nodes can benefit equally from hormone therapy with a luteinizing hormone-releasing hormone (LHRH) agonist and tamoxifen or chemotherapy
  ○ After chemotherapy, the addition of an LHRH agonist to tamoxifen is actively being studied but is not yet considered to be standard of care.
  ○ Women with high-risk disease should receive chemotherapy (see Tables 76–1 and 76–2).
  ○ Most premenopausal women who receive adjuvant chemotherapy become permanently amenorrheic and have improved outcomes compared to those women who continue to menstruate.

- Tamoxifen is considered the standard of care in premenopausal women.
- The role of aromatase inhibitors in this population has not been determined.
- Postmenopausal women with ER positive/PR positive tumors benefit from a number of different agents.
  ○ The selective aromatase inhibitors include anastrozole, letrozole, and exemestane. These drugs inhibit the aromatase enzyme in normal tissues (such as fat) and tumor.
  ○ When compared to tamoxifen, 5 years of letrozole or anastrozole provide an improved disease-free survival and decreased incidence of contralateral breast cancers compared with 5 years of tamoxifen. Superior overall survival has yet to be demonstrated.[14,15]
  - Women on aromatase inhibitors have a higher incidence of bone fractures, osteopenia, and osteoporosis.
  - Adjuvant letrozole has been associated with an increased incidence of heart disease.[15]

TABLE 76–2   Adjuvant Systemic Treatment Options for Women with Axillary Node-Negative Breast Cancer

PATIENT GROUP	LOW RISK	INTERMEDIATE RISK	HIGH RISK
Premenopausal ER+ or PR+	None or tamoxifen	Tamoxifen plus chemotherapy, tamoxifen alone, ovarian ablation, GnRH analog	Chemotherapy plus tamoxifen, chemotherapy plus ablation or GnRH analog, chemotherapy plus tamoxifen plus ovarian ablation or GnRH analog, or ovarian ablation alone or with tamoxifen or GnRH analog alone or with tamoxifen
Premenopausal, ER– or PR–			Chemotherapy
Postmenopausal, ER+ or PR+	None or tamoxifen	Hormonal therapy plus chemotherapy, hormonal therapy alone	Hormonal therapy plus chemotherapy, hormonal therapy alone
Postmenopausal, ER– or PR–			Chemotherapy
Older than 70 years of age	None or hormonal therapy	Hormonal therapy alone, hormonal therapy plus chemotherapy	Hormonal therapy; consider chemotherapy if ER– or PR–

ER+, estrogen receptor positive; ER–, estrogen receptor negative; GnRH, gonadotropin-releasing hormone; PR+, progesterone receptor positive; PR–, progesterone receptor negative.

TABLE 76–3 Treatment Options for Women with Axillary Node-Positive Breast Cancer

PATIENT GROUPS	TREATMENT
Premenopausal, ER+ or PR+	Chemotherapy plus tamoxifen, chemotherapy plus ovarian ablation/GnRH analog, chemotherapy plus tamoxifen plus ovarian ablation/GnRH analog, ovarian ablation alone or with tamoxifen or GnRH alone or with tamoxifen
Premenopausal, ER− or PR−	Chemotherapy
Postmenopausal, ER+ or PR+	Hormonal therapy plus chemotherapy, hormonal therapy alone
Postmenopausal, ER− or PR−	Chemotherapy
Older than 70 years of age	Hormonal therapy alone; consider chemotherapy if receptor-negative

ER+, estrogen receptor positive; ER−, estrogen receptor negative; GnRH, gonadotropin-releasing hormone; PR+, progesterone receptor positive; PR−, progesterone receptor negative.

- Arthralgias commonly occur with all aromatase inhibitors (20%–30%) and can necessitate switching to another hormonal agent such as tamoxifen.
  - After 5 years of tamoxifen, the addition of 5 years of letrozole has been shown to further decrease the recurrence rate, with the benefit largely confined to node-positive patients.[16]
  - Trials that compared 2 to 3 years of tamoxifen followed by 2 to 3 years of anastrozole or exemestane show superiority to 5 years of tamoxifen, with improvement in both disease-free survival and overall survival.[17,18]

TREATMENT OF METASTATIC BREAST CANCER

- Treatment of metastatic disease is based on menopausal status, hormone receptor status, and HER2 status.
  - Hormonal therapy will produce tumor regression or disease stabilization for at least 6 months in 50% to 60% of women with hormone-sensitive disease.
    - Tumors that are also HER2 positive can be less responsive to tamoxifen than the selective aromatase inhibitors
    - In premenopausal women with ER and/or PR positive disease, an LHRH agonist with tamoxifen has been shown to be superior to tamoxifen alone.[19]
    - For postmenopausal women, the selective aromatase inhibitors are considered first-line therapy, and the three agents appear comparable in their efficacy.
  - With progression of disease after an initial response to hormonal therapy, additional hormonal therapies

can also produce disease regression (eg, other aromatase inhibitor, fulvestrant, progestational agents, fluoxymesterone).
  - When advanced hormone-sensitive breast cancer does not respond to hormonal therapy, chemotherapy is recommended.
- Chemotherapy achieves palliation in women with advanced disease.
  - Combinations of chemotherapy can be associated with a greater likelihood of tumor regression than single agents, but without improvement in survival.[20]
  - Serial single agents are generally considered the standard of care.
  - The most active agents include: anthracyclines, taxane, vinorelbine, capecitabine, gemcitabine; cyclophosphamide.
- HER2-positive, hormone-resistant breast cancer should be treated with chemotherapy and the humanized monoclonal antibody trastuzumab.
  - The addition of trastuzumab to initial chemotherapy is associated with an improved survival compared with chemotherapy alone.
    - Trastuzumab is associated with an incidence of cardiac dysfunction, therefore, the patient's cardiac ejection fraction should be monitored every 3 months.
    - Trastuzumab should be discontinued if the ejection fraction becomes abnormal or declines by ≥10% from baseline.
    - Cardiac function should continue to be monitored as it can return to normal; trastuzumab can be resumed in select patients.
  - Lapatinib is a dual kinase inhibitor of both epidermal growth factor receptor (EGFR) and HER2 that is approved for the treatment of advanced HER2-positive breast cancer that has progressed after initial therapy with a trastuzumab-containing regimen.[21]
    - Clinical trials demonstrated that capecitabine with lapatinib produced longer remissions compared to capecitabine alone.
    - Cardiac dysfunction may occur less often with lapatinib than trastuzumab.
    - Data suggest that brain metastases may be less common in women who have been treated with lapatinib.
- Women with one or more bone metastasis should be initiated on monthly bisphosphonates, which have been shown to decrease skeletal related events (fracture, spinal cord compression, hypercalcemia, and need for surgery or radiation therapy).
  - Zoledronate may be superior to pamidronate in the prevention of skeletal-related events.
  - Monthly bisphosphonates are often continued indefinitely, although the available data supporting the

use of bisphosphonates in this setting is for 2 years of treatment.

○ The use of intravenous (IV) bisphosphonates has been associated with osteonecrosis of the jaw following dental extraction.

○ Attention to good dentition is recommended for patients on intravenous bisphosphonates.

MANAGEMENT OF NONINVASIVE CANCERS

• Ductal carcinoma in situ is most often diagnosed by biopsy of microcalcifications on mammography.

• Following lumpectomy, whole-breast radiation therapy is associated with a decreased incidence of in-breast recurrences; at 5 years 16% compared with 7%.[22]

○ Smaller radiation fields are being studied in this setting but are not considered standard of care.

○ It has yet to be proven that radiation can be eliminated in low-grade, small lesions that have been completely removed.

• In ER and/or PR positive ductal carcinoma in situ (DCIS), adjuvant tamoxifen will decrease the incidence of ipsilateral recurrences and new contralateral breast primaries.[23]

• Lobular carcinoma in situ (LCIS) is generally not palpable nor is it identified on mammography. It is usually diagnosed as an incidental finding on biopsy.

○ The lifetime risk for development of invasive breast cancer is approximately 30%.

○ Women treated with 5 years of tamoxifen are less likely to develop invasive breast cancer.[24]

○ In contrast to DCIS, postoperative radiation therapy to the breast is not indicated.

NEOADJUVANT THERAPY

• Systemic therapy administered prior to surgical removal of the primary tumor (neoadjuvant therapy) is indicated in patients with unresectable disease and inflammatory breast cancer.

○ The definition of unresectable is somewhat controversial but usually includes primary tumors that are ulcerated, attached to the chest wall, >6 cm in size, or are characterized by the presence of firm, fixed, axillary nodes.

○ Systemic therapy with hormonal agents or chemotherapy will produce tumor regression after which surgery and radiation therapy are indicated.

○ In unresectable disease and inflammatory breast cancer, neoadjuvant therapy can result in improved outcomes.

• Neoadjuvant therapy may be indicated in women with tumors confined to the breast.

○ Neoadjuvant therapy is equivalent to adjuvant therapy in disease free and overall survivals.

○ Breast conservation therapy can be achieved more often following neoadjuvant therapy.[25]

SCREENING

• Screening mammography with two views of the breast has been recommended for all women older than 40 years of age.

○ In women age ≥50 years, screening mammography results in a survival benefit.

○ The data for screening mammography in women age 40 to 49 years does not consistently show a survival advantage. However, given the low risk of the procedure it is generally recommended.

○ Little data exist for screening mammography in older women. The American Geriatric Society has recommended that an annual or biannual examination be performed in women who are expected to live for more than 2 years.

• Annual screening MRI of the breast can be of benefit in women who are at high risk for heritable breast cancer; it should be used in conjunction with annual mammography.

BREAST CANCER PREVENTION

• Women who are carriers of BRCA1 or BRAC2 mutations have a high enough risk for developing breast cancer that aggressive surveillance or prophylactic surgeries can be considered.

○ Prophylactic oophorectomy has been shown to decrease the incidence of breast cancer for both BRCA1 and BRCA2 mutation carriers.[26]

○ BRCA1 and BRCA2 mutation carriers who undergo prophylactic bilateral mastectomy have a decreased incidence of breast cancer compared to women who elected to perform regular breast exams and annual mammography.[27]

• In a randomized, double-blind, placebo-controlled trial, tamoxifen has been shown to decrease the incidence of breast cancer in women who are at high risk for development of breast cancer. High risk includes any woman with LCIS or a Gail Risk Assessment score of more than 1.67% over 5 years.[24] The Gail Risk Model determines the 5-year and lifetime risks for developing breast cancer according to known risk factors (www.cancer.gov/bcrisktool/Default.aspx).

- ○ Overall, the incidence of breast cancer was decreased by 53% in the tamoxifen arm.
- ○ The incidence of hormone-receptor–positive breast cancers was decreased by 62%. However, hormone-receptor–negative breast cancers developed equally in the tamoxifen and placebo arms.
- ○ Women on tamoxifen have an increased incidence of thromboembolic complications, cataracts, and uterine cancer.
- • Raloxifene has been shown to be comparable to tamoxifen as a chemopreventive agent. In a randomized double-blind study, raloxifene was as effective as tamoxifen in preventing invasive breast cancers in postmenopausal women at increased risk for developing breast cancer.[28]
  - ○ Fewer thromboembolic events and cataracts were reported with raloxifene than tamoxifen. Other side effects were comparable.
  - ○ Although not statistically significant there were more noninvasive cancers in women treated with raloxifene.

REFERENCES

1. Shen Y, Yang Y, Inoue LYT, Munsell MF, Miller AB, Berry DA. Role of detection method in predicting breast cancer survival: Analysis of randomized screening trials. *J Natl Cancer Inst.* 2005;97:1195–1203.
2. Jatoi I, Chen BE, Anderson WF, Rosenberg PS. Breast cancer mortality trends in the United States according to estrogen receptor status and age at diagnosis. *J Clin Oncol.* 2007;25:1683–1690.
3. Writing Group for the Women's Health Initiative I. Risks and benefits of estrogen plus progestin in healthy post-menopausal women: Principal results from the Women's Health Initiative randomized controlled trial. *JAMA.* 2002;288:321–333.
4. Women's Health Initiative Steering C. Effects of conjugated equine estrogen in postmenopausal women with hysterectomy: The Women's Health Initiative randomized controlled trial. *JAMA.* 2004;291:1701–1712.
5. Lehman CD, Gatsonis C, Kuhl CK, et al. MRI evaluation of the contralateral breast in women with recently diagnosed breast cancer. *N Engl J Med.* 2007;356:1295–1303.
6. Fisher B, Anderson S, Bryant J, et al. Twenty-year follow-up of a randomized trial comparing total mastectomy, lumpectomy, and lumpectomy plus irradiation for the treatment of invasive breast cancer. *N Engl J Med.* 2002;347:1233–1241.
7. Veronesi U, Cascinelli N, Mariani L, et al. Twenty-year follow-up of a randomized study comparing breast-conserving surgery with radical mastectomy for early breast cancer. *N Engl J Med.* 2002;347:1227–1232.
8. Edge SB, Niland JC, Bookman MA, et al. Emergence of sentinel node biopsy in breast cancer as standard-of-care in academic comprehensive cancer centers. *J Natl Cancer Inst.* 2003;95:1514–1521.
9. Lyman GH, Giuliano AE, Somerfield MR, et al. American Society of Clinical Oncology guideline recommendations for sentinel lymph node biopsy in early-stage breast cancer. *J Clin Oncol.* 2005;23:7703–7720.
10. Ragaz J, Jackson SM, Le N, et al. Adjuvant radiotherapy and chemotherapy in node-positive premenopausal women with breast cancer. *N Engl J Med.* 1997;337:956–962.
11. Overgaard M, Hansen PS, Overgaard J, et al. Postoperative radiotherapy in high-risk premenopausal women with breast cancer who receive adjuvant chemotherapy. *N Engl J Med.* 1997;337:949–955.
12. Romond EH, Perez EA, Bryant J, et al. Trastuzumab plus adjuvant chemotherapy for operable HER2-positive breast cancer. *N Engl J Med.* 2005;353:1673–1684.
13. Piccart-Gebhart MJ, Procter M, Leyland-Jones B, et al. Trastuzumab after adjuvant chemotherapy in HER2-positive breast cancer. *N Engl J Med.* 2005;353:1659–1672.
14. Howell A, Cuzick J, Baum M, et al. Results of the ATAC (Arimidex, tamoxifen, alone or in combination) trial after completion of 5 years' adjuvant treatment for breast cancer. *Lancet.* 2005;365:60–62.
15. Breast International Group (BIG) 1–98 Collaborative Group; Thurlimann B KA, Coates AS, Mouridsen H, et al. A comparison of letrozole and tamoxifen in postmenopausal women with early breast cancer. *N Engl J Med.* 2005;353:2747–2757.
16. Goss PE, Ingle JN, Martino S, et al. Randomized trial of letrozole following tamoxifen as extended adjuvant therapy in receptor-positive breast cancer: Updated findings from NCIC CTG MA 17. *J Natl Cancer Inst.* 2005;97:1262–1271.
17. Coombes RC, Hall E, Gibson LJ, et al. A randomized trial of exemestane after two to three years of tamoxifen therapy in postmenopausal women with primary breast cancer. *N Engl J Med.* 2004;350:1081–1092.
18. Jakesz R, Jonat W, Gnant M, et al. Switching of post-menopausal women with endocrine-responsive early breast cancer to anastrozole after 2 years' adjuvant tamoxifen: combined results of ABCSG trial 8 and ARNO 95 trial. *Lancet.* 2005;366:455–462.
19. Klijn JGM, Blamey RW, Boccardo F, Tominaga T, Duchateau L, Sylvester R. Combined tamoxifen and luteinizing hormone-releasing hormone (LHRH) agonist versus LHRH agonist alone in premenopausal advanced breast cancer: A meta-analysis of four randomized trials. *J Clin Oncol.* 2001;19:343–353.
20. Sledge GW, Neuberg D, Bernardo P, et al. Phase III trial of doxorubicin, paclitaxel, and the combination of doxorubicin and paclitaxel as front-line chemotherapy for metastatic breast cancer: an intergroup trial (E1193). *J Clin Oncol.* 2003;21:588–592.
21. Geyer CE, Forster J, Lindquist D, et al. Lapatinib plus capecitabine for HER2-positive advanced breast cancer. *N Engl J Med.* 2006;355:2733–2743.
22. Fisher B, Costantino J, Redmond C, et al. Lumpectomy compared with lumpectomy and radiation therapy for the treatment of intraductal breast cancer. *N Engl J Med.* 1993;328:1581–1586.

23. Fisher B DJ, Wolmark N, Wickerham DL, et al. Tamoxifen in treatment of intraductal breast cancer: National Surgical Adjuvant Breast and Bowel Project B-24 randomised controlled trial. *Lancet.* 1999;353:1993–2000.

24. Fisher B, Costantino JP, Wickerham DL, et al. Tamoxifen for the prevention of breast cancer: Current status of the National Surgical Adjuvant Breast and Bowel Project P-1 Study. *J Natl Cancer Inst.* 2005;97:1652–1662.

25. Fisher B, Brown A, Mamounas E, et al. Effect of preoperative chemotherapy on local-regional disease in women with operable breast cancer: Findings from National Surgical Adjuvant Breast and Bowel Project B-18. *J Clin Oncol.* 1997;15:2483–2493.

26. Rebbeck TR, Lynch HT, Neuhausen SL, et al. Prophylactic oophorectomy in carriers of BRCA1 or BRCA2 mutations. *N Engl J Med.* 2002;346:1616–1622.

27. Meijers-Heijboer H, van Geel B, van Putten WLJ, et al. Breast cancer after prophylactic bilateral mastectomy in women with a BRCA1 or BRCA2 mutation. *N Engl J Med.* 2001;345:159–164.

28. Vogel VG, Costantino JP, Wickerham DL, et al. Effects of tamoxifen vs raloxifene on the risk of developing invasive breast cancer and other disease outcomes: The NSABP study of tamoxifen and raloxifene (STAR) P-2 trial. *JAMA.* 2006; 295:2727–2741.

77 LUNG CANCER

Vamsidhar Velcheti and
Ramaswamy Govindan

EPIDEMIOLOGY

- Lung cancer is the leading cause of cancer related deaths in the United States. It is estimated that over 200,000 people will be diagnosed with lung cancer and more than 75% of them will die of lung cancer in the year 2007.
- The median age at diagnosis of lung cancer is approximately 70 years.
- The epidemiology of lung cancer follows the changes in patterns of cigarette smoking over time with a 10- to 20-year lag time.
- Tobacco smoking is by far the most important risk factor for lung cancer; however, several other environmental and biological factors contribute to the onset and progression of lung cancer.
- Although a biological predisposition to lung cancer is not clearly established, genetic risk factors associated with metabolism of the carcinogens in tobacco smoke could determine the susceptibility to lung cancer.

PATHOLOGY OF LUNG CANCER

- The histologic types of lung cancer are based on analysis with light microscopy and with standard staining techniques.
- Broadly speaking, there are two types of lung cancer: small cell lung cancer (SCLC) and non–small cell lung cancer (NSCLC). NSCLC accounts for approximately 85% of all lung cancers. There has been a significant decline in the incidence of SCLC over the past three decades in the United States.
- The three main cell types of NSCLC are squamous cell carcinoma, adenocarcinoma, and large-cell carcinoma
- The incidence of squamous cell carcinoma is on the decline. Adenocarcinoma now accounts for approximately 50% of all NSCLC in the United States. Adenocarcinoma is particularly common in females, persons who never smoked, and younger patients.
- Adenocarcinomas and large-cell cancers are predominantly peripheral, and squamous cell carcinomas are central tumors.

CLINICAL PRESENTATION

- A majority of patients diagnosed with lung cancers are symptomatic at the time of diagnosis; only a few are discovered incidentally on a chest radiograph.
- The clinical symptoms and signs in patients with lung cancer result from (1) the local tumor growth, (2) tumor metastasis, and (3) paraneoplastic syndromes
- Clinical manifestations of lung cancer caused by local tumor growth and intrathoracic spread include cough, shortness of breath, chest pain, hemoptysis, and obstructive pneumonia.
- Vocal cord paralysis and superior vena cava syndrome (SVCS) are symptoms of locally advanced disease.
- Approximately two-thirds of the patients diagnosed with SCLC and one-third of the patients diagnosed with NSCLC present with distant disease.
- The most common sites of metastases are mediastinal lymph nodes, pleura, bones, liver, adrenal glands, and brain.
- The signs and symptoms resulting from CNS involvement range from vague nonspecific headaches or mental status changes to focal or generalized seizures and localized weakness. Epidural and intramedullary spinal cord metastases are not uncommon in patients with lung cancer.
- Numerous paraneoplastic syndromes have been identified in patients with lung cancer. The major categories of paraneoplastic syndromes include endocrine, neurologic, and cutaneous manifestations.

- The most common paraneoplastic syndrome in patients with lung cancer is the syndrome of inappropriate secretion of antidiuretic hormone (SIADH). SIADH is most frequently reported in patients with SCLC.
- SIADH results from the inappropriate secretion of arginine vasopressin. It manifests as hyponatremia (<130 MEq/L). It is essential to rule out other nonmalignant causes of SIADH (like pulmonary infections, central nervous system trauma, infection, or space-occupying lesions). The severity or the presence of SIADH does not correlate with the prognosis of the patient.
- Humoral hypercalcemia of malignancy results from the secretion of a parathyroid hormone (PTH)-related protein. This is most commonly seen in patients with squamous cell carcinoma (in about 15% of the patients). This is the most common cause of hypercalcemia in NSCLC.
- Eaton-Lambert syndrome (from SCLC) is a pseudomyasthenic syndrome, which presents with proximal limb muscle weakness and fatigue. This results from an antibody-mediated impairment of presynaptic neuronal calcium channel activity, causing a decreased release of acetylcholine.
- Hypertrophic pulmonary osteoarthropathy is characterized by the formation of new periosteal bone in the digits and clubbing of the digits.

WORKUP AND STAGING

- As with any patient with cancer, the workup starts with a thorough physical examination of the axillary, cervical, supraclavicular, and scalene regions for possible lymphadenopathy; the chest for signs of airway obstruction or pleural effusion; and the abdomen for any organomegaly.

IMAGING

- Chest radiograph: All patients with a presentation suspicious for lung cancer need to be evaluated by a chest x-ray (CXR). Lung cancer can present as a mass, peripheral nodule, hilar or mediastinal changes suggestive of lymphadenopathy, pleural effusions, or as metastatic disease.
- It is essential to distinguish benign lesions based on the radiographic appearance to avoid unnecessary invasive and expensive procedures. Previous chest x-rays should be sought to see the temporal progression of the lesions. A nodule that is stable over a period of 2 years is unlikely to be malignant. The presence of certain patterns of calcification within the lesion (bulls-eye, popcorn, or multipunctate foci) are suggestive of benign lesions. CXR may reveal areas of atelectasis suggesting an endobronchial lesion, and pneumonic infiltrates may be seen in association with obstructing lesions. Plain chest radiographs have a low predictive value (sensitivity of approximately 60%) in the determination of mediastinal nodal metastases.
- Computed tomography (CT): Any suspicious lesion on a chest radiograph needs to be evaluated by a CT scan of the chest and upper abdomen. CT offers better visualization of the nodule and more sensitive detection of mediastinal lymph node involvement, and it also can help identify local invasion of the chest wall and pleura. However, the sensitivity of CT when done alone is only 79% for detecting mediastinal lymph nodes and 62% for detecting chest wall or soft tissue invasion.
- Positron emission tomography (PET): PET is a useful adjunct tool to complete the staging workup in patients with recently diagnosed NSCLC. PET added to CT increases the sensitivity (89%–93%) and specificity (94%–100%) of noninvasive staging of lung cancer significantly. The role of a PET scan in staging workup of patients with SCLC is controversial at this time.
- Magnetic resonance imaging (MRI): MRI of the chest is not routinely used in the staging workup of patients with lung cancer. It is particularly helpful in the setting of suspected spinal cord, vascular, or chest wall involvement.

PATHOLOGICAL DIAGNOSIS

- Sputum cytologic examination: Sputum cytology is a very simple test with a positive predictive value that can approach 100%, but with a very low sensitivity rate of only 10%. This is most useful in patients with centrally located tumors. Up to 80% of central tumors can be diagnosed with three sputum samples, compared with 20% of peripheral nodules larger than 3 cm. However, sputum cytology is seldom used these days to diagnose lung cancer.
- Flexible fiberoptic bronchoscopy (FFB): FFB is very helpful in determining the endobronchial extent of disease. An accurate histological diagnosis can be established in over 95% of tumors that are visible by FFB. The diagnosis of peripheral tumors can be established in over 50% of patients by cytological studies of brushings and bronchioloalveolar lavage.
- Mediastinoscopy: Mediastinoscopy is indicated for preoperative mediastinal nodal assessment (in patients with nodes >1cm on CT). Cervical mediastinoscopy is more accurate for staging superior mediastinal lymph nodes, whereas extended or anterior (Chamberlain)

approach is better for anterior mediastinal lymph nodes, and left-sided lesions. Increasingly endoscopic ultrasound (EUS) and endobronchial ultrasound (EBUS) are used to biopsy some of the mediastinal lymph glands and left-sided lesions.

STAGING

NON–SMALL CELL LUNG CANCER

- The International Staging System uses the TNM description system and is shown in Table 77–1.
- Stage-specific survival is outlined in Table 77–2.

TABLE 77–1   TNM Descriptors

STAGE GROUPING: TNM SUBSETS	
STAGE	TNM SUBSET
Stage 0	Tis: Carcinoma in situ
Stage IA	T1 N0 M0
Stage IB	T2 N0 M0
Stage IIA	T1 N1 M0
Stage IIB	T2 N1 M0
	T3 N0 M0
Stage IIIA	T3 N1 M0
	T1 N2 M0, T2 N2 M0, T3 N2 M0
Stage IIIB	T4 N0 M0, T4 N1 M0, T4 N2 M0
	T4 N3 M0
	T1 N3 M0, T2 N3 M0, T3 N3 M0
Stage IV	Any T, any N, M1

M, distant metastasis; M1, distant metastasis present including separate metastatic tumor nodule(s) in the ipsilateral non-primary tumor lobe(s) of the lung; M0, no distant metastasis; MX, Presence of distant metastasis cannot be assessed; N, regional lymph nodes; N1, metastasis to ipsilateral peribronchial and/or ipsilateral hilar lymph nodes, and intrapulmonary nodes involved by direct extension of the primary tumor; N2, metastasis to ipsilateral mediastinal and/or subcarinal lymph node(s); N3, metastasis to contralateral mediastinal, contralateral hilar, ipsilateral or contralateral scalene, or supraclavicular lymph node(s); N0, no regional lymph node metastasis; NX, regional lymph nodes cannot be assessed; T, primary tumor; T1, tumor <3 cm in greatest dimension, surrounded by lung or visceral pleura, without bronchoscopic evidence of invasion more proximal than the lobar bronchus a (ie, not in the main bronchus); T2, tumor with any of the following features of size or extent: >3 cm in greatest dimension; involves main bronchus, >2 cm distal to the carina; invades the visceral pleura; associated with atelectasis or obstructive pneumonitis that extends to the hilar region but does not involve the entire lung; T3, tumor of any size that directly invades any of the following: chest wall (including superior sulcus tumors), diaphragm, mediastinal pleura, parietal pericardium; or tumor in the main bronchus <2 cm distal to the carina, but without involvement of the carina; or associated atelectasis or obstructive pneumonitis of the entire lung; T4, tumor of any size that invades any of the following: mediastinum, heart, great vessels, trachea, esophagus, vertebral body, carina; or tumor with a malignant pleural or pericardial effusion, or with satellite tumor nodule(s) within the ipsilateral primary-tumor lobe of the lung; Tis, carcinoma in situ; T0, no evidence of primary tumor; TX, Primary tumor cannot be assessed, or tumor proven by the presence of malignant cells in sputum or bronchial washes but not visualized with imaging or bronchoscopy.

TABLE 77–2   Expected Five-Year Survival with Treatment

STAGE	TNM SUBSET	AVERAGE 5-YEAR SURVIVAL
Stage IA	T1 N0 M0	82%
Stage IB	T2 N0 M0	68%
Stage IIA	T1 N1 M0	52%
Stage IIB	T2 N1 M0	
	T3 N0 M0	40%
Stage IIIA	T3 N1 M0	
	T1–3 N2 M0	9%-15%, depending on subset
Stage IIIB	T4 N0-2 M0	
	T1–4 N3 M0	<5%
Stage IV	Any T, any N, M1	NA

NA, not applicable

SMALL CELL LUNG CANCER

- The Veterans Administration Lung Group staging system categorizes patients into limited-stage and extensive-stage disease. SCLC is classified as limited stage when the tumor is confined to one hemithorax and regional lymph nodes. Presence of disease extending beyond one hemithorax (able to be encompassed by radiation) or in distant organs would constitute extensive-stage disease. Over 70% of patients with SCLC present with extensive-stage disease.

THERAPY AND PROGNOSIS

NON–SMALL CELL LUNG CANCER

- The general overview of the management of NSCLC is summarized in Table 77–3.

STAGE I AND II

- Surgery: Stages I and II NSCLC are treated surgically whenever complete resection is possible. Preoperative assessment should determine stage (for potential resection), cardiopulmonary reserve (whether intended

TABLE 77–3   Overview of Management of Non–Small Cell Lung Cancer

STAGE	TREATMENT
Stage I A	Surgical resection
Stage I B	Surgical resection + Adjuvant chemotherapy
Stage II B	Surgical resection + Adjuvant chemotherapy
Stage III A T3N1	Surgical resection + Adjuvant chemotherapy
Stage III A T3N2	Chemoradiation
Stage III B (No pleural effusion)	Chemoradiation
Stage III B (pleural effusion)	Chemotherapy
Stage IV	Chemotherapy

resection is possible), and perioperative risk of the intended procedure. Adequate pulmonary function (estimated postpneumonectomy forced expiratory volume at one second [FEV1]>1.2 L) and a maximal O_2 consumption greater than 15 cc/kg/min are prerequisites for surgical resection. Smoking cessation programs should be initiated at least 2 weeks prior to surgery. Perioperative mortality is determined by the patient's age, comorbid conditions, and extent of resection. Lobectomy is the most commonly used procedure and the results are equivalent to pneumonectomy when complete resection is achieved. Local recurrence is twice as common with segmentectomy and wedge resection and should be reserved for those who cannot tolerate lobectomy. Tumor or lymph nodes involving the proximal bronchus or pulmonary artery or tumor crossing the major fissures are indications for pneumonectomy.

- Patients with extensive comorbid conditions who are poor surgical candidates can be treated with definitive radiation therapy. Survival after radiation therapy depends on the performance status, radiation dose, tumor size, and complete response by 6 months after completion of RT.
- Cisplatin-based adjuvant chemotherapy improves survival in patients with resected stage I-III NSCLC. The majority of patients included in these studies had stage II or III disease. Adjuvant chemotherapy is typically not recommended for patients with stage IA disease. The 5-year survival advantage with adjuvant chemotherapy is between 4% and 15%.

Stage III

- Stage IIIA includes T3 Nl or N2 nodal disease with a significant difference in prognosis, with the latter being worse. Surgical resection followed by adjuvant chemotherapy with a platinum based regimen is an option for patients with T3N1 disease followed by adjuvant chemotherapy.
- The role of surgery is not well defined in stage III A patients involving the mediastinal nodes (N2). A large intergroup study comparing chemoradiation with chemoradiation followed by surgery did not show any survival advantage with the addition of surgery. The majority of patients with stage III A disease are treated with definitive chemoradiation
- Patients with mediastinal involvement detected at the time of resection should be considered for platinum based adjuvant chemotherapy. The role for postoperative radiation therapy (PORT) in this setting is unclear.
- Combined-modality therapy with chemotherapy and radiation is indicated in the treatment of patients with stage IIIB disease (except those with malignant pleural effusion).

- Currently, concurrent chemoradiation with a cisplatin-based doublet is recommended in patients with good performance status and unresected stage III disease. However, the role of consolidation chemotherapy and the optimal dosing of the regimen remain undetermined. For patients with poor performance status, radiation and chemotherapy may be administered for symptom palliation.

Stage IV

- Initial therapy
  - Systemic chemotherapy for advanced NSCLC has been shown to improve the quality of life and survival compared to best supportive care. Some of the commonly used combination regimens in the treatment of NSCLC are listed in Table 77–4.
  - There appears to be no significant difference in the overall survival among the commonly used platinum-based chemotherapy regimens. Therefore, the treatment of stage IV disease should be individualized and take into consideration the performance status of the patient and any comorbid conditions. The addition of bevacizumab (an inhibitor of vascular endothelial growth factor) to platinum-based chemotherapy in the first-line setting is associated with better response and improved survival in a selected subgroup of patients with metastatic NSCLC.
  - Patients with poor performance status should be considered for single-agent chemotherapy such as vinorelbine as supportive care.
  - Patients with metastatic NSCLC are treated with four to six cycles of adjuvant chemotherapy. There is no role for maintenance chemotherapy.
- Second-line therapy
  - Docetaxel improves survival compared to best supportive care in patients who have progressive disease following platinum-based therapy.
  - Pemetrexed has been shown to be equivalent to docetaxel in terms of response rate and survival; however, pemetrexed is associated with significantly less myelosuppression than docetaxel.
  - The epidermal growth factor receptor tyrosine kinase (EGFR-TK) inhibitor erlotinib improves survival in the second-line/third-line setting when compared with placebo.

SMALL CELL LUNG CANCER

Limited-Stage Disease

- Combination chemotherapy (with cisplatin and etoposide), along with thoracic radiation therapy, is the treatment of choice for limited-stage disease. Concurrent chemoradiation therapy appears to be

TABLE 77–4 Chemotherapy for Lung Cancer

DRUG	TYPE OF AGENT	MAJOR ADVERSE EFFECTS	COMMENTS
Cisplatin (Platinol)	Atypical alkylator	Nausea and vomiting (common), nephrotoxicity,[a] ototoxicity, neuropathy, myelosuppression (mild), electrolyte wasting (potassium and magnesium)	Hydration required before administration
Carboplatin (Paraplatin)	Atypical alkylator	Myelosuppression,[a] nausea and vomiting (mild), neurotoxicity (rare), nephrotoxicity	Dose usually determined by area under the curve, taking renal function into account with use of the Calvert formula
Nonplatinum agents			
Etoposide (VePesid)	Topoisomerase II inhibitor	Myelosuppression,[a] nausea and vomiting, stomatitis, diarrhea	Stomatitis and diarrhea rare with normal function
Topotecan (Hycamtin)	Topoisomerase I inhibitor	Myelosuppression,[a] nausea and vomiting, diarrhea, headache	Increased monitoring of liver function necessary
Irinotecan (Camptosar)	Topoisomerase I inhibitor	Myelosuppression,[a] nausea and vomiting, diarrhea	
Gemcitabine (Gemzar)	Antimetabolite	Myelosuppression,[a] nausea and vomiting, diarrhea, edema, influenza-like syndrome	Increased monitoring of liver function necessary
Paclitaxel (Taxol)	Microtubule inhibitor	Myelosuppression,[a] mucositis, peripheral neuropathy, hyper sensitivity reaction, nausea and vomiting	Requires pretreatment with dexamethasone, diphenhydramine, ranitidine
Docetaxel (Taxotere)	Microtubule inhibitor	Myelosuppression,[a] edema and fluid retention, diarrhea, nausea and vomiting,	Requires treatment with dexamethasone before, during, and after infusion
Vinorelbine (Navelbine)	Microtubule inhibitor	Myelosuppression,[a] nausea and vomiting,	Mild vesicant
Vincristine (Oncovin)	Microtubule inhibitor	Neuropathy,[a] constipation	Vesicant
Pemetrexed	Antimetabolite	Rash, fatigue, low incidence of myelosuppression	

[a]Principles of cancer chemotherapy: use drugs active against the cancer to be treated, use drugs with different mechanism of action, use drugs with different toxicity profile and use each drug at their maximal effective dose.
SOURCE: From Spira A, Ettinger DS. Multidisciplinary management of lung cancer. *N Engl J Med.* 2004;350:379–392.

more beneficial than sequential chemoradiation. Twice daily radiation appears to be more beneficial but is associated with significant toxicities.

• Surgical resection after chemoradiation does not appear to improve survival in patients with SCLC.
• Prophylactic cranial irradiation has demonstrated significant reduction in CNS relapse and also increase in overall survival by 5%.

EXTENSIVE-STAGE DISEASE

• The current standard of care is combination chemotherapy with a platinum agent (cisplatin or carboplatin) and etoposide. There is no role for thoracic irradiation in this stage except for palliation of symptoms. Chemotherapy improves survival in patients with extensive-stage disease; the overall response rate is 60% to 80%. Maintenance chemotherapy has not been shown to improve overall survival. However, almost all the patients with extensive-stage disease will die from relapsed SCLC. Topotecan has been approved for use in patients with relapsed SCLC. However, it is only modestly effective. Several ongoing studies will determine the utility of antiangiogenic agents in SCLC.

BIBLIOGRAPHY

American Society of Clinical Oncology. Clinical practice guidelines for the treatment of unresectable non-small-cell lung cancer. Adopted on May 16, 1997 by the American Society of Clinical Oncology. *J Clin Oncol.* 1997;15:2996–3018.

Ettinger D, Johnson B. Update: NCCN small cell and non-small cell lung cancer Clinical Practice Guidelines. *J Natl Compr Canc Netw.* 2005;3(Suppl 1):S17–21.

Faivre-Finn C, Lee LW, Lorigan P, et al. Thoracic radiotherapy for limited stage small cell cancer: Controversies and future developments. *Clin Oncol (R Coll Radiol).* 2005;17:591–598.

Osterland K. Chemotherapy in small cell lung cancer. *Eur Respir J.* 2001;18:1026–1043.

Penland SK, Socinski MA. Management of unresectable stage III non small cell lung cancer: The role of combined chemoradiation. *Semin Radiat Oncol.* 2004;14:326–34.

Pfister DG, Johnson DH, Azzoli CG, et al. American Society of Clinical Oncology treatment of unresectable non small cell lung cancer guideline: Update 2003. *J Clin Oncol.* 2004;22:330–53.

Schrump AN, Altorki NK, Henschke CL. Non small cell lung cancer. In: DeVita VT, Hellman S, Rosenberg SA, eds. *Cancer: Principles and Practice of Oncology.* 7th ed. Philadelphia, PA: Lippincott Williams & Wilkins; 2005.

Spira A, Ettinger DS. Multidisciplinary management of lung cancer. *N Engl J Med.* 2004;350:379–92.

Turrisi AT, Kim K, Blum R, et al. Twice-daily compared with once-daily thoracic radiotherapy in limited small-cell lung cancer treated concurrently with cisplatin and etoposide. *N Engl J Med.* 1999;340:265–71.

78 GASTROINTESTINAL CANCERS

Rami Owera

COLORECTAL CANCER

EPIDEMIOLOGY

- Colorectal cancer (CC) is the third most common malignancy in the United States and the fourth in the world.
- Despite significant improvements in adjuvant and palliative treatment, it remains the second most common malignancy-related death in the United States, exceeded only by lung cancer.
- An estimated 148,000 new cases of CC are diagnosed annually in the United States.
- Approximately 56,000 individuals die annually of CC.
- Colon cancer incidence and prevalence is approximately equal in males and females, whereas rectal cancer is more frequent in males (1.7:1 ratio).
- The risk of CC increases with age, with more than 90% of cases diagnosed after age 50 years.
- Industrial societies (United States, Canada, and Western Europe) have a higher incidence than developing countries because of higher consumption of saturated fat and red meat.
- Immigrants from low-incidence regions assume the risk of their adopted country.

RISK FACTORS

- Although no specific risk factors have been clearly elucidated, CC remains largely a disease of the elderly and middle aged population (it is rarely diagnosed before the age of 40) and, accordingly age is an important determinant of the development of CC. Other risk factors which appear to contribute to the development of CC include: smoking, alcohol abuse, and obesity.

- CC tends to cluster in families (25% of cases). In addition, the number of family members affected, their age of onset, and relationship to the patient (first-degree relative) increases the overall risk of CC. Accordingly, the family history influences the timing and frequency of screening.
- Adenomatous polyps found during routine colonoscopy increase the risk of CC.
- Inflammatory bowel disease, especially ulcerative colitis, increases the risk of developing CC. The risk of CC in patients with inflammatory bowel disease exceeds that of age-matched controls beginning approximately 10 years after the onset of pancolitis. Left-sided colitis carries a lower risk.
- Dietary factors have been implicated in the development of CC: increased risk with high intake of red meat and fatty food, decreased risk with high intake of fruits, vegetables and vitamins. Considerable controversy exists regarding the exact role of diet in CC.
- Sedentary lifestyles have also been associated with a higher risk of CC.
- Alcohol and tobacco use appear to directly correlate with the incidence of CC.
- Prior radiation for the treatment of prostate cancer is associated with an increased risk of rectal cancer.

HEREDITARY SYNDROMES

- Sporadic colon cancers comprise approximately 80% to 85% of all cases, with the remaining 15% to 20% attributed to inherited syndromes.
- Familial adenomatous polyposis (FAP) is caused by a mutation of tumor suppressor gene APC (adenomatous polyposis coli) located at 5q21. Innumerable polyps (polyposis) begin in the late teens and the median age of onset of untreated CC is 42 years. Screening should begin by age 15, and prophylactic resection of the entire colon and rectum should be performed at the time of polyposis formation.
- Hereditary nonpolyposis colorectal cancer (HNPCC), also known as Lynch syndrome, is caused by mutations in DNA mismatch repair genes. HNPCC affects at least three relatives, one of whom should be a first-degree relative and at least one person should have developed the disease before age 50 years. HNPCC accounts for approximately 5% to 10% of all colon cancer cases.
  - Gardner's syndrome is a variant of FAP associated with adenomatous polyps and extracolonic manifestations: skull osteomas, upper gastrointestinal polyps, and neoplasms of the thyroid, liver, and biliary tract.

○ Turcot's syndrome is a variant of FAP associated with brain tumors.
○ Peutz-Jeghers syndrome is associated with polyps in the small intestine.
○ Cowden syndrome is associated with multiple hamartomas involving the breast, thyroid, skin, central nervous system, and gastrointestinal tract.
○ Juvenile polyposis syndrome is characterized by multiple hamartomatous/juvenile polyps with a predilection for the colon and stomach.

PATHOLOGY

- Approximately 95% of colon cancers are adenocarcinomas; a small number are mucinous and signet-ring cell carcinomas.
- Neuroendocrine carcinomas tend to be more aggressive and respond poorly to therapy.
- Most malignant colon lesions are preceded by adenomas. The malignant potential of adenomas correlates with size, histopathology, and degree of dysplasia. Villous and tubulovillous adenomas are associated with a higher incidence of malignant transformation than tubular adenomas.
- Although polyps larger than 2 cm have a transformation rate of approximately 40%, those smaller than 1 cm have a risk of less than 1%.

SCREENING

- For the general population, an annual fecal occult blood test and flexible sigmoidoscopy every 3 to 5 years or colonoscopy every 10 years, beginning at age 50, is recommended.
- Almost all rectal cancers but only one-half to two-thirds of colon cancers can be detected by sigmoidoscopy.
- Double contrast barium enema (BE) every 5 to 10 years is also used for screening but is of limited value in patients with ulcerative colitis or HNPCC patients.
- FAP screening should start at puberty.
- Hereditary nonpolyposis colorectal cancer screening should start at age 21 years.
- For inflammatory bowel disease, screening should start 8 years after pancolitis and 12 to 15 years after left-sided colitis.
- For individuals with first-degree family members (also consider screening for individuals with multiple CC risk factors: smoking, alcohol, obesity), screening should start at age 40.

CLINICAL PRESENTATION

- Patients with right-sided colon lesions usually present with vague abdominal pain, acute or chronic gastrointestinal bleeding, anemia, fatigue, and bloating.
- Patients with left-sided colon cancers frequently present with changes in bowel habit, obstruction, melena, and hematochezia.
- Constitutional symptoms such as malaise, weight loss, and early satiety are common in colon cancer, especially in the advanced and metastatic stages.
- Rarely patients present with fever, bacteremia, and sepsis secondary to *Streptococcus bovis.*

DIAGNOSTIC WORK UP
- Colonoscopy with biopsy of suspicious lesions.
- Computed tomography (CT) scan of the abdomen and pelvis (primarily for staging).
- Chest x-ray (staging).
- CT scan of the chest for patients with rectal cancer is indicated, since these patients have a higher incidence of pulmonary metastasis.
- Serum CEA levels are useful to detect recurrent disease.
- Double-contrast BE in patients who cannot undergo full-length colonoscopy.

STAGING
The TNM classification is the preferred staging system for CC, however the venerable Duke's classification system is perhaps the best known. The TNM features used to stage CC are outlined below:
- In situ: intraepithelial or invasion of the lamina propria
- T1: invades the submucosa
- T2: invades the muscularis propria
- T3: penetrates through the muscularis propria into the subserosa, or into nonperitonealized pericolic or perirectal tissues
- T4: directly invades other organs or structures, and/or perforates the visceral peritoneum
- N1: 1 to 3 regional nodes
- N2: 4 or greater regional lymph nodes
- MS: Distant metastasis

STAGE GROUPINGS
- *Stage I*
  ○ T1 N0 M0
  ○ T2 No M0
- *Stage II*
  ○ T3 N0 M0
  ○ T4 N0 M0
- *Stage IIIA*
  ○ T1,2 N1 M0
- *Stage IIIB*
  ○ T3,4 N1 M0
- *Stage IIIC*
  ○ Any T N2 M0
- *Stage IV*
  ○ Any T, Any N, M1

TREATMENT

GENERAL CONSIDERATIONS

- The usual therapy for CC involves laparoscopic laparotomy with en bloc resection of the involved bowel segment and pericolic lymphadenectomy. At least 12 lymph nodes must be examined to rule out locally advanced disease.
- There is no role for adjuvant chemotherapy in stage I or low-risk stage II disease. High-risk stage II (T3, T4, bowel obstruction or perforation) should be considered for adjuvant chemotherapy. Adjuvant chemotherapy improves survival and reduces recurrence in high-risk stage II lesions and in locally advanced disease (stage III). Palliative chemotherapy improves survival in metastatic disease.
- Solitary metastatic lesions to the liver occur in 15% to 20% of patients with CC. Surgical resection of solitary hepatic metastatic foci should be considered, since the 5-year relapse free survival is approximately 30%.
- Neoadjuvant chemoradiation therapy is recommended in T3, T4, or node positive rectal cancers.

SURGERY FOR CC

- Wide margins are essential: 5 cm on either side with removal of the lymphatic drainage of the tumor and the adjacent mesentery is recommended. Cecal cancers require resection of the terminal ileum and its associated mesentery. Tumors located in the ascending colon are resected with a standard right hemicolectomy. Tumors at the hepatic flexure may require an extended right hemicolectomy. Tumors in the midtransverse colon are usually resected from the hepatic flexure to the splenic flexure. Rectal lesions require a low anterior resection with total mesorectal excision.

CHEMOTHERAPY

- 5-Fluorouracil (5-FU) and leucovorin were the first drugs to show improvement in disease-free survival in the adjuvant setting for high-risk stage II and locally advanced stage III lesions.
- An impressive list of new agents has been approved for use in CC in both the adjuvant and metastatic settings. Several studies are ongoing to determine the optimal regimen in advanced CC (high-risk stage II and greater)
- 5-FU and leucovorin in combination with oxaliplatin (FOLFOX) or irinotecan (FOLFIRI) are considered the standard first-line therapy in metastatic colon cancer. Oxaliplatin is associated with a sensory neuropathy that may limit its long-term use.
- Bevacizumab (Avastin) is a vascular endothelial growth factor inhibitor that is also being used in combination with chemotherapy in the metastatic setting.
- Cetuximab (Erbitux) and panitumumab (Vectibix) are anti-epithelial growth factor receptors that may improve survival in combination with chemotherapy as second-and third-line agents in the metastatic setting.

ESOPHAGEAL CANCER

EPIDEMIOLOGY

- Approximately 15,000 new cases of esophageal cancer occur annually with 13,800 deaths.
- Esophageal cancer is at least three times more common in men than women.
- Esophageal cancer is more common in Asia.
- Adenocarcinomas are more common in whites, whereas squamous cell carcinomas are more common in African Americans.
- There has been a rise in the number of adenocarcinomas reported in the past two decades believed to be secondary to a parallel increase in chronic gastroesophageal reflux disease (GERD).

RISK FACTORS

- Alcohol and tobacco use are the most common risk factors associated with esophageal squamous cell carcinoma.
- High-fat/low-protein, high-calorie diets also appear to increase the risk of developing esophageal carcinoma.
- Barrett esophagus, usually caused by chronic GERD, results in replacement of the squamous epithelium at the distal esophagus by columnar intestinal epithelium and is associated with an increased risk of developing esophageal adenocarcinoma (incidence of 1% to 2% over 10 years).

PATHOLOGY

- Adenocarcinomas are more prevalent in Western societies (approximately 60% of all esophageal tumors) and are usually located in the distal one-third of the esophagus.
- Squamous cell tumors are the most common histology worldwide and usually arise from the proximal two-thirds of the esophagus.

CLINICAL PRESENTATIONS

- Dysphagia is the most common symptom. Other symptoms include anorexia, weight loss, fatigue, cough, sore throat, heartburn, hoarseness, and odynophagia.

DIAGNOSIS

- The gold standard to establish the diagnosis is endoscopy with biopsy of a suspicious lesion.
- CT of the chest and abdomen is useful to stage the disease.
- Endoscopic ultrasound helps to evaluate the depth of the lesion and the involvement of regional lymph nodes.

STAGING

- *T Stages*
  - Tis: carcinoma in situ (the tumor has not invaded beyond the epithelium, the first or innermost layer of the esophagus)
  - T1: tumor invades the lamina propria (second layer) or submucosa (third layer)
  - T2: tumor invades the muscularis propria (fourth layer)
  - T3: tumor invades the adventitia (fifth and outermost layer)
  - T4: tumor invades nearby structures
- *N Stages*
  - N0: no spread to nearby lymph nodes
  - N1: spread to nearby lymph nodes
- *M Stages*
  - M0: no spread to distant organs
  - M1a: spread to distant lymph nodes
  - M1b: spread to distant organs

STAGE GROUPINGS
- Stage I: T1 N0 M0
- Stage IIA: T2 N0 M0 or T3 N0 M0
- Stage IIB: T1 N1 M0 or T2 N1 M0
- Stage III: T3 N1 M0 or T4 any N M0
- Stage IV: any T any N M1

TREATMENT

- Surgical resection remains the primary therapy for early stage esophageal tumors. Unfortunately, most patients present with locally advanced or metastatic disease.
- Chemoradiotherapy, with or without surgery, is used for locally advanced tumors.
- 5-Fluorouracil and cisplatin are the most common chemotherapy agents used. Palliative chemotherapy or best supportive care is standard for metastatic tumors.

- The overall 5-year survival for locally advanced disease is approximately 30% and is slightly improved in selected patients when concurrent chemoradiation therapy is used preoperatively.
- The life expectancy for patients with metastatic esophageal cancer is measured in months.

SURVIVAL RATES BY STAGE

- The survival of 11,154 patients with esophageal cancer based on stage is summarized below (data extracted from the 2005 National Cancer Data Base):

STAGE	PERCENT OF PATIENTS	5-YEAR RELATIVE SURVIVAL RATE
0	1%	52%
I	10%	41%
II	21%	26%
III	18%	13%
IV	26%	3%
Unknown	25%	–

GASTRIC CANCER

EPIDEMIOLOGY

- It is estimated that 22,000 new cases of gastric cancer will be diagnosed annually in the United States. Of these, approximately 12,000 individuals will die of gastric cancer.
- Gastric cancer is much more common in Japan and Russia and still ranks as one of the leading causes of cancer-related deaths worldwide.
- The median age at the time of diagnosis is 70 years.

RISK FACTORS

- Increased consumption of processed/preserved foods increases the risk of developing gastric cancer. *Helicobacter pylori* infection plays an important role in the development of gastric adenocarcinoma. Importantly, the WHO has classified *H. pylori* as a definite carcinogen.

PATHOLOGY

- Adenocarcinomas account for 95% of all gastric tumors. The remaining 5% are carcinoids, lymphomas, and leiomyosarcomas.
- There are two main categories of gastric cancer: diffuse (more aggressive) and intestinal (ulcerative).

CLINICAL PRESENTATION

- Symptoms include abdominal pain, nausea, emesis, fatigue, anorexia, and weight loss.
- Other features include occult and occasionally overt gastrointestinal bleeding.
- Dysphagia is more common in proximal gastric tumors.
- Most patients present with locally advanced or metastatic disease.

DIAGNOSIS

- Upper endoscopy with biopsy.
- Upper gastrointestinal series and barium swallow.
- CT scan of the abdomen and pelvis to evaluate local tumor extent and to rule out distant metastasis.

STAGING

- The 1997 American Joint Committee on Cancer *Staging Manual* utilizes the following tumor, node, metastasis classification system for staging gastric carcinoma:

PRIMARY TUMOR
- TX: primary tumor cannot be assessed
- T0: no evidence of primary tumor
- Tis: carcinoma in situ, intraepithelial tumor without invasion of the lamina propria
- T1: tumor invades the lamina propria or submucosa
- T2: tumor invades the muscularis propria or subserosa
- T3: tumor penetrates the serosa (ie, visceral peritoneum) without invasion of adjacent structures
- T4: tumor invades the adjacent structures

REGIONAL LYMPH NODES
- NX: regional lymph nodes cannot be assessed
- N0: no regional lymph node metastases
- N1: metastasis in 1 to 6 regional lymph nodes
- N2: metastasis in 7 to 15 regional lymph nodes
- N3: metastasis in more than 15 regional lymph nodes

DISTANT METASTASIS
- MX: distant metastasis cannot be assessed
- M0: no distant metastasis
- M1: distant metastasis

STAGE GROUPING
- Stage 0: Tis N0 M0
- Stage IA: T1 N0 M0
- Stage IB: T1 N1 M0, T2 N0 M0
- Stage II: T1 N2 M0, T2 N1 M0, T3 N0 M0
- Stage IIIA: T2 N2 M0, T3 N1 M0, T4 N0 M0
- Stage IIIB: T3 N2 M0
- Stage IV: T4 N1-3 M0, T1-3 N3 M0, Any T Any N M1

TREATMENT

- Surgery represents the only viable chance of cure for localized disease. Curative resection involves tumor removal along with regional lymph node dissection. Neoadjuvant chemotherapy should be considered prior to surgery.
- Adjuvant chemotherapy and radiation therapy improve survival in selected patients. Chemotherapy usually consists of a combination regimen that can include: 5-fluorouracil, doxorubicin, mitomycin, methotrexate, cisplatin, etoposide, paclitaxel, and/or docetaxel. Although, some patients may initially respond, there is little evidence to suggest that survival is prolonged.

PANCREATIC CANCER

EPIDEMIOLOGY

- Approximately 35,000 new cases are reported annually. Importantly, since 32,500 deaths are also reported annually, pancreatic cancer is one of the most fatal malignancies.
- Pancreatic cancer is the fourth leading cause of cancer related death in the United States.
- The median age at the time of diagnosis is 55 years.
- Pancreatic cancer is slightly more common in African Americans than whites.

RISK FACTORS

- Tobacco use appears to be responsible for approximately one-third of all cases in the United States.
- High-fat and red meat consumption, obesity, and decreased physical activity increase the risk for pancreatic cancer.
- Chronic pancreatitis as a result of alcohol abuse may also confer additional risk.
- Exposure to chemicals and toxins such as petroleum increases pancreatic cancer risk.
- Familial cases have been reported but are rare.

PATHOLOGY

- Adenocarcinomas account for more than 95% of all pancreatic cancers. Sarcomas and lymphomas account for the remainder and carry a similar poor prognosis.

CLINICAL PRESENTATION

- Nausea, emesis, and vague abdominal pain with radiation to the back are among the most common symptoms. Most patients experience anorexia and weight loss that can be profound.

- Jaundice (painful or painless) with or without pruritus is typical of pancreatic head lesions.
- Some patients present with an acute thromboembolic event, and occasionally disseminated intravascular coagulation or Trousseau's syndrome.

DIAGNOSIS

- Most are diagnosed via CT scan of the abdomen. Endoscopic retrograde cholangiopancreatography (ERCP) or endoscopic ultrasound with biopsy is used to confirm the diagnosis.
- Magnetic resonance imaging (MRI) of the abdomen is gaining popularity, particularly for patients with a high clinical suspicion and a negative CT scan.
- Serum cancer antigen (CA) 19-9 is usually, but not always, elevated. CA 19-9 can be elevated in other benign or malignant disorders; therefore, it is neither sensitive nor specific for pancreatic cancer.

STAGING

PRIMARY TUMOR
- TX: Primary tumor cannot be assessed
- T0: No evidence of primary tumor
- Tis: Carcinoma in situ
- T1: Tumor limited to the pancreas, 2 cm or less in greatest dimension
- T2: Tumor limited to the pancreas, more than 2 cm in greatest dimension
- T3: Tumor extends beyond the pancreas but without involvement of the celiac axis or the superior mesenteric artery
- T4: Tumor involves the celiac axis or the superior mesenteric artery (unresectable primary tumor)

REGIONAL LYMPH NODES
- NX: Regional lymph nodes cannot be assessed
- N0: No regional lymph node metastasis
- N1: Regional lymph node metastasis

DISTANT METASTASIS
- M0: No distant metastasis
- M1: Distant metastasis

STAGE GROUPING
- Stage 0: Tis N0 M0
- Stage IA: T1 N0 M0
- Stage IB: T2 N0 M0
- Stage IIA: T3 N0 M0
- Stage IIB: T1 N1 M0, T2 N1 M0, T3 N1 M0
- Stage III: T4 Any N M0
- Stage IV: Any T Any N M1

TREATMENT

RESECTABLE DISEASE
- The standard surgical treatment is pancreaticoduodenectomy (Whipple's procedure). The procedure itself is associated with a high morbidity and mortality. Only 20% to 30% of patients are candidates for this type of surgery eg, do not have locally advanced tumors.
- Adjuvant chemotherapy with gemcitabine or 5-FU with or without radiation therapy may improve disease free and overall survival.

LOCALLY ADVANCED AND METASTATIC DISEASE
- Systemic chemotherapy with gemcitabine is the standard therapy for patients with good performance status.
- The objective response rate is less than 20%.
- Historically, adding a second agent to gemcitabine has failed to improve survival.
- Recently, erlotinib (Tarceva) (an epidermal growth factor receptor inhibitor) has been shown to slightly improve survival when combined with gemcitabine. The one-year survival increased from 17% to 23%.

PROGNOSIS

- Patients with resectable disease have an overall 5-year survival of 20% to 30% for node negative disease and less than 10% for node positive disease.
- Locally advanced or unresectable patients have a median survival of 8 to 10 months.
- Patients with metastatic pancreatic cancer have a median survival of only 4 to 6 months.

HEPATOCELLULAR CARCINOMA

EPIDEMIOLOGY

- In the United States 20,000 new cases of hepatocellular carcinoma (HCC) are estimated annually.
- The incidence continues to increase because of increased numbers of patients with chronic hepatitis C.
- HCC is the fifth most common tumor in the world and is one of the most common causes of cancer related deaths worldwide.
- It is more common in males than females, with an approximate ratio of 3:1.
- HCC is more common in African Americans, Hispanics, and Asians than whites.

RISK FACTORS

- Chronic hepatitis B or C viral infections are the most common risk factors associated with the development

of HCC. Chronic hepatitis C alone accounts for approximately 40% of all cases.
- Alcoholic cirrhosis accounts for approximately 15% of all cases.
- Liver cirrhosis secondary to hemochromatosis, primary biliary cirrhosis, and Wilson's disease also increase the risk of developing HCC.
- Tobacco use and oral contraceptive pills may increase the risk as well.

CLINICAL PRESENTATION

- Right upper quadrant abdominal pain, nausea, anorexia, early satiety, and weight loss
- Jaundice, ascites, and complications related to ascites
- Easy bruising and bleeding secondary to thrombocytopenia and coagulopathy

DIAGNOSIS

- CT scan or MRI of the abdomen. CT or ultrasound guided biopsy to confirm the diagnosis.
- Serum alpha-fetoprotein (AFP) tends to be elevated in approximately two-thirds of all cases.
- Abdominal ultrasound with a serum AFP has been useful to screen for HCC in high-risk individuals.

STAGING

- Tumor, node, metastasis staging criteria for HCC:
- T1: solitary tumor without vascular invasion
- T2: solitary tumor with vascular invasion or multiple tumors (none more than 5 cm)
- T3: multiple tumors more than 5 cm in diameter or tumor involving a major branch of the portal or hepatic vein(s)
- T4: tumor(s) with direct invasion of adjacent organs other than the gallbladder or with perforation of the visceral peritoneum
- N0: indicates no nodal involvement
- N1: indicates regional nodal involvement
- M0: indicates no distant metastasis
- M1: indicates metastasis beyond the liver

STAGE GROUPING
- Stage 0: Tis N0 M0
- Stage II: T2 N0 M0
- Stage IIIA: T3 N0 M0
- Stage IIIB: T4 N0 M0
- Stage IIIC: Any T N1 M0
- Stage IV: Any T Any N M1

TREATMENT

- Surgical resection is the definitive treatment, if feasible.
- Less than one-third of all patients are surgical candidates.
- Patients who undergo partial hepatic resection and liver transplantation have a 5-year overall survival of 30% to 40%. Importantly, HCC accounts for almost 20% of liver transplant recipients in the United States.
- Until recently, adjuvant or neoadjuvant systemic therapy failed to improve disease-free progression or survival. Recently, sorafenib (a tyrosine kinases receptor inhibitor) was found to improve survival in patients with HCC.

BILIARY TRACT CANCERS

- Estimated incidence of 8000 annually in the United States. Gallbladder carcinomas are the most common type of biliary tract cancer. Almost all biliary tract cancers are adenocarcinomas. Patients usually present with obstructive jaundice and pain and locally advanced disease. An ERCP with biopsy of a suspicious lesion is the gold standard for diagnosis.
- Surgical resection is usually palliative (approximately 10% to 20% cure rate).
- Adjuvant systemic chemotherapy and radiation therapy are currently investigational and the overall, long-term survival for locally advanced and metastatic disease remains poor.

BIBLIOGRAPHY

American Cancer Society. *American Cancer Society Figures and statistics.* Atlanta, GA: American Cancer Society; 2005.

Desch CE, Benson AB 3rd, Somerfield MR, et al. Colorectal cancer surveillance: 2005 update of an American Society of Clinical Oncology practice guideline. J Clin Oncol 2005 Nov 20; 23(33):8512–9.

Devesa SS, Blot WJ, Fraumeni JF Jr. Changing patterns in the incidence of esophageal and gastric carcinoma in the United States. *Cancer.* 1998;83:2049–2053.

Fush CS, Mayer RJ. Gastric carcinoma. *N Engl J Med.* 1995;333: 32–41.

Jean-François Bosset, M.D., Marc Gignoux, M.D., Jean-Pierre Triboulet, M.D., et al. Chemoradiotherapy followed by surgery in squamous cell carcinoma of the esophagus. *N Engl J Med.* 1997;337:161–167.

Jemal A, et al. Cancer Statistics, *CA Cancer J Clin.* 2006;56: 106–130.

Jürgen Weitz, Moritz Koch, Jürgen Debus, et al. Colorectal Cancer. The Lancet - Vol. 365, Issue 9454, 8 January 2005, Pages 153–165.

Kelly H, Goldberg R. Systemic therapy for metastatic colorectal cancer: current options, current evidence. *J Clin Oncol.* 2005; 23: 4553–4560.

Konner J, O'Reilly E. Pancreatic cancer: epidemiology, genetics and approaches to screening. *Oncology.* 2002;16:1615–1622.

Larsson, SC. *JNCI.* 2005;97:1679.

Meyerhardt J, Mayer R. Systemic therapy for colorectal cancer. *N Engl J Med.* 2005;352:476–487.

Sun W., Haller DG. Adjuvant therapy of colon cancer. *Semin Oncol.* 2005 Feb;32(1):95–102.

Thierry André, M.D., Corrado Boni, M.D., Lamia Mounedji-Boudiaf, M.D., et al. Oxaliplatin, fluorouracil, and leucovorin as adjuvant treatment for colon cancer.

Van Cutsem E, Labianca R, Hossfeld D, et al. Randomized phase III trial comparing infused irinotecan/5-fluorouracil (5-FU)/folinic acid (IF) versus 5-FU/FA (F) in stage III colon cancer patients. Proceedings from the 41st annual meeting of the American Society of Clinical Oncology. Orlando, FL: 2005; Abstract #LBA8.

79 GENITOURINARY ONCOLOGY

Noah M. Hahn

PROSTATE CANCER

EPIDEMIOLOGY

- In 2007, physicians will diagnose more than 218,000 new cases of prostate cancer. In addition, 27,000 men will die because of prostate cancer.[1]
- Prostate cancer ranks second among causes of cancer-related deaths in the United States.[1]
- One in six men will be diagnosed with prostate cancer in their lifetime.[1]
- Risk factors for prostate cancer include age, family history, African American race, and high-fat diets.[2]
- African American men are 60% more likely to be diagnosed with prostate cancer in their lifetime and 2.4 times more likely to die of prostate cancer when they are diagnosed compared to white age-matched controls.[3]

CLINICAL PRESENTATION, DIAGNOSIS, AND STAGING

- The median age at diagnosis is 68 years.[4]
- Presenting signs can include urinary tract obstructive symptoms, a palpable prostate nodule on digital rectal examination, erectile dysfunction, or pelvic pain; however, most men are asymptomatic and are diagnosed via an elevated prostate-specific antigen (PSA) test.

- Nonmalignant etiologies (ie, benign prostatic hyperplasia [BPH], prostatitis, etc) can also cause an elevated PSA. Confirmation of malignancy requires a prostate biopsy.
- The tumor, node, metastasis (TNM) staging of prostate cancer is summarized in Table 79–1.[5]
- The risk of metastatic disease at diagnosis is determined by assessment of clinical risk factors that include clinical stage, PSA level, and prostate biopsy Gleason grade.[6]
- The Gleason grade is a histologic assessment of the degree of differentiation of prostate cancer present in a biopsy specimen. The most prevalent histologic pattern is scored on a scale from 1 (representing a very well differentiated malignancy) to 5 (representing poorly differentiated anaplastic malignancy). The same method is used to score the second most prevalent histologic pattern. The two scores are summed to give the composite Gleason grade (ie, a cancer composed of 50% Gleason grade 4 and 30% Gleason grade 3 is scored as a composite Gleason grade of 4 + 3 = 7).
- For patients with low risk of metastatic disease defined as Gleason grade <7, PSA <10, and clinical stage T1–T2, the risk of metastatic disease is small and no further staging studies are necessary. In other patients, bone scan and computed tomography (CT) scan of the abdomen and pelvis should be considered to rule out metastatic disease.[7]
- Only 5% of new prostate cancer cases present with metastatic disease at the time of diagnosis.[4]

LOCALIZED DISEASE

- Localized prostate cancer is defined as prostate cancer confined to the prostate, peri-prostate tissues, or seminal vesicles without metastatic spread to pelvic lymph nodes or distant sites. Cure is possible in these men.
- Current options for men with localized prostate cancer include: watchful waiting, prostatectomy, radiation, or primary hormonal therapy.
- Each therapy presents unique risks, benefits, and side-effect profiles as described below.
- **Watchful waiting**
  - Because of the significant side affects associated with treatment and the frequency of concurrent medical comorbidities, watchful waiting is an attractive option for many men with prostate cancer.
  - In men with a Gleason score of 7 or less, the 10-year cancer specific survival rate with watchful waiting is 87%. For men with a Gleason score of 8 to 10; the 10-year cancer specific survival falls to 34%.[8]
  - Watchful waiting in young healthy patients requires frequent reassessments by a urologist, monitoring of PSA values, repeated clinical examinations, and

TABLE 79–1   Prostate Cancer TNM Staging

CLINICAL T STAGE		REGIONAL LYMPH NODES	
Tx	Primary tumor cannot be assessed	Clinical	
T0	No evidence of primary tumor	Nx	Regional lymph nodes were not assessed
T1	Clinically inapparent tumor neither palpable nor visible by imaging	N0	No regional lymph node metastasis
T1a	Tumor incidental histologic finding in 5% or less of tissue resected	N1	Metastases in regional lymph node(s)
T1b	Tumor incidental histologic finding in more than 5% of tissue resected	Pathologic	
T1c	Tumor identified by needle biopsy (eg, because of elevated PSA)	pNx	Regional lymph nodes not sampled
T2	Tumor confined within the prostate (tumor found in one or both lobes by needle biopsy, but not palpable or reliably visible by imaging, is classified as T1c)	pN0	No regional lymph nodes
T2a	Tumor involves one-half of one lobe or less	pN1	Metastases in regional node(s)
T2b	Tumor involves more than one-half of one lobe but not both lobes		
T2c	Tumor involves both lobes	**Distant metastasis**	
T3	Tumor extends through the prostate capsule (Invasion into the prostatic apex or into (but not beyond) the prostatic capsule is classified not as T3 but as T2)	Mx	Distant metastasis cannot be assessed (not evaluated by any modality)
T3a	Extracapsular extension (unilateral or bilateral)	M0	No distant metastasis
T3b	Tumor invades seminal vesicle(s)	M1	Distant metastasis
T4	Tumor is fixed or invades adjacent structures other than seminal vesicles: bladder neck, external sphincter, rectum, levator muscles, and/or pelvic wall	M1a	Nonregional lymph node(s)
		M1b	Bone(s)
Pathologic T stage		M1c	Other site(s) with or without bone disease
pT2	Organ confined (there is no pathologic T1 classification)		
pT2a	Unilateral, involving one-half of one lobe or less	**Stage groupings**	
pT2b	Unilateral involving more than one-half of one lobe but not both lobes		
pT2c	Bilateral disease	Stage I	T1a N0 M0 G1
pT3	Extraprostatic extension	Stage II	T1a N0 m0 G2,3–4
			T1b N0 M0 Any G
			T1c N0 M0 Any G
			T1 N0 M0 Any G
			T2 N0 M0 Any G
pT3a	Extracapsular extension (positive surgical margin should be indicated by an R1 descriptor [residual microscopic disease])	Stage III	T3 N0 M0 Any G
pT3b	Seminal vesicle invasion	Stage IV	T4 N0 M0 Any G
			Any T N1 M0 Any G
			Any T Any N M1 Any G
pT4	Invasion of bladder, rectum		
Histologic grade			
Gx	Grade cannot be assessed		
G1	Well differentiated (slight anaplasia) (Gleason 2–4)		
G2	Moderately differentiated (moderate anaplasia) (Gleason 5–6)		
G3–4	Poorly differentiated (marked anaplasia) (Gleason 7–10)		

PSA, prostate-specific antigen.

Source: Used with the permission of the American Joint Committee on Cancer (AJCC), Chicago, Illinois. The original source for this material is the *AJCC Cancer Staging Manual*. 6th ed. New York, NY; Springer; 2002. www.springeronline.com.5.

periodic rebiopsy of the prostate to monitor for disease progression.

○ The risks associated with watchful waiting include: urinary tract obstruction, pelvic pain, and spread to distant sites.

• **Prostatectomy**

○ In healthy patients, prostatectomy provides a curative surgical treatment option.

○ In appropriately selected patients, cure is possible in 75% of patients.[9]

○ A single randomized controlled Scandinavian study of men with low- to intermediate-grade tumors detected by digital rectal examination demonstrated a small overall survival advantage for prostatectomy when compared to watchful waiting. Overall quality of life scores were similar with both approaches.[10,11] This survival advantage was limited to men younger than 65 years of age.

○ Major side effects of surgery include incontinence (8.7% severe, 21.6% still require diapers), and erectile dysfunction (30%–90% depending on preoperative age, preoperative potency, and nerve-sparing prostatectomy vs non–nerve-sparing).[12,13]

• **Radiation**

○ External beam radiation therapy (EBRT) also provides a curative treatment option for men who wish to avoid surgery or who are not surgical candidates.

○ In appropriately selected patients, EBRT compares well to prostatectomy and provides cure rates approaching 75%.[14]

○ No large randomized trials comparing prostatectomy directly to EBRT have been performed.

○ Side effects of EBRT include chronic urinary frequency or incontinence (10%), erectile dysfunction (68% when the dose exceeds 75 Gy), and chronic proctitis or rectal bleeding (10%).[15]

○ Brachytherapy (BRT) is a radiation technique in which radioactive "seeds" are placed directly into the prostate tumor allowing higher radiation doses to be delivered to the tumor while reducing radiation exposure to surrounding normal tissues. For low-risk patients (low tumor grade and low tumor volume), BRT appears to provide rates of cancer control equivalent to prostatectomy.

• **Primary hormonal therapy**

○ For patients who decline or are not candidates for definitive local therapy with surgery or EBRT, the use of hormone therapy alone as a primary treatment for prostate cancer has become increasingly common.[16]

○ Testosterone stimulates prostate cancer growth. Hormone therapy options include bilateral orchiectomy or injections with leuteinizing hormone-releasing hormone (LHRH) agonists (ie, leuprolide, goserelin acetate, etc). These hormonal therapies exert their antineoplastic effect by causing serum testosterone levels to decline to castrate levels.

○ At 5 years, continued control of prostate cancer growth as assessed by stable PSA levels has been reported at 74% with primary hormonal therapy.[17]

○ Side effects include decreased libido (90%–100%), hot flashes (50%–70%), fatigue, loss of bone density, and muscle atrophy.

ADJUVANT THERAPY

• In prostatectomy patients with spread of cancer to the pelvic lymph nodes, an improvement in overall survival from 45% to 64% at a median of 11.9 years of follow-up has been shown with the use of adjuvant hormonal therapy compared to delaying hormone therapy until symptoms develop.[18]

• The addition of adjuvant EBRT in patients with positive surgical margins, seminal vesical involvement, high Gleason grade, or T3/T4 tumors has been shown to decrease the rate of local tumor recurrence and rates of PSA relapse; however no improvement in overall survival has been seen.[19,20]

• In patients with Gleason grades from 8 to 10 or high-volume Gleason grade 7 disease, the addition of hormonal therapy to EBRT has demonstrated a 10% absolute improvement in overall survival compared to EBRT alone.[21–23]

METASTATIC DISEASE

• In the modern PSA era, biochemical relapse of prostate cancer following prostatectomy, as detected by a rising PSA only, predates the appearance of radiographic (ie, on bone scan or CT scan) metastatic disease by a median of 8 years. Factors that predict a shorter time period until appearance of metastatic disease include: Gleason grade from 8 to 10, an interval of less than 2 years between prostatectomy and biochemical relapse, and a PSA doubling time of less than 10 months.[24]

• For patients with radiographic metastatic disease, hormonal therapy via orchiectomy or LHRH agonist therapy can significantly alleviate symptoms and delay progression.

• Androgen-independent prostate cancer (AIPC) is defined by progression of radiographic disease or a rising PSA while receiving hormonal therapy with a documented castrate level serum testosterone.

• Secondary hormone therapies such as antiandrogen drugs (ie, bicalutamide, flutamide, nilutamide) and anti-adrenal drugs (ie, ketoconazole) are options for men with disease that progresses in spite of castrate serum levels of testosterone. PSA responses are seen in 20% to 30% of men, generally lasting only 3 to 6 months; however, a prolonged response can be seen in a small subset of patients. These responders are thought to have disease responsive to circulating adrenal androgens.

- Hormone-refractory prostate cancer (HRPC) is defined by disease that is unresponsive to all hormone manipulations.
- Docetaxel-based chemotherapy has demonstrated a modest improvement in overall survival in HRPC patients compared to prior palliative mitoxantrone based chemotherapy.[25,26]
- Bisphosphonate therapy with zoledronic acid is a standard supportive-care agent for HRPC patients with bone metastases because of its ability to decrease the rate of skeletal fractures.[27]

BLADDER CANCER

EPIDEMIOLOGY

- More than 67,000 new cases of bladder cancer will occur in 2007, with more than 12,000 deaths.[1]
- Bladder cancer is the fifth most common new cancer diagnosed in the United States.[1]
- Smoking is by far the most significant risk factor for bladder cancer in the United States. Other risk factors include: male gender, white race, exposure to arylamine toxins (aniline dyes, leather tanning agents, rubber industry, etc), chronic schistosomal infection, chronic indwelling Foley catheters, and certain drugs (phenacetin and cyclophosphamide).[28]

CLINICAL PRESENTATION, DIAGNOSIS, AND STAGING

- Bladder cancer is a disease that occurs in older individuals with a median age at diagnosis of 73 years.[4]
- Hematuria is the most common presenting symptom. Dysuria, pelvic pain, urinary obstruction, fatigue, and weight loss can also be present.
- Bladder cancer should be considered in all males with microscopic hematuria.
- Malignancy can be confirmed by urine cytology. Direct visualization of the bladder mucosa by cystoscopy with transurethral resection of bladder tumor (TURBT) is needed to determine the depth of tumor invasion.
- Transitional cell carcinoma (also referred to as urothelial cell carcinoma) accounts for more than 90% of bladder cancers. Other rare histologic forms of bladder cancer include squamous cell, adenocarcinoma, small cell, and sarcomatoid variants.
- Superficial bladder cancer is defined as disease that does not penetrate the muscular layer of the bladder wall eg, known as the muscularis propria. No additional staging studies are required in patients with superficial disease.

- A summary of bladder cancer TNM staging is provided in Table 79–2.[5]
- Patients with muscle invasive bladder cancer (T2–T4) should have a chest x-ray as well as a CT scan of the abdomen and pelvis to rule out distant metastases.

LOCALIZED DISEASE

- **Superficial bladder cancer**
  - The clinical course of superficial bladder cancer is characterized by frequent recurrences requiring repeat cystoscopies with TURBT.
  - High-risk patients include those with multiple or recurrent high-grade Ta/T1 tumors or patients with de-novo carcinoma in situ. In such patients, recurrence is common. Progression to the muscle-invasive stage can occur in 40% of these patients, with death occurring in 20% to 30% of patients.[29–32]
  - Intravesical administration of Bacille Calmette-Guérin (BCG) decreases the frequency of tumor recurrences in high-risk patients, and slightly delays progression of disease to the muscle-invasive stage.[33,34] BCG has not shown an improvement in overall survival.
  - BCG-refractory patients with superficial bladder cancer can be treated with other intravesical agents such as mitomycin C, gemcitabine, or interferon. However, cystectomy provides the best chance for long-term cure.
- **Muscle invasive bladder cancer**
  - The presence of muscle-invasive disease on TURBT mandates aggressive treatment plans for optimal tumor control.
  - For select patients with a small bladder tumor and no evidence of carcinoma in situ, bladder-sparing approaches (ie, partial cystectomy, concurrent chemotherapy and EBRT) can be considered.
  - Most patients with muscle-invasive disease are best served by cystectomy.
  - Postcystectomy prognosis is highly dependent on final pathologic staging with a 5-year disease-free survival of 85% for organ-confined and lymph-node negative disease (T0–T3a), 58% for extravesical extension and lymph node negative disease (T3b–T4), and 35% for lymph node positive disease.[35]

ADJUVANT THERAPY

- The addition of adjuvant cisplatin-based chemotherapy following cystectomy in patients with positive lymph nodes or extravesical extension of tumor (T3–T4) provides an improved disease free survival.[36] A recent meta-analysis suggests a 9% absolute

TABLE 79–2 Bladder Cancer TNM Staging

T STAGE		DISTANT METASTASIS	
Tx	Primary tumor cannot be assessed	Mx	Distant metastasis cannot be assessed
T0	No evidence of primary tumor	M0	No distant metastasis
Ta	Noninvasive papillary carcinoma	M1	Distant metastasis
Tis	Carcinoma in situ: "flat tumor"		
T1	Tumor invades subepithelial connective tissue	**Stage groupings**	
T2	Tumor invades muscle		
T2a	Tumor invades superficial muscle (inner half)	Stage 0a	T1 N0 M0
T2b	Tumor invades deep muscle (outer half)	Stage 0is	Tis N0 M0
T3	Tumor invades perivesical tissue	Stage I	T1 N0 M0
T3a	Microscopically	Stage II	T2a N0 M0
			T2b N0 M0
T3b	Macroscopically (extravesical mass)	Stage III	T3a N0 M0
			T3b N0 M0
			T4a N0 M0
T4	Tumor invades any of the following: prostate, uterus, vagina, pelvic wall, abdominal wall	Stage IV	T4b N0 M0
			Any T N1 M0
			Any T N2 M0
			Any T N3 M0
			Any T Any N M1
T4a	Tumor invades prostate, uterus, vagina		
T4b	Tumor invades pelvic wall, abdominal wall		
Regional lymph nodes			
Nx	Regional lymph nodes cannot be assessed		
N0	No regional lymph node metastasis		
N1	Metastasis in a single lymph node, 2 cm or less in greatest dimension		
N2	Metastasis in a single lymph node, more than 2 cm but not more than 5 cm in greatest dimension; or multiple lymph nodes, none more than 5 cm in greatest dimension		
N3	Metastases in a lymph node, more than 5 cm in greatest dimension		

SOURCE: Used with the permission of the American Joint Committee on Cancer (AJCC), Chicago, Illinois. The original source for this material is the *AJCC Cancer Staging Manual*. 6th ed. New York, NY; Springer; 2002. www.springeronline.com.5.

improvement in overall survival with cisplatin-based adjuvant chemotherapy.[37]

• However, adjuvant chemotherapy studies have been small and underpowered. Therefore, these results should be viewed with caution. Larger more definitive studies are underway in Europe to confirm or refute these earlier studies.

• In the neoadjuvant setting, two meta-analyses have confirmed a 5% overall survival advantage with cisplatin based chemotherapy compared to cystectomy alone.[38,39]

METASTATIC DISEASE

• For patients with metastatic disease, standard therapy consists of cisplatin-based chemotherapy.

• Poor prognostic features for metastatic bladder cancer include a Karnofsky performance status (KPS) below 80 and the presence of visceral metastases (ie, lung, liver, bone).[40]

• In patients with lymph-node only metastatic disease with a KPS of 80 or above, 5-year overall survival approaches 21% with cisplatin and gemcitabine chemotherapy.[41]

KIDNEY CANCER

EPIDEMIOLOGY

• In 2007, more than 51,000 cases of new kidney cancer and more than 12,000 deaths caused by kidney cancer will occur in the United States.[1]

• The incidence of kidney cancer has steadily increased by 2% to 3% each year since the mid-1970s.[4]

• Risk factors for kidney cancer include: smoking, obesity, hypertension, chronic hemodialysis, and acquired cystic kidney disease.[42]

• Kidney cancer is associated with specific gene mutations found in several familial cancer syndromes including: von Hippel-Lindau syndrome (*VHL* gene chromosome 3p), hereditary papillary renal cancer syndrome (*MET* oncogene chromosome 7p), and Birt-Hogg-Dube syndrome (folliculin gene chromosome 17p11.2).[42]

- Aberrations in the *VHL* gene have also been noted in as many as 70% of sporadic kidney cancers.[43]

CLINICAL PRESENTATION, DIAGNOSIS, AND STAGING

- Similar to other urologic malignancies, kidney cancer affects older individuals with a median age at diagnosis of 65 years.[4]
- Common presenting symptoms include hematuria, flank pain, weight loss, shortness of breath, or fatigue.

- Kidney cancer can present with the manifestations of a paraneoplastic syndrome including: hypercalcemia, erythrocytosis, hypertension, and elevated liver function tests in the absence of liver metastases (Stauffer syndrome).
- Many kidney cancers today are initially discovered incidentally on CT scan imaging for other purposes. The standard staging studies for kidney cancer include a CT scan of the abdomen and pelvis and a chest x-ray. If the primary tumor extends beyond the renal capsule, a CT of the chest should also be included.
- Biopsy of a suspicious renal mass should not be performed as part of the standard workup. Surgical candidates should proceed directly to nephrectomy.
- A summary of kidney cancer staging is provided in Table 79–3.[5]

TABLE 79–3 Kidney Cancer TNM Staging

T STAGE		DISTANT METASTASIS	
Tx	Primary tumor cannot be assessed	Mx	Distant metastasis cannot be assessed
T0	No evidence of primary tumor	M0	No distant metastasis
T1	Tumor 7 cm or less in greatest dimension, limited to the kidney	M1	Distant metastasis
T1a	Tumor 4 cm or less in greatest dimension, limited to the kidney	**Stage groupings**	
T1b	Tumor more than 4 cm but not more than 7 cm in greatest dimension, limited to the kidney		
T2	Tumor more than 7 cm in greatest dimension, limited to the kidney	Stage I	T1 N0 M0
T3	Tumor extends into major veins or invades adrenal gland or perinephric tissues but not beyond Gerota fascia	Stage II	T2 N0 M0
T3a	Tumor directly invades adrenal gland or perirenal and/or renal sinus fat but not beyond Gerota fascia	Stage III	T1 N1 M0
			T2 N1 M0
			T3 N0 M0
			T3 N1 M0
			T3a N0 M0
			T3a N1 M0
			T3b N0 M0
			T3b N1 M0
			T3c N0 M0
			T3c N1 M0
T3b	Tumor grossly extends into the renal vein or its segmental (muscle-containing) branches, or vena cava below the diaphragm	Stage IV	T4 N0 M0
			T4 N1 M0
			Any T N2 M0
			Any T Any N M1
T3c	Tumor grossly extends into vena cava above diaphragm or invades the wall of the vena cava		
T4	Tumor invades beyond Gerota fascia		
Regional lymph nodes			
Nx	Regional lymph nodes cannot be assessed		
N0	No regional lymph node metastases		
N1	Metastases in a single regional lymph node		
N2	Metastases in more than one regional lymph node		

SOURCE: Used with the permission of the American Joint Committee on Cancer (AJCC), Chicago, Illinois. The original source for this material is the *AJCC Cancer Staging Manual.* 6th ed. New York, NY; Springer; 2002. www.springeronline.com.5.

- Histologically, clear cell renal cell carcinoma is the most common form (~70%), with papillary renal cell carcinoma (~10%–15%), chromophobe renal cell carcinoma (~5%), oncocytoma (~1%–2%), collecting duct carcinoma (~1%), and medullary carcinoma (~1%) occurring less frequently.[44]
- The clinical management of kidney cancer has been best defined for clear cell renal cell carcinomas.

LOCALIZED DISEASE

- For disease confined to the kidney, radical nephrectomy is the treatment of choice and provides a 5-year cancer specific survival rate of 74% to 91%. Even for disease that extends beyond the renal capsule, 5-year overall survival rates of 42% are achieved with surgical resection.[45]
- The role of extended lymph node dissection remains controversial.
- For high-risk surgical patients, tumors less than 3.5 cm in size can be managed with close observation with a low risk of metastases.[46]

ADJUVANT THERAPY

- Traditional cytotoxic chemotherapy agents provide no benefit in the adjuvant or neoadjuvant setting.
- Immunotherapeutic agents (ie, interleukin-2 [IL-2], interferon-alpha [IFN-α], vaccines) given as postnephrectomy adjuvant therapy have failed to demonstrate an advantage over nephrectomy alone.
- An intergroup study investigating the adjuvant role of antiangiogenic therapy (sunitinib, sorafenib) is ongoing.[47]

METASTATIC DISEASE

- Common sites of kidney cancer metastases include retroperitoneal and mediastinal lymph nodes, lung, bone, and brain.
- Metastatic tumors are often hypervascular and can cause significant bleeding.
- The prognosis of metastatic renal cell carcinoma is extremely variable. Poor prognostic factors include: anemia, hypercalcemia, no history of prior nephrectomy, KPS less than 80, and elevated lactate dehydrogenase. A median overall survival of 20 months, 10 months, and 4 months is observed in patients with zero, less than three, and three or more risk factors respectively.[48]
- Conventional chemotherapeutic agents have minimal activity.

- In rare cases (<5%), spontaneous regression of metastatic lesions has been documented suggesting a potential therapeutic role for immunotherapy.[49]
- Both IFN-α and IL-2 have been studied extensively. Partial responses are seen in 10% to 20% of patients. Both agents produce significant side effects including fever, fatigue, myalgias, cytopenias, depression, and edema. Although rare (~5%), only high-dose IL-2 has been shown to produce durable responses.
- Nephrectomy followed by IFN-α has been shown to provide a modest overall survival advantage (11 months vs 8 months) compared to IFN-α monotherapy.[50]
- In 2006, the oral vascular endothelial growth factor receptor (VEGFR) tyrosine kinase inhibitors, sorafenib and sunitinib, were approved for use in metastatic kidney cancer. Sunitinib demonstrated a progression-free survival advantage compared to IFN-α as a first-line agent.[51] Sorafenib has demonstrated a progression-free survival advantage compared to placebo as second-line therapy.[52] In addition, a new agent targeting the mammalian target of rapamycin (mTOR) named temsirolimus demonstrated an overall survival advantage compared to IFN-α in the first-line setting for poor risk metastatic renal cell carcinoma patients.[53] New treatment regimens combining immunotherapy and antiangiogenic agents are under intense investigation.

TESTICULAR CANCER

EPIDEMIOLOGY

- Testicular cancer is the most common malignancy among males between the ages of 20 and 44 years. In relation to all cancers, however, testicular cancer remains a rare malignancy with only 7900 new cases and 390 deaths expected in 2007.[4]
- Testicular cancer arises from embryologic germ cells that also reside in the gonads, retroperitoneum, anterior mediastinum, and pineal gland.
- Risk factors associated with testicular cancer include cryptorchidism, family history, Klinefelter syndrome, western European ancestry, and prior history of testicular cancer.[54–58]

CLINICAL PRESENTATION, DIAGNOSIS, AND STAGING

- Testicular cancer most commonly presents in young men as a painless testicular nodule or mass. Less often, patients can present with testicular pain, back pain, fatigue, shortness of breath, or hemoptysis.

- All testicular masses should be evaluated by testicular ultrasound and serum levels of α-fetoprotein (AFP) and β-human chorionic gonadotropin (β-hCG).
- Testicular biopsy is not routinely performed. The diagnosis should be confirmed by orchiectomy and pathologic examination of the affected testis. In extragonadal cases, a core biopsy of a retroperitoneal or mediastinal mass can also suffice. In difficult cases where AFP and β-hCG are normal, biopsy cytogenetics and fluorescent in situ hybridization (FISH) can be performed to identify an isochrome 12p [i(12p)] abnormality. This molecular signature is pathognomonic for germ cell tumors and is present in 85% of cases.[59]
- Patients should complete their staging with a CT scan of the abdomen and pelvis and a chest x-ray.
- Clinically, testicular cancers are grouped and managed as either seminoma (ie, pure seminoma on orchiectomy specimen or extragonadal core biopsy) or nonseminoma (can have a component of seminoma on biopsy, but other histologies are also present). The presence of an elevated AFP level confirms that a nonseminoma component is present, even if the original orchiectomy failed to demonstrate a nonseminoma histology.
- Several clinical staging systems have been proposed for testicular cancer. In simplest terms, stage I refers to disease confined to the testicle with normal serum markers following orchiectomy, stage II refers to disease that has spread to the retroperitoneal lymph nodes, and stage III refers to disease that has spread to distant organs (ie, lung, liver, bone). A summary of the American Joint Committee on Cancer (AJCC) staging of testicular cancer is shown in Table 79–4.[5]

CLINICAL STAGE I MANAGEMENT

- The prognosis for patients with clinical stage I disease is excellent with cure rates exceeding 95%.
- The treatment decisions following orchiectomy for clinical stage I disease must consider both patient concerns about potential relapse and the risk of subjecting patients to unnecessary treatment.
- For seminoma patients, postorchiectomy options include surveillance, prophylactic radiation, and prophylactic chemotherapy. With surveillance, 20% of patients will experience relapsed disease.[60] Risk factors for relapse include a tumor larger than 4 cm and invasion into the rete testis in the orchiectomy

specimen. Treatment with conventional platinum-based chemotherapy will cure almost all clinical stage I seminoma relapses. Both prophylactic para-aortic radiation and a single cycle of carboplatin chemotherapy have been shown to decrease the relapse rate to less than 5%.[61,62]
- For nonseminoma patients, postorchiectomy options include surveillance, retroperitoneal lymph node dissection, and prophylactic chemotherapy. With surveillance, 30% of patients will relapse.[60] Risk factors for recurrent disease include a predominance of embryonal carcinoma or lymphovascular invasion on orchiectomy specimen.[63] As in the case of seminoma, relapsed nonseminoma patients can expect excellent cure rates with traditional chemotherapy administered at the time of relapse. Retroperitoneal lymph node dissection provides cure in two-thirds of patients who have microscopic stage II disease.[64] More recently, the administration of one cycle of prophylactic bleomycin, etoposide, and cisplatin has been shown to decrease the relapse rate to 1%.[65]

ADVANCED DISEASE MANAGEMENT

- Advanced disease refers to testicular cancer that has spread beyond the testis to the retroperitoneal lymph nodes or distant organs.
- For nonbulky stage II seminoma (lymph nodes less than 5 cm), radiation therapy can provide cure in nearly 85% of cases.[66]
- For all other patients, systemic chemotherapy with three to four cycles of bleomycin, etoposide, and cisplatin (with or without bleomycin) is the standard of care.
- Advanced disease patients are risk-stratified based on several clinical features including: tumor marker levels, presence of nonpulmonary visceral metastases (ie, liver, brain, etc), and the presence of a nonseminoma primary mediastinal tumor.
- Even in patients with advanced disease, cure is possible in 92%, 80%, and 48% of patients in good-, intermediate-, and poor-risk categories, respectively.[67]
- For patients who relapse after systemic chemotherapy, high-dose chemotherapy with autologous stem cell transplant can cure up to 60% of patients.[68]
- For patients who achieve a complete response to chemotherapy, late relapse (recurrence more than 2 years from completion of therapy) occurs in 2% to 3% of patients. These patients are chemorefractory; some can still achieve cure with surgical resection of all remaining disease.[69]

TABLE 79–4   Testicular Cancer TNM Staging

T STAGE		DISTANT METASTASIS	
pTx	Primary tumor cannot be assessed	Mx	Distant metastasis cannot be assessed
pT0	No evidence of primary tumor (eg, histologic scar in testis)	M0	No distant metastasis
pTis	Intratubular germ cell neoplasia (carcinoma in situ)	M1	Distant metastasis
pT1	Tumor limited to the testis and epididymis without vascular/lymphatic invasion; tumor may invade into the tunica albuginea but not the tunica vaginalis	M1a	Nonregional nodal or pulmonary metastasis
pT2	Tumor limited to the testis and epididymis with vascular/lymphatic invasion, or tumor extending through the tunica albuginea with involvement of the tunica vaginalis	M1b	Distant metastasis other than nonregional lymph nodes and lungs
pT3	Tumor invades the spermatic cord with or without vascular/lymphatic invasion		
pT4	Tumor invades the scrotum with or without vascular/lymphatic invasion	**Serum tumor markers**	
		Sx	Marker studies not available or not performed
Regional lymph nodes		S0	Marker study levels within normal limits
Clinical		S1	LDH $<1.5 \times$ ULN and HCG <5000 (mIU/mL) and AFP <1000 (ng/mL)
Nx	Regional lymph nodes cannot be assessed	S2	LDH $1.5–10 \times$ ULN or HCG 5000–50,000 (mIU/mL) or AFP 1000–10,000 (ng/mL)
N0	No regional lymph node metastasis	S3	LDH $>10 \times$ ULN or HCG $>50,000$ (mIU/mL) or AFP $> 10,000$ (ng/mL)
N1	Metastasis with a lymph node mass 2 cm or less in greatest dimension; or multiple lymph nodes, none more than 2 cm in greatest dimension		
N2	Metastasis with a lymph node mass more than 2 cm but not more than 5 cm in greatest dimension; or multiple lymph nodes, any one mass greater than 2 cm but not more than 5 cm in greatest dimension		
N3	Metastasis with a lymph node mass more than 5 cm in greatest dimension		
Pathologic			
pNx	Regional lymph nodes cannot be assessed		
pN0	No regional lymph node metastasis		
pN1	Metastasis with a lymph node mass 2 cm or less in greatest dimension and less than or equal to 5 nodes positive, none more than 2 cm in greatest dimension		
pN2	Metastasis with a lymph node mass more than 2 cm but not more than 5 cm in greatest dimension; or more than 5 nodes positive, none more than 5 cm; or evidence of extranodal extension of tumor		
pN3	Metastasis with a lymph node mass more than 5 cm in greatest dimension		
Stage groupings			
Stage 0	pTis N0 M0 S0	Stage III	Any pT/Tx Any N M1 Sx
Stage I	pT1–4 N0 M0 Sx	Stage IIIA	Any pT/Tx Any N M1a S0
			Any pT/Tx Any N M1a S1
Stage IA	pT1 N0 M0 S0	Stage IIIB	Any pT/Tx N1–3 M0 S2
			Any pT/Tx Any N M1a S2
Stage IB	pT2 N0 M0 S0	Stage IIIC	Any pT/Tx N1–3 M0 S3
	pT3 N0 M0 S0		Any pT/Tx Any N M1a S3
	pT4 N0 M0 S0		Any pT/Tx Any N M1b Any S

(Continued)

TABLE 79–4 Testicular Cancer TNM Staging (Continued)

T STAGE		DISTANT METASTASIS
Stage IS	Any pT/Tx N0 M0 S1–3	
Stage II	Any pT/Tx N1–3 M0 Sx	
Stage IIA	Any pT/Tx N1 M0 S0	
	Any pT/Tx N1 M0 S1	
Stage IIB	Any pT/Tx N2 M0 S0	
	Any pT/Tx N2 M0 S1	
Stage IIC	Any pT/Tx N3 M0 S0	
	Any pT/Tx N3 M0 S1	

AFP, α-fetoprotein; HCG, human chorionic gonadotropin; LDH, lactate dehydrogenase; ULN, upper limits of normal.
SOURCE: Used with the permission of the American Joint Committee on Cancer (AJCC), Chicago, Illinois. The original source for this material is the *AJCC Cancer Staging Manual*. 6th ed. New York, NY; Springer; 2002. www.springeronline.com.5.

REFERENCES

1. Jemal A, Siegel R, Ward E, Murray T, et al. Cancer statistics, 2007. *CA Cancer J Clin.* Jan-Feb 2007;57(1):43–66.

2. Routh JC, Leibovich BC. Adenocarcinoma of the prostate: Epidemiological trends, screening, diagnosis, and surgical management of localized disease. *Mayo Clin Proc.* Jul 2005;80(7):899–907.

3. American Cancer Society. *Cancer Facts & Figures for African Americans 2005–2006.* Atlanta, GA: American Cancer Society; 2005.

4. Ries L, Harkins D, Krapcho M, et al. SEER Cancer Statistics Review, 1975–2003. http://seer.cancer.gov/csr/1975_2003/. Accessed November, 2005.

5. Greene F, Page D, Fleming I. *AJCC Cancer Staging Manual.* 6th ed. New York, NY: Springer; 2002.

6. Partin AW, Kattan MW, Subong EN, et al. Combination of prostate-specific antigen, clinical stage, and Gleason score to predict pathological stage of localized prostate cancer. A multi-institutional update [see comment][erratum appears in JAMA 1997;278(2):118]. *JAMA.* May 14, 1997;277(18):1445–1451.

7. NCCN Clinical Practice Guidelines in Oncology Prostate Cancer v 1.2007. Accessed February 3, 2007, 2007. www.nccn.org

8. Chodak GW, Thisted RA, Gerber GS, et al. Results of conservative management of clinically localized prostate cancer [see comment]. *N Engl J Med.* Jan 27, 1994;330(4):242–248.

9. Hull GW, Rabbani F, Abbas F, et al. Cancer control with radical prostatectomy alone in 1,000 consecutive patients. *J Urol.* Feb 2002;167 (2 pt 1):528–534.

10. Bill-Axelson A, Holmberg L, Ruutu M, et al. Radical prostatectomy versus watchful waiting in early prostate cancer [see comment]. *N Engl J Med.* May 12, 2005;352(19):1977–1984.

11. Steineck G, Helgesen F, Adolfsson J, et al. Quality of life after radical prostatectomy or watchful waiting [see comment]. *N Engl J Med.* Sep 12, 2002;347(11):790–796.

12. Stanford JL, Feng Z, Hamilton AS, et al. Urinary and sexual function after radical prostatectomy for clinically localized prostate cancer: The Prostate Cancer Outcomes Study [see comment]. *JAMA.* Jan 19, 2000;283(3):354–360.

13. Rabbani F, Stapleton AM, Kattan MW, et al. Factors predicting recovery of erections after radical prostatectomy.[see comment]. *J Urol.* Dec 2000;164(6):1929–1934.

14. Shipley WU, Thames HD, Sandler HM, et al. Radiation therapy for clinically localized prostate cancer: A multi-institutional pooled analysis. *JAMA.* May 5, 1999;281(17):1598–1604.

15. Zelefsky MJ, Cowen D, Fuks Z, et al. Long-term tolerance of high dose three-dimensional conformal radiotherapy in patients with localized prostate carcinoma. *Cancer.* Jun 1, 1999;85(11):2460–2468.

16. Cooperberg MR, Grossfeld GD, Lubeck DP, Carroll PR. National practice patterns and time trends in androgen ablation for localized prostate cancer [see comment]. *J Natl Cancer Inst.* Jul 2, 2003;95(13):981–989.

17. Janoff DM, Peterson C, Mongoue-Tchokote S, et al. Clinical outcomes of androgen deprivation as the sole therapy for localized and locally advanced prostate cancer. *BJU Int.* Sep 2005;96(4):503–507.

18. Messing EM, Manola J, Yao J, et al. Immediate versus deferred androgen deprivation treatment in patients with node-positive prostate cancer after radical prostatectomy and pelvic lymphadenectomy. *Lancet Oncology.* Jun 2006; 7(6):472–479.

19. Bolla M, van Poppel H, Collette L, et al. Postoperative radiotherapy after radical prostatectomy: A randomised controlled trial (EORTC trial 22911) [see comment]. *Lancet.* Aug 13–19, 2005;366(9485):572–578.

20. Thompson IM, Jr., Tangen CM, Paradelo J, et al. Adjuvant radiotherapy for pathologically advanced prostate cancer: A randomized clinical trial. *JAMA.* Nov 15, 2006;296(19):2329–2335.

21. Bolla M, Gonzalez D, Warde P, et al. Improved survival in patients with locally advanced prostate cancer treated with radiotherapy and goserelin.[see comment]. *N Engl J Med.* Jul 31, 1997;337(5):295–300.

22. Hanks GE, Pajak TF, Porter A, et al. Phase III trial of long-term adjuvant androgen deprivation after neoadjuvant hormonal cytoreduction and radiotherapy in locally advanced carcinoma of the prostate: the Radiation Therapy Oncology Group Protocol 92–02 [erratum appears in *J Clin Oncol.* 2004; 22(2):386]. *J Clin Oncol.* Nov 1, 2003;21(21):3972–3978.

23. Pilepich MV, Winter K, Lawton CA, et al. Androgen suppression adjuvant to definitive radiotherapy in prostate carcinoma—long-term results of phase III RTOG 85–31.[see comment]. *Int J Radiat Oncol Biol Phys.* Apr 1, 2005;61(5):1285–1290.

24. Pound CR, Partin AW, Eisenberger MA, et al. Natural history of progression after PSA elevation following radical prostatectomy [see comment]. *JAMA.* May 5, 1999;281(17): 1591–1597.

25. Petrylak DP, Tangen CM, Hussain MHA, et al. Docetaxel and estramustine compared with mitoxantrone and prednisone for advanced refractory prostate cancer [see comment]. *N Engl J Med.* Oct 7, 2004;351(15):1513–1520.

26. Tannock IF, de Wit R, Berry WR, et al. Docetaxel plus prednisone or mitoxantrone plus prednisone for advanced prostate cancer [see comment]. *N Engl J Med.* Oct 7, 2004;351(15):1502–1512.

27. Saad F, Gleason DM, Murray R, et al. Long-term efficacy of zoledronic acid for the prevention of skeletal complications in patients with metastatic hormone-refractory prostate cancer.[see comment]. *J Natl Cancer Inst.* Jun 2, 2004;96(11): 879–882.

28. Ross RK, Yu MC, Yuan J-M. The epidemiology of bladder cancer. In: Vogelzang NJ, Scardino PT, Shipley WU, Debruyne FM, Linehan WM, eds. *Comprehensive Textbook of Genitourinary Oncology.* 3rd ed. Philadelphia, PA: Lippincott Williams & Wilkins; 2006:357–363.

29. Cookson MS, Herr HW, Zhang ZF, et al. The treated natural history of high risk superficial bladder cancer: 15-year outcome. *J Urol.* Jul 1997;158(1): 62–67.

30. Heney NM, Ahmed S, Flanagan MJ, et al. Superficial bladder cancer: Progression and recurrence. *J Urol.* Dec 1983;130(6): 1083–1086.

31. Kurth KH, Denis L, Bouffioux C, et al. Factors affecting recurrence and progression in superficial bladder tumours. *Eur J Cancer.* Oct 1995;31A(11):1840–1846.

32. Millan-Rodriguez F, Chechile-Toniolo G, Salvador-Bayarri J, et al. Primary superficial bladder cancer risk groups according to progression, mortality and recurrence [see comment]. *J Urol.* Sep 2000;164(3 pt 1):680–684.

33. Bohle A, Bock PR. Intravesical bacille Calmette-Guérin versus mitomycin C in superficial bladder cancer: Formal meta-analysis of comparative studies on tumor progression [see comment]. *Urology.* Apr 2004;63(4):682–686; discussion 686–687.

34. Sylvester RJ, van der Meijden APM, Lamm DL. Intravesical bacillus Calmette-Guérin reduces the risk of progression in patients with superficial bladder cancer: A meta-analysis of the published results of randomized clinical trials. *J Urol.* Nov 2002;168(5):1964–1970.

35. Stein JP, Lieskovsky G, Cote R, et al. Radical cystectomy in the treatment of invasive bladder cancer: Long-term results in 1,054 patients. *J Clin Oncol.* Feb 1, 2001;19(3):666–675.

36. Kruz M, Sasse E, Sasse A, et al. Adjuvant chemotherapy for muscle invasive bladder cancer: A systematic review and meta-analysis. *J Clin Oncol.* Jun 1, 2005;23(suppl 16S pt I): 4733.

37. Advanced Bladder Cancer Meta-Analysis C. Adjuvant chemotherapy in invasive bladder cancer: A systematic review and meta-analysis of individual patient data Advanced Bladder Cancer (ABC) Meta-analysis Collaboration. *Euro Urol.* Aug 2005;48(2):189–199; discussion 199–201.

38. Advanced Bladder Cancer Meta-Analysis C. Neoadjuvant chemotherapy in invasive bladder cancer: A systematic

39. Advanced Bladder Cancer Meta-Analysis C. Neoadjuvant chemotherapy in invasive bladder cancer: Update of a systematic review and meta-analysis of individual patient data advanced bladder cancer (ABC) meta-analysis collaboration. *Eur Urol.* Aug 2005;48(2):202–205; discussion 205–206.

40. Bajorin DF, Dodd PM, Mazumdar M, et al. Long-term survival in metastatic transitional-cell carcinoma and prognostic factors predicting outcome of therapy. *J Clin Oncol.* Oct 1999; 17(10):3173–3181.

41. von der Maase H, Sengelov L, Roberts JT, et al. Long-term survival results of a randomized trial comparing gemcitabine plus cisplatin, with methotrexate, vinblastine, doxorubicin, plus cisplatin in patients with bladder cancer. *J Clin Oncol.* Jul 20, 2005;23(21):4602–4608.

42. Chow W-H, Devesa SS, Moore LE. Epidemiology of renal cell carcinoma. In: Vogelzang NJ, Scardino PT, Shipley WU, Debruyne FM, Linehan WM, eds. *Comprehensive Textbook of Genitourinary Oncology.* 3rd ed. Philadelphia, PA: Lippincott Williams & Wilkins; 2006:669–679.

43. Clifford SC, Prowse AH, Affara NA, et al. Inactivation of the von Hippel-Lindau (VHL) tumour suppressor gene and allelic losses at chromosome arm 3p in primary renal cell carcinoma: Evidence for a VHL-independent pathway in clear cell renal tumorigenesis. *Genes Chromosomes Cancer.* Jul 1998;22(3): 200–209.

44. Murphy WB, Grignon DJ, Perlman EJ. Tumors of the kidney, bladder, and related urinary structures. In: *AFIP Atlas of Tumor Pathology.* Vol fascicle 1. Washington, DC: American Registry of Pathology; 2004:101–175.

45. Tsui KH, Shvarts O, Smith RB, et al. Prognostic indicators for renal cell carcinoma: A multivariate analysis of 643 patients using the revised 1997 TNM staging criteria. *J Urol.* Apr 2000;163(4):1090–1095; quiz 1295.

46. Bosniak MA, Birnbaum BA, Krinsky GA, et al. Small renal parenchymal neoplasms: Further observations on growth [see comment]. *Radiology.* Dec 1995;197(3): 589–597.

47. Wood CG. Multimodal approaches in the management of locally advanced and metastatic renal cell carcinoma: Combining surgery and systemic therapies to improve patient outcome. *Clin Cancer Res.* Jan 15, 2007;13(2):697s–702.

48. Motzer RJ, Mazumdar M, Bacik J, et al. Survival and prognostic stratification of 670 patients with advanced renal cell carcinoma. *J Clin Oncol.* Aug 1, 1999;17(8): 2530–2543.

49. Oliver RT, Nethersell AB, Bottomley JM. Unexplained spontaneous regression and alpha-interferon as treatment for metastatic renal carcinoma. *Br J Urol.* Feb 1989;63(2): 128–131.

50. Flanigan RC, Salmon SE, Blumenstein BA, et al. Nephrectomy followed by interferon alfa-2b compared with interferon alfa-2b alone for metastatic renal-cell cancer. *N Engl J Med.* Dec 6, 2001;345(23):1655–1659.

51. Motzer RJ, Hutson TE, Tomczak P, et al. Sunitinib versus interferon alfa in metastatic renal-cell carcinoma. *N Engl J Med.* Jan 11, 2007;356(2):115–124.

52. Escudier B, Eisen T, Stadler WM, et al. Sorafenib in advanced clear-cell renal-cell carcinoma. *N Engl J Med.* Jan 11, 2007;356(2):125–134.

53. Hudes G, Carducci M, Tomczak P, et al. A phase III randomized, three-arm study of temsirolimus (TEMSR) or interferon-alpha (IFN) or the combination of TEMSR + IFN in the treatment of first-line, poor-risk patients with advanced renal cell carcinoma (adv RCC). *J Clin Oncol.* Jun 20, 2006;24(18S suppl pt 1):LBA4.

54. Parkin DM, Bray F, Ferlay J, et al. Global cancer statistics, 2002. *CA Cancer J Clin.* Mar 1, 2005;55(2):74–108.

55. Rapley EA, Crockford GP, Easton DF, et al. International testicular cancer linkage C. Localisation of susceptibility genes for familial testicular germ cell tumour. *APMIS.* Jan 2003; 111(1):128–133; discussion 133–125.

56. Strader CH, Weiss NS, Daling JR, et al. Cryptorchism, orchiopexy, and the risk of testicular cancer. *Am J Epidemiol.* May 1988;127(5):1013–1018.

57. Volkl TMK, Langer T, Aigner T, et al. Klinefelter syndrome and mediastinal germ cell tumors. *Am J Med Gen A.* Mar 1, 2006;140(5):471–481.

58. Wanderas EH, Fossa SD, Tretli S. Risk of a second germ cell cancer after treatment of a primary germ cell cancer in 2201 Norwegian male patients. *Eur J Cancer.* Feb 1997;33(2): 244–252.

59. Houldsworth J, Bosl GJ, Chaganti R. Biology and genetics of adult male germ cell tumors. In: Vogelzang NJ, Scardino PT, Shipley WU, Debruyne FM, Linehan WM, eds. *Comprehensive Textbook of Genitourinary Oncology.* 3rd ed. Philadelphia, PA: Lippincott Williams & Wilkins; 2006:563–571.

60. Hahn NM, Sweeney CJ. Germ cell tumors: An update of recent data and review of active protocols in stage I and metastatic disease. *Urol Oncol.* Jul-Aug 2005;23(4):293–302.

61. Jones WG, Fossa SD, Mead GM, et al. Randomized trial of 30 versus 20 Gy in the adjuvant treatment of stage I testicular seminoma: A report on Medical Research Council Trial TE18 European Organisation for the Research and Treatment of Cancer Trial 30942 (ISRCTN18525328) [see comment]. *J Clin Oncol.* Feb 20, 2005;23(6):1200–1208.

62. Oliver RTD, Mason MD, Mead GM, et al. Radiotherapy versus single-dose carboplatin in adjuvant treatment of stage I seminoma: A randomised trial [see comment]. *Lancet.* Jul 23–29, 2005;366(9482):293–300.

63. Leibovitch I, Foster RS, Kopecky KK, et al. Identification of clinical stage A nonseminomatous testis cancer patients at extremely low risk for metastatic disease: A combined approach using quantitative immunohistochemical, histopathologic, and radiologic assessment. *J Clin Oncol.* Jan 1998;16(1):261–268.

64. Sweeney CJ, Hermans BP, Heilman DK, et al. Results and outcome of retroperitoneal lymph node dissection for clinical stage I embryonal carcinoma-predominant testis cancer. *J Clin Oncol.* Jan 14, 2000;18(2):358–366.

65. Albers P, Siener R, Krege S, et al. One course of adjuvant PEB chemotherapy versus retroperitoneal lymph node dissection in patients with stage I non-seminomatous germ-cell tumors (NSGCT): Results of the German Prospective Multicenter Trial (Association of Urological Oncology [AUO]/German testicular cancer study group [GTCSG] Trial 01–94). *J Clin Oncol.* Jun 20, 2006;24(pt 1 suppl 18S):4512.

66. Zagars GK, Pollack A. Radiotherapy for stage II testicular seminoma. *Int J Radiat Oncol Biol Phys.* Nov 1, 2001;51(3):643–649.

67. International Germ Cell Cancer Collaborative Group. International Germ Cell Consensus Classification: A prognostic factor- based staging system for metastatic germ cell cancers. *J Clin Oncol.* Feb 1, 1997;15(2):594–603.

68. Einhorn L, Williams S, R A. Salvage chemotherapy with high dose carboplatin + etoposide (HDCE) and peripheral blood stem cell transplant (PBSCT) in patients with germ cell tumors (GCT). *J Clin Oncol.* Jun 20, 2006;24(pt I suppl 18S):4549.

69. Baniel J, Foster RS, Einhorn LH, Donohue JP. Late relapse of clinical stage I testicular cancer [see comment]. *J Urol.* Oct 1995;154(4):1370–1372.

80 GYNECOLOGIC CANCERS

Sara E. Crowder and Michael C. Perry

There are three gynecologic malignancies likely to be seen by primary care physicians: ovarian cancer, endometrial cancer, and cervical cancer. Gestational trophoblastic disease and vulvar cancer, rarer problems, will not be discussed.

OVARIAN CANCER

Ovarian cancer is the second most common gynecologic malignancy, the most common cause of death among women with gynecologic malignancies, and the fifth leading cause of cancer death in women in the United States.[1] Approximately 22,430 American women will be diagnosed with ovarian cancer during 2007, and an estimated 15,280 will die of their disease. Because of the vague nature of its symptoms, and the lack of a useful screening regimen, most patients are diagnosed in late stages and the cure rate is correspondingly low.

Ovarian cancer patients are typically older than 50 years of age and the incidence increases with age, with a peak incidence of 54 per 100,000 in patients 75 to 79 years of age. Older women have poorer outcomes, perhaps due to less aggressive treatment.

Although there are no specific symptoms to suggest ovarian cancer, most affected patients have nonspecific symptoms such as lower abdominal pressure or discomfort, gas, bloating, constipation, menstrual irregularities, low back pain, nausea, or fatigue. Since these symptoms are nonspecific, ovarian cancer is likely missed during the initial evaluation.

Epithelial ovarian cancers typically spread intraperitoneally with drop metastases and carcinomatosis, but they can also undergo lymphatic and occasionally hematogenous spread. The majority of the patients present with a distended abdomen and omental caking.

Physical examination may reveal a solid, fixed mass, and if tumor has spread, ascites, and/or pleural effusions. Computed tomography (CT) scans of the abdomen and pelvis are also helpful to delineate the extent of disease prior to surgery. Evaluation should include a serum CA-125 level, imaging with CT and/or ultrasound and prompt referral to a gynecologic oncologist.

Ovarian cancers may arise from four different cell lines: (1) Epithelial ovarian cancers (serous [75% of all ovarian cancers], mucinous, endometrioid, clear cell, Brenner tumors, and carcinosarcomas [mixed Müllerian tumors]) arise from the epithelial lining covering the ovary and are contiguous with the parietal peritoneum, (2) Nonepithelial tumors arise from the germ cells (dysgerminoma, yolk sac, embryonal carcinoma, choriocarcinoma, teratoma), (3) gonadal stroma (granulosa cell, thecoma, fibroma, Sertoli cell, Sertoli-Leydig, steroid), and (4) the nonspecific mesenchyme. Nonepithelial tumors require more specialized management.

The ovary may also be the site of metastases from other primary sites such as the stomach (Krukenberg tumors), colon, breast, and endometrium, or from non-Hodgkin lymphomas.

There are three special circumstances in the differential diagnosis of ovarian cancer that must be considered.

(1) Low malignant potential or borderline tumors may resemble ovarian carcinomas, although they often present at a younger age and a lower stage. They may be treated conservatively with preservation of the uterus and contralateral ovary. Full surgical staging is frequently performed when the diagnosis is acquired on a frozen section, because up to half will actually have invasive pathology on permanent sections. Borderline tumors usually do not require adjuvant therapy, but may present with late recurrences 10 to 20 years later.

(2) Primary peritoneal carcinoma, arising from the coelomic epithelium of the peritoneum, presents like ovarian cancer, and can occur even when the ovaries have been removed. Staging, treatment, and prognosis are the same as epithelial ovarian cancer.

(3) Fallopian tube cancers are rare, present much like ovarian cancer, and are treated in an identical fashion.

The diagnosis of ovarian cancer is established by pathologic examination of a surgical specimen. Patients who present with ascites may be diagnosed via paracentesis but will usually require surgery as a component of definitive therapy. Transcutaneous needle biopsy of a pelvic mass is discouraged because of the risk of abdominal wall seeding or tumor spread.

Staging is carried out with CT scans of the abdomen and pelvis, serum CA-125 tumor marker levels, and by surgical exploration.

The primary treatment of epithelial ovarian cancer is surgical resection (debulking) followed by chemotherapy. In selected cases, there may be a role for neoadjuvant chemotherapy. The surgery should be performed by a gynecologic oncologist. The surgery typically involves a total abdominal hysterectomy, bilateral salpingo-oophorectomy, omentectomy, washings, peritoneal biopsies, and pelvic and paraaortic node sampling with a concerted effort to debulk the tumor to the smallest residual disease. Those patients who have no single residual tumor mass greater than two centimeters are considered optimally debulked, and carry an improved prognosis.

Properly staged IA or IB, histologic grade 1 or 2 patients only require surgical excision. All others should receive postoperative chemotherapy. Chemotherapy is usually comprised of the combination of paclitaxel and carboplatin (or cisplatin) and may include intraperitoneal chemotherapy. Follow-up is performed every 3 months, with serum CA-125 levels as an adjunct to physical examination and CT scans of the abdomen and pelvis.

Most patients will initially respond to chemotherapy and then relapse, and thus be candidates for second-line chemotherapy. If the relapse occurs within 6 months of platinum based therapy the disease is considered platinum-resistant. If longer than 6 months has elapsed since chemotherapy, the disease may be considered platinum sensitive and the patient retreated with a platinum containing regimen. Second-line chemotherapy includes gemcitabine, topotecan, liposomal doxorubicin, oral etoposide, vinorelbine, and hexamethylmelamine; but the likelihood of a prolonged response is <10%. Many patients receive multiple different chemotherapeutic agents in succession.

Over the last 25 years, the 5-year survival rate has improved modestly from 37% in the early 1970s to 44% by year 2000.[1] Five-year survival rates by stage are: stage I-76% to 93%, stage II-60% to 74%, stage IIA-41%, stage IIIB-25%, stage IIIC-23%, and stage IV 11% (see Table 80–1).[2]

ENDOMETRIAL CANCER

Cancer of the endometrium is the most common gynecologic cancer and the fourth most common cancer in women. In 2007, it is estimated that there will be 39,080 cases and 7400 deaths. Since postmenopausal vaginal bleeding is a common symptom, many women are diagnosed early and cured with appropriate therapy. Endometrial cancer is a disease of middle-aged or older

TABLE 80–1 FIGO Staging for Primary Carcinoma of the Ovary*

Stage I	Growth limited to the ovaries
Stage IA	Growth limited to one ovary; no ascites containing malignant cells. No tumor on the external surface; capsule intact.
Stage IB	Growth limited to both ovaries; no ascites containing malignant cells. No tumor on the external surfaces; capsules intact.
Stage IC[a]	Tumor either stage Ia or Ib but with tumor on the surface of one or both ovaries; or with capsule ruptured; or with ascites present containing malignant cells or with positive peritoneal washings.
Stage II	Growth involving one or both ovaries with pelvic extension.
Stage IIA	Extension and/or metastases to the uterus and/or tubes.
Stage IIB	Extension to other pelvic tissues.
Stage IIC[a]	Tumor either stage IIa or IIb, but with tumor on the surface of one or both ovaries; or with capsule(s) ruptured; or with ascites present containing malignant cells or with positive peritoneal washings.
Stage III	Tumor involving one or both ovaries with peritoneal implants outside the pelvis and/or positive retroperitoneal or inguinal nodes. Superficial liver metastasis equals stage III. Tumor is limited to the true pelvis, but with histologically proven malignant extension to small bowel or omentum.
Stage IIIA	Tumor grossly limited to the true pelvis with negative nodes but with histologically confirmed microscopic seeding of abdominal peritoneal surfaces.
Stage IIIB	Tumor of one or both ovaries with histologically confirmed implants of abdominal peritoneal surfaces, none exceeding 2 cm in diameter. Nodes negative.
Stage IIIC	Abdominal implants >2 cm in diameter and/or positive retroperitoneal or inguinal nodes.
Stage IV	Growth involving one or both ovaries with distant metastasis. If pleural effusion is present, there must be positive cytologic test results to allot a case to stage IV. Parenchymal liver metastasis equals stage IV.

*These categories are based on findings at clinical examination or surgical exploration. The histological characteristics are to be considered in the staging, as are results of cytologic testing as far as effusions are concerned. It is desirable that a biopsy be performed on suspect areas outside the pelvis.

[a]To evaluate the impact on prognosis of the different criteria for allotting cases to stage IC or IIC, it would be of value to know if rupture of the capsule was (a) spontaneous or (b) caused by the surgeon, and if the source of malignant cells detected was (a) peritoneal washings or (b) ascites.

Used with the permission of the American Joint Committee on Cancer (AJCC), Chicago, Illinois. The original source for this material is the *AJCC Cancer Staging Manual*. 6th ed. (2002) published by Springer-Verlag New York, Inc.

woman and the median age at diagnosis is 61 years: 75% of patients are postmenopausal.

Hyperestrogenism is believed to be responsible for most endometrial cancers, whether derived from obesity, early menarche, late menopause, nulliparity, or a history of anovulatory menstrual cycles. Diabetes mellitus appears to confer a separate risk. The use of the antiestrogen tamoxifen for breast cancer increases the risk of developing endometrial cancer. Endometrial cancer may be hereditary, associated with the breast cancer antigen genes, BRCA1 or BRCA2, or as part of the Lynch Syndrome, (hereditary nonpolyposis colorectal cancer [HNPCC], Cancer Family Syndrome)

The most common histology is endometrioid adenocarcinoma. The rarer papillary serous and clear cell carcinomas do not appear to be estrogen dependent and carry a worse prognosis. Papillary serous carcinomas may present with a metastatic pattern mimicking ovarian cancer.

The typical clinical scenario involves an obese white woman with postmenopausal bleeding. Up to 20% of postmenopausal bleeding, unrelated to hormonal therapy is due to endometrial cancer. Premenopausal

women are more likely to have a history of endometrial hyperplasia and present with dysfunctional uterine bleeding. Metastases to the vagina, adnexa, pelvic and paraaortic lymph nodes, and lungs may occur.

The diagnosis is established by histologic examination of an endometrial curetting, from either office sampling with a Pipelle or a dilation and curettage.

Staging is done using the Federation Internationale de Gynecologie et d'Obstetrique (FIGO) system (Table 80–2). At surgery total abdominal hysterectomy and bilateral salpingo-oophorectomy is performed with peritoneal washings, as a minimum. Lymph node sampling may be done depending upon the tumor grade, histologic type, extent of the tumor spread, depth of invasion, and involvement of the uterine cervix. CT scans are not required, but a CA-125 level may be useful to assess and monitor the extent of the disease.

Surgery may be considered even when there is metastatic disease to improve local control of symptoms such as pain or bleeding. Adjuvant radiation therapy may be of benefit to those patients with localized disease and high-risk disease such as grade 3 histology, positive lymph nodes, and deep invasion. Radiation

TABLE 80–2   Staging of Endometrial Cancer

TNM STAGE	FIGO[a] STAGES	DEFINITION
TX		Primary tumor cannot be assessed
T0		No evidence of primary tumor
Tis		Carcinoma in situ
T1	I	Tumor confined to corpus uteri
T1a	IA	Tumor limited to endometrium
T1b	IB	Tumor invades up to or less than one-half of the myometrium
T1c	IC	Tumor invades to more than one-half of the myometrium
T2	II	Tumor invades cervix but does not extend beyond uterus
T2a	IIA	Endocervical glandular involvement only
T2b	IIB	Cervical stromal invasion
T3	III	Local and/or regional spread as specified in T3a, b, and/or N1 and FIGO IIIA, B, and C below
T3a	IIIA	Tumor involves uterine serosa and/or adnexa (direct extension or metastasis) [often termed stage IIIA2] and/or cancer cells in ascites or peritoneal washings [stage IIIA1]
T3b	IIIB	Vaginal involvement (direct extension or metastasis)
N1	IIIC	Metastasis to the pelvic and/or paraaortic lymph nodes
T4	IVA	Tumor invades bladder mucosa and/or bowel mucosa (Bullous edema is not sufficient to classify a tumor as T4)
M1	IVB	Distant metastasis. (Excluding metastasis to vagina, pelvic serosa, or adnexa. Including metastasis to intraabdominal lymph nodes other than paraaortic, and/or inguinal lymph nodes)

[a]FIGO, Federation Internationale de Gynecologie et d'Obstetrique.
Used with the permission of the American Joint Committee on Cancer (AJCC), Chicago, Illinois. The original source for this material is the *AJCC Cancer Staging Manual*. 6th ed. New York: Springer-Verlag; 2002.

therapy is also the treatment of choice for surgically or medically inoperable patients.

Chemotherapy is used for recurrent or metastatic disease, and has an emerging role as adjuvant therapy. Well differentiated tumors and/or those positive for estrogen and progesterone receptors may respond to progestins. Although there are several single agents with activity against endometrial cancer, chemotherapy is usually given in combination, particularly paclitaxel/ carboplatin or doxorubicin/cisplatin.

The prognosis of most endometrial cancer patients is good when the diagnosis is established early. Typical 5-year survival rates are 94% for stage IA, 95% for stage IB, 75% for stage IC, 60% for stage II, 40% for stage III, and 5% for stage IV.

CERVICAL CANCER

While there will be approximately 11,150 cases of cervical cancer in the United States this year with about 3670 deaths, cervical cancer is a considerably larger problem world-wide, especially in underdeveloped countries where routine Pap smears are not performed. Almost all cervical cancers are caused by the human papilloma virus (HPV), which is transmitted through sexual intercourse. High-risk HPV subtypes such as 16 and 18 have been linked to premalignant and malignant lesions, while low risk subtypes cause benign lesions such as genital warts. The typical patient is a woman age 45 to 55 years of age who has had multiple sexual partners, often from an early age, and is of lower socio-economic class. Smoking and chronic immunosuppression are also risk factors.

Nearly 90% of cervical cancers are squamous cell cancers, while the remaining 10% are adenocarcinomas. Most patients are diagnosed via an abnormal Pap smear. More advanced lesions may be associated with a vaginal discharge or abnormal bleeding. The tumor typically spreads by direct extension; lymphatic dissemination or hematogenous dissemination is infrequent. Advanced lesions that have spread to the pelvic sidewall produce pelvic pain, dyspareunia, sciatica, leg edema, or flank pain from hydronephrosis. More extensive disease may involve the bladder or rectum.

The diagnosis is established by histologic evaluation of a cervical biopsy specimen, usually following the finding of an abnormal Pap smear. Staging may be established on physical examination, routine x-rays, colposcopy, cystoscopy, proctosigmoidoscopy, intravenous pyelography (IVP) or barium enema (Table 80–3). An abdominal-pelvic CT scan is the standard method for initial staging.

Treatment for early stage disease may include either radiation therapy (teletherapy plus brachytherapy) or surgery (radical hysterectomy), with similar cure rates, but differing acute and late toxicities. The disease-remission

TABLE 80–3   Staging for Cervical Cancer

TNM STAGE	FIGO[a] STAGE	DEFINITION
TX		Primary tumor cannot be assessed
T0		No evidence of primary tumor
Tis	0	Carcinoma in situ
T1	I	Cervical carcinoma confined to uterus (extension to corpus should be disregarded)
T1a	A	Invasive carcinoma diagnosed only by microscopy.
		All macroscopically visible lesions—even with superficial invasion—are T1b/1B. Stromal invasion with a maximal depth of 5.0 mm measured from the base of the epithelium and a horizontal spread of 7.0 mm or less. Vascular space involvement, venous or lymphatic, does not affect classification
T1a1	IA1	Measured stromal invasion 3 mm or less in depth and 7 mm or less in lateral spread
T1a2	IA2	Measured stromal invasion more than 3.0 mm and not more than 5.0 mm with a horizontal spread 7.0 mm or less
T1b	IB	Clinically visible lesion confined to the cervix or microscopic lesion greater than IA2
T1b1	IB1	Clinically visible lesion 4.0 cm or less in greatest dimension
	IB2	Clinically visible lesion more than 4.0 cm
T2	II	Cervical carcinoma invades beyond uterus but not to pelvic wall or to the lower third of vagina
T2a	IIA	Tumor without parametrial invasion
T2b	IIB	Tumor with parametrial invasion
T3	II	Tumor extends to the pelvic wall, and/or involves the lower third of the vagina, and/or causes hydronephrosis or nonfunctioning kidney
T3a	IIIA	Tumor involves lower third of the vagina, no extension to pelvic wall
T3b	IIIB	Tumor extends to pelvic wall and/or causes hydronephrosis or nonfunctioning kidney
	IV	Cervical carcinoma has extended beyond the true pelvis or has involved (biopsy proven) the bladder mucosa or rectal mucosa. Bullous edema does not qualify as a criterion for stage IV disease.
T4	IVA	Spread to adjacent organs (bladder, rectum, or both)
M1	IVB	Distant metastasis
NX[b]		Regional lymph nodes cannot be assessed
N0[b]		No regional lymph nodes metastasis
N1[b]		Regional lymph node metastasis
AJCC stage grouping		
Stage 0 Tis N0 M0		
Stage IA1 T1a1 N0 M0		
Stage IA2 T1a2 N0 M0		
Stage IB1 T1b1 N0 M0		
Stage IB2 T1b2 N0 M0		
Stage IIA T2a N0 M0		
Stage IIB T2b N0 M0		
Stage IIIA T3a N0 M0		
Stage IIIB T1 N1 M0		
T2 N1 M0		
T3a N1 M0		
T3b Any N M0		
Stage IVA T4 Any N M0		
Stage IVB Any T Any N M1		

[a]Federation Internationale de Gynecologie et d'Obstetrique.
[b]Regional lymph nodes (N), AJCC staging only: Include paracervical, parametrial, hypogastric (obturator), common, internal and external iliac, presacral and sacral.
Source: Used with the permission of the American Joint Committee on Cancer (AJCC), Chicago, IL. The original source for this material is the *AJCC Cancer Staging Manual*. 6th ed. New York: Springer-Verlag; 2002.

rates of radiation therapy have been improved by the addition of adjuvant chemotherapy with cisplatin, used as a radiosensitizer.

Adjuvant chemo-radiation may be used for high-risk postsurgical patients, defined as those with positive lymph nodes, positive or close surgical margins, lymphovascular space invasion, large tumors, and deep invasion.

Patients with recurrent disease after surgery may be candidates for chemo-radiation, while those who recur after chemo-radiation may be candidates for radical surgery with exenteration only if the disease is limited to the central pelvis. Chemotherapy may be used for patients who are not candidates for surgery or radiation therapy, but response rates with cisplatin are only about 20%, with few cures.

Five-year survival rates are 85% for FIGO stage I, 60% to 80% for stage II, 35% to 45% for stage III, and 2% to 15% for stage IV.

REFERENCES

1. Jemal A, Siegel R, Ward E, et al. Cancer statistics, 2007. *CA Cancer J Clin.* 2007;57:43–66.
2. Berek, JS, Hacker, NF, eds. *Practical Gynecologic Oncology.* 4th ed. Philadelphia, PA: Lippincott Williams & Wilkins; 2005.

81 SARCOMAS

Nancy F. McKinney

GENERAL

- Sarcomas are a heterogeneous group of tumors that arise from embryonic mesoderm. These include bone sarcomas (osteosarcomas and chondrosarcomas), Ewing sarcomas, peripheral primitive neuroectodermal tumors, and soft tissue sarcomas.
- Soft tissue sarcomas are the most frequent sarcoma but are rare (comprising less than 1% of all cancers). Approximately 11,000 new cases are diagnosed annually in the United States; however, the incidence appears to be increasing.

SOFT TISSUE SARCOMA

EPIDEMIOLOGY AND PATHOGENESIS

- The etiology of sarcomas is poorly understood, and the vast majority of cases are sporadic.
- There is an increased incidence (8- to 50-fold) after therapeutic irradiation for other kinds of cancers such as lymphomas, cervical cancer, ovarian cancer, testicular cancer, and breast cancer.
- Sarcomas have also been associated with rare genetic disorders, such as neurofibromatosis type I, hereditary retinoblastoma, and Li-Fraumeni syndrome.
- Exposure to chemical agents such as pesticides, vinyl chloride, arsenic, dioxins (agent orange), and chlorophenols (wood preservatives) have been associated with the development of sarcomas.

CLINICAL PRESENTATION

- Sarcomas can originate in any area of the body. Approximately 60% arise in the extremities, 30% in the trunk, and 10% in the head and neck region.
- The most common presentation is a painless, enlarging mass.
- Sarcomas enlarge in a spherical fashion, rarely infiltrating the surrounding structures.
- They may cause site-dependent symptoms of paresthesias or distal edema.

DIAGNOSIS

- The work-up of a suspected sarcoma involves radiographs of the involved limb to determine if it is a bone neoplasm, and a computed tomography of the lungs to evaluate for lung metastasis. Computed tomography is an excellent test for evaluating intraabdominal sarcomas, whereas magnetic resonance imaging is better suited for evaluating sarcomas of the extremities, head and neck, and pelvis. The routine use of positron emission tomography in the diagnosis of sarcoma is not recommended at this time.
- Once a sarcoma is suspected, a biopsy should be obtained. Percutaneous core needle biopsy is preferable to fine needle aspiration because this technique provides a larger sample on which pathologic interpretation can be performed. In addition, a core needle biopsy permits administration of neoadjuvant therapy (chemotherapy and/or radiation therapy before surgery) if desired.

HISTOLOGY

- Soft tissue sarcomas are heterogeneous and more than 70 histologic subtypes have been described.
- Histologic grade is determined by several features including degree of cellularity, cellular pleomorphism, mitotic activity, presence of necrosis, and infiltrative or invasive growth pattern.
- The clinical aggressiveness of sarcomas tends to correspond with histologic grade. High-grade sarcomas are generally aggressive, fast growing, and metastasize early. Conversely, low-grade sarcomas tend to be indolent with little capacity to metastasize. Intermediate-grade sarcomas tend to have an intermediate biological aggressiveness.

STAGE

- The staging system created by the American Joint Committee on Cancer in 2002 is widely used (Table 81–1). This system incorporates the following prognostic values:
  - Grade (differentiation)
  - Depth (deep or superficial to deep fascia)
  - Size (less than or greater than 5 cm)

TABLE 81–1 American Joint Committee on Cancer Staging System for Soft Tissue Sarcoma

Primary tumor (T)

TX	Primary tumor cannot be assessed
T0	No evidence of primary tumor
T1	Tumor 5 cm or less in greatest dimension
T1a	Superficial tumor[1]
T1b	Deep tumor
T2	Tumor more than 5 cm in greatest dimension
T2a	Superficial tumor[1]
T2b	Deep tumor

Regional lymph nodes (N)

NX	Regional lymph nodes cannot be assessed
N0	No regional lymph node metastasis
N1	Regional lymph node metastasis

Distant metastasis (M)

MX	Distant metastasis cannot be assessed
M0	No distant metastasis
M1	Distant metastasis
	Biopsy of metastatic site performed _____ □Y _____ □N
	Source of pathologic metastatic specimen _____

Stage grouping

I	T1a	N0	M0	G1–2	G1	Low
	T1b	N0	M0	G1–2	G1	Low
	T2a	N0	M0	G1–2	G1	Low
	T2b	N0	M0	G1–2	G1	Low
II	T1a	N0	M0	G3–4	G2–3	High
	T1b	N0	M0	G3-4	G2–3	High
	T2a	N0	M0	G3–4	G2–3	High
III	T2b	N0	M0	G3–4	G2–3	High
IV	Any T	N1	M0	Any G	Any G	High or Low
	Any T	N0	M1	Any G	Any G	High or Low

Histologic grade (G)

GX	Grade cannot be assessed
G1	Well differentiated
G2	Moderately differentiated
G3	Poorly differentiated
G4	Poorly differentiated or undifferentiated (four-tiered systems only)[2]

Resldual tumor (R)

RX	Presence of residual tumor cannot be assessed
R0	No residual tumor
R1	Microscopic residual tumor
R2	Macroscopic residual tumor

Additional descriptors

For identification of special cases of TNM or pTNM classifications, the "m" suffix and "y," "r," and "a" prefixes are used. Although they do not affect the stage grouping, they indicate cases needing separate analysis.

m suffix indicates the presence of multiple primary tumors in a single site and is recorded in parentheses: pT(m)NM.

y prefix indicates those cases in which classification is performed during or following initial multimodality therapy. The cTNM or pTNM category is identified by a "y" prefix. The ycTNM or ypTNM categorizes the extent of tumor actually present at the time of that examination. The "y" categorization is not an estimate of tumor prior to multimodality therapy.

r prefix indicates a recurrent tumor when staged after a disease-free interval, and is identified by the "r" prefix: rTNM.

a prefix designates the stage determined at autopsy aTNM.

TNM, tumor, node, metastasis,

NOTES:
1. Superficial tumor is located exclusively above the superficial fascia without invasion of the fascia deep tumor is located either exclusively beneath the superficial fascia, superficial to the fascia with invasion of or through the fascia, or both superficial yet beneath the fascia. Hetropetioneal, mediaslinal, and pelvic sarcomas are classified as deep tumors.
2. Ewing's sarcoma is classified as G4.

Additional descriptors

Lymphatic vessel invention (L)

LX	Lymphatic vessel invasion cannot be assessed
L0	No lymphatic vessel invasion
L1	Lymphatic vessel invasion

Venous invasion (V)

VX	Venous invasion cannot be assessed
V0	No venous invasion
V1	Microscopic venous invasion
V2	Microscopic venous invasion

SOURCE: Adapted with permission from Greene FL, Compton CC, Fritz AG, eds. *AJCC Cancer Staging Atlas*. Chicago IL: Springer, 2006.

○ Presence of distant or nodal metastases
○ One limitation of this staging system is that it does not take into consideration the anatomic site of the sarcoma, which is also a prognostic indicator.

SURVIVAL

- Approximately 40% to 50% of patients diagnosed with soft tissue sarcoma die of their disease. Despite much research in this field, the outcome has changed little in the last 30 years.
- Survival depends on the location, size, and histology of the tumor; the age and health of the patient; the presence of distant metastasis; and the completeness of the surgical resection.
- The presence of distant metastasis is a poor prognostic indicator in sarcomas. Nodal metastasis is rare (<5%), and the most common site of distant metastasis is the lung (70%–80%), followed by bone, brain, and liver. Some patients have had long-term survival following surgical excision of all metastatic disease.

TREATMENT

- Surgical excision is the treatment of choice for sarcomas. Radiation therapy can complement surgery, allowing for less invasive procedures. The role of chemotherapy in soft tissue sarcoma is controversial, but emerging.

SURGERY

- In localized disease, surgical resection with wide margins (1–2 cm), with or without radiation therapy, offers the best chance for cure. It is important to obtain adequate margins, because sarcomas compress tissue planes, creating a *pseudocapsule* of the surrounding tissue. Malignant cells penetrate this pseudocapsule, and simple "shelling out" of the sarcoma leaves microscopic disease in 66% to 90% of cases. Margin status is an independent prognostic factor for local recurrence.
- Wide local resection is often used in conjunction with preoperative or postoperative radiation therapy. This is especially important with close or positive margins.

RADIATION THERAPY

- In the 1970s, one-half of all patients with extremity sarcomas underwent limb amputation. Today amputation is required in <10%, primarily because of adjunctive radiation therapy.

- Radiation therapy should be considered for all high-grade extremity soft tissue sarcomas (unless there are large, clear margins), and for intermediate-grade extremity tumors with close or positive margins. There is no clear role for radiation therapy in low-grade soft tissue sarcomas (except possibly in recurrence).
- Adjuvant radiation may be given pre- or postoperatively, although the optimal timing remains controversial.
- With preoperative radiation therapy, lower doses of radiation may be given and the radiation fields are typically smaller. In addition, radiation may debulk the tumor, thus facilitating complete surgical resection in previously unresectable or poorly resectable tumors. However, with preoperative radiation therapy, it is more difficult to assess the surgical margins and there is twice the rate of wound complications.
- Brachytherapy, also known as interstitial implant therapy, is an alternative to standard external beam radiation therapy. With this procedure, seeds or catheters are implanted into the tumor bed, which increases the dose of radiation to the tumor. The seeds are left in situ for 4 to 6 days and then removed. Brachytherapy has been associated with local control rates of approximately 90%. However, head-to-head studies have not been performed comparing this with conventional radiation therapy. Brachytherapy may also be used in combination with a large external beam radiation field, with a brachytherapy boost to a specific area.

CHEMOTHERAPY

- Soft tissue sarcomas are generally considered chemoresistant. However, several recent studies have suggested a role for chemotherapy. The re-emergence of chemotherapy is fueled by the observation that metastatic disease is common even if local control is obtained.
- The aim of chemotherapy is to eradicate micrometastasis, as well as to reduce the risk of local recurrence. Chemotherapy may be administered in either the adjuvant or palliative setting.
- The decision to utilize chemotherapy should be established on an individualized basis. Most experts recommend treatment only in clinical trials, at a center experienced in the management of sarcomas.
- The two chemotherapeutic agents that appear most active in soft tissue sarcoma are doxorubicin and ifosfamide. Gemcitabine and docetaxel have also been shown to have modest efficacy.
- Histologic classification is an important predictor of response to chemotherapy. Synovial sarcomas and angiosarcomas are highly chemosensitive; liposarcomas and leiomyosarcomas are less chemosensitive;

and gastrointestinal stromal tumors (GISTs), clear cell sarcomas, and alveolar soft part sarcomas are chemoresistant.

- Similarly, histologic grade can predict chemosensitivity. High-grade tumors are more chemosensitive, and low- and intermediate-grade sarcomas are chemoresistant.

RECURRENT OR METASTATIC DISEASE

- Despite optimal multimodality therapy, at least 20% to 40% of patients with soft tissue sarcoma develop recurrent disease, with a median disease-free interval of 18 months.
- Distant pulmonary metastases are the most common site of recurrence for extremity sarcomas. Patients with retroperitoneal or intraabdominal sarcomas tend to have local recurrences.
- Less common sites of metastasis are bone (7%), liver (4%), and lymph nodes (4%).
- Early surgical and/or radiation therapy of recurrent local or metastatic disease can prolong survival.
- Isolated local recurrence should be treated with margin negative resection if possible. This may require amputation, but radiation therapy with or without chemotherapy engenders acceptable local control with limb sparing surgery, even with recurrence.
- If isolated pulmonary recurrence is identified, complete pulmonary resection can achieve long-term survival in 15% to 40% of patients with resectable disease (small, less than 4 metastases, no endobronchial invasion, and a long disease-free interval). It is unclear if the addition of chemotherapy will prolong survival.
- Unfortunately, most patients with recurrent or metastatic disease are not candidates for radical surgery, and therefore, chemotherapy is the only viable option. The prognosis in these patients is very poor. Doxorubicin and ifosfamide are the most active agents for metastatic soft tissue sarcomas, with response rates of 16% to 36%.
- Combination regimens that contain an anthracycline such as doxorubicin (Adriamycin) (AI, [Adriamycin and ifosfamide] and MAID [mesna, Adriamycin, ifosfamide, dacarbazine]) are considerably more toxic but have higher response rates (35%–60%).
- The Cochrane Database Review in 2003 performed a meta-analysis of 2281 participants from eight randomized controlled trials comparing single-agent doxorubicin versus doxorubicin-based combination chemotherapy. There was a marginal increase in response rates, significant increase in toxicity, and no improvement in overall survival at 1 year with the combination.

GASTROINTESTINAL STROMAL TUMORS

- Gastrointestinal stromal tumors (GISTs) are rare tumors, comprising approximately 5% of soft tissue sarcomas. They are the most common sarcoma of the gastrointestinal tract. Recently, GISTs have become an area of considerable interest in oncology because these tumors possess unique immunophenotypical markers, which have been targeted by specific therapeutic agents, thus serving as a exciting paradigm for the treatment of other cancers.
- GISTs originate from the interstitial cells of Cajal, which are believed to act as intestinal pacemaker cells which regulate intestinal motility.
- Historically, GISTs were believed to be derived from smooth muscle, and were often misclassified as leiomyomas or leiomyosarcomas. However, these tumors are now known to possess unique ultrastructural features and immunophenotypical markers. Most GISTs express the KIT (CD117) receptor kinase tyrosine, and a minority are platelet-derived growth factor-α (PDGF-α) positive. Mutations in c-KIT or PDGF-α result in constitutive kinase activity. The specific mutation may predict the tumor behavior and certainly predicts its response to therapy.
- Although GISTs may arise anywhere in the gastrointestinal tract, they most commonly arise in the stomach, small intestine, and colon. There is an equal male to female ratio, and the incidence is estimated between 3000 to 5000 cases per year. GISTs have been reported in people of all ages; however, most patients are between 40 and 80 years. The median age at diagnosis is 60 years.
- Surgical resection is the only chance for cure in patients with primary, localized GIST. Wedge resection is generally sufficient. Negative margins are desirable; but unlike other soft tissue sarcomas, they need not be wide, because GISTs tend to merely displace adjacent tissues and not invade. Gross total resection is possible in approximately 85% of patients, and of these only approximately 70% to 90% have negative microscopic margins. The 5-year survival is approximately 50% following complete resection.
- Although surgery is the treatment of choice for surgically resectable disease, one-half of all patients with resected GIST develop disease recurrence or metastasis. In addition, approximately one-third of patients present with unresectable or metastatic disease at diagnosis, and surgery is not an option for curative intent. The most common sites of recurrence or metastasis are the liver, peritoneal surfaces, lung, and bone.
- Historically, treatment of GISTs involved surgery and observation, because they were not believed to be

radiosensitive or chemosensitive. However, with the development of targeted tyrosine kinase inhibitors, the treatment of GIST tumors has been revolutionized.

- The use of the specific tyrosine kinase inhibitor imatinib mesylate (Gleevec) was first reported in GIST in 2000. Importantly, the administration of imatinib has significantly improved progression free and overall survival in patients with unresectable or metastatic GIST.
- Sunitinib malate (Sutent) is a multikinase inhibitor that has been shown to improve time to progression and overall survival in patients with metastatic GIST who are intolerant of or resistant to imatinib.
- Although GIST is an uncommon tumor, it serves as a model for treating solid tumors with targeted agents. Understanding the molecular biology of the tumor has led to exciting and promising treatment modalities.

BONE SARCOMA

- Sarcomas of the bone are rare and occur primarily in children. Osteosarcoma is the most common form of bone sarcoma, followed by chondrosarcoma, and the Ewing/Pediatric neuroendocrine tumor family of tumors.
- The clinical presentation of bone sarcomas depends on the bone involved, and these sarcomas can affect any bone. The most common symptoms are pain and a soft tissue mass.
- Survival of patients with bone sarcomas has improved dramatically over the last 30 years, in concert with a dramatic increase in the number of limb-sparing operations. These improvements can be attributed to multimodal therapy with chemotherapy, radiation therapy, and surgery.

OSTEOSARCOMA

- Most osteosarcomas occur at the metaphyseal region of the long bones, most commonly around the knee joint or elbow joint. The age at diagnosis is typically 10 to 20 years, and there is a slight male predominance.
- On radiograph, osteosarcomas have a characteristic sunburst appearance.
- Histologically, osteosarcomas may be divided into three categories: conventional, fibroblastic, and chondroblastic osteosarcoma, albeit they are clinically similar.
- Treatment involves aggressive chemotherapy and surgery. Patients generally undergo preoperative chemotherapy. Postoperative chemotherapy is commonly given as well. Chemotherapy agents active in osteosarcoma include doxorubicin, cisplatin, ifosfamide, bleomycin, cyclophosphamide, dactinomycin, and methotrexate. Several different combinations of

drugs have proven useful. Osteosarcomas are not radiation sensitive, and accordingly radiation therapy is not generally advised.

CHONDROSARCOMA

- Chondrosarcomas more commonly occur in flat bones and are classically discovered in the shoulder or pelvic girdle. Adults and children alike may develop these tumors, and there is an equal male-to-female ratio. In patients greater than 60 years of age chondrosarcomas are associated with Paget disease or with prior therapeutic irradiation.
- On radiographs, chondrosarcomas show a characteristic *lobulated* appearance.
- Histologically, they are characterized by cartilaginous proliferation that permeates into the bone marrow.
- Chondrosarcomas are generally chemoresistant and radiation resistant, and the treatment of choice is surgery alone.

EWING SARCOMA/PEDIATRIC NEUROENDOCRINE TUMOR

- Ewing sarcoma/pediatric neuroendocrine tumor of the bone tend to occur in the diaphyses of the bone. This is a disease of childhood, and there is a slight male predominance. On radiographs they reveal a characteristic onionskin appearance.
- Treatment involving preoperative and postoperative systemic chemotherapy with a multidrug regimen such as vincristine, doxorubicin, cyclophosphamide, ifosfamide, and etoposide in combination with surgery and radiation therapy has increased the cure rate from less than 10% to greater than 60%. Unlike osteosarcoma, Ewing sarcoma/pediatric neuroendocrine tumors are highly radiation sensitive, and consolidation radiation therapy is part of the standard approach.

BIBLIOGRAPHY

Blakely LJ, Trent JC, Patel S. Soft tissue and bone sarcomas. In: Kantarjain, H, Wolff, R, Koller, C, eds. *MD Anderson Manual of Medical Oncology.* New York, NY: McGraw-Hill; 2006: 879–902.

Casas-Ganem J, Healey JH. Advances that are changing the diagnosis and treatment of malignant bone tumors. *Curr Opin Rheum.* 2005;17(1):79–85.

Demetri GT, Van Oosterom AT, Blackstein M, et al. Phase 3 multicenter, randomized, double-blind, placebo-controlled trial of SU11248 in patients following failure of imatinib for metastatic GIST. *J Clin Oncol,* 2005;23(16 suppl):4000.

Ginsberg JP, Woo S, Johnson ME. Ewing's sarcoma family of tumors. In: Pizzo PA, Poplack DG, eds. *Principles and Practice of Pediatric Oncology.* Philadelphia, PA: Lippincott-Raven Publishers; 2002:973–1016.

Gold JS, DeMatteo RP. Combined surgical and molecular therapy: The gastrointestinal stromal tumor model. *Ann Surg.* 2006;244: 176–184.

Greene FL, Compton CC, Fritz AG, eds, *AJCC Cancer Staging Atlas.* Chicago, Springer IL: 2006.

Maki RG, Fletcher JA, Heinrich MC, et al. Results from a continuation trial of SU11248 in patients with imatinib-resistant GIST. *J Clin Oncol.* 2005;23(16 suppl):9011.

Paolo GG, Piero P. Adjuvant chemotherapy for soft tissue sarcoma. *Curr Opin Oncol.* 2005;17:361–365.

Rubin BP. Gastrointestinal stromal tumours: An update. *Histopathology.* 2006;48:83–96.

Shinomura Y, Kazuo K, Shusaku T, et al. Pathophysiology, diagnosis, and treatment of gastrointestinal stromal tumors. *Gastroenterol J.* 2005;40:775–780.

Tornillo L, Terracciano LM. An update on molecular genetics of gastrointestinal stromal tumors *J Clin Pathol.* 2006;59:557–563.

82 CARCINOMA OF UNKNOWN PRIMARY

C. Daniel Kingsley

The diagnosis of cancer in a patient without a known primary is a relatively common event, accounting for up to 5% of all cancers. The patient usually presents with symptoms related to the area of metastatic tumor. The diagnosis of carcinoma of unknown primary (CUP) is only considered after a thorough evaluation including history, physical, imaging, blood tests, and pathologic evaluation fails to reveal the primary origin of the malignancy. Although most patients with advanced or metastatic cancer do not respond well to therapy (median survival of 3 to 4 months), there are subgroups, comprising approximately 40% of patients, that have a more favorable outcome.

EPIDEMIOLOGY

Cancers of unknown primary occur with equal frequency in men and women and the incidence tends to increase with age, with most patients presenting at approximately 60 years of age. Prior to the advent of modern imaging, autopsy series identified the primary site in only 70% to 80% of patients with an unknown primary. The usual primary site for lesions above the diaphragm was the lung, and the usual primary site for lesions below the diaphragm was the gastrointestinal tract. The wide-spread use of computed tomography (CT) has been associated with an earlier diagnosis of cancer which, in turn, has broadened the distribution for cancers of unknown primary.

DIAGNOSIS

As with all cancers, the diagnosis should be established via direct tissue examination by an experienced pathologist. The initial pathological evaluation by light microscopy can divide these tumors into four broad categories, consisting of adenocarcinoma (~60%), poorly differentiated adenocarcinoma/carcinoma (~20%), squamous cell cancer (~10%), and poorly differentiated neoplasm (~5%). Immunohistologic techniques can help to further delineate the cancer subtype and facilitate prediction of chemotherapy responsiveness. For example, identification of a cancer of unknown primary as either a sarcoma, carcinoma, or lymphoma can dramatically alter the therapeutic approach and efficacy (with cures being noted in some subgroups). Prostate-specific antigen (PSA) should be stained for in males, and estrogen receptors (ERs), progesterone receptors (PRs), and HER2-neu should be analyzed in women. Leukocyte common antigen (LCA) may be positive in patients with anaplastic lymphomas. Melanomas are often positive for S-100, vimentin, and hydroxy-β-methylbutyrate 45 (HMB-45). Vimentin, von Willebrand antigen, and desmin are often positive in sarcomas. Human chorionic gonadotropin (hCG) and α-fetoprotein (AFP) can prove useful in the diagnosis of extragonadal germ cell tumors. Neuron-specific enolase, chromogranin, and synaptophysin are suggestive of neuroendocrine tumors. Cytokeratins (CKs) 7 and 20 have been extensively used in the evaluation of cancers of unknown primary. Characteristic CK7 and CK20 patterns have been described in specific tumors. For example, a CK7+/CK20+ tumor is most consistent with a urothelial, mucinous ovarian, pancreatic, or biliary tumor whereas a CK7−/CK20+ tumor is likely to be either a colorectal or Merkel cell tumor. The use of electron microscopy has permitted identification of neuroendocrine tumors and melanomas by confirming the presence of granules and premelanosomes, respectively.

Patients with cancer of unknown primary usually present with symptoms related to the tumor involvement. In addition, a careful history will also identify systemic constitutional symptoms such as anorexia, fatigue, weakness, or weight loss. A careful history, review of symptoms, and complete physical examination, coupled with the site of known disease and the pathologic diagnosis can direct the astute oncologist to the most likely primary.

Routine laboratory tests should include a complete blood count, comprehensive metabolic panel, hemoccult stool testing, chest x-ray, urinalysis, symptom-directed endoscopy, and CT of the abdomen and pelvis. In general, random radiographic imaging has not proven useful in identifying asymptomatic primaries, although recent small series looking at positron emission tomography (PET) or fused PET/CT revealed a 30% rate of identifying the primary site and were particularly useful in cervical node CUPs.

Certain subsets of patients should undergo further testing depending on their demographics or location of known disease. A mammogram or breast magnetic resonance imaging (MRI) should be performed in women with adenocarcinoma and axillary lymphadenopathy or ER/PR positivity. A serum PSA should be done in males. Young males with a poorly differentiated carcinoma should have a serum hCG and AFP checked. Squamous cell carcinoma in a high or mid-cervical lymph node should prompt thorough endoscopic examination of the oropharynx, nasopharynx, hypopharynx, larynx, and upper esophagus with blind biopsies throughout. A low-cervical or supraclavicular lymph node would require the addition of a bronchoscopy in the workup. Patients with squamous cell cancer in an inguinal node should have a thorough evaluation of the perineum (penis/scrotum or vulva/vagina/cervix) and anus.

Genetic testing can also help to classify and identify unknown cancers. Isochromosome (i12p) is positive in a large percentage of men with germ cell tumors. Ewing sarcoma and most peripheral neuroepitheliomas are positive for chromosomal translocations, t(11;22). Epstein-Barr virus can be detected in most patients with nasopharyngeal carcinomas.

THERAPY

Patients can be divided into two main groups—those with a favorable subtype of CUP and those without a favorable subtype. For the 60% without favorable subtyping, various empiric regimens have been attempted, but the response rates are poor and long-term survival is dismal. As new chemotherapy is introduced, results appear to be improving in these patients. For example, the combination of paclitaxel and cisplatin has increased the response rate to 40%. The combination of paclitaxel, carboplatin, and etoposide has become the latest first-line, standard therapy with 50% response rates being reported and 3-year survivals of 14%. The remaining 40% with a favorable subtype is discussed below.

Women with isolated axillary adenopathy and an adenocarcinoma of the axilla should be treated for locally advanced breast cancer. Mammography and/or breast MRI are useful for identifying tumors, however, up to 60% of patients in this group will only exhibit evidence of tumor in their mastectomy specimens. Testing for ER/PR and HER2-neu is imperative to direct therapy. These patients receive either a modified radical mastectomy or axillary node dissection plus radiation therapy to the breast, followed by adjuvant therapy for stage II breast cancer. This combination of therapy has resulted in significant long-term survival.

Women with peritoneal carcinomatosis should be treated as if they have stage III ovarian cancer. They will often have a suggestive pathology (papillary adenocarcinoma or serous cystadenocarcinoma) and should undergo cytoreductive surgery followed by a taxane/platinum combination. CA-125, if elevated, could be followed as a tumor marker. Five-year survival rates of up to 25% have been reported.

Men with blastic bony metastasis or an elevated PSA can be treated for metastatic prostate cancer. They would initially be treated with hormonal manipulation and the response rates are generally good.

Patients with only a single metastatic site can be treated with either radiation therapy or surgical excision of the solitary lesion with reports of long disease free intervals in some patients.

Patients with squamous cell carcinoma and cervical lymphadenopathy should be treated for head and neck cancer using combined modality (chemotherapy and radiation) therapy. The bilateral neck, nasopharynx, oropharynx, and hypopharynx are included in the field, which has increased the 5-year survival from 30% to 60%.

Patients with squamous cell carcinoma and inguinal lymphadenopathy are usually treated with resection and possibly radiation therapy with long-term remission rates approaching 25%.

Patients with poorly differentiated carcinomas seem to have highly responsive tumors with cisplatin alone, having a 64% overall response rate and a 27% complete response rate.

Young men with retroperitoneal or mediastinal masses are treated as extragonadal germ-cell tumors. They should receive four cycles of bleomycin, etoposide, and cisplatin followed by surgical resection of any residual disease. This therapy produces cures in up to 40% of patients.

Young women with lung nodules and a history of recent pregnancy, miscarriage, or missed menses could have an underlying choriocarcinoma; their serum hCG levels will always be elevated. These patients often respond to chemotherapy and resection of residual disease.

Patients with poorly differentiated carcinomas with neuroendocrine features almost always present with multiple liver metastasis. This disease is very sensitive to chemotherapy and is treated with an etoposide/platinum based regimen, with up to 70% response rates and long-term survival as high as 20%.

BIBLIOGRAPHY

Gatter KC, Alcock C, et al. Clinical importance of analyzing malignant tumors of uncertain origin with immunohistological techniques. *Lancet.* 1985;1:1302.

Greco FA, Burris HA III, Erland JB, et al. Carcinoma of unknown primary site. Long term follow-up after treatment with paclitaxel, carboplatin, and etoposide. *Cancer.* 2000;89: 2655.

Gutzeit A, Antoch G, Kuhl H, et al. Unknown primary tumors: Detection with dual-modality PET/CT- initial experience. *Radiology.* 2004;234:227.

Hainsworth JD, Greco FA. Treatment of patients with cancer of an unknown primary site. *N Engl J Med.* 1993;329: 257.

Hainsworth JD, Greco FA. Management of patients with cancer of unknown primary. *Oncology.* 2000;14:563.

Horning SJ, Carrier EK, Rouse RV, et al. Lymphomas presenting as histologically unclassified neoplasms: Characteristics and response to treatment. *J Clin Oncol.* 1989;7:1281.

National Cancer Institute. Carcinoma of unknown primary: Treatment—health professional information [NCI PDQ]; 9/20/2005.

Pavlidis N, Briasoulis E, et al. Diagnostic and therapeutic management of cancer of an unknown primary. *Eur J Cancer.* 2003; 39:1990.

Varadhachary GR, Abbruzzese JL, Lenzi R. Diagnostic strategies for unknown primary cancer. *Cancer.* 2004;100:1776.

Wong WL, Saunders M. The impact of FDG PET on the management of occult primary head and neck tumors. *J Clin Oncol.* 2003;15:461.

83 ONCOLOGIC EMERGENCIES
C. Daniel Kingsley

The oncologic emergencies are acute, potentially life-threatening events arising in patients with cancer or as consequence of its treatment, which if not anticipated, diagnosed, and treated may result in significant morbidity or mortality.

EPIDURAL SPINAL CORD COMPRESSION

EPIDEMIOLOGY

Epidural spinal cord compression (ESCC) occurs in 5% to 10% of cancer patients, but has been estimated to occur in as many as 30% with widely metastatic cancer. It has been described in most cancers, but most commonly occurs with lung (24%), breast (21%), and prostate (20%). In 10% to 20% of patients, ESCC is the presenting symptom of their cancer. The distribution of the lesions are as follows: 10% cervical, 60% thoracic, and 30% lumbosacral; 10% to 40% are multifocal.

PATHOPHYSIOLOGY

85% to 90% of ESCCs are secondary to bony metastasis of the vertebrae extending into the epidural space. The tumor directly compresses the spine eliciting neurologic symptoms and signs in dermatomes of the affected tracts. Compressive lesions could also arise because of vertebral body collapse. Nonmalignant causes of ESCC include abscess, disc herniation, vertebral hemangioma, hematoma, syrinx, radiation myelopathy, or arachnoiditis.

DIAGNOSIS

Patients with ESCC present with neurologic symptoms attributed to the level of cord involvement; 96% of patients will complain of pain, exacerbated by percussion, and localizing to the site of involvement. The pain increases with the supine position, which tends to distinguish ESCC from benign disk disease. Weakness is present in 60% to 85% of patients and paraplegia can develop in a matter of hours. Patients can exhibit radicular symptoms, sensory loss, and bowel or bladder dysfunction. A positive Lhermitte sign with passive neck flexion may be elicited and decreased sphincter tone may be discovered on rectal examination. Magnetic resonance imaging (MRI) of the spine is the imaging modality of choice to diagnose ESCC. Plain radiographs are positive in 80% to 90% of patients, revealing erosion of the pedicles, vertebral collapse, or evidence of a paravertebral mass. Computed tomography (CT) and myelography are less sensitive compared to MRI.

THERAPEUTIC APPROACH

80% of patients that are ambulatory at the time of diagnosis will remain ambulatory if treatment is initiated immediately. In contrast, patients presenting with paraplegia rarely respond. Steroids should be initiated without delay. They are believed to reduce vasogenic edema and acutely reduce the mass-like effect associated with ESCC. Dexamethasone 10 mg intravenous (IV) as a bolus followed by 4 mg every 6 hours is the usual dose employed. One study suggested that high dose dexamethasone (96 mg IV followed by 24 mg every 6 hours) may be preferable, although randomized trials have not been performed. A neurosurgical consult in concert with radiation therapy should be sought. If surgery is performed, the traditional approach has been through a posterior incision, although recent studies suggest that improved results are obtained with the anterior approach. Regardless, surgery tends to be reserved for patients who are medically fit, have a good life expectancy, with well localized radioresistant tumors, or who require a biopsy for diagnosis.

Radiation therapy generally consists of 30 to 50 Gy, administered over 2 to 4 weeks. The radiation window typically involves two adjacent vertebral bodies above and below the affected area, and is delayed until 2 weeks after the surgery. Radiation therapy alone is reserved for those not medically fit for surgery, with a poor life expectancy, or with multiple sites of involvement. A notable exception to the use of radiation therapy or surgery applies to lymphomas which are highly chemosensitive tumors and, thus may be treated with chemotherapy alone.

Patients who can realistically expect to fully recover are those whose lesions have been symptomatic for less than 24 hours and exhibit good neurologic function at the time of treatment. The median survival after diagnosis is 6 months with longer survival rates observed in patients with good neurologic function. Approximately 10% of patients will relapse within months. Patients surviving longer than a year will almost always experience a relapse.

SUPERIOR VENA CAVA SYNDROME

EPIDEMIOLOGY

Superior vena cava syndrome (SVCS) was originally described in patients with syphilitic aneurysms of the ascending aorta. Cancer is currently responsible for more than 90% of SVCS, with small cell lung, diffuse large B cell lymphoma, lymphoblastic lymphomas, breast, germ cell, and thymomas predominating. Lung cancer is responsible for the majority (65% to 85%) of SVCS related to malignancy. 2.4% to 4.2% of patients with lung cancer (and 20% of patients with small cell lung cancer) will experience an SVCS. Thrombosis due to long-term indwelling catheters is a growing cause of SVCS in patients receiving chemotherapy. Importantly, SVCS is the presenting feature in up to 60% of patients with an underlying malignancy.

PATHOPHYSIOLOGY

The superior vena cava (SVC) is the major draining vein for blood derived from the head, neck, upper extremities, and upper thorax. The SVC resides in the middle mediastinum and is surrounded by the aorta, pulmonary arteries, trachea, right bronchus, perihilar and paratracheal lymph nodes. Obstruction of the SVC can be due to thrombosis, extrinsic compression, or direct tumor invasion. Collateral flow to the right atrium is established over a period of weeks to months, mainly through the azygous vein, but also through the internal mammary, lateral thoracic, paraspinal, and esophageal veins. The rate at which the SVC is occluded, relative to the development of collateral flow, will determine the extent and severity of symptoms. Because collateral flow can minimize the serious complications associated with SVCS, most patients do not require emergent relief of the obstruction. Nonetheless, laryngeal edema with stridor is a life-threatening complication which requires emergent radiotherapy.

DIAGNOSIS

The diagnosis can usually be established clinically. Patients complain of dyspnea (most common), cough, head fullness, hoarseness, headache, nasal congestion, epistaxis, dizziness, dysphagia, hemoptysis, or syncope. Physical examination reveals facial, neck, or arm swelling that is exacerbated by leaning forward or lying down. Patients may also develop telangiectasias of the chest, neck, and upper back, as well as proptosis, stridor, plethora, cyanosis, tachypnea, or confusion. Up to 20% of patients will present with neurologic abnormalities because of increased intracranial pressure. These patients will manifest papilledema, agitation, confusion, or seizures. Chest x-rays are abnormal in 84% of patients and are characterized by mediastinal widening, a right hilar mass, or pleural effusion. CT scans are helpful in distinguishing between thrombosis and external compression. In addition, the CT scan delineates the level of SVC obstruction, provides an assessment of collateral circulation, and identifies mediastinal adenopathy.

THERAPEUTIC APPROACH

Unless the patient is experiencing a life-threatening symptom (stridor), immediate treatment is directed at comfort and safety. The patient is placed on supplemental oxygen, the head is elevated, and a reduced sodium diet is prescribed. Some patients may benefit from diuretic administration and corticosteroids (especially effective in steroid responsive tumors eg, lymphomas).

Since most patients presenting with an SVCS have undiagnosed cancer, efforts are directed toward establishing a tissue diagnosis. Radiation therapy (RT) is utilized for most tumors that are associated with SVCS. Typically RT is administered over 7 to 10 days. Some tumors (small cell lung cancer, lymphomas, and germ cell tumors) that are highly chemosensitive are treated with chemotherapy alone. Anticoagulation may be indicated for patients that develop a catheter-associated thrombus.

If contraindications to therapy exist or standard therapy fails, an endovascular stent can be inserted into the SVC to restore venous return. Endovascular stenting provides excellent results in patients with external compression as compared to patients with intraluminal pathology. The majority of patients will experience relief within 2 to 4 days of initiating appropriate therapy (RT, steroids, chemotherapy) and some may exhibit improvement within 24 hours. 89% will experience objective relief within 14 days. Unfortunately, the RT failure rate is 10% to 20% and the overall relapse rate is as high as 50%. Moreover, the mean survival after treatment of malignancy-associated SVCS is only 6 to 7 months.

FEBRILE NEUTROPENIA

EPIDEMIOLOGY

Febrile neutropenia (FN) is responsible for 60,000 hospitalizations each year at a cost of over $13,000 per hospitalization. FN is responsible for the majority of deaths attributable to acute leukemia, and half of all deaths related to lymphoma. The cancers associated with the highest incidence of FN are leukemia (8.45% of patients) and non-Hodgkin lymphomas (NHL) (3.36%). The highest incidence rates for solid tumors are seen with pancreatic (2.45%), lung (1.81%), ovary (1.01%), and stomach (1%).

PATHOPHYSIOLOGY

FN is associated with an extraordinary risk of infection in cancer patients. Common sources of bacterial seeding are derived from the respiratory tract, oropharynx, sinuses, urinary tract, gastrointestinal tract, skin, and venous catheter sites.

Importantly, most cases of FN are culture negative. Indeed, microbiologically documented infections are identified in less than 20% of cases. Positive cultures reveal gram-positive organisms (mainly *Staphylococcus aureus*, *Staphylococcus epidermidis*, and *Streptococcus viridans*) in 70% of cases. Gram-negative organisms are also cultured but are less common that gram-positive organisms. *Candida* and *Aspergillus* should be considered in all patients with FN.

DIAGNOSIS

FN is defined as a single temperature of $\geq 101°F$ or a sustained temperature of $\geq 100.4°F$ one hour apart, in concert with an absolute neutrophil count (ANC) of 500 cells/mm^3 (or less than 1000 cells/mm^3 but expected to drop below 500 cells/mm^3 within the next 48 hours). The evaluation of FN must proceed without delay and requires a minimum of two blood cultures, urinalysis with culture, complete blood count with differential, complete metabolic panel, chest x-ray, and site-specific cultures.

THERAPEUTIC APPROACH

Once cultures are obtained, antibiotics at full dose should be initiated without delay. Delays in therapy have been associated with mortality rates that exceed 70%. In contrast, survival is greater than 90% if antibiotics are initiated without delay. Empiric intravenous broad-spectrum antibiotic therapy is appropriate in all patients considered to be at high risk. Low-risk patients include individuals with an expected length of neutropenia that is less than 7 days, good performance status, absence of comorbid conditions, and normal hepatic and renal function.

Low risk adults may be treated with oral ciprofloxacin and amoxicillin/clavulanate as outpatients.

- Antibiotic choice is the subject of considerable controversy, however monotherapy appears as effective as combination therapy. In all cases, antibiotic choices should be driven by the constellation of clinical, laboratory and microbiology data, if available. The principle concern regarding monotherapy is the emergence of antibiotic resistance. Monotherapy with cefepime, meropenem, imipenem, or ceftazidime has been employed. Combination therapy typically includes an aminoglycoside (amikacin, gentamicin, or tobramycin) plus either an antipseudomonal penicillin (piperacillin-tazobactam or ticarcillin-clavulanate), extended release cephalosporin (cefepime, or ceftazidime), or a carbapenem (imipenem or meropenem) Vancomycin is added if there is clinical evidence of a catheter-related infection, mucositis, history of antibiotic use, known colonization or exposure to methicillin-resistant *S. aureus*, or hypotension/shock before culture results are known.
- If the patient defervesces within 3 to 5 days and no specific etiology is uncovered, low-risk patients can be discharged on an oral fluoroquinolone to complete 7 to 10 days of therapy, while high-risk patients should receive the initial regimen for a full 7 to 10 days.

If there is persistent fever after 3 to 5 days, the patient should be reassessed for new sites of infection or development of drug-resistant organisms. If there is no new cause found, antifungal therapy should be initiated. Early guidelines recommended adding amphotericin B with or without changing the antibiotics. Recently, several studies examining the efficacy of newer antifungal agents (voriconazole, caspofungin, and itraconazole) have revealed similar response rates with a lower incidence of toxicity.

Therapy can be discontinued if: (1) no specific infection is documented; (2) the patient has been afebrile for at least 2 days, and (3) the neutrophil count has been ≥500 cells/mm^3 for 3 days.

Granulocyte-colony stimulating factor (GCSF) is recommended in very high-risk patients, such as patients expected to experience prolonged (>10 d) and profound (≤100 cells/mm^3) neutropenia, have uncontrolled primary disease, age greater than 65 years, lobar pneumonia, invasive fungal disease, hypotension, or multiorgan dysfunction. It may also be considered in patients that develop FN during hospitalization (nosocomial infection).

• Respiratory isolation should be employed for all patients with FN. The patient's meals should be well cooked, with no fresh fruit, and no flowers in the room. The equipment in the room should remain with the patient, and strict hand washing should be observed by all. When the patient has recovered, GCSF should be considered for all future chemotherapy cycles, or chemotherapy dose modifications as the patients risk for subsequent episodes of FN is markedly increased.

HYPERCALCEMIA OF MALIGNANCY

EPIDEMIOLOGY

Primary hyperparathyroidism is responsible for approximately 90% of patients with hypercalcemia in the ambulatory setting, whereas malignancy is responsible for the majority of hypercalcemia occurring in the hospitalized patient (65%). Up to 30% of cancer patients will develop hypercalcemia, with non–small cell lung (35%), breast (25%), multiple myeloma/lymphoma (14%), gastrointestinal (6%), head and neck (6%), and renal cell (3%) predominating. Approximately 50% of patients with cancer-associated hypercalcemia die within 30 days.

PATHOPHYSIOLOGY

Multiple factors are involved in the development of hypercalcemia in the cancer patient. Parathyroid hormone-related peptide (PTHrP) stimulates bone resorption and elevates serum calcium in many patients, particularly patients with squamous cell carcinomas. Breast cancer

with bony metastasis and multiple myeloma are relatively common causes of hypercalcemia. The mechanism responsible for hypercalcemia in these settings is incompletely understood, but is though to occur via a local osteolytic effect induced by osteoclast activating factors such as tumor necrosis factor, interleukin-1, and interleukin-6. Tumoral synthesis of calcitriol (1,25-OH vitamin D) causes the vast majority of hypercalcemia's associated with Hodgkin lymphomas and up to one-third of hypercalcemia associated with the NHLs. Rarely, ectopic production of parathyroid hormone (PTH) causes hypercalcemia. This phenomenon has been described with ovarian, lung, and pancreatic cancers. Severe hypercalcemia is associated with a very poor prognosis.

DIAGNOSIS

Patients with hypercalcemia usually complain of nausea, vomiting, constipation, anorexia, abdominal pain, dyspepsia, polyuria, polydipsia, fatigue, pruritus, or weight loss. They may develop CNS-like symptoms including lethargy and coma. Additional clinical manifestations include dehydration, paralytic ileus, pancreatitis, renal insufficiency, proximal muscle weakness, depression, seizures, and electrocardiographic (ECG) findings including a short QT interval, wide T waves, prolonged PR interval, and virtually any arrhythmia.

Since roughly 40% of calcium is bound to albumin, an ionized (free) calcium should be obtained. Hypercalcemia is generally grouped into three categories that reflect the overall severity, mild (10.5–12 mg/dL), moderate (12.1–13.5 mg/dL), and severe (>13.5 mg/dL). A characteristic laboratory feature of the hypercalcemia of malignancy is a marked depression of intact parathyroid hormone level except in rare instances of ectopic production or concurrent hyperparathyroidism. If the hypercalcemia is due to PTHrP, hypophosphatemia, hyperchloremia, and a mild metabolic acidosis are observed. Conversely when calcitriol is responsible for the hypercalcemia, the serum phosphate is usually normal (or mildly increased) and hypercalciuria is prominent.

THERAPEUTIC APPROACH

Several strategies have been employed in the management of the hypercalcemia of malignancy: (1) augmenting urinary calcium excretion (loop diuretics and saline); (2) reducing bone resorption (calcitonin), (3) decreasing intestinal calcium absorption (corticosteroids), (4) chelation of ionized calcium, and (5) hemodialysis. Typically patients with hypercalcemia are dehydrated (calcium interferes with urinary concentration), therefore administration of 2-6 L (pending examination of the patients volume status) of isotonic saline is essential. Maintenance intravenous saline is then administered at a rate of 200 mL to 300 mL/h (rate adjustments are based on the volume assessment). Hydration alone can reduce the serum calcium by 20% to 40%, but will rarely normalize the calcium. Once patients are sufficiently hydrated, a loop diuretic can be adminstered to further increase the urinary calcium excretion.

Multiple agents are available that impair bone resorption and decrease the serum calcium. Zoledronate (4 mg IV over 15 min) is considered the bisphosphonate of choice as it is more effective and longer acting than pamidronate (60–90 mg over 2 to 4 h). It is effective in 60% to 90% of cases but requires 24 to 48 hours to elicit a response. Calcitonin (4 mg/kg subQ or IM every 12 h) is useful in patients with severe or symptomatic hypercalcemia as it exerts its effect within 4 to 6 hours after administration. Unfortunately tachyphylaxis occurs rapidly with calcitonin and, therefore, it is usually not effective after 48 hours. Mithramycin is effective in 80% of patients but exhibits significant nephrotoxicity and, accordingly, is of limited use since most patients with hypercalcemia present with renal insufficiency. For patients who do not respond to zoledronate, gallium nitrate (100–200 mg/m²/d for 5 d) can be administered and is effective in 70% to 90% of patients. Steroids are employed in patients with hypercalcemia secondary to calcitriol secretion. Dialysis should be considered in patients with oliguria secondary to heart failure or kidney injury.

Importantly, treatment of the underlying malignancy is necessary to effectively manage the hypercalcemia over time.

TUMOR LYSIS SYNDROME

EPIDEMIOLOGY

Tumor lysis syndrome (TLS) is seen more frequently in patients with rapidly proliferating malignancies, high tumor burden, elevated lactate dehydrogenase (LDH), preexisting renal insufficiency, chemotherapy sensitive tumors, or dehydration. High-grade NHL and acute lymphoblastic leukemias (ALL) are the malignancies most commonly associated with TLS, but it has been described with most solid tumors. There are rare reports of TLS occurring spontaneously as a result of necrosis or after surgical manipulation of large tumor masses. TLS usually occurs 1 to 5 days after chemotherapy, or after steroid administration in NHL and ALL. Prior to allopurinol premedication, up to 10% of patients with ALL experienced TLS. Salicylates, radiographic contrast dye, ethambutol, probenecid, and thiazide diuretics have all been reported to worsen the metabolic derangements of TLS.

PATHOPHYSIOLOGY

The destruction of a large number of rapidly proliferating cells causes the release of intracellular protein and electrolytes, which if untreated may result in life threatening metabolic derangements and acute renal failure. Elevated uric acid can precipitate in the kidneys causing renal failure. Hyperkalemia can induce arrhythmias. Hyperphosphatemia elicits a fall in the serum calcium and can promote deposition of calcium phosphate in the kidneys resulting in kidney injury. Hypocalcemia can induce neuromuscular irritability and possibly tetany.

DIAGNOSIS

Patients present with nausea/vomiting, fatigue, weakness, myalgias, progressive oliguria, uremia, fluid overload, hypertension, neuromuscular irritability, arrhythmias, seizures or sudden death. Laboratory testing reveals hyperuricemia, hyperphosphatemia, hyperkalemia, hypocalcemia, and lactic acidosis. The Cairo-Bishop definition of TLS requires abnormalities in at least two of the following within 3 days before until 7 days after chemotherapy:
- Uric acid >8 mg/dL or a 25% increase over baseline
- Potassium >6 mEq/L or a 25% increase over baseline
- Phosphate 4.5 mg/dL or a 25% increase over baseline
- Calcium <7 or a 25% decrease over baseline

Clinical TLS requires the diagnosis of laboratory TLS plus a serum creatinine at least 1.5× the upper limit of normal, seizure, cardiac arrhythmia, or sudden death. An ultrasound of the kidneys should be performed to rule out obstruction or hydronephrosis.

THERAPEUTIC APPROACH

The best treatment for TLS is to prevent it from occurring. Patients should receive (intravenously or orally) 300 to 600 mg/daily of allopurinol for 1 to 2 days prior to receiving chemotherapy. Hydration with saline plus sodium bicarbonate (added to increase the solubility of uric acid in the urine) to maintain a urine output of 2 to 5 L/day and a urine pH of 7 or greater is recommended. Chemistries should be obtained every 6 to 12 hours in high-risk patients. Rasburicase (recombinant urate oxidase) can be given in lieu of allopurinol for high-risk patients or those not responsive to allopurinol. If TLS occurs, patients should be observed in the intensive care unit and all metabolic abnormalities should be corrected. Dialysis should be considered if the patient has life-threatening electrolyte abnormalities (potassium is

>6, uric acid >10, phosphate >10) or there is symptomatic hypocalcemia.

SYNDROME OF INAPPROPIRATE ANTIDIURETIC HORMONE

EPIDEMIOLOGY

The syndrome of inappropriate antidiuretic hormone secretion (SIADH) is observed in 1% of patients with cancer. Small cell lung cancer is responsible for 60% of the cases. Roughly 10% of patients with small cell lung cancer will develop SIADH. Hyponatremia is the most common electrolyte abnormality in cancer patients.

PATHOPHYSIOLOGY

Elevated levels of arginine vasopressin (ADH), either secreted by the posterior pituitary or produced ectopically by tumor cells, induces reabsorption of water in the collecting duct and concentrates the urine. If the intake of water is not correspondingly reduced, the serum osmolality and serum sodium concentration will fall. Occasionally SIADH worsens after chemotherapy because of drug toxicity or release of ADH from the dying tumor cells.

DIAGNOSIS

Most patients with SIADH are asymptomatic. The clinical symptoms depend upon both the absolute fall in serum sodium concentration and rate of decrease. Symptoms include anorexia, malaise, nausea, vomiting, and apathy. Advanced symptoms include headache, confusion, lethargy, altered mental status, seizure, and coma. The diagnosis of SIADH is established via the pertinent laboratory and clinical information (also shown in Fig. 119-1).

THERAPEUTIC APPROACH

Water restriction is the mainstay of therapy. Typically water intake is reduced to <500 mL/day. Patients who are refractory to fluid restriction can be treated with oral demeclocycline (300–600 mg twice daily). This therapy requires up to 3 days to elicit a response. Patients presenting with life-threatening symptoms (coma or seizure) should be treated with hypertonic saline. However, rapid correction (>2 mEq/L/h) may produce central pontine myelinolysis.

PERICARIDAL TAMPONADE

EPIDEMIOLOGY

Pericardial tamponade (PT) has been described in 2% to 30% of cancer patients at autopsy. Half of the cases are secondary to pericardial metastasis with 75% of those associated with lung cancer, breast cancer, esophageal cancer, melanoma, or lymphomas. Radiation pericarditis can develop weeks to months after radiotherapy and can spontaneously resolve. In rare instances, radiation pericarditis (chronic effusion and thickened pericardium) has been described up to 20 years after exposure.

PATHOPHYSIOLOGY

Fluid accumulates in the pericardium from altered vascular permeability, localized bleeding, or lymphatic obstruction. The fluid increases the intrapericardial pressures which decrease diastolic filling and cardiac output.

DIAGNOSIS

Up to two-thirds of patients with PT are asymptomatic. The remainder will complain of dyspnea (87%), chest pain, orthopnea, or generalized weakness. Other findings include tachycardia, hypotension, jugular venous distention, edema, cyanosis, diminished cardiac sounds, pulsus paradoxus, or a pericardial friction rub. The ECG reveals low voltage in all the limb leads and electrical alternans (cyclic beat to beat shifts in the QRS axis due to the mechanical swinging of the heart to and fro). Chest x-ray can reveal an enlarged cardiac silhouette, pleural effusions, or pulmonary congestion. Echocardiography establishes the diagnosis. Pericardial fluid cytology should be obtained to confirm the diagnosis, but false-negatives do occur.

THERAPEUTIC APPROACH

Asymptomatic patients can be observed. Symptomatic patients usually require pericardiocentesis to relieve their symptoms; regardless 60% will reaccumulate. Sclerosing agents have been used to permanently seal the pericardial sac and prevent recurrences (73% to 94% success rate), but pain and atrial arrhythmias limit the usefulness of this approach. A pericardial window (subxiphoid pericardiotomy and pericardial stripping), which permits unimpeded fluid drainage into the thoracic cavity, is an option in patients that have failed pericardiocentesis. Chemotherapy reduces the primary tumor and metastatic tumor burden and, hence the likelihood of recurrence.

BIBLIOGRAPHY

Ahmann FR. A reassessment of the clinical implications of the superior vena caval syndrome. *J Clin Oncol.* 1984;2:961-969.

Arrambide K, Toto RD. Tumor lysis syndrome. *Semin Nephrol.* 1993;13:273-299.

Caggiano V, Weiss RV, et al. Incidence, cost, and mortality of neutropenia hospitalization associated with chemotherapy. *Cancer.* 2005;103:1916-1928.

Cervantes A, Chirivella I. Oncological emergencies. *Ann Oncol.* 2004;15(Suppl 4):iv299–306.

Daw HA, Markman M. Epidural spinal cord compression in cancer patients: Diagnosis and management. *Cleve Clin J Med.* 2000;67:497–512.

Del Toro G, Morris E, Cairo MS. Tumor lysis syndrome: Pathophysiology, definition, and alternative treatment approaches. *Clin Adv Hematol Oncol.* 2005;3:54–67.

Dempke W, Firusian N. Treatment of malignant pericardial effusion with ^{32}P-colloid. *Br J Cancer.* 1999;80:1955–1966.

Feusner J, Farber MS. Role of intravenous allopurinol in the management of acute tumor lysis syndrome. Semin Oncol 2001;28(Suppl 5):13–22.

Flombaum CD. Metabolic emergencies in the cancer patient. *Semin Oncol.* 2000;27:322–334.

Freifeld A, Marchigiani D, Walsh T, et al. A double-blind comparison of empirical oral and intravenous antibiotic therapy for low-risk febrile patients with neutropenia during cancer chemotherapy. *N Engl J Med.* 1999;341:305–312.

Higdon ML, Higdon JA. Treatment of oncologic emergencies. *Am Fam Physician.* 2006;74:1873–1899.

Krimsky WS, Behrens RJ, Kerkvliet GJ. Oncologic emergencies for the internist. *Cleve Clin J Med.* 2002;69:209–215.

Lo N, Cullen M. Antibiotic prophylaxis in chemotherapy-induced neutropenia: Time to reconsider. *Hematol Oncol.* 2006;24:120.

Loblaw DA, Perry J, Chambers A, Lapierre NJ. Systematic review of the diagnosis and management of malignant extradural spinal cord compression: The Cancer Care Ontario Practice Guidelines Initiative's Neuro-Oncology Disease Site Group. *J Clin Oncol.* 2005;23:2028–2037.

Lonardi F, Gioga G, Agus G, et al. Double-flash, large-fraction radiation therapy as palliative treatment of malignant superior vena cava syndrome in the elderly. *Support Care Cancer.* 2002;10:156.

Mundy GR, Guise TA. Hypercalcemia of malignancy. *Am J Med.* 1997;103:134.

Poortmans P, Vulto A, Raaijmakers E. Always on a Friday? Time patterns of referral for spinal cord compression. *Acta Oncol.* 2001;40:88.

Quinn JA, DeAngelis LM. Neurologic emergencies in the cancer patient. *Semin Oncol.* 2000;27:311–321.

Rolston KV. The Infectious Diseases Society of America 2002 guidelines for the use of antimicrobial agents in patients with cancer and neutropenia: Salient features and comments. *Clin Infect Dis.* 2004;39(Suppl 1):s44.

Shepherd FA. Malignant pericardial effusion. *Curr Opin Oncol.* 1997;9:170.

Silverman P, Distelhorst CW. Metabolic emergencies in clinical oncology. *Semin Oncol.* 1989;16:504.

Smith TJ, Khatcheressian J, Lyman G, et al. 2006 update of recommendations for the use of white blood cell growth factors: An evidence-based clinical practice guideline. *J Clin Oncol.* 2006;24:3187.

Stewart AF. Clinical practice. Hypercalcemia associated with cancer. *N Engl J Med.* 2005;352:373.

Tangiawa N, Sawada S, Mishima K, et al. Clinical outcome of stenting in superior vena cava syndrome associated with malignant tumors. *Acta Radiol.* 1998;39:669.

84 THE RISK OF THERAPY-RELATED ORGAN DAMAGE IN LONG-TERM SURVIVORS OF CANCER TREATMENT

Michael C. Perry

At current rates, nearly 1 million cancer patients are added to the list of those cured every year. Many survivors bear some mark of their diagnosis and therapy, and experience a variety of long-term complications, ranging from medical problems to psychosocial disturbances to sexual dysfunction to inability to find employment or insurance. A recent study reviewed the Childhood Cancer Survivor population and found a high incidence of chronic health conditions years after treatment. This chapter deals with the medical problems produced by chemotherapy, radiation therapy, or their combination.

In 1982, the idea of using timing as a means of classifying chemotherapeutic toxicity was advanced, dividing side effects into immediate (onset in hours to days), early (onset in days to weeks), delayed (onset in weeks to months), and late (onset in months to years). The latter group is the subject of this chapter.

There are several requirements for detecting late consequences. There must be a sizable population of long survivors, which implies effective therapy. For many solid tumors (colorectal cancer, breast cancer, lung cancer), effective therapy has only recently been available. The population of survivors with childhood malignancies has provided much information. Many common adult cancers, when advanced, are refractory to current therapies; and therefore there are few long-term survivors of metastatic breast, lung, pancreatic, ovarian, and colon cancer. To accurately assess side effects, a fairly uniform treatment schedule must be followed, such as radiation therapy for early stage Hodgkin disease (or a standard chemotherapy for non-Hodgkin lymphomas). Although varying doses and fields of radiation may have been used, the therapy must be sufficiently similar to permit analysis. Careful long-term follow-up is, of course, essential to detect any future abnormalities. Finally, it is important to appreciate that therapy may produce subclinical damage that may only become relevant in the presence of a second inciting factor, such as the development of a coexisting disease or advancing age.

Using the aforementioned definition, the diseases primarily studied for long-term organ damage include pediatric malignancies (acute lymphoblastic leukemia, Ewing sarcoma, neuroblastoma, osteogenic sarcoma, rhabdomyosarcoma, and Wilms tumor), Hodgkin and non-Hodgkin lymphomas, testicular cancer, early stage breast cancer, and the small proportion of lung cancer patients with limited stage, small-cell lung cancer.

Perhaps the best-known late consequence of chemotherapy is anthracycline-induced congestive heart failure, which was recognized very early in the doxorubicin (Adriamycin) era. A dose-dependent dropout of myocardial cells was seen on endomyocardial biopsy, and eventually ventricular failure ensued. Coexisting cardiac disease, concurrent medications, and thoracic radiation therapy may hasten the onset of congestive heart failure. Other related drugs share the potential for cardiac toxicity. The development of dexrazoxane may permit the use of doxorubicin (Adriamycin) for longer periods of time and hence higher cumulative doses without congestive heart failure.

Other chronic cardiac complications include premature coronary artery disease or pericarditis from mediastinal radiation therapy (as for Hodgkin disease or left-sided breast cancer).

Pulmonary fibrosis associated with bleomycin was recognized as dose-dependent, and exacerbated by age, preexisting lung disease, radiation to the chest, high concentrations of inhaled oxygen, and the concomitant use of other chemotherapeutic agents. Several other chemotherapy agents can cause pulmonary fibrosis, and at least five can promote pulmonary venoocclusive disease, especially following high-dose therapy; such as that utilized in peripheral blood/bone marrow transplantation.

Clinically significant long-term damage to the liver from standard-dose chemotherapy is relatively infrequent and mostly confined to patents who have received chronic methotrexate for maintenance therapy of acute lymphoblastic leukemia. Although rarely seen with standard-dose chemotherapy, hepatic venoocclusive disease is more common with high-dose therapy, such as autologous bone marrow transplantation.

Cisplatin is capable of producing reduced renal function, which is usually asymptomatic. It does render the patient more susceptible to acute renal injury (sometimes requiring dialysis or transplantation) if other renal insults are incurred. Cyclophosphamide cystitis may eventually lead to the development of bladder cancer. Ifosfamide produces a Fanconi-like syndrome, which is usually, but not always, reversible. An unusual side effect of chemotherapy for testicular cancer is the development of Raynaud phenomenon, seen in up to 40% of patients. The pathologic mechanism is unknown, but bleomycin has been used in most patients. The severity can vary from minor to debilitating.

Dose-related hearing loss can occur with the administration of cisplatin, usually with doses in excess of 400 mg/m^2. This is irreversible and patients should be screened with audiometric exams periodically during such therapy.

Cataracts are associated with chronic corticosteroid use, radiation therapy to the head, and rarely tamoxifen.

Thyroid disease is common in patients who have received radiation therapy to the neck, especially patients with Hodgkin disease treated with mantle radiation therapy. In one study of 1677 patients whose thyroid was irradiated, the incidence of thyroid disease was 52% at 20 years after treatment and 67% at 26 years. Hypothyroidism was the most common abnormality, followed by Graves disease, thyroiditis, and thyroid cancer. Any patient whose neck has been irradiated should be closely followed for the development of hypothyroidism and other thyroid abnormalities.

The late consequences of radiation therapy on the musculoskeletal system are related to the radiation dose, volume of tissue irradiated, and the age of the child at the time of therapy. Damage to the microvasculature of the epiphyseal growth zone may result in leg-length discrepancy, scoliosis, and short stature.

Although many patients experience peripheral neuropathy during chemotherapy, only a few have chronic problems, such as patients with coexisting medical diseases such as diabetes mellitus. Neurocognitive sequelae from intrathecal chemotherapy, with or without radiation therapy, are recognized complications of successful therapy of childhood acute lymphoblastic leukemia.

Prophylactic cranial radiation, used in the treatment of limited stage small-cell lung cancer can produce long-term neuropsychiatric effects, and the risk of toxicity must be balanced against the high probability of brain metastases in untreated patients.

Reversible azoospermia can be caused by many chemotherapy agents. The gonads may be permanently damaged by radiation therapy or by chemotherapeutic agents, particularly the alkylating agents. The extent of the damage depends on the patient's age and the total dose administered. As a woman nears menopause, smaller doses of chemotherapy cause ovarian failure. In men, chemotherapy may produce infertility, but male sex hormone production is not usually affected. However, women commonly lose both fertility and hormone production. The premature induction of menopause in a young woman can have serious medical and psychologic consequences.

Second malignancies are becoming a major concern for those cured of cancer. These cancers include myelo-dysplasia and acute myelogenous leukemia from chemotherapy, non-Hodgkin lymphomas from chemotherapy and radiation therapy, and sarcomas, melanomas, and breast cancer from radiation therapy. Tamoxifen-induced endometrial cancer is an example of a hormonally induced second cancer.

In the future, with the use of new chemotherapeutic agents, and newer techniques of radiation therapy and combined modality treatment, we can perhaps anticipate a lower incidence of chronic side effects or second malignancies. Additional populations at risk include cancers responsive to newer chemotherapy such as ovarian cancer, and cancers where chemotherapy and radiation therapy are used in an organ-sparing approach to avoid disfiguring surgery such as bladder cancer, anal cancer, and laryngeal cancer.

BIBLIOGRAPHY

Beaty O, Hudson MM, Greenwald C, et al. Subsequent malignancies in children and adolescents after treatment for Hodgkin's disease. *J Clin Oncol.* 1995;13:603–609.

Bines J, Oleske DM, Cobleigh M. Ovarian function in premenopausal women treated with adjuvant chemotherapy for breast cancer. *J Clin Oncol.* 1996;14:1718–1729.

Bjergaard JP, Osterlind K, Hansen M, et al. Acute nonlymphocytic leukemia, preleukemia, and solid tumors following intensive chemotherapy of small cell carcinoma of the lung. *Blood.* 1985;66:1393–1397.

Byrd R. Late effects of treatment of cancer in children. *Pediatr Clin North Am.* 1985;32:835–857.

Chatterjee R, Goldstone AH. Gonadal damage and effects on fertility in adult patients with haematological malignancy undergoing stem cell transplantation. *Bone Marrow Transplant.* 1996;17:5–11.

Curtis RE, Rowlings PA, Deeg HJ, et al. Solid cancers after bone marrow transplantation. *N Engl J Med.* 1997;336:897–904.

Dang SP, Liberman BA, Shepherd FA, et al. Therapy-related leukemia and myelodysplasia in small-cell lung cancer.

DeLaat CA, Lampkin BC. Long-term survivors of childhood cancer: evaluation and identification of sequelae of treatment. *CA Cancer J Clin.* 1992;42:263–282.

Diller L. Rhabdomyosarcoma and other soft tissue sarcomas of childhood. *Curr Opin Oncol.* 1992;4:689–695.

Doll DC, Shauab N. Vascular toxicity. In: Perry MC. *The Chemotherapy Sourcebook.* 4th ed. Philadelphia, PA: Wolters Kluwer; 2008:245–258.

Ewer MS, Benjamin RS. Cardiotoxicity of chemotherapeutic drugs. In: Perry MC. *The Chemotherapy Sourcebook.* 2nd ed. Baltimore, MD: Williams and Wilkins; 1996:649–663.

Fisher B, Costantino JP, Redmond CK, Fisher ER, Wickerham DL, Cronin WM. Endometrial cancer in tamoxifen-treated breast cancer patients: Findings from the National Surgical Adjuvant Breast and Bowel project (NSABP) B-14. *JNCI.* 1994;86:527–537.

Forbes JF. Long-term effects of adjuvant chemotherapy in breast cancer. *Acta Oncol.* 1992;31:243–250.

Green DM, Donckerwolcke R, Evans A, D'Angio GJ. Late effects of treatment for Wilms tumor. *Hematol Oncol Clin North Am.* 1995;9:1317–1327.

Hancock S, Tucker M, Hoppe R. Factors affecting late mortality from heart disease after treatment of Hodgkin's disease. *JAMA.* 1993;270:1949–1955.

Hancock SL, Cox RS, McDougall IR. Thyroid diseases after treatment of Hodgkin's disease. *N Engl J Med.* 1991;325:599–605.

Hancock SL, Donaldson SS, Hoppe RT. Cardiac disease following treatment of Hodgkin's disease in children and adolescents. *J Clin Oncol.* 1993;11:1208–1215.

Henry-Amar M, Hayat M, Meerwaldt JH, et al. Causes of death after therapy for early stage Hodgkin's disease entered on EORTC protocols. *Int J Radiat Oncol Biol Phys.* 1990;19:1155–1157.

Johnson DH, Porter LL, List AF, et al. Acute nonlymphocytic leukemia after treatment of small cell lung cancer. *Am J Med.* 1986;81:962–968.

Morgenstern D and Govindeem R. Pulmonary toxicity of chemotherapeutic drugs. In: Perry MC. *The Chemotherapy Sourcebook.* 4th ed. Philadelphia, PA: Wolters Kluwer; 2008:191–196.

Lange BJ, Meadows AT. Late effects of Hodgkin's disease treatment in children. *Cancer Treat Res.* 1989;41:195–220.

Le Chevalier T. Review of toxicity and long-term sequelae in lung cancer. *Antibiot Chemother.* 1998;41:199–203.

Li F. *Cancer survivors: Future Clinical and Research Issues.* ASCO Education Book; 1998.

Lipshultz S, Colan S, Gelber R, et al. Late cardiac effects of doxorubicin therapy for acute lymphoblastic leukemia in childhood. *N Engl J Med.* 1991;324:808–815.

Lipshultz S, Lipsitz S, Mone S, et al. Female sex and higher drug dose as risk factors for late cardiotoxic effects of doxorubicin therapy for childhood cancer. *N Engl J Med.* 1995;332: 173801743.

Marina N. Long-term survivors of childhood cancer: The medical consequences of cure. *Pediatr Clin North Am.* 1997;44: 1021–1042.

Meister LA, Meadows AT. Late effects of childhood cancer therapy. *Curr Probl Pediatr.* 1993;23:102–131.

Mohn A, Chiarelli F, DiMarzio A, Impicciatore P, Marisico S, Angrilli F. Thyroid function in children treated for acute lymphoblastic leukemia. *J Endocrinol Invest.* 1997;20:215–219.

Morris Jones PH. The late effects of cancer therapy in childhood [editorial]. *Br J Cancer.* 1991;64:1–2.

Neglia JP, Nesbitt ME. Care and treatment of long-term survivors of childhood cancer. *Cancer.* 1993;71:3386–3391.

Nicholson HS, Byrne J. Fertility and pregnancy after treatment for cancer during childhood or adolescence. *Cancer.* 1993;71:3392–3399.

Nicholson HS, Mulvihill JJ. Late effects of therapy in survivors of childhood and adolescent osetosarcoma. *Cancer Treatment Research.* 1992;62:45–48.

Ochs J, Mulhern R. Long-term sequelae of therapy for childhood acute lymphoblastic leukaemia. *Bailli'ere's Clinical Hematology.* 1994;7:365–376.

Ochs J, Mulhern RK. Late effects of antileukemic treatment. *Pediatr Clin North Am.* 1988;35:815–833.

Oeffinger K, Mertens AC, Sklar CA, et al. Chronic health conditions in adult survivors of childhood cancer. *N Engl J Med.* 2006;355:1572–1582.

Osanto S, Bukman A, Van Hoek F, Sterk PJ, De Laat JAPM, Hermans J. Long-term effects of chemotherapy in patients with testicular cancer. *J Clin Oncol.* 1992;10:574–579.

Perry MC, Longo DL. Late consequences of cancer and its treatment. In *Harrison's 16th Edition of Principles of Internal Medicine.* McGraw-Hill Medical Publishing Division; 2005:583–586.

Perry MC, Yarbro JW. Complications of chemotherapy: An overview. In: *Toxicity of Chemotherapy.* Grune and Stratton; 1984:1–19.

Perry MC. Chemotherapy, toxicity, and the clinician. *Semin Oncol.* 1982;9:1–4.

Ratain MJ, Kaminer LS, Bitran JD, et al. Acute nonlymphocytic leukemia following etoposide and cisplatin combination chemotherapy for advanced non-small cell carcinoma of the lung. *Blood.* 1987;70:1412–1417.

Reid HL, Jaffe N. Radiation-induced changes in long-term survivors of childhood cancer after treatment with radiation therapy. *Semin Roentgenol.* 1994;29:6–14.

Rowland KM, Murthy A. Hodgkin's disease: Long term effects of therapy. *Med Pediatr Oncol.* 1986;14:88–96.

Schellong G. The balance between cure and late effects in childhood Hodgkin's lymphoma: the experience of the German-Austrian Study Group since 1978. *Ann Oncol.* 1996;7: S67–S72.

Schenkein DP, Schwartz RS. Neoplasms and transplantation-trading swords for plowshares (editorial). *N Engl J Med.* 1997;336:949–950.

Shapiro CL, Henderson IC. Adjuvant therapy of breast cancer. *Hematol Oncol Clin North Am.* 1994;8:213–231.

Shapiro CL, Recht A. Late effects of adjuvant therapy for breast cancer. *JNCI Monographs.* 1994;16:101–112.

Steinherz L. Steinherz R, Tan C, et al. Cardiac toxicity 4 to 20 years after completing anthracycline therapy. *JAMA.* 1991;266:1672–1677.

Valagussa P, Santoro A, Bonnadonna G. Thyroid, pulmonary, and cardiac sequelae after treatment for Hodgkin's disease. *Ann Oncol.* 1992;3:S111–S115.

Van Basten JP, Koops HS, Slijfer DT, Pras E, van Driel NF, Hoekstra HJ. Current concepts about testicular cancer. *Eur J Surg Oncol.* 1997;23:354–366.

Van Leeuwem F, Klokman W, Hagenbeek A, et al. Second cancer risk following Hodgkin's disease: A 20-year follow-up study. *J Clin Oncol.* 1194;12:312–325.

Van Leeuwen FE. Risk of acute myelogenous leukaemia and myelodysplasia following cancer treatment. *Bailli'ere's Clinical Hematology.* 1996;7:57–84.

Vogelzang NJ, Bosl GJ, Johnson K, et al. Raynaud's phenomenon: A common toxicity after combination chemotherapy for testicular cancer. *Ann Intern Med.* 1981;95:288–292.

Von Hoff DD, Rozencweig M, Layard M, Slavik M, Muggia F. Daunomycin-induced cardiotoxicity in children and adults: A review of 110 cases. *Am J Med.* 1977;62:200–208.

85 FEVER OF UNKNOWN ORIGIN

Musab U. Saeed and Donald J. Kennedy

DEFINITION AND CLASSIFICATION

- The archetypical definition of a fever of unknown origin (FUO) includes: (1) temperature >38.3°C (101°F) on multiple occasions, (2) duration of fever for at least 3 weeks, and (3) uncertain diagnosis after at least 1 week of investigation of pertinent clinical findings.
- The classic definition has undergone revision and is currently subdivided into four categories:
  1. Classic FUO: >3 weeks duration, >2 outpatient visits for evaluation or 3 days of hospitalization.
  2. Nosocomial FUO: hospital-acquired fever and uncertain diagnosis after 3 days of investigation.
  3. Immunodeficient FUO: >3 days duration with an uncertain diagnosis after 48 hours of evaluation in an immunocompromised host.
  4. Human immunodeficiency virus (HIV) associated FUO: >3 weeks duration (as an outpatient) or >3 days duration as an inpatient in a confirmed HIV infected patient.

ETIOLOGY

CLASSIC FEVER OF UNKNOWN ORIGIN

- A classic FUO is usually caused by one of the following conditions:
  - Infections (23%–36%): Tuberculosis, endocarditis, local suppurative process (eg, biliary tract, kidney), septic thrombophlebitis, cytomegalovirus, and Epstein-Barr virus

  - Neoplastic (7%–31%): Lymphoma, leukemia, renal cell carcinoma, and gastrointestinal tumors
  - Collagen vascular diseases (9%–20%): systemic lupus erythematosus, rheumatoid arthritis, mixed connective tissue disease, temporal arteritis
  - Miscellaneous (17%–24%): Drug fever, deep vein thrombosis, pulmonary emboli, sarcoidosis, factitious or fraudulent fever

NOSOCOMIAL FEVER OF UNKNOWN ORIGIN

- The most common causes of nosocomial FUO include pneumonia, urinary tract infection, surgical site infection, catheter-related infections, *Clostridium difficile* colitis, and drugs.

IMMUNODEFICIENCY- AND HUMAN IMMUNODEFICIENCY VIRUS–ASSOCIATED FEVER OF UNKNOWN ORIGIN

- In addition to the causes of classic FUO, consider opportunistic infections caused by *Mycobacterium tuberculosis*, atypical mycobacteria, *Pneumocystis jirovecii*, and fungi (*Histoplasma capsulatum*, *Cryptococcus neoformans*, and *Coccidioides immitis*). Malignancies such as Kaposi sarcoma and primary brain lymphoma should also be entertained.

CLINICAL FEATURES

- The initial evaluation should include a comprehensive history with emphasis on recent travel, exposure to pets and sick contacts, work environment, family history of fevers (familial Mediterranean fever), and a complete list of medication used by the patient.
- On examination special attention should be directed toward identification of a rash or other skin lesion. Fungal infections, HIV, measles, rubella, Epstein-Barr

509

virus, hepatitis B virus, and ehrlichiosis usually present with a maculopapular rash. Herpes simplex virus and varicella-zoster virus present with a vesicular rash, whereas patients with *Rickettsiae,* yellow fever, viral hemorrhagic fever, and coxsackievirus may develop a petechial rash. A careful funduscopic, otoscopic, genital, and rectal examination should also be performed.

- Lymphadenopathy may provide a vital clue to the underlying condition. Importantly, affected lymph nodes can be easily biopsied.
- Nosocomial FUO requires special attention to all intravascular devices, previous surgical procedure sites, evidence of pneumonia, and medications.

DIAGNOSIS

- The diagnostic investigation should be guided by the history and physical examination.
- Complete blood count with manual differential, blood smear, erythrocyte sedimentation rate, blood cultures for bacteria, fungi, acid-fast bacilli (AFB), and fungal serologies may point toward the underlying diagnosis.
- Bone marrow aspiration and biopsy should be considered in patients with suspected hematologic or granulomatous diseases.
- Imaging studies such as computed tomography scan, magnetic resonance imaging, and ultrasound may prove useful when evaluating an affected organ system. Although highly sensitive, radiolabeled imaging is not very specific and its role in the evaluation of FUO is yet to be determined.

MANAGEMENT

- Empiric therapeutic trials pose significant risks and are usually met with limited success. As a general rule, treatment should be withheld whenever possible until the etiology can be determined.
- Hospitalized patients who are neutropenic or septic are an exception because of a high prevalence of serious bacterial infections. These patients should receive empiric broad spectrum antibiotics after obtaining appropriate cultures. β-lactam-aminoglycoside combinations, piperacillin with ciprofloxacin, or a single agent antipseudomonal cephalosporin or carbapenem are among several options available. Vancomycin should be considered for patients with indwelling vascular catheters or those at risk for resistant gram-positive pathogens.
- With the exception of the fever that accompanies primary HIV infection, a fever that develops in a patient with known HIV is usually the result of an underlying infection.
- Medications which have been associated with fever include, but is not limited to, atropine, amphotericin B, antihistamines angiotensin-converting enzyme inhibitors, barbiturates, cephalosporins, diuretics, heparin, nonsteroidal antiinflammatory drugs, macrolides, phenytoin, and penicillins.

BIBLIOGRAPHY

Hashmey HR, Roberts NJ Jr. Fever and fever of unknown etiology. In: Betts RF, Chapman SW, Penn RL, eds. *A Practical Approach to Infectious Disease.* 5th ed. Philadelphia, PA: Lippincott Williams & Wilkins; 2003:1.

Mackowiak PA, Durack DT. Fever of unknown origin. In: Mandell GL, Bennett JE, Dolin R, eds. *Principles and Practice of Infectious Diseases.* 6th ed. Philadelphia: Elsevier Churchill Livingstone; 2005:718.

Norman DC. Fever in the elderly. *Clin Infect Dis.* 2000;31:148–151.

86 CENTRAL NERVOUS SYSTEM INFECTIONS

Musab U. Saeed and Donald J. Kennedy

ACUTE BACTERIAL MENINGITIS

ETIOLOGY

- The most common causes of bacterial meningitis in the adult are *Neisseria meningitis* and *Streptococcus pneumoniae.* Among newborns the most common pathogens include group B streptococcus (70%), *Listeria monocytogenes* (20%), and *Streptococcus pneumonia* (10%). The frequency of meningitis caused by *Haemophilus influenzae* has decreased substantially since the introduction of a conjugated vaccine. *Listeria monocytogenes* is also a common pathogen in the cell mediated immunodeficient host and in patients >60 years of age.
- Patients with head trauma, recent neurosurgic procedures, immunosuppression, and gram-negative septicemia may develop infection with gram-negative bacilli (*Klebsiella* spp., *Escherichia coli, Serratia marcescens, Pseudomonas aeruginosa,* and *Salmonella* spp.).

CLINICAL FEATURES

- Patients may present with fever, headaches, meningismus, altered mental status, vomiting, photophobia, and focal neurologic deficits (10%–20%).
- On examination, nuchal rigidity is present in up to 90% of patients and may persist for several weeks despite clinical improvement. A positive Kernig and Brudzinski sign may be elicited. Increased intracranial pressure may lead to severe hypertension, bradycardia, photophobia, papilledema, and cranial nerve palsies.

DIAGNOSIS

- Lumbar puncture should be performed promptly before initiating antibiotics in all suspected cases of meningitis. Cerebrospinal fluid (CSF) analysis is invaluable in establishing an early diagnosis (Table 86–1). Gram stain of the CSF may identify the causative pathogen in 60%–90% of cases. Blood cultures should be obtained in all suspected cases of bacterial meningitis.
- Computed tomography (CT) scan or magnetic resonance imaging (MRI) should be performed in patients with clinical evidence of increased intracranial pressure. However, diagnostic imaging should not delay initial antibiotic treatment. Importantly, a screening CT is not necessary in the vast majority of patients unless there is evidence of mass effect (previous history of CNS disease, new onset seizure, papilledema, altered mental status, or focal neurologic deficits).

MANAGEMENT

- Treatment of acute bacterial meningitis *must* begin without delay. A reasonable empiric antibiotic regimen includes a third-generation cephalosporin (ceftriaxone) combined with vancomycin. Ampicillin should be added to the regimen for patients at high-risk for infection

TABLE 86–1   Cerebrospinal Fluid Analysis in Meningitis

STUDIES	BACTERIAL	VIRAL	CHRONIC
WBC/mm^3	100–10,000	100–1000	100–1000
Predominant cells	PMNs	Lymphocytes	Lymphocytes
Glucose (45–85 mg/dL)	<45	Normal or low	<45
Protein (15–45 mg/dL)	>50	>50	>50
Opening pressure (70–180 mm H$_2$O)	↑↑↑	↑↑	↑

PMN, polymorphonuclear neutrophil; WBC, white blood cell.

with *L. monocytogenes*. Once a pathogen is identified, antibiotics should be modified accordingly. The duration of therapy is usually 10 to 14 days.

ASEPTIC MENINGITIS AND VIRAL ENCEPHALITIS

ETIOLOGY

- Aseptic meningitis is characterized by meningeal inflammation with negative bacterial cultures and Gram stain of the blood and CSF.
- Aseptic meningitis and encephalitis are usually the result of viral infection.
- Enterovirus (echoviruses, coxsackie viruses) and herpes viruses are the most common pathogens depending on the clinical setting. For example, in the summer and fall enteroviruses are the most common pathogens.
- Viral encephalitis is associated with a wide variety of pathogens including, but not limited to, Herpesviridae, Flaviviridae (St. Louis encephalitis virus, West Nile virus, Dengue fever virus), Togaviridae (Eastern, Western, and Venezuelan equine encephalitis virus), Colorado tick fever, Paramyxoviridae (mumps virus), and Poxviridae.

CLINICAL FEATURES

- Viral meningitis may initially present with nonspecific complaints including fever, headaches, rash, diarrhea, upper respiratory tract findings, myalgias, and conjunctivitis. The time of year (summer versus winter), history of mosquito (West Nile virus) or tick bites (ehrlichia), and risk factors for human immunodeficiency virus (HIV) are important historical findings.
- There is considerable variability in the natural history of viral meningoencephalitis, depending on the etiologic agent. Rabies virus is almost always fatal, whereas, enteroviruses are self-limited without sequelae. Herpes simplex encephalitis develops rapidly and is associated with changes in the patients personality, hallucinations, and aphasia (caused by temporal lobe involvement). Imaging studies may reveal focal abnormalities in the temporal lobes.
- The geographic location and the mode of entry (Table 86–2) may prove useful in identifying the causative pathogen.
- Viral encephalitis is characterized by headache, fever, nuchal rigidity, altered level of consciousness, lethargy, confusion, seizures, stupor, and coma. Patient may develop focal neurologic signs (cranial

TABLE 86–2 **Viral Causes of Meningeal Inflammation and Encephalitis and Their Portal of Entry**

PORTAL OF ENTRY	VIRUS
Respiratory tract	Measles, mumps, VZV, adenovirus
Gastrointestinal tract	Enteroviruses, echovirus, poliovirus
Genital tract	HSV
Skin subcutaneous tissue (e.g. mosquitoes, tick bites)	Flaviviruses,(West Nile, Dengue fever virus, St. Louis and Japanese encephalitis)

HSV, herpes simplex virus; VZV, varicella-zoster virus.

nerve involvement), aberrant motor activity, tremors, and an abnormal plantar response. Spinal involvement can induce flaccid paralysis with depression of the deep tendon reflexes.

DIAGNOSIS

- Enterovirus and herpes simplex virus (HSV) can be detected by polymerase chain reaction (PCR), or viral culture.
- In viral meningoencephalomyelitis, the CSF is characterized by variable pleocytosis (10–2000 cells/mm^3), with a predominance of mononuclear cells. The CSF fluid may also be associated with an increased number of red blood cells, especially with herpes simplex encephalitis. Cerebrospinal fluid PCR is available for some viruses including herpes viruses, enteroviruses, and polyomavirus, however, PCR is not routinely performed considering the wide-range of potential viral etiologies.

MANAGEMENT

- Viral meningitis requires supportive care since most viruses do not respond to antiviral therapy.
- Treatment with intravenous acyclovir for HSV encephalitis should be initiated promptly after the initial evaluation of the lumbar puncture. Meningitis associated with either primary or reactivation of HSV-2 is usually self-limited, but acyclovir may hasten recovery.
- Meningitis associated with either primary or cytomegalovirus encephalitis can be treated with ganciclovir or foscarnet. Neurologic disease–associated HIV may improve with antiretroviral treatment.

CHRONIC MENINGITIS

ETIOLOGY

- If neurologic symptoms and signs persist and the CSF remains abnormal for 4 or more weeks, a diagnosis of chronic meningitis should be considered. The most

common pathogens isolated in this setting include mycobacteria, fungi (*Cryptococcus neoformans, Coccidioides immitis, Candida* spp., *Histoplasma capsulatum*), and spirochetes (*Treponema pallidum, Borrelia burgdorferi*).

CLINICAL FEATURES

- A careful history detailing travel (coccidioidomycosis), exposure to sexually transmitted diseases, exposure to animals (rodents), occupational exposure to infectious agents, and medication use (NSAIDs) should be obtained. The physical examination should include a careful skin examination for lesions (rashes consistent with connective tissue disease), subcutaneous nodules, and lymphadenopathy (fungal and TB); ophthalmologic and otoscopic examination should also be performed.
- Tuberculous and cryptococcal meningitis may manifest symptoms and signs of slowly progressive hydrocephalus, including headache, nausea, vomiting, and mental deterioration.

DIAGNOSIS

- Repeated lumber puncture may be required to establish the diagnosis. Cerebrospinal fluid cytology, VDRL/RPR, fungal and acid-fast bacilli stains, and cultures should be obtained. Crytococcal antigen, serum antibodies to *Histoplasma capsulatum, Brucella* species, and *Toxoplasma gondii* in the appropriate clinical setting may also prove valuable. A meningeal and brain biopsy should be considered in patients that continue to deteriorate and the diagnosis has not been established.
- Chronic fungal or bacterial meningitis is associated with moderate mononuclear pleocytosis in the CSF. Meningoencephalitis caused by *Nocardia, Actinomyces, Candida,* or *Aspergillus* elicits a polymorphonuclear response and coccidioidomycosis may be associated with CSF and peripheral eosinophils.
- Tests for specific immunoglobulin M in serum and CSF may be especially useful when evaluating *Mycoplasma* and Epstein-Barr virus.

MANAGEMENT

- Tuberculosis (TB) is the most common cause of chronic meningitis. Empiric treatment with antituberculous drugs is appropriate in patients with severe symptoms or a deteriorating clinical course.

- Meningitis caused by fungi (*C. neoformans*, coccidioides, or *Candida* spp) should be treated with appropriate anti-fungals (amphoterecin B, 5-fluctytocine, or fluconazole).
- Neurosyphilis is treated with intravenous penicillin G, 12 to 24 million units daily in four divided doses for 10 to 14 days.

BRAIN ABSCESS, SUBDURAL EMPYEMA, AND EPIDURAL ABSCESSES

ETIOLOGY

- Brain abscess are frequently polymicrobial and include Streptococcus species such as *Streptococcus anginosus, Streptococcus constellatus,* and *Streptococcus intermedius* (30%–60%). Patients with penetrating cranial trauma or infective endocarditis may develop *S. aureus* infections (10%–15%). Gram-negative bacilli such as *Escherichia coli, Klebsiella* species, and *Pseudomonas* species are seen in patents with an otogenic focus. Immunocompromised patients are at risk for fungal infections (*Candida* spp., *Aspergillus* spp.) and toxoplasmosis. Mucormycosis should be considered in the diabetic.
- Subdural empyema is a complication of otorhinologic infections with paranasal sinus involvement. Polymicrobial infections are common with these infections and include streptococci, staphylococci, anaerobes, and gram-negative bacilli.
- Epidural abscess is usually hematogenous in origin but can also occur after penetrating trauma or craniotomy. The most commonly isolated organism is *S. aureus* (50%–90%), followed by streptococci and gram-negative bacilli.

CLINICAL FEATURES

- Patients with brain abscess may present with clinical findings of an acute infection, such as fevers, headache, and mental status changes, or with symptoms of an expanding intracranial mass lesion such as nausea, vomiting, seizures, and focal neurologic deficits.
- Subdural empyema is characterized by high fevers, headaches, vomiting, altered mental status which quickly progresses to obtundation.
- Because of its location between dura and surrounding vertebrae, epidural abscess is more insidious in onset and progression than a subdural empyema. The symptoms of a spinal epidural abscess include back pain and spinal cord dysfunction (lower extremity weakness and incontinence).

DIAGNOSIS

- Computed tomography (CT) scan or MRI are the imaging studies of choice for identification of a brain abscess. CT scan with contrast reveals hypodense areas within the brain coupled with a uniform ring enhancement signifying brain edema. MRI provides somewhat better definition of the lesion, and is particularly valuable to assess the epidural and subdural space. Subdural empyema is characterized by a crescentic hypodense appearance, whereas epidural abcesses appear as superficial circumscribed hypointense lesions.
- CT guided aspiration of the suspected abscess should be performed for Gram stain, aerobic and anaerobic cultures, and cultures for AFB and fungi.

MANAGEMENT

- Lesions greater than 2.5 cm in diameter should be excised or aspirated, and empiric antibiotics should be initiated after obtaining appropriate stains and cultures. Empiric antibiotics are chosen based on clinical features (Table 86–3).
- Fungal brain abscess carries a high mortality rate in the immunocompromised patient. The antifungal treatment of choice is combined therapy with amphotericin B and 5-flucytosine.

TABLE 86–3 Antibiotic Recommendations for Therapy Based on Predisposing Conditions and the Most Likely Organism

ANTIBIOTIC OF CHOICE	PREDISPOSING CONDITION (LIKELY ORGANISM)
Vancomycin + metronidazole + third-generation cephalosporin	Unknown
Metronidazole + third-generation cephalosporin	Ear or sinus infections (gram-negatives rods, anaerobes)
Penicillin + metronidazole	Dental abscesses (streptococci, oral cavity anaerobes)
Vancomycin or nafcillin + gentamicin	Bacterial endocarditis (gram-positive cocci)
Penicillin + metronidazole + sulfonamide	Lung abscess or empyema (gram-positive cocci, anaerobes, nocardia)
Vancomycin + third-generation cephalosporin	Trauma/recent neurosurgery (MRSA, gram-negative rods)

MRSA, methicillin-resistant *Staphylococcus aureus*.

- Antibiotic recommendations for epidural and subdural abscesses are similar to brain abscess (see Table 86–3). Both conditions require prompt surgical drainage and prolonged antibiotic administration (4 to 6 weeks). In the presence of concurrent osteomyelitis the treatment duration may need to be extended.

BIBLIOGRAPHY

Choi C. Bacterial meningitis in aging adults. *Clin Infect Dis.* 2001;33:1384.

Quagliarello VJ, Scheld WM. Treatment of bacterial meningitis. *N Engl J Med.* 1997;336:708.

Roos KL, Tyler KL. Meningitis encephalitis, brain abscess and empyema. In: Kasper DL, Braunwald E, Fauci AS, et al, eds. *Harrison's Principles of Internal Medicine.* 16th ed. New York: McGraw-Hill; 2005:2471.

87 RESPIRATORY TRACT INFECTIONS

Musab U. Saeed and Donald J. Kennedy

PHARYNGITIS, LARYNGITIS AND TONSILLITIS

ETIOLOGY

- Inflammation of the pharynx, larynx, and tonsils is usually associated with a viral etiology (adenovirus, influenza A and B, parainfluenza virus, rhinovirus, Epstein-Barr virus, cytomegalovirus, human immunodeficiency virus [HIV]). Laryngotracheobronchitis (croup) is usually caused by parainfluenza type 1 or 3.
- Bacterial etiologies of pharyngitis include Group A (*Streptococcus pyogenes*), C, and G streptococci, *Neisseria gonorrhea,* and less commonly *Corynebacterium diphtheriae.* Inflammation of these structures can also constitute an early expression of *Mycoplasma pneumoniae* and *Chlamydia pneumoniae* infections.

CLINICAL FEATURES

- The history should focus on exposure to sick contacts, recent travel, vaccination, unprotected sexual activity (HIV, herpes simplex virus II), and exposure to oral secretions (Epstein-Barr virus, herpes simplex virus I, varicella-zoster virus).
- Viral pharyngitis usually presents with symptoms of upper respiratory infection including sore throat, rhinorrhea, cough, conjunctivitis, hoarseness (more common in laryngitis), and enlarged tonsils. Epstein-Barr virus, cytomegalovirus, and primary HIV can present with similar symptoms it is vitally important to differentiate between them.
- Group A *Streptococcus* (GAS) should be identified early to avoid complications such as rheumatic fever, toxic shock syndrome, and glomerulonephritis. GAS typically presents as a febrile illness in children characterized by sore throat, headache, pharyngeal erythema, swelling of the uvula, painful enlarged cervical lymph nodes, skin rash, and abdominal pain.
- Diphtheria is rarely seen in the United States because of widespread vaccination. It presents with low-grade fever, pharyngeal inflammation, and a characteristic grey membrane on the oropharyngeal mucosa, which firmly adheres to the surface and bleeds if scraped.
- Laryngitis (regardless of the etiology) may reveal hyperemia and vascular engorgement of vocal cords by indirect laryngoscopy.

DIAGNOSIS

- A rapid strep test is useful but can be negative in up to 10% to 20 % of GAS infections; thus if negative, throat cultures should be obtained.
- Patients who present with fever, adenopathy, pharyngitis, myalgias, and erythematous maculopapular rash should be evaluated for an infectious mononucleosis syndrome (Monospot test, Epstein-Barr virus serology), and HIV (polymerase chain reaction).

TREATMENT

- Viral pharyngitis should be managed with supportive care; however, administering antiviral agents (amantadine for influenza A; zanamivir or oseltamivir for influenza A or B) may reduce the duration of symptoms in influenza. Herpes simplex virus ulcerative infections of the oropharynx may be treated with acyclovir, valacyclovir, and famciclovir, especially in immunocompromised patients.
- Pharyngitis caused by *S. pyogenes* should be treated with a 10 day course of penicillin or a macrolide (azithromycin, clarithromycin, or erythromycin).
- Patients with recurrent pharyngitis and tonsillitis may benefit from tonsillectomy.

- Treatment of diphtheria requires antibiotics and anti-toxin. Active immunization is available and is recommended for all individuals.

ACUTE BRONCHITIS

ETIOLOGY

- Acute bronchitis is usually a self-limited inflammatory disease of the tracheobronchial segment of the respiratory tract.
- Influenza virus, adenovirus, rhinovirus, and respiratory syncytial virus are the most commonly involved pathogens. Nonviral pathogens include *Bordetella pertussis, Mycoplasma pneumoniae,* and *Chlamydia pneumoniae.*

CLINICAL FEATURES

- Patients usually present with fever, cough associated with sputum production, and chest pain. Chest auscultation my reveal harsh breath sounds with crackles or wheezes. Attention should be paid to travel history, exposure to sick contacts, vaccination, and cigarette use.

DIAGNOSIS

- Radiographic imaging of the chest is required in patients in whom pneumonia is suspected. The presence of pulmonary infiltrates indicates pneumonia rather than bronchitis.
- Productive respiratory secretions should be submitted for Gram stain and culture. Rapid diagnostic tests for influenza virus may be helpful. Patients with suspected *M. pneumoniae* should have antibody titers obtained.
- Patients in whom cough persists beyond the expected duration of the acute illness should undergo a more extensive evaluation, including repeat chest x-ray and appropriate sputum stains (acid-fast bacilli, fungal), and cultures. Bronchoscopy may be required to exclude foreign body aspiration, tuberculosis, tumors, and other noninfectious diseases of the tracheobronchial tree and lungs.

TREATMENT

- Treatment of most cases of acute bronchitis is symptomatic and does not require antimicrobial agents unless there is evidence to support a diagnosis of *Bordetella pertussis,* mycoplasma, or chlamydial bronchitis.

- Amantadine (only active against influenza A), zanamivir and oseltamivir are helpful in cases of influenza if administered within the first 48 hours of symptoms. Annual vaccination for influenza prevents infection in populations at risk (health care personnel, chronic illness, etc.).

COMMUNITY-ACQUIRED PNEUMONIA

ETIOLOGY

- Pneumonia is the most common cause of infection-related deaths in the United States.
- The most commonly isolated bacterial pathogens are *S. pneumoniae* (50%) and *Haemophilus influenzae* (3%–38%), followed by *Staphylococcus aureus* (2%–5%) especially in older adults (>65 years of age) and those with recent influenza infection. Gram-negative bacilli should also be considered in older adults with chronic medical problems and a recent hospitalization.
- Atypical pneumonia is caused by *M. pneumoniae, C. pneumoniae, Legionella pneumophila,* and a variety of viral pathogens (influenza A and B, adenovirus, parainfluenza virus, and respiratory syncytial virus). Other rare pathogens that can cause atypical pneumonia include *Chlamydia psittaci, Coxiella burnetii,* and *Francisella tularensis.*
- *Legionella* species should be considered in patients with multiple organ system involvement.

CLINICAL FEATURES

- Most patient are adults older than age 50 years with underlying chronic medical conditions (chronic obstructive pulmonary disease, cardiovascular disease, neurologic diseases, diabetes, alcohol abuse, immunosuppression, malignancy, chronic use of steroids, and HIV).
- Patients with typical community-acquired pneumonia present with acute onset fever, productive cough, chills, fatigue, sweating, and pleuritic chest pain. Physical examination may reveal tachypnea, tachycardia, and crackles on chest auscultation.
- Atypical pneumonia usually begins as a mild respiratory tract illness with a minimally productive cough, which advances to produce fevers, chills, night sweats, myalgias, weakness, conjunctivitis, nausea, and vomiting.
- Aspiration pneumonia should be considered in patients who are at risk for aspiration and present with

necrotizing pneumonia, cavitations, or empyema. Risk factors include age older than 70 years, mechanical ventilation, malnutrition, altered mental status, chronic obstructive pulmonary disease and alcoholism.

DIAGNOSIS

- Patients usually present with leukocytosis; however, when present, leukopenia is a poor prognostic sign. In patients with a productive cough, sputum Gram stain can reveal neutrophils with bacteria, often with a single organism predominating. Blood cultures should be obtained.
- A chest x-ray may be negative early in the disease. Lobar consolidation and pleural effusions are seen more commonly with bacterial involvement, whereas bilateral diffuse infiltrates occur in atypical pneumonia.

MANAGEMENT

- Selection of empiric therapy depends on the most likely pathogen, antibiotic resistance in the geographic location, history of recurrent infections, severity of illness and need for hospitalization.
- Guidelines have been developed by the American Thoracic Society and Infectious Diseases Society of America, which uses age, comorbidities, severity of disease, and clinical findings to determine the optimal management strategy. These guidelines are useful but are not a substitute for clinical judgment. A reasonable empiric antimicrobial approach for the treatment of pneumonia as an outpatient is summarized in Table 87–1.
- Patients who require hospitalization at the outset, who fail outpatient treatment, or who have a history of recent hospitalization, may have drug resistant *S. pneumoniae,*

TABLE 87–2   Antibiotic Recommendations for Hospitalized Patients

PATIENTS	ANTIBIOTIC RECOMMENDATIONS
No recent antibiotic therapy	Quinolones or a macrolide +β-lactam
Recent antibiotic therapy	Macrolide + β-lactam or quinolones
Intensive care unit:	
Pseudomonas is not a concern	β-lactam + macrolide or quinolones
Pseudomonas is a concern	Piperacillin-tazobactam or carbapenem or cefepime + ciprofloxacin or aminoglycoside + macrolide

gram-negative bacilli (*Pseudomonas aeruginosa*) or *Legionella*. (Table 87–2).

NOSOCOMIAL PNEUMONIA

ETIOLOGY

- Nosocomial pneumonia is an important cause of hospital acquired infection and is associated with a high mortality.
- Ventilator-associated pneumonia is a subcategory of nosocomial pneumonia, which is associated with protracted use of mechanical ventilation (>48 hours). Mechanical ventilation is the single greatest risk factor involved in the development of hospital-acquired pneumonia.
- The most common pathogens isolated are gram-negative bacilli (*K. pneumoniae, Pseudomonas* spp., *Escherichia coli, Serratia marcescens, Enterobacter* spp.), anaerobes, and *S. aureus.*

CLINICAL FEATURES

- The clinical presentation is characterized by fever, productive cough, hypoxia, and tachypnea.

TABLE 87–1   Empiric Antibiotic Therapy for Treatment of Pneumonia as an Outpatient

PATIENT POPULATION	ANTIBIOTIC RECOMMENDATIONS
Previously healthy:	
No recent antibiotic therapy	Macrolide (erythromycin, azithromycin, clarithromycin) or doxycycline
Recent antibiotic therapy	Quinolones or macrolide + amoxicillin-clavulanic acid
Comorbidities (COPD, diabetes, renal or heart failure, malignancy):	
No recent antibiotic therapy	Macrolide or quinolones
Recent antibiotic therapy	Quinolones or macrolide + β-lactam

COPD, chronic obstructive pulmonary disease.

- In ventilator-associated pneumonia, patients develop purulent secretions, increased ventilator requirements, and develop new pulmonary infiltrates.

DIAGNOSIS

- White blood cell counts usually reveal leukocytosis with neutrophil predominance. Sputum Gram stain and culture should be obtained as they may aid in identification of the pathogen.
- Chest radiographs can reveal new or changing infiltrates. Computerized tomography (CT) scan may differentiate between pneumonia, secondary lung abscesses, and other lung processes (pulmonary emboli).
- Bronchoscopy is useful when investigating aspiration and ventilator-associated pneumonia. Bronchoalveolar lavage (BAL), bronchial brush, and transbronchial biopsy with histopathological staining, cytology, and microbiological culture, should be obtained.
- Open lung biopsy may be required to establish a diagnosis in the immunosuppressed host.

MANAGEMENT

- Therapy should be initiated without delay when nosocomial pneumonia is suspected. Empiric antibiotic therapy for patients at low risk for *Pseudomonas aeruginosa* (<5 days of hospitalization, not intubated) includes a β-lactam antibiotic plus a macrolide or a quinolone if *Legionella* is a consideration. If the patient is at risk for aspiration, anaerobic coverage should be included.
- With prolonged hospitalization and intubation, an antibiotic with activity against *Pseudomonas aeruginosa* such as piperacillin-tazobactam, imipenem, or cefepime should be employed. Methicillin-resistant *Staphylococcus aureus* should also be considered and appropriate coverage instituted.

CHRONIC PNEUMONIA

ETIOLOGY

- The most common etiology of chronic pneumonia is tuberculosis, followed by atypical mycobacteria, fungi (*Histoplasma, Coccidioides, Blastomyces,* and *Paracoccidioides*), *Actinomyces,* or a mixed aerobic and anaerobic infection.
- In immunocompromised patients, in addition to the aforementioned common pathogens, opportunistic infections

such as cryptococcosis, aspergillosis, and pneumocystis should be considered.

CLINICAL FEATURES

- The usual presentation is characterized by a protracted fever, chills, malaise, anorexia, weight loss, persistent cough, hemoptysis, chest pain, and dyspnea. A careful skin and mucus membrane examination may reveal lesions which aid in the diagnosis. Chest examination may reveal crackles and wheezes.

DIAGNOSIS

- Standard laboratory data may reveal anemia of chronic disease, and leukocytosis. Polymorphonuclear cell predominance is suggestive of a bacterial etiology, while a leukemoid reaction can develop in disseminated mycobacterial and fungal infections. Pancytopenia should suggest miliary tuberculosis, invasive fungal infections, HIV infection, or hematologic disorders.
- Sputum Gram stain and culture, arterial blood gas analysis, pulmonary function tests, and fungal serologies may provide important clues to the underlying diagnosis.
- The chest radiograph is usually obtained initially, although CT scanning provides more detailed images. Upper lobe involvement is more commonly seen in mycobacterial infections and histoplasmosis. Calcification is more typical for tuberculosis, histoplasmosis, and coccidioidomycosis. Fibrocavitary lesions may suggest tuberculosis or atypical mycobacterial diseases, histoplasmosis, coccidioidomycosis, aspergillosis, and sporotrichosis. Abscess of the chest wall or osteomyelitis of a rib adjacent to the pneumonia or pleural effusion may be seen with actinomycosis, nocardiosis, and tuberculosis.
- Transbronchial or open lung biopsy with appropriate stains and cultures are the procedures of choice to establish a diagnosis.

MANAGEMENT

- Ideally a definitive diagnosis should be established before starting antimicrobial therapy. If immediate empirical therapy is required, the decision should be based on epidemiologic, clinical, and microbiologic information.
- Bronchoscopy may be used to remove thick secretions, mucus plugs, or foreign bodies as well as to expand a collapsed lung.

• Lobectomy or pneumonectomy is considered in patients with chronic destructive pneumonia and concurrent abscess formation.

PLEURAL EFFUSION AND EMPYEMA

ETIOLOGY

• Empyema is most commonly a sequela to bacterial pneumonia; however, it can develop after trauma, esophageal rupture, and a thoracotomy.
• Empyema secondary to pneumonia is usually caused by a mixture of organisms, which includes anaerobes (*Bacteroides* spp., *Prevotella* spp., *Fusobacterium* spp., *and Peptostreptococcus* spp.) and pyogenic bacteria (*S. aureus, S. pneumoniae,* and *S. pyogenes*).
• Immunocompromised patients (eg, organ transplant, HIV, steroid dependent) have a higher incidence of empyema since fungi and gram-negative bacilli or more commonly associated with pneumonia in these individuals.

CLINICAL FEATURES

• The history should document risk factors for aspiration, recent surgeries or trauma, and poor oral hygiene.
• Patients usually present with fevers, chills, shortness of breath, cough, and chest pain. Physical examination may reveal decreased breath sounds, dullness to percussion, and crackles over the involved area.

DIAGNOSIS

• Chest radiographs should be obtained as the initial diagnostic evaluation. A lateral decubitus film may reveal as little as 50 mL of fluid.
• A CT scan of the chest can differentiate between simple versus complicated fluid collections. On the CT scan, an empyema is usually characterized by a smooth contour, whereas a lung abscess reveals irregular margins.
• Pleural fluid analysis, Gram stain, culture, and cytology may reveal the primary etiology. Exudative pleural effusion usually points toward an infectious cause (Table 87–3).

TREATMENT

• Empiric antibiotics should be selected based on Gram stain, most likely organism involved, history of presentation, and the antibiotics, pharmacokinetic properties

TABLE 87–3 Exudative Versus Transudative Pleural Effusions

LAB STUDIES	TRANSUDATE	EXUDATE
Appearance	Clear	Opaque
White blood cell count	<10.000/mm³	>50,000/mm³
pH	>7.2	<7.2
Pleural fluid–to–serum protein ratio	< 0.5	> 0.5
Lactate dehydrogenase	<200 IU/L	>200 IU/L
Glucose	>60 mg/dL	<60 mg/dL

(penetration into the pleural space). A third-generation cephalosporin (eg, ceftriaxone, cefepime) with either clindamycin or metronidazole, β-lactam antibiotics with a β-lactamase inhibitor (amoxicillin/clavulanate, ampicillin/ sulbactam, piperacillin/tazobactam), or a carbapenem (imipenem, ertapenem) provide excellent aerobic and anaerobic coverage.
• Complicated pleural effusions generally require chest tube drainage and lung reexpansion. Fibrinolytic therapy with intrapleural thrombolytics may improve drainage and is useful for patients with loculated effusions.
• Surgical management with video-assisted thoracoscopic surgery or thoracotomy is used for decortications and empyema drainage especially with multiloculated complex effusions.

LUNG ABSCESS

ETIOLOGY

• Lung abscess is usually a complication of aspiration pneumonia and therefore is a polymicrobial infection. The most commonly isolated organisms are mouth flora anaerobes (*Prevotella melaninogenica, Fusobacterium nucleatum, Peptostreptococcus* spp.) mixed with microaerophilic organisms and viridans streptococci. Less commonly isolated organisms include *S. aureus,* streptococcal species, gram-negative bacilli (*Klebsiella* spp., *P. aeruginosa, Burkholderia pseudomallei*), and *Actinomyces* species.
• In the immunocompromised host, opportunistic organisms such as mycobacteria, *Nocardia, Aspergillus,* Zygomycetes, and other fungi should be considered.

CLINICAL FEATURES

• Patients with a lung abscess usually present with a protracted indolent course characterized by fevers, night sweats, purulent productive cough, pleuritic chest pain, and weight loss.

DIAGNOSIS

- Sputum should be obtained for Gram stain and cultures; however, negative cultures are not uncommon. Acid-fast bacilli and fungal stains and cultures are useful in the appropriate clinical setting.
- Bronchoscopy with BAL and bronchial brushings aid in establishing a definitive diagnosis.
- Chest radiographs typically reveal a thick-walled, irregularly shaped, fluid-filled cavity with surrounding infiltrates. A CT scan offers greater sensitivity than a chest radiograph and can detect small cavities and endobronchial obstructions; a CT scan may also be used to guide needle aspirations of an affected site.

TREATMENT

- Because most lung abscesses are polymicrobial in nature (often head and neck flora), a combination of penicillin and β-lactamase inhibitor, clindamycin or a carbapenem for 6 to 8 weeks are acceptable therapies.
- Surgical intervention is reserved for patients who do not improve with antibiotic therapy.

BIBLIOGRAPHY

American Thoracic Society, Infectious Diseases Society of America. Guidelines for the management of adults with hospital-acquired, ventilator-associated, and healthcare-associated pneumonia. *Am J Respir Crit Care Med.* 2005;171:388–416.

Betts RF, Chapman SW, Penn RL, eds. *A Practical Approach to Infectious Disease.* 5th ed. Philadelphia: Lippincott Williams & Wilkins; 2003.

Mandell GL. In Bennett JE, Dolin R, eds. *Principles and Practice of Infectious Diseases.* 6th ed. Philadelphia: Elsevier Churchill Livingstone; 2005.

Mandell LA, Bartlett JG, Dowell SF, et al. Update of practice guidelines for the management of community-acquired pneumonia in immunocompetent adults. *Clin Infect Dis.* 2003; 37:1405–1433.

Marrie TJ, Campbell GD, Walker DH. Pneumonia. In: Kasper DL, Braunwald E, Fauci AS, et al, eds. *Harrison's Principles of Internal Medicine.* 16th ed. New York: McGraw-Hill; 2005; 1529.

Niederman MS, Mandell LA, Anqueto A, et al. Guidelines for the management of adults with community-acquired pneumonia. Diagnosis, assessment of severity, antimicrobial therapy and prevention. *Am J Respir Crit Care Med.* 2001;163:1730.

88 CARDIOVASCULAR INFECTIONS

Mary Abigail C. Dacuycuy and Donald J. Kennedy

INFECTIVE ENDOCARDITIS

EPIDEMIOLOGY AND ETIOLOGY

- Infective endocarditis (IE) is characterized by infection of the endocardial surface, most frequently the valves, of the heart.
- Risk factors for IE include structural heart disease, prosthetic valves and other intracardiac devices, injection drug use (IDU), intravascular catheters, and hemodialysis shunts or fistulas.
- The mitral valve is most commonly affected, followed by the aortic valve and a combination of both the mitral and aortic valve. In general, tricuspid valve IE is infrequent and is seen almost exclusively with IDU.
- Streptococci (most commonly viridans streptococci) and staphylococci (most commonly *Staphylococcus aureus*) account for 80% to 90% of IE, whereas enterococci are responsible for 5% to 18%. IE in IDU is usually caused by *S. aureus.*
- The HACEK group (*Haemophilus aphrophilus, Actinobacillus actinomycetemcomitans, Cardiobacterium hominis, Eikenella corrodens, Kingella kingae,* and *Kingella denitrificans*) of organisms consists of fastidious gram-negative bacilli that cause 5% to 10% of IE.
- Infective endocarditis caused by non-HACEK gram-negative aerobic bacilli (eg, Enterobacteriaceae and *Pseudomonas*) is uncommon. Other uncommon organisms that can cause IE include *Neisseria gonorrhoeae,* gram-positive bacilli, anaerobic bacteria, *Bartonella* species, *Coxiella burnetii,* or fungi.

CLINICAL FEATURES

- Patients frequently present with fever, anorexia, weight loss, malaise, fatigue, chills, weakness, nausea, vomiting, night sweats, and arthralgias.
- Physical examination commonly reveals a heart murmur usually caused by valvular regurgitation. Skin and mucosal manifestations may include petechiae on the conjunctivae, buccal mucosa, palate, and extremities; painful, inflammatory nodules on fingers and toes (Osler nodes); and hemorrhagic, macular, painless

TABLE 88–1 Diagnosis of Infective Endocarditis According to the Modified Duke Criteria

Definite IE	**Pathologic criteria:**
	Microorganisms shown by culture or histological examination of a vegetation, a vegetation that has embolized, or an intracardiac specimen *or*
	Pathologic lesions: vegetation or intracardiac abscess confirmed by histologic examination showing active IE
	Clinical criteria:
	2 major criteria *or*
	1 major criterion and 3 minor criteria *or*
	5 minor criteria
Possible IE	1 major criterion and 1 minor criterion *or*
	3 minor criteria
Rejected	Firm alternative diagnosis explaining evidence of IE *or*
	Resolution of IE syndrome with antibiotic therapy for <4 days *or*
	No pathologic evidence of IE at surgery or autopsy, with antibiotic therapy for <4 days *or*
	Does not meet criteria for possible IE

IE, infective endocarditis.
SOURCE: Adapted from Badour LM, Wilson WR, Bayer AS, et al. Infective endocarditis: diagnosis, antimicrobial therapy, and management of complications: a statement for healthcare professionals from the Committee on Rheumatic Fever, Endocarditis, and Kawasaki Disease, Council on Cardiovascular Disease in the Young, and the Councils on Clinical Cardiology, Stroke, and Cardiovascular Surgery and Anesthesia, American Heart Association: Endorsed by the Infectious Diseases Society of America. *Circulation.* 2005;111:394–434.

plaques on palms and soles (Janeway lesions). Oval, pale, retinal lesions surrounded by hemorrhage (Roth spots) may also be present.

- Coronary artery emboli may arise from aortic valve vegetations and cause myocardial infarction. When tricuspid valve IE is present, multiple septic pulmonary emboli are common.
- The kidneys may be affected by embolic infarcts, immune complex glomerulonephritis, and abscesses. Splenic involvement may present as splenomegaly, infarctions, and abscesses.
- Neurologic complications include cerebral emboli (most common) and mycotic aneurysms, which can rupture.
- Anemia of chronic disease is almost always present as is an elevated erythrocyte sedimentation rate. Urinalysis frequently shows proteinuria and hematuria.

DIAGNOSIS

- Blood cultures are positive in most cases of IE, and at least three sets of blood cultures should be obtained in the first 24 hours. If the patient has received antibiotics, more cultures should be obtained as previous antibiotic therapy reduces the likelihood of obtaining a positive culture.
- Special diagnostic tests (eg, lysis-centrifugation blood cultures, serology) may be performed if the blood cultures are negative. For slow-growing organisms, incubating the blood cultures for 4 weeks may increase the recovery rate.
- Echocardiography (both transesophageal and transthoracic) should be performed in all patients as

early as possible. These studies allow visualization of valvular vegetations which help in establishing the diagnosis and provide images for follow-up during the course of treatment. A negative echocardiogram cannot exclude a diagnosis of IE.

- The modified Duke criteria (Tables 88–1 and 88–2) is a useful tool for evaluating a patient suspected of IE; however, it should not usurp sound clinical judgment.

MANAGEMENT

- The management of patients with endocarditis should involve an infectious diseases specialist, cardiologist, and cardiovascular surgeon.
- Antimicrobial therapy is the mainstay of treatment for IE, and current recommended regimens are based on the following general principles:
  ○ Parenteral antibiotics are essential for sustained antibacterial activity.
  ○ Prolonged treatment is necessary (ie, a minimum of 4 to 6 weeks in most cases).
  ○ Bactericidal antibiotics should be administered whenever possible.
  ○ Synergistic antibiotic combinations are highly desirable to elicit an effective and rapid bactericidal effect (eg, ampicillin plus an aminoglycoside for enterococcal endocarditis).
- Badour and colleagues detailed the treatment of endocarditis in the American Heart Association Scientific Statement on Infective Endocarditis—Diagnosis, Antimicrobial Therapy, and Management of Complications.

TABLE 88–2   Terminology Used in to Calculate the Modified Duke Score

Major criteria	**Blood culture positive for IE:**
	Typical microorganisms consistent with IE from two separate blood cultures: *Viridans streptococci, Schistosoma bovis,* HACEK Group, *Staphylococcus aureus,* or community-acquired enterococci in the absence of a primary focus *or*
	Persistently positive blood cultures for any microorganism: at least two positive blood cultures drawn >12 h apart; or all of three or a majority of at least four separate blood cultures (with first and last sample drawn at least 1 h apart)
	Single positive blood culture for *Coxiella Burnetii* or antiphase 1 IgG antibody titer >1:800
	Evidence of endocardial involvement:
	Echocardiogram findings positive for IE: oscillating intracardiac mass on valve or supporting structures, in the path of regurgitant jets, or on implanted material in the absence of an alternative anatomic explanation; *or*
	Abscess; *or*
	New partial dehiscence of prosthetic valve
	New valvular regurgitation (worsening or change in preexisting murmur not sufficient)
Minor criteria	Predisposition: predisposing heart condition, or IDU
	Fever: >38°C (>100.4°F)
	Vascular phenomena: arterial embolism, septic pulmonary infarcts, mycotic aneurysm, intracranial and conjunctival hemorrhage, Janeway lesions
	Immunologic phenomena: glomerulonephritis, Osler nodes, Roth spots, rheumatoid factor
	Microbiologic evidence: positive blood culture but not meeting a major criterion as above or serologic evidence of active infection with organism consistent with IE

IE, infective endocarditis; HACEK, *Haemophilus* species, *Actinobacillus actinomycetemcomitans, Cardiobacterium hominis, Eikenella corrodens, Kingella kingae,* and *Kingella denitrificans;* IDU, injection drug use; IgG, immunoglobulin G.
SOURCE: Adapted from Badour LM, Wilson WR, Bayer AS, et al. Infective endocarditis: diagnosis, antimicrobial therapy, and management of complications: a statement for healthcare professionals from the Committee on Rheumatic Fever, Endocarditis, and Kawasaki Disease, Council on Cardiovascular Disease in the Young, and the Councils on Clinical Cardiology, Stroke, and Cardiovascular Surgery and Anesthesia, American Heart Association: Endorsed by the Infectious Diseases Society of America. *Circulation.* 2005;111:394–434.

- Clinical indications for surgery include refractory congestive heart failure; highly-resistant organisms (eg, fungal IE); persistent infection while on therapy; more than one serious systemic embolic episode during effective antimicrobial therapy; and prosthetic valve IE.
  - Echocardiographic findings that usually require surgical intervention include evidence of valve dehiscence, perforation, rupture, fistula, or a large perivalvular abscess; acute aortic or mitral insufficiency with ventricular failure; new heart block; anterior mitral leaflet vegetation with a diameter >10 mm; persistent vegetation after systemic embolization; and an increase in vegetation size despite appropriate antimicrobial therapy.

PREVENTION

- Measures to prevent IE include treatment of predisposing cardiac conditions (eg, surgical repair of anatomical risk factors such as a ventricular septal defect); elimination of portals of entry of organisms (eg, prompt treatment of dental abscess); and antibiotic prophylaxis for transient bacteremia during surgical procedures.
- Prophylaxis is recommended in individuals who have cardiac conditions that confer a higher risk for developing endocarditis than the general population and are undergoing procedures that are associated with bacteremia (especially organisms commonly associated with endocarditis).
- High-risk cardiac conditions include prosthetic cardiac valves, previous bacterial endocarditis, complex cyanotic congenital heart diseases, or surgically constructed systemic pulmonary shunts or conduits. Moderate-risk cardiac conditions include other uncorrected congenital malformations (eg, patent ductus arteriosus, ventricular septal defect, primum atrial septal defect, coarctation of the aorta, or bicuspid aortic valve), acquired valvular dysfunction (eg, rheumatic heart disease), hypertrophic cardiomyopathy, and mitral valve prolapse with valvular regurgitation and/or thickened leaflets.
- Surgical procedures that are associated with significant bacteremia are as follows:
  - Oral and dental: procedures with significant bleeding from hard or soft tissues, periodontal surgery, scaling, professional teeth cleaning, tonsillectomy, or adenoidectomy
  - Respiratory: surgical operations that involve the respiratory mucosa, bronchoscopy with a rigid bronchoscope
  - Gastrointestinal: sclerotherapy for esophageal varices, esophageal stricture dilation, endoscopic retrograde cholangiography with biliary obstruction, biliary tract surgery, surgical operations that involve intestinal mucosa
  - Genitourinary: prostatic surgery, cystoscopy, urethral dilation

• Antibiotics should be administered 30 to 60 minutes before the procedure; a single dose of antibiotic suffices in most cases. Specific endocarditis prophylactic regimens are summarized in the recommendations of the American Heart Association on prevention of bacterial endocarditis (www.circ.ahajournals.org/cgi/reprint/CIRCULATIONAHA.106.183095v1).

INFECTIONS OF PROSTHETIC VALVES AND OTHER CARDIOVASCULAR DEVICES

EPIDEMIOLOGY AND ETIOLOGY

• Infection may complicate the use of cardiovascular devices such as prosthetic valves (16% to 32% among all cases of IE), pacemakers, defibrillators, left ventricular assist devices, intra-aortic balloon pumps, or vascular grafts.
• Infections of cardiovascular devices may occur by any of the following routes: microbial contamination at the time of surgery; hematogenous dissemination; or contiguous infection.
• Staphylococci (most commonly coagulase-negative staphylococci) are the major pathogens in prosthetic valve endocarditis, especially during the first year after valve replacement surgery.

CLINICAL FEATURES

• Signs and symptoms depend, in part, on the location of the infected portion of the device and the virulence of the infecting organism.
• Bloodstream infections present with fever, weight loss, malaise, and myalgias, and are complicated by sepsis, shock, and organ dysfunction. Embolic events may lead to stroke, myocardial or bowel infarction, or ischemia of the skin and muscle.
• Signs of inflammation are usually apparent at the site of device placement with or without purulent drainage.

DIAGNOSIS

• Blood cultures should be obtained and an echocardiogram should be performed. Imaging studies (eg, ultrasound, computed tomography scan, or magnetic resonance imaging) may reveal fluid collections around the device, which in turn can be aspirated for microbiologic and histopathologic studies.

• The modified Duke criteria should be employed in patients suspected of prosthetic valve endocarditis.

MANAGEMENT

• The management team should include an infectious diseases specialist, cardiologist, and cardiovascular surgeon.
• The principles of treatment include administration of pathogen-specific antimicrobial therapy and device removal. Bactericidal antibiotics given parenterally for an extended duration (frequently 6 to 8 weeks) are necessary for most infections. Because many of these devices are life sustaining, device replacement is usually required. If device removal is not feasible, an attempt to control the acute infection is required followed by lifelong oral suppressive therapy.

MYOCARDITIS

EPIDEMIOLOGY AND ETIOLOGY

• Inflammation of the myocardium may be secondary to infectious and noninfectious causes. Viruses (especially coxsackie B virus) are the most common etiology of infectious myocarditis.
• Myocarditis is usually suspected when unexplained heart failure or arrhythmias occur with an associated systemic febrile illness or after an upper respiratory tract infection. In some cases the antecedent illness may not be apparent.

CLINICAL FEATURES

• Patients with myocarditis can be asymptomatic or develop rapidly progressive fatal disease with congestive heart failure and arrhythmias.
• Patients complain of fatigue, dyspnea, chest pain, and palpitations. The physical examination reveals tachycardia; gallops; murmurs of mitral or tricuspid insufficiency; or, rarely, a pericardial friction rub (if there is a concomitant pericarditis).

DIAGNOSIS

• The diagnosis of myocarditis is challenging and requires a high index of suspicion, usually in consultation with a cardiologist.
• Cardiac enzymes may be elevated, and the electrocardiogram may show nonspecific ST-T wave changes

and conduction abnormalities. The chest x-ray may demonstrate cardiomegaly and echocardiography may detect systolic dysfunction, wall motion abnormalities, and ventricular dilatation.
- Patients with progressive clinical deterioration require endomyocardial biopsy to establish a definitive diagnosis.

MANAGEMENT

- Most cases of acute viral myocarditis are self-limited, and patients recover completely. Patients with persistent wall motion abnormalities and ventricular dilatation may develop dilated cardiomyopathy.
- If a specific infection is identified (such as *Toxoplasma* or *Trypanosoma*), antimicrobial therapy should be directed at the causative pathogen.

PERICARDITIS

EPIDEMIOLOGY AND ETIOLOGY

- Inflammation of the pericardium may be idiopathic or caused by infectious and noninfectious causes.
- Idiopathic and viral pericarditis predominate and usually follow a benign and self-limited course. The enteroviruses, especially the coxsackie viruses, are the most frequent causes of viral pericarditis.
- Purulent bacterial pericarditis is uncommon and is usually derived from a contiguous infected region (such as from the head and neck) or from postoperative infections.
- Acute or chronic pericarditis may occur in up to 1% of patients with pulmonary tuberculosis and may progress to chronic and constrictive pericarditis. Fungi and parasites are rare causes of pericarditis.

CLINICAL FEATURES

- Pericarditis can be clinically silent or be associated with severe hemodynamic derangements and death.
- Typically, patients develop fever and complain of chest pain that is retrosternal; radiating to the shoulder and neck; and worsened by breathing, swallowing, and lying.
- The classic physical exam finding is a high-pitched, scratching, or grating friction rub, which is often evanescent and variable in quality.
- In the presence of a large pericardial effusion and cardiac tamponade, there may be dyspnea, jugular venous distension, and a pulsus paradoxus.

DIAGNOSIS

- Chest x-ray may reveal cardiomegaly. The electrocardiogram typically reveals diffuse ST-segment elevation without a change in QRS morphology or reduced QRS voltage and electrical alternans if there is a large pericardial effusion.
- Echocardiography is important in confirming the presence of pericardial effusion and characterizing the cardiac hemodynamics.
- Pericardial biopsy and drainage may be required to establish the etiology in patients with persistent symptoms or clinical deterioration.

MANAGEMENT

- The mainstay for patients with suspected viral or idiopathic pericarditis includes bed rest and symptomatic pain relief with close monitoring for the development of hemodynamic compromise. Nonsteroidal anti-inflammatory agents may be administered (they should be avoided if concomitant myocarditis exists). Pericardiocentesis or pericardiotomy is performed when there is cardiac tamponade.
- Patients with purulent bacterial pericarditis almost always rquire surgical intervention in combination with systemic antibiotics. Patients with tuberculous pericarditis require antituberculous therapy and may benefit from corticosteroid therapy or surgical drainage.

BIBLIOGRAPHY

Badour LM, Wilson WR, Bayer AS, et al. Infective endocarditis: diagnosis, antimicrobial therapy, and management of complications: a statement for healthcare professionals from the Committee on Rheumatic Fever, Endocarditis, and Kawasaki Disease, Council on Cardiovascular Disease in the Young, and the Councils on Clinical Cardiology, Stroke, and Cardiovascular Surgery and Anesthesia, American Heart Association: Endorsed by the Infectious Diseases Society of America. *Circulation.* 2005;111:394–434.

Dajani AS, Taubert KA, Wilson W, et al. Prevention of bacterial endocarditis: recommendations by the American Heart Association. *Circulation.* 1997;96:358–366.

Mandell GL, Bennett JE, Dolin R, eds. *Mandell, Douglas, and Bennett's Principles and Practice of Infectious Diseases.* 6th ed. Philadelphia: Elsevier; 2005.

89 INTRAABDOMINAL INFECTIONS

Mary Abigail C. Dacuycuy and Donald J. Kennedy

PERITONITIS

EPIDEMIOLOGY AND ETIOLOGY

- Infectious peritonitis is classified as secondary peritonitis (associated with an intraabdominal process); spontaneous bacterial peritonitis (no other intraabdominal abnormalities); or peritonitis complicating peritoneal dialysis (PD).
- Secondary peritonitis is usually caused by a breach in the mucosal barrier (eg, perforation of a peptic ulcer or ruptured appendix) leading to spillage of gastrointestinal or genitourinary microorganisms into the peritoneal cavity. Typically, a mixture of aerobic (*Escherichia coli, Klebsiella/Enterobacter* spp., *Proteus* spp., and enterococci) and anaerobic organisms (*Bacteroides fragilis, Prevotella melaninogenica, Peptococcus, Peptostreptococcus, Fusobacterium, Eubacterium lentum,* and *Clostridium*) are isolated.
- Spontaneous bacterial peritonitis (SBP) or primary peritonitis usually occurs in patients with cirrhosis and ascites. Infection may result from hematogenous or lymphogenous spread, transmural migration from the intestine, or ascending infection from the genital tract. Usually, SBP is monomicrobial (*E. coli* is most frequently isolated, followed by *Klebsiella pneumoniae, Streptococcus pneumoniae,* and other streptococcal species including enterococci).
- In peritonitis complicating PD, skin flora (*Staphylococcus epidermidis, Staphylococcus aureus, Streptococcus* spp., diphtheroids) are the usual agents of infection. Less frequently, gram-negative organisms (*E. coli, Klebsiella/Enterobacter, Proteus,* and *Pseudomonas* spp.) may be isolated. It is typically a monomicrobial infection.

CLINICAL FEATURES

- The manifestations of secondary peritonitis include abdominal pain and distension, fever, chills, anorexia, nausea, vomiting, and changes in bowel habits. Physical findings may reveal abdominal tenderness, abdominal rigidity, and hypoactive or absent bowel sounds.

- Usually, SBP presents with fever, with or without abdominal complaints. Bacteremia is present in 75% of patients with SBP caused by aerobic bacteria.

DIAGNOSIS

- In secondary peritonitis, computed tomography (CT) of the abdomen and pelvis should be performed to visualize intraabdominal anatomy. Paracentesis may be helpful, but an unsuccessful paracentesis cannot exclude secondary peritonitis.
- In SBP, paracentesis should be performed; and peritoneal fluid should be examined for cell count with differential, Gram stain, and culture. Peritoneal neutrophil counts >250 cells/mm^3, positive Gram stain, or a positive culture are considered diagnostic for SBP. A primary intraabdominal source of infection must be excluded before diagnosing SBP.
- In peritonitis associated with PD, the dialysate is almost always cloudy, and microscopic examination reveals a leukocyte count greater than 100 cells/mm^3 with neutrophils predominating. The dialysate should be examined with Gram stain and culture.

MANAGEMENT

- Secondary peritonitis requires a combination of surgical intervention and antimicrobial therapy. Antimicrobial therapy should be initiated with carbapenems, third-generation cephalosporin plus metronidazole, fluoroquinolones plus metronidazole, or β-lactam/β-lactamase inhibitor combinations, immediately after appropriate specimens (blood and, if possible, peritoneal fluid) are obtained. The duration of treatment is usually 5 to 7 days after successful surgery. Persistent evidence of infection warrants reevaluation.
- Spontaneous bacterial peritonitis may be treated empirically with a third-generation cephalosporin, β-lactam/β-lactamase combination (eg, piperacillin-tazobactam), carbapenem, or a quinolone. Antimicrobial therapy should be continued even when the cultures are sterile if there is a strong clinical suspicion of SBP. Clinical improvement together with a decline in the ascitic fluid leukocyte count of greater than 25% should occur within 48 to 72 hours of appropriate antimicrobial therapy; if there is no improvement, other diagnoses should be considered. The usual duration of treatment is 10 to 14 days.
- Peritonitis associated with PD may be treated with antibiotics administered via the parenteral or intraperitoneal route. After cultures are obtained, an appropriate

initial empirical regimen would include a combination of vancomycin and gentamicin. The duration of antibiotic therapy ranges from 10 days to 3 weeks. If the signs and symptoms of peritonitis persist beyond 96 hours of therapy, reevaluation is warranted. Indications for catheter removal include skin exit-site or tunnel infection; fungal, fecal, mycobacterial, or *Pseudomonas* peritonitis; persistent or recurrent peritonitis with the same organism; and concomitant intraabdominal abscess.

INTRAABDOMINAL ABSCESS

EPIDEMIOLOGY AND ETIOLOGY

- Intraabdominal abscess is usually a complication of processes causing secondary peritonitis, SBP, or peritonitis complicating PD.
- It is frequently polymicrobial with anaerobic (*B. fragilis,* clostridia) and aerobic organisms (*E. coli, Klebsiella/ Enterobacter* group, *Proteus* spp., *Pseudomonas aeruginosa,* and enterococci).

CLINICAL FEATURES

- Patients usually present with high-grade fever, intermittent fever, shaking chills, abdominal pain, and tenderness over the affected area.

DIAGNOSIS

- Computed tomography and magnetic resonance imaging can accurately identify and localize abscesses. CT scan may show a low-density mass with a defined capsule; CT is also useful in guiding percutaneous drainage.

MANAGEMENT

- Intraabdominal abscesses require early and adequate drainage. Importantly, specimens should be sent for histopathologic and microbiologic studies. Percutaneous drainage is initially performed; however, surgery may be necessary when there is loculated, poorly organized, multiple, or extensive collections, or failure to respond to the initial intervention.
- Antimicrobial therapy should be started immediately after blood cultures are obtained even before drainage is performed. Empiric antibiotic therapy should be directed at both aerobes and anaerobes and should be adjusted based on the organisms isolated.

LIVER ABSCESS

EPIDEMIOLOGY AND ETIOLOGY

- Liver abscesses may be classified as either pyogenic or amebic.
- Pyogenic liver abscesses may arise from several sources:
  - Biliary tree (ie, cholangitis)
  - Bacteremia (eg, endocarditis)
  - Portal vein (eg, drainage from diverticulitis)
  - Direct extension from a contiguous focus of infection (eg, perinephric abscess)
  - Trauma
  - Cryptogenic
- *Escherichia coli, K. pneumoniae,* enterococci, and viridans streptococci are commonly isolated in pyogenic liver abscesses. *S. aureus* is often present in monomicrobial abscesses secondary to bacteremia.
- Amoebic liver abscess is caused by the protozoan *Entamoeba histolytica.* In the United States it is rare and found in travelers and immigrants from endemic areas. Infection with *E. histolytica* results from ingestion of cysts in contaminated food or water.

CLINICAL FEATURES

- Fever and right upper quadrant abdominal pain are common symptoms, whereas jaundice is infrequently seen. Amebic abscess is indistinguishable from pyogenic abscess based on clinical presentation alone.
- Leukocytosis and elevated alkaline phosphatase are common. Blood cultures are positive in patients with pyogenic abscess half of the time.

DIAGNOSIS

- Ultrasonography and CT scanning are useful for identifying and guiding percutaneous drainage of abscesses. Aspirates should be sent for the appropriate stains and cultures.
- In the appropriate clinical setting, a presumptive diagnosis of amebic liver abscess can be established based on serology and radiographic imaging. Antiamebic antibodies have a high sensitivity and specificity for *E. histolytica* infection, but they cannot distinguish colitis from extraintestinal disease or old from new infection. *E. histolytica* antigen may also be detected in serum and stool samples. Examination of the stool for cysts is less helpful because one cannot distinguish *E. histolytica* from *Entamoeba dispar* (an avirulent commensal).

MANAGEMENT

- Pyogenic liver abscesses usually require drainage. Empiric antimicrobial therapy should immediately be administered after blood cultures are obtained. Abscesses arising from a biliary source require antibiotics against enterococci and aerobic gram-negative bacilli, whereas abscesses from a colonic or pelvic source should be treated with a regimen that has activity against aerobic gram-negative bacilli and anaerobes. If a hematogenous source is suspected, the antimicrobial regimen should include an antibiotic with activity against *S. aureus*. The duration of antibiotics is usually 4 to 6 weeks and should be based on the patient's clinical response and follow-up imaging.
- Uncomplicated amebic liver abscesses may be treated with medical therapy alone. Metronidazole is given for 7 to 10 days and paromomycin is also administered to eliminate *E. histolytica* that colonize the bowel lumen. Indications for drainage include poor response to appropriate therapy after 3 to 5 days; exclusion of pyogenic liver abscess, bacterial superinfection, and other diagnoses; and large lesions, particularly left-sided abscesses that can rupture into the pericardium.

INFECTIONS OF THE BILIARY SYSTEM

EPIDEMIOLOGY AND ETIOLOGY

- Acute cholecystitis usually follows obstruction of the cystic duct by a gallstone. Infection is a complication in 25% to 50% of cases and may lead to emphysematous or gangrenous cholecystitis, gallbladder empyema, perforation, pyogenic liver abscess, and bacteremia.
- In some patients with severe underlying illness (eg, burns, sepsis), gallbladder inflammation may occur in the absence of gallstones and is termed *acalculous cholecystitis.*
- Cholangitis is usually secondary to obstruction of bile flow by a common bile duct stone. Bacteria may ascend the biliary tract and cause infection.
- Gastrointestinal flora is commonly isolated from the bile of patients with biliary tract infection. These include gram-negative bacilli (*E. coli, Klebsiella* spp., and *Enterobacter* spp.), anaerobes (*Bacteroides* spp., *Fusobacterium* spp., and clostridia), and enterococci.
- Parasites (eg, *Clonorchis, Ascaris,* and *Echinococcus*) may also cause obstruction and infection of the biliary tree.

CLINICAL FEATURES

- Patients frequently complain of right upper quadrant abdominal pain, which may radiate to the infrascapular region. On physical examination, there usually is tenderness in the right upper quadrant and pain during inspiration (Murphy sign). Fever, tachycardia, and leukocytosis are common findings.
- Ascending cholangitis may present with right upper quadrant pain, fever, jaundice, hypotension, and altered mental status.

DIAGNOSIS

- Findings on ultrasonography that are suggestive of acute cholecystitis include gallstones, gallbladder wall thickening of >2 mm, pericholecystic fluid, intramural gas, or ductal dilatation. Hepatoiminodiacetic acid scanning has greater sensitivity than ultrasound and failure of the gallbladder to accumulate the radiolabeled marker is highly suggestive of acute cholecystitis. Magnetic resonance cholangiography can visualize the bile ducts and detect stones.

TREATMENT

- Definitive treatment of infections of the biliary system consists of removal of the obstruction and the infected material surgically, percutaneously, or endoscopically. Antimicrobial therapy is an adjunctive measure.
- Empiric coverage should be directed against gram-negative bacilli and anaerobes with piperacillin-tazobactam, third-generation cephalosporins plus metronidazole, fluoroquinolones plus metronidazole, or carbapenems.

PANCREATIC INFECTIONS

EPIDEMIOLOGY AND ETIOLOGY

- Pancreatic infections usually occur as a complication of acute pancreatitis caused by noninfectious etiologies (eg, gallstones, alcohol, endoscopic retrograde cholangiography). Severe pancreatitis, which is characterized by multiple organ failure and pancreatic necrosis, is associated with a high mortality rate.
- Infections may be monomicrobial or polymicrobial and organisms are usually derived from the gastrointestinal flora. Gram-negative bacteria (most commonly *E. coli* and *Klebsiella* spp.), gram-positive bacteria (enterococcal, streptococcal, and staphylococcal species), and anaerobes may be isolated.
- Between 4 and 7 weeks after the onset of acute pancreatitis, necrotic tissue may liquefy into pseudocysts, which are sterile, or pancreatic abscesses. Pseudocysts may subsequently become superinfected and develop into abscesses.

CLINICAL FEATURES

- Pancreatic abscess typically manifests fever, abdominal pain, and leukocytosis in patients recovering from acute pancreatitis.

DIAGNOSIS

- The presence or absence of infection in acute pancreatitis is difficult to establish because both entities may present with a systemic inflammatory response syndrome and multiple organ failure.
- In the presence of infection, CT scan of the abdomen may show gas within and surrounding necrotic pancreatic tissue. Later in the course, pseudocysts or abscesses may be visualized.
- Pancreatic tissue sampling and aspiration of fluid collections are recommended when there is persistent systemic toxicity or organ failure despite aggressive supportive care. Specimens should be sent for microbiologic and histologic examination.

MANAGEMENT

- Treatment of infected pancreatic necrosis consists of either percutaneous or open drainage in combination with appropriate antibiotics.
- Antibiotics should be started early in patients with necrotizing pancreatitis if there is associated fever, leukocytosis, and/or organ failure, while appropriate cultures (including pancreatic tissue culture) are obtained.
- Antimicrobial regimens must have activity against aerobes and anaerobes. Carbapenem monotherapy, a quinolone plus metronidazole, or a third-generation cephalosporin plus metronidazole, are usually given for 14 days; however some patients may require extended therapy based on their clinical course.

DIVERTICULITIS

EPIDEMIOLOGY AND ETIOLOGY

- Inflammation and infection of bowel wall = diverticul is most commonly located in the sigmoid and descending colon.
- Acute diverticulitis is a polymicrobial infection with mixed aerobes and anaerobes. Organisms that are commonly isolated include Enterobacteriaceae, *Bacteroides* species, *Peptostreptococcus* species, viridans streptococci, and enterococci.

CLINICAL FEATURES

- Patients with diverticulitis may complain of recurrent abdominal pain that begins in the hypogastric area then localizes to the left lower quadrant area. Patients also develop fever, nausea and vomiting, changes in bowel habits, and urinary symptoms. Hematochezia is uncommon.
- On physical examination there may be abdominal tenderness and guarding in the left lower quadrant and suprapubic area. Bowel sounds may be hypoactive, and an abdominal mass may be palpated. High-grade fever and abdominal rigidity suggest peritonitis secondary to perforation.

DIAGNOSIS

- The diagnosis of diverticulitis is based on clinical presentation; however, imaging studies are recommended to exclude other diagnoses (eg, tumors, inflammatory bowel disease) and complications. Computed tomography is the diagnostic procedure of choice. It may reveal diverticui, pericolic fat stranding, bowel wall thickening, or abscess formation.
- Colonoscopy is avoided in the initial work-up of diverticulitis because of the risk of perforation.

MANAGEMENT

- Most patients with acute diverticulitis can be treated successfully with antibiotics, bowel rest, and analgesics. Antimicrobial regimens should have activity against both aerobic and anaerobic organisms as in secondary peritonitis.
- If there is no improvement within 48 to 72 hours, the patient should be reevaluated for perforation, obstruction, development of abscess, and fistula formation; for which surgical intervention may be indicated.

BIBLIOGRAPHY

Kasper DL, Braunwald E, Fauci AS, et al, eds. *Harrison's Principles of Internal Medicine*. 16th ed. McGraw-Hill Professional; 2004.

Mandell GL, Bennett JE, Dolin R, eds. *Mandell, Douglas, and Bennett's Principles and Practice of Infectious Diseases*. 6th ed. Philadelphia: Elsevier; 2005.

Solomkin JS, Mazuski JE, Baron EJ, et al. IDSA guidelines for the selection of anti-infective agents for complicated intraabdominal infections. *Clin Infect Dis.* 2003;37:997–1005.

90 HEPATITIS

Musab U. Saeed and Donald J. Kennedy

INTRODUCTION

- Inflammation of the liver can be caused by several infectious and noninfectious etiologies. Viruses are the most common cause of infectious hepatitis.
- Primary liver viruses include hepatitis A virus (HAV), hepatitis B virus (HBV), hepatitis C virus (HCV), hepatitis D virus (HDV), and hepatitis E virus (HEV).
- Epstein-Barr virus, cytomegalovirus, varicella-zoster virus, herpes simplex, adenovirus, and Coxsackie virus infection may also be associated with mild hepatitis.
- In all forms of acute viral hepatitis, alanine aminotransferase and aspartate aminotransferase levels are initially elevated, followed by an elevated bilirubin.

HEPATITIS A AND E VIRUSES

ETIOLOGY

- Both HAV and HEV are RNA viruses that are very similar in their transmission, clinical presentation, and management.
- Transmission for both viruses is most commonly via the fecal-oral route. Hepatitis A virus has been associated with ingestion of contaminated food (shellfish, clams, mussels, and oysters), water, or milk. Oral-anal transmission is seen mostly in sexually active gay men. Hepatitis E virus infections in the United States are usually reported in patients with a travel history to endemic areas (eg, India, Mexico, Middle East, and Northeast Africa).

CLINICAL FEATURES

- Both viruses have an incubation period of 15 to 50 days, which is followed by an acute phase characterized by anorexia, malaise, nausea, vomiting, abdominal pain, and fever. Some patients also develop jaundice.
- Most patients resolve their infection without development of chronic disease. Rarely, fulminant hepatic failure occurs, particularly in pregnancy complicated by HEV infection.

DIAGNOSIS

- Anti-HAV immunoglobulin M (IgM) becomes detectable before symptoms start, peaks during the acute phase, and is undetectable by 6 months. Anti-HAV immunoglobulin G (IgG) indicates prior infection or vaccination and implies protection.
- Anti-HEV IgM, which is used to diagnosis acute hepatitis E, remains detectable for 3 to 4 months.

MANAGEMENT

- Both infections require symptomatic management and supportive care.
- Active immunization for HAV is established with a two-dose regimen at 0 and 6 to 12 months. Vaccination is recommended for children living in endemic areas; travelers to endemic areas; food handlers; sexually active gay men; patients with HBV, HCV, human immunodeficiency virus; and intravenous drug users. There is no vaccination available for HEV.
- Postexposure prophylaxis for HAV involves administration of a single dose of immunoglobulin, which confers immunity for 6 months. It is recommended for household contacts of patients with acute HAV or individuals who have ingested food prepared by an infected individual. Unimmunized travelers to high-risk areas of the world should receive the immunoglobulin 2 weeks before departure.

HEPATITIS B AND D VIRUSES

ETIOLOGY

- Hepatitis B virus is a DNA virus with a worldwide distribution exceeding 400 million people.
- Hepatitis D virus requires HBV for its assembly and replication.
- The route of transmission for both HBV and HDV is through direct physical contact of mucous membranes (unprotected sexual activity), blood (intravenous drug use), or inoculation via infected body fluids.

CLINICAL FEATURES

- Hepatitis B has an incubation period of 1 to 4 months. Patients usually present with malaise, nausea, vomiting, fever, arthritis, urticaria, and right upper quadrant tenderness. Eventually, 30% of patients with hepatitis B infection develop jaundice.
- Overall, 5% to 7% of adult patients with acute HBV develop chronic heaptitis, and less than 1% develop fulminant hepatitis. Chronic HBV is inversely proportional to the age of onset (eg, 90% of infants infected at birth versus 5% of infected adults develop chronic disease). Chronic infection may lead to cirrhosis, end-stage liver disease, and hepatocellular carcinoma.

- There are two clinical presentations associated with HDV infection: (1) an acute coinfection superimposed on HBV; which is usually a self-limited disease, and (2) a superinfection, which arises in patients previously infected with HBV who acquire HDV; this type of infection is associated with a more aggressive course than coinfection and, accordingly, is complicated by the development of chronic hepatitis with greater frequency.

DIAGNOSIS

- Hepatitis B virus serology and antigen status are the cornerstones of differentiating among the different stages of the disease.
- Hepatitis B surface antigen (HBsAg) is detectable 2 to 6 weeks before the onset of clinical symptoms; and should be cleared in 6 months if the patient fully recovers. Persistence of HBsAg beyond 6 months implies chronic infection.
- Hepatitis B surface antibody (HBsAb) indicates recovery from an acute infection or active immunization and, therefore, correlates with immunity.
- Hepatitis B core antibody (HBcAb) IgM can be detected within 1 month of the initial infection. The development of anti-HBc IgG antibodies in concert with anti-HBsAb implies recovery from a previous infection, however, the presence of anti-HBc IgG with HBsAg implies chronic HBV infection.
- Hepatitis B early antigen (HBeAg) is a marker of intact virus (viral replication) and, thus implies a high degree of infectivity.
- In acute hepatitis D, anti-HDV IgM levels rise transiently. Sustained high titers of anti-HDV correlate with chronic disease.

MANAGEMENT

- Acute hepatitis B is treated with supportive care.
- In chronic hepatitis B the primary goal is to suppress HBV replication, manifested by a negative HBV viral load and HBeAg.
- Pegylated interferon (IFN)-α is administered weekly for 4 months. A sustained virologic response rate of 15% to 30% is observed.
- Lamivudine treatment for 1 year confers a similar viral response rate as IFN-α, but its use is limited by the development of resistance. Adefovir is an alternative for lamivudine resistant cases.
- Patients that develop end-stage liver disease can undergo successful liver transplantation but HBV recurs in the transplanted liver (the effects of HBV recurrence in the transplanted liver significantly worsens the prognosis of the graft).

- Hepatitis B virus immunization of all newborn children is administered at 0, 1, and 6 months. Additional doses are recommended for nonconverters. Successful immunization against HBV confers protection against HDV.
- Postexposure prophylaxis with a single dose of hepatitis B immunoglobulin is recommended for individuals who have never been vaccinated, nonresponders to vaccination and vaccinated individuals with anti-HB viral titers less than 10 U/mL.
- There is no specific treatment for HDV, except to prevent HBV infection.

HEPATITIS C VIRUS

ETIOLOGY

- Hepatitis C virus is a RNA virus transmitted by intravenous drug use; unprotected sexual activity (but less common than hepatitis B); and, rarely, transmission occurs from occupational needle puncture.

CLINICAL FEATURES

- Acute hepatitis C is usually asymptomatic; however, it may present with jaundice, fatigue, lethargy, myalgias, and right upper quadrant pain 2 to 12 weeks after exposure.
- Between 70% and 80% of HCV infections become chronic, and 25% develop cirrhosis and end-stage liver disease after 20–25 years of infection.

DIAGNOSIS

- Antibodies to Hepatitis C are detectable after 8 to 9 weeks by enzyme-linked immunosorbent assay and can be confirmed by a recombinant immunoblot assay. Antibodies are not a marker of immunity.
- Hepatitis C virus polymerase chain reaction (PCR) is used to confirm viremia after infection and should be monitored in 2 to 4 months after the initial infection. Persistently elevated hepatitis C PCR is associated with the development of chronic hepatitis. Hepatitis C virus genotyping may aid in determining the optimal therapy and response.

MANAGEMENT

- Ribavirin with pegylated INF-α is the treatment of choice for patients with chronic infection and elevated liver enzymes without end stage liver cirrhosis.
- Interferon-α should not be used in patients with severe depression, bipolar disorder, and active drug or

alcohol use. Ribavirin is contraindicated in anemia, hemolysis, advanced renal insufficiency, cerebral vascular disease, and pregnancy (teratogenic effects).

- Transplant is the only option in end-stage liver disease but the infection recurs after transplantation (the effects of HCV recurrence in the transplanted liver slightly worsens the prognosis of the graft).

BIBLIOGRAPHY

Burton JR, Shaw-Stiffel TA. Hepatitis viruses. In: Betts RF, Chapman SW, Penn RL, eds. *A Practical Approach to Infectious Disease.* 5th ed. Philadelphia: Lippincott Williams Wilkins; 2003:477.

Centers for Disease Control and Prevention. CDC MMWR Hepatitis home page: http://www.cdc.gov/ncidod/diseases/hepatitis/ index.htm.

Curry MP, Choppa S. Acute viral hepatitis. In: Bennett JE, Dolin R, eds. *Principles and Practice of Infectious Diseases.* 6th ed. Philadelphia: Elsevier Churchill Livingstone; 2005:1426.

Dienstag JL. Chronic viral hepatitis. In: Mandell GL, Bennett JE, Dolin R, eds. *Principles and Practice of Infectious Diseases.* 6th ed. Philadelphia: Elsevier Churchill Livingstone; 2005:1441.

91 GENITOURINARY TRACT INFECTIONS

Mary Abigail C. Dacuycuy and Donald J. Kennedy

DEFINITIONS

- The term *urinary tract infection* (UTI) denotes the presence of infected urine in the bladder. *Significant bacteriuria* is defined as the presence of ≥10^5 bacteria/mL of urine. *Asymptomatic bacteriuria* refers to significant bacteriuria in a patient without symptoms.
- Urinary tract infections may be subdivided into lower tract infections (urethritis and cystitis) and upper tract infections (acute pyelonephritis, prostatitis, and intrarenal and perinephric abscesses).
- *Uncomplicated UTI* is an infection in a structurally and neurologically normal urinary tract. *Complicated UTI* is an infection in a urinary tract with functional or structural abnormalities (including indwelling catheters and calculi). Urinary tract infections in men, pregnant

women, children, and hospitalized patients are considered complicated.

URETHRITIS

- Urethritis is discussed in Chap. 94 on Sexually Transmitted Infections.

ACUTE CYSTITIS

EPIDEMIOLOGY AND ETIOLOGY

- Adult women have a higher incidence of UTI than men. Colonization of the female urinary tract by uropathogens is facilitated by the short length of the female urethra and the proximity of the female urethra to the anus. In males, UTI is usually associated with abnormalities of the urinary tract.
- More than 95% of uncomplicated cystitis is caused by a single organism. The most common pathogens are the gram-negative bacilli, which include *Escherichia coli* (80% to 90%), *Proteus, Pseudomonas, Klebsiella,* and *Enterobacter. Staphylococcus saprophyticus* accounts for 10% to 15% of acute cystitis in young females. Enterococci, yeast, or multiple organisms may be isolated in complicated UTIs.
- Cystitis is almost always caused by an ascending infection from the urethra.
- Hematogenous infection is rare. Isolation of *Staphylococcus aureus* from the urine should arouse suspicion of bacteremic infection of the urinary tract including the kidney.

CLINICAL FEATURES

- Irritative voiding symptoms (dysuria, frequency, urgency) and suprapubic discomfort are common. Occasionally, hematuria is present. Fever is usually absent and the physical examination is often unremarkable.

DIAGNOSIS

- A presumptive diagnosis can be made in the presence of typical clinical features and pyuria, which is defined as ≥10 leukocytes per high power field on microscopic examination of the urine.
- The diagnosis can be proven by urine culture, and patients with infection usually have ≥10^5 bacteria/mL in midstream clean-catch voided urine. Bacterial growth in urine obtained by suprapubic aspiration would be considered significant even if less than 10^5 colonies per mL.

MANAGEMENT

- All symptomatic UTIs should be treated.
- All men, children, and infants with UTI require an evaluation of the urinary tract including a urine culture, renal ultrasound, plain abdominal radiograph, and/or an intravenous urogram.
- Women with their first episode of uncomplicated acute bacterial cystitis should receive 3 days of therapy (short-course therapy). Trimethoprim-sulfamethoxazole (TMP-SMX) is the antibiotic of choice, but quinolones are acceptable alternatives (eg, for *E. coli* resistant to TMP-SMX). Women with treatment failure, persistent microscopic hematuria or pyuria at follow-up, or recurrent UTIs also require further evaluation of the urinary tract.
- All men, and women who have a history of previous UTI caused by antibiotic-resistant organisms or more than 7 days of symptoms, should receive 7 to 10 days of therapy.
- Asymptomatic bacteriuria is often best left untreated except in pregnancy and in patients who will undergo urologic procedures.
- Other agents that have been used with varying degrees of success include amoxicillin-clavulanic acid, cephalosporins, and nitrofurantoin.

ACUTE PYELONEPHRITIS

EPIDEMIOLOGY AND ETIOLOGY

- Pyelonephritis is an acute bacterial infection of the kidney and renal pelvis that usually arises via an ascending route of infection. Microorganisms are similar to those causing acute cystitis, with *E. coli* being the most common.

CLINICAL FEATURES

- Symptoms include fever and flank pain, often associated with dysuria, urgency, and frequency. Nausea, vomiting, and diarrhea may also be present.
- Signs include fever, tachycardia, and costovertebral angle tenderness.

DIAGNOSIS

- Urinalysis shows pyuria, bacteriuria, and occasionally, hematuria and white cell casts. Urine culture almost always demonstrates the pathogen and blood cultures may also be positive.

MANAGEMENT

- Urinalysis, urine culture, and blood cultures should be obtained before instituting empiric antimicrobial therapy.
- Most patients with acute pyelonephritis should be hospitalized. Empiric antimicrobial therapy for hospitalized patients includes third-generation cephalosporins, parenteral fluoroquinolones, piperacillin-tazobactam, aminoglycosides, aztreonam, or imipenem.
- Patients with mild to moderate illness and no nausea or vomiting who are considered reliable and compliant may be managed with outpatient therapy. Oral quinolones, TMP-SMX, and amoxicillin-clavulanic acid may be administered.
- Therapy is modified based on the organism isolated and its antibiotic susceptibility. Duration of therapy is usually 14 days.
- Imaging studies such as computed tomography and ultrasonography should be performed to exclude an abscess or obstruction, especially in patients who fail to respond appropriately to therapy (no bacteriologic response by 48 hours and persistent systemic toxicity beyond 3 days), or if the initial diagnosis is unclear.

PROSTATITIS

EPIDEMIOLOGY AND ETIOLOGY

- Prostatitis refers to various inflammatory conditions affecting the prostate gland. The National Institutes of Health consensus classification of prostatitis syndromes is comprised of acute bacterial prostatitis (ABP), chronic bacterial prostatitis (CBP), chronic nonbacterial prostatitis, and asymptomatic inflammatory prostatitis.
- Gram-negative organisms, most commonly *E. coli,* are the most frequent pathogens associated with ABP and CBP. Chronic bacterial prostatitis is a frequent cause of relapsing UTI in men.

CLINICAL FEATURES

- Acute bacterial prostatitis is characterized by high fevers, chills, irritative voiding symptoms, and perineal and back pain. The prostate gland is warm, swollen, and extremely tender on rectal examination. Massage of the acutely infected prostate gland is contraindicated because it can precipitate bacteremia.
- Many men with CBP are asymptomatic, but some may complain of irritative voiding symptoms and perineal and low back pain. The prostate may feel normal or boggy.

DIAGNOSIS

- ABP is essentially a clinical diagnosis based on symptoms and physical examination of the prostate. Urinalysis may show pyuria and bacteriuria, and urine cultures usually demonstrate the infecting organism. Blood cultures may also be positive.
- The method of choice for an accurate diagnosis of CBP is the Meares and Stamey localization technique, which requires simultaneous quantitative cultures of the urethral urine (first voided bladder specimen [VB_1]), second midstream bladder specimen (VB_2), prostatic secretions expressed by massage (EPS), and the urine voided after massage (first voided bladder specimen [VB_3]). If CBP is present, the number of bacteria in EPS or ejaculate and VB_3 will exceed those in VB_1 or VB_2 by at least 10-fold.

MANAGEMENT

- In patients with ABP, empiric antimicrobial treatment with a quinolone or a β-lactam with an aminoglycoside should be initiated immediately after urinalysis and urine and blood cultures are obtained. Duration of therapy is usually 4 to 6 weeks.
- Chronic bacterial prostatitis is difficult to cure because few antimicrobial agents penetrate well into the noninflamed prostate. Long-term cure rates of 60% to 70% may be obtained with a quinolone or TMP-SMX given for 6 to 12 weeks. If therapy fails with these regimens, recurrent episodes of CBP may be managed by either continuous low-dose suppressive therapy or treatment of exacerbations of symptomatic UTI.

PERINEPHRIC AND INTRARENAL ABSCESS

EPIDEMIOLOGY AND ETIOLOGY

- Perinephric abscess usually occurs secondary to a mechanical obstruction of the urinary tract which precipitates acute pyelonephritis or occasionally secondary to bacteremia. The etiologic organisms are usually gram-negative enteric bacilli and occasionally gram-positive cocci when the infection is of hematogenous origin.
- Intrarenal abscesses usually occur as a consequence of hematogenous spread of bacteria, often *S. aureus*, from a primary focus of infection elsewhere in the body. The primary focus of infection is not apparent in one-third of patients. Intrarenal abscess may also

occur as a complication of acute pyelonephritis and may be located in the renal cortex or medulla, or both.

CLINICAL FEATURES

- Patients with perinephric or intrarenal abscess may complain of fever, chills, and abdominal and flank pain. Patients with perinephric abscess may also have irritative voiding symptoms. The diagnosis should be strongly considered in any patient with a febrile illness and unilateral flank pain who does not respond to therapy for acute pyelonephritis.

DIAGNOSIS

- Patients with perinephric abscess frequently manifest pyuria and proteinuria. Urinalysis is usually normal, and blood cultures are generally negative in patients with intrarenal abscess.
- Renal ultrasonography and computed tomography scans enable the early detection of lesions.

MANAGEMENT

- Intrarenal and perinephric abscesses are managed with antimicrobial therapy with or without percutaneous drainage and/or surgery.
- Duration of therapy must be individualized, taking into consideration underlying host status, the nature of the abscess, adequacy of drainage (if undertaken), and response to therapy (both clinical and as revealed by serial imaging studies). Antimicrobial therapy is usually given for at least 2 to 4 weeks.

BIBLIOGRAPHY

Dembry LM, Andriole VT. Renal and perirenal abscesses. *Infect Dis Clin North Am.* 1997;11:663–680.

Sobel JD, Kaye D. Urinary tract infections. In: Mandell GL, Bennett JE, Dolin R, eds. *Mandell, Douglas, and Bennett's Principles and Practice of Infectious Diseases.* 6th ed. Philadelphia: Elsevier; 2005:875.

Warren JW, Abrutyn E, Hebel JR, et al. Guidelines for antimicrobial treatment of uncomplicated acute bacterial cystitis and acute pyelonephritis in women. *Clin Infect Dis.* 1999;29: 745–758.

92 SKIN AND SOFT TISSUE INFECTIONS

*Mary Abigail C. Dacuycuy
and Donald J. Kennedy*

IMPETIGO

EPIDEMIOLOGY AND ETIOLOGY

- Impetigo is a superficial infection of the epidermis that frequently occurs in children and is nearly always caused by Group A *Streptococcus* (GAS) and/or *Staphylococcus aureus.*
- In streptococcal impetigo, responsible organisms initially colonize the unbroken skin and inoculation originates at minor breaks in the skin. In staphylococcal impetigo, nasal colonization precedes cutaneous disease.

CLINICAL FEATURES

- Nonbullous impetigo begins as vesicles that evolve into pustules, which readily rupture. The purulent discharge dries and forms thick, golden-yellow, crusts. Pruritus is common, and scratching of lesions can spread the infection.
- Bullous lesions appear as vesicles coalesce to form bullae containing clear yellow or slightly turbid fluid. Lesions decompress with rupture.
- Ecthyma is a deeply ulcerated form of impetigo.

DIAGNOSIS

- Diagnosis is established by clinical findings and confirmed by Gram stain of smears of vesicles showing gram-positive cocci. Culture of exudate beneath an unroofed crust reveals *S. aureus*, GAS, or a mixture of streptococci and *S. aureus.*

MANAGEMENT

- Untreated lesions of impetigo can be complicated by suppurative lymphadenitis, cellulitis, and bacteremia. Another complication of GAS infection is poststreptococcal glomerulonephritis.
- Community-acquired (CA) methicillin-resistant *S. aureus* (MRSA) is emerging as a frequent cause of

skin and soft tissue infections and should be considered in the selection of empiric antimicrobial therapy. Vancomycin, linezolid, daptomycin, trimethoprim-sulfamethoxazole, clindamycin, minocycline, and fluoroquinolone have activity against most strains of CA-MRSA. There may be inducible resistance to clindamycin if erythromycin resistance is present.
- Daily cleansing and prompt care of minor skin wounds prevents recurrence.

CUTANEOUS ABSCESS, FURUNCLE, AND CARBUNCLE

EPIDEMIOLOGY AND ETIOLOGY

- Cutaneous abscesses are infections within the dermis and deeper skin tissues characterized by collections of polymorphonuclear leukocytes.
- Folliculitis, furuncles, and carbuncles represent a continuum of severity of infection.
- Folliculitis is a pyoderma located within hair follicles and the apocrine gland regions.
- A furuncle is a deep inflammatory nodule that usually develops from preceding folliculitis and occurs in areas that are subject to friction and perspiration such as the neck, face, axillae, and buttocks.
- A carbuncle is a deeper infection composed of interconnecting abscesses usually arising in several contiguous hair follicles.
- *Staphylococcus aureus* is the usual etiologic agent. Predisposing factors include chronic *S. aureus* carrier state, obesity, diabetes mellitus, and poor hygiene.

CLINICAL FEATURES

- Lesions are warm, erythematous, and tender.
- A furuncle is initially a firm tender nodule with a central necrotic plug, which becomes fluctuant. An abscess forms below the necrotic plug, often topped by a central pustule.
- A carbuncle is composed of multiple, adjacent, coalescing furuncles with superficial pustules, necrotic plugs, and sievelike openings draining pus.

DIAGNOSIS

- Clinical diagnosis is based on the morphologic features of the lesion.
- Laboratory examinations include Gram stain and culture of purulent material.

MANAGEMENT

- Most small furuncles can be treated by application of moist heat, which promotes drainage. Large furuncles and carbuncles that are fluctuant require incision and drainage.
- Systemic antibiotics should be given if there is surrounding cellulitis or systemic symptoms of fever, chills, and leukocytosis. Antibiotics should be continued until evidence of acute inflammation has subsided, usually for 7 to 10 days.
- Recurrent furunculosis is managed by eradication of staphylococcal carriage. This involves several measures:
  ◦ Systemic antibiotics for the most recent episode.
  ◦ Intranasal application of 2% mupirocin ointment to eliminate nasal carriage.
  ◦ Rifampin (together with the systemic antibiotic) to eradicate nasal carriage.
  ◦ Four percent chlorhexidine bath to decrease skin colonization. Resistance to rifampin emerges if used alone.

CELLULITIS AND ERYSIPELAS

EPIDEMIOLOGY AND ETIOLOGY

- Cellulitis is a cutaneous infection that involves the dermis and subcutaneous tissues and is most commonly caused by GAS and *S. aureus.* Cellulitis occurs most frequently on the lower extremities.
- Erysipelas is an infection involving the upper dermis and superficial lymphatics. It is more common in infants, young children (<10 years of age), and older adults (>55 years of age) and is almost always caused by GAS. Sites of predilection include the lower legs, face, areas of preexisting lymphedema, and the umbilical stump.
- Previous trauma or an underlying skin lesion (eczematous lesion, fungal infection, and furuncle) predisposes to the development of these infections.

CLINICAL FEATURES

- The involved area is erythematous, warm, edematous, and tender. Systemic manifestations such as fever, chills, and malaise may develop; and bacteremia may be present.
- Erysipelas is distinguished from cellulitis by the sharply demarcated and elevated border of the lesion. Cellulitis may progress to lymphangitis and lymphadenitis.

DIAGNOSIS

- Clinical diagnosis is based on morphologic features of the lesion.

MANAGEMENT

- Antimicrobial therapy with a penicillinase-resistant penicillin or a first-generation cephalosporin is reasonable. Patients with life-threatening penicillin allergies can be treated with clindamycin or vancomycin. In cases of uncomplicated cellulitis, 5 days of antibiotic treatment is as effective as a 10-day course.
- Antibiotics with activity against MRSA should be given if the infection is hospital acquired, the patient is not improving, or CA-MRSA is suspected.
- Elevation of the affected area, which is frequently overlooked, hastens improvement by promoting mobilization of the edema and decreasing the intensity of the inflammatory response.

NECROTIZING FASCIITIS

EPIDEMIOLOGY AND ETIOLOGY

- Necrotizing fasciitis is an uncommon, severe, rapidly progressive infection characterized by extensive necrosis involving the subcutaneous soft tissues (particularly the superficial and often the deep fascia) and overlying skin.
- The monomicrobial form of this infection is usually community acquired and may be caused by GAS, *Clostridium perfringens, S. aureus, Vibrio vulnificus, Aeromonas hydrophila,* and anaerobic streptococci. It is most commonly seen in the lower extremities. Risk factors include diabetes, peripheral vascular disease, or venous insufficiency with edema. Mortality may approach 50% to 70%.
- In the polymicrobial form, anaerobic and aerobic organisms, most of which originate from bowel flora, may be cultured. Clinical settings in which this infection may develop include bowel surgery with peritoneal soiling, decubitus ulcers, at the site of parenteral drug abuse, and spread from a perianal or groin abscess.
- Fournier's gangrene is a form of necrotizing fasciitis occurring in males that involves the scrotum, perineum, penis, and abdominal wall. Risk factors include diabetes mellitus, local trauma, paraphimosis, perirectal or perianal infection, and surgery in the region.

CLINICAL FEATURES

- The initial presentation is characterized by erythema, swelling, induration, warmth, and exquisite tenderness, which progresses into bullae containing red-black fluid, and frank cutaneous gangrene. At this point the area may be numb or anesthetic. With progression, there is high-grade fever and severe systemic toxicity.

DIAGNOSIS

- Diagnosis is primarily based on clinical findings. Signs of severe sepsis or no improvement of symptoms, despite antimicrobial therapy, are highly suggestive of the disease.
- A blunt instrument or a finger through an open wound or a limited incision easily dissects through tissue planes into the deep fascia.
- Computed tomography scan or magnetic resonance imaging may show fascial plane infection or gas; however therapy should not be delayed pending imaging.
- Samples for culture are best obtained from deep tissues during surgery. Blood cultures are often positive.

MANAGEMENT

- Immediate and complete surgical debridement of necrotic tissue is essential.
- Empiric antimicrobial therapy must cover both aerobes and anaerobes (piperacillin-tazobactam, carbapenem, cefotaxime plus clindamycin or metronidazole). Methicillin-resistant *S. aureus* must also be considered given its increasing prevalence.
- The antibiotic regimen should be modified when the pathogen is identified. Group A *Streptococcus* should be treated with penicillin and clindamycin. Clindamycin is given to suppress streptococcal toxin production. Intravenous immunoglobulin may be administered to treat streptococcal toxic shock syndrome.

BIBLIOGRAPHY

Stevens DL, Bisno AL, Chambers HF, et al. Practice guidelines for the diagnosis and management of skin and soft-tissue infections. *Clin Infect Dis.* 2005;41:1377–1406.

Swartz MN, Pasternack MS. Cellulitis and subcutaneous tissue infections. In Mandell GL, Bennett JE, Dolin R, eds. *Mandell, Douglas, and Bennett's Principles and Practice of Infectious Diseases*, 6th ed. Philadelphia: Elsevier; 2005:1172.

Wolff K, Johnson, RA, Suurmond D. *Fitzpatrick's Color Atlas & Synopsis of Clinical Dermatology*. 5th ed. New York: McGraw-Hill; 2005.

93 BONE AND JOINT INFECTIONS

Musab U. Saeed and Donald J. Kennedy

OSTEOMYELITIS

- Infection of bone and bone marrow is most commonly caused by bacteria and less often by fungi and mycobacteria.

CLASSIFICATION

- Osteomyelitis is classified based on the origin and duration of the infection: (1) hematogenous osteomyelitis, (2) contiguous osteomyelitis, and (3) chronic osteomyelitis.

HEMATOGENOUS OSTEOMYELITIS

ETIOLOGY

- *Staphylococcus aureus* is the most common pathogen (40%–60%) followed by *Staphylococcus epidermidis*. *Streptococci* are more common in children and diabetic patients while gram-negative bacilli (*Escherichia coli, Salmonella,* and *Klebsiella*) (10%–15%) are more common in patients with chronic renal disease, diabetes, alcoholism, and cancer.
- Some organisms are characteristically identified in special patient populations; for example, *Salmonella* is seen more commonly in sickle cell disease and *Pseudomonas* is prevalent in intravenous drug users.

CLINICAL FEATURES

- Patients with osteomyelitis usually develop bone pain, fevers, rigors, diaphoresis, with local swelling, erythema, warmth and point tenderness adjacent to the affected site. The symptoms are of a subacute nature and typically less than 3 weeks in duration. However some individuals present exclusively with bone pain and lack other signs of infection.

DIAGNOSIS

- Two to four sets of blood cultures should be obtained in patients with suspected osteomyelitis. The cultures are positive in 50% of patients.

- The erythrocyte sedimentation rate (ESR) and C-reactive protein increase with disease progression and are useful to monitor therapeutic response.
- Although radiologic findings lag behind the clinical presentation by weeks, x-rays are, nonetheless, valuable. Radiographic findings suggestive of osteomyelitis include subperiosteal elevation, lytic bone lesions, and eventually, sclerotic changes.
- Bone scans are highly sensitive but lack specificity. A three-phase technetium scan or an indium scan may be positive as early as 24 hours after seeding the bone, however these studies are expensive, nonspecific, and positive in a variety of other conditions including cancers and traumatic injuries.
- Magnetic resonance imaging (MRI) is extremely useful as it provides detailed anatomical information and serves to distinguish between soft tissue and bone marrow involvement. Computed tomography (CT) scanning also provides excellent images of the bone cortex and is valuable for biopsy localization.
- A bone biopsy should be considered in all patients in whom the diagnosis is suspected but unconfirmed; or in whom fungal infection, mycobacteria, or malignancy is suspected.

MANAGEMENT

- Intravenous (IV) antibiotics are directed at known or suspected pathogens for 4 to 6 weeks. Penicillins, cephalosporins (eg, ceftriaxone), gentamicin, clindamycin, and quinolones are all acceptable antibiotics. IV therapy may be followed by oral therapy with TMP-SMX, quinolones, clindamycin, or linezolid in patients that respond quickly to parenteral therapy or to avoid the risks associated with prolonged use of indwelling vascular catheters. While there is less experience with oral therapy, the long-term response appears similar to those attained with parenteral therapy.
- Surgery may be indicated to confirm the diagnosis, to remove the nidus of infection in patients responding poorly to therapy, or if concomitant joint infection is suspected.

CONTIGUOUS OSTEOMYELITIS

ETIOLOGY

- Contiguous osteomyelitis occurs when tissue infection spreads to adjacent bone. A polymicrobial infection is common in this setting. *Staphylococcus aureus* (50%–60%), *S. epidermidis*, gram-negative bacilli (eg, *Pseudomonas aeruginosa*), and anaerobes are the most likely pathogens.

- In open fractures, environmental organisms (*Nocardia, Bacillus, Aeromonas*, fungi, and atypical mycobacteria) should be considered and treated appropriately.

CLINICAL FEATURES

- Most patients have a history of an open fracture, recent surgery, diabetic ulceration, or animal bites with soft tissue infection of the surrounding area.
- Patients present with soft tissue swelling, pain, and erythema with constitutional symptoms of fever and malaise.

DIAGNOSIS

- Leukocytosis with an elevated ESR and C-reactive protein is expected but their absence does not necessarily exclude an infection. Blood cultures should be obtained as early as possible.
- X-rays generally prove useful, however, the overlying skin infection may interfere with the interpretation. Bone scans, while quite sensitive, are of limited use because they cannot distinguish between trauma, tumor, and infection.
- Superficial wound and sinus tract cultures are not particularly useful as they do not correlate with pathogens identified by bone biopsy. The bone biopsy is an essential tool to establish the underlying disease process and identify the pathogen(s). Histopathology, smear, and cultures should be obtained.

MANAGEMENT

- The antibiotics of choice are similar to the agents used for hematogenous osteomyelitis but therapy should be based on the results of intraoperative cultures.
- Meticulous wound care, surgical debridement, and amputation are a pivotal component of management, as relapse rates are between 40% and 50% of cases.
- In general, 4 to 6 weeks of IV antibiotics are administered after debridement is completed; however, the duration may be modified based on the response. An oral antibiotic after completing IV antibiotics is sometimes considered in patients that are at high-risk for recurrence (diabetes).

CHRONIC OSTEOMYELITIS

ETIOLOGY

- Recurrent or persistent osteomyelitis at the site of previous treatment.

- Chronic osteomyelitis commonly develops in diabetic patients because of peripheral neuropathy, microvascular disease and poor foot care. Mild non–limb-threatening infections are usually caused by *S. aureus,* gram-negative bacilli or anaerobic organisms. Severe limb threatening infections are usually polymicrobial.

CLINICAL FEATURES

- Patients present with localized swelling, sinus tract formation, and drainage from the wound site. Fever and constitutional symptoms are rarely seen.
- A limb-threatening diabetic foot infection is usually associated with a full thickness ulcer that is contiguous with the bone; the patient has evidence of local soft tissue infection. Pain is usually absent because of neuropathy.

DIAGNOSIS

- White blood cell (WBC) counts are usually normal; ESR and C-relative protein may be elevated but are nonspecific.
- Radiographs may be useful if previous films are available for comparison. Bone scans may be useful if negative, but a positive scan is not particularly helpful since it remains positive for months after treatment.
- CT and MRI provide greater detail of the local anatomy and are useful in guiding bone biopsies.
- A bone biopsy with histopathology and cultures is required to establish a definitive diagnosis. The biopsy must be performed prior to administering antimicrobial therapy. Bacterial, mycobacterial, and fungal cultures should also be requested.

MANAGEMENT

- Surgical debridement in concert with 4 to 6 weeks of IV antibiotics directed at the known or suspected pathogen(s) is recommended.
- Without surgical intervention, the role of antimicrobial therapy is limited. Patients who are poor surgical candidates may require long-term (3–6 mo), even lifelong, suppression with antibiotics. Oral quinolones have been used to treat chronic osteomyelitis caused by gram-negative bacilli.
- Most patients with diabetes who develop osteomyelitis require surgical intervention. Infections are usually polymicrobial and require broad spectrum antibiotics. Piperacillin-tazobactam, ampicillin and sulbactam, a cephalosporin or a quinolone with metronidazole or clindamycin are all acceptable regimens.

INFECTIOUS ARTHRITIS

ETIOLOGY

- Infectious inflammation of the joint is usually monoarticular and often due to hematogenous spread from another site (50%–75%).
- The most common pathogen in the young adult (15–40 y) is *Neisseria gonorrhea,* whereas S. *aureus* (37%–65%) and *Streptococcus* species are seen more commonly in patients older than 40 years of age. Intravenous drug users, patients who are immunocompromised, or patients with chronic debilitating diseases may develop infection with gram-negative organisms (eg, *E. coli, P. aeruginosa*). Lyme disease should also be considered in the appropriate clinical setting.
- The most common pathogens involved in prosthetic joint infections are coagulase-negative staphylococci (22%), *S. aureus* (22%), streptococci and gram-negative bacilli (20%–25%).
- Viruses that produce inflammation of the joints include rubella, hepatitis B virus (HBV), hepatitis C virus (HCV), and human parvovirus.

CLINICAL FEATURES

- Patients with chronic joint damage (osteoarthritis, rheumatoid arthritis), sickle cell disease, immunosuppression, prosthetic joints, intravenous drug use, and sexually transmitted disease are at a higher risk of infection. The joints most commonly affected are the knees, elbows, wrists, and shoulders.
- Usual presentation is characterized by, erythema and warmth followed by fever, chills, and decreased range of motion coupled with severe pain.
- Early prosthetic joint infection may mimic a typical surgical site wound infection with dehiscence, drainage, and joint pain. Delayed presentations are characterized by mild joint pain and drainage and less frequently fever, soft tissue swelling, or constitutional symptoms.

DIAGNOSIS

- Synovial fluid should be aspirated and analyzed in all cases of suspected infectious arthritis (Table 93–1). The Gram stains are positive in 35% to 65% of cases.

TABLE 93–1 Joint Fluid Analysis

STUDIES	SEPTIC ARTHRITIS	REACTIVE ARTHRITIS	NONINFECTIOUS ARTHRITIS
Clarity/color	Opaque/Yellow	Clear/Yellow	Clear/Colorless
WBC/mm^3	>100,000 (range 25,000–250,000)	2000–100,000	200–2000
PMN	≥75%	≥50%	>25%
Cultures/smears	(+)	(−)	(−)
Glucose	↓↓↓	↓	Normal
Crystals	(−)	(−)	(−)

PMN, polymorphonuclear neutrophils; WBC, white blood cell.

In patients with chronically infected joints, fungal and mycobacterial smears and cultures should be obtained. Blood cultures are positive in approximately 10% of cases.

- Initial radiologic findings demonstrate increase volume of the joint space which may evolve to frank joint erosions in 2 to 4 weeks. The MRI is very sensitive and specific for septic arthritis, however the CT is usually used for guided needle aspiration.

MANAGEMENT

- Antibiotics should be initiated after joint drainage. Importantly, many patients may require repeated drainage. Antibiotics are chosen based the clinical picture and Gram stain results (Table 93–2) and are subsequently modified, based on cultures. The duration of treatment is usually 4 weeks.
- Early postoperative prosthetic joint infection (<1 mo) may be treated without removal of the prosthesis with a prolonged (3 to 6 mo) course of antibiotics. In infections that develop >1 month after surgery, a two-stage surgical procedure with explantation of the prosthesis, followed by 6 weeks of IV antibiotics, and then reimplantation of a new prosthesis provides a reasonable chance of cure.

TABLE 93–2 Treatment Recommendations Based on the Organism Seen on Gram Stain

GRAM STAIN	ANTIBIOTICS
Gram-positive cocci	Nafcillin, cefazolin, clindamycin Vancomycin (risk of MRSA)
Gram-negative cocci	Ceftriaxone
Gram-negative rods	Cefepime, piperacillin-tazobactam, carbapenem
Gram stain negative	Add ceftazidime, quinolones, aminoglycoside to gram positive coverage regimen above

MRSA, Methicillin-resistant *Staphylococcus aureus.*

BIBLIOGRAPHY

Madeoff LC, Thaler SJ, Maguire JH, Infectious arthritis. In: Kasper DL, Braunwald E, Fauci AS, et al, eds. *Harrison's Principles of Internal Medicine.* 16th ed. New York: McGraw-Hill; 2005:2050.

Mandell GL. In; Bennett JE, Dolin R, eds. *Principles and Practice of Infectious Diseases.* 6th ed. Philadelphia: Elsevier Churchill Livingstone; 2005.

Nolan RL, Chapman SW. Bone and joint infections. In: Betts RF, Chapman SW, Penn RL, eds. *A Practical Approach to Infectious Disease.* 5th ed. Philadelphia: Lippincott Williams & Wilkins; 2003: 127.

94 SEXUALLY TRANSMITTED INFECTIONS

Mary Abigail C. Dacuycuy and Donald J. Kennedy

GENITAL HERPES

ETIOLOGY

- Genital herpes is caused by herpes simplex virus type 1 (HSV-1) and type 2 (HSV-2). Most cases of genital herpes are caused by HSV-2.
- Transmission of genital herpes is through close contact with a person who is shedding virus in genital or oral secretions or at a mucosal surface. HSV-2 remains latent in sensory neurons of presacral ganglia and can reactivate and cause recurrent disease.

CLINICAL FEATURES

- Typical lesions are multiple, painful, grouped vesicles usually located on the penis or on the labia or vulva. Vesicles rupture to form ulcers that heal by crusting over.

- A manifestation of primary infection may include aseptic meningitis.
- Asymptomatic shedding is common and can cause transmission of infection.

DIAGNOSIS

- Diagnosis is usually established clinically when characteristic lesions are present.
- HSV infection is best confirmed by isolation of HSV in cell culture or by demonstration of HSV DNA in scrapings from lesions.

MANAGEMENT

- Therapeutic options for active infection and suppression include acyclovir, valacyclovir, and famciclovir. Primary infection is usually treated for 7 to 10 days; recurrences may be treated for 1 to 3 days, depending on the agent used.
- Suppressive therapy reduces the frequency of genital herpes recurrences by 70% to 80% in patients who have six or more recurrences per year.
- Intravenous acyclovir should be administered to patients who have severe HSV disease or complications (eg, meningitis, encephalitis, pneumonitis, hepatitis).
- All persons should abstain from sexual activity when lesions or prodromal symptoms are present.

SYPHILIS

ETIOLOGY

- Syphilis is a systemic disease caused by the spirochete *Treponema pallidum* which is transmitted by sexual contact or other close contact with an active lesion.

CLINICAL FEATURES

- Primary syphilis consists of one or more painless ulcers (chancres) that appear at the site of inoculation and resolve spontaneously.
- Secondary syphilis occurs approximately 3 to 6 weeks after the appearance of the chancre. Signs and symptoms include: (1) generalized maculopapular rash on the palms and soles, oral mucous membranes, and genitalia; (2) patchy alopecia; (3) generalized lymphadenopathy; (4) condylomata lata (hypertrophic lesions resembling flat warts) in moist areas and painless shallow ulcers on mucous membranes that are highly contagious; and (5) constitutional symptoms such as fever and malaise. Manifestations resolve without treatment.

- Latent syphilis is clinically silent and is diagnosed only on the basis of serologic tests. Early latent syphilis (<1 year) must be distinguished from late latent disease (≥1 year) because the therapeutic approach differs.
- Late (tertiary) syphilis occurs in approximately one-third of infected patients 2 to 60 years after infection. CNS involvement may present as meningovascular syphilis, general paresis, tabes dorsalis, or dementia. Cardiovascular involvement consists of aortitis, aortic insufficiency, saccular aneurysms and coronary ostial stenosis. Late benign gummatous lesions which are granulomatous lesions usually involving the skin, mucous membranes, and bones may occur.

DIAGNOSIS

- Darkfield examination and direct fluorescent antibody (DFA) tests of lesion exudate or tissue are the definitive methods for establishing diagnosis in primary and secondary syphilis.
- The nontreponemal (eg, VDRL and RPR) tests are used for screening but are nonspecific. Nontreponemal antibody titers usually correlate with disease activity and become nonreactive after successful treatment of syphilis.
- The treponemal tests (eg, FTA-ABS and TP-PA) detect antibodies against specific *T. pallidum* antigens and are used to confirm a positive nontreponemal test result. These tests can remain positive for life.
- The VDRL-CSF (Venereal Disease Research Laboratory-cerebrospinal fluid) is highly specific but insensitive and, when reactive, is considered diagnostic of neurosyphilis. The CSF FTA-ABS is less specific but is highly sensitive, and when negative, can exclude neurosyphilis in patients with late disease but not in patients with early disease.

MANAGEMENT

- Penicillin G, administered parenterally, is the preferred drug for treatment of all stages of syphilis (Table 94–1).
- Individuals who were sexually exposed within 90 days preceding the diagnosis of primary, secondary, or early latent syphilis in a sex partner should be treated presumptively as early syphilis.
- Patients should be informed about the Jarisch-Herxheimer reaction which is a self-limited acute febrile reaction that usually occurs within the first 24 hours after therapy for syphilis.
- All patients who have syphilis should be offered testing for HIV infection.

TABLE 94–1   Antimicrobial Therapy for Syphilis

STAGE	RECOMMENDED REGIMENS FOR ADULTS
Primary, secondary, and early latent syphilis (<1 y)	Benzathine penicillin G 2.4 million units IM in a single dose
Late latent syphilis or latent syphilis of unknown duration and tertiary syphilis (gumma and cardiovascular syphilis)	Benzathine penicillin G 7.2 million units total, administered as 3 doses of 2.4 million units IM each at 1-week intervals
Neurosyphilis	Aqueous crystalline penicillin G 18–24 million units per day, administered as 3–4 million units IV every 4 hours or continuous infusion for 10–14 days

SOURCE: Adapted from the Centers for Disease Control and Prevention: Sexually transmitted diseases treatment guidelines, 2006. *MMWR Recomm Rep.* 2006;55:1–94.

URETHRITIS AND CERVICITIS

ETIOLOGY

- *Neisseria gonorrhoeae* and *Chlamydia trachomatis* are the most common causes of urethritis and cervicitis that are sexually transmitted.

CLINICAL FEATURES

- In men, symptoms of urethritis include mucopurulent urethral discharge, dysuria, or urethral pruritus. Approximately 2% to 3% of men acquiring urethral gonococcal infection are asymptomatic. Women are usually unaware of the urethral discharge, and urethritis presents as dysuria and frequency.
- Cervicitis is frequently asymptomatic. Mucopurulent endocervical exudate and endocervical bleeding may be present on pelvic examination.

DIAGNOSIS

- In men with symptoms, a Gram stain of urethral discharge or swab that demonstrates polymorphonuclear leukocytes with gram-negative intracellular diplococci (GNID) is >99% specific and >95% sensitive for diagnosing gonococcal urethritis. In asymptomatic men, a negative Gram stain cannot exclude infection.
- Culture and nucleic acid amplification tests (NAATs) are available for the detection of genitourinary infection with *N. gonorrhoea* and *C. trachomatis.* Culture requires female endocervical or male urethral swab specimens. NAAT is FDA-approved for use with endocervical swabs, vaginal swabs, male urethral swabs, and female and male urine.

MANAGEMENT

- Patients infected with *N. gonorrhoeae* frequently are coinfected with *C. trachomatis,* therefore if chlamydial test results are not available, patients should be treated for both gonorrhea and chlamydia.
- All patients tested for gonorrhea and chlamydia should be tested for other STDs, including syphilis and HIV. All partners should be evaluated for sexually transmitted disease and be treated for gonococcal and/or chlamydial infection.
- See Table 94–2 for treatment of chlamydial and gonococcal urethritis and cervicitis.

BACTERIAL VAGINOSIS

ETIOLOGY

- Bacterial Vaginosis (BV) is a clinical syndrome resulting from replacement of the normal *Lactobacillus* sp. in the vagina with high concentrations of anaerobic bacteria, *Gardnerella vaginalis*, and *Mycoplasma hominis.* Whether BV results from a sexually transmitted pathogen remains unclear.

CLINICAL FEATURES

- Affected women usually are sexually active and may complain of a mild to moderate vaginal discharge with a fishy odor.

DIAGNOSIS

- Clinical diagnosis can be established by the presence of at least three of the following signs or symptoms: (1) homogeneous, thin, white, nonfloccular discharge that smoothly coats the vaginal walls; (2) presence of clue cells (vaginal epithelial cells studded with coccobacilli) on microscopy; (3) vaginal fluid pH > 4.5; and (4) a fishy odor in the vaginal discharge before or after addition of 10% KOH (ie, the whiff test).

MANAGEMENT

- Therapeutic options include oral or intravaginal metronidazole and intravaginal clindamycin. Patients should be advised to avoid consuming alcohol during treatment with metronidazole and for 24 hours thereafter.
- Routine treatment of sex partners is not recommended.

TABLE 94–2 Therapy for Chlamydial and Gonococcal Urethritis and Cervicitis

DISEASE	RECOMMENDED REGIMENS
Chlamydial urethritis and cervicitis	Azithromycin 1 g orally in a single dose OR
	Doxycycline 100 mg orally twice a day for 7 d
Uncomplicated gonococcal urethritis and cervicitis	Ceftriaxone 125 mg IM in a single dose OR
	Cefixime 400 mg orally in a single dose OR
	Ciprofloxacin 500 mg orally in a single dose[a] OR
	Ofloxacin 400 mg orally in a single dose[a] OR
	Levofloxacin 250 mg orally in a single dose[a]
	PLUS
	TREATMENT FOR CHLAMYDIA IF CHLAMYDIAL
	INFECTION IS NOT EXCLUDED
Gonococcal infection in MSM[b] or heterosexuals with a history of recent travel[a]	Ceftriaxone 125 mg IM in a single dose OR
	Cefixime 400 mg orally in a single dose
	PLUS
	TREATMENT FOR CHLAMYDIA IF CHLAMYDIAL
	INFECTION IS NOT EXCLUDED

SOURCE: Adapted from the Centers for Disease Control and Prevention: Sexually transmitted diseases treatment guidelines, 2006. *MMWR Recomm Rep.* 2006;55:1–94.
[a] Quinolones should not be used for infections in MSM or in those with a history of recent foreign travel or partners' travel, infections acquired in California or Hawaii, or infections acquired in other areas with increased quinolone-resistant *N. gonorrhoeae* (QRNG) prevalence.
[b] MSM: men who have sex with men

TRICHOMONIASIS

ETIOLOGY

- Trichomoniasis is caused by the protozoan *Trichomonas vaginalis* and is almost always sexually transmitted. It is the most common curable STD in young, sexually active women.

CLINICAL FEATURES

- Most women complain of profuse, yellow-green, malodorous vaginal discharge with vulvar irritation, dysuria, and dyspareunia. Lower abdominal pain is uncommon and should prompt evaluation of a secondary process. Most men who are infected are asymptomatic.
- Examination usually reveals pooling in the posterior vaginal fornix of a yellow-green or grayish-white discharge. There is diffuse vulvar erythema in severe cases. The vaginal walls are inflamed and in severe cases may appear granular. Punctate hemorrhages (colpitis macularis) of the cervix may result in a strawberry-like appearance. The vaginal pH is almost always greater than 5.0

DIAGNOSIS

- Saline wet mount of vaginal secretions demonstrating motile, flagellated trichomonads may establish a diagnosis but has a sensitivity of approximately 60%–70%.

MANAGEMENT

- Therapeutic options include metronidazole or tinidazole.
- Sex partners should be treated and patients should abstain from sexual intercourse until they and their partners are treated and asymptomatic.

HUMAN PAPILLOMAVIRUS

ETIOLOGY

- Human Papillomavirus (HPV) is a double-stranded DNA virus. Benign genital warts are usually caused by HPV types 6 or 11. Persistent infection with high-risk HPV types 16, 18, 31, 33, and 35 is strongly associated with the development of cervical cancer.
- HPV infection is common and is frequently sexually transmitted. HPV infection is usually self-limited.

CLINICAL FEATURES

- The majority of HPV infections are asymptomatic.
- Genital warts usually appear as flat, papular, or pedunculated lesions on the penis, vulva, scrotum, perineum, and perianal skin. They may also be located on the uterine cervix and in the vagina, urethra, anus, and mouth. Genital warts can be painful and friable depending on their size and location.

DIAGNOSIS

- The diagnosis of genital warts is based on clinical findings. Biopsy to detect HPV viral DNA or RNA or capsid protein in lesions may be performed if the diagnosis is uncertain.

MANAGEMENT

- The goal of treatment is the removal of warts and relief of symptoms. No therapy has been proven to eradicate HPV.
- Genital warts may be treated with podofilox, imiquimod, cryotherapy, podophyllin, trichloroacetic or bichloracetic acid, or surgical removal depending on the location of the lesion. Management of cervical warts should include consultation with a specialist.
- Use of condoms reduces transmission of HPV infection.
- A quadrivalent HPV vaccine is available for females and administered intramuscularly in a three-dose schedule.

BIBLIOGRAPHY

1. Centers for Disease Control and Prevention. Sexually transmitted diseases treatment guideline, 2006. *MMWR Recomm Rep.* 2006;55:1–94.
2. Tramont EC. *Treponema pallidum* (Syphilis). In: Mandell GL, Bennett JE, Dolin R, eds. *Mandell, Douglas, and Bennett's Principles and Practice of Infectious Diseases*, 6th ed. Philadelphia: Elsevier; 2005:2768.
3. Wolff K, Johnson RA, Suurmond D. *Fitzpatrick's Color Atlas & Synopsis of Clinical Dermatology*. 5th ed. New York: McGraw-Hill; 2005.

95 HUMAN IMMUNODEFICIENCY VIRUS AND ACQUIRED IMMUNODEFICIENCY SYNDROME

Musab U. Saeed and Donald J. Kennedy

EPIDEMIOLOGY AND ETIOLOGY

- As of 2005 according to the Joint United Nations Programme on HIV/AIDS, there are approximately 33 to 46 million people in the world with HIV/AIDS.

TABLE 95–1   Case Defining Illnesses in AIDS

Fungi	Candidiasis, PCP, cryptococcosis, histoplasmosis (extrapulmonary), and coccidioidomycosis
Viruses	CMV (any organ other than liver, spleen, lymph nodes or eye), HHSV 8 (Kaposi sarcoma), HSV (bronchitis, pneumonitis, esophagitis of any duration or >1 month of mucocutaneous ulcer), JC virus (progressive multifocal leukoencephalopathy)
Mycobacteria	*M. tuberculosis* (extrapulmonary or pulmonary), *M. avium* (disseminated)
Parasites	Toxoplasmosis of internal organ, cryptosporidiosis isoporosis (diarrhea >1 month)
Bacteria	*Salmonella* (septicemia), recurrent bacterial pneumonia
Tumors	Cervical cancer, Hodgkin and non-Hodgkin lymphoma, Burkitt lymphoma, primary CNS lymphoma
Others	HIV-associated wasting, dementia

Of these 70% are living in Africa, where the adult prevalence is 7.2%. According to a recent CDC estimate, there are currently 850,000 to 950,000 cases in the United States.
- HIV is an RNA virus with a envelope glycoprotein (GP120). The virus attaches to CD4 receptors, which induces a conformational shift in GP120 which in turn binds to a coreceptor, either CCR5 or CRCX4 (chemokine receptors) that promote entry into host cells. The HIV RNA is assimilated into the host's genome and utilizes reverse transcriptase to transcribe new DNA. These infected host cells then are capable of producing intact HIV.
- AIDS is the most severe manifestation of a clinical spectrum of HIV illness caused by progressive immunosuppression induced by HIV. AIDS is usually characterized by opportunistic infections, neoplasms, or other manifestations referred to as AIDS defining illnesses (Table 95–1).

CLINICAL FEATURES

- Transmission: The major modes of HIV transmission are summarized in Table 95–2. It is important to obtain a detailed sexual history and to explore risk factors for HIV transmission.
- Incubation period: After exposure to the virus, there is a 2- to 3-week incubation period prior to viral symptoms.
- Acute retroviral syndrome: Primary HIV infection presents as a clinical spectrum that encompasses asymptomatic seroconversion to a mononucleosis type syndrome characterized by fever, adenopathy, pharyngitis, erythematous maculopapular rash on the face and trunk, and myalgias. Less commonly headaches, nausea, vomiting, diarrhea, and weight

TABLE 95–2 Mode of Transmission for HIV

MODE OF TRANSMISSION	COMMENTS
Homosexual anal intercourse	More commonly seen in North America and Europe. Receptive partner at higher risk
Heterosexual contact	More commonly seen in Africa, South America, and Caribbean. Receptive partner at higher risk
IV drug use	Higher rates with cocaine and heroine use
Blood transmission	Uncommon in the US since screening was started (1985)
Perinatal transmission	Transmission can take place during gestation, delivery, or postpartum
Heath care setting	Percutaneous injury by a contaminated hollow needle

loss may develop during the initial presentation. During this time the CD4 count decreases and the HIV viral load concentration is high. Some patients may present with an opportunistic infection, including but not limited to aphthous ulcers, *PCP*, cryptococcal meningitis, and *Candida* esophagitis.

- The acute clinical syndrome resolves in 2 to 3 weeks and is accompanied by a reduction of viral load as an anti-HIV immune response is mounted. The viral load usually stabilizes between 6 and 12 months.
- Clinical latency: Many HIV-infected patients develop persistent generalized lymphadenopathy, involving the cervical, submandibular, occipital, and axillary lymph nodes.
- CD4 counts decline slowly over a period of years (the rate of decline of CD4 cells is variable among individual patients but tends to correlate with the viral load).
- In most untreated patients, the patient's immune system becomes sufficiently compromised predisposing to a variety of opportunistic infections.
- Opportunistic infections and late-stage disease are characterized by CD4 counts below 200 cells/mm^3. The incidence (and to some extent type) of opportunistic

TABLE 95–3 Opportunistic Infections Correlating with CD4 Counts

CD4 COUNT	OPPORTUNISTIC INFECTIONS
500 cells/mm^3	*Candida* vaginitis
500–200 cells/mm^3	Bacterial pneumonia, herpes zoster, thrush, cryptosporidiosis Kaposi sarcoma
200–100 cells/mm^3	PCP, histoplasmosis, coccidioidomycosis, tuberculosis, PML
100–50 cells/mm^3	Toxoplasmosis, cryptococcosis, microsporidiosis, candida esophagitis
<50 cells/mm^3	Disseminated CMV, *Mycobacterium avium* complex

infection correlates with the severity of immunosuppression (Table 95–3). The median survival without treatment after the CD4 count has decreased to <200cells/mm^3 is approximately 3.7 years.

DIAGNOSIS

- The current CDC recommendations for HIV screening were revised in 2006 to include routine voluntary HIV screening of all patients aged 13 to 64 years as a normal part of medical care. Importantly, early diagnosis is essential to optimize therapy and prevent transmission of HIV to uninfected individuals. Clearly, physicians should have a high level of suspicion for acute HIV infection in any patient presenting with a compatible clinical syndrome that reports exposure to HIV or exhibits high-risk behavior. All patients diagnosed with tuberculosis (TB) or sexually transmitted diseases (STDs) should be screened for HIV.
- Antibodies to HIV become detectable in 2 to 3 months after acquiring primary HIV infection, although there can be a delay of up to 6 months. An HIV polymerase chain reaction (PCR) test may be employed to screen for HIV infection during the acute phase.
- HIV is usually diagnosed by detection of antibodies to the viral antigens with an enzyme-linked immunosorbent assay (ELISA), which is 99% sensitive and 90% specific. A positive ELISA is confirmed with a Western blot assay which has a specificity of greater than 99%.
- The absolute CD4 count is the most widely used marker for prognosis and monitoring therapy. However, the CD4 count is inherently variable, especially among individuals and, therefore, must be interpreted in the context of the complete clinical and laboratory picture.
- The viral load measures the quantity of actively replicating HIV virus and correlates well with the rate of disease progression and response to antiretroviral therapy (ART). For example, manifesting a high viral load early in the course of HIV infection is a poor prognostic indicator and an indication to initiate ART.
- Genotypic and phenotypic analysis is used to identify resistance against ART. Testing is more reliable in treatment naive patients than patients that have received treatment in the past. For example, detection of a K103N mutation excludes utility of non-nucleoside reverse transcriptase inhibitors (NNRTIs).
- Initial laboratory tests for patients with newly diagnosed HIV usually include a complete blood count, basic metabolic panel, screening for STDs (*Chlamydia, N. gonorrhea,* and syphilis), tuberculosis, Pap smear for women; serologies for cytomegalovirus (CMV), hepatitis A virus (HAV), hepatitis B virus (HBV), hepatitis C

TABLE 95–4 Screening Tests, Preventive Measures, and Prophylaxis Recommendations for HIV-Positive Patients

DISEASE	SCREENING TEST/CD4 COUNT	PREVENTION AND PROPHYLAXIS
Hepatitis A	Anti HAV antibody (IgG)	Vaccination
Hepatitis B	Anti HBs antibody (IgG)	Vaccination
Hepatitis C	Anti HCV antibody (IgG)	None
Tuberculosis	PPD > 5mm	INH × 9 mo
CMV	Anti-CMV antibody (IgG)	
Syphilis	VDRL/RPR	PCN
Toxoplasmosis	Anti-toxoplasma antibody (IgG) CD4 count<100 cells/mm^3	TMP-SMX
PCP	CD4< 200 cells/mm^3	TMP SMX
VZV	Anti-Varicella antibody(IgG)	Vaccination
HPV	PAP smear	
N. gonorrhoeae	DNA prob test	Azithromycin +Ceftriaxone
C. trachomatis		
S. Pneumoniae		Vaccination every 5 y
Influenza		Vaccination every y
MAC	CD4 count< 50 cells/mm^3	Azithromycin

virus (HCV), and toxoplasmosis. Table 95–4 lists the screening tests, appropriate prophylaxis, and immunization recommendations.

MANAGEMENT

- Prevention of HIV transmission is one of the most important aspects of HIV care. Patient education regarding safe sexual practices and risks of sharing needles should be done regularly. HIV patients need to be counseled about their moral obligation to inform their partner of their HIV status, encourage them to undergo testing regularly, and use barrier techniques to prevent transmission.
- Before starting ART, compliance issues need to be discussed in detail with the patient. The clinical goals of ART include prolongation of life, improvement in quality of life, and reduction of HIV transmission. The laboratory goals include the greatest possible reduction of viral load (preferably <20–50 copies/mL), CD4 counts within the normal range, and minimize drug toxicity.
- Indications for initiating ART includes symptomatic disease or presence of AIDS defining illnesses, CD4 count <200/mm^3 (though many experts recommend offering therapy when the CD4 count is 250–350 cells/mm^3), or a viral load of >100,000 copies/mL.
- Treatment needs to be individualized for patients based on genotyping (eg, resistance testing), comorbid conditions, tolerance of side effects, and ease of administration to maximize compliance. There are four major groups of medications available (Table 95–5). It is recommended that ART should be initiated with a minimum of three medications. Preferred combinations include two nucleoside/nucleotide reverse transcriptase inhibitors (NRTI) with protease inhibitors (PI) or two NRTI with nonnucleoside reverse transcriptase inhibitors (NNRTI).

- With the initiation of ART, the patient's immune recovery may trigger a systemic inflammatory response, known as immune reconstitution syndrome (IRS). Immune reconstitution syndrome may also signal a previously occult opportunistic infection. Accordingly, the astute clinician must consider infections due to mycobacteria, herpes simplex virus, cytomegalovirus or chronic hepatitis B or C, particularly when IRS is exaggerated. In most cases the symptoms of IRS resolve in a few weeks.
- Perinatal transmission can be substantially reduced with proper perinatal care including treatment with ART, cesarean section, and avoidance of breast feeding. The guidelines for treatment of the mother are the same as that for the general population with the exception of avoiding medications that are potentially harmful during pregnancy (eg, EFV, TDF and D4t+ddI).
- It is recommended that all babies born to HIV positive mothers receive a 6-week course of oral AZT to reduce mother-to-child transmission of HIV. Some experts recommend that AZT be given in combination with other anti-HIV medications. In addition to HIV treatment, the neonate should also receive treatment to prevent *P. carinii/jiroveci* pneumonia (PCP), with sulfamethoxazole and trimethoprim until the child is confirmed as HIV negative.
- Postexposure prophylaxis for HIV transmission is based on the type of exposure, HIV risk status of the source and nature of exposure. In occupational exposure the highest risk is with large bore needles, deep tissue injury, visible blood on the device, and blood from a patient with a high viral load. Diagnostic testing for HIV should be done at the time of exposure, 6 weeks, 3 months, and 6 months later.

TABLE 95–5 Major Antiretroviral Therapeutic Agents and Their Common Side Effects

Nucleoside/Nucleotide Reverse Transcriptase Inhibitors NRTIs

Zidovudine (AZT)
Didanosine (ddI)
Tenofovir (TDF)
Emtricitabine (FTC)
Zalcitabine (ddC)
Stavudine (d4T)
Lamivudine (3TC)
Abacavir (ABC)

Common Side Effects Associated with NRTIs

Lactic acidosis	AZT, ddI, ddC, d4T
Lipoatrophy	AZT, ddC, d4T
Peripheral neuropathy	ddI, ddC, d4T
Pancreatitis	ddI, ddC
Anemia, neutropenia	AZT
Nephrotoxicity	TDF
Hypersensitivity	ABC

Non-Nucleoside Reverse Transcriptase Inhibitors NNRTIs

Efavirenz Nevirapine Delavirdine

Common Side Effects Associated with NNRTIs

Rash	All NNRTIs
Elevated AST, ALT	All NNRTIs
CNS symptoms, teratogenic	Efavirenz

Protease Inhibitors (Pis)

Indinavir (IDV)
Ritonavir (RTV)
Saquinavir (SQV)
Nelfinavir Tipranavir (TPV)
Lopinavir (LPV)
Atazanavir (ATV)
Fosamprenavir (FPV)

Common Side Effects Associated with PIs

Fat accumulation	All PIs
Insulin resistance	All PIs
Hyperlipidemia	All PIs
Nephrolithiasis	IDV
Diarrhea	RTV, LPV, TPV

Fusion Inhibitors

Enfuvirtide (ENF)

Common Side Effects Associated with Fusion Inhibitors

Local pain	Enfuvirtide (ENF)

OPPORTUNISTIC INFECTIONS AND OTHER COMPLICATIONS ASSOCIATED WITH HIV INFECTION

• Patients with HIV infection develop a variety of nonopportunistic diseases and opportunistic infections. A wide range of pathogens are encountered depending on the extent and severity of immunosuppression, geographic location, and environmental exposures.

PCP (PNEUMOCYSTIS JIROVECI)

• PCP presents as a pulmonary disease in patients with HIV. Initial symptoms may include chest tightness, dry cough, and shortness of breath during exercise. On further evaluation a chest radiograph may show diffuse infiltrates, pulmonary function tests may be abnormal and arterial blood gases reveal hypoxemia. The causative organism can be recovered from sputum or bronchoalveolar lavage. Trimethoprim/sulfamethoxazole (TMP-SMX) is the treatment of choice; however dapsone, pentamidine and atovaquone are possible alternatives. Corticosteroid therapy has been shown to reduce the incidence of acute respiratory failure in patients whose initial room air Po_2 is lower than 70 mm Hg. Patients with CD4 counts <200/mm^3 should receive prophylaxis against PCP with TMP-SMX (patients who are intolerant of TMP-SMX can be treated with dapsone or atovaquone).

TOXOPLASMA GONDII

• *Toxoplasma gondii* infection in patients with advanced HIV (CD4 cell count <100 cells/mm^3) is usually a reactivation of latent disease rather than a primary process. In patients with HIV, toxoplasmosis presents as focal neurological deficits, retinochoroiditis, pneumonitis, and rarely as a disseminated disease. Computed tomography (CT) or magnetic resonance imaging (MRI) of the brain may reveal multiple, space-occupying ring enhancing lesions that involve the corticomedullary junction or basal ganglia. Serologic testing for antibodies only establishes past exposure. A brain biopsy may be necessary to establish a definitive diagnosis. Recommended treatment includes pyrimethamine plus sulfadiazine. Primary prophylaxis is recommended for patients with a CD4 count <100 cells/mm^3 with TMP-SMX.

MYCOBACTERIUM TUBERCULOSIS

• Tuberculosis in patients with HIV usually manifests as pulmonary disease, although extrapulmonary manifestations are seen more frequently than in immunocompetent patients. The diagnosis is established by identification of *M. tuberculosis* in respiratory secretions, tissue, or blood by AFB stain or culture. Therapy consists of isoniazid, rifampin, pyrazinamide, and ethambutol for 2 months followed by isoniazid plus rifampin for an additional 4 months. Prophylaxis with 9 months of isoniazid is recommended for patients with HIV and a PPD skin test induration diameter of >5 mm.

MYCOBACTERIUM AVIUM COMPLEX (MAC)

• Disseminated MAC usually presents with fever, weight loss, diarrhea, elevated serum alkaline phosphatase levels, and anemia. Positive blood culture or biopsy of affected tissue is diagnostic. A positive culture from the respiratory secretions, stool, or urine does not necessarily imply infection, however, and clinical correlation is required. Treatment regimens usually include clarithromycin or azithromycin plus ethambutol. Prophylaxis for MAC with clarithromycin or azithromycin is recommended in HIV patients with CD4 counts <50 cells/mm³.

CHRONIC DIARRHEA

- HIV patients with chronic diarrheal syndromes are often infected with protozoan pathogens (eg, *Cryptosporidia, Isospora, Cyclospora,* and *Microsporidia*). Cryptosporidiosis improves with ART therapy. *Isospora* and *Cyclospora* can be treated with TMP-SMX. Albendazole and fumagillin are used to treat *Microsporidia* infections.

KAPOSI SARCOMA

- Kaposi sarcoma (KS) is caused by Human Herpes Virus 8 (HHV8). It is characterized by a painless, cutaneous, nodular lesion that is usually red, purple, brown, or black in color. In severe cases KS can cause obstruction of a vital structure such as the larynx, bronchi, biliary tract, or bowel. In these life-threatening situations, either radiation therapy or cytotoxic chemotherapy can be used to produce a rapid and sustained response.

CRYPTOCOCCUS NEOFORMANS

- Cryptococcal infection in patients with HIV is usually characterized by meningoencephalitis. Initial symptoms include headaches, confusion, lethargy or obtundation. The diagnosis is based on CSF analysis which reveals increased opening pressure, decreased glucose, elevated protein, and lymphocytic pleocytosis. A CSF India ink or Gomori methenamine-silver stain; and cryptococcal polysaccharide antigen test are particularly useful in arriving at a diagnosis. Initial treatment usually employs amphotericin B (with or without flucytosine) for at least 2 weeks; followed by fluconazole, daily for an extended duration (2-4 months).

CYTOMEGALOVIRUS (CMV)

- HIV-infected patients with CD4 counts <50 cells/mm³ are at risk for developing CMV infections. Retinitis is the most commonly recognized CMV manifestation in HIV patients however; esophagitis, enteritis, colitis, pneumonitis, and encephalitis have been documented.
- Treatment options include ganciclovir, valganciclovir, or foscarnet.

PROGRESSIVE MULTIFOCAL LEUKOENCEPHALOPATHY

- Progressive multifocal leukoencephalopathy (PML) presents as a unifocal or multifocal demyelinating process, caused by JC virus (a human polyoma virus). Detection of JC virus in the cerebrospinal fluid by PCR is helpful in establishing a diagnosis.
- No effective therapy has been identified other than ART.

LYMPHOMA AND OTHER NEOPLASTIC DISEASES

- Patients with HIV may develop Hodgkin, non-Hodgkin, or Burkitt's lymphoma. Primary central nervous system lymphoma (PCNSL) in HIV-infected individuals is 1000-fold higher than that in the general population. EBV is identified in virtually all PCNSLs. Chemotherapy and radiation therapy is employed if indicated. Drug interactions between antiretroviral and antineoplastic agents should be carefully reviewed.

COGNITIVE OR MOTOR DISORDER

- CNS complications are seen in approximately 15% of patients with HIV/AIDS. Clinical characteristics of these disorders can involve cognitive, behavioral, and motor systems. CT and MRI may show subcortical or cortical atrophy. No specific therapy has been identified, although patients treated with zidovudine and indinavir had a greater improvement in neuropsychologic scores compared to those treated with other drugs.

BIBLIOGRAPHY

Bartlett JG, Gallant JE. *Medical Management of HIV Infection.* 2005–2006 Edition. John Hopkins University Press; 2005.

Branson BM, Handsfield H, Lampe MA, et al. Revised recommendations for HIV testing of adults, adolescents, and pregnant women in health-care settings. *MMWR Recomm Rep.* 2006;55:1–17.

Fauci AS, Lane HC. Human immunodeficiency virus disease: AIDS and related disorders. In: Kasper DL, Braunwald E, Fauci AS, et al, eds. *Harrison's Principles of Internal Medicine.* 16th ed. New York, NY: McGraw-Hill, 2005;1076.

Mandell GL, Bennett JE, Dolin R, et al. *Mandell, Douglas, and Bennett's Principles and Practice of Infectious Diseases.* 6th Ed. Philadelphia: Elsevier Churchill Livingstone; 2005.

Zolopa AR, Katz MH. Infectious diseases: HIV. In: Tierney LM Jr, McPhee SJ, Papadakis MA, eds. *Current Medical Diagnosis & Treatment.* New York: McGraw-Hill; 2006.

96 MYCOBACTERIA

Musab U. Saeed, Mary Abigail C. Dacuycuy, and Donald J. Kennedy

TUBERCULOSIS

ETIOLOGY AND EPIDEMIOLOGY

- It is estimated that one-third of the world's population is infected by *Mycobacterium tuberculosis,* which is responsible for approximately two million deaths each year.
- Tuberculosis (TB) encompasses a variety of diseases caused by *M. tuberculosis* and less commonly *Mycobacterium bovis.*
- The mode of transmission is predominantly inhalation of aerosolized pulmonary secretions. Transmission depends on the concentration of bacilli, duration of exposure, and host immunity.

CLINICAL FEATURES

- Pulmonary TB is a common manifestation of this disease. Primary pulmonary TB is usually asymptomatic; however, patients may complain of nonspecific constitutional symptoms such as fever, lassitude, regional lymphadenitis, and rarely erythema nodosum. If the primary infection progresses, it may produce a cavitary lesion or disseminated infection.
- Mycobacteria = enter a latent phase after resolution of the primary infection which may last from months to years. Reactivation is usually characterized by fever, night sweats, malaise, weight loss, and as the disease progresses, blood streaked sputum, and hemoptysis. Tuberculous pleurisy is seen in patients >65 years of age and is due to breakdown of a subpleural focus, whereas tuberculous empyema may develop because of a bronchopleural fistula.
- Miliary TB implies hematogenous spread which can occur in a newly acquired infection as well as reactivation of latent disease.

- Extrapulmonary TB most commonly involves lymph nodes, pleura, genitourinary tract, meninges, pericardium, bones, and joints. Lymphatic TB is found most commonly in children, women, and individuals from underserved countries.

DIAGNOSIS

- Pulmonary TB is transmitted by inhalation and patients with active respiratory tract infection should be placed in respiratory isolation. Chest x-ray findings in active pulmonary TB usually include upper lobe infiltrates or cavitary lesions, although any pattern may be seen.
- Sputum, fluid, or biopsy of the involved tissue should be sent for appropriate stains (acid-fast, fluorescent and auramine-rhodamine) and cultures. Blood cultures should be obtained in patients with HIV. The sputum should be obtained early in the morning and a minimum of three separate samples procured. Sputum induction with nebulized saline may aid in obtaining an adequate specimen. Bronchoscopy with a bronchial wash, BAL, and biopsy may be required if sputa fail to yield the diagnosis.
- Fine-needle aspiration of an affected area may reveal epithelioid cells and granuloma, but acid-fast bacillus (AFB) stains are usually negative.
- Mycobacterial culture requires only 10 to 100 organisms to produce a positive result, and thus cultures can be revealing even in the presence of a negative smear. Newer automated liquid culture systems can detect growth in 1 to 3 weeks. Genetic probes may be able to rapidly confirm Mycobacterium after sufficient growth.
- In the presence of adenopathy, a lymph node biopsy should be considered as it may reveal caseating granulomas, positive acid-fast smears, and positive cultures.
- A purified protein derivative (PPD) skin test is useful in screening for prior mycobacterial infection. After an intradermal inoculation into the forearm, the maximum diameter of the induration is measured transversely to the long axis of the forearm. Table 96–1 summarizes the induration size that is considered positive in different patient populations.

TREATMENT

- A comprehensive approach with the assistance of the public health department is required to manage different aspects of this disease. Treatment of TB requires monitoring for drug adherence, toxicity, and response; identifying contacts and evaluating home risks; and surveillance for outbreaks and drug resistance.

TABLE 96–1 Induration Size Considered Positive in Different Patient Populations

INDURATION SIZE	PATIENT POPULATION
≥5 mm	Patients with HIV Close contacts of patients with tuberculosis Patients with fibrotic changes on chest x-ray Organ transplant recipients Patients receiving prednisone (≥15mg/day) chronically
≥10 mm	Recent immigrants (within 5 y) from high prevalence areas Diabetics, IV drug users, homeless Residents and employees of nursing homes, hospitals, and jails
≥15 mm	Population with no risk factors for tuberculosis

HIV, human immunodeficiency virus; PPD, purified protein derivative.

- Active pulmonary TB is usually treated with isoniazid (INH), rifampin, pyrazinamide, and ethambutol for 2 months followed by INH and rifampin for an additional 4 months. Vitamin B6 should be added to prevent peripheral neuropathy associated with INH.
- Drug resistance is becoming a growing concern especially in third world countries. Risk factors for developing resistance include erratic adherence to therapy, suboptimal dosing, malabsorption of drugs, or the failure to identify a partially resistant organism (which typically require multiple agents for successful therapy). At least three active new agents should be initiated when multidrug-resistant (MDR) TB is suspected. Therapy for proven MDR TB should continue for an extended course.
- Recent skin test conversion (usually within a 12 month period) and patients at high risk for developing active TB (immunocompromised host) require treatment with INH for 9 months.
- From an infection control aspect, the length of time required for isolation precautions is based on whether the patient is considered an infection risk. For example, patients who are improving may be released from isolation with positive smear results if public health authorities have completed their household evaluation, there is no continued contact with individuals at risk for TB (eg, immunosuppressed hosts or infants), and arrangements for directly observed therapy (DOT) and follow-up have been completed.

INFECTIONS CAUSED BY NONTUBERCULOUS MYCOBACTERIA (NTM)

EPIDEMIOLOGY AND ETIOLOGY

- NTM are composed of species other than *M. tuberculosis, M. africanum, M. bovis, M. caprae, M. microti,* and *M. leprae.*

- Based on their growth rates on agar plates, NTM generally may be classified as
  - Rapidly growing (growth within 7 days)—eg, *M. fortuitum*
  - Slowly growing (growth after 7 d)—eg, *M. avium* and *M. intracellulare* (MAC), *M. kansasi*
  - Intermediately growing (growth in 7 to 10 d)—eg, *M. marinum*
- Most NTM species are recovered from the environment (eg, soil, water, animals, plant material). Tap water is a major reservoir for common human NTM pathogens, in particular, *M. kansasii, M. xenopi,* and MAC.

CLINICAL FEATURES

- NTM may produce pulmonary disease, lymphadenitis, cutaneous and musculoskeletal infections, and disseminated disease.

CHRONIC PULMONARY DISEASE
- Chronic bronchopulmonary disease is the most common localized infection caused by NTM in the immunocompetent host. In the United States, the most common cause is MAC followed by *M. kansasii.*
- Patients often complain of chronic productive cough and fatigue. Other less common symptoms include malaise, dyspnea, fever, hemoptysis, and weight loss.
- The diagnosis is established by examining microbiologic stains and performing cultures for acid-fast bacilli (AFB), chest imaging, and/or lung biopsy (granulomatous inflammation and/or AFB).

LYMPHADENITIS
- Localized lymphadenitis is the most common presentation of NTM in children, with a peak incidence between 1 and 5 years of age. In the United States 80% of culture-positive cases in children are caused by MAC.
- Lymph nodes of the anterior cervical chain are usually affected and are unilateral and painless. The nodes may enlarge and erode through the skin (fistulization). Purulent drainage is common in this setting.
- A definitive diagnosis is established via culture of the etiologic organism from lymph node drainage.

CUTANEOUS AND MUSCULOSKELETAL INFECTIONS
- Localized cutaneous and soft tissue infections are most commonly caused by *M. marinum* and rapidly growing NTM. *M. marinum* infection is commonly referred to as *swimming pool* or *fish tank granuloma.* The infection may occur in either an immunocompetent or an immunocompromised host. The diagnosis is established via culture of specific NTM from open wounds or tissue biopsy.

- Infection of tendon sheaths, bones, bursae, and joints may be caused by both rapidly growing and slowly growing NTM through direct inoculation of the pathogen (eg, trauma, surgical incisions, puncture wounds, or injections). Surgical debridement is often necessary for both diagnosis and therapy.

DISSEMINATED DISEASE
- Disseminated NTM infection almost exclusively occurs in the immunosuppressed patient (human immunodeficiency virus [HIV]-positive host, organ transplant recipient, or patients receiving chronic steroids).
- In the HIV-positive patient, disseminated disease is most commonly caused by *M. avium.*

MANAGEMENT

- Specific treatment regimens are based on the NTM cultured, the organ system involved, and susceptibility testing. Combination regimens are generally administered for an extended course.

BIBLIOGRAPHY

Kasper DL, Braunwald E, Fauci AS, et al. *Harrison's Principles of Internal Medicine*. 16th ed. New York: McGraw-Hill; 2005.

Mandell GL, Bennett JE, Dolin R, eds. *Mandell, Douglas, and Bennett's Principles and Practice of Infectious Diseases*. 6th ed. Philadelphia: Elsevier; 2005.

Wallace RJ Jr, Cook JL, Glassroth J, et al. Diagnosis and treatment of disease caused by nontuberculous mycobacteria. American Thoracic Society Statement. *Am J Respir Crit Care Med*. 1997;156(Suppl):S1–S25.

97 FUNGAL INFECTIONS
Mary Abigail C. Dacuycuy and Donald J. Kennedy

INTRODUCTION

- Most fungi are categorized as yeasts or molds. Yeastlike fungi (eg, *Candida* spp., *Penicillium marneffei*) are typically round or oval, unicellular, and reproduce by budding. Molds (eg, *Aspergillus* spp.,

Zygomycetes) are composed of tubular structures called hyphae and grow by branching and longitudinal extension. Some fungi do not fall neatly in either category (eg, *Pneumocystis jiroveci*) while others can grow in either fashion. The dimorphic fungi grow in the host as yeasts but grow at room temperature in the laboratory as molds (eg, *Histoplasma capsulatum*, *Blastomyces dermatitidis*, *Sporothrix schenckii*, *Coccidioides* spp., and *Paracoccidioides brasiliensis).*
- Fungi may be identified in specimens by staining with Gomori methenamine-silver, periodic acid-Schiff (stains the polysaccharide cell wall in viable fungi), or calcofluor (fungi appear white under the fluorescent microscope), and a presumptive diagnosis is based on the characteristic appearance on microscopy. A definitive diagnosis requires culture of the fungi from affected tissue.
- The mycoses study group of the Infectious Diseases Society of America has published practice guidelines for the treatment of fungal infection.

CANDIDIASIS

EPIDEMIOLOGY AND ETIOLOGY

- *Candida* organisms are yeasts that are human commensals and are commonly found throughout the entire gastrointestinal tract, in the female genital tract, and on the skin.
- Most infections are endogenous in origin and are promoted by the following conditions: antibiotic suppression of normal bacterial flora allowing *Candida* organisms to proliferate; disruption of normal biologic barriers (eg, indwelling intravenous catheters, abdominal surgery, burns); and immune suppression (eg, diabetes mellitus, renal failure, human immunodeficiency virus (HIV), neutropenia, hematologic malignancies, solid or stem cell transplantation, corticosteroid use).
- Though *Candida* organisms have been recovered from the environment and inanimate objects, *Candida* spp. are rarely laboratory contaminants.

CLINICAL FEATURES

- *Candida* infections have a large number of manifestations that can be subdivided based on organ involvement.
- Mucous membrane infections include thrush, esophagitis, non-esophageal gastrointestinal involvement (with ulceration as the most common lesion), and vulvovaginitis.

- Cutaneous candidiasis syndromes include generalized cutaneous candidiasis (widespread eruptions over the entire body); erosio interdigitalis blastomycetica (infection between fingers or toes); folliculitis; balanitis (vesicles on the penis); cutaneous lesions of disseminated candidiasis; intertrigo (infection in warm, moist skin surfaces that are in close proximity); paronychia and onychomycosis; and perianal candidiasis.
- Deep organ involvement may affect the following areas: central nervous system (eg, meningitis or abscess); respiratory tract (usually from dissemination); cardiovascular system (eg, endocarditis, myocarditis, or pericarditis); urinary tract; musculoskeletal system (eg, arthritis, osteomyelitis, costochondritis, myositis); abdominal viscera (eg, peritoneum, liver, spleen, or gallbladder); vasculature; and ocular system.
- *Candida* infection may also present as a syndrome of disseminated candidiasis and candidemia.

DIAGNOSIS

- A definitive diagnosis requires culture of the fungi from clinically relevant tissue. Colonization must be differentiated from infection especially when *Candida* is isolated from the urine or sputum.

MANAGEMENT

- Treatment is based on the specific *Candida* species isolated and organ system involved.
- Antifungal therapy includes amphotericin B, azoles (eg, fluconazole or voriconazole), and echinocandins (eg, caspofungin).
- *Candida glabrata* are frequently resistant to the azoles, and some *Candida tropicalis* are also resistant to azoles. *Candida krusei* have intrinsic resistance to azoles, whereas *Candida lusitaniae* have intrinsic resistance to amphotericin.
- In candidemia or invasive candidiasis associated with intravascular catheters and/or foreign body, the intravascular catheter or foreign body must be removed.

ASPERGILLOSIS

EPIDEMIOLOGY AND ETIOLOGY

- Worldwide, aspergillosis is the most common invasive mold infection and is caused by *Aspergillus* spp. *Aspergillus* is a mold that is characterized by septated hyphae with 40 degree angle branching. It is found ubiquitously in organic debris (hay, decaying vegetation, soil, and potted plants), pepper and spices, and construction sites. *Aspergillus fumigatus* and *Aspergillus flavus* account for the majority of all infections while others are caused by *Aspergillus niger, Aspergillus terreus*, and *Aspergillus nidulans*.
- The main route of infection is inhalation of spores which colonize the lungs, nose, and paranasal sinuses. *Aspergillus* spp. cause disease in humans by tissue invasion, colonization, and subsequent allergic reaction (ie, allergic bronchopulmonary aspergillosis or ABPA); and colonization of preexisting cavities (fungus ball or aspergilloma).
- The main risk factors that promote invasive aspergillosis are: (1) prolonged and profound neutropenia (< 500/μL) especially in bone marrow transplant recipients; (2) high dose corticosteroid therapy; (3) broad-spectrum antibiotic therapy; (4) chronic granulomatous disease; (5) acquired immune deficiency syndrome (AIDS) with CD4 counts <50 cells/mm^3; and (6) treatment with immunosuppressive agents.

CLINICAL FEATURES

- Invasive aspergillosis with pulmonary involvement may present as acute bronchopneumonia with cavitation on imaging, or slowly progressive bronchopneumonia.
- Invasive aspergillosis may also present with extrapulmonary involvement of the central nervous system, heart, bone, or skin. Virtually any organ can be infected but the most common sites of infection are the lung and brain.
- Individuals with ABPA may present with symptoms of asthma, peripheral blood eosinophilia, and elevated serum IgE levels.
- Aspergillomas may cause m̲a̲s̲s̲i̲v̲e̲ ̲h̲e̲m̲o̲ptysis or chronic invasive necrotizing asper̲g̲i̲l̲l̲o̲s̲i̲s̲.

DIAGNOSIS

- Due to the ubiquitous na̲t̲u̲r̲e̲ ̲o̲f̲ ̲A̲s̲p̲e̲r̲g̲i̲l̲l̲u̲s̲, ̲e̲s̲t̲a̲b̲lishing a definitive diag̲n̲o̲s̲i̲s̲ ̲o̲f̲ ̲a̲s̲p̲e̲r̲g̲i̲l̲l̲o̲s̲i̲s̲ is difficult. Aspergilli ca̲n̲ ̲b̲e̲ ̲i̲s̲o̲l̲a̲t̲e̲d̲ ̲i̲n̲ ̲5̲% of healthy individuals a̲n̲d̲ ̲i̲n̲ ̲m̲a̲n̲y̲ ̲p̲a̲t̲i̲e̲nts with chronic lung disease a̲n̲d̲ ̲o̲r̲g̲a̲n̲ ̲f̲a̲i̲l̲u̲r̲e̲. On the other hand, in immunocompromised patients with appropriate clinical findings, positive sputum cultures have a high positive predictive value.
- In invasive aspergillosis, positive blood cultures are rare and contamination of blood specimens may occur.
- The diagnosis of invasive aspergillosis is ideally established based on a combination of culture results and histologic proof of tissue invasion.

MANAGEMENT

- Corticosteroid therapy is the mainstay of therapy for ABPA but there is a paucity of data concerning its use.

- In aspergilloma, the goal of therapy is to prevent life-threatening pulmonary hemorrhage either by surgical resection or bronchial artery embolization. Therapy must be individualized and the morbidity must be weighed against the clinical benefit.
- Due to the high mortality from invasive aspergillosis among immunocompromised patients, aggressive evaluation is imperative and empiric therapy is often necessary. Antifungal therapies that are employed include voriconazole (recommended primary therapy), amphotericin B, or caspofungin. The optimal duration of therapy is unknown, but likely depends on the extent and severity of invasive aspergillosis, response to therapy, and the patient's underlying disease or immune status.

MUCORMYCOSIS

EPIDEMIOLOGY AND ETIOLOGY

- *Mucormycosis* is the common name given to several different diseases caused by fungi—most commonly *Rhizopus*, *Rhizomucor*, and *Cunninghamella*—of the order Mucorales, class Zygomycetes. The Mucoraceae are molds with broad, ribbon-shaped, nonseptate hyphae with right-angle branching. They are ubiquitous and grow in decaying organic material.
- Mucormycosis is a rare disease and occurs almost exclusively in patients with underlying disease such as diabetes mellitus (typically uncontrolled and ketosis-prone), hematologic disease especially neutropenia, immunosuppression especially chronic corticosteroid administration, iron overload, intravenous drug use (IVDU), repeated skin trauma, or kwashiorkor.
- Infection with Mucorales occurs via inhalation of spores, deposition of spores in nasal turbinates, or direct inoculation of abraded skin.
- The hallmark of the disease is angio-invasion (with predilection for veins over arteries) resulting in thrombosis and tissue necrosis.

CLINICAL FEATURES

- The clinical manifestations depend on the underlying organ system involved.
- The major forms of mucormycosis are rhinocerebral (common in diabetes), disseminated disease (common in neutropenic, leukemic patients), pulmonary, cutaneous (common in skin trauma), gastrointestinal (common in kwashiorkor), central nervous system (common in IVDU), and miscellaneous (bones, kidney, heart, mediastinum).

DIAGNOSIS

- In general, clues to the diagnosis include signs of vasculitis with tissue necrosis such as necrotic appearing drainage or eschar on the involved tissue. Infected tissues have an unusually low tendency to bleed during surgery.
- Diagnosis is established by biopsy of appropriate tissue with culture and microscopic evaluation. The fungi can be visualized by staining with PAS, GMS, and hematoxylin and eosin (H&E). They are identified near blood vessels and surrounded by neutrophilic infiltrate in tissue samples.

MANAGEMENT

- Mucormycosis is a rapidly progressive disease with an overall mortality rate as high as 50%. Immediate aggressive combination of surgical debridement of necrotic tissue and antifungal treatment as well as treatment of the underlying disease is warranted.
- Amphotericin B is the antifungal agent of choice.

BLASTOMYCOSIS

EPIDEMIOLOGIC AND ETIOLOGY

- Blastomycosis is a systemic infection caused by inhalation of spores of *Blastomyces dermatitidis*. From the lung, the organisms disseminate to other organs.
- *Blastomyces dermatitidis* is a dimorphic fungus. The yeast form is large (8–15 µm in diameter), thick-walled, spherical, multinucleated, and usually produces single broad-based buds.
- The natural habitat of the organism has not been resolved.
- Areas endemic for blastomycosis in the United States include Illinois, Wisconsin, Minnesota, Ohio, the Atlantic coastal states and the Southeastern states, with the exception of Florida.

CLINICAL FEATURES

- Blastomycosis usually presents with pulmonary involvement, and may progress to disseminated disease. The most common findings on pulmonary imaging studies include focal pneumonia, nodules, and areas of cavitation.
- The most common extrapulmonary sites involved are the skin, bones, CNS, genitourinary tract, and spleen.
- Chronic cutaneous blastomycosis usually present as one or more subcutaneous nodules that eventually ulcerate on the face, hands, wrist, or lower leg.

DIAGNOSIS

- Infection is best diagnosed by direct examination or positive culture of sputa, skin lesions, or other specimens. Fungi may be visualized by staining with calcofluor, GMS, and PAS. Fungal cultures should be incubated for at least 4 weeks.
- Identification in culture is confirmed by detection of exoantigen A, by demonstration of conversion of mold to yeast, or by hybridization with a specific DNA probe.

MANAGEMENT

- Acute pulmonary blastomycosis in immunocompetent individuals may undergo spontaneous resolution and not require therapy. However, these patients need to be observed for at least 2 years for the possibility of reactivation, disease progression, or dissemination.
- All patients who are immunocompromised, have progressive pulmonary disease, or have extrapulmonary disease should be treated. Treatment options include amphotericin B, itraconazole (preferred azole), or fluconazole (has better CNS penetration than itraconazole).

COCCIDIOIDOMYCOSIS

EPIDEMIOLOGY AND ETIOLOGY

- Coccidioidomycosis is a systemic infection caused by inhalation of spores of *Coccidioides immitis* or *Coccidioides posadasii*.
- The *Coccidioides* are dimorphic fungi confined to the Southwestern United States (California, Arizona, New Mexico, Nevada, Utah, and Texas), contiguous regions of Northern Mexico, and specific areas of Central and South America.
- In nature and in the laboratory, the fungi appear as molds with septate branching hyphae; in tissue they appear as spherules which are spherical thick-walled structures with hundreds of endospores.
- The majority of infections are benign and self-limited. One percent of cases will develop progressive pulmonary disease, dissemination or both. Risk factors for disseminated disease include: extremes of age, male gender, certain ethnic groups (Filipino > African American > Native American > Hispanic > Asian), late pregnancy and postpartum, and depressed cell-mediated immunity (patients with malignancy, patients receiving chemotherapy or steroids, or patients with HIV).
- The organism can be isolated from soil, and individuals who are exposed to the soil in endemic areas (eg, construction workers) are at risk for infection.

CLINICAL FEATURES

- Primary coccidioidomycosis following inhalation is asymptomatic and infection usually resolves without complications; but others may develop flu-like symptoms. Radiographic imaging may show nodules, cavities, or calcifications. Endogenous reactivation of residual pulmonary lesions is rare in immunocompetent individuals.
- Up to 20% of patients with primary pulmonary coccidiomycosis may have associated erythema nodosum or erythema multiforme. These lesions are very painful, persist for 1 week, and are associated with strong immunity and a good long-term prognosis.
- Secondary or disseminated coccidioidomycosis usually develops within a few months as a complication of primary infection. It may present as a chronic and progressive pulmonary disease, with extrapulmonary involvement (mostly meninges, skin, or bone), or as a generalized systemic infection.

DIAGNOSIS

- Definitive diagnosis is established by finding spherules of *Coccidioides* in sputum, draining sinuses, or tissue specimens. The spherules can be visualized by staining with calcofluor, PAS, GMS, and H&E.
- Cultures must be done under a biosafety hood. Colonies develop within 1 to 2 weeks and culture identification is confirmed by production of spherules *in vitro* or by production of exoantigen F. Positive blood cultures are infrequent and are associated with dissemination and high mortality.
- The complement fixation (CF) test measures IgG antibodies to the coccidioidin antigen and correlates with disease activity. The CF titer declines with recovery and eventually disappears; rises with active, uncontrolled infection (poor prognosis); or remains stable or fluctuates with a recalcitrant or stabilized lesion.

MANAGEMENT

- Patients with localized acute pulmonary infections and no risk factors for dissemination often require only periodic reassessment to demonstrate resolution of their self-limited process.
- Patients with extensive infection or who are at high risk for complications because of immunosuppression or other preexisting factors have several treatment options that may include antifungal drug therapy, surgical debridement, or a combination of both.
- Fluconazole and itraconazole are the initial therapy of choice for most chronic pulmonary or disseminated

infections. Amphotericin B is administered to patients with respiratory failure or rapidly progressive coccidioidal infections, or women during pregnancy. Duration of antifungal therapy often ranges from many months to years, and some patients may require lifelong suppressive therapy to prevent relapses.

HISTOPLASMOSIS

EPIDEMIOLOGY AND ETIOLOGY

- Histoplasmosis is caused by the thermally dimorphic fungus *Histoplasma capsulatum*. It occurs worldwide and infection is initiated by inhalation of the organism. Ninety-five percent of infections are inapparent and are detected only by residual lung calcification.
- *Histoplasma capsulatum* lives in soil with high nitrogen content and is associated with bat and avian habitats (eg, chicken houses or bat caves). In the United States, histoplasmosis is endemic in the Ohio and Mississippi Valleys (Missouri, Kentucky, Tennessee, Indiana, Ohio, and southern Illinois).

CLINICAL FEATURES

- Initial pulmonary episodes may be acute or chronic and dissemination may occur by hematogenous or lymphatic spread from lungs to other organs (most commonly to the spleen, liver, lymph nodes, and bone marrow).
- Ninety-five percent of all persons with acute primary histoplasmosis with or without dissemination are asymptomatic and most individuals are able to contain the infection. Granulomatous responses from previous lesions may undergo fibrosis and leave residual scars or calcification in the lungs, liver, or spleen. Resolution confers some immunity to reinfection.
- Chronic pulmonary histoplasmosis may develop immediately after primary inhalation or after years of apparent quiescence usually in males with underlying chronic obstructive pulmonary disease with emphysema. Lesions are usually apical in location and may result in cavitation.
- Disseminated histoplasmosis may also be acute and fulminant and rapidly fatal in patients with compromised cell-mediated immunity (patients with AIDS, on immunosuppressive drugs, or with lymphomatous neoplasia). In most cases, this condition is a reactivation of a quiescent lesion acquired years earlier.
- Other forms of involvement include ocular histoplasmosis, granulomatous or fibrosing mediastinitis, and pericarditis.

DIAGNOSIS

- Diagnosis is established by identifying the yeast cells inside macrophages in sputa, tissue from biopsy or surgery, CSF, blood, or bone marrow. Lysis centrifugation is the most sensitive and rapid method to recover *Histoplasma* from blood. The fungi can be visualized with the Wright or Giemsa stain.
- The fungi characteristically grow slowly in culture and sometimes require an incubation period of 8 to 12 weeks. In culture, the diagnosis is confirmed by conversion of the mold to yeast form, by detection of specific exoantigens, or by specific DNA probe.
- Antibodies to histoplasmin (mycelial) and yeast antigen are measured by complement fixation while precipitins of serum and histoplasmin are detected by immunodiffusion.
- Radioimmunoassay test for polysaccharide antigen is positive in serum (79%) and urine (97%) in disseminated histoplasmosis. This test has prognostic value in that titers decrease with successful treatment and increase with relapse. However, the test lacks optimal specificity and the urine antigen is positive in patients with other systemic mycoses.

MANAGEMENT

- Most primary pulmonary infections go undetected and require no treatment. Symptoms in immunocompetent persons however may be alleviated with itraconazole.
- Treatment is required in patients with chronic pulmonary or disseminated infection and immunocompromised hosts. Treatment options include amphotericin B and itraconazole.

CRYPTOCOCCOSIS

- Cryptococcosis is a systemic infection caused by the encapsulated yeast-like fungus *Cryptococcus neoformans*.
- Cryptococcosis is discussed in Chap. 95 (HIV and AIDS).

BIBLIOGRAPHY

Chapman SW, Bradsher RW Jr, Campbell GD Jr, et al. Practice guidelines for the management of patients with blastomycosis. Infectious Diseases Society of America. *Clin Infect Dis.* 2000;30(4):679–683.

Galgiani JN, Ampel NM, Blair JE, et al. Infectious diseases society of america. Coccidioidomycosis. *Clin Infect Dis.* 2005;41(9):1217–1223.

Mandell GL, Bennett JE, Dolin R, eds. *Mandell, Douglas, and Bennett's Principles and Practice of Infectious Diseases*, 6th ed. Philadelphia: Elsevier; 2005.

Pappas PG, Rex JH, Sobel JD, et al. Infectious Diseases Society of America Guidelines for treatment of candidiasis. *Clin Infect Dis.* 2004;38(2):161–189.

Stevens DA, Kan VL, Judson MA, et al. Practice guidelines for diseases caused by aspergillus. Infectious Diseases Society of America. *Clin Infect Dis.* 2000;30(4):696–709.

Wheat J, Sarosi G, McKinsey D, et al. Practice guidelines for the management of patients with histoplasmosis. Infectious Diseases Society of America. *Clin Infect Dis.* 2000; 30(4):688–695.

98 NOCARDIA

*Mary Abigail C. Dacuycuy
and Donald J. Kennedy*

EPIDEMIOLGY AND ETIOLOGY

- *Nocardia* are aerobic, gram-positive, branching, beaded, filamentous rods that are found in soil, plants and decomposing organic material; they are also present in the gastrointestinal tract, oropharynx, and skin of animals.
- *Nocardia asteroides* accounts for the vast majority of clinical nocardial infections in humans. Cell-mediated immunosuppression (patients with systemic lupus erythematosus, transplant recipients, HIV-positive patients) is a major predisposing factor for infection.

CLINICAL MANIFESTATIONS

- Clinical manifestations may vary from localized to disseminated disease.
- Pulmonary nocardiosis may present with nodules, cavitations, consolidation, or pleural thickening on imaging.
- Neurologic involvement may manifest as abscesses, or granulomas.
- Primary cutaneous infection commonly occurs in immunocompetent patients and results from traumatic inoculation. Lesions are characteristically painless, slowly progressive, and localized.
- Disseminated infection may spread to the bones, heart, kidneys, and retina.

DIAGNOSIS

- Diagnosis of invasive nocardial infection usually requires demonstration of the organism in affected specimens. Sputum, bronchial wash, exudates, tissue biopsy, or cerebrospinal fluid (CSF) should be collected for culture and staining (both Gram stain and modified acid-fast bacilli smear) in suspected cases.

MANAGEMENT

- Management is based on the host factors, the site of the disease, and in vitro activity of antibiotics.
- The majority of infections can be treated effectively with antibiotic therapy.
- The most active parenteral agents for *N. asteroides* are trimethoprim-sulfamethoxazole (TMP-SMX), amikacin, imipenem, ceftriaxone, and cefotaxime. The most active oral agents include TMP-SMX, minocycline, and amoxicillin.
- Less seriously ill patients may be treated with oral antibiotics whereas seriously ill patients are treated with combination regimens parenterally, for an extended duration.
- Nocardial brain abscess and other extrapulmonary lesions may require surgical debridement or drainage in addition to antibiotic therapy.

BIBLIOGRAPHY

Forbes BA, Sahm DF, Weissfeld AS, eds. *Bailey and Scott's Diagnostic Microbiology*, 11th ed. St. Louis: Mosby; 2002.

Mandell GL, Bennett JE, Dolin R, eds. *Mandell, Douglas, and Bennett's Principles and Practice of Infectious Diseases*. 6th ed. Philadelphia: Elsevier; 2005.

99 RICKETTSIOSES AND EHRLICHIOSIS

*Mary Abigail C. Dacuycuy
and Donald J. Kennedy*

INTRODUCTION

- Rickettsioses and ehrlichiosis are infections that are caused by fastidious obligate intracellular gram-negative bacteria that belong to the order Rickettsiales. Patients generally complain of fever, headache, with or without rash. Common laboratory abnormalities include neutropenia, thrombocytopenia, and a mild increase in serum hepatic transaminases. Culture of the pathogens is extremely difficult and diagnosis is usually established by serology or polymerase chain reaction (PCR). Doxycycline is generally the treatment of choice.

ROCKY MOUNTAIN SPOTTED FEVER (RMSF)

EPIDEMIOLOGY AND ETIOLOGY

- RMSF is caused by *Rickettsia rickettsii*. The dog tick (*Dermacentor*) and the wood tick (*Amblyomma*) are the vectors and main reservoirs of the disease.
- Endemic areas include east of the Rocky Mountains, most commonly Oklahoma, the Carolinas, Virginia, Maryland, Montana, and Wyoming. Infections are seasonal occurring primarily from May to September.
- After skin inoculation of the *R. rickettsii*, the organism spreads via lymphatics and small blood vessels into the systemic and pulmonary circulation and proliferates in the vascular endothelial cell. There is subsequent cell-to-cell spread and endothelial cell injury.

CLINICAL FEATURES

- The incubation period ranges from 2 to 14 days with a median of 7 days.
- RMSF usually begins with fever, myalgia, headache, and gastrointestinal complaints.
- Petechial rash usually appears 3 to 5 days after the onset of fever in 84% to 91% of cases and typically begins around the wrists and ankles. Involvement of the palms and soles is characteristic (36% to 82%) but appears late in the course.
- Neurologic involvement may present as meningitis or meningoencephalitis and is associated with a worse prognosis. Patients may develop renal failure and noncardiogenic pulmonary edema that may progress to acute respiratory distress syndrome (ARDS). In severe untreated RMSF, death may occur within the first 5 days.
- Laboratory abnormalities can also include hyponatremia (SIADH) and increased lactate dehydrogenase (LDH) or creatine kinase (CK) from diffuse tissue injury.
- Patients who survive RMSF usually have solid immunity to *R. rickettsii*.

DIAGNOSIS

- *Rickettsia rickettsii* may be isolated from the blood by centrifugation-enhanced cell culture systems and can be demonstrated in cutaneous biopsy specimens by immunohistochemistry.
- Serum antibodies become detectable during convalescence. A diagnostic titer of 1:64 by indirect immunofluorescence assay (IFA) is the most sensitive and specific test.

MANAGEMENT

- Since there is the potential for rapidly lethal illness and difficulty in establishing the diagnosis, presumptive therapy with doxycycline must be started immediately in the appropriate clinical setting. Doxycycline is usually given for 7 days and is continued for 2 days after the patients fever defervesces.

HUMAN MONOCYTOTROPIC ERLICHIOSIS (HME)

EPIDEMIOLOGY AND ETIOLOGY

- HME is caused by *Ehrlichia chaffeensis* and the major target cells are the macrophages or monocytes.
- Peak incidence of the disease occurs in May to July and is seen mostly in areas from New Jersey to Illinois and Texas.
- The tick vectors include *Amblyomma americanum* (southcentral and southeastern states), and *Dermacentor variabilis* and *Ixodes pacificus* (western states).

CLINICAL FEATURES

- Median incubation period is 7 days.
- Immunocompetent patients may present with mild to severe multisystemic illness with a median duration of 23 days whereas in immunocompromised patients the disease can be fatal.
- Patients often complain of fever, flu-like illness, headache, nausea, vomiting, and abdominal pain. A maculopapular rash may be present in 30% of cases.
- Severe complications of the disease include ARDS, acute renal failure, meningoencephalitis, coagulopathy, gastrointestinal hemorrhage, and death.
- Important laboratory features include thrombocytopenia, leukopenia, and elevated serum hepatic transaminases.
- Morulae (clusters of multiplying organisms in host cell vacuoles that form large aggregates that are mulberry shaped) are seen in the cytoplasm of infected cells after 5 to 7 days in a small number of cases.

DIAGNOSIS

- The major diagnostic criterion is serologic via IFA with *E. chaffeensis*-infected cells. There should be a fourfold rise in antibody titer during the disease with a minimal peak titer of 1:64.

- Polymerase chain reaction (PCR) of blood is the most sensitive test for timely diagnosis but may not be readily available.

MANAGEMENT

- Doxycycline is the standard treatment and is administered empirically if HME is suspected.

HUMAN GRANULOCYTOTROPIC ANAPLASMOSIS (HGA)

EPIDEMIOLOGY AND ETIOLOGY

- HGA is caused by *Anaplasma phagocytophila* and the principal target cells are the granulocytes.
- The major tick vector is the *Ixodes scapularis* in the Eastern United States. Other endemic areas include mid-Atlantic and upper Midwestern United States.
- There is a bimodal distribution of occurrence with a peak in July and November corresponding to the adult and nymphal stages.

CLINICAL FEATURES

- Incubation period ranges from 1 to 2 weeks.
- Clinical presentation is similar to that of HME but rash is seen in only 10% of cases.
- Morulae are observed in 20% to 80% of the cases.
- The presence of neutropenia may distinguish HGA from HME.

DIAGNOSIS

- Diagnosis is confirmed by serology with a fourfold increase in antibody titer by IFA; PCR of blood; presence of morulae; and culture.

MANAGEMENT

- Doxycycline is the mainstay of empirical treatment.

BIBLIOGRAPHY

Forbes BA, Sahm DF, Weissfeld AS, eds. *Bailey and Scott's Diagnostic Microbiology*, 11th ed. St. Louis: Mosby; 2002.

Mandell GL, Bennett JE, Dolin R, eds. *Mandell, Douglas, and Bennett's Principles and Practice of Infectious Diseases*. 6th ed. Philadelphia: Elsevier; 2005.

100 PROTOZOAN AND HELMINTHIC INFECTIONS

Musab U. Saeed and Donald J. Kennedy

- A diversity of protozoa and helminths may cause infections in humans and are responsible for considerable morbidity, especially in children and immunocompromised patients.

HELMINTH INFECTIONS

- Parasitic helminths include nematodes (roundworms), platyhelminths (flatworms), cestodes (tapeworms), and trematodes. The helminthiases are among the most common infections in the world with a variable geographic distribution.
- The life cycles of these organisms vary in their complexity, number of hosts required to complete the life cycle, and clinical manifestations; however the basic stages consists of an egg form, one or more larval stages, and the adult worm. Transmission may occur by ingestion of the egg or larvae, penetration of intact skin by larvae, or via a biological vector.
- The diagnosis requires knowledge of the typical clinical presentation and geographic distribution of the organism. While obtaining a history, the clinician should obtain a detailed travel and diet history, exposure to animals, and access to appropriate hygiene. Microscopic examination of stool, urine, blood, and tissue may reveal eggs, larvae or the adult organism.
- Most helminthic infections can be treated successfully with medications and have an excellent prognosis. Table 100–1 summarizes the clinical features of several important helminthic infections.

PROTOZOAL DISEASES

- Protozoa are generally unicellular organisms with a diverse epidemiology, and are responsible for many infections with a variety of clinical presentations.
- Protozoans have been classified as Mastigophora (flagella), Sarcodina (pseudopodia), Apicomplexa (sporozoa), and Ciliophora (ciliates).
- The diagnosis and therapy can be challenging unless the physician is experienced with these infectious diseases. Table 100–2 summarizes the clinical features of several important protozoan pathogens in humans.

TABLE 100–1 Common Infections Caused By Helminthics

ORGANISM/DISEASE	MODE OF TRANSMISSION/ CLINICAL FEATURES	DIAGNOSIS	TREATMENT
Ascaris lumbricoides (roundworm)/Ascariasis	Ingestion of eggs/ Abdominal pain, intestinal obstruction	Eggs in stool	Mebendazole, albendazole
Trichuris trichiura/Trichuriasis	Ingestion of eggs/Mostly asymptomatic	Adult worm or eggs in stool	Mebendazole, albendazole
Necator americanus (hookworm)	Penetration of skin by larva/ Iron deficiency anemia, abdominal pain	Eggs or larvae in stool	Mebendazole, albendazole
Strongyloides stercoralis/ Strongyloidosis	Penetration of skin by larva/ skin pruritus, cough erythema, abdominal pain	Larvae in stool	Mebendazole, albendazole
Enterobius vermicularis (pin worm)	Ingestion of eggs/Perianal pruritus	Eggs from perianal skin on cellulose acetate tape	Mebendazole, albendazole pyrantel pamoate
Wuchereria bancrofti, *Brugia Malayi* (Filariasis)	Mosquito bite/Lymphatic inflammation, lymphedema, epididymitis	Microfilaria in blood, body fluid. ELISA	Diethylcarbamazine, albendazole
Taenia solium (pork tapeworm)	Ingestion of eggs/Epigastric pain, weight loss, diarrhea, seizures with CNS involvement (Neurocysticercosis)	Eggs or proglottids in stool; CT or MRI brain	Praziquantel, niclosamide
Tenia Saginata (beef tapeworm)	Ingestion of eggs/Usually asymptomatic, abdominal pain	Proglottids or eggs in stool	Praziquantel
Diphyllobothrium latum (fish tapeworm)	Ingestion of cyst in raw fish/Vitamin B12 deficiency		Niclosamide. praziquantel
Schistosoma haematobium/ Schistosomiasis	Penetration of skin by larva/Dermatitis, dysuria, frequency, hematuria, (Squamous cell cancer of bladder)	FAST-ELISA, EITB	Praziquantel
Paragonimus westermani/ Paragonimiasis	Ingestion of crustaceans/ abdominal pain, diarrhea, chest pain cough	Eggs in sputum, feces or biopsy	Praziquantel

CNS, Central nervous system; CT, computed tomography; EITB, enzyme-linked immunoelectrotransfer blot; FAST-ELISA, fast enzyme-linked immunoabsorbent assay; MRI, magnetic resonance imaging.

TABLE 100–2 Common Protozoan Infections

DISEASE/ ORGANISM	MODE OF TRANSMISSION/ CLINICAL FEATURES	DIAGNOSIS	TREATMENT
Malaria/ *Plasmodium* spp. (*falciparum, vivax, ovale, malaria*)	Transmitted by *Anopheles* mosquitoes bite/Paroxysms of fever, chills, rigors, fatigue, muscle aches, jaundice, alt. mental status, hepatosplenomegaly	Thick and thin blood films shows trophozoite or gametophyte	Quinine, chloroquine, mefloquine, amodiaquine, primaquine
Babesiosis/ *Babesia microti*	Transmitted by ticks/ Irregular fever, chills, fatigue, muscle pain, hepatosplenomegaly	Thick and thin blood film (Giemsa-stained)	Quinine, atovaquone, clindamycin
Leishmaniasis/ *Leishmania donovani*	Transmitted by sandflies/Has a prolonged incubation period followed by cachexia, fever, maculopapular skin lesions, lymphadenopathy and splenomegaly	Demonstrate the parasite on stained slide or culture	Amphotericin B, paromomycin, pentamidine
Trypanosomiasis./ *Trypanosoma cruzi*, *Trypanosoma gambiense*	Transmitted by Tsetse fly/ lymphadenopathy, periocular edema hepatosplenomegaly, myocarditis, and megacolon	Demonstration of parasite in blood or tissue. PCR	Nifurtimox, benznidazole
Amebiasis/ *Entamoeba histolytica*	Transmitted by fecal-oral route/ Intestinal disease (dysentery, colitis) extraintestinal disease (liver abscess, brain abscess)	Demonstration of cyst or trophozoites in stool); endoscopy	Metronidazole or tinidazole, add paromomycin for extraintestinal disease
Giardia lamblia	Transmitted by fecal-oral route/ Diarrhea, foul-smelling stools, abdominal pain	Demonstration of oval and parasite in stool; Antigen detection	Metronidazole, quinacrine
Toxoplasmosis gondii	Transmitted by ingestion of uncooked meat, cat feces/Lymphadenopathy, fever, malaise, maculopapular rash, hepatosplenomegaly and seizures (encephalitis)	Isolation of organism in blood, or body fluid; PCR	Pyrimethamine + leucovorin + sulfadiazine or clindamycin
Cryptosporidia, Isospora, Cyclospora, and *Microsporidia*	Ingestion of eggs /Chronic diarrhea in immunocompromised patients	Isolation of cyst or organism in stool	(*Cryptosporidia*) (antiretroviral therapy, ART). (*Isospora* & *Cyclospora*) TMP-SMX. (*Microsporidia*) Albendazole

BIBLIOGRAPHY

Kasper DL, Braunwald E, Fauci AS, et al. *Harrison's Principles of Internal Medicine.* 16th ed. New York: McGraw-Hill; 2005.

Mandell GL, Bennett JE, Dolin R, et al. *Principles and Practice of Infectious Diseases.* 6th ed. Philadelphia: Elsevier Churchill Livingstone; 2005.

World Health Organization, Division of Partners for Parasite Control (PPC), available at: http://www.who.int/wormcontrol/en/. 2006.

James Sl: Emerging parasitic infections. *FEMS Immunol Med Microbiol.* 1997;18:313–19.

101 CEREBROVASCULAR DISEASE

Paisith Piriyawat

EPIDEMIOLOGY

- Stroke is the third leading cause of death and the number one cause of long-term disability in the United States.
- A large majority of strokes, 80% to 85%, are ischemic due to a thrombus or embolus.
- Hemorrhagic stroke is either intraparenchymal (10%) or subarachnoid (5%) in location.
- Stroke prevalence is higher in the southern states (stroke belt) such as Georgia, Alabama, Mississippi, and Louisiana.
- Asians, blacks and Hispanic whites develop hemorrhagic stroke more frequently than non-Hispanic whites.

PATHOPHYSIOLOGY

Ischemia rapidly develops after a decrease in blood flow. Neurons in the center of a hypoperfused area lose function which may evolve to irreversible injury within minutes. Neurons on the edge of the affected region are functionally impaired but salvageable. The center region is referred to as the umbra, and the surrounding area the penumbra. The penumbra is the principal target of treatment. Cerebral blood flow of the penumbra is approximately 10 to 20 mL/100 g per minute, while that in the adjacent normal area is 50 to 55 mL/100 g per minute. The earlier blood flow is restored to the penumbra, the better the neurological outcome.

ETIOLOGICAL CLASSIFICATION

ISCHEMIC STROKE

- In situ thrombosis usually secondary to disease of the arterial wall (eg, vascular stenosis/intimal thickening, vasculitis/arteritis, vasospasm, venous thrombosis, hypercoagulable states).
- Embolism (eg, atheromatous ulcer, cardiac arrhythmia, intracardiac disease).
- Systemic hypotension.

HEMORRHAGIC

- Intraparenchymal hemorrhage (eg, hypertensive microaneurysms, amyloid angiopathy)
- Subarachnoid hemorrhage (eg, cerebral aneurysm, arteriovenous malformation)

CLINICAL MANIFESTATIONS

Once critical interruption of the cerebral blood flow occurs, neuronal dysfunction begins almost immediately, producing sudden neurologic deficits. The symptoms and signs vary depending upon the size and vascular territory of the jeopardized area and are summarized below:
- Major artery occlusion
  - Anterior circulation
    - Middle cerebral artery (MCA)
      - Contralateral differential hemiparesis and hemiparesthesia (ascending severity: face < arm < leg)
      - Contralateral homonymous hemianopia
      - Gaze deviation
      - Aphasia if the dominant hemisphere is involved and extinction if nondominant

- Anterior cerebral artery (ACA)
  - Contralateral differential hemiparesis and hemiparesthesia (descending severity: face > arm > leg)
  - Urinary incontinence
- Ophthalmic artery (OA)
  - Ipsilateral blindness
- Internal carotid artery (ICA)
  - All of the symptoms noted above
  - Posterior circulation
    - Posterior inferior cerebellar artery (PICA) (lateral medullary or Wallenberg syndrome)
      - Ipsilateral hemifacial numbness
      - Contralateral hemibody numbness
      - Vertigo and ipsilateral hemiataxia
      - Ipsilateral Horner syndrome
    - Basilar artery (BA)
      - Altered mental status
      - Unilateral or bilateral weakness and numbness
      - Abnormal ocular movement on pupillary examination
      - Ataxia
    - Posterior cerebral artery (PCA)
      - Contralateral hemianopia
- Penetrating artery occlusion
  - Deep-seated infarcts
  - Classic syndromes (depending on infarct location)
    - Pure motor deficit
    - Pure sensory deficit
    - Ataxic hemiparesis
    - Dysarthria-clumsy-hand syndrome
    - Mixed motor-sensory deficit
- Intracerebral hemorrhage
  - Clinical features (altered level of consciousness, contralateral hemiparesis, hemisensory deficit) depend on the size and location of the hematoma.
  - The putamen, thalamus, pons and cerebellum are commonly involved with severe hypertension
  - Lobar hemorrhages are typical in patients older than 65 years of age
  - Increased intracranial pressure results from expanding hematomas and hydrocephalus from obstructed flow of the cerebrospinal fluid.
- Subarachnoid hemorrhage
  - Sudden severe headache, altered consciousness, focal deficits

DIAGNOSIS

The diagnosis of cerebrovascular disease is based principally on clinical and radiographic information. Typical patients with ischemic stroke present with sudden-onset neurological deficits referable to a specific vascular territory. Frequently, multiple vascular risk factors are present.

In patients with hemorrhage, the clinical manifestations depend on hematoma location and concomitant increased intracranial pressure.

Standard neuroimages usually confirm the diagnosis:
- Acute ischemic change (within 24 hours)
  - Computed tomography (CT): usually subtle findings
    - Loss of gray-white differentiation
    - Cortical effacement
    - Loss of basal ganglion signals
    - Occasionally, hyperdensity of the MCA or BA signifying clot or thrombosis
  - Magnetic resonance imaging (MRI)
    - Hyperintensity on diffusion-weighted imaging (DWI) appears within 1 hour
- Subacute ischemic change (24–72 hours)
  - CT: hypodense lesion
  - MRI: hyperintensity on DWI, T2-weighted or fluid attenuated inversion recovery (FLAIR) imaging
- Old infarct (months)
  - Persistent changes on CT, T2-weighted and FLAIR
  - Loss of DWI hyperintensity between 2 and 4 weeks
- Acute intraparenchymal hematoma
  - CT: hyperdense mass
- Subarachnoid hemorrhage
  - CT: hyperdensity in the basal cisterns and/or ventricles

Classically, transient ischemic attacks (TIAs) are sudden, reversible focal neurological deficits that last 24 hours or less. DWI usually reveals small infarcts in the territories in which the symptoms occurred. Thus, some patients with presumed transient ischemia actually exhibit small infarcts.

INVESTIGATION

The initial evaluation is directed at confirming the site of the infarct or hemorrhage. Attention is then directed to the etiology of the stroke and consideration is directed to diseases of the blood, blood vessel or heart or causes of ruptured arteries contributing to intraparenchymal hematomas or subarachnoid hemorrhages.

- Confirmation of diagnosis and evaluation of the cerebral vasculature
  - CT is rapid and identifies bleeding (Fig. 101–1)
  - MRI of the brain is the most sensitive imaging technique
    - DWI identifies an infarct within approximately 1 hour (Fig. 101–2A)
    - Perfusion weighted images (PWI) with DWI defines the penumbra.
  - MRA identifies pertinent stenosis of intracranial arteries or notable disease within cervical arteries (Fig. 101–2B)

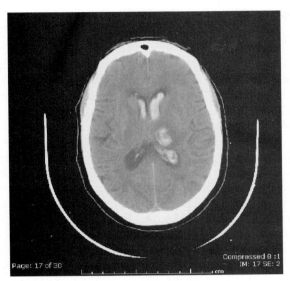

FIG. 101–1 Computed tomography in a patient with stroke symptoms within 2 hours. Note hyperdense (blood) areas in the ventricles.

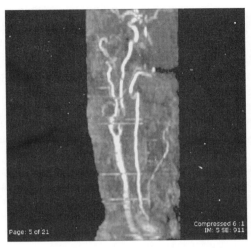

FIG. 101–2B MRA revealing intracranial vascular stenosis in a patient with ischemic stroke.

- Complete blood count (CBC), prothrombin time (PT), partial thromboplastin time (PTT), platelets, glucose, lipid profile, glycosylated hemoglobin A_{1c}.
- Toxic drug screen if drug abuse is suspected.
- 12 Lead electrocardiogram (ECG) to identify coronary artery disease and cardiac arrhythmia, especially atrial fibrillation.
- Carotid ultrasound is useful to identify plaques and critical stenosis.
- Echocardiography is used to identify settings at risk for cardioembolism (eg, intracardiac clot, patent foramen ovale, poor left ventricular systolic function)
- Angiography is useful to confirm the location, extent, and severity of a vascular stenosis (Fig. 101–2C)

TREATMENT

To successfully restore blood flow to the brain, intravenous thrombolytic therapy must be administered within 3 hours of onset. Accordingly, careful pretreatment evaluation with special attention directed to the time of onset is of utmost importance. A variety of clinical conditions preclude the administration of thrombolytic therapy (stroke within the preceding 3 months, major surgery within the preceding 14 days, gastrointestinal bleeding within the preceding 21 days, lumbar puncture within the preceding 7 days, rapidly improving symptoms, minor symptoms, suspected subarachnoid hemorrhage, pericarditis, severe hypertension [>185/110 mm Hg], pregnancy,

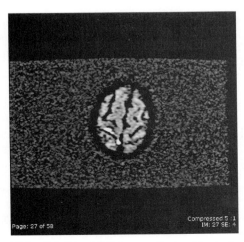

FIG. 101–2A MRI in a patient with stroke symptoms within 1 hour. Note hyperdense lesions in the occipital region.

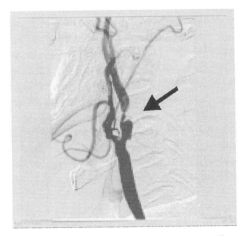

FIG. 101–2C Carotid arteriogram revealing an area of significant stenosis in a patient with ischemic stroke.

thrombocytopenia, elevated international normalized ratio [INR], diffuse swelling or bleeding on CT scan). The risk for intracranial hemorrhage increases 3 hours after the onset. Importantly, the earlier treatment is administered, the better the neurological recovery/outcome. Alteplase is currently the only thrombolytic agent approved for acute occlusive ischemic stroke.

- Concurrent medical management is also required. Patients with blood pressures exceeding 220/120 mm Hg are excluded from thrombolytic therapy until a target blood pressure of <185/110 mm Hg is achieved. Recommended antihypertensives for acute stroke include intravenous labetalol or infusions of nicardipine or nitroprusside. Adequate oxygenation and reasonable blood glucose level are necessary to avoid intracellular lactic acidosis from anaerobic respiration in ischemic neurons.
- Risks of stroke complications should be minimized.
- Swallowing is evaluated by bedside examination or modified barium swallowing to prevent aspiration pneumonia. Deep vein thrombosis is lessened by using subcutaneous heparin or leg compressive devices. Early ambulation reduces atelectasis and avoids pressure sores. Indwelling catheters are used only when necessary to minimize infectious complications.
- Summary of treatment for acute ischemic stroke include:
  - Airway maintenance.
  - Intravenous thrombolytic therapy
    - Onset-to-treatment time: unequivocally <3 hours
    - Thorough review of contraindications
      - Unclear onset
      - Serious head injury
      - Major surgery within 2 weeks
      - Systolic blood pressure >185 mm Hg or diastolic >110 mm Hg
      - Suspected subarachnoid hemorrhage
      - Gastrointestinal or genitourinary hemorrhage within 21 days
      - Seizure at onset
      - Elevated partial thromboplastin or PT
      - Platelet count <100,000/mm3
      - Glucose <50 or >400 mg/dL
  - Alteplase: 0.9 mg/kg (max 90 mg)
    - 10% of the total dose is administered as a bolus over 1 minute
    - The remainder is administered over 60 minutes
  - Oxygen supplementation
  - Adequate nondextrose fluid administration
  - Prevention of complications
    - Close blood glucose monitoring
    - Aspiration precautions
    - Feeding tube placement if necessary
    - Frequent repositioning and early ambulation
  - Rehabilitation: physical, occupational, and speech therapies

PREVENTION

Atherosclerosis plays an important role in both primary and secondary prevention of ischemic stroke. Therefore, the risk factors which promote atherosclerosis (high blood pressure, diabetes, and elevated cholesterol) must be controlled. Angiotensin-converting enzyme inhibitors (ACEI) and the HMG-CoA reductase inhibitors may confer additional protection against recurrent stroke in addition to their effects on blood pressure and cholesterol, respectively. Patients should refrain from smoking and a cessation program, if available, should be offered. Antithrombotic agents, either antiplatelet or anticoagulant, are generally prescribed for secondary stroke prevention. Both are equally effective except for atrial fibrillation where anticoagulant therapy to maintain an INR between 2.0 and 3.0 is preferred. Neither is recommended for primary prevention. Corrective procedures for internal carotid stenosis are indicated in symptomatic patients with areas of stenosis that exceed 70%. Preventive strategies are summarized below:

- Control or modification of atherosclerotic risk factors is strongly recommended for both primary and secondary prevention.
- ACEI and statins are associated with vascular protection besides their principal pharmacological properties.
- Available antiplatelet agents include: aspirin 81 to 325 mg/day, clopidogrel, and a combination of aspirin and extended-release dipyridamole. Ticlopidine is less frequently used because of the infrequent complication of thrombotic thrombocytopenic purpura.
- Anticoagulant therapy with a target INR of 2.0 to 3.0 is indicated in patients with atrial fibrillation and one of the following: congestive heart failure, hypertension, age >75 years, diabetes, and previous stroke or TIA.
- No antithrombotic drug is currently recommended for primary prevention.
- Carotid endarterectomy is generally recommended for patients with >70% symptomatic stenosis. The endovascular approach is reasonable for patients with unacceptable perioperative risk.

BIBLIOGRAPHY

Adams H, Adams R, Del Zoppo G, Goldstein LB. Guidelines for the early management of patients with ischemic stroke: 2005 guidelines update a scientific statement from the Stroke Council of the American Heart Association/American Stroke Association. *Stroke.* 2005;36:916–921.

Brott T, Broderick J, Kothari R, et al. Early hemorrhage growth in patients with intracerebral hemorrhage. *Stroke.* 1997; 28:1–5.

Executive Committee for the Asymptomatic Carotid Atherosclerosis Study. Endarterectomy for asymptomatic carotid artery stenosis. *JAMA*. 1995;273:1421–1428.

Goldstein LB, Adams R, Alberts MJ, et al. Primary Prevention of Ischemic Stroke A Guideline From the American Heart Association/American Stroke Association Stroke Council: Cosponsored by the Atherosclerotic Peripheral Vascular Disease Interdisciplinary Working Group; Cardiovascular Nursing Council; Clinical Cardiology Council; Nutrition, Physical Activity, and Metabolism Council; and the Quality of Care and Outcomes Research Interdisciplinary Working Group: the American Academy of Neurology affirms the value of this guideline. *Stroke*. 2006;37:1583–1633.

North American Symptomatic Carotid Endarterectomy Trial Collaborators. Beneficial effect of carotid endarterectomy in symptomatic patients with high-grade carotid stenosis. *N Engl J Med*, 1991;325:445–453.

The National Institute of Neurological Disorders and Stroke rt-PA Stroke Study Group. Tissue plasminogen activator for acute ischemic stroke. *N Engl J Med*. 1995;333:1581–1587.

Sacco RL, Adams R, Albers G, et al. Guidelines for prevention of stroke in patients with ischemic stroke or transient ischemic attack: A statement for healthcare professionals from the American Heart Association/American Stroke Association Council on Stroke: Co-sponsored by the Council on Cardiovascular Radiology and Intervention: The American Academy of Neurology affirms the value of this guideline. *Stroke*. 2006;37:577–617.

102 MOVEMENT DISORDERS

Francis A. Mithen

ACTION TREMOR

- Action tremors comprise the largest group of movement disorders and are characterized by rhythmic and oscillatory movement of a body part with a relatively constant frequency and variable amplitude. The tremor is increased during activity and, accordingly, may be disabling. Essential tremor or enhanced physiologic tremor are the most common action tremors. The etiology remains incompletely understood but an autosomal dominant pattern of inheritance has been described in up to 50% of patients with essential tremor. Action tremors progress slowly, usually affect the limbs, but less often effect the voice or head. Action tremors are suppressed briefly with ethanol and are sometimes associated with a hearing disorder. Unlike Parkinsonian tremor, action tremors are not present at rest.

MEDICATIONS

- *Primidone*: Effective for limb tremor but not for voice or head tremor.
- *β-Blockers*: Benefit similar to primidone but limited by orthostasis and dyspnea.
- *Benzodiazepines*: Effective for voice, head, and limb tremor but limited by sedation. Modafinil can counteract the drowsiness.
- *Topiramate*: Effective for voice, head, and limb tremor but associated with renal stones, paresthesias, weight loss, and cognitive side effects.

OTHER TREATMENTS

- Botulinum toxin or deep brain stimulation is effective in select patients.

ATAXIA

- Ataxia or clumsiness may be caused by sensory, motor, basal ganglia, or cerebellar dysfunction. Cerebellar ataxia occurs with various medications; cerebrovascular disease; acute or chronic use of ethanol; vitamin deficiencies (thiamine, B_{12}, and E); hypothyroidism; autoimmune disorders; posterior fossa masses; occult nonneurological malignancy; multiple sclerosis (MS); neurodegenerative diseases; neurological malformations; or genetic disorders.[1]

MANAGEMENT

- Assessment should generally include brain computed tomography (CT) or magnetic resonance imaging (MRI); cardiovascular risk factor assessment; serum methylmalonic acid as well as vitamin E and B_{12} levels; evoked potential studies; thyroid studies; evaluation for an occult malignancy; and, occasionally, genetic testing.
- Physical and occupational therapy as well as various prosthetic devices stabilize or improve function. Specific causes of ataxia require appropriate treatment such as risk factor reduction and antiplatelet agents for cerebrovascular disease, surgery for posterior fossa tumors, or thyroid replacement for hypothyroidism. Patients with certain hereditary ataxias (eg, Refsum disease) may benefit from dietary modification. Carbonic anhydrase inhibitors and increased intake of fat-soluble vitamins are also helpful in select patients.

DYSKINESIAS

- Dyskinesias are abnormal involuntary movements caused by basal ganglia dysfunction. Dyskinesias are classified as follows:
  - *Athetosis*: slow, writhing movements
  - *Ballism*: flailing, proximal limb movements
  - *Chorea*: rapid, random, jerky movements involving a succession of different body parts[2,3]
  - Choreoathetotic movements are intermediate in speed between chorea and athetosis.[2,3]
- Dyskinesias have been described in a variety of conditions:
  - Structural lesions involving the brain: stroke, tumor
  - Metabolic disturbances: hyperthyroidism
  - Hereditary diseases: Huntington disease (HD)
  - Autoimmune disorders: systemic lupus erythematosus
  - Multiple sclerosis
  - Following streptococcal infection: Sydenham's chorea
  - During pregnancy
  - During or following the use of various medications including anticonvulsants, sympathomimetic agents, lithium, dopamine agonists, and dopamine antagonists.[3–6]

Rarely, dyskinesias are paroxysmal and, therefore, may be confused with seizure disorders. Paroxysmal dyskinesias are often familial but may be secondary to other clinical disorders (multiple sclerosis and hypoparathyroidism).[7] Paroxysms are triggered by sudden movement (paroxysmal kinesigenic dyskinesias [PKDs]); ethanol, caffeine, or stress (paroxysmal nonkinesigenic dyskinesias [PNKDs]); or exercise (paroxysmal exertional dyskinesias [PEDs]).[7] Paroxysms include both dyskinetic and dystonic movements.[7]

MANAGEMENT

- Because dyskinesias are symptoms of other conditions, the cause(s) should be sought and managed appropriately. Moreover, some dyskinesias are self-limited (eg, chorea gravidarum), or insufficiently bothersome to warrant suppression.

MEDICATIONS

NONPAROXYSMAL DYSKINESIAS

- *Dopamine antagonists*: effective but limited by Parkinsonism, tardive dyskinesias, acute and tardive dystonias, and tardive tics.
- *Dopamine depleting agents*: reserpine and tetrabenazine (not Food and Drug Administration approved) are effective, but limited by Parkinsonism, depression, and orthostasis.

- *Other agents*: benzodiazepines, ondansetron, or anticonvulsants (eg, valproic acid, carbamazepine) may be helpful.

PAROXYSMAL DYSKINESIAS

- Sometimes PKDs respond to various anticonvulsants, PNKDs and PEDs improve with benzodiazepines, carbonic anhydrase inhibitors, or anticholinergic agents.[7]

DYSTONIAS

- Dystonias are characterized by episodic, involuntary, repetitive contraction of one or more muscles.[2,8] Except for blepharospasm and spasmodic dysphonia, dystonic spasms produce an abnormal, often *twisting* posture of the affected body area that last seconds to days.[2,8] The longer the abnormal posture exists, the more likely fixed contractures develop.
- Dystonia is classified according to the anatomic distribution of the spasms, age of onset, or underlying etiology.[8] Focal dystonias affect isolated body areas:
  - Blepharospasm: blinking or eyelid closure
  - Spasmodic dysphonia: contraction of laryngeal muscles
  - Oromandibular dystonia: protracted mouth opening or closure with or without contraction of lower face and tongue muscles
  - Spasmodic torticollis: head turning or tilting as well as neck flexion or extension
  - Limb dystonia: writer's cramp[8]
- Segmental dystonias affect two or more adjacent body regions; for example, Meige syndrome comprises blepharospasm and oromandibular dystonia.[8] Multifocal dystonias affect nonadjacent body areas, such as hemidystonia involving the limbs on one side.[8] Generalized dystonias affect several body regions including dystonia musculorum deformans.[8] The probability of dystonias becoming generalized over time is inversely related to the age of onset.[8]
- Although several gene abnormalities are associated with dystonias, there are many other causes to consider including the use of medications such as anticonvulsants, dopamine antagonists, and dopaminergic agents; structural brain lesions; brain infection; MS; cervical myelopathy; exposure to manganese or carbon monoxide; and other genetic neurogenerative diseases, such as HD and Wilson disease.[8]

MANAGEMENT

- The cause(s) of various dystonias should be sought and managed appropriately. Physical and occupational therapy as well as various prosthetic devices are used to stabilize or improve function and prevent contractures. Some patients effectively utilize *sensory tricks* to control focal dystonias (eg, touching the chin may temporarily lessen torticollis).[8]

MEDICATIONS

- *Anticholinergic agents*: Effective, but high doses are often required.[8] Children usually tolerate effective doses better than adults.
- *Dopamine antagonists*: Effective, but have significant side effects.
- *Dopamine depleting agents*: Effective, but have significant side effects.
- *Botulinum toxin*: Many focal dystonias and selected aspects of generalized dystonias are reduced for weeks to months with botulinum toxin injections.
- *Dopaminergic agents*: Dopamine agonists or levodopa produce marked benefit in patients with familial dopa-responsive dystonia.[8] Accordingly, a trial of low-dose dopamine agonists or levodopa should be considered in patients with dystonias, except perhaps those with isolated blepharospasm or dysphonia.[8]
- *Other agents*: Carbamazepine is useful. High-dose benzodiazepines and baclofen are often effective and surprisingly well-tolerated, but abrupt cessation of these agents produces a dramatic withdrawal syndrome characterized by acute agitation and seizures.
- *Surgery*: Denervation of affected muscles or deep brain stimulation is used in selected patients.[8]

PARKINSONISM

- Parkinsonism is characterized by rest tremor, *lead pipe* rigidity, bradykinesia, and a gait disturbance. Parkinsonism is associated with a variety of clinical syndromes and medications. For example, metoclopramide, amiodarone, and several neuroleptic agents commonly induce Parkinsonism. Parkinson disease (PD) is idiopathic Parkinsonism. PD typically begins after the age of 50 years, however, familial forms tend to begin earlier in life, sometimes before 30 years of age. Although PD progresses more rapidly than does action tremor, it is usually not disabling until 10 to 15 years after onset of symptoms.
- Nonmotor symptoms of PD (constipation, urinary abnormalities, sleep disturbance, panic attacks, depression, dementia) often become more troublesome than the motor symptoms in PD, particularly as the diseaase progresses. Dementia substantially increases the risk of psychiatric side effects associated with anti-Parkinson medications.

- Numerous disorders including Alzheimer disease, cervical myelopathy, strokes, and depression may be characterized by Parkinsonian features; but generally these disorders are not associated with a tremor. Given the absence of tremor, these disorders have been referred to as *Parkinsonism Minus* syndromes.

MANAGEMENT OF PARKINSON DISEASE

- An MRI of the brain and cervical cord should be performed in patients who present without a tremor to exclude other clinical conditions that may mimic PD. Physical and occupational therapy as well as emotional support are extremely important. Hypophonation, dysarthria, and dysphagia benefit from speech therapy. Psychosis is a side effect of most of the anti-PD medications. Importantly, demented patients are more likely to be afflicted than are patients with normal cognition. As is true of any incurable, progressive illness, management of PD becomes more challenging and less satisfactory over time.

MEDICATIONS FOR MOTOR SYMPTOMS

- *Amantadine*: An effective dose is attainable within several days to a few weeks but limited by constipation, urinary retention, memory loss, and psychosis.
- *Anticholinergic agents*: An effective dose is reachable within several days to a few weeks but also limited by constipation, urinary retention, memory loss, and psychosis.
- *Dopamine agonists*: Bromocriptine, pergolide, pramipexole, and ropinirole require slow titration over several weeks to minimize side effects. Although dopamine agonists are less potent than levodopa, side effects are similar (orthostasis, dyskinesias, psychosis, sedation, sleep attacks). Bromocriptine and pergolide are rarely associated with heart valve abnormalities and retroperitoneal fibrosis.
- *Monoamine oxidase type B inhibitors*: Amphetamine-like side effects limit the use of selegiline. Rasagiline possibly has neuroprotective effects.
- *Levodopa*: Levodopa is the most potent anti-PD medication (and, hence, the drug of choice) available and is also believed to be neuroprotective. A significant problem with levodopa is the loss of sustained, intraday benefit as PD progresses. Levodopa is usually given with carbidopa to reduce nausea and is often provided with entacapone to reduce motor fluctuations.
- *Dopaminergic side effects*: Orthostasis is reduced by several measures:

○ Support garments (usually not tolerated because of their inconvenience).

○ Fludrocortisone (promotes congestive heart failure and hypertension).

○ Indomethacin (ineffective when used alone).

○ Midodrine (ineffective when used alone and can worsen benign prostatic hyperplasia).

○ Quetiapine and clozapine are useful for drug-induced psychosis, but clozapine requires close hematological monitoring.

○ Amantadine is effective in reducing drug-induced dyskinesias. However, severe dyskinesias and painful dystonias require a substantial dose reduction of dopaminergic agents or deep brain stimulation.

○ Modafinil is useful for sedation in some patients.

• *Apomorphine*: Subcutaneous formulation is available as *rescue therapy*. Unfortunately, patients with advanced PD, who might benefit the most, are also the patients most likely to develop unacceptable side effects.

• *Surgery*: Deep brain stimulation is helpful in select patients.

RESTLESS LEGS SYNDROME

• Restless legs syndrome (RLS), a fairly common disorder, characterized by one or more of the following: urge to move the lower extremities (LEs), temporary reduction of symptoms with LE exercise, onset or worsening of symptoms during rest, and onset or worsening of symptoms during the evening or night hours.[9] Patients with idiopathic RLS often have affected relatives that exhibit periodic limb movements during sleep.[9] RLS is also associated with advancing age; pregnancy; renal failure; peripheral neuropathy; iron deficiency with or without anemia; and the use of ethanol, caffeine, nicotine, antidopaminergic agents, antihistamines, and various antidepressants.[9]

MANAGEMENT

• Secondary causes should be sought and treated appropriately. Patients with iron deficiency are given supplemental iron. All patients should limit the use of ethanol, caffeine, and nicotine for several hours before bedtime.

MEDICATIONS

• *Dopamine agonists*: Agents of choice for patients with moderate to severe symptoms are less likely than levodopa to produce rebound (return of symptoms during sleep caused by declining drug levels) and

augmentation (temporal escalation of symptoms, increase in severity of symptoms, and possible spread of symptoms to other body regions).[9]

• *Levodopa*: Rebound and augmentation restrict use to patients with intermittent symptoms.

• *Other agents*: Benzodiazepines, opiates, baclofen, carbamazepine, or clonidine are useful.[9]

TICS AND TOURETTE SYNDROME

• Tics are compulsive, usually brief, stereotyped behaviors or vocalizations preceded by an urge to act and followed by transient relief for having done so.[10,11] Motor tics are oftentimes simple movements (eg, blinking), or complex (eg, touching body parts). Vocal tics are also simple, such as sniffing, or complex such as echolalia.[10,11] Motor tics change in anatomic distribution and severity over time. Nearly 10% of individuals have tics temporarily during childhood, but most affected children do not need treatment.[10] Tics occur in various genetic neurodegenerative disorders, eg, HD, or result from the use of stimulant medications, eg, methylphenidate.[10,11]

• Tourette syndrome, considered to be a genetic disorder, has the following features: motor tics, vocal tics, onset before age 18, and tics for at least 1 year.[10,11] Most Tourette syndrome patients also have symptoms of obsessive-compulsive disorder (OCD) or attention deficit disorder (ADD).[10,11]

MANAGEMENT

• Unless another neurological disorder is suspected, extensive diagnostic testing is usually not needed to assess tic disorders. Supportive counseling, psychological care of co-morbid conditions (eg, cognitive therapy for OCD), and environmental modifications are vital adjuncts to medical treatment and obviate the need for medications.

MEDICATIONS

• *α-agonists*: Clonidine, by pill or transdermal patch, suppresses tics and also reduces symptoms of ADD, but is limited by sedation, hypotension, and irritability.[10,11] Guanfacine is longer acting and less sedating than clonidine.[10,11] Either agent may take several weeks to exert maximum benefit.[10,11]

• *Dopamine antagonists*: Effective, but are associated with significant side effects as noted above.

• *Tetrabenazine*: Effective, but are associated with significant side effects as described above.

- *Other agents*: Clonazepam or botulinum toxin are helpful in select patients.[10,11] Selective serotonin reuptake inhibitors, such as citalopram, alleviate coincidental symptoms of OCD.

WILSON DISEASE

- Wilson disease is a rare, potentially treatable, autosomal recessive disorder in which copper accumulates and injures the brain, liver, and other organs.[12] Initial symptoms and signs are usually secondary to hepatic involvement or neuropsychiatric (Parkinsonism, dystonia, ataxia, proximal *wing beating* tremor, psychosis).[12] The following support the diagnosis:
  - Slit-lamp examination reveals Kaiser-Fleischer rings (brownish or gray-green rings that represent granular deposits of copper in Descemet membrane in the cornea)
  - Decreased serum ceruloplasmin (90% have a serum concentration < 20 mg/dL)
  - Increased urinary copper (usually > 100 mcg/day)
  - Abnormal copper accumulation in the liver (considered the gold standard)
  - CT or MRI abnormalities in the basal ganglia and brainstem[12]

MANAGEMENT

- *Diet*: Avoidance of copper-rich foods and beverages is essential.
- *Liver transplantation*: Although potentially curative, transplantation is usually reserved for patients with significant liver dysfunction.[12]

MEDICATIONS

- Penicillamine is effective but limited by skin reactions as well as worsening of neurologic symptoms, bone marrow suppression, myasthenia, and systemic lupus erythematosus.[12]
- Trientine is less effective but better tolerated.[12] Optimal doses for either penicillamine or trientine are established by monitoring urinary copper excretion (>2000mcg/day for 6 months, then 200-500 mcg/day for 1-5 years).
- Zinc acetate promotes copper uptake by intestinal mucosa cells.[12] The cells, and accumulated copper, are eliminated in the feces following the 6-day life span of the these lining cells.[12] Zinc is used following chelation therapy to reduce copper absorption, as the sole agent for pregnant or pediatric patients, or for patients intolerant of chelating agents.[12]

REFERENCES

1. www.wemove.org/ataxia. 2007.
2. Fahn S. Overview of movement disorders. In: Noseworthy JH, ed. *Neurological Therapeutics Principles and Practice.* 2nd ed. Abingdon, UK: Informa Healthcare; 2006:2741–2765.
3. www.wemove.org/choreoathetosis. 2006.
4. www.wemove.org/hd. 2006. (accessed December 29, 2007).
5. www.wemove.org/syd. 2006. (accessed December 29, 2007).
6. www.wemove.org/td. 2006. (accessed December 29, 2007).
7. www.wemove.org/pdys. 2006. (accessed December 29, 2007).
8. www.wemove.org/dys. 2006. (accessed December 29, 2007).
9. www.wemove.org/rls. 2006. (accessed December 29, 2007).
10. www.wemove.org/tics. 2006. (accessed December 29, 2007).
11. www.wemove.org/ts. 2006. (accessed December 29, 2007).
12. www.wemove.org/wil. 2006. (accessed December 29, 2007).

103 NEUROMUSCULAR DISORDERS
Ghazala Hayat

MYASTHENIA GRAVIS

EPIDEMIOLOGY

- The prevalence of myasthenia gravis (MG) is 1 per 10,000.
- There is a bimodal distribution with a female predominance in the younger age group (15–30 years of age) and male predominance in the older age group (60–75 years of age).

ETIOLOGY

- MG is an autoimmune, anti-acetylcholine receptor (AchR) antibody disorder. The auto-antibodies are directed against nicotinic AchRs in the muscle membrane.
- Antibodies block the binding of acetylcholine and decrease AchRs on postsynaptic membranes.
- Recently antibodies against muscle-specific kinase have been identified. These antibodies interfere with regulation and maintenance of AchRs.

PATHOPHYSIOLOGY

- The AchR consists of five subunits; α, β, γ, Δ, and ϵ around a central ion channel. The most common antibodies are directed against the α-subunit.
- AchR antibodies lead to decreased density and number of AchRs. This impairs the ability of the muscle membrane to reach the threshold for contraction and results in clinical weakness.
- The pathogenesis involves activated B and T cells. The thymus gland is abnormal histologically in most patients. Approximately 15% have a lymphoepithelial thymoma, and 70% show follicular hyperplasia.

CLINICAL PRESENTATION

- The hallmark of MG is fluctuating, fatigable weakness, usually affecting the ocular, bulbar, and proximal muscles.
- Approximately 60% of patients present with ocular symptoms, including ptosis and diplopia. Approximately 90% of these patients will eventually develop generalized weakness. Neck drop because of weakness in the neck flexors and extensors and rapidly progressive dysarthria, dysphagia, and dyspnea occurs in some patients.
- Increased ambient temperature, many drugs, and infection alter neuromuscular transmission and exacerbate the symptoms.

DIAGNOSIS

- MG is a clinical diagnosis assisted by laboratory testing. A history of fluctuating and fatigable weakness, especially affecting ocular and bulbar muscles suggest the diagnosis.
- AchR binding, modulating, and blocking antibodies and muscle-specific kinase antibody assays should be performed.
- Antistriated muscle antibodies are found in high titers in patients with a thymoma.
- Approximately 10% of the patients are seronegative.
- Electrodiagnosis shows >10% decrement on repetitive nerve stimulation test at a low frequency (<5 Hz). The decrement increases with postexercise exhaustion. This test is approximately 75% sensitive in generalized MG.
- Single-fiber electromyography is a more sensitive (>90%) but nonspecific test that shows jitter and blocking and manifestations of neuromuscular junction blockade.
- Intravenous edrophonium assists in the diagnosis by inducing transient improvement.
- Computed tomography (CT) imaging of the chest is indicated to detect thymic enlargement and possible tumor.

THERAPEUTIC INTERVENTIONS

- Targeted improvement of neuromuscular transmission
  - Anticholinesterase agents
    - Pyridostigmine, physostigmine
  - Corticosteroids
- Antibody suppression
  - Azathioprine
  - Mycophenolate mofetil
  - Cyclosporin A
  - Intravenous immunoglobulin (IVIG)
- Antibody removal
  - Plasma exchange
- Thymectomy is a safe procedure and contributes to remission in up to 37% of patients.

MYASTHENIC CRISIS

- Presents as rapidly progressive respiratory distress.
  - Obtain pulmonary function studies
- Monitor for cardiac arrhythmias.
- IVIG and plasma exchange reverses weakness in several days to weeks.

PREGNANCY

- Approximately one-third of patients experience exacerbation of symptoms.
- Some patients worsen after delivery.
- Neonates can experience transient respiratory distress, feeding difficulties, and generalized weakness because of transplacental diffusion of antibodies.

DRUGS LEADING TO EXACERBATION

- Neuromuscular-blocking agents
- Aminoglycosides
- Antiarrhythmics
- Phenytoin

ACUTE INFLAMMATORY DEMYELINATING POLYRADICULOPATHY (GUILLAIN-BARRÉ SYNDROME)

EPIDEMIOLOGY

- Incidence ranges from 0.6 to 2.4 per 100,000 per year.
- Any age is affected with a slight male predominance.
- Occurrence is worldwide.

- Approximately 70% of cases occur after a viral infection or after infection with *Campylobacter jejuni*
- Also encountered after vaccination, surgery, and epidural anesthesia.

ETIOLOGY

- It is likely a cell-mediated autoimmune process, but the antigen is not known. Anti-GM1 ganglioside antibodies develop and decline with clinical recovery.

PATHOPHYSIOLOGY

- Increased titers of immunoglobulin G (IgG) anti-GM1 antibodies occur, especially with *C. jejuni* infection.
- The peripheral nerves are characterized by segmental demyelination with mononuclear infiltration. If severe, axonal damage results.
- The motor nerves are preferentially affected compared to the sensory nerves.
- Inflammatory infiltrates also develop in the sympathetic and dorsal root ganglia.

CLINICAL PRESENTATION

- Acute inflammatory demyelinating polyradiculopathy (AIDP) is a diverse disorder that usually presents as a motor, mixed sensory motor, or cranial nerve neuropathy. Prognosis depends on the extent of demyelination and axonal damage.
- The most common presentation is ascending weakness with minimal sensory symptoms. The weakness plateaus after 2 to 3 weeks.
- Areflexia or hyporeflexia, especially in the lower extremities, is an early finding.
- Cranial neuropathies especially involving the facial nerve (50%), can also occur.
- Abnormalities of autonomic nerve function is underscored by cardiac arrhythmias and intestinal ileus.
- Progressive weakness of respiratory muscles may require intubation.

VARIANTS OF GUILLAIN-BARRÉ SYNDROME

- Acute motor axonal neuropathy is usually associated with high titers of *C. jejuni*. These patients have a relatively aggressive course.
- Patients can also present with primarily axonal motor-sensory involvement and a fulminant course.
- Miller-Fisher syndrome presents with ophthalmoplegia, ataxia, and areflexia. High titers of anti-GQ1b antibodies are detected in the serum.

DIAGNOSIS

- Cerebrospinal fluid shows cytoalbuminologic dissociation, that is, no or low cells with high protein. The elevated protein develops 1 to 2 weeks after the onset of symptoms.
- Human immunodeficiency virus (HIV) testing is indicated because of its known association with an acute inflammatory neuropathy.
- Electrophysiologic studies reveal evidence of demyelination and slowing of nerve conduction studies with conduction block. Depending on the severity of the process, evidence of axonal involvement leading to denervation can occur.

THERAPEUTIC INTERVENTION

- Patients are closely monitored for cardiac arrhythmias and respiratory distress.
- Respiratory parameters, for example, inspiratory and expiratory pressures and forced vital capacity, are obtained three or four times a day.
- Plasma exchange is beneficial.
- Intravenous immunoglobulin therapy accompanies plasma exchange.
- Patients with extensive axonal injury require long-term rehabilitation.

PROGNOSIS

- Most patients have a favorable prognosis and recover completely.
- Patients with extensive axonal damage have residual weakness.
- Approximately 3% to 5% of patients experience relapses over years.

DIABETIC NEUROPATHY

EPIDEMIOLOGY

- Occurs in 10% to 100% of diabetic patients; the incidence varies depending on the criteria used for establishing diabetic neuropathy (DN).
- Several different types of DN are encountered clinically (see below).

ETIOLOGY

- Direct glucose neurotoxicity.
- Increased polyol pathway activity with accumulation of fructose and sorbitol and reduced nerve inositol.

- Reduced sodium-potassium-adenosine triphosphatase (Na^+-K^+-ATPase) activity.
- Decreased axonal transport.
- Intracellular oxidative stress with accelerated apoptosis.

PATHOPHYSIOLOGY

- Microvascular abnormalities accompanied by depressed prostaglandins, decreased nerve blood flow, and endoneurial ischemia.
- Trophic compound (nerve growth factor) deficiency.
- Abnormal glycosylation of proteins resulting in accumulation of advanced glycation end products.
- Autoimmune-mediated neurotoxicity has been described.

CLINICAL MANIFESTATIONS

- Length-dependent DN commences in the toes and progresses in a stocking-glove fashion.
- The neuropathy involves segmental thoracic and abdominal nerves that produce symptoms that mimic many cardiac or gastrointestinal disorders.
- Motor weakness occurs distally in the involved nerve distribution.
- Sensory symptoms consist of numbness, tingling, burning, and knife-like sensations.
- Ataxia has been described.
- Cranial neuropathies, especially cranial nerves III, V, and VII.
- Autonomic neuropathy is common and affects the pupils, lacrimal nerve, baroreceptor reflex, and thermoregulatory system.
- Focal-limb neuropathies such as carpal tunnel syndrome, ulnar neuropathy, and lateral femoral cutaneous neuropathy can occur.
- Lumbosacral plexopathy is often bilateral, but asymmetrical; pain, oftentimes severe, typically accompanies the weakness.

LABORATORY INVESTIGATIONS

- Serum glucose; glycosylated hemoglobin (HbA_{1c})
- Electrophysiological studies (neurovascular checks [NVC]; electromyelography [EMG])
- Autonomic testing (Tilt table)
- Sensory nerve (sural or radial) or distal skin biopsy

THERAPEUTIC INTERVENTIONS

- Optimal glucose control
- Treatment of hypertension (HTN) and dyslipidemia

- Pancreatic transplant will reverse the neuropathy in many.
- Relief of neuropathic pain
  - Tricyclic agents
  - Anticonvulsants, for example, carbamazepine, gabapentin, lamotrigine, topiramate, and oxcarbazepine
- IVIG is used in rapidly progressive DN.
- Local agents: lidocaine patches and capsaicin ointment.
- Symptomatic treatment of autonomic neuropathy.
- Foot care.

PROGNOSIS

- Slow progression over years
- Foot ulcers are common and potentially life threatening
- Chronic pain, particularly in the lower extermities

IMMUNE-MEDIATED INFLAMMATORY MYOPATHIES

Three conditions will be discussed in this chapter:
- Polymyositis (PM)
- Dermatomyositis (DM)
- Inclusion body myositis (IBM)

EPIDEMIOLOGY

- Inflammatory myopathies occur in 1:100,000 adults.
- IBM is more common in men.
- More women than men are affected by DM.

ETIOLOGY

- PM is usually associated with other autoimmune disorders, especially systemic lupus erythematosus, rheumatoid arthritis, and Sjögren's syndrome.
- DM often presents as an *overlap syndrome*, (with features of scleroderma and mixed connective tissue disease).
- Viral infection often antedates the clinical syndrome.
- The incidence of cancer is increased in DM and to a lesser extent in PM.
- BM is presumably autoimmune in nature, but responds poorly to immune-modulating therapy.

PATHOPHYSIOLOGY

- In PM and IBM, a T-cell–mediated cytotoxic process is likely. Class I major histocompatibility complex (MHC) antigen expression is increased and CD8+ cells have been characterized in the inflammatory area.

- Complement-dependent endothelial injury of the microvasculature has been described in DM.
- Autoantibodies, especially anti-JO1, have been detected in sera. Howeever, these antibodies are relatively non-specific and have been noted in other clinical conditions eg, interstitial lung disease.
- A T-cell mediated inflammatory response has been well characterized in IBM.

CLINICAL PRESENTATION

- PM, DM, and IBM are characterized by bilateral motor weakness
- The diagnosis of PM is one of exclusion. These patients typically develop proximal weakness and dysphagia in an insidious fashion.
- DM is suspected in patients that present with a heliotrope rash surrounding the eyes, face, upper body, and knuckles.
- Inflammatory myopathy is characterized by cardiac arrhythmias, for example, A-V conduction delays.
- Interstitial lung disease is seen with increased frequency in DM and PM.
- IBM features distal and proximal weakness, especially of the quadriceps and finger flexors.

LABORATORY INVESTIGATIONS

- Serum creatine phosphokinase (CPK) is usually elevated 50 to 100 times above normal.
- Electrodiagnostic studies show evidence of myopathy and insertional irritability consistent with an inflammatory process.
- A muscle biopsy is diagnostic in inflammatory myositis. A biopsy should be performed on affected muscle, although severely atrophic muscle should be avoided.
- In DM and PM, a complete evaluation for an occult malignancy should be carried out. At a minimum, a thorough physical examination of breast, rectum, and pelvis should be performed. In addition, mammography, pelvic ultrasonography, and serum CA-125 levels should be performed in women and stool for occult blood in men. Whether CT scan of chest, abdomen, or pelvis is routinely obtained remains controversial.

THERAPEUTIC INTERVENTIONS

- High-dose corticosteroids are effective in many patients, resulting in improved strength and preserved muscle function. The duration of therapy remains controversial, but most clinicians will administer corticosteroids for at least 9-12 months. Initially administered at a dose of 1mg/kg/day, the steroid is tapered to approximately 5 mg/day at 6 months.
- Methotrexate, azathioprine, and mycophenolate mofetil have been utilized as steroid-sparing agents or reserved for use in patients refractory to steroids alone.
- IVIG, plasmapheresis, or rituximab may prove useful in patients with recurrent disease or those refractory to standard immunosuppression.

BIBLIOGRAPHY

Asbury AK, Cornblath DR. Assessment of current diagnostic criteria for Guillain-Barré syndrome. *Ann Neurol.* 1990;27(suppl): S21–24.

Bech E, Orntoft TF, Andersen LP, et al. IgM anti-GM1 antibodies in the Guillain-Barré syndrome: A serological predictor of the clinical course. *J Neuroimmunol.* 1997;72:59–66.

Berrih-Aknin S, Cohen Kaminsky S, Newmann D, et al. Cellular aspects of myasthenia gravis. *Immunol Res.* 1988;7:189–199.

Boulton AJ, Vinik AI, Arezzo JC, et al. Diabetic neuropathies: A statement by the American Diabetes Association. *Diabetes Care.* 2005;28(4):956–962.

Brannagan TH. Peripheral neuropathy pain: Mechanisms and treatment. *J Clin Neuromuscular Dis.* 2003;5:61–71.

Buchbinder R, Forbes A, Hall S, et al. Incidence of malignant disease in biopsy-proven inflammatory myopathy. A population-based cohort study. *Ann Intern Med.* 2001;134:1087–1095.

Callen JP. Dermatomyositis. *Lancet.* 2000;355(9197):53–57.

Cornblath DR, Mellits ED, Griffin JW, et al. Motor conduction studies in Guillain-Barré syndrome: Description and prognostic value. *Ann Neurol.* 1988;23:354–359.

Dalakas MC. The molecular and cellular pathology of inflammatory muscle diseases. *Curr Opin Pharmacol.* 2001;1:300–306.

Dalakas MC. Therapeutic approaches in patients with inflammatory myopathies. *Semin Neurol.* 2003;23:199–206.

Diabetes Control and Complications Trial Research Group. The effect of intensive treatment of diabetes on the development and progression of long-term complications in insulin-dependent diabetes mellitus. *N Engl J Med.* 1993;329(14):977–986.

Drachman DB, McIntosh KM, Reim J, et al. Strategies for treatment of myasthenia gravis. *Ann N Y Acad Sci.* 1993;681:515–528.

Dyck PJ, Davies JL, Wilson DM, et al. Risk factors for severity of diabetic polyneuropathy. *Diabetes Care.* 1999b;22:1479–1486.

Dyck PJ, Windebank AJ. Diabetic and nondiabetic lumbosacral radiculoplexus neuropathies: New insights into pathophysiology and treatment. *Muscle Nerve.* 2002;25(4):477–491.

Evoli A, Tonali P, Bartoccioni E, et al. Ocular myasthenia: Diagnostic and therapeutic problems. *Acta Neurol Scand.* 1988;77:31.

Evoli A, Tonali PA, Padua L, et al. Clinical correlates with anti-MuSK antibodies in generalized seronegative myasthenia gravis. *Brain.* 2003;126(pt 10):2304–2311.

French Cooperative Group on Plasma Exchange in Guillain-Barré syndrome. Appropriate number of plasma exchanges in Guillain-Barré syndrome. *Ann Neurol.* 1997;41:298–306.

Hafer-Macko C, Hsieh ST, Li CY, et al. Acute motor axonal neuropathy: An antibody-mediated attack on axolemma. *Ann Neurol.* 1996;40:635–644.

Hiraga A, Mori M, Ogawara K, et al. Differences in patterns of progression in demyelinating and axonal Guillain-Barré syndromes. *Neurology.* 2003;61(4):471–474.

Howard FM, Lennon VA, Finley J, et al. Clinical correlations of antibodies that bind, block or modulate human acetylcholine receptors in myasthenia gravis. *Ann N Y Acad Sci.* 1987;505: 526–538.

Jury EC, D'Cruz D, Morrow WJ. Autoantibodies and overlap syndromes in autoimmune rheumatic disease. *J Clin Pathol.* 2001;54:340–347.

Krendel DA, Costigan DA, Hopkins LC. Successful treatment of neuropathies in patients with diabetes mellitus. *Arch Neurol.* 1995;52:1053–1061.

Low PA, Benrud-Larsen LM, Sletten DM, et al. Autonomic symptoms and diabetic neuropathy: A population-based study. *Diabetes Care.* 2004;27(12):2942–2947.

Mastaglia FL, Garlepp MJ, Phillips BA, et al. Inflammatory myopathies: Clinical, diagnostic and therapeutic aspects. *Muscle Nerve.* 2003;27:407–425.

Mulder D, Graves M, Hermann C. Thymectomy for myasthenia gravis: Recent observations and comparisons with past experience. *Ann Thorac Surg.* 1989;48:551–555.

Phillips LH, Melnick PA. Diagnosis of myasthenia gravis in the 1990s. *Semin Neurol.* 1990;10:62–69.

104 SPINAL CORD AND NERVE ROOT DISORDERS

Florian P. Thomas and Robert M Woolsey

INTRODUCTION

A hallmark of many but not all cord diseases is a *level* below which sensory, motor, or reflex functions are affected and above which they are intact. Clinical features often indicate that the cord is involved primarily dorsally, ventrally, laterally, centrally, or totally. Syndromes can be complete or incomplete with some preservation of function. This chapter focuses on entities that primary care physicians are likely to encounter. Acute traumatic conditions will not be discussed since they are typically triaged in emergency rooms and often quickly evaluated in specialized trauma centers. For some formerly important diseases, such as tabes dorsalis and poliomyelitis readers are referred to other standard texts. Hereditary conditions are only discussed if they are relevant in the different diagnosis of more common conditions.

SYMPTOMS AND SIGNS OF SPINAL CORD DYSFUNCTION

MOTOR ABNORMALITIES

Motor abnormalities result from dysfunction of *upper motor neuron* (UMN) pathways that mediate voluntary movement and target the anterior horn cells (AHC). Early features include loss of dexterity, weakness, and paralysis occurs when 50% and 90%, respectively, of the UMNs ceased functioning. Acute UMN paralysis or spinal shock presents with hypotonia and areflexia.[4] Over days to weeks, tone and reflexes return, and muscles often become hypertonic and stiff with hyperactive tendon reflexes (spasticity). In slowly progressive conditions, spasticity develops gradually without initial spinal shock. Spasms are a phenomenon related to, but not identical, with spasticity, in which activation of small dorsal root afferents excites AHCs in adjacent spinal segments and promote contraction of synergistic muscles. Spastic paralysis is often associated with extensor plantar responses (Babinski sign). Weakness caused by AHC or *lower motor neuron* (LMN) dysfunction reflects loss of ~50% of LMNs.[3] Such conditions cause more severe muscle atrophy than UMN dysfunction, and are often accompanied by fasciculations.

SENSORY ABNORMALITIES

All sensory information passing from the periphery to the brain, except from the head, traverses the dorsal columns or the spinothalamic tracts. The former convey joint position, vibration and touch sensation from the ipsilateral body, and information about visceral distention. The lateral spinothalamic tract mediates temperature and pain sensation from the opposite side. The anterior spinothalamic tract is involved in touch sensation.

Dorsal column disease causes gait ataxia because the brain is deprived of conscious knowledge regarding leg position. If the lesion affects the cervical cord, there is also upper limb ataxia. Vision compensates for loss of proprioception to a great degree. Dorsal column disease also causes paresthesias described as tingling, numbness, crawling, or deadness mainly in the distal limbs. Lhermitte phenomenon, originating in the dorsal columns, is an electric shock sensation over the neck that extends into the back and sometimes the limbs. Position sense is lost when ~75% of dorsal column axons have ceased working. Lateral spinothalamic tract dysfunction reduces pain and temperature perception on the contralateral side of the body, one or two dermatomes below the level of the lesion, but rarely causes paresthesia. Bilateral lesions affect erection, ejaculation, and orgasm.

PAIN

Several types of pain occur in cord and root disorders. Local and radicular pain is nociceptive, ie, generated from pain receptors that travel through spinothalamic pathways. Central neuropathic pain results from damage to spinal cord pain transmission pathways.

Local pain arises from pain receptors in the blood vessels of the paravertebral muscles, the cord, and bones or ligaments of the spine. It is the most intense over its source and often extends laterally to the shoulders, trunk, and hips. Less than 5% of local back or neck pain originates from the cord or cauda equina itself. Approximately 20% is caused by conditions of the spine. In 75%, no cause is identified. Local pain of cord origin is usually associated with mass lesions (tumor, abscess, hematoma) or acute processes, eg, transverse myelitis or infarction.

Radicular pain results from involvement of or traction on dorsal root ganglia. It radiates into the peripheral distribution of the root involved, ie, arms, trunk, or legs.

Central pain is common with trauma and intramedullary tumors but rare in other cord disorders. Onset is frequently months or years after injury. It is characterized by burning or lancinating features and occurs in an area of impaired sensation.

Neurogenic intermittent claudication, a form of peripheral neuropathic pain, occurs in lumbar stenosis and spinal vascular abnormalities. Standing and walking causes dull back and leg pain, and sometimes numbness and weakness. Signs of vascular insufficiency are typically missing: Standing without walking causes symptoms with neurogenic, but not with vascular claudication.

SPHINCTER SYMPTOMS

The bladder is affected by spinal shock. Thus, incontinence occurs in almost all acute bilateral cord conditions with leg weakness. The detrusor and sphincter muscles eventually become hypertonic and hyperreflexic, and reflex voiding is provoked by bladder distention. If the conus medullaris or cauda equina are involved, flaccidity persists.

With conditions of slower onset, hyperreflexic sphincter symptoms develop over time, with small-capacity bladder, frequency, urgency, and urge incontinence. If the conus medullaris or cauda equina is affected, the bladder and sphincter muscles slowly become atonic and hyporeflexic, producing symptoms of infrequent urination, urinary retention, and overflow incontinence.

The gastrointestinal system is affected in an analogous fashion. LMN lesions result in slow stool propulsion and low anal sphincter tone. With UMN lesions, fecal retention develops because of anal external sphincter contraction.

SPINAL CORD AND CAUDA EQUINA SYNDROMES

The syndromes are summarized in Table 104–1. The clinical presentations describe typical and complete involvement of pathways. Atypical presentations occur, and often presentations are incomplete.

COMMON NEUROLOGICAL SPINAL CORD AND NERVE ROOT CONDITIONS

MULTIPLE SCLEROSIS

Relapsing-remitting spinal multiple sclerosis (MS) is the most common cause of an acute spontaneous cord syndrome in patients aged 15 to 50. MS plaques have a predilection for the dorsal cord and cervical and upper thoracic segments and commonly occur bilaterally. MS attacks typically evolve from onset to maximal deficit over 1 day to 1 week, although onset may be faster or slower. Recovery from maximal deficit to maximal improvement usually occurs over 1 to 3 months, but sometimes is slower or faster. Most commonly, patients have an attack about every 2 years. Some MS symptoms are more likely to improve than others: Sensory symptoms remit completely in over 75%, but only 50% of patients with mono- or hemiparesis remit completely; fewer than 20% of those with quadriparesis or paraparesis do so, and even fewer with bladder symptoms. After 5 to 10 years, attacks become less common, less distinct, and recovery from attacks is more limited; this marks the transition to *secondary progressive MS*. Approximately 15% of MS patients progress without remissions or exacerbations; ie, *primary progressive MS*. Of these, 30% to 50% develop a progressive myelopathy which culminates in wheelchair dependency after 20 years.

When cord symptoms occur in a case of known MS, there is no diagnostic problem. In 30% to 60%, cord symptoms herald the onset of the disease. Spinal MRI shows discrete or diffuse lesions. Gadolinium contrast reveals enhancement with recent lesions. Oftentimes *silent* lesions are found in the brain by MRI. The cerebrospinal fluid (CSF) reveals selective oligoclonal bands or elevated immunoglobulins in 80%. Evoked potential studies are typically abnormal.

For disabling attacks, high-dose methylprednisolone is used to reduce the inflammatory reaction and accelerate recovery. Subcutaneous interferon-β-1b (Betaseron), intramuscular (Avonex) or subcutaneous (Rebif) interferon-β-1a, and subcutaneous glatiramer acetate (Copaxone) decrease the frequency of exacerbations and the rate of disease progression. Treatment options are not well established for PPMS.

TABLE 104–1 Spinal Cord and Cauda Equina Syndromes

SYNDROME	AFFECTED PATHWAYS	FEATURES	CAUSES
Dorsal cord bilateral	Dorsal columns: Corticospinal tracts: Descending autonomic tracts to sacral segments:	Gait ataxia/paresthesia Acute: Flaccid, hyporeflexia Chronic: Hypertonia, hyperreflexia, Babinski sign Incontinence	Acute: Multiple sclerosis Chronic: Friedreich ataxia, B12 deficiency, vascular malformation, epidural tumors, HIV, cervical spondylosis, atlantoaxial subluxation
Anterior or ventral cord bilateral	Anterior two-thirds of cord: Spinothalamic tracts Corticospinal tracts Descending autonomic tracts to sacral segments	Loss of pain/temperature sensation Weakness and reflex changes Incontinence	Acute: Cord infarction (anterior spinal artery syndrome), disk herniation Chronic: Radiation myelopathy disk herniation
Central cord bilateral	Disruption of crossing fibers: Spinothalamic tract: Dorsal columns spared: Reflex arch: Large lesions involving anterior horns or corticospinal tracts	Impaired pain/temperature at the level of the lesion, but normal above/below Proprioception, vibration intact Reflex loss in the analgesic area Weakness	Acute: Neck hyperextension in presence of spondylosis Chronic: Syringomyelia, intramedullary tumor
Lateral cord brown-séquard unilateral	Spinothalamic tract: Dorsal columns: Corticospinal tract:	Contralateral: Impaired pain/temperature sensation Ipsilateral: Paresthesias (often spared) Ipsilateral: Weakness	Acute: Cord infarction Chronic: Intramedullary or intradural extramedullary tumors
Total cord bilateral	All pathways	Complete or near complete loss of strength, sensation and sphincter control below the level of the lesion	Acute: Vascular malformation Decompression sickness intramedullary abscess, transverse myelitis, nonorganic, cord hemorrhage
Cauda equina unilateral or bilateral	5 lumbar, 4 sacral pairs of roots supplying the legs & perineum	L5-S1 involvement: Lower back pain radiating to posterior thighs and calves, weak foot plantar flexion, loss of ankle jerks, incontinence. Lesions at higher levels add higher level motor, sensory and reflex loss.	Acute: Disk herniation Chronic: Disk herniation, spondylosis, arachnoiditis, intradural, extramedullary or extradural tumors
Pure motor syndrome bilateral	Upper motor neuron Lower motor neuron Upper and lower motor neuron	Incoordination, weakness, hyperreflexia, Babinski sign Weakness, atrophy, fasciculations Combination of both	HTLV-1 or HIV-1 associated myelopathy, spondylosis, hereditary spastic paraplegia, post-polio syndrome, electric shock

ACUTE TRANSVERSE MYELITIS

Acute transverse myelitis (ATM) manifests with generally symmetrical weakness and sensory loss below the affected spinal segment. Symptoms evolve over hours to weeks. A few or many spinal cord segments are involved by demyelination or necrosis of all cord elements. Generally, patients present with paresthesias in the legs, and approximately 30% have pain over the involved cord segments. Weakness and incontinence follow. ATM can be complete or incomplete. Because it is often preceded by a vaccination or viral illness, an immunologically mediated mechanism is presumed. Although rare, when ATM occurs in the immunocompromised host, it is caused by cord infection due to herpes simplex virus (HSV), varicella-zoster virus (VZV), cytomegalovirus (CMV), or Epstein-Barr virus (EBV). CSF is sometimes normal, but often shows lymphocytic pleocytosis and increased protein and immunoglobulins. Magnetic resonance imaging (MRI) is normal or reveals nonspecific intramedullary swelling, signal changes, and contrast enhancement. Patients may recover completely, incompletely, or not at all. In 5% of patients, ATM evolves into MS. Clinical features in ATM are more often symmetrical than in MS. Abnormal visual or auditory evoked potentials or brain MRI suggest MS.

SPONDYLOSIS WITH COMPRESSION OF THE SPINAL CORD, NERVE ROOTS, OR CAUDA EQUINA

With a prevalence of 50% at age 45 and 90% at 60 years of age, age-related spondylosis is essentially universal. As intervertebral disks lose height, the surrounding annulus fibrosis becomes slack, bulges outward, and calcifies to form *spurs* that intrude into the anterior spinal canal or intervertebral foramen. Usually, multiple levels are involved. A similar process affects the posterior vertebral articular facets. With severe spondylosis, compression occurs of the cord, cauda equina, or nerve roots. In rheumatoid arthritis, the transverse atlantal ligament that holds the odontoid process of C1 (axis) against the anterior arch of C1 (atlas) often becomes disrupted, allowing forward movement of C1 and atlantoaxial subluxation.

Cervical cord compression produces gait ataxia with hyperreflexia, weakness, sensory deficit, and bladder symptoms. Arm involvement depends on the level of the lesion. Some patients show a pure motor syndrome that may be mistaken for ALS. Traumatic neck hyperextension with canal narrowing causes severe cord compression and produces a central cord syndrome (Table 104–1). Cauda equina compression results in neurogenic intermittent claudication (see above). Patients show only minor abnormalities on neurologic examination or none at all, so the history is crucial. Root compression by osteophytes intruding into the intervertebral canal in the cervical or lumbar intervertebral spaces produces neurologic features similar to those caused by disk herniation.

MRI reveals loss of height of intervertebral discs, disc desiccation, degenerative spondylolisthesis, scoliosis, spur formation with annular bulges, and tears within the posterior annulus. Reduction in the diameter of the neural foramina and spinal canal with narrowing of the thecal sac is sometimes present. Changes in the articular facets and facet joints also occur. Later the spinal cord atrophies and shows signal changes indicative of myelomalacia.

Although it is difficult to anticipate disease progression, patients with more severe deficits are frequently treated with surgical decompression using an anterior or posterior approach. About two-thirds of patients improve.

INTERVERTEBRAL DISK HERNIATION

Disks usually protrude dorsolaterally into the nerve root canal, because the annulus fibrosis is reinforced in the midline by the posterior longitudinal ligament. However, at times a herniating disk detaches the ligament from the vertebral body and pushes it into the spinal canal or tears through the ligament, compressing the cord or cauda equina. Herniations are more common in the lower cervical, lower half of the thoracic, or lower lumbar spine. They are sudden, or the disk is slowly extruded resulting in a chronic progressive syndrome. Moderate to severe back pain usually occurs at the herniation site. Compression of the cervical or thoracic cord results in unilateral or bilateral weakness and sensory loss below the lesion with variable sphincter dysfunction.

Almost all lumbar herniations producing a cauda equina syndrome occur between the L5-S1 or the L4–5 disk space and cause localize spinal pain and bilateral sciatica. L5-S1 herniation causes sensory deficits related to the compression of all sacral roots and motor deficit related to the S1 compression. Ankle reflexes are diminished or absent. Urinary retention and overflow incontinence are usually present.

MRI typically reveals a soft tissue mass of disc intensity protruding posteriorly and compressing roots, caudal sac, or spinal cord. However, desiccated or calcified disks, scar tissue, or disk migration renders these interpretations less obvious. Furthermore, since 15% to 20% of asymptomatic individuals have ruptured disks, the correlation between MRI and clinical presentation is challenging. Treatment options include removal of the disk material, though spontaneous recovery occurs. Outcomes are typically very good with lumbar disk herniations, less so with cervical or thoracic lesions.

SPINAL TUMORS

Spinal epidural tumors are almost always malignant. Most originate from metastatic lesions in the vertebrae that extend into the epidural space and compress the cord or cauda equina. Only 5% spread hematogenously to the epidural space itself. The lung and breast are sites of origin in approximately 50%. Some cases occur in patients with known cancer, but epidural metastasis is not infrequently the presenting feature. Rarely, the cord itself is the site of a metastasis, usually from the lung.

Local and simultaneous or subsequent radicular pains are common first symptoms. After a variable interval, myelopathy develops with weakness and sensory loss below the lesion. Bladder symptoms occur in more than 50%. Untreated, these features progress to anesthetic paraplegia or tetraplegia with loss of sphincter function. Metastatic epidural and intramedullary tumors are treated with emergent high-dose corticosteroids and radiation. Although patients may not improve, deterioration is halted or slowed. Many patients die within 6 months of diagnosis.

Intradural extramedullary tumors, or tumors in the subarachnoid space, unlike epidural tumors, are benign, slow growing, and surgically curable. Two common tumors are meningiomas arising from arachnoidal cells near the dentate ligament and neurofibromas (schwannomas) that originate from spinal root Schwann cells. Both affect any cord segment. They present with local neck or back pain and frequently with radicular pain. Because of slow growth, cord symptoms are delayed for months or years, but weakness (ipsilateral at first) and sensory loss below the lesion ensue and sphincter dysfunction follows. Surgery is often curative.

Intramedullary tumors, commonly ependymomas or astrocytomas, arise in the cord itself; the former often occur in the cauda equina and lower half of the cord, while the latter mostly involve the upper spinal axis. Ependymomas are usually well demarcated and histologically benign. Astrocytomas are more infiltrative and malignant in 25%. With ependymomas and benign astrocytomas, patients are often symptomatic months or years before the tumor is found. Local neck or back pain is a common first symptom, followed by weakness and sensory symptoms below the lesion. A lateral or central cord syndrome is present in some patients (see Table 104–1). Fifty percent of ependymomas arise from the filum terminale and produce a cauda equina syndrome. Surgery is often curative for ependymomas and benign astrocytomas, with a 10-year postoperative survival of approximately 80%; with malignant astrocytomas, this figure is only 15%.

MRI typically reveals T1 and T2 prolongation in lesions and enhancement. Metastatic tumors often show bone destruction and marrow replacement. Such lesions must be separated from osteoporotic compression fractures. Intradural-extramedullary tumors remodel the adjacent bone but do not destroy it. Typically, they grow through the neural foramen and exhibit a *dumbbell* shape. Dural vascular malformations simulate extramedullary-intradural masses. Intramedullary tumors are associated with syrinxes or have cystic components.

SUBACUTE COMBINED DEGENERATION

Subacute combined degeneration (SCD) is a neuromyeloencephalopathy caused by vitamin B12 (cobalamin) deficiency. Although young individuals are occasionally involved, almost all patients are older than 40 years and most are older than 60 years. B12 deficiency causes degenerative changes that begin in the myelin of the upper thoracic dorsal column. The cause of cobalamin deficiency in most patients is secondary to deficiency of gastric *intrinsic factor*. Inactivation of B12 by recreational (*whippets* or *whippits*) or iatrogenic N_2O use, dietary deficits, achlorhydria, infections (*Helicobacter pylori*, fish tapeworm, blind loop syndrome) and medications (metformin, proton pump inhibitors, colchicine, neomycin) must also be considered.

Frequently it is difficult to tease apart the relative contribution of PNS and CNS features. Onset is often characterized by numbness or paresthesias in the feet, impaired position and vibration sense, and gait ataxia. Tendon jerks are increased at the knees and decreased at the ankles. Weakness and Babinski signs are less common and late features. Autonomic dysfunction is rare.

While B12 is used for erythrocytic and granulocytic maturation, restoration of blood counts can occur because of folate supplements in many processed food items. Consequently, hematological abnormalities secondary to B12 deficiency are rare in the United States. However, folate does not compensate for B12 in CNS or PNS pathways.

The diagnosis rests on the demonstration of a low serum B12. However, clinical B12 deficiency, evidenced by methylmalonic acid (MMA) accumulation, may occur with *normal* B12 levels (300 to 400 pg/mL). Thus, MMA should be measured whenever B12 levels are below this range. Abnormal B12 or MMA levels warrant determination of intrinsic factor (IF) or parietal cell antibodies, whose presence confirms the diagnosis of pernicious anemia. A Shilling test is less frequently used. B12 deficiency is treated with oral B12, 1000 µg daily for life, of which even in the absence of IF, 1% or 10 µg is absorbed. This is adequate since the the daily requirement of B12 is only 2 mcg. Alternatively B12 may be administered intramuscularly, subcutaneously, or intranasally. Parenteral B12 is preferable in patients after barosurgery

Many patients with SCD recover completely when treated in a timely fashion, but complete recovery is unlikely with severe or longstanding deficits prior to treatment.

SPINAL ABSCESS

Spinal epidural abscess is a collection of pus within the spinal canal external to the dura. The source of the infection is usually extension from vertebral osteomyelitis or hematogenous spread from a distant site. Often no cause is found. *Staphylococcus aureus* is the most common pathogen. At the onset, there is fever and local pain. As the abscess enlarges, root involvement produces pain radiating into the limbs or around the trunk. With cord or cauda equina compression, sensory and motor function below the level of compression is affected. Onset is over days to weeks, but in some cases, symptoms evolve slowly with no or inconspicuous fever, raising suspicion of a tumor, until at surgery or autopsy the diagnosis is established.

Leucocytosis is common. CSF examination yields pleiocytosis, high protein, and normal glucose. However, lumbar puncture should be avoided if possible, because neurological deterioration sometimes follows drainage of fluid from below the lesion. MRI often shows changes in the adjacent disc or vertebra, in disc height, and in the vertebral endplates. The spinal abscess itself reveals T1 and T2 prolongation with contrast enhancement.

Treatment is tightly linked to outcome: Patients treated before the onset of paralysis usually recover completely. Patients who are paraplegic for more than 48 hours often remain so. Treatment consists of decompression and antibiotics.

INTRASPINAL HEMORRHAGE

Intraspinal hemorrhage occurs in the epidural, subdural, or subarachnoid spaces, or into the cord (hematomyelia). Causes include trauma (10%), bleeding from a vascular malformation or tumor (5%), anticoagulants or coagulopathy (25%); in 60% the cause remains unknown. Features include acute back pain at onset over the area of hemorrhage, followed rapidly by weakness and sensory loss below the lesion, and sphincter dysfunction. CT or MRI images are influenced by location and state of oxygenation and age of the blood. Treatment relies on urgent surgical evacuation of the hematoma. Approximately 50% of patients with total loss of sensory and motor function at the time of operation recover to some degree; approximately 10% recover completely.

VASCULAR MALFORMATIONS OF THE SPINAL CORD

Extramedullary malformations arise from fistulas between an artery supplying the cord and a vein draining it. Shunting of high pressure blood into veins causes dilatation and elongation. The result is a tangle of vessels along the nerve root or on the dorsal lower thoracic or lumbar cord. When the anterior spinal artery is involved, the abnormal vessels are on the ventral or lateral surface. Cord symptoms are produced by compression from the venous mass or by a *steal* phenomenon. Most patients are middle-aged or older men with progressive leg weakness and sensory loss, moderate back pain, bladder symptoms, and neurogenic claudication exaggerated by walking.

The less common intramedullary malformations usually become symptomatic in childhood or young adult life. Although they may also have a chronic progressive course, 30% present as a sudden, at times catastrophic, spinal cord event because of hemorrhage or infarction.

MRI shows signal changes within the cord and/or flow voids within dilated vessels. Definitive diagnosis is established via spinal angiography.

Treatment involves fistula obliteration by surgical or embolization techniques; this halts neurologic deterioration and 50% improve.

BIBLIOGRAPHY

Noseworthy JH, Lucchinetti C, Rodriguez M, Weinshenker BG. Multiple sclerosis. *N Engl J Med.* 2000;343(13):938–952.

Transverse Myelitis Consortium Working Group. Proposed diagnostic criteria and nosology of acute transverse myelitis. *Neurology.* 2002;59(4):499–505.

McCormack BM, Weinstein PR. Cervical spondylosis. An update. *West J Med.* 1996;43–51.

Schiff D, O'Neill BP. Intramedullary spinal cord metastases: Clinical features and treatment outcome. *Neurology.* 1996;47(4): 906–912.

Diamond AL, Diamond R, Freedman SM, Thomas FP. "Whippets"-induced cobalamin deficiency manifesting as cervical myelopathy. *J Neuroimaging.* 2004;14(3):277–80.

Mackenzie AR, Laing RB, Smith CC, Kaar GF, Smith FW. Spinal epidural abscess: The importance of early diagnosis and treatment. *J Neurol Neurosurg Psychiatry.* 1998;65(2): 209–212.

Wisoff HS. Spontaneous intraspinal hemorrhage. In: Wilkins RH, Rengarchary SS, eds. *Neurosurgery.* 2nd ed. New York, NY: McGraw-Hill; 1996:2559–2565.

Detweiler PW, Porter RW, Spetzler RF. Spinal arteriovenous malformations. *Neurosurg Clin N Am.* 1999;10(1):89–100.

105 EPILEPSY

Jayant N. Acharya

TERMINOLOGY

- The term *seizure* refers to the transient occurrence of signs and/or symptoms caused by abnormal excessive or synchronous neuronal activity in the brain.
- *Epilepsy* is a chronic brain disorder of various etiologies characterized by recurrent, unprovoked seizures. Traditionally, patients with single or only provoked seizures are not considered to have epilepsy. Epilepsy is not a single disease but is divided into various epileptic syndromes.
- *Epileptic syndromes* are groups of epileptic patterns, consisting of one or more seizure types, with similar clinical courses and response to treatment.
- *Convulsions* are seizures with prominent motor activity (eg, generalized tonic-clonic seizures). Seizures may also be *nonconvulsive,* manifested only by altered consciousness (eg, absence or complex partial seizures).

EPIDEMIOLOGY

- Epilepsy affects approximately 1% of Americans, and approximately 200,000 new cases are diagnosed each year in the United States.
- The cumulative lifetime incidence of seizures, including patients who have had at least one seizure in their entire lives, is 9% to 11%. The cumulative adjusted lifetime incidence of epilepsy is approximately 3% by age 80 years.[1]
- The incidence of epilepsy is higher in neonates, infants, and adolescents followed by a relative plateau during most of adulthood. The incidence again increases sharply after age 60 years.[1]

CLASSIFICATION OF SEIZURES

- The 1981 International Classification of Epileptic Seizures (ICES, Table 105–1)[2] is currently used worldwide, although alternative approaches to classification are also available (eg semiologic seizure classification[3]). The ICES classifies seizures based on seizure symptomatology and electroencephalograph (EEG) findings into partial and generalized seizures.

PARTIAL SEIZURES

- The initial clinical and EEG findings indicate activation of a part of one cerebral hemisphere. Based on the level of consciousness, the partial seizures are classified further into simple and complex partial seizures.

TABLE 105–1 International Classification of Epileptic Seizures (1981)

Partial Seizures

Simple partial (consciousness preserved)
Motor
Sensory: somatosensory or special sensory
Autonomic
Psychic
Complex partial (consciousness impaired)
With automatisms
Without automatisms
Simple partial seizures followed by impaired consciousness
Partial seizures evolving to secondarily generalized tonic-clonic seizures

Generalized Seizures

Absence
Tonic-clonic
Myoclonic
Atonic

Unclassified Seizures

SOURCE: Modified with permission from Hauser WA, Hesdorffer DC. *Epilepsy: Frequency, causes and consequences.* New York, NY: Demos; 1990.

- *Simple partial seizures* are characterized by preserved consciousness. They are divided into those with *motor* (tonic or clonic activity, usually unilateral), *sensory* (somatosensory or special sensory-olfactory, gustatory, visual, auditory, vertiginous), *autonomic* (vomiting, pallor, flushing, sweating, pupillary dilatation), and *psychic* (aphasia, déjà vu, fear) manifestations. Motor or somatosensory seizures may remain focal or spread to contiguous cortical areas leading to sequential involvement of body parts (*Jacksonian march*). Following a motor seizure, patients may experience transient weakness of the affected region (*Todd palsy*).
- *Complex partial seizures*: The hallmark of complex partial seizures is impairment of consciousness that is defined as the inability to respond normally to stimuli because of *altered awareness* (demonstrated by amnesia for ictal events) *and/or responsiveness* (inability of the patient to carry out simple commands or willed movements). Patients with complex partial seizures also have *automatisms* (more or less coordinated motor activity) such as lip smacking, chewing, and picking at clothes or objects. Complex partial seizures often begin with a motionless stare and usually last a few seconds to 3 minutes. After the seizure, patients are confused and drowsy for a variable period. Most complex partial seizures originate in the temporal lobe, but they also arise from the frontal lobe.
- A seizure *aura* occurs before consciousness is lost and for which memory is retained afterwards. Conventionally, the term is restricted to the initial sensations of seizures without objective signs. Thus, simple partial seizures, except motor and some autonomic seizures, are auras.
- Any partial seizure can evolve into a generalized tonic-clonic (GTC) seizure. The generalized seizure is then called a *secondarily GTC seizure,* which must be distinguished from a primary GTC seizure. Clues indicating a partial onset are the presence of an aura, focal motor or complex partial features prior to generalization, and postictal Todd palsy or aphasia.

GENERALIZED SEIZURES

- The initial clinical and EEG changes indicate involvement of both hemispheres. Consciousness is usually impaired and motor manifestations are bilateral. They are divided into the following categories:
- *Absence (petit mal) seizures* are characterized by abrupt interruption of ongoing activity with a blank stare, unresponsiveness, and, sometimes, eye blinking. Attacks typically last a few seconds, and there

is no postictal confusion. Ictal EEG reveals a generalized 3 Hz spike-wave pattern.

○ *Tonic-clonic (grand mal) seizures*: These are characterized by abrupt loss of consciousness, sometimes preceded by a vague ill-described warning. The patient becomes stiff (tonic phase) and respiration is inhibited, sometimes accompanied by cyanosis. Tongue biting and urinary and fecal incontinence can occur. This stage is followed by generalized rhythmic, unidirectional jerky activity (clonic phase). Saliva often froths from the mouth. At the end of this stage, deep respiration occurs and all the muscles relax. The patient remains unconscious for a variable duration and then awakens with musculoskeletal aches. The mean duration (excluding the postictal state) is approximately 1 minute.

○ *Myoclonic seizures*: These consist of sudden, brief, shocklike contractions that are generalized, focal, or segmental. Consciousness is preserved.

○ *Atonic seizures*: These are characterized by a sudden, transient decrease in muscle tone leading to a head drop, dropping of a limb, or loss of all muscle tone and slumping to the ground. If consciousness is lost, it is usually brief.

• *Status epilepticus* is defined as two or more seizures without intervening recovery of consciousness or a single seizure lasting 20 to 30 minutes. Status epilepticus presents as recurrent generalized convulsive seizures; nonconvulsive seizures (complex partial/absence), which produce a continuous *epileptic twilight state*; or as continuous simple partial seizures (*epilepsia partialis continua*).

CLASSIFICATION OF EPILEPTIC SYNDROMES

• Clinically, epileptic syndrome classification is more useful than seizure classification for prognosis and treatment. In addition to seizure symptomatology and EEG findings, the international classification of epileptic syndromes[4] considers age of onset, intellectual development, findings on neurologic examination, results of neuroimaging studies, and etiology.

• Epileptic syndromes are divided into *localization-related* (partial, focal), *generalized,* and *undetermined* epilepsies as well as *special syndromes* based on anatomical origin. Within each category, based on etiology, syndromes are further divided into *idiopathic* (arising from an unknown cause except a possible hereditary predisposition, with the additional implication of underlying normal neurologic status), *symptomatic* (of known etiology), and *cryptogenic* (presumably symptomatic; but the exact etiology is not known) epilepsies.

• The most common epileptic syndromes are *benign childhood epilepsy with centrotemporal spikes (benign Rolandic epilepsy), temporal lobe epilepsy, childhood absence epilepsy (pyknolepsy), juvenile myoclonic epilepsy, West syndrome, and Lennox-Gastaut syndrome.*

• *Febrile seizures* typically occur between the ages of 6 months and 5 years and are characterized by generalized seizures occurring during an acute febrile illness. There are two types: (1) *simple* (80%–90% of patients), with a single, generalized seizure lasting <15 minutes, and (2) *complex* (10%–20% of patients), with focal seizures, duration >15 minutes, and more than one seizure in a day or postictal signs. Overall, the risk of developing epilepsy (particularly temporal lobe epilepsy) later in life is <4%, but it is greater with complex than with simple febrile seizures.

ETIOLOGY

GENETICS

• Familial epilepsy usually presents as childhood-onset epilepsy without evidence of underlying brain disease. A genetic basis is more likely in patients with generalized rather than partial epilepsies, but a number of genetic partial epilepsies have been recently described (eg, autosomal dominant nocturnal frontal lobe epilepsy). In general, although there is evidence for a familial tendency of seizures in relatives of patients with epilepsy, there is no single epilepsy gene. However, a number of epileptic syndromes have been mapped to specific chromosomal locations (eg, autosomal dominant nocturnal frontal lobe epilepsy: 20q). The gene product has also been determined in some of these conditions. The relationship between the genetic abnormality and the epilepsy is not yet clear, but an emerging theme is that the genetic defects cause abnormalities of ion channels and/or key structural membrane proteins.

SECONDARY CAUSES

• Secondary causes include the following:

○ *Congenital*: cortical dysplasia, heterotopias

○ *Infectious*: meningitis, encephalitis including herpes simplex, abscess, cysticercosis, toxoplasmosis, rubella, neurosyphilis, tuberculosis

○ *Neoplastic*: meningiomas, gliomas, metastatic tumors, hamartomas

○ *Traumatic*: prenatal and perinatal injuries, head injury

○ *Vascular*: stroke (especially embolic), arteriovenous malformations, Sturge-Weber syndrome, subarachnoid hemorrhage, cerebral venous thrombosis
○ *Degenerative*: Alzheimer disease
○ *Metabolic*: hypoglycemia, hyponatremia, hypocalcemia, hypoxia, hyperglycemia, pyridoxine deficiency, hypomagnesemia, porphyria, thyrotoxicosis, uremia
○ *Toxic*: psychotropic drugs, high doses of antihistaminics, lead, mercury, carbon monoxide, withdrawal from alcohol
○ *Demyelinating*: multiple sclerosis

APPROACH TO THE PATIENT WITH SEIZURES

- If the patient presents shortly after a seizure, stabilize the vital signs; provide cardiovascular and respiratory support; and treat acute problems such as infections, metabolic abnormalities and drug toxicity. When the patient is stable, every effort should be made to determine if the patient had a previous history of seizures.
- Obtain all possible clinical details about the seizure including auras, if present. Since the patient may have been unresponsive during the seizure, eyewitnesses, if available, should be carefully questioned. Identify risk factors such as a history of febrile seizures, prior seizures, family history of seizures, or previous head trauma or other structural brain disease. Obtain a developmental history in children. Determine if there was a precipitating factor for the seizure such as sleep deprivation, systemic disease, infection, metabolic derangements, or drug use or withdrawal.
- On physical examination, observe for signs of infection, systemic illness, skin changes suggestive of neurocutaneous syndromes (eg, tuberous sclerosis), organomegaly, and signs of trauma or vascular disease. Perform a complete neurologic examination.

INVESTIGATIONS
- Routine blood studies: complete blood count (CBC), metabolic profile, liver function tests, serum and urine toxicology screen
- Consider a lumbar puncture if central nervous system infection is suspected.
- An *EEG* should be performed in all patients. It assists in establishing the diagnosis of epilepsy, classifying the seizure type and identifying a specific epileptic syndrome. The EEG may also reveal other abnormalities suggestive of the etiology (eg, focal slowing suggesting a structural lesion). The EEG hallmark of epilepsy is an interictal spike (epileptiform discharge),

but this is present only at brief intervals. Therefore, it is common for a standard 30-minute record to show no abnormalities in the presence of epilepsy. Only 50% to 60% of EEGs obtained after a seizure in patients later diagnosed as having epilepsy show epileptiform discharges. The diagnostic yield is increased by obtaining EEGs after sleep deprivation and with multiple (up to four) or prolonged (2-hour) monitoring. Thus, *an abnormal EEG helps to confirm the diagnosis of epilepsy, but a normal EEG does not rule out epilepsy.*

- *Neuroimaging* studies are necessary in all patients with new-onset seizures except children with a clinical evaluation indicating a benign form of epilepsy such as childhood absence epilepsy. Magnetic resonance imaging is more sensitive than computed tomography and is the imaging method of choice. It identifies lesions such as hippocampal atrophy and subtle cortical dysplasia that cannot be seen on computed tomography, as well as larger lesions such as tumors or vascular lesions. Functional imaging studies such as positron emission tomography and single-photon emission computed tomography are used in patients being evaluated for epilepsy surgery.

DIFFERENTIAL DIAGNOSIS

- Disorders mimicking seizures include the following:
  ○ Syncope
  ○ Transient ischemic attack
  ○ Psychogenic seizures
  ○ Sleep disorders: periodic leg movements of sleep, cataplexy
  ○ Movement disorders: tremor, nonepileptic myoclonus, chorea, tics
  ○ Migraine: confusional, basilar
  ○ Metabolic disturbances: hypoglycemia, hypoxia
  ○ Vestibular disorders
- These conditions are usually distinguished from seizures by a careful history and relevant laboratory studies. Occasionally, video-EEG monitoring, sleep studies, tilt table testing, or cardiac electrophysiology may be required.

TREATMENT

- It is important to treat underlying conditions such as metabolic abnormalities, medication abuse or withdrawal, and structural brain lesions as well as to instruct the patient to avoid precipitating factors, if possible. In addition, many patients require antiepileptic drug (AED) therapy

ANTIEPILEPTIC DRUG THERAPY

INITIATION

- *Single seizure*: Whether or not to initiate treatment is controversial. Estimates of recurrence risk in patients with unprovoked or idiopathic seizures range from 34% to 71%. Treatment should probably be initiated in the presence of one or more of the following: family history of epilepsy (particularly in a sibling), EEG with definite epileptic pattern, presence of a structural lesion (tumor, arteriovenous malformation, or infection), history of prior acute seizure, status epilepticus at onset, postictal Todd palsy, and abnormal neurologic examination. The consequences of seizure recurrence to the patient are also important. For instance, withholding treatment from an adult in a high-risk occupation may expose the patient to far greater risk than would result from AED use. Each patient's circumstances must be individualized and the options discussed in detail with the patient and family before a decision is made.
- *Two or more unprovoked seizures*: The recurrence risk increases to 70% or more, therefore, all patients should be treated.

AVAILABLE ANTICONVULSANTS

- The older, established AEDs include phenytoin; carbamazepine; valproic acid; phenobarbital; primidone; ethosuximide; and the benzodiazepines diazepam, clonazepam, and lorazepam (Table 105-2). These are available in a variety of formulations and have been the mainstay of epilepsy treatment for many years. Many new AEDs are available in the United States. These include gabapentin, lamotrigine, topiramate, tiagabine, felbamate, levetiracetam, oxcarbazepine, zonisamide, and pregabalin. These agents are still mainly used as second-line therapies in addition to one or more of the older drugs (adjunctive therapy); but they are likely to be increasingly used in the future not only for refractory epilepsy, but also for initial treatment because they appear equally efficacious, better tolerated, and have fewer drug interactions.[5,6] In addition, clobazam and vigabatrin are available in other parts of the world.

CHOICE OF ANTIEPILEPTIC DRUG

- Choosing the appropriate drug in a patient depends on the type of seizure (Table 105–3), relative convenience of dosing schedule, potential side effects and interactions, and economic considerations.

PRINCIPLES OF TREATMENT WITH ANTIEPILEPTIC DRUGS

- Use a single drug (monotherapy) whenever possible.
- Start with a low dose, increase gradually until seizures are controlled or adverse effects appear. Some AEDs, including phenytoin, diazepam, lorazepam, phenobarbital, and valproic acid are given intravenously in a *loading dose* to achieve therapeutic blood levels quickly for acute control of seizures and in the management of status epilepticus.
- If one drug fails, switch to another drug and gradually increase the dosage.
- Monitoring AED blood levels can be useful for establishing dosage schedule, treatment of recurrence, and monitoring compliance with medications.
- There are *therapeutic ranges* of blood levels for most AEDs, but blood levels should serve only as a guideline. Patients may exhibit seizure control with no signs of toxicity at drug levels that would otherwise be considered toxic. *Treat the patient, not the level.*
- Use two drugs when monotherapy fails. Observe for interactions.
- Be aware of differing pharmakokinetics in children, the elderly, pregnant women, and patients with hepatic or renal disease.

DISCONTINUING THERAPY

- Overall, approximately 70% of children and 60% of adults eventually discontinue therapy. The clinical profile suggesting the greatest likelihood of remaining seizure-free consists of complete control of seizures for 1 to 5 years, single seizure type, normal neurologic examination, and normal EEG. Withdrawal may be attempted after 2 years but should be gradual. Patients with juvenile myoclonic epilepsy require lifelong treatment.

MANAGEMENT OF STATUS EPILEPTICUS

- Generalized convulsive status epilepticus is a medical emergency because it leads to cardiorespiratory dysfunction, hyperthermia, metabolic derangements, and irreversible neuronal injury. Nonconvulsive status is subtle and often missed clinically until an EEG is performed. The most common causes of status are AED withdrawal or noncompliance, metabolic disturbances, drug toxicity, central nervous system infection, tumors, and head trauma.
  - First confirm the presence of status epilepticus, assess cardiovascular and respiratory status (*a*irway, *b*reathing, *c*irculation), perform a brief medical and neurologic examination, establish venous access, and obtain laboratory studies (rapid blood glucose, CBC, electrolytes, calcium, arterial blood gas, liver and renal function studies, toxicology, and AED levels).
  - Administer thiamine (100 mg) and 50 mL of 50% dextrose intravenously (IV).

TABLE 105–2 Clinical Aspects of the Antiepileptic Drugs Available in the United States

DRUG	FORMS	INITIAL DOSE IN MG (ADULTS)	MAINTENANCE DOSE IN MG (ADULTS)	DOSING SCHEDULE	THERAPEUTIC LEVEL (MG/L)	COMMON ADVERSE EFFECTS	MAJOR INTERACTIONS
PHT	Oral, IV	200	200–700	tid–qd	10–20	Gum hypertrophy, hirsutism, diplopia, dysarthria, ataxia	Warfarin, OCP, CBZ, PB, VPA, FBM, salicylates, antacids, alcohol
CBZ	Oral	200–400	600–1600	bid–tid	4–12	Leucopenia, hyponatremia, diplopia, dysarthria, ataxia	Erythromycin, propoxyphene, warfarin, OCP, cimetidine, PHT, PB, PRM
VPA	Oral, IV	500	500–3000	qd–tid	50–100	Weight gain, alopecia, sedation, hepatotoxicity, tremor, pancreatitis, gastric disturbance	FBM, PHT, CBZ, PB, PRM, LTG, salicylates, warfarin
PB	Oral, IV	60	60–240	qd	15–40	Drowsiness, cognitive problems, hyperkinesis, respiratory depression	PHT, VPA, CBZ, propoxyphene, warfarin
PRM	Oral	125	250–1500	bid–tid	5–12	Drowsiness, nausea, dizziness	PHT, CBZ, VPA, propoxyphene
ESX	Oral	500	500–2000	qd–bid	40–100	Nausea, vomiting, gastric distress, ataxia, drowsiness	PHT, CBZ, PB, PRM, VPA, Isoniazid
GBP	Oral	300	1200–4800	tid	Not done	Dizziness, edema drowsiness, fatigue	None
LTG	Oral	12.5–50	100–700	qd, bid	2–20	Rash, ataxia, dizziness, insomnia	OCP, VPA, PHT, CBZ, PB, OXC
TPM	Oral	25–50	100–400	qd, bid	9–12	Weight loss, mental slowing, dysnomia, kidney stones	OCP (>200 mg), PHT, CBZ, PB, VPA
OXC	Oral	150–600	900–1800	bid–tid	10–35	Hyponatremia, rash, ataxia	OCP, PHT, CBZ, PB, LTG
LEV	Oral	500–1000	2000–3000	bid	Not done	Somnolence, asthenia, psychosis	None
ZNS	Oral	100	200–400	qd, bid		Kidney stones, mental slowing, hypohidrosis	PHT, CBZ, PB
TGB	Oral	4–12	12–48	bid–qid	0.001–0.234	Dizziness, somnolence, fatigue	PHT, CBZ, PB
FBM	Oral	1200	1800–4800	tid	30–100	Aplastic anemia, hepatotoxicity	PHT, CBZ, PB, VPA, OCP
PGB	Oral	150	300–600	bid	Not done	Dizziness, edema drowsiness, weight gain, fatigue	None

CBZ, carbamazepine; ESX, ethosuximide; FBM, felbamate; GBP, gabapentin IV, intravenous; LEV, levetiracetam; LTG, lamotrigine; OCP: oral contraceptive pills; OXC, oxcarbazepine; PB, phenobarbital; PGB, pregabalin; PHT, phenytoin; PRM, primidone; TGB, tiagabine; TPM, topiramate VPA, valproic acid; ZNS, zonisamide.

TABLE 105–3 Choice of Antiepileptic Drug Based on Seizure Type

SEIZURE TYPE	FIRST LINE	SECOND LINE
Partial	Phenytoin Carbamazepine Valproic acid	Oxcarbazepine Lamotrigine Topiramate Levetiracetam Zonisamide Pregabalin
Generalized tonic-clonic	Valproic acid Topiramate	Lamotrigine Levetiracetam Zonisamide
Absence	Valproic acid Ethosuximide	Lamotrigine
Myoclonic	Valproic acid Benzodiazepines	Levetiracetam Zonisamide Lamotrigine Topiramate
Atonic	Valproic acid Benzodiazepines	Levetiracetam Zonisamide Lamotrigine Topiramate

○ Antiepileptic drugs should be instituted promptly when a seizure lasts >5 minutes and are administered sequentially if seizures are not controlled.[7]

- Start with lorazepam 0.1 mg/kg IV at 2 mg/min.
- If seizures continue, administer phenytoin (20 mg/kg IV at 50 mg/min) or fosphenytoin (20 mg/kg phenytoin equivalents IV at 150 mg/min). Fosphenytoin, a modified form of phenytoin, is water soluble, and can be administered IV or intramuscularly (IM) (phenytoin should not be given IM), has a lower incidence of cardiac complications, and is not associated with the thrombophlebitis that occurs with IV phenytoin but is considerably more expensive.
- Additional 5 to 10 mg/kg of phenytoin or fosphenytoin if seizures persist.
- If seizures continue, the patient often needs endotracheal intubation followed by phenobarbital (20 mg/kg IV at 50 to 75 mg/min).
- For refractory seizures, administer additional phenobarbital (5–10 mg/kg) and/or anesthesia with midazolam or propofol in the intensive care unit, usually with continuous EEG monitoring.
- Nonconvulsive status often responds to small doses of lorazepam or diazepam IV but, when refractory, requires additional AEDs. Anesthetics should be avoided.

MANAGEMENT OF REFRACTORY EPILEPSY

- Approximately 60% to 70% of patients become seizure-free with AED therapy. For the remaining patients with medically refractory epilepsy, treatment options include the following:

○ *Surgical treatment*: The most common type of epilepsy surgery performed is *anterior temporal lobectomy*. In some patients *lesionectomy* (tumors, vascular malformations), *hemispherectomy* (Sturge-Weber syndrome, Rasmussen disease), or *corpus callosotomy* (for atonic seizures in Lennox-Gastaut syndrome) is necessary. Before surgery, patients undergo extensive presurgical evaluation to determine if they are suitable candidates for surgery, localize the epileptic focus, and map functional areas of the brain.[8]

○ *Vagus nerve stimulation*: Intermittent electrical stimulation of the left cervical vagus nerve in combination with AED is often useful in reducing seizure frequency in patients with refractory partial onset seizures.[9] The mechanism of action is unknown. The device includes a pacemaker-like generator as well as a bipolar lead with two stimulating electrodes and is subcutaneously implanted by a surgeon.

○ *Dietary treatment*: The ketogenic diet (high in fat as well as low in protein and carbohydrate, producing an increase in ketone bodies) has been used for several decades in patients with refractory partial seizures or the Lennox-Gastaut syndrome. As with vagus nerve stimulation, the exact mechanism of action is unclear.

REFERENCES

1. Hauser WA, Hesdorffer DC. *Epilepsy: Frequency, Causes and Consequences.* New York, NY: Demos; 1990.
2. Commission on Classification and Terminology of the International League Against Epilepsy. Proposal for revised clinical classification of epileptic seizures. *Epilepsia.* 1981;22:489–501.
3. Lüders HO, Acharya JN, Baumgartner C, et al. Semiological seizure classification. *Epilepsia.* 1998;39:1006–1013.
4. Commission on Classification and Terminology of the International League Against Epilepsy. Proposal for revised clinical classification of epileptic syndromes. *Epilepsia.* 1989;30:389–399.
5. French JA, Kanner AM, Bautista J, et al. Efficacy and tolerability of the new antiepileptic drugs I. Treatment of new onset epilepsy. *Neurology.* 2004;62:1252–1260.
6. French JA, Kanner AM, Bautista J, et al. Efficacy and tolerability of the new antiepileptic drugs II. Treatment of refractory epilepsy. *Neurology.* 2004;62:1261–1273.
7. Lowenstein DH, Alldredge BK. Status epilepticus. *N Engl J Med.* 1998;338:970–976.
8. Rosenow F, Luders H. Presurgical evaluation of epilepsy. *Brain.* 2001;124:1683–1700.
9. Schachter SC, Schmidt D. *Vagus Nerve Stimulation.* 2nd ed. London, UK: Martin Dunitz; 2003.

106 HEADACHE

David J. Walsh

INTRODUCTION

Headache is one of the most common medical complaints, with a lifetime prevalence of 69% to 93% in men and 84% to 99% in women. The predominance of women with headache is largely because of their higher incidence of migraine.

The International Headache Society classifies headaches into 13 main categories with 65 subdivisions. However, for routine, clinical purposes the most common and important headaches are highlighted in this chapter.

EVALUATION

Headaches are classified according to the features that accompany them. Therefore, the history is essential in establishing the type of headache. This is quickly accomplished by noting each of the following:

- Onset (ie, When did the first headache begin?)
- Location (eg, unilateral, bilateral, ocular)
- Character of pain (eg, aching, stabbing, pressure-like, throbbing)
- Severity at onset (eg, instant, subacute, gradual)
- Intensity (eg, effect on functional activities)
- Associated symptoms (eg, nausea, vomiting, flashing lights, paresthesias, tearing, rhinorrhea)
- Duration (ie, seconds, minutes, hours, days)
- Provocations (eg, exercise, foods)
- Means of relief (eg, sleep, medications)

Recording the patient's responses to these questions is a practical and remarkable accurate approach to establish the etiology of a headache. A complete physical examination with special attention to the patients mental status, cranial nerve function, ocular fundus, strength, balance, and coordination should follow.

Routine complete blood count (CBC), urinalysis, and chemical profile in the absence of additional symptoms or signs of an underlying disease are not usually helpful. A sedimentation rate to screen for temporal arteritis, however, is an important test for patients older than 50 years of age with new onset head or neck pain. Neuroimaging is highly advised in specific circumstances (Table 106–1). Lumbar puncture (LPs) is necessary in patients with fever, chills, nuchal rigidity, immunosuppressed state, or meningeal enhancement by neuroimaging.

TABLE 106–1   Indications for Neuroimaging

Sudden onset and/or extreme worsening of pain
Change in pattern, frequency, severity of headache
Progressive headache
Headache that awakens from sleep
Impaired consciousness
Neurologic signs
Persistent localized pain
Comorbidity, eg, AIDS, malignancy, VP shunt

AIDS, acquired immunodeficiency syndrome; VP, ventriculoperitoneal.

Effective treatment is dependent on an accurate diagnosis. Multiple medications are readily available and should be promptly provided. Adequate relief should not be left to chance. Attention to dose, route of administration, frequency of use, effectiveness, and interference with daily life is necessary.

MIGRAINE HEADACHE

Migraine headache is believed to be a genetically based disorder that is more common in women. A diagnosis of migraine is suggested by the following:

- Pattern of recurrent, similar (stereotypic) headaches
- Duration of pain lasting 4 to 72 hours
- No other readily explainable etiology
- Two or more of the following characteristics:
  - Hemicranial location
  - Throbbing character
  - Interference with daily activities
  - Photophobia or phonophobia
  - Unexplained nausea and vomiting.

Migraine headache with aura consists of the above findings plus at least one reversible sign of focal neurologic dysfunction such as visual, sensory, or speech disturbances that develop over 5 or more minutes and last less than 60 minutes.

The management of migraine headache includes:

- Patient education as to nature of the headaches with assurance regarding the excellent prognosis
- Focused strategy (medications, avoidance of precipitants) for treating acute episodes and decreasing recurrence
- Developing a strategy to minimize the headaches' interference with activities of daily life

Prompt treatment of an acute migraine headache increases the likelihood of remission. Mild to moderate migraine headaches respond to a number of over-the-counter preparations (Table 106–2). The most effective, safe dose is employed and repeated as necessary. Failure to employ adequate doses of the medication is a common cause of failure. Severe migraine headaches require specific agents that have been developed in the

TABLE 106–2   Drugs for Mild to Moderate Migraine

FIRST LINE

Acetaminophen
Acetaminophen + aspirin + codeine
Aspirin
Ibuprofen
Naproxen

SECOND LINE

Acetaminophen + codeine
Chlorpromazine
Isometheptene
Ketorolac

TABLE 106–3   Specific Agents for Treatment of Migraine

Sumatriptan
Naratriptan
Rizatriptan
Zolmitriptan (± choice from Table 106–4)

TABLE 106–4   Drugs for Treating Nausea ± Vomiting in Migraine

Chlorpromazine
Metoclopramide
Odansetron
Prochlorperazine

TABLE 106–5   Migraine Rescue Medicines

Butalbital + aspirin + caffeine
Butorphanol nasal spray
Opiates

TABLE 106–6   Headache Prophylaxis

Tricyclic antidepressants
Antiepileptics (eg, valproate, topiramate)
NSAIDs
β-Blockers
Calcium channel blockers

NSAIDs, nonsteroidal antiinflammatory drugs.

TABLE 106–7   Differential Diagnosis of Thunderclap Headache

Subarachnoid hemorrhage
Pituitary hemorrhage
Intracranial hemorrhage
Cerebral venous-sinus, thrombosis
Arterial dissection
Acute hypertension
Acute glaucoma
Acute obstructive hydrocephalus

past decade (Table 106–3). A single medicine may not be consistently effective, so barring unacceptable side effects, several trials of the same medication should be utilized before changing the treatment regimen. Limitations on analgesic use should be established to minimize side effects and medication abuse.

Nausea with or without vomiting is occasionally debilitating and may interfer with medication administration. Such patients benefit from antiemetic drugs, even in the absence of vomiting (Table 106–4).

A "rescue" medication should be available for severe headaches when the usual regimen fails (Table 106–5). The ultimate goal is to minimize pain and suffering while decreasing the time to remission and recurrence rates.

Prophylactic therapy is employed when headache frequency regularly interferes with daily life or medication abuse leads to analgesic-induced headaches. Prophylactic therapy should be considered when headaches occur more often than once per week. A variety of preventive agents are available to reduce headache frequency and severity (Table 106–6).

THUNDERCLAP HEADACHE

Thunderclap headache is an excruciatingly painful headache (often described as the "worst headache in my life") that reaches its zenith within 1 minute and persists for many hours. This type of headache is seen following a subarachnoid hemorrhage (SAH) and frequently is associated with nausea, vomiting, nuchal rigidity, and impaired consciousness. Smaller SAH are associated with less severe headaches, and the examination can be normal. Nevertheless, these less severe headaches have the telltale features of abruptness and persistence and are usually bilateral. In either event, a computed tomography (CT) scan is mandatory, and, if the scan is unrevealing, a lumbar puncture is required. Not infrequently, several days or weeks before a sentinel headache, an *early warning leak* precedes the headache. These also are typically sudden, but much less severe. A majority occur while the patient is engaged in some type of physical activity. The newness, suddenness, and persistence of these headaches should alert the astute clinician to a possible subarachnoid leak. Other types of sudden onset headache should be considered once a SAH is excluded. These are summarized in Table 106–7.

TENSION-TYPE HEADACHE

Tension-type headaches are defined as lasting 30 minutes to 7 days with pain characterized by two or more of the following:

• Tight or pressing feeling
• Mild or moderate severity

- Bilateral location
- Not exacerbated by daily activities
- Nausea and/or vomiting are absent.

Unless accompanying symptoms and signs point to an underlying disease or condition, diagnostic testing is unlikely to reveal a cause. However, a change in the profile of the headache, especially the frequency, character, or intensity warrants consideration of a new or superimposed condition.

Tension headaches are often treated with the same pharmacological agents used for mild to moderate migraine headaches (see Table 106–2). Frequent or chronic tension-type headaches are better managed with a combination of prophylactic agents (see Table 106–6). The combination approach is more likely to be effective while avoiding overuse headaches and other side effects. Relaxation therapies with or without biofeedback and cognitive-behavioral techniques are also helpful for recurrent tension-type headaches.

SELECT HEADACHES

Chronic daily headache can represent chronic migraine, tension-type headache, or medication-overuse headache. The latter should be suspected when the headache occurs at least 15 days per month preceded by a 3 month history of simple analgesic use for 15 days per month, or after the use of combination analgesics or narcotics for 10 days per month. Treatment is challenging, and requires medication withdrawl, the use of prophylactic agents, attention to mood and emotional disorders, and empathy. Any patient with a chronic headache disorder should periodically be reassessed for new symptoms and signs, possible headache reclassification, or unsuspected underlying pathology.

Exertion headache is characterized by an intense, often throbbing headache that typically lasts several minutes to an hour during or after physical exercise or exertion. Exertion headaches are often prevented by β-blockers at doses used for preventing migraine. Both pre-exercise medication administration and daily regimens have been advocated. These headaches are usually short lived and remit completely.

Cluster headache is characterized by attacks of severe, piercing pain occurring unilaterally around or above the orbit or temple. One or more autonomic symptoms such as conjunctiva injection, tearing, rhinorrhea, eyelid edema, pupil changes, forehead perspiration, and marked restlessness are typically present. Cluster headache lasts 15 minutes to 3 hours and recurs several times a day or week. Recurrent

attacks persist for weeks or months and are separated by symptom-free periods. The acute attack is treated similarly to migraine headache. Oxygen at 5 to 6 L/min via a face mask for 10 to 15 minutes is also useful in terminating an attack. Verapamil is frequently effective in prevention.

Temporal arteritis is characterized by a *new* headache in a patient older than 50, often 65, years of age. Additional symptoms are oftentimes insidious and may present years before the diagnosis of temporal arteritis. These include amaurosis, diplopia, jaw claudication, neck ache, fever, malaise, weight loss, muscle aches or stiffness, and arthralgias. Examination of the temporal and other cephalic arteries for edema, tenderness and loss of pulse is essential. The sedimentation rate and C-reactive protein are frequently elevated. The diagnosis is established with a biopsy of the superficial temporal artery. Treatment with corticosteroids is important for both relief and prevention of blindness.

Postlumbar puncture headache is a headache that develops in the upright position after a lumbar puncture. The mechanism is believed to involve leakage of spinal fluid out of the punctured dura. It occurs in 13% to 32% of patients, and is minimized by using a smaller bore lumbar puncture (LP) needle (24–26 gauge), parallel insertion of the needle (bevel parallel to the long axis of the spine), replacement of the stylet before withdrawal of the needle and use of nontraumatic needles (eg, Whitacre, Sprotte). The amount of cerebral spinal fluid (CSF) removed, duration of the supine position post-LP, and increased fluid intake have not been shown to reduce the incidence of post-LP headaches. Treatment consists of bed rest. Caffeine sodium benzoate (500 mg in 1000 mL of lactated Ringer's intravenous (IV) solution) over several hours sometimes helps. Epidural blood patching is the most successful intervention.

Trigeminal neuralgia (tic douloureux) is characterized by a sudden, lancinating pain lasting seconds to minutes involving one or more distributions of the trigeminal nerve. Triggering movements or events (eg, cold breeze on cheek, brushing of the teeth) are common. Dental disease presents in a similar fashion and must be excluded. Trigeminal neuralgia commonly develops in patients after the age of 60 years. Remissions may occur, but permanent resolutions are rare. Treatment with carbamazepine, gabapentin, lamotrigine, and pregabalin is helpful. There are several surgical options in the event of medication failure.

Short duration, unilateral, neuralgic, conjunctival injection, and tearing **(SUNCT)** headaches are short (seconds to a few minutes), frequently recurring, unilateral pains around an eye or temporal region. They are frequently accompanied by red eye, tearing, and rhinorrhea and can represent an unusual presentation of a common headache disorder. Lamotrigine is thought to be the treatment of choice.

PATIENT EDUCATION

American Council for Headache Education	www.achenet.org
American Headache Society	www.ahsnet.org
National Headache Foundation	www.headaches.org

BIBLIOGRAPHY

Evans RW, Armon C, Frohman EM, Goodin DS. Assessment: Prevention of post-lumbar puncture headaches: Report of the therapeutics and technology assessment subcommittee of the American Academy of Neurology. *Neurology.* 2000;55:909–914.

Headache Classification Subcommittee of the International Headache Society. The international classification of headache disorders: 2nd ed. *Cephalgia.* 2004;24(suppl 1):1–160.

Silbestein SD. Practice parameter: Evidence-based guidelines for migraine headache (an evidence-based review): Report of the quality standards subcommittee of the American Academy of Neurology. *Neurology.* 2000;55:754–762.

Swannell AJ. Polymyalgia rheumatica and temporal arteritis: diagnosis and management. *BMJ.* 1997;314:1329–1332.

107 PERSONALITY DISORDERS

Miggie Greenberg and Mehret Gebretsadik

DEFINITIONS

- **Personality** is a stable set of intrapsychic (internal) characteristics and tendencies that determines the behavior of people. The behavior determined by personality is relatively consistent over time.
- **Personality traits** are enduring patterns of perception relating to, and thinking about the environment and oneself that are exhibited in a wide range of social and personal contexts.
- **Personality disorder** is defined in the *Diagnostic and Statistical Manual of the American Psychiatric Association, Fourth Edition (DSM-IV)*, as follows:
  ○ An enduring pattern of inner experience and behavior that differs markedly from the expectations of the individual's culture.
  ○ Long-standing and maladaptive patterns of perceiving and responding to other people and to stressful circumstances.
  ○ Pervasive and inflexible across many situations.
  ○ Has an onset in adolescence or early adulthood, is stable over time, and leads to distress or impairment
  ○ Patients with personality disorders must exhibit behavioral patterns that cause significant distress or impairment in personal, social, and/or occupational situations.

CLASSIFICATION

The DSM-IV classifies ten personality disorders, grouped into three clusters (A, B, and C). Others are classified as personality disorders not otherwise specified or secondary to general medical condition.

CLUSTER A: ODD OR ECCENTRIC

- Paranoid personality disorder: pervasive pattern of mistrust and suspiciousness.
- Schizoid personality disorder: detachment from social relationships and restricted emotional expression.
- Schizotypal personality disorder: cognitive/perceptual distortions and eccentricities; social and interpersonal deficits.

CLUSTER B: DRAMATIC, EMOTIONAL, ERRATIC

- Antisocial personality disorder: disregard for and violations of the rights of others; lack of empathy and remorse for wrongdoing.
- Borderline personality disorder: instability of interpersonal relationships, self image and affect; marked impulsivity.
- Histrionic personality disorder: excessive emotionality and attention-seeking behavior.
- Narcissistic personality disorder: grandiosity, need for admiration, and sense of entitlement.

CLUSTER C: ANXIOUS OR FEARFUL

- Avoidant personality disorder: social inhibition, feelings of inadequacy, and hypersensitivity to criticism.
- Dependent personality disorder: excessive need to be cared for, submissive behavior, and fear of separation.
- Obsessive-compulsive personality disorder: preoccupation with orderliness and perfectionism; mental and interpersonal control.

Personality disorder secondary to general medical condition: personality disorder caused by a medical condition that antedates the onset of the personality disorder.

Personality disorder not otherwise specified: a disorder that does not fulfill criteria for the above with features of one or more personality disorders.

ETIOLOGY

- Genetic: Cluster A personality disorders are more common in relatives of schizophrenia patients, cluster B in family members with mood disorders, and cluster C patients have first-degree relatives with anxiety disorders.
- Biological: evidence of abnormalities in neurotransmitter and brain area function, and personality change resulting from medical causes.
- Environmental: evidence of increased prevalence of personality disorders in individuals with dysfunctional early life experiences.

EPIDEMIOLOGY

- Personality disorders affect 10% to 15% of the adult US population. Individuals may have more than one personality disorder. The prevalence rate is higher in the clinical setting and highest in the outpatient/inpatient psychiatric setting. The following are prevalence data for specific personality disorders in the general population
  - Paranoid personality disorder: 0.5% to 2.5%
  - Schizotypal personality disorder: 3%
  - Schizoid personality disorder: perhaps as high as 7.5%.
  - Antisocial personality disorder: 3% of men, 1% of women; 75% of prisoners exhibit the features of this disorder.
  - Borderline personality disorder: 2% overall most prevalent personality disorder in general clinical settings (12–15%), accounting for 51% of all inpatients and 27% of outpatients with a personality disorder.
  - Dependent personality disorder: 2% to 4%
  - Histrionic personality disorder: 2% to 3%
  - Narcissistic personality disorder: Less than 1%
  - Avoidant personality disorder: 1% to 10%
  - Obsessive-compulsive personality disorder: 1%
- Race
  - No differences in prevalence across the races have been noted.
- Sex
  - Cluster A: Schizoid personality disorder is slightly more common in males than in females. Both paranoid and schizotypal personality disorders are more frequent in males.
  - Cluster B: Antisocial personality disorder is three times as prevalent in men as in women. Borderline personality disorder is three times as common in women as in men. Of patients with narcissistic personality disorder, 50% to 75% are male. Dependent personality is more common in women than men.
  - Cluster C: Obsessive-compulsive personality disorder is diagnosed twice as often in men than in women. Histrionic personality is more often diagnosed in women than men.
- Age
  - Personality disorders generally should not be diagnosed in children and adolescents less than 18 years of age because personality development is not complete and symptomatic traits may not persist into adulthood.
  - Because the criteria for diagnosis of personality disorders are closely related to behaviors of young and middle adulthood, DSM-IV diagnoses of personality disorders are unreliable in the elderly population.
- Mortality/Morbidity
  - Patients with personality disorders have increased morbidity/mortality due to increased rates of suicide, substance abuse, accidental injury, depression, homicide (hence legal problems), poor coping/interpersonal skills (hence poor support system and therapeutic alliance), and treatment noncompliance.

CLINICAL FEATURES

The clinical presentation varies among individuals based on the specific patients profile, comorbid psychiatric illnesses including substance abuse, past treatment history, and existing psychosocial stressors. Some are readily apparent while others are noted through a course of time. However, the core clinical features are generally consistent. A patient may fulfill the criteria for more than one personality disorder.

CLUSTER A: ODD OR ECCENTRIC

- Paranoid personality disorder: marked distrust of others, including the belief, without reason, that others are exploiting, harming, or trying to deceive them; lack of trust; belief of others' betrayal; belief in hidden meanings; unforgiving and grudge holding.
- Schizoid personality disorder: primarily characterized by a very limited range of emotion, both in expression and experience; indifferent to social relationships.
- Schizotypal personality disorder: peculiarities of thinking, odd beliefs, and eccentricities of appearance, behavior, interpersonal style, and thought (eg, belief in psychic phenomena and magical powers).

CLUSTER B: DRAMATIC, EMOTIONAL, ERRATIC

- Antisocial personality disorder: lack of regard for the moral or legal standards in the local culture, marked

social impairment, and a disregard for societal norms or rules. Sometimes called psychopaths or sociopaths.
- Borderline personality disorder: Lack of one's own identity, with rapid changes in mood, intense unstable interpersonal relationships, marked impulsively, instability in affect and in self-image.
- Histrionic personality disorder: exaggerated and often inappropriate displays of emotional reactions, approaching theatricality, in everyday behavior.
- Narcissistic personality disorder: Behavior or a fantasy of grandiosity, a lack of empathy, a need to be admired by others, an inability to see the viewpoints of others, and hypersensitive to the opinions of others.

CLUSTER C: ANXIOUS OR FEARFUL

- Avoidant personality disorder: marked social inhibition, feelings of inadequacy, and extremely sensitive to criticism.
- Dependent personality disorder: extreme dependence on others, to a point where the individual is incapable of making decisions or taking an independent position. Fear of separation and submissive behavior. Marked lack of decisiveness and self-confidence.
- Obsessive-compulsive personality disorder: characterized by perfectionism and inflexibility; preoccupation with uncontrollable patterns of thought and action.

PERSONALITY DISORDER NOT OTHERWISE SPECIFIED

- Personality disorders that do not fit in to any of the above personality categories or with features of more than one personality disorder but without the complete criteria of any one disorder.
- Personality disorders characterized by passive aggressive and depressive behavior or personality traits such as masochism, sadism, and oppositional behavior are included under this category.

PERSONALITY DISORDER SECONDARY TO GENERAL MEDICAL CONDITION

- Marked change in personality style and traits from a previous level of functioning.
- Evidence of a causative organic factor antedating the onset of the personality change.
- Structural damage to the brain is usually the cause, and head injury is the most common cause.
- Other causes include cerebrovascular disease, cerebral tumors, epilepsy (partial complex), Huntington

disease, multiple sclerosis, endocrine disorders, heavy metal poisoning, neurosyphilis, and AIDS.
- The cardinal features include emotional lability and impaired impulse control, however the sensorium remains intact and patients have minimal cognitive deficits, if at all.
- Course and prognosis depends on the cause and severity of injury. Psychopharmacological symptomatic treatment is occasionally helpful.

PHYSICAL EXAMINATION AND LABORATORY WORKUP

No specific physical findings are associated with personality disorders. The physical examination may reveal findings related to the sequelae of various personality disorders.
- Patients (particularly those with cluster B disorders) may show signs of previous suicide attempts or stigmata of substance abuse.
- Substance abuse is a common comorbidity and may be reflected in the physical stigmata of alcoholism or drug abuse.
- Suicide attempts may be accompanied by residual scars from self-inflicted wounds.

MENTAL STATUS FINDINGS

- Patients with histrionic personality disorder may display *la belle indifference*; an apparently indifferent detachment while describing dramatic physical symptoms.
- Patients with antisocial personality disorder often have hostile or oppositional behavior.
- Patients with cluster B personality disorders, principally borderline personality disorder, commonly display a labile affect.
- Patients with a paranoid personality disorder describe persecutory themes without the formal thought disorder observed in psychotic disorders such as schizophrenia.
- Patients with schizotypal personality disorder characteristically speak in odd or idiosyncratic language.

LABORATORY EVALUATION

- Toxicology screen: substance abuse is common in patients with personality disorder and substance intoxication can alter the personality of a patient.
- Screening for human immunodeficiency virus (HIV) and other sexually transmitted diseases is recommended, because these illnesses may elicit personality changes.

- Brain imaging to rule out organic causes.
- Psychological testing may prove useful as a support-ive tool or to direct the clinician toward an alternate clinical diagnosis.

COMORBIDITIES AND DIFFERENTIAL DIAGNOSIS

COMORBIDITIES

Patients with personality disorders are at higher risk than the general population for (axis I) psychiatric disorders and mood disorders. Some comorbidities are more spe-cific to particular personality disorders and clusters.

CLUSTER A

- Paranoid personality disorder can represent a prodrome to delusional disorder or frank schizophrenia. These indi-viduals are at risk for agoraphobia, major depression, obsessive-compulsive disorder, and substance abuse.
- Individuals with schizoid personality disorder may develop major depression.
- Patients with schizotypal personality disorder may develop brief psychotic disorder, schizophreniform disorder, or delusional disorder.

CLUSTER B

- Antisocial personality disorder is associated with a risk for anxiety disorders, substance abuse, somatiza-tion disorder, and pathological gambling.
- Borderline personality disorder is associated with a risk for substance abuse, eating disorders (particularly bulimia), and post-traumatic stress disorder. Suicide is a particular risk in borderline patients.
- Histrionic personality disorder is associated with somatoform disorders.
- Narcissistic personality disorder is at risk for anorexia nervosa and substance abuse as well as depression.

CLUSTER C

- Avoidant personality disorder is associated with anxi-ety disorders (especially social phobias).
- Dependent personality disorder carries a risk for anx-iety disorders and adjustment disorder.
- Individuals with obsessive-compulsive personality dis-order may be at risk for myocardial infarction because of their type A lifestyle. They may also be at risk for anxiety disorders. Notably, they are probably not at increased risk for obsessive-compulsive disorder.

DIFFERENTIAL DIAGNOSIS

- One must consider adjustment reaction, axis 1 psychi-atric disorders, central nervous system disorders, med-ical disorders, medication use, and substance abuse/dependence

THERAPEUTICS AND PREVENTION

The treatment of personality disorders is approached in the context of individual patient's dominating symp-toms, severity of illness, type of disorder, and comorbid psychiatric conditions. While psychotherapy is the main-stay of intervention for long-term improvement, biolog-ical treatments are often used to alleviate distress and acute decompensations.

Psychotherapy is at the core of care for personality disorders. Because most personality disorders induce symptoms as a result of poor or limited coping skills, psychotherapy aims to improve perceptions of and responses to social and environmental stressors.

- Psychodynamic psychotherapy examines the ways that patients perceive events, based on the assumption that perceptions are shaped by early life experiences. Psychotherapy aims to identify perceptual distortions and their historical sources and to facilitate the devel-opment of more adaptive modes of perception and response. Treatment is usually extended over a course of several years at a frequency from several times a week to once a month.
- Cognitive behavior therapy (CBT) is based on the con-cept that cognitive errors arising out of long-standing beliefs influence the meaning attached to interpersonal events. CBT examines the manner in which an indi-vidual views their world and perception of it. This very active form of therapy identifies the distortions and engages the patient in efforts to reformulate percep-tions and behaviors. This therapy is typically limited to treatment periods of 6 to 20 weeks, once weekly. In the case of personality disorders, the treatment periods are repeated often over the course of several years.
- Interpersonal therapy (IPT) identifies patients' difficul-ties as resulting from a limited range of interpersonal problems including such issues as role definition and grief. Current problems are interpreted narrowly through the screen of these formulations, and solutions are framed in interpersonal terms. Therapy is offered weekly for a period of 6 to 20 sessions.
- Group psychotherapy: interpersonal psychopathology is demonstrated during interaction with peer patients, whose feedback is used by the therapist to identify and correct maladaptive ideas, communication, and behavior. Therapy typically occurs once weekly over a course of several months to years.

- Dialectical behavior therapy (DBT) is a skill-based therapy that can be used in both individual and group formats. Primarily applied to borderline personality disorder, the emphasis of this manual-based therapy is on the development of coping skills to enhance affective stability and impulse control and on reducing self-destructive behavior. Other cluster B personality disorders with impulsive behavior can greatly benefit from this approach.

PHARMACOTHERAPY

Recent developments in neuropsychobiology and neurotransmitter biology and its relationship to the development of personality disorders has important implications for pharmacotherapy. The following neuropsychobiological concepts have emerged as the basis for pharmacotherapeutic approaches in the management of personality disorders.

- Dopamine: cognitive/perceptual distortions in schizotypal and paranoid personality disorders with high novelty-seeking behavior.
- Serotonin: impulsivity/aggression in antisocial and borderline personalities with low harm avoidance and increased risk-taking behavior.
- Noradrenaline: affect dysregulation due to low adrenergic activity in borderline personality disorder patients.
- Adrenaline: anxious and avoidant personality disorders with low threshold for activation of sympathetic arousal system.

The most effective strategies however, have been symptom based, and time limited. Symptomatic treatment focuses in three core areas including affect dysregulation, cognitive/perceptual distortion, and impulsive/behavioral dyscontrol.

- Cognitive/perceptual distortions: characterized by symptoms such as suspiciousness, paranoid ideation, ideas of reference, odd communication, muddled thinking, magical thinking, episodic distortions of reality, derealization, depersonalization, illusions, stress-induced hallucinations—treat with typical/atypical antipsychotics
- Affective dysregulation: characterized by symptoms such as lability of mood, *rejection sensitivity*, mood crashes, inappropriate intense anger, temper outbursts, chronic emptiness, dysphoria, loneliness, anhedonia, social anxiety and avoidance—treat with mood stabilizers, selective serotonin reuptake inhibitors (SSRIs), serotonin-norepinephrine reuptake inhibitors (SNRIs) and monoamine oxidase inhibitors (MAOIs).
- Impulse/behavior dyscontrol: characterized by symptoms such as sensation seeking, risky or reckless behavior, no reflective delay, low frustration tolerance, impulsive aggression, recurrent assaultive behavior, threats, property destruction, impulsive binges (drugs, alcohol, food, sex, spending), recurrent suicidal threats and behavior, self-mutilation—treat with mood stabilizers and SSRIs.

ELECTROCONVULSIVE THERAPY

- Electroconvulsive therapy (ECT) is used in personality disorders when severe depression and acute suicidality are unresponsive to other treatment options or when a rapid improvement is required to restore the patient to a reasonably functional status; typically applied to the cluster B personalities (especially borderline personality disorder).

PREVENTION

There is no proven method of preventing personality disorders. Some of the consequences and complications are avoidable if there is consideration of the following:

- Inquiries about suicidal ideation with subsequent inquiry about firearms, lethal medications, and other available means of suicide should be regularly assessed.
- Drugs with potential for dependency, such as benzodiazepines and narcotic analgesics should be used rarely and with great caution.
- Patients with personality disorder who have children should be asked frequently and in detail about their parenting practices. Their low frustration tolerance, externalization of blame for psychological distress, and impaired impulse control put the children of these patients at risk for neglect or abuse.

COURSE AND PROGNOSIS

- Personality disorders are lifelong conditions.
- Attributes of cluster A and B personality disorders tend to become less severe in middle age and late life.
- Patients with cluster B personality disorders are particularly susceptible to substance abuse, impulse control, and suicidal behavior, which may shorten their lives.
- Cluster C characteristics tend to become exaggerated in later life.
- Complications of personality disorders include suicide, substance abuse, accidental injury, depression, and homicide (a potential complication, particularly in paranoid and antisocial personality disorders)

BIBLIOGRAPHY

Personality disorders: In Sadock BJ, Sadock VA, eds. *Kaplan and Sadock's Synopsis of Psychiatry.* 9th ed. Philadelphia, PA: Lippincott Williams & Wilkins; 2003;800–821.

Smallwood P. Personality disorders. In: Stern TA, Herman JB, eds. *Massachusetts General Hospital Psychiatry Update and Board Preparation.* 2nd ed. New York, NY: McGraw-Hill; 2004: 187–194.

Tyrer P, Bateman AW. Drug treatment for personality disorders. *Advances in Psychiatry Treatment.* 2004;10:389–398.

Ward RK. Assessment and management of personality disorders. *Am Fam Physician.* 2004;70:1505–12.

108 SEXUAL AND GENDER IDENTITY DISORDERS

Sundeep Jayaprabhu and George T. Grossberg

SEXUAL DEVELOPMENT

- Sexuality is influenced by four factors:
  1. Sexual identity in all mammalian embryos is anatomically female during early fetal life; fetal androgens are responsible for the differentiation of male from female.
  2. Gender identity is established by the age of 2 to 3 years.
     - *Gender role* is defined as the speech or actions that one uses to disclose himself or herself as a boy, man, girl, or woman, largely derived from gender identity.
  3. Sexual orientation is defined by the object of sexual impulses: heterosexual, homosexual, or bisexual.
  4. Sexual behavior is a psychophysiologic experience; according to Diagnostic and Statistical Manual of Mental Disorders, 4th edition, Text Revision (DSM-IV-TR) the four-phase sexual response cycle includes desire, excitement, orgasm, and resolution.

SEXUAL DISORDERS

- Sexual disorders are divided by the DSM-IV-TR into two major categories:
  1. *Sexual dysfunction*: an impairment of the sexual response cycle.
  2. *Paraphilias*: intense and recurrent sexual urges or behavior that involve unusual activities or objects and are associated with marked distress.

SEXUAL DYSFUNCTION

- Sexual dysfunction is a psychophysiological impairment of sexual desire and/or of the sexual response cycle.
  - General categorizations include lifelong versus acquired type, generalized versus situational type, psychologic factors versus physiologic versus combined type.
  - DSM-IV-TR classifies seven major types of sexual dysfunction:
    1. Sexual desire disorders
    2. Sexual arousal disorders
    3. Orgasmic disorders
    4. Sexual pain disorders
    5. Sexual dysfunction secondary to general medical condition
    6. Substance-induced sexual dysfunction
    7. Sexual dysfunction not otherwise specified
  - Table 108–1 summarizes the sexual response cycle and associated dysfunctions.
  - Meta-analysis reveals that sexual dysfunction is higher in women (43%) than men (31%).[1]

SEXUAL DESIRE DISORDERS

- Hypoactive sexual desire disorder:
  - A deficiency or absence of sexual fantasies and the desire for sexual activity, diagnosis should only be considered when it is distressing to the patient.
  - More common than sexual aversion disorder, more common among women, prevalence of low levels of sexual interest among women is between 17% and 55%.[2]
  - Sample of 1493 women revealed that 71% were sexually active in the past year with a sexual activity frequency of monthly or less in 37%, weekly in 33% and daily in 1%.[1]
- Sexual aversion disorder:
  - An aversion to and avoidance of genital sexual contact with a sexual partner; severity and duration of symptoms should be taken into consideration.
  - Lack of desire is a common complaint among married couples seeking sex therapy, usually affecting women more than men.
  - Inhibition of desire may be a defense for unconscious fears about sex.

SEXUAL AROUSAL DISORDERS

- A chronic or recurrent inability to attain or maintain an adequate erection in males and adequate lubrication or swelling response in females until sexual activity is completed.
  - Female sexual arousal disorder:
    - Prevalence is likely underestimated but is approximated at between 8% to 15% with at least three studies reporting a prevalence of 21% to 28%.[2]

TABLE 108–1   Sexual Response Cycle and Associated Pathology

PHASES	CHARACTERISTICS	DYSFUNCTIONS
1. Desire	Involves patient's motivations, personality, and drives; distinct in the lack of physiologic descriptions	Hypoactive sexual desire disorder, sexual aversion disorder, hypoactive sexual desire caused by a general medical condition, substance-induced sexual dysfunction with impaired desire
2. Excitement	Sense of sexual pleasure with associated physiologic changes	Female sexual arousal disorder, male erectile disorder, male erectile disorder caused by a general medical condition, substance-induced sexual dysfunction with impaired arousal
3. Orgasm	Climax of sexual pleasure associated with a rhythmic contraction of perineal muscles and pelvic reproductive organs as well as release of sexual tension	Female orgasmic disorder; male orgasmic disorder, premature ejaculation, other sexual dysfunction caused by a general medical condition, substance-induced sexual dysfunction with impaired orgasm
4. Resolution	A feeling of general well-being and muscle relaxation; males have a refractory period that increases in length with age during which orgasms are not possible; females, however, may have multiple orgasms without a refractory period	Postcoital dysphoria, postcoital headache

SOURCE: Adapted from Sadock B, Sadock V. Sexual dysfunctions, paraphilias, and gender identity disorders. In Sadock B, Sadock V. *Kaplan & Sadock's Pocket Handbook of Clinical Psychiatry.* 3rd ed. New York, NY: Lippincott Williams & Wilkins; 2001:188.

- Psychologic causes include guilt, anxiety, and fears.
- Physiologic causes include hormonal abnormalities (testosterone, estrogen, and prolactin), increased serotonin, decreased dopamine, low thyroxin levels, and the use of drugs with anticholinergic activity.
- Hormonal imbalances may induce excitement phase dysfunction.
- A study by Masters and Johnson found that woman had increased sexual desire prior to onset of menses.[3]
- Male erectile disorder (ED):
  - Random worldwide prevalence rates of ED in men younger than 40 years of age is 1% to 9%, 40 to 59 years of age 2% to 9% with some studies revealing rates as high as 20% to 30%, 60 to 69 years of age 20% to 40%, and men 70 to 90 years of age have a prevalence of 50% to 75%.[2] Lifelong ED is rare, occurring in approximately 1% of males younger than age 35.[3]
  - The causes of ED are generally classified into organic versus psychologic, or a combination of both.
  - History of spontaneous erections, morning erections, or erections at times other than with the subjects partner suggest a functional/psychologic etiology.
  - The best test to discriminate between a psychological or organic etiology is via monitoring of *nocturnal penile tumescence,* during rapid eye movement sleep.

ORGASMIC DISORDERS
- In females, characterized by the inability to achieve orgasm by either masturbation or coitus.
  - Kinsey reports that only 5% of married women older than age 35 years have never achieved orgasm; moreover, the first orgasm achieved occurs during adolescence in 50% while masturbating. Other studies report that 46% of women have difficulty achieving orgasm.[3]

- Reported prevalence rates in the United States, Australia, England, and Sweden are approximately 25% in women ages 8 to 74 years.[2]
  - Conscious or unconscious factors may contribute to orgasmic disorders including fears of rejection by the partner, damage to the vagina, and impregnation; anger toward males; and guilty feelings about the subjects sexual desires.
- In males, orgasmic disorders are characterized by failed or difficult ejaculation during coitus.
  - Considered lifelong if a male has never achieved ejaculation; while acquired if the disorder occurs after a normal period of functioning.
  - Prevalence rates in United States and France are between 7% and 8%.[2]

PREMATURE EJACULATION
- Premature ejaculation is defined as orgasm and ejaculation earlier then desired by the male.
- Prevalence rates for early ejaculatory disturbances range from 9% to 31%,[2] and is more common among college-educated males.[3]
- Premature ejaculation is the chief complaint in 35% to 40% of males treated for sexual disorders.[3]
- Psychologic considerations include fear of the vagina, anxiety about intercourse, negative cultural influences, and stressors in the patient's life.

SEXUAL PAIN DISORDERS
- Vaginismus:
  - Involuntary muscle contractions of the outer third of the vagina that interferes with penile insertion and intercourse.
  - More commonly described in women with higher education or in higher socioeconomic groups.

○ Causes include conscious or unconscious fears of the penis, views on sex, traumatic sexual experiences in the past, or life stressors.

• Dyspareunia:

○ Persistent or recurrent genital pain in either sex that occurs during or around the time of intercourse.

○ Characterized by similar psychodynamic factors as described with vaginismus.

○ Rarely occurs in males; usually associated with an organic condition (prostatitis, Peyronie disease, or herpes).

○ Repeated episodes of dyspareunia may precipitate vaginismus and vice versa.

SEXUAL DYSFUNCTION CAUSED BY A GENERAL MEDICAL CONDITION

• Male ED can be caused by several general medical conditions

○ Between 20% and 50% of men with ED have an organic/medical basis.[3]

○ Organic conditions (Table 108–2) and numerous medications have been implicated in ED.

○ Procedures used to differentiate organically induced impotence from psychologic or functional impotence include the following:

 ▪ Monitoring nocturnal penile tumescence.

 ▪ Using a strain gauge to monitor tumescence.

 ▪ Performing penile plethysmography or ultrasonography to measure the blood pressure in the penis.

 ▪ Nerve conduction studies to determine the pudendal nerve latency time.

○ Other labs/tests useful during the evaluation include: glucose tolerance test; plasma hormone assays; liver function tests; thyroid function tests; prolactin levels follicle-stimulating hormone levels; cystometric studies; testosterone levels.

• Dyspareunia:

○ Approximately 30% of all genital surgical procedures in women result in temporary dyspareunia, and 30% to 40% of women attending sex therapy clinics for dyspareunia reveal pelvic pathology.[3]

○ A recent analysis revealed that 29% of women and 45% of men report that rectal surgery impaired their sexual lives and the most common reported

TABLE 108–2   Medical Disorders Implicated in Erectile Dysfunction

Cardiovascular diseases:	**Infectious and parasitic diseases:**
Atherosclerosis	Elephantiasis
Aortic aneurysm	Mumps
Leriche syndrome	**Genetic disorders:**
Cardiac failure	Klinefelter syndrome
Neurologic disorders:	Congenital penile vascular/structural abnormalities
Multiple sclerosis	**Nutritional disorders:**
Transverse myelitis	Malnutrition
Parkinson disease	Vitamin deficiencies
Temporal lobe epilepsy	**Pharmacologic agents:**
Traumatic and neoplastic spinal cord diseases	Alcohol and other dependence-inducing substances (heroin, methadone, morphine, cocaine, amphetamines, and barbiturates)
Central nervous system tumor	Prescribed medications (psychotropic, antihypertensive, estrogens, and antiandrogens)
Amyotrophic lateral sclerosis	**Poisoning:**
Peripheral neuropathy	Lead
General paresis	Herbicides
Tabes dorsalis	**Surgical procedures:**
Endocrine disorders:	Perineal prostatectomy
Diabetes mellitus	Abdominal-perineal colon resection
Dysfunction of pituitary-adrenal-testis axis	Sympathectomy
Acromegaly	Aortoiliac surgery
Addison disease	Radical cystectomy
Chromophobe adenoma	Retroperitoneal lymphadenectomy
Adrenal neoplasia	**Miscellaneous:**
Myxedema	Radiation therapy
Hyperthyroidism	Pelvic fracture
Renal and urologic disorders	Any severe systemic disease or debilitating condition
Peyronie disease	
Chronic renal failure	
Hydrocele and varicocele	
Pulmonary disorders:	
Respiratory failure	
Hepatic disorders:	
Cirrhosis	

SOURCE: Adapted from Sadock B, Sadock V. Sexual dysfunctions, paraphilias, and gender identity disorders. In Sadock B, Sadock V. *Kaplan & Sadock's Pocket Handbook of Clinical Psychiatry.* 3rd ed. New York, NY: Lippincott Williams & Wilkins; 2001:191.

problem was lubrication for women (56%) and impotence for men (52%); both genders reported a negative body image.[4]

- Vulvar vestibulitis and interstitial cystitis may cause dyspareunia but without obvious physical findings.
- Hypoactive sexual desire disorder caused by a general medical condition:
  - Sexual desire commonly decreases after major illness or surgery, especially if body image suffers (eg, mastectomy, prostatectomy).
  - Some studies suggest abnormalities in biochemical markers; one study found lower serum testosterone levels in men with decreased sexual desire compared to controls.[3]
- Other female sexual dysfunctions caused by a general medical condition:
  - Medical conditions implicated in female sexual dysfunction include hypothyroidism, diabetes mellitus, and primary hyperprolactinemia.
  - Medications that may interfere with a normal orgasm in females include antihypertensives, central nervous system stimulants, tricyclic drugs, selective serotonin reuptake inhibitors (SSRIs), monoamine oxidase inhibitors, and dopamine receptor antagonists.
- Other male sexual dysfunctions caused by a general medical condition:
  - Organic causes implicated in male orgasmic disorder include genitourinary surgery (prostatectomy), Parkinson disease, and other neurologic disorders.
  - Medications which have been implicated in failed ejaculation include guanethidine monosulfate (Ismelin®), phenothiazines, methyldopa (Aldomet®), tricyclic medications, and SSRIs.
  - *Retrograde ejaculation* should be considered in the differential of failed ejaculation. Importantly, retrograde ejaculation is always secondary to an organic cause; for example, anticholinergic medications including thioridazine (Mellaril®) and phenothiazines are relatively common causes of retrograde ejaculation.

SUBSTANCE-INDUCED SEXUAL DYSFUNCTION

- Initially, small doses of some agents may enhance sexual performance, but continued use generally impairs sexual performance.
- Alcohol increases desire by removing inhibition but impairs performance.
- Cocaine and amphetamines produce similar effects as alcohol with an initial increase in energy and desire but eventual dysfunction; men experience prolonged erections without ejaculation but sustained cocaine use is associated with ED.
- Substances of abuse also interfere with relationships and impair social and sexual skills.

SEXUAL DYSFUNCTION NOT OTHERWISE SPECIFIED

- Include sexual dysfunctions not described by the aforementioned categories.
- In men, this may include orgasmic anhedonia and in women one may encounter a condition similar to premature ejaculation in men.
- Can include compulsive or coitus/genital pain with masturbation.

TREATMENTS

- Analytically oriented sex therapy:
  - Analytically oriented sex therapy is one of the most effective treatment modalities especially when integrated with sex therapy.
  - Fears and desires are considered similarly in both psychodynamic/psychoanalytic therapy and sex therapy.
- Behavioral techniques and exercises:
  - The goal of therapy is to gain verbal and sexual communication between the patient and his/her partner and increase intimacy.
  - Techniques should not be performed in the presence of a therapist.
  - Behavioral techniques are successful 40% to 85% of the time.[3]
  - Dysfunction-specific techniques and exercises:
    - Vaginismus: The woman is instructed to use her fingers or dilator to gently dilate the vaginal orifice
    - Premature ejaculation: The coronal ridge of the glans is squeezed during impending ejaculation.
    - Female orgasmic disorder (primary anorgasmia): The woman is encouraged to employ fantasies as she masturbates or uses a vibrator.
    - Male erectile disorder: The subject is encouraged to masturbate to demonstrate that erection is possible.
    - Retarded ejaculation: Extravaginal masturbation leading to ejaculation followed by a gradual introduction into the vaginal orifice and vaginal ejaculation.
- Biological therapy:
  - Pharmacotherapy.
    - Erectile disorder/premature ejaculation: Sildenafil (Viagra) augments penile blood flow via an increased synthesis of nitrous oxide; oral prostaglandins (Vasomax), injectable phentolamine alprostadil (Caverject), and transurethral alprostadil suppository (Muse) are also used; consider leveraging the side-effect profile of SSRIs and antidepressants which are associated with ED and retarded ejaculation.
    - Sexual aversion disorder: SSRIs and tricyclic antidepressants have proven useful.
  - Surgical options include penile implants and revascularization.

PARAPHILIAS

- Paraphilias are defined as abnormal expressions of sexuality that can range from near normal to destructive behavior (Table 108–3).
- The DSM-IV-TR characterizes these impulses as clinically significant only if they are associated with significant emotional distress, impairment of relationships, or if the subject has acted on these impulses.
- Pedophilia is the most common, with a high risk of repeat offenses; studies suggest that more than 50% of women and 20% of men in the United States will be sexually assaulted some time in their life.[5]
- Treatment includes the following:
  - Self-help groups are based on the 12-step concept of Alcoholics Anonymous (AA), and include Sexaholics Anonymous (SA), Sex and Love Addicts Anonymous (SLAA), and Sex Addicts Anonymous (SAA).
  - Insight-oriented and supportive psychotherapy, cognitive behavioral therapy, and couples therapy aid in understanding and repairing psychological damage.
  - The routine use of pharmacotherapy is not recommended because substance dependence is a common comorbid condition; SSRIs may reduce libido and assist with the compulsive aspect of illness, eg, medroxyprogesterone acetate decreases libido in men.

GENDER IDENTITY DISORDERS

- Gender identity is defined as the innate consciousness of being male or female and, usually, corresponds to one's biological sex.
- Limited information is available regarding epidemiology, but trends point toward a greater vulnerability to gender identity problems in males.
- Diagnosis of gender identity disorder according to the DSM-IV-TR focuses on persistent and intense distress about one's gender assignment or the insistence that he/she is of the opposite sex.
- In children with gender identity disorder, their manner of play is commonly typical of that of the opposite sex.

TABLE 108–3   Paraphilias

DISORDER	DEFINITION	GENERAL CONSIDERATIONS	TREATMENT
Exhibitionism	Exposing genitals in public	Often desire is to shock a female and reaffirm that his penis is present and/or intact	Insight-oriented psychotherapy; aversive conditioning
Fetishism	Sexual arousal with inanimate objects	Usually in men; accompanied by guilt	Insight-oriented psychotherapy; aversive conditioning, implosion (eg, masturbatory satiation)
Frotteurism	Rubbing genitals against female to achieve arousal and orgasm	Usually performed by passive men in crowded places	Insight-oriented psychotherapy; aversive conditioning; group therapy
Pedophilia	Sexual activity with children younger than age 13	Most common paraphilia; 95% heterosexual, 5% homosexual; high risk of repeat offenses; often accompanied by fear of adult sexuality and low self-esteem	Place patient in treatment unit; group therapy; insight-oriented therapy; antiandrogen medication
Sexual masochism	Sexual pleasure with humiliation or from being physically/emotionally abused	Defense against guilt about sex; punishment turned inward	Insight-oriented therapy; group therapy
Sexual sadism	Sexual arousal with inflicting physical or mental pain/suffering to another person	Named after Marquis de Sade; can progress to rape	Insight-oriented psychotherapy; aversive conditioning
Transvestic fetishism	Cross-dressing	Often used in heterosexual arousal; not the same as trans-sexualism: wanting to be opposite sex	Insight-oriented psychotherapy
Voyeurism	Sexual arousal by watching sexual acts; variant is scatologia	Masturbation occurs during voyeurism	Insight-oriented psychotherapy; aversive conditioning
Other paraphilias:			
Excretory paraphilias	Coprophilia or urophilia on partner or vice versa	Fixation at anal stage; may use enemas-klismaphilia	Insight-oriented psychotherapy
Zoophilia	Sex with animals	More common in rural areas	Behavior modification; insight-oriented psychotherapy

SOURCE: Adapted from Sadock B, Sadock V. Sexual dysfunctions, paraphilias, and gender identity disorders. In Sadock B, Sadock V. *Kaplan & Sadock's Pocket Handbook of Clinical Psychiatry.* 3rd ed. New York, NY: Lippincott Williams & Wilkins; 2001:199.

- In adolescents and adults, the expression of gender identity disorder may extend from wearing clothes and engaging in activities of the opposite sex to seeking surgery to alter physical characteristics to that of the opposite sex.
- Course and prognosis depends on the age of onset and intensity of symptoms.
  - Homosexuality is encountered in one-third to two-thirds of gender identity disorder cases.[3]
  - Homosexuality is more common in males than females for unclear reasons.
- Treatment is complex and controversial.
  - Sex-reassignment surgery:
    - A permanent procedure, therefore, appropriate preparations are recommended prior to undergoing surgery, in particular, cross-gender living for 3 to 12 months.
    - Approximately 50% who satisfy criteria follow through with surgery.[3]
    - One study suggests satisfaction rates with surgery of 87% in males converting to female and 97% in females converting to male.[6]
    - Suicide has been reported in up to 2% of subjects postsurgery.[3]
  - Hormonal treatment:
    - Estrogen for biological males, testosterone for biological females.
    - Clinicians should monitor for the development of hypertension, hyperglycemia, hepatic dysfunction, and thromboembolic disease while on hormonal therapy.
  - Controversial issues include consent to treatment in intersex infants, societal norms, and transference/countertransference.

REFERENCES

1. Sadock B, Sadock V. Sexual dysfunctions, paraphilias, and gender identity disorders. In Sadock B, Sadock V. *Kaplan & Sadock's Pocket Handbook of Clinical Psychiatry*. 3rd ed. New York, NY: Lippincott Williams & Wilkins; 2001:187.
2. Addis I, Van Den Eeden S, Wassel-Fyr CL, et al. Sexual activity and function in middle-aged and older women. *Obstet Gynecol*. 2006;107:4.
3. Lewis R, Fugl-Meyer K, et al. Epidemiology/risk factors of sexual dysfunction. *J Sex Med*. 2004;1:1.
4. Hendren S, O'Connor B, et al. Prevalence of male and female sexual dysfunction is high following surgery for rectal cancer. *Ann Surg*. 2005;242:2.
5. Grossman L, Martis B, Fichtner C. Are sex offenders treatable? A research overview. *Psychiatr Serv*. 1999;50:3.
6. Wylie K. ABC of sexual health: gender related disorders. *BMJ*. 2004;329:615–617.

109 MOOD, ANXIETY, SLEEP, AND EATING DISORDERS

Stacy Neff

MOOD DISORDERS

A person's emotional state can vary from day to day depending on various circumstances (eg, weather, stressors, financial issues, etc). When these variations cause marked distress or dysfunction they can lead to pathological states characterized by disturbances in mood. Mood disorders can vary from deeply depressed to exorbitantly elevated. The major subclassifications of mood disorders include unipolar depression, bipolar affective disorder, dysthymia, and cyclothymia.

LIFETIME PREVALENCE

- Major depressive disorder (MDD): 10% to 25% for women, 5% to 12% for men
- Dysthymic disorder: 6%
- Bipolar type I disorder: 0.4% to 1.6%
- Bipolar type II disorder: 0.5%
- Cyclothymic disorder: 0.4 to 1.0%

The diagnosis of a mood disturbance is established by confirming specific symptoms and signs through a detailed history and physical examination. There are several screening instruments (eg, Beck Depression Inventory), but these are generally not used to diagnose depression, but rather establish the severity and extent of symptoms. The history should elicit the following:

- Onset and duration of symptoms.
- Job stressors.
- Relationships and losses.
- Financial stressors.
- Past psychologic history.
- Family psychologic history.
- Importantly, remediable causes of depression such as adrenal or thyroid dysfunction must be ruled out.
- Substance use.

Medical conditions that are commonly associated with depression include:

- Hypothyroidism
- Fibromyalgia
- Chronic pain syndromes
- Diabetes mellitus
- Chronic fatigue syndrome
- Corticosteroid use
- Hypercalcemia

- Chronic, sustained illness of almost any type (cancer, connective tissue diseases, arthritis, heart failure, etc.)

The risk factors associated with the development of depression include:

- Female gender.
- Previous history or family history of depressive illness.

Several neurologic conditions that promote depression, include:

- Parkinson disease
- Dementia
- Seizure disorders
- Cerebrovascular disease
- Cancers

The most common feature of the mood disorders is depression; a persistent lowering of mood with loss of interest in outside activities and decreased ability to experience pleasure. The major feature(s) that distinguishes the different mood disorders is the severity of the depression and the presence of manic episodes.

EPIDEMIOLOGIC FACTORS

- The female-to-male ratio for MDD is 2:1.
- No difference is noted between gender for the bipolar disorders.
- The peak onset of depression is between the ages of 20 to 50 years. Depression also occurs in the geriatric population and is often undiagnosed; however, the incidence is lower in persons older than age 65 years.
- Manic symptoms usually develop by age 45 years (organic causes should be considered if mania occurs at a later age, the average onset for a bipolar disorder is 30 years of age).
- No differences are noted between races.
- There is a higher incidence in those without close interpersonal relationships and those that are either divorced or separated.
- There is *no* correlation between MDD and socioeconomic status.
- There *does* appear to be a higher incidence of bipolar type I disorder in upper socioeconomic groups.

MAJOR DEPRESSIVE DISORDER

Criteria for the diagnosis of MDD is based on the *Diagnostic and Statistical Manual of Mental Disorders, 4th edition, Text Revision (DSM-IV-TR)*. At least five symptoms listed below during the same 2-week period must be present and be associated with either depressed mood or loss of interest or pleasure. The following mnemonic, SIG E CAPS (Give Energy CAPSules is useful.

- (S) change in sleep (insomnia or hypersonic)
- (I) decreased interest

- (G) inappropriate guilt or feelings of worthlessness
- (E) decreased energy or fatigue
- (C) decreased concentration
- (A) change in appetite (decreased or increased)
- (P) psychomotor agitation (observed by others, not self-reported)
- (S) recurrent thoughts of death

Treatment can include psychotherapy, pharmacotherapy, or a combination of both. Antidepressants can require up to 4 to 6 weeks to achieve a maximal effect on mood.

- First-line agents include the selective serotonin reuptake inhibitors (SSRIs) (fluoxetine, paroxetine, sertraline, citalopram, and escitalopram) and should be selected primarily on the basis of their side-effect profile and duration of action (long-acting vs short acting). For example, fluoxetine (Prozac) has a long half-life and has a stimulant effect; therefore it is an excellent choice for a patient who is poorly compliant. Conversely, fluoxetine would be less desirable in a patient exhibiting anxiety.
- Other antidepressants include tricyclic antidepressants (TCAs), monoamine oxidase inhibitors (MAOIs), serotonin-norepinephrine reuptake inhibitor (SNRIs) (venlafaxine and duloxetine), bupropion, and mirtazapine.
- When one class of antidepressant fails to improve symptoms, a different class should be considered. If a partial response with one class is attained, adding an agent from a different class may induce an additive effect.
- Patients with refractory depression or those that cannot tolerate pharmacotherapy can benefit greatly from electroconvulsive therapy (ECT). ECT is sometimes initiated in patients with severe depression while awaiting for the full effects of pharmacotherapy.

DYSTHYMIC DISORDER

Dysthymia is common in the general population and is more common in younger, unmarried, and lower socioeconomic individuals. It can coexist with other disorders, including MDD. Dysthymia is considered a subclinical variant of depression that must persist for at least 2 years and be associated with an insidious onset and progression. Patients often complain that they have been depressed for years. Psychotherapy is the mainstay of treatment, however, pharmacotherapy with antidepressants can offer benefit to select patients.

MINOR DEPRESSIVE DISORDER

Those patients who do not meet the full diagnostic criteria for MDD (less than five but at least two of the nine symptoms) and exhibit symptoms for at least 2 weeks, are diagnosed with minor depression. Atypical depressives often experience hypersomnia and hyperphagia rather than insomnia and loss of appetite. Patients with atypical depression may respond well to the MAOIs or bupropion.

When patients present with depression, the clinician **must screen for suicidal risk**.

- Inquire about suicidal ideation and specific plans (the more lethal, the greater the risk).
- Determine if the patient has the means to carry out the act and the lethality of the method (Example: If a patient states that they are going to shoot themselves, ask if they possess a firearm).
- Determine whether psychotic symptoms are also present?
- Substance abuse is more commonly associated with suicide.
- Establish whether previous suicide has been attempted and the details of the event.
- Establish a family history or recent exposure to suicide.
- Suicidal risk is sometimes difficult to establish. In general, patients with an elaborate and lethal plan, those with psychotic symptoms (auditory hallucinations) and those who are noncompliant with their medications or have had a previous unsuccessful attempt should be considered at the highest risk. Such patients should be immediately hospitalized and aggressively managed with cognitive therapies and pharmacologic interventions.

BIPOLAR AFFECTIVE DISORDER

This disorder is characterized by a fluctuation in mood between the extremes of mania and major depression. According to the *DSM-IV-TR,* manic features include the following (note the mnemonic, DIG FAST):

- (D) distractibility
- (I) increase in goal-directed activity (eg, cleaning, writing a book, painting, etc.)
- (G) grandiosity or self-inflated esteem
- (F) flight of ideas or subjective experience of racing thoughts
- (A) activities: excessive involvement in pleasurable activities that have a high potential for painful consequences (eg, sexual indiscretions, gambling, reckless driving)
- (S) decreased need for sleep (awakening after only 2- to-3 hours of sleep)
- (T) more talkative or pressure to continue talking
- These symptoms must cause significant impairment in social, occupational, or other functioning.

Bipolar disorder cannot be diagnosed with the first episode of depression as it cannot be differentiated from MDD. Therefore, the diagnosis can only be established after the first manic episode. The disturbed mood must persist for at least 1 week. When the severity and duration of the manic symptoms do not meet *DSM-IV-TR* criteria, then the mania is known as hypomania and the patient is considered to have type II bipolar disorder.

Treatment includes the use of the mood stabilizer class of drug.

- Mood stabilizers include lithium, divalproex, aborigine, topiramate, and carbamazepine.
- Lithium, divalproex, and olanzapine (an antipsychotic) are standard treatments for the mania phase.
- Adjunctive therapies for the mania phase include sedatives such as clonazepam, lorazepam, haloperidol, olanzapine, and risperidone.
- The use of antidepressants without a mood stabilizer or antipsychotic agent could lead to a manic episode.

CYCLOTHYMIA

Cyclothymia is considered a less severe variant of bipolar disorder type II, characterized by a mania phase alternating with mild depression. Patients with cyclothymia often have multiple interpersonal difficulties. *DSM-IV-TR* criteria indicate that the symptoms must be present for at least 2 years, and patients must experience alternating periods of hypomania and depression, without criteria for MDD. The symptoms cannot be absent for more than 2 months at time.

Other less common mood disorders highlighted in the *DSM-IV-TR* include:

- Minor depressive disorder: fewer than five of the nine symptoms for MDD for at least 2 weeks.
- Recurrent brief depressive disorder (sometimes precipitated by life stressors).
- Premenstrual dysphonic disorder.
- Mood disorder caused by a general medical condition (eg, Parkinson systemic lupus erythematosus [SLE], hypothyroidism).
- Substance-induced mood disorder.
- Mood disorder not otherwise specified (NOS).

PSYCHOSIS

Psychosis is defined as a disturbance in one's perception of reality. These patients can experience hallucinations (auditory, visual, or tactile), delusions, or thought disorganization. They can easily be agitated and become aggressive. Psychosis can be present in either major depressive disorder or bipolar affective disorder.

ANXIETY DISORDERS

The most common anxiety disorders and their lifetime prevalence are as follows:
- Generalized anxiety disorder (GAD): 5%
- Panic disorder: 1.5% to 5%
- Social phobia: 3% to 13%
- Specific phobia: 11%
- Obsessive-compulsive disorder (OCD): 2% to 3%
- Post-traumatic stress disorder (PTSD): 8% of the general population (up to 75% in high-risk groups such as war veterans)

EPIDEMIOLOGY

- There is a 2:1 female-to-male ratio in GAD.
- Social phobia has a 3:2 female-to-male ratio.
- Specific phobias have a 2:1 female-to-male ratio.
- Social phobia rarely presents after age 25 with a peak incidence between the ages of 11 and 15 years.
- There is a 3:1 female-to-male ratio in panic disorder (possibly because men are less likely to report the symptoms).
- Panic disorder can occur at any age, but the mean age of presentation is 25 years.
- OCD occurs equally among adults, but in adolescence is more common in boys.
- The mean age of onset for OCD is approximately age 20 years.

Anxiety disorders are extremely common and can cause marked distress which interferes with daily activities.

GENERALIZED ANXIETY DISORDER

A detailed history should focus on the following:
- Possible medical causes (hyperthyroidism, pheochromocytoma, SLE, congestive heart failure [CHF], cerebrovascular disease, substance abuse or withdrawal, side effects of medications).
- Comorbid psychiatric disorders.
- Detailed social history including stressful events and possible abuse.

The Diagnostic criteria for GAD includes excessive anxiety occurring more often than not for at least 6 months, that is difficult to control and causes marked distress or impairment in social, occupational, or other areas of functioning. The anxiety must be associated with three or more of the following symptoms:
- Restlessness
- Easily fatigued
- Difficulty with concentration
- Irritability

- Muscle tension
- Sleep disturbance (other than hypersomnia)

The treatment of GAD consists of psychotherapy, pharmacotherapy, or both. First-line psychotherapy involves cognitive behavioral therapy. Pharmacotherapy includes:
- Antidepressants: SNRIs (venlafaxine, duloxetine), SSRIs (paroxetine, sertraline, citalopram, escitalopram, fluoxetine), and TCAs (imipramine, nortriptyline). Importantly, the maximal effects of these agents may require several weeks to manifest. In addition, the side effects of these drugs can mimic the symptoms of anxiety; therefore, the dose should be titrated slowly.
- Venlafaxine, paroxetine, escitalopram are the only antidepressants that are approved by the Food and Drug Administration (FDA) for the treatment of GAD. However, many other agents appear to exert beneficial effects on the symptoms of anxiety. In general, the selection of a particular agent is based on its side-effect profile.
- Benzodiazepines: Not considered first-line agents for long-term therapy because of abuse potential; can be useful in the short-term because other medications require up to 6 weeks to exert their maximal effect.
  - Short-acting benzodiazepines can cause rebound anxiety between doses.
- Buspirone: Can be effective for anxiety, however, it requires 4 to 6 weeks to exert its maximal effect.
- Medication selection should also be based on the presence of comorbid conditions. For example, the antidepressants would be a good choice in patients who are depressed. Conversely, benzodiazepines should be used cautiously in patients with a substance-abuse history.

PANIC DISORDER

One panic attack does not constitute panic disorder. The *DSM-IV-TR* criteria for the disorder consist of the following:
- Recurrent attacks.
- Fear of a recurrent attack for at least 30 days following at least one attack.
- Cannot be attributed to a medical condition or substance abuse.
- Causes a significant change in behavior specifically during the attacks.

The symptoms of panic attack consist of a discrete period of intense fear or discomfort with at least four of the following symptoms, occurring abruptly and peaking within 10 minutes:
- Palpitations
- Diaphoresis

- Trembling
- Shortness of breath
- Sensation of choking
- Chest pain or discomfort
- Nausea or abdominal pain
- Feeling dizzy, unsteady, or lightheaded
- Feelings of unreality or feeling detached from oneself
- Fear of losing control
- Fear of dying or impending sense of doom
- Paresthesias
- Chills or hot flushes

Panic disorder can be diagnosed with or without agoraphobia.

The *DSM-IV-TR* criteria for agoraphobia include:
- Anxiety about being in a place or situation where escape may be difficult or embarrassing in the event of panic-like symptoms.
- Behavior modified to avoid situations.
- The anxiety cannot be attributed to another mental disorder.

Panic attacks can occur spontaneously or can be precipitated by excitement, physical exertion, sexual activity, or emotional trauma.

Treatment involves the use of pharmacotherapy and cognitive- behavioral therapy. Pharmacotherapy includes:
- SSRIs: All are effective for panic disorder but require several weeks to exert their maximal effect.
- TCAs: Less widely used than SSRIs because of their adverse effects.
- Benzodiazepines: Rapid onset of action, therefore they are useful to alleviate symptoms acutely. However, the benzodiazepines have significant abuse potential. Tapering off the benzodiazepine must occur slowly or a withdrawal syndrome associated with increased anxiety may be precipitated.

Cognitive-behavioral therapy includes the following:
- Educating the patient to identify and respond to dysfunctional thoughts. A variety of techniques (relaxation, biofeedback) are used to facilitate improved understanding that permits an awareness of aberrant thoughts coupled with coping mechanisms to deal with disordered thoughts and beliefs.

SOCIAL PHOBIA

The criteria for a social phobia are as follows:
- Specific phobia in which a patient has marked distress or fear for one or more social situations in which the person may be scrutinized or surrounded by unfamiliar people.
- Exposure to the situation causes severe anxiety and results in avoidance of the situation or engenders significant distress at or during the situation.
- The patient must recognize this fear as unjustified, and that this belief interferes with the individuals normal routine.

- The duration of the phobia must exceed at least 6 months in patients younger than 18 years of age.
- This fear or anxiety cannot be attributed to another medical or other mental disorder.
- If a medical or mental disorder is present, the fear must be clearly unrelated.

Panic attacks frequently occur in concert with phobias, but unlike panic disorder, social phobias are anticipated.

The treatment for social phobia includes both psychotherapy and pharmacotherapy. The same medications used in GAD can be effective for social phobia. Additionally, when the social phobia is associated with performing (such as public speaking), β-blockers administered just prior to the performance reduce symptoms. The most commonly used agents are atenolol and propranolol.

SPECIFIC PHOBIAS

Specific phobias are characterized by intense fear that is precipitated by specific objects or situations and have been grouped into five categories: (1) animal type, (2) natural environment type (heights), (3) blood-injection-injury type (injections), (4) situational type (planes), and (5) other.
- Natural environment type are more common in children younger than 10 years of age.
- Situational type occurs in patients in their early 20s.
- Blood-injection-injury type is often characterized by autonomic dysfunction (bradycardia and hypotension preceded by tachycardia) at the onset of anxiety.

Some specific phobias include:
  ◦ Acrophobia, fear of heights
  ◦ Agoraphobia, fear of open places
  ◦ Ailurophobia, fear of cats
  ◦ Hydrophobia, fear of water
  ◦ Claustrophobia, fear of closed spaces
  ◦ Cynophobia, fear of dogs
  ◦ Mysophobia, fear of dirt and germs
  ◦ Pyrophobia, fear of fire
  ◦ Xenophobia, fear of strangers
  ◦ Zoophobia, fear of animals

The most effective treatment for phobias is behavioral therapy. Other potential therapeutic treatments include hypnosis, supportive therapy, and family therapy.

OBSESSIVE-COMPULSIVE DISORDER

- This disorder is characterized by recurrent obsessions or compulsions that cause severe distress.
- The obsession or compulsions are time consuming and interfere with daily living.
- Patients may have an obsession, compulsion, or both.

- Obsessions are linked to a patients thoughts, feelings, or sensations. They are recurrent and intrusive. By *DSM-IV-TR* criteria, the patient attempts to ignore or suppress these thoughts, impulses, or images.
- Compulsions are behaviors that are conscious and recurrent. These behaviors are aimed at reducing anxiety.
- OCD has four major symptom patterns:
  - Contamination: There is an obsession to avoid a contaminated object or a compulsion to cleanse (washing hands).
  - Pathological doubt: The obsession is doubt (eg, locked door), followed by the compulsion to repeatedly examine.
  - Intrusive thoughts: These thoughts are often about acts of aggression or sex that the person finds repulsive. They are not accompanied by compulsions to act.
  - Symmetry: The obsession about symmetry or precision followed by the compulsion to organize.
- Other patterns include religious obsessions and hoarding.
- Treatment for OCD includes pharmacotherapy, behavioral therapy, psychotherapy, and for extreme or treatment-resistant cases, ECT and psychosurgery.
- ECT is not considered as effective as psychosurgery, but because it is less invasive, it is often utilized prior to surgery.
- The surgical procedure of choice for OCD is a cingulotomy, which can be successful in up to 30%.
- Some patients will notice a relief of symptoms immediately following surgery, but symptoms may recur after several months.

POST-TRAUMATIC STRESS DISORDER

There are several factors that appear to predispose to PTSD.
- Presence of childhood trauma.
- Personality disorders: borderline, paranoid, dependent, and antisocial.
- Poor family or social support system.
- Female gender.
- Other psychiatric illnesses in the family or genetic vulnerability.
- Recent stressful life changes.
- External locus of control rather than an internal locus of control.
- Alcohol abuse.
  There are four major components of PTSD as follows:
- Traumatic event: The person must have either experienced or witnessed an event that involved either actual or threatened death or injury and reacted with intense fear, helplessness, or horror.

- The traumatic event is experienced again via intrusive recollections, dreams, feeling as if the event were recurring, or exposure to events similar to the initial event that causes intense psychologic distress or physiologic reactions.
- Avoidance of stimuli associated with the trauma: includes avoidance of thoughts or feelings, activities, loss of recall regarding important aspects of the trauma, diminished interest in activities, feeling of detachment, restricted affect, or sense of foreshortened future.
- Increased arousal: difficulty falling or staying asleep, irritability or outbursts of anger, difficulty with concentration, hypervigilance, or exaggerated startle response.
- The duration of the above symptoms must be present for at least 1 month and cause significant distress in functioning. When a person has experienced these symptoms but does not meet the timeline (>1 month), the diagnosis is consistent with acute stress disorder.
  Treatment involves primarily psychotherapy. Therapeutic approaches include behavior therapy, cognitive therapy, supportive therapy, and hypnosis. Abreaction can also be useful. This is a technique that encourages the patient to experience the emotions associated with the traumatic event. Pharmacotherapy can be used to reduce the associated anxiety and depression that accompanies the disorder.

SLEEP DISORDERS

Sleep disorders are primarily classified into two categories: dyssomnias and parasomnias. By definition, primary disorders cannot be caused by another mental disorder, physical condition, or substance. These disorders are caused by an abnormal sleep-wake mechanism.

DYSSOMNIAS

- Primary insomnia: difficulty initiating or maintaining sleep for at least 1 month, occurring at least three times per week.
- Primary hypersomnia: Excessive somnolence for at least 1 month; patients do not complain about the quality of sleep or daytime sleepiness. There is no evidence of an abnormal sleep-wake cycle or aberrant sleep architecture.
- Narcolepsy: Excessive daytime sleepiness and abnormal manifestations of rapid eye movement (REM) sleep occurring daily for at least 3 months. The attacks can last up to 20 minutes and occur two to six times a day. This includes hypnologic (predormital) and hypnopompic (postdormital) hallucinations, cataplexy, and sleep paralysis. Onset of REM sleep occurs within 10 minutes.

- Breathing-related sleep disorder: any breathing disorder that results in disruption of the normal sleep pattern, such as obstructive or central sleep apnea, and central alveolar hypoventilation syndrome.

Treatment is directed at correcting the underlying disturbance. Patients should be educated regarding effective sleep hygiene including:
- Retiring to sleep at the same time (especially important for those working odd shifts) every day.
- Awakening at the same time every day.
- Avoid stimulating activities near bedtime (heavy exercise).
- Avoid stimulants (caffeine and alcohol).
- Avoid daytime napping.
- Eliminate distracting noises.
- Darken the bedroom.

Pharmacologic treatment of insomnia includes agents specifically designed for inducing sleep. Medications associated with sedation are appropriate in select patients. The following drugs are useful in the management of insomnia:
- Zolpidem
- Zaleplon
- Trazodone
- Mirtazapine
- TCAs
- Temazepam
- Chlorohydrate
- Anticonvulsants
- Atypical antipsychotics
- Antihistamines

Pharmacologic treatment of hypersomnia includes the use of stimulants.

Breathing disorders should be evaluated with sleep studies and treated accordingly (see Chapter 117).

PARASOMNIAS

The most common parasomnias include nightmare disorder, sleep terror disorder, and sleepwalking disorder.
- Nightmare disorder consists of nightmares occurring during REM sleep.
- Sleep terror disorder occurs early (usually during the first third of the sleep cycle) and during nonrapid eye movement (NREM) sleep. Patients afflicted will often scream and have intense anxiety. They often fall back to sleep immediately, but occasionally will remain awake and disoriented. They will not remember the episode. This occurs more often in children.
- Sleepwalking disorder (somnambulism) occurs during the first third of the night during NREM sleep. The sleepwalker will often go about performing ordinary tasks (walking, talking, driving, cooking, and eating)

during the episode. The person may awaken during the event with some confusion, but typically will return to bed without any awareness of his or her activities.

EATING DISORDERS

EPIDEMIOLOGY

- Eating disorders can occur in as many as 4% of adolescent and teenage students.
- The age of onset is almost always in the mid-teens; however, up to 5% can present in their early 20s.
- Anorexia nervosa can occur in as many as 0.5% to 1% of adolescent girls.
- The female-to-male ratio in anorexia nervosa is 10 to 20:1.
- Anorexia nervosa is more common in developed countries.
- Bulimia nervosa is more common than anorexia nervosa and occurs in 1% to 3% of young women.
- The female-to-male ratio in bulimia nervosa is 10:1.
- Bulimia nervosa occurs in later adolescence compared to anorexia nervosa.
- The percentage of females that do not meet the full criteria for either anorexia nervosa or bulimia nervosa is estimated to be 5% and 40%, respectively.

ANOREXIA NERVOSA

- Often associated with other mental disorders: depression, 65%; social phobia, 34%; OCD, 26%.
- Some studies have shown that administration of opioid antagonists result in dramatic weight gain, suggesting that endogenous opioids influence satiety.
- Multiple factors influence the incidence of anorexia: biologic, social, psychologic, and psychodynamic factors.
  - Biologic factors include: endogenous opioids (as noted above); hypothalamic-pituitary axis dysfunction eg., dysfunction in serotonin, dopamine, and norepinephrine (involved in regulating eating behavior in the par ventricular nucleus of the hypothalamus).
  - Social factors include peer pressure with an emphasis on appearance and thinness.
  - Psychologic and psychodynamic factors suggest that anorexia may reflect the adolescents desire to establish independence. These patients tend to lack autonomy and view self-starvation as a mechanism to gain control.
- The *DSM-IV-TR* criteria for establishing the diagnosis of anorexia nervosa are as follows:
  - Failure to maintain 85% of expected body weight.
  - Intense fear of gaining weight or appearing overweight.

○ Impaired view of one's own body, low self-esteem usually related to the patients perception of their body, and denial of the serious consequences of a very low body weight.
○ Amenorrhea.
○ Subtypes include restricting type and binge-eating/purging type:
  ▪ Restricting type: no binge-eating or purging behavior.
  ▪ Binge-eating/purging type: during the episode, binge/ purging behavior has occurred.
  ▪ Patients with restricting type are more likely to have obsessive-compulsive traits.
  ▪ Patients with binge/purging type are more likely to be involved with substance abuse and prone to poor impulse control and personality disorders.

• The objective signs and medical complications are as follows:
○ Cachexia
○ Hypothermia
○ Dependent edema
○ Bradycardia
○ Hypotension
○ Lanugo
○ Hypokalemic alkalosis (because of self-induced vomiting)
○ Electrocardiographic (ECG) changes include: flattening or inversion of T waves, ST-segment depression, and lengthening of the QT interval (likely as a result of the associated electrolyte disorders)
○ Erosion of dental enamel (because of induced vomiting)
○ Seizures (because of large fluid shifts and electrolyte disturbances)
○ Mild neuropathies
○ Fatigue and weakness
○ Mild cognitive disorder
○ Amenorrhea
○ Leukopenia
○ Osteoporosis

• Course and prognosis of anorexia nervosa:
○ Restricting type is less likely to be associated with spontaneous recovery.
○ Short-term response to hospitalization is good, however, most patients continue their previous preoccupation with food and weight.
○ Mortality is 5% to 18%.
○ One-half of those with anorexia will develop symptoms of bulimia.

• Treatment consists of the following:
○ Hospitalize to treat medical complications (dehydration, hypokalemia).
○ Treatment of the underlying condition should be focused on psychotherapy, both individual and family.

○ Medications have a limited, but important role. Some medications that have been employed include: cyproheptadine, amitriptyline, clomipramine, pimozide, chlorpromazine, and flextime.

BULIMIA NERVOSA

• Bulimia refers to binge eating.
• Patients with bulimia are similar to patients with anorexia (they are concerned about appearance and weight gain); however, unlike anorexics; they tend to maintain normal body weight.
• Patients will often binge eat and then participate in compensatory behaviors (eg, induced vomiting, laxative use, diuretics, enemas or other medications, fasting, and excessive exercise).
• The binge eating and compensatory behavior occur approximately twice per week for 3 months.
• Postbinge anguish (depression) often follows a purging episode.
• Unlike anorexics, bulimics may still be sexually active.
• Those that engage in purging activities are at risk for metabolic disturbances, as well as gastric and esophageal tears.

Treatment involves cognitive-behavioral therapy, dynamic psychotherapy, and pharmacotherapy. Compared to anorexia nervosa, antidepressants such as the SSRIs, TCAs, and MAOIs are reasonably effective in patients with bulimia nervosa. Other medications that have been found to be helpful in bulimia include topiramate and odansetron. Lithium and naltrexone have been recently studied, but have not been successful compared to placebo.

BIBLIOGRAPHY

Ciechanowski P, Katon W. Overview of generalized anxiety disorder. www.uptodate.com.

Ciechanowski P, Katon W. Overview of phobic disorders. www.uptodate.com.

Rosenbaum J, Arana G, Hyman S, et al. *Handbook of Psychiatric Drug Therapy.* 5th ed. Philadelphia, PA: Lippincott Williams & Wilkins; 2005.

Sadock B, Sadock V. Anxiety disorders. In Edmondson J, Gabbard G, Grebb J, et al, eds. *Kaplan & Sadock's Synopsis of Psychiatry Behavioral Sciences/Clinical Psychiatry. 9th ed.* Philadelphia, PA: Lippincott Williams & Wilkins; 2003: 591–642.

Sadock B, Sadock V. Eating disorders. In Edmondson J, Gabbard G, Grebb J, et al, eds. *Kaplan & Sadock's Synopsis of Psychiatry Behavioral Sciences/Clinical Psychiatry. 9th ed.* Philadelphia, PA: Lippincott Williams & Wilkins; 2003:739–755.

Sadock B, Sadock V. Mood disorders. In Edmondson J, Gabbard G, Grebb J, et al, eds. *Kaplan & Sadock's Synopsis of Psychiatry Behavioral Sciences/Clinical Psychiatry. 9th ed.* Philadelphia, PA: Lippincott Williams & Wilkins; 2003:534–590.

Sadock B, Sadock V. Normal sleep and sleep disorders. In Edmondson J, Gabbard G, Grebb J, et al, eds. *Kaplan & Sadock's Synopsis of Psychiatry Behavioral Sciences/Clinical Psychiatry. 9th ed.* Philadelphia, PA: Lippincott Williams & Wilkins; 2003:739–755.

Stovall, Jeffrey M.D. Bipolar Disorder. www.uptodate.com.

110 SCHIZOPHRENIA AND OTHER PSYCHOTIC DISORDERS

Harmeeta K. Singh and Jothika N. Manepalli

INTRODUCTION

The major symptom of these disorders is *psychosis*, which encompasses disorders of thought, delusions, and/or hallucinations, these symptoms lead to impairment of reality. Psychotic disorders include *schizophrenia, brief psychotic disorder, schizophreniform disorder, schizoaffective disorder, delusional disorder,* and *shared psychotic disorder.*

DISORDERS OF THOUGHT

DISRUPTION IN THE THOUGHT PROCESS
• Illogical ideas.
• Thought blocking (abrupt halt in train of thought, often caused by hallucinations).
• Deficiencies in thought or content of speech.
• Impaired abstraction ability.
• Neologisms.

DISRUPTION IN THE FORM OF THOUGHT
• Incoherence.
• Word salad (unrelated combinations of words/phrases).
• Loose associations (ideas shift from one subject to another in an unrelated fashion).
• Paucity of speech.
• Echolalia (parroting a word just spoken by someone else).

DELUSIONS

Delusions are *fixed false beliefs* that are not correctable by reason or logic and are not based on simple ignorance or shared by a culture/subculture. These false beliefs significantly hinder a person's ability to function. (eg, believing that people are trying to inflict harm when there is no objective evidence to support the belief; believing oneself to be a famous or powerful individual, such as Jesus Christ or the president).

HALLUCINATIONS

Hallucinations are *false perceptions*. They can be *visual* (seeing shadows of dead people), *auditory* (hearing voices), *olfactory* (smelling odors), *tactile* (a sensation of bugs crawling on the body), or *cenesthetic* (sensations from the viscera).

SCHIZOPHRENIA

DSM-IV-TR CLASSIFICATION

• A. *Characteristic symptoms*: two or more of the following symptoms present for 1 month:
  ◦ *Delusions*
  ◦ *Hallucinations*
  ◦ *Disorganized speech* (frequent derailment or incoherence)
  ◦ *Grossly disorganized* or *catatonic behavior*
  ◦ *Negative symptoms* (affective flattening, alogia, or avolition)
  NOTE: *Only 1 Criterion A symptom is required if delusions are bizarre or hallucinations consist of a voice maintaining a running commentary of the person's behavior or thoughts, or 2 or more voices conversing with each other.*
• B. Decline in social and/or occupational functioning.
• C. Continuous signs of the disturbance for at least 6 months with at least 1 month of active symptoms.
• D. Schizoaffective/mood disorder has been excluded.
• E. Substance abuse/general medical condition has been excluded.
• F. If there is a history of autistic disorder or another pervasive development disorder, the additional diagnosis of schizophrenia is made only if prominent delusions or hallucinations are present for at least 1 month.

SCHIZOPHRENIA SUBTYPES

Subtypes are defined by the *predominant symptomatology* at the time of the evaluation.
• Paranoid type: Preoccupation with 1 or more *delusions* or frequent *auditory hallucinations* with none of the

following predominant: disorganized speech, disorganized or catatonic behavior, or flat or inappropriate affect.

- Disorganized type: *All* of the following are prominent—*disorganized, speech, disorganized behavior, and flat or inappropriate affect.* Criteria are not met for catatonic type.
- Catatonic Type—Characterized by at least *two* of the following:
  1. Motor immobility characterized by *catalepsy, waxy flexibility,* or *stupor.*
  2. *Excessive purposeless motor activity* which is not influenced by internal stimuli.
  3. *Extreme negativism* (motiveless resistance to all instructions or maintenance of rigid posture against attempts to be moved) or *mutism.*
  4. Peculiarities of voluntary movement as seen in *posturing* (voluntary assumptions of inappropriate or bizarre postures), stereotyped movements, prominent mannerisms, or prominent grimacing.
  5. *Echolalia* or *echopraxia*
- Undifferentiated type: schizophrenia in which symptoms that meet *Criterion A* are present, but criteria are *not* met for paranoid, disorganized or catatonic types.
- Residual type:
  1. *Absence* of prominent delusions, hallucinations, disorganized speech, and grossly disorganized or catatonic behavior, with
  2. *Continuing* evidence of the disturbance, as indicated by the presence of negative symptoms or 2 or more symptoms listed in Criterion A for schizophrenia, present in an *attenuated* form (eg, odd beliefs/unusual perceptual experiences).

PREVALENCE OF SCHIZOPHRENIA

- 50% for monozygotic twins suggesting a genetic predisposition.
- 40% for individuals with two parents with a previous diagnosis of schizophrenia.
- 12% for first-degree relatives of schizophrenic patients.
- 1% of the world's population is affected by schizophrenia.
- 2.5 million Americans have the disease; it has no gender, racial, cultural, or economic boundaries.
- *Age of onset:* Symptoms appear between the ages of 13 and 35 years, often earlier in males compared to females (ages 25–35).
- 10% to 13% suicide rate—Similar to the suicide rate in depressive illnesses (schizophrenia is associated with *comorbid depression* which can be severe and debilitating).
- *Life expectancy:* 10-year shorter lifespan than the general population related to lifestyle issues (poor nutrition, lack of exercise, smoking, substance abuse, decreased access to medical care, and higher suicide rate).

CAUSES OF SCHIZOPHRENIA

The etiology, although incompletely understood, likely involves a combination of genetic and environmental factors. Hyperactive dopaminergic systems have long been implicated in the development of schizophrenia. Nonetheless, there is little other than circumstantial evidence to support this hypothesis. Other theories have implicated brain structure (perhaps occurring during development) and various comorbid conditions such as antecedent *viral infections* and *immune-mediated disorders.* Internal or external stress may precipitate relapses and exacerbations of the illness.

EARLY WARNING SIGNS OF SCHIZOPHRENIA

Highly individualized symptoms may develop slowly over months or years, or may appear abruptly. The disease may be characterized by cyclic patterns with many relapses followed by remissions. Specific early warning signs include:

- Hearing or seeing something that is not confirmed by others.
- Constant sensation of being watched.
- Peculiar or nonsensical manner of speaking or writing.
- Strange body positioning.
- Feeling indifferent toward important situations.
- Deterioration of academic or work performance.
- Change in personal hygiene and appearance.
- Change in personality.
- Withdrawal from social situations.
- Irrational, angry or fearful response to loved ones.
- Inability to sleep or concentrate.
- Inappropriate or bizarre behavior.
- Extreme preoccupation with religion or the occult.

POSITIVE SYMPTOMS OF SCHIZOPHRENIA

Characterized by *excessive function* which respond to atypical and traditional antipsychotic medications. These symptoms are not unique to schizophrenia and may be indistinguishable from drug withdrawal or psychosis associated with manic- depressive illness. Positive symptoms include:

- *Delusions:* Delusions are the most common positive symptom (60–70%); themes of *persecution* are especially common.

- *Hallucinations*—visual, emotional, gustatory, auditory, or odor perception. Auditory hallucinations are the most common and are often characterized by voices that communicate *commands* or *comments* to the individual.
- *Disorganized thought process and speech:* Moving from one topic to another in a nonsensical fashion. Individuals often craft their own words/sounds (*neologisms*).
- *Strange behavior.*
- *Psychomotor activity/agitation.*

NEGATIVE SYMPTOMS

Characterized by *loss of function;* these symptoms respond better to atypical antipsychotics.
- *Social withdrawal*
- *Extreme apathy*
- *Amotivation/avolition*
- *Emotional unresponsiveness*
- *Thought blocking*
- *Flattened affect*
- *Cognitive disturbances*
- *Poor grooming/hygiene*

DIFFERENTIAL DIAGNOSES

MEDICAL
- Temporal lobe epilepsy: prominent *visual* and *gustatory* hallucinations associated with an *aura*.
- Neurological disease/trauma: prominent *visual* hallucination associated with *delirium* features.
- Poisoning: visual and tactile hallucinations, delirium features are possible.
- Endocrine disorders: hypothyroidism/pheochromocytoma.

PSYCHIATRIC
- *Brief psychotic disorder:* duration of symptoms is 1 day to 1 month.
- *Schizophreniform disorder:* symptoms last at least 1 month (but less than 6 months).
- *Schizoaffective disorder:* psychosis associated with mood symptoms.
- *Manic phase of bipolar disorder:* grandiose delusions with mood congruent auditory hallucinations.
- *Delusional disorder:* Nonbizarre delusions which involve situations that occur in real life (eg, being followed, poisoned, having an illness, deceived by spouse/lover) lasting at least 1 month.
- *Schizoid and schizotypal personality disorder:* psychotic features are absent.

OTHERS
- *Substance abuse* (hallucinogens/amphetamines).

BRAIN PATHOLOGY ASSOCIATED WITH SCHIZOPHRENIA

- Decreased size of the amygdala, hippocampus, and parahippocampal gyrus.
- Movement problems implicate the basal ganglia.
- Lateral and third ventricular enlargement have been characterized.
- Abnormal cerebral symmetry.
- Changes in brain density.
- Abnormalities of the frontal lobes as evidenced by decreased uptake of glucose in the prefrontal cortex on positron-emission scanning.

NEUROTRANSMITTERS IMPLICATED IN SCHIZOPHRENIA

- Dopamine: associated with hyperactivity
  - Increased number of dopaminergic receptors
  - Increased dopamine concentration
  - Hypersensitivity of receptors to dopamine
- Serotonin: associated with hyperactivity
  - Hallucinogens that increase serotonin levels cause psychotic symptoms
  - Atypical antipsychotics have antiserotonergic activity (5HT-2)
- Norepinephrine: associated with hyperactivity
  - Implicated in paranoid type
- γ-aminobutyric acid (GABA): Patients with schizophrenia have a decreased number of GABA-ergic neurons in the hippocampus
- Glutamate
  - Glutamate antagonists increase the symptoms of schizophrenia
  - Glutamate agonists decrease the symptoms of schizophrenia

TREATMENT OF SCHIZOPHRENIA

PHARMACOLOGICAL TREATMENT
- *Traditional/Conventional Antipsychotics:* (also known as neuroleptics) are D-2 receptor antagonists. Please see Table 110–1 below for the common agents in this group and Table 110–2 for side-effect profiles. These agents can produce sedation, orthostatic hypotension, anticholinergic side-effects, such as urinary retention, constipation, and mental confusion. Other side effects include weight gain, type 2 diabetes mellitus, leukopenia, elevated liver enzymes, jaundice, tachycardia, and QT abnormalities.

TABLE 110–1 Conventional and Atypical Antipsychotics

AGENTS	DOSE RANGES (MG/DAY)	
Conventional High Potency		
Haloperidol (Haldol)	2–100 mg	Depot preparation 50–100 mg once a month
Fluphenazine[a]	5–60 mg	Depot preparation 12.5–100 mg every 3–6 wk
Thiothixene (Navane)	5–60 mg	
Trifluoperazine[a]	5–40 mg	
Conventional Medium Potency		
Perphenazine[a]	8–64 mg	
Loxapine (Loxitane)	30–250 mg	
Molindone (Moban)	50–225 mg	
Conventional Low Potency		
Chlorpromazine[a]	100–800 mg	
Thioridazine[a]	100–800 mg	
Atypical		
Risperidone (Risperdal)	0.5–6 mg	
Olanzapine (Zyprexa)	5–30 mg	
Quetiapine (Seroquel)	25–800 mg	
Ziprasidone (Geodon)	40–160 mg	Start with 20–40 mg twice daily
Aripiprazole (Abilify)	5–30 mg	
Clozapine (clozaril)		
First of atypicals, used for refractory schizophrenia	25–900 mg	-Restricted access in U.S. -Agranulocytosis and seizures are serious reactions

[a]Available as generic only.

- Hyperprolactinemia is common and causes amenorrhea, galactorrhea, and sexual dysfunction (such as impotence and decreased libido). Most distressing are the extrapyramidal symptoms (EPS).
- Low-potency agents have prominent anticholinergic and antihypertensive side-effects; whereas high potency agents are associated with prominent EPS. Employing the smallest effective dose and monitoring closely for complications is advisable.
- Extrapyramidal symptoms:
  ○ Parkinsonian symptoms: resting tremor, akinesia, and rigidity
  ○ Acute dystonia: slow, prolonged muscular spasms most commonly seen in males younger than 40 years of age.
  ○ Akathisia: subjective feeling of motor restlessness
  ○ Neuroleptic malignant syndrome (NMS): High fever, sweating, confusion, increased blood pressure and pulse, muscular rigidity, high creatine phosphokinase (CPK), and renal failure. NMS has a 20% mortality rate; it is more common in males and tends to develop early in the course of pharmacotherapy.
  ○ Tardive dyskinesia (TD): writhing (choreoathetoid) movements of tongue, head, face, and mouth. TD is more common in older females and does not generally occur in the first *6 months* of antipsychotic treatment.
- *Second generation/atypical antipsychotics:* These agents are now considered first-line drugs because of their favorable side effect profile (little anticholinergic-like activity, lower incidence of EPS symptoms, and

TABLE 110–2 Side Effect Profile of Available Antipsychotics

SIDE EFFECT	NEUROLEPTIC	CLOZAPINE	RISPERIDONE	OLANZAPINE	QUETIAPINE	ZIPRASIDONE	ARIPIPRAZOLE
Anticholinergic	+/− to +++	+++	+/−	+	+/−	+/− to +	+/−
EPS	+/− to +++	0 to +/−	0 to +/−	0 to +/−	0 to +/−	0 to +/−	0 to +/−
Orhtostatic hypotension	+ to −++	+++	++	+	+ to ++	+ to +++	+
Prolactin elevation	++ to +++	0	++	0 to +/−	0 to +/−	0 to +/−	0 to +/−
Sedation	+ to +++	+++	+	++	+ to ++	+ to ++	0
Seizures	+/− to ++	++	+/−	+/−	+/−	+/−	+/−
Weight gain	+ to ++	+++	++	++ to +++	++	+/− to ++	0 to +/−

TABLE 110–3   Receptor Binding Profile of Atypical Antipsychotics (* = lease, **** = greatest)

DRUG	DOPAMINE D1	D2	SEROTONIN 5 HT - 1A	5 HT - 2A	MUSCARINIC M1	ADRENERGIC a1	HISTAMINIC H1	NOREPINEPHRINE NE
Clozapine	***	***	*	****	****	****	****	0
Risperidone	***	****	**	****	0	****	***	0
Olanzapine	****	****	*	****	****	****	****	0
Quetiapine	*	****	****	****	0	****	****	0
Ziprasidone	**	****	**	****	0	****	***	***
Aripiprazole	*	****	**	****	0	**	**	0

little effect on prolactin levels). These agents ameliorate both positive and negative symptoms associated with schizophrenia. These agents are referred to as atypical because they interfere with neurotransmitter systems other than the dopaminergic system. Table 110–3 summarizes the receptor-binding characteristics of these agents.

- Risperidone at higher doses can cause EPS. Ziprasidone is associated with a mean QTc increase of 21 milliseconds. Table 110–4, shows the mean increases in QTc of various agents. Accordingly, these agents must be used with caution in patients with underlying cardiac disease or rhythm disturbances.
- Atypical agents are metabolized via the cytochrome P450 isoenzyme system, and accordingly may interact with many other medications. They have also been associated with hypercholesterolemia, hyperglycemia, and weight gain. It is advisable to educate the patient on dietary control and to monitor weight, serum glucose and lipid panels periodically.
  ○ *Clozapine (Clozaril):* first *atypical antipsychotics* approved.
    ▪ Indications: Treatment-resistant schizophrenia and patients who are considered at high risk for suicidal behavior.
    ▪ Black Box Warning and side effects: Black Box Warning for *drug-induced agranulocytosis* (1%). The *National Clozapine Registry* monitors patients on Clozapine. Weekly blood cell counts are advised for patients for 6 months then biweekly thereafter. Clozapine also carries a Black Box Warning for seizures and myocarditis.

TABLE 110–4   QTc Interval of Various Agents

DRUG	DOSE (mg)	INCREASE IN QTc (msec)
Thioridazine	300	36
Ziprasidone	160	20
Quetiapine	800	14.5
Risperidone	16	11.6
Olanzapine	20	6.8
Haloperidol	15	4.7

ELECTROCONVULSIVE THERAPY

- Electroconvulsive therapy (ECT) is the treatment of choice in the following settings:
  ○ Severe psychosis requiring rapid control.
  ○ Patient's exhibiting significant side-effects or are otherwise sensitive to standard medications.
  ○ Patient that are intolerant of medications.

PSYCHOLOGICAL TREATMENT STRATEGIES

- Case management
- Family education
- Psychosocial rehabilitation programs
- Self-help groups
- Housing programs
- Employment programs
- Therapy/counseling
- Crisis services

CAUSES FOR RELAPSE IN SCHIZOPHRENIA

The most common cause of a relapse in the schizophrenic patient is noncompliance with the medication and follow-up regimen. Individuals who suffer from this illness lack insight and therefore often feel that they do not require medications. Auditory hallucinations may promote noncompliance by suggesting that the patient discontinue medications (because they are "poisons" or simply not necessary). Depot injections are available with haloperidol (Haldol) decanoate (monthly), fluphenazine (Prolixin) decanoate (monthly), and risperidone (Risperdal) Consta (biweekly). The depot formulations minimize noncompliance and simplifies the medication regimen. Depot injections are especially useful for long-term maintenance therapy.

PROGNOSIS FOR SCHIZOPHRENIA

- Chronic, life-long impairment is the rule.
- While no cure currently exists, patients with this illness can lead productive and fulfilling lives with the proper treatment including medications and rehabilitation programs.
- *Improved prognosis:* Female patients, prominence of mood symptoms, older age of onset, married with

social support, good employment history, positive symptoms, and few relapses.

INDICATIONS FOR HOSPITALIZATION

- Psychotic symptoms that prevent the patient from caring for his/her basic needs.
- Suicidal ideation: usually secondary to psychosis or comorbid depression.
- Command-type hallucinations to harm oneself or others should be hospitalized especially if patient has a history of acting on the hallucinations.
- Danger to themselves or others.

BRIEF PSYCHOTIC DISORDER

DSM-IV-TR CRITERIA

- A. At least 1 of the following:
  - *Delusions*
  - *Hallucinations*
  - *Disorganized speech*
  - *Grossly disorganized or catatonic behavior*
- B. *Duration of Symptoms*: At least 1 day to 1 month after which the individual returns to their previous level of functioning.
- C. Mood disorder with psychotic features, substance abuse, schizoaffective disorder, schizophrenia, or other medical conditions have been ruled out.

This is a *rare* disorder that has a sudden onset usually precipitated by a psychosocial stressor and is seen in the younger age group (25–35 years of age). Brief psychotic disorder has a higher incidence in patients with borderline and histrionic personality disorders. Mood and affect may be labile and associated with higher risk for suicide. The treatment usually involves brief hospitalization and a short course of neuroleptics to control psychosis (eg, risperidone 2-4 mg) with benzodiazepines as an adjunct (lorazepam). Supportive psychotherapy is beneficial in conjunction with psychopharmacology. 50% to 80% of individuals recover completely whereas 20% to 50% may ultimately develop classic schizophrenia or a mood disorder.

SCHIZOPHRENIFORM DISORDER

DSM-IV-TR CRITERIA

- A. Individual meets *Criterion A* for schizophrenia with at least 2 of the following:

- Delusions, hallucinations, disorganized speech, grossly disorganized or catatonic behavior, or negative symptoms.
- B. *Duration of symptoms*: At least *1 month* but *less than 6 months* duration.
- C. Schizoaffective disorder, mood disorder with psychotic features, substance abuse, and general medical conditions must be excluded.

Schizophreniform disorder is characterized by similar negative/positive symptoms observed with schizophrenia and carries a lifetime prevalence of 0.2%. Social and occupational functioning may or may not be impaired with this illness. Good prognostic indicators include an onset of psychosis within 4 weeks of a behavioral change in the absence of a flat or blunted affect.

Depression often coexists resulting in an increased risk for suicide among individuals with this disorder. Treatment is similar to that of brief psychotic disorder involving brief hospitalization, neuroleptics in conjunction with psychotherapy. Antidepressants may be added for comorbid depression. Early and aggressive treatment is associated with a better prognosis. About 33% recover completely, whereas, 66% progress to schizoaffective disorder or schizophrenia.

SCHIZOAFFECTIVE DISORDER

DSM-IV-TR CRITERIA

- A. This disorder meets criteria for schizophrenia and concurrently meets criteria for a major depressive disorder, manic episode, or mixed episode.
- B. The associated delusions and hallucinations must be present for at least 2 weeks without significant mood symptoms.
- C. Mood symptoms must be present for a significant portion of the illness.

Schizoaffective disorder is characterized by the clinical features of schizophrenia in concert with chronic and recurrent mood symptoms. The lifetime prevalence of this condition is less than 1% with an increased prevalence among first-degree relatives. Schizoaffective disorder is subclassified based on the nature of the concomitant mood disorder into bipolar type or depressed type. This disorder carries a better prognosis when compared to schizophrenia.

Treatment includes hospitalization and psychopharmacologic agents based on the dominant symptoms, such as antipsychotics, mood stabilizers (lithium), and antidepressants. ECT has been proven beneficial in individuals with refractory psychosis, mania, or depression.

DELUSUIONAL DISORDER

DSM-IV-TR CRITERIA

* A. Nonbizarre delusions at least 1 month in duration.
* B. These patients do not exhibit hallucinations, disorganized thought or speech, disorganized or catatonic behavior, negative symptoms of schizophrenia (gustatory and tactile hallucinations may be seen if congruent with the delusion).

The characteristic features of delusional disorder are the nonbizarre plausible nature of the delusions, such as a delusion that they are being followed. Cognition and sensorium remains intact with generally no social or occupational impairment. The disorder usually affects patients between 35 and 45 years of age. Delusional disorder is refractory to antipsychotic medication, whereas psychotherapy is of some benefit.

SHARED PSYCHOTIC DISORDER

Shared psychotic disorder is characterized by the development of delusional symptoms in a previously healthy patient while involved with another person (eg, spouse, family member) with a similar delusional symptom (the *inducer*). The psychotic symptoms only occur after exposure to the inducer. This illness is seen more commonly in women. Treatment involves removing the individual from the influence of the inducer. Social and psychotherapy, and antipsychotic medications may also be used. From 10% to 40% of cases resolve with separation from the inducer.

OTHER PSYCHOTIC DISORDERS

PSYCHOTIC DISORDERS DUE TO GENERAL MEDICAL CONDITION

Medical conditions that can cause psychosis include hyperthyroidism, stroke, malignancies, electrolyte imbalances, and renal failure. These conditions should be sought and treated appropriately. The associated psychosis usually resolves with suitable medical therapy.

SUBSTANCE-INDUCED PSYCHOTIC DISORDER

Substances of abuse including alcohol, methamphetamines, cocaine, lysergic acid diethylamide (LSD), phencyclidine (PCP), have been associated with the development of psychosis. Removal of the offending agent and/or treatment of withdrawal symptoms is associated with improvement or resolution of the psychosis.

PSYCHOTIC DISORDER NOT OTHERWISE SPECIFIED

These include disorders where no specific diagnosis can be made (eg, postpartum psychosis).

BIBLIOGRAPHY

American Psychiatric Association. *Quick Reference to the Diagnostic Criteria. from DSM-IV-TR.* Arlington, VA: American Psychiatric Association; 2000.

American Psychiatric Association. *The Practice of ECT: Recommendations for Treatment, Training, and Privileging.* Washington, DC: American Psychiatric Press; 2001:5–25.

Fadem B, Simring S. *Psychiatry Recall: Second Edition.* Baltimore, MD: Lippincott Williams & Wilkins; 2004.

Hahn RK, Albers LJ, Reist C. *Psychiatry: 2006 Edition.* Laguna Hills, CA: Current Clinical Strategies Publishing; 2006.

111 SUBSTANCE-RELATED DISORDERS

Jeffrey Kao and George T. Grossberg

INTRODUCTION

* Recent studies indicate that 25% to 40% of hospital admissions are related to substance abuse, and as many as 20% of outpatients seen in a general medicine practice are suffering from problems related to addiction.

DEFINITIONS

* Substance intoxication:
  ○ Characterized by reversible maladaptive behavior or psychological changes caused by recent ingestion of a substance.
* Substance abuse:
  ○ Maladaptive pattern of substance use leading to significant impairment over a 12-month period, characterized by at least one of the following:
    ▪ Failure to fulfill obligations at work, school, or home.
    ▪ Recurrent use in settings that could lead to physical injury (eg, while driving).

- Incurring legal action because of substance use.
- Continued use despite recurrent social, legal, or physical problems incurred by using the substance.
- Substance dependence:
  ○ Maladaptive pattern of use leading to impairment over a 12-month period characterized by three or more of the following:
  ○ Tolerance (diminution in the psychophysiologic response to a drug after continued use).
  ○ Withdrawal (the signs and symptoms that appear when a drug that causes physical dependence is suddenly discontinued or decreased in dosage).
  ○ A substance use pattern that escalates (larger quantities over longer period than intended).
  ○ Unsuccessful efforts to reduce or eliminate the drug.
  ○ Significant time devoted to procuring, recovering, or using a substance.
  ○ Social, occupational, and recreational activities are curtailed or abandoned.
  ○ Continued use despite recognition that the drug can engender significant harm.

ALCOHOL

OVERVIEW

- The third largest health problem in the United States, after heart disease and cancer; alcohol use or abuse is associated with 100,000 deaths annually.[1]
- Eight million alcohol-dependent individuals reside in the United States.[2]
- Approximately 10% of women and 20% of men meet criteria for alcohol abuse during their lifetime, whereas, 5% of women and 10% of men meet criteria for alcohol dependence during their lifetime.[3]
- Approximately one-third of individuals with an alcohol disorder also exhibit the signs and symptoms of an additional psychiatric disorder (eg, depression, anxiety, abuse of other substances).
- Lifetime suicide risk among alcohol-dependent individuals is 5 to 10 times greater than the general population.[3]

BIOLOGICAL BASIS FOR ALCOHOL ABUSE

- Alcohol directly activates γ-aminobutyric acid (GABA) receptors and inhibits N-methyl-D-aspartate (NMDA) receptors. Alcohol also interacts with a variety of other neurotransmitter systems including, opioid, dopaminergic, and the serotonergic systems. Several of these neurotransmitter systems are believed to promote alcohol craving.[4]

- A genetic basis for alcohol dependency has also been proposed. For example, first-degree relatives of habitual alcohol users have a four fold higher incidence of alcohol abuse than the general population. Genetic factors also appear to influence the response to an alcohol load, with some patients exhibiting a reduced sensitivity to the effects of alcohol. The biological response to an alcohol load is thought to depend on polymorphisms in genes which encode for central nervous system proteins, or proteins involved in alcohol metabolism (alcohol dehydrogenase)

EVALUATION OF ALCOHOL-RELATED DISORDERS

- Obtain a detailed history of alcohol use:
  ○ Determine the age when alcohol was first used, the quantity, frequency of use, and longest sobriety period. Screen for use of other drugs and substances.
    - According to the National Institute on Alcohol Abuse and Alcoholism, a person at high risk for adverse consequences from alcohol consumes more than 14 drinks per week or 4 drinks per occasion for men and more than 7 drinks per week or 3 drinks per occasion for women.[5]
  ○ Perform a comprehensive psychiatric evaluation for comorbid psychiatric disorders, such as mood disorders. Inquire about legal issues, history of violence, employment history, history of physical abuse, marital history, and family history.
  ○ Distinguishing between primary psychiatric and substance-induced psychiatric disorders is sometimes difficult during the initial evaluation. Substance-induced psychiatric disorders typically resolve within 2 weeks. Therefore, a psychiatric disorder likely exists if the condition has not resolved after 2 weeks of sobriety.
- Obtain a detailed physical examination:
  ○ Observe for the signs of intoxication including slurred speech, disinhibition, ataxia, and disorientation.
  ○ Examine the patient for evidence of liver disease (alcoholic hepatitis or cirrhosis): hepatomegaly, jaundice, tender/full abdomen, ascites, spider angiomata, gynecomastia, and palmar erythema.
  ○ Observe for alcohol withdrawal symptoms which include tremulousness, insomnia, anxiety, autonomic instability, and diaphoresis.
  ○ Wernicke encephalopathy (common neurological disorder secondary to thiamine deficiency) includes the triad of ataxia, confusion, and ophthalmoplegia.
    - Intravenous administration of thiamine is safe and effective, although residual deficits are common (ataxia and nystagmus). If left untreated, patients

may progress to Korsakoff syndrome (disorder of selective anterograde and retrograde amnesia).
  ○ Korsakoff amnestic syndrome is chronic and rarely reversible.
• Alcohol can injure several organ systems (other than the brain):
  ○ Inquire about sleep difficulties (sleep apnea), peripheral neuropathy (direct toxicity or nutritional deficiencies such as B12), cirrhosis or hepatitis, high blood pressure (prominent during withdrawal), cancers (esophagus, colon and breast), cardiomyopathy, and anemia (vitamin deficiency).
• Laboratory tests:
  ○ The liver function tests typically reveal an increase in aspartate aminotransferase which is roughly two times greater than the elevation in alanine aminotransferase. *Chronic* alcohol abuse may not be associated with an elevation in the standard liver function tests, however an increase in γ-glutamyltransferase is usually detected.
  ○ Anemia can be secondary to chronic disease or vitamin deficiencies (folate and B12).
  ○ Alcohol-induced hypoglycemia has been described in the acute setting. Perhaps because of impaired hepatic gluconeogenesis and malnutrition.

TREATMENT OF PATIENTS WITH ALCOHOL DISORDERS

• Acamprosate, a structural analog of GABA, decreases glutamergic neurotransmission during alcohol withdrawal and reduces craving.
  ○ A major side effect of this agent is diarrhea.
• Naltrexone, an opiate antagonist, although contraindicated in patients on opiates, decreases craving and reduces the pleasurable effects associated with ongoing alcohol use. It should not be used in patients with alcoholic hepatitis or cirrhosis because of hepatotoxicity a long-acting intramuscular form is available.
• Disulfiram inhibits alcohol dehydrogenase and, therefore, promotes an increase in circulating acetaldehyde. Acetaldehyde accumulation leads to tachycardia, dyspnea, skin flushing, nausea, and vomiting if the patient continues to drink alcohol. Accordingly, the drug serves as a deterrent for ongoing alcohol use.
  ○ Disulfiram is effective in highly motivated patients. Liver function tests must be monitored carefully because of the risk of drug-induced hepatitis. Disulfiram may trigger a violent reaction if taken with some cough syrups and certain foods. Accordingly, a careful review of potential interactions must be performed by the clinician before initiating therapy with this agent.

• Topiramate increased abstinence in at least one clinical trial; although significant weight loss is a common problem with this agent.
• Counseling includes motivational enhancement therapy, Alcoholics Anonymous, cognitive behavioral therapy, group therapy, self-help programs, and family counseling.

MANAGEMENT OF ALCOHOL WITHDRAWAL

• Symptoms of withdrawal:
  ○ Minor withdrawal: insomnia, irritability, anxiety, nausea, headache, diaphoresis, and palpitations; occurs within 6 hours of the last drink; can occur while the blood alcohol level is elevated, albeit, falling.
  ○ Withdrawal seizures: can occur from 2 to 48 hours after the last drink; usually generalized (tonic-clonic)
    ▪ Risk factors include previous withdrawal seizures or a history of a seizure disorder; more than one-third of patients later develop delirium tremens.
  ○ Alcoholic hallucinosis occurs within 12 to 24 hours of the last drink and resolves in 1 to 2 days; they are generally characterized by auditory hallucinations but any level of the sensory system may be affected (visual or tactile). However, the sensorium remains intact.
  ○ Delirium tremens occur in 5% of patients undergoing withdrawal; the symptoms include hallucinations, disorientation, autonomic instability, agitation, and diaphoresis. Delirium tremens begin 48 to 96 hours after the last drink and last 1 to 5 days.
    ▪ Risk factors include a history of sustained drinking, previous delirium tremens, age younger than 30 years, and concurrent illness.
    ▪ Mortality rate associated with delirium tremens can exceed 10%. Death is usually caused by arrhythmias or aspiration pneumonia.

TREATMENT OF ALCOHOL WITHDRAWAL

• The Clinical Institute Withdrawal Assessment is a tool used to measure the severity of alcohol withdrawal. The instrument assesses the severity of nausea, tremor, autonomic hyperactivity, agitation, hallucinations, and disorientation. A maximum score is 67. Administration of a scheduled dose of a benzodiazepine is employed when the score is greater than 8. If less than 8, benzodiazepines can be used as needed[6] (see Table 111–1).
• Providing a quiet, safe environment is important.
• Electrolyte disturbances (hypokalemia, hypomagnesemia, and hypophosphatemia) should be monitored and treated promptly.

TABLE 111–1 Clinical Institute Withdrawal Assessment for Alcohol (CIWA-Ar) Scale

NAUSEA AND VOMITING—0 no nausea and no vomiting **1** mild nausea with no vomiting **2 3 4** intermittent nausea with dry heaves **5 6 7** constant nausea, frequent dry heaves and vomiting

TREMOR—0 no tremor **1** not visible, but can be felt fingertip to fingertip **2 3 4** moderate, with patient's arms extended **5 6 7** severe, even with arms not extended

PAROXYSMAL SWEATS—0 no sweat visible **1** barely perceptible sweating, palms moist **2 3 4** beads of sweat obvious on forehead **5 6 7** drenching sweats

ANXIETY—0 no anxiety, at ease **1** mildly anxious **2 3 4** moderately anxious, or guarded, so anxiety is inferred **5 6 7** equivalent to acute panic states as seen in severe delirium or acute schizophrenic reactions

AGITATION—0 normal activity **1** somewhat more than normal activity **2 3 4** moderately fidgety and restless **5 6 7** paces back and forth during most of the interview, or constantly thrashes about

TACTILE DISTURBANCES—0 none **1** very mild itching, pins and needles, burning or numbness **2** mild itching, pins and needles, burning or numbness **3** moderate itching, pins and needles, burning or numbness **4** moderately severe hallucinations **5** severe hallucinations **6** extremely severe hallucinations **7** continuous hallucinations

AUDITORY DISTURBANCES—0 not present **1** very mild harshness or ability to frighten **2** mild harshness or ability to frighten **3** moderate harshness or ability to frighten **4** moderately severe hallucinations **5** severe hallucinations **6** extremely severe hallucinations **7** continuous hallucinations

VISUAL DISTURBANCES—0 not present **1** very mild sensitivity **2** mild sensitivity **3** moderate sensitivity **4** moderately severe hallucinations **5** severe hallucinations **6** extremely severe hallucinations **7** continuous hallucinations

HEADACHE, FULLNESS IN HEAD—0 not present **1** very mild **2** mild **3** moderate **4** moderately severe **5** severe **6** very severe **7** extremely severe

ORIENTATION AND CLOUDING OF SENSORIUM—0 oriented and can do serial additions **1** cannot do serial additions or is uncertain about date **2** disoriented for date by no more than 2 calendar days **3** disoriented for date by more than 2 calendar days **4** disoriented for place and/or person

Total CIWA-Ar score: _____Rater's initials: _____Maximum possible score: 67

SOURCE: Adapted from http://www.agingincanada.ca/CIWA.HTM.

- Benzodiazepines: Longer acting benzodiazepines such as Librium are preferred. Patients with liver cirrhosis should receive lorazepam or oxazepam, since these agents have a shorter half-life.[7] Oral therapy is preferred, but parenteral administration may be required to prevent seizures and delirium tremens.
- Thiamine is administered intravenously to prevent Wernicke syndrome. Thiamine administration should precede intravenous glucose containing replacement/maintenance fluids. The glucose in these solutions can precipitate an acute Wernicke or Korsakoff syndrome.
- β-Blockers are useful for controlling blood pressure and tachyarrhythmias; however, they do not prevent progression to more serious symptoms of withdrawal. β-Blockers must be used in conjunction with benzodiazepines.[6]
- Anticonvulsant use is controversial. Most seizures are self-limited. In status epilepticus, phenytoin can be used in conjunction with benzodiazepines. Long-term prophylaxis is not recommended.
- Refractory delirium tremens should be managed with phenobarbital or propofol. Most patients will require mechanical ventilation for airway control.

NARCOTIC ABUSE

OVERVIEW

- Lifetime prevalence is approximately 1%. Current users are estimated between 600,000 and 800,000. Male-to-female ratio is 3:1, and it is most common in the 20- to 40-year age group.[3]
- Between 80% and 90% of addicts develop a co-morbid psychiatric disorder during their lifetime. Common psychiatric disorders that accompany narcotic abuse include major depressive disorder and antisocial personality disorder.[4]

MECHANISM OF ACTION

- Narcotics bind to three endogenous opioid receptors in the brain
  1. μ: induces peripheral analgesia, respiratory depression, constipation, physical dependence, and euphoria.
  2. δ: spinal analgesia, modulates μ receptor function
  3. κ: spinal analgesia, miosis, and diuresis
- Narcotics exert significant effects on the ventral segmental reward area of the brain.

EVALUATION OF NARCOTIC-ABUSING PATIENTS

- Obtain a detailed history of the pattern, habit, route of administration, use of other substances, and psychiatric history.
- Physical examination:
  ○ Intoxication is characterized by pinpoint pupils, lethargy, mental clouding, psychomotor retardation, and slurred speech.
  ○ Withdrawal symptoms include sweating, piloerection, yawning, lacrimation, rhinorrhea, muscle twitching, irritability, muscle aches, dilated pupils, autonomic instability, diarrhea, and stomach cramps.
  ○ Overdoses are characterized by impaired respiratory drive, pinpoint pupils, bradycardia, coma, pulmonary edema, and hypothermia.
  ○ The examination should also focus on the heart (exclude subacute bacterial endocarditis), lymph nodes (may be enlarged suggesting an underlying infection such as human immunodeficiency virus), liver (hepatomegaly suggesting infection from hepatitis A, B, or C, and skin (abscesses and cellulites from parenterals).

TREATMENT OF NARCOTIC-ABUSING PATIENTS

- Overdose: Naloxone is administered intravenously, multiple doses or a continuous drip may be required because of naloxone's short half-life.
- Methadone maintenance therapy: Methadone is a long-acting synthetic narcotic that is administered in a dosage of between 20 and 80 mg daily. It is administered once daily and is associated with minimal euphoria. Importantly, methadone maintenance programs have been associated with a reduction in criminal activity as well as human immunodeficiency virus infection.[8]

- L-Alpha-acetyl-methadol is a longer acting opioid than methadone, requiring administration only three times weekly. The usual dose is 30 to 80 mg three times a week. Potential side effects include QT prolongation and precipitation of cardiac arrhythmias.[9]
- Buprenorphine: A partial μ-agonist, buprenorphine causes fewer withdrawal symptoms, is safe in overdose, and has little potential for abuse.[10]
- Clonidine: This centrally-acting a$_2$-agonist suppresses tachycardia and reduces blood pressure but has no effect on craving.
- Naltrexone: An opioid antagonist, naltrexone should only be used in highly motivated patients as a deterrent. It may precipitate withdrawal symptoms.
- Counseling or abstinence-based therapies (Narcotics Anonymous, residential treatment, and aftercare).
- Importantly, consider other substances that might interfere with the results of the urine drug screen. (Table 111–2)

STIMULANTS (COCAINE AND AMPHETAMINE)

OVERVIEW

- Ten percent of the population has used cocaine at least once during their lifetime. Fifty-five percent of drug-abusing patients are dependent on cocaine.[3]
- Highest use is among persons in the age range between 18 and 34 years of age. Males are more likely to use cocaine than females.[3]

TABLE 111–2   Urine Drug Screen

DRUG	DURATION OF DETECTABILITY	POTENTIAL SUBSTANCES THAT MAY CAUSE FALSE POSITIVES IN DRUG SCREEN
Amphetamines	2–4 days	OTC cold medicines that contain ephedrine, pseudoephedrine; phenylephrine, selegiline, stimulants used in ADHD, trazodone, bupropion, desipramine, amantadine
Benzodiazepines	Less than or equal to 30 days	Prescribed sleep aids and antianxiety medications
Cocaine	2–3 days	anesthetics containing cocaine, certain antibiotics such as amoxicillin
Marijuana	up to 30 days with chronic heavy use	NSAIDs, dronabinol, efavirenz, hemp seed oil, promethazine (Phenergan)
Opiates	1–3 days	Rifampin, fluoroquinolones, poppy seeds, prescribed pain killers
Phencyclidine	Up to 30 days with heavy use	Ketamine, dextromethorphan

ADHD, attention deficit hyperactivity disorder; NSAID, nonsteroidal antiinflammatory drug; OTC, over-the-counter.
SOURCE: Modified from Up To Date, originally from *The Medical Letter.* 2002;44:71

MECHANISM OF ACTION

- Competitively inhibits the reuptake of dopamine, serotonin, and norepinephrine.[4]
  - Elicits a profound effect on the reward circuit of the corticomesolimbic dopaminergic system.

EVALUATION OF STIMULANT-ABUSING PATIENTS

- Obtain a detailed history of pattern, habit, route, use of other substances, and psychiatric history.
- Physical examination:
  - In the acute setting: observe for arrhythmias; hypertension; chest pain; mydriasis; hyperreflexia; hyperpyrexia; diaphoresis; anorexia; hypersexuality; and psychosis, including formication (belief that bugs are crawling on the body).
  - Associated medical sequelae include pulmonary edema, myocardial infarction, cardiomyopathy, intestinal ischemia, ischemic stroke, cerebral atrophy, and preterm labor/spontaneous abortion in pregnant patients.[4]
  - Cocaine withdrawal can be indistinguishable from clinical depression: dysphoria, fatigue, paranoia, insomnia, agitation, and psychomotor retardation.

TREATMENT FOR COCAINE CRAVING AND WITHDRAWAL

- Currently, no uniformly effective pharmacologic treatment is available.
  - Tapering is not required for acute detoxification.
  - Use of dopamine agonists may reduce the craving sensation.
    - Bromocriptine or amantadine have been used with some success, but no medication is FDA approved for this indication.
  - Treat underlying depression with a selective serotonin reuptake inhibitor after the patient has been detoxified.
- Counseling and therapy should involve individual, family, and group therapy as well as Cocaine Anonymous.

BENZODIAZEPINE

- Most commonly prescribed for its anxiolytic and sedative-hypnotic properties.[3]
- Intoxication and withdrawal are similar to alcohol:
  - Intoxication presents as slurred speech, disinhibition, and ataxia.
  - Withdrawal is characterized by autonomic instability, tremulousness, hyperreflexia, insomnia, and seizures in severe cases.

TREATMENT OF OVERDOSE

- Flumazenil: benzodiazepine-receptor antagonist
  - Initial dose of 0.2 mg of Flumazenil is administered intravenously over 30 seconds, followed by a second 0.2 mg intravenous dose if there is no response after at least 30 seconds. Repeat at 60-second intervals up to total dose of 5 mg.[4]
  - Flumazenil is short acting and may precipitate withdrawal seizures.
  - It is contraindicated in patients dependent on benzodiazepines or those receiving tricyclic antidepressants, flumazenil may unmask cardiac arrhythmias (caused by tricyclic antidepressants) that were previously suppressed by a benzodiazepine.

DETOXIFICATION

- Convert from a short-acting benzodiazepine to a long-acting benzodiazepine, such as clonazepam (Klonopin®) and taper slowly over the course of several weeks.

MISCELLANEOUS DRUGS

ECSTASY, 304 METHYLENEDIOXYMETHAMPHETAMINE

- Both a hallucinogen and a stimulant, ecstasy causes neurotoxicity of serotonergic neurons. It is associated with fulminant hepatic failure.[11]

MARIJUANA

- Marijuana is the most frequently used illicit drug in the United States. It induces euphoria, time distortion, anxiety, depression, and paranoia. There is a high prevalence of marijuana abuse in patients involved in motor vehicle accidents. Marijuana is associated with an increased prevalence of schizophrenia and depression. Nonetheless, marijuana has multiple potential medicinal uses including the treatment of nausea/vomiting, glaucoma, and pain.[12]

PHENCYCLIDINE

- Phencyclidine is an NMDA receptor antagonist. It is associated with vertical nystagmus (pathognomonic feature), confusion, and ataxia; high doses can induce seizures, hyperthermia, and hypertensive emergencies. The drug has been associated with dissociation and violent behavior. The acute psychosis can be managed with haloperidol.[3]

REFERENCES

1. Kenna GA, McGeary JE, Swift RM. Pharmacotherapy, pharmacogenomics, and the future of alcohol dependence treatment, part 1. *Am J Health Syst Pharm.* 2004;61:2272.
2. Kosten TR, O'Connor PG. Management of drug and alcohol withdrawal. *N Engl J Med.* 2003;348:1786.
3. Sadock BJ, Sadock VA. *Synopsis of Psychiatry.* Philadelphia, PA: Lippincott Williams & Wilkins; 2003.
4. Stern TA. *The Ten-Minute Guide to Psychiatric Diagnosis and Treatment.* New York, NY: Professional Publishing Group; 2005.
5. National Institute on Alcohol Abuse and Alcoholism. *The Physicians' Guide to Helping Patients With Alcohol Problems.* Washington, DC: Government Printing Office; 1995.
6. Carlson RW, Keske B, Cortez A. Alcohol withdrawal syndrome: alleviating symptoms, preventing progression. *J Trauma.* 1998; 13:311.
7. Saitz R, O'Malley SS. Pharmacotherapies for alcohol abuse. Withdrawal and treatment. *Med Clin North Am.* 1997;81:881.
8. Effective medical treatment of opiate addiction. National Consensus Development Panel on Effective Medical treatment of Opiates Addiction. *JAMA.* 1998;280:1936.
9. Schwetz BA. From the Food and Drug Administration. *JAMA.* 2001;285:2705.
10. Fischer G, Gombas W, Eder H, et al. Buprenorphine versus methadone maintenance for the treatment of opioid dependence. *Addiction.* 1999;94:1337.
11. Dndrew V, Mas A, Bruguera M, et al. Ecstasy: A common cause of severe acute hepatotoxicity. *J Hepatol.* 1998;29:394.
12. Clark PA. The ethics of medical marijuana: government restrictions vs medical necessity. *J Public Health Policy.* 2000;21:40.

112 CHRONIC OBSTRUCTIVE PULMONARY DISEASE

Joseph Roland D. Espiritu and George M. Matuschak

DEFINITION

- Chronic obstructive pulmonary disease (COPD) is a preventable and treatable disease state characterized by airflow limitation that is not fully reversible.[1,2] The airflow limitation is usually both progressive and associated with an abnormal response of the lungs to noxious particles and gases, primarily caused by cigarette smoking.
- COPD encompasses the clinical disorders of chronic bronchitis and emphysema, occasionally with elements of bronchiectasis. Cystic fibrosis is a "chronic obstructive pulmonary disease" but is not grouped under the COPD spectrum because of its unique genetic etiology (ie, mutations in the cystic fibrosis transmembrane conductance regulator [CFTR] protein that affect the chloride channel in exocrine cells).
- *Chronic bronchitis* is clinically defined by a mucus-producing cough most days of the month, 3 months of a year for 2 successive years without other underlying disease to explain the cough.
- *Emphysema* is anatomically defined by abnormal enlargement and inflammatory destruction of the alveolar walls, ducts, and sacs distal to the small-airway terminal bronchioles.
- Each lung lobule contains approximately 5000 alveoli. The commonest form of emphysema is the centrilobular (centriacinar) pattern primarily involving the upper lung lobes. Panlobular (panacinar) emphysema is an anatomical variant involving destruction of alveolar structures throughout lung lobules in all lung fields, particularly the bases and is common in smoking subjects with α_1-antitrypsin (AAT) deficiency.
- Bronchiectasis is characterized by abnormal dilation of the central and/or peripheral airways, generally with associated abnormalities in mucociliary clearance.

EPIDEMIOLOGY

- COPD is the fourth leading cause of death in subjects >45 years of age in the United States and the fourth most frequent cause of death worldwide.[1,2] Compared with declining age-adjusted mortality rates from 1965–1998 for other major chronic diseases such as coronary heart disease and stroke, COPD-related mortality increased by 163%.[1]
- Smoking is the commonest risk factor for COPD; approximately 80% to 90% of COPD deaths are caused by smoking. Female smokers are nearly 13 times as likely to die from COPD as women who never smoked. In 2000, for the first time, the number of deaths in the United States from COPD was greater in women than in men. Male smokers are nearly 12 times as likely to die from COPD as men who never smoked.[3]
- In 2003, 10.7 million U.S. adults were estimated to have COPD.[3] However, close to 24 million U.S. adults with active or previous smoking histories have evidence of obstructive lung dysfunction, suggesting that COPD is underdiagnosed.
- Inhaled tobacco smoke causes airway and lung inflammation. However, clinically overt, progressive COPD does not develop in approximately 60% of patients with significant smoking histories. As approximately 40% of those with previous or ongoing tobacco abuse do not develop COPD, diagnostic spirometry and/or additional pulmonary function tests of bronchodilator responsiveness, lung volume determinations, and diffusion

capacity are recommended to characterize lung pathophysiologic responses to smoking.

- Chronic bronchitis affects people of all ages, but is higher in those >45 years old. Females are more than twice as likely to be diagnosed with chronic bronchitis as males.[3]
- Chronic bronchitis is the most frequent cause of hemoptysis in the United States, particularly during symptomatic episodes of lower respiratory tract infection.
- The Global Initiative for Chronic Obstructive Lung Disease (GOLD) has defined severity criteria for spirometric evidence of COPD (Table 112–1). In American adults aged 25–75 years, prevalence rates are 6.9% for mild COPD and 6.6% for moderate COPD according to the National Health and Nutrition Examination Survey III (NHANES-III).[3]
- Risk factors for COPD include host and environmental factors (Table 112–2). Exposure to tobacco smoke is the most important predisposing factor, followed by AAT (α_1-antiproteinase) deficiency and indoor air pollution in developing countries. Smokers have more respiratory symptoms, a faster decline in lung function, and higher death rates because of COPD.
- There is a strong interaction between smoking and airway hyper-responsiveness (AHR) as determined by clinical findings of bronchospasm and/or positive methacholine bronchoprovocation test results. AHR is a risk factor for mortality in COPD.[2,3]
- AAT deficiency is the best characterized genetic predisposition to COPD. Most cases occur in whites with a

TABLE 112–1   Spirometric Classification of COPD Severity by the Global Initiative for Chronic Obstructive Lung Disease (GOLD)[a]

Stage I: Mild

FEV_1:FVC ratio <0.70
FEV_1 ≥80% predicted

Stage II: Moderate

FEV_1:FVC ratio <0.70
50% ≤ FEV_1 < 80% predicted

Stage III: Severe

FEV_1:FVC ratio <0.70
30% ≤ FEV_1 <50% predicted

Stage IV: Very severe

FEV_1:FVC ratio <0.70
FEV_1 <30% predicted *or*
FEV_1 <50% predicted *plus* chronic respiratory failure

FEV_1, forced expiratory volume at one second; FVC, forced vital capacity.
[a]Criteria reflect post-bronchodilator values during pulmonary function testing.
SOURCE: From National Heart, Lung and Blood Institute (NHLBI)/World Health Organization (WHO) Workshop. Global strategy for the diagnosis and management and prevention of chronic obstructive pulmonary disease. 2006 update. http://www.goldcopd.org.

TABLE 112–2   Risk Factors for COPD

HOST FACTORS	EXPOSURES
Genetic factors	Smoking
Gender	Socioeconomic status
Airway reactivity	Occupation
IgE and asthma	Environmental pollution
	Perinatal events and childhood illness
	Recurrent bronchopulmonary infections
	Diet

COPD, chronic obstructive pulmonary disease; IgE, immunoglobulin E.
SOURCE: From Mannino DM, Homa DM, Akinbami LJ, Ford ES, Redd SC. Chronic obstructive pulmonary disease surveillance—United States, 1971–2000. *MMWR Surveill Summ.* 2002;51:1–16.

prevalence of approximately 1% in COPD populations; however, existing prevalence data are likely underestimates as AAT deficiency is as common as cystic fibrosis, and occurs in approximately 1 in every 3000 births. Thus, only 5% to 6% of the estimated 100,000 AAT-deficient patients in the United States are currently diagnosed by blood screening. The mean delay between presentation of AAT deficiency-related complaints and diagnosis of AAT deficiency by blood testing is nearly 6 years.

- Abnormal homozygous Pi (protein inhibitor)*ZZ or Pi*Null phenotypes cause severely reduced blood AAT levels. Severe panacinar emphysema is especially likely in smokers or ex-smokers at younger ages, in whom obstructive pulmonary symptoms generally develop between ages 32 and 42 years.
- AAT deficiency is also a risk factor for chronic bronchitis, bronchiectasis, and asthma in the absence of overt emphysema.

PATHOPHYSIOLOGY

RESPIRATORY SYSTEM

- Pathophysiologic changes in the lungs of COPD patients occur in the proximal airways, peripheral airways, lung parenchyma, and pulmonary vasculature.
- Within proximal and peripheral airway lumens, increased numbers of neutrophils accumulate in patients with COPD; activated macrophages are also increased in airway lumens in addition to their infiltration of airway walls. In contrast, CD8+ (suppressor) T lymphocytes predominate in the lung parenchyma of COPD patients.[1–4] This inflammatory cellular phenotype in COPD differs from asthmatic patients, in which a predominance of eosinophils and CD4+ (helper) T lymphocytes occurs.
- The number of neutrophils in the air spaces of nonsmokers is normally <3% to 5% on differential counts

of bronchoalveolar lavage fluid (BALF), whereas smokers have increased numbers of BALF neutrophils. Smoking induces alveolar macrophages to release neutrophil chemotactic factors, such as interleukin-8, thus amplifying neutrophil recruitment. Nicotine is also chemotactic for neutrophils and smoke activates the alternative complement pathway.

- Elastase, a potent protease, is secreted by neutrophils and macrophages. Elastase degrades parenchymal elastin even as inflammation is further promoted by the strongly pro-oxidative effects of inhaled tobacco smoke and other noxious gases and particulates.

- Lung inflammation is promoted by two mechanisms leading to an oxidant/antioxidant imbalance: (1) activation of oxidation-reduction (redox)-sensitive transcription factors such as nuclear factor-κB (NF-κB), which bind to and activate cytokine and chemokine inflammatory genes; and (2) oxidative inactivation of antiinflammatory proteins such as AAT. Inflammatory responses are exaggerated in smokers or patients exposed to air pollution who develop COPD, particularly with AAT deficiency.

- Airway inflammation causes hypertrophy and hyperplasia of mucus-secreting goblet cells, as well as repeated injury and repair of the respiratory epithelium and related structures. Airway remodeling involving collagen deposition produced fixed airways obstruction.

- Traditionally, COPD was viewed as large airway chronic bronchitis versus emphysema involving parenchymal destruction distal to terminal bronchioles. Recent data indicate that COPD actually encompasses varying combinations of small airways inflammatory disease (obstructive bronchiolitis) as well as lung parenchymal destruction (Fig. 112–1).[4]

- Chronic bronchitis is characterized by hypertrophy and inflammation of airway mucus glands including goblet cells, leading to increased mucus secretion. Impaired mucociliary clearance and thickened, inflamed bronchial walls contribute to pathologic airway remodeling and luminal narrowing, whereas chronic bacterial colonization of the airways is associated with frequent infections.

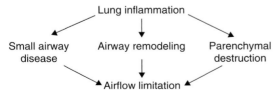

FIG. 112–1 Pathophysiology of chronic obstructive pulmonary disease (COPD). Small airway disease, neutrophilic airway inflammation and remodeling, as well as lung parenchymal destruction typified by emphysema with accompanying loss of alveolar attachments and reduced elastic recoil all contribute to expiratory airflow limitation.

Tobacco smoke also interferes with the ciliary action of the respiratory epithelium.

- Small peripheral airways <2 mm in diameter normally account for 10% to 15% of the total airway resistance; inflammation of these structures in COPD, typified by obstructive bronchiolitis, causes increased airway resistance, even as expiratory emptying of distal lung units is impaired from elastin fiber degradation and abnormal dilation of distal airspaces that culminate in reduced elastic recoil pressure.

- The thickness of the walls of small airways in COPD, reflecting inflammation and remodeling, correlates with physiological measures of reduced expiratory airflow such as the forced expiratory volume in 1 second (FEV_1).

- Progressive expiratory airflow limitation in COPD and dyspnea on exertion reflect an accelerated annual rate of decline in the FEV_1. Normally the rate of FEV_1 loss is approximately 30 mL/y in normal adults >30 years of age; however in COPD patients the rate of FEV_1 loss is nearly 60 mL/y.

- Lung hyperinflation is defined by an elevated residual volume (RV), total lung capacity (TLC), and RV:TLC ratio during pulmonary function testing. In moderate-severe COPD, hyperinflation develops during exercise (ie, dynamic hyperinflation) from the combined effects of increased breathing frequency and minute ventilation, early closure of small airways, and reduced elastic recoil. Hyperinflation places the diaphragm and other muscles of respiration at a mechanical disadvantage by reducing their radius of curvature and thus, force generation according to the length-tension relationship. The work of breathing is therefore increased, leading to exercise intolerance. An increasingly sedentary lifestyle produces respiratory muscle weakness and deconditioning, which augment exertional dyspnea for any level of lung function.

- Reductions in the diffusing capacity of lung for carbon monoxide (DLCO) characterize emphysematous COPD. The DLCO is a measure of the conductance of carbon monoxide (CO) from alveolar gas to hemoglobin in pulmonary capillary blood.

- The pulmonary capillary blood volume is normally approximately 75 mL. Alveolar capillary loss and destruction in moderate-severe emphysema reduce capillary blood volume and thus, the DLCO Increases in ventilation-perfusion ratio (V:Q) mismatching ensue; most notably, an increase in dead space ventilation from ventilation of alveoli without corresponding alveolar capillary perfusion. The DLCO may not be a sensitive measure of milder degrees of emphysema.

- Exertional oxygen (O_2) desaturation in COPD is increasingly common as the patient's DLCO falls below 40% of predicted values, as in sleep-related O_2 desaturation.

- Arterial hypoxemia along with acidosis are potent stimuli for pulmonary vasoconstriction, which over time results in abnormal vascular remodeling, luminal narrowing, and an increased pressure gradient for pulmonary venous blood flow (ie, mean pulmonary artery pressure—pulmonary capillary wedge pressure). The associated increases in pulmonary vascular resistance predispose to progressive secondary pulmonary hypertension and right ventricular hypertrophy (cor pulmonale).

- Despite similar degrees of expiratory airflow limitation in COPD as reflected by decreased forced vital capacity (FVC) and FEV_1 values, wide ranges in partial pressure of carbon dioxide ($PaCO_2$) are observed. Two main determinants affect arterial $PaCO_2$ levels in COPD: (1) reductions in the FEV_1 of ≥60% to 70%, and (2) the ventilatory drive (more specifically, the hypercapnic ventilatory response to $PaCO_2$).

- COPD patients who require intubation and mechanical ventilatory support for acute or acute-on-chronic respiratory failure are at risk for auto–positive end-expiratory pressure (PEEP). Predisposing factors for auto–PEEP include tachypnea, which reduces the length of each respiratory cycle (ie, a respiratory rate of 20 breaths/min equals a 3-second respiratory cycle length), lower ventilator peak inspiratory flow rates (which prolong the duration of the inspiratory phase within each respiratory cycle), and bronchospasm, which predisposes to incomplete expiratory lung emptying and higher end-expiratory lung volumes.

- Pathophysiologic hemodynamic consequences of auto–PEEP include arterial hypotension secondary to decreased venous return and cardiac output. Overestimation of central venous and/or pulmonary artery pressures also occurs, as these pressure are routinely referenced to atmospheric pressure rather than intrathoracic pressure. Of note, hemodynamic consequences of auto–PEEP result from parallel elevations in intrathoracic or intrapleural pressure; elevated airway pressure per se causes no hemodynamic effects.

- Adverse respiratory consequences of auto–PEEP include increased work of breathing during inspiration because of the patient's need to generate greater negative inspiratory pressures to trigger the ventilator, and the augmented expiratory work of breathing.

- Auto–PEEP cannot be determined by visualizing displays of the peak inspiratory pressure because the ventilator circuit is open to atmosphere. However, the presence of auto–PEEP can be suspected by inspection of the airway pressure waveforms. Definitive measurement of auto–PEEP is performed with an end-expiratory pause or brief occlusion, which causes the ventilator manometer or digital readout to record the actual end expiratory pressure.

- In certain patients, judicious application of external PEEP can offset auto–PEEP. More reliable methods to reduce auto–PEEP involve pharmacologic treatment of bronchospasm and airway inflammation, limiting tachypnea by increasing each respiratory cycle length via sedation and other measures, and increasing ventilator peak expiratory flow rates to shorten the inspiratory phase and lengthen the expiratory phase of each respiratory cycle.

SYSTEMIC INFLAMMATORY EFFECTS

- Markers of systemic inflammation such as circulating tumor necrosis factor α (TNF-α), soluble tumor necrosis factor receptor 55 (sTNFR-55), interleukin (IL)-1β, IL-6, C-reactive protein (CRP), fibrinogen, and other acute-phase reactants are all elevated in patients with COPD. This suggests that COPD is a systemic disease affecting multiple organs.

- Weight loss with reduced skeletal muscle mass frequently complicate COPD and is associated with a worse prognosis. Elevation of high-sensitivity blood CRP concentrations correlate with body mass indices in COPD patients in GOLD stages II and III and with postbronchodilator FEV_1 values.[5]

DIAGNOSIS

- COPD is suspected in patients with progressive exertional dyspnea, chronic daily cough productive of variable amounts of sputum (usually greatest in the morning), wheezing, a history of recurrent lower respiratory tract infections, and/or hemoptysis, especially in the context of current or previous cigarette smoking.

- The duration and intensity of exposure to tobacco smoke in the form of cigarette packs per year should be documented in all smokers and ex-smokers. In never-smokers, determination of passive smoking (ie, second-hand smoke) at home or work is especially important.

- Substantial deterioration in expiratory airflow to <50% of predicted FVC and FEV_1 flow rates can occur by the time patients with COPD present with respiratory symptoms such as exertional dyspnea.[3,4] However, factors modifying symptoms in individual patients include the degree of airflow limitation, level of physical exertion, extent of deconditioning, and presence of other cardiopulmonary diseases.

- Cigarette smoking is a risk factor for coronary artery disease; exertional dyspnea can therefore reflect multiple causes including COPD, angina without chest pain, pulmonary hypertension, and physical deconditioning.

- COPD and asthma both cause wheezing and can coexist. Certain clinical features are useful in distinguishing the predominant condition (Table 112–3).

- Poor sleep quality and depression are common in patients with advanced COPD. A comprehensive sleep history should be obtained in all such patients. Overnight pulse oximetry and/or polysomnographic testing are indicated to exclude sleep-disordered breathing and nocturnal O_2 desaturation, particularly in subjects with complaints of daytime sleepiness.

- Physical examination has low diagnostic sensitivity and specificity in ambulatory patients with COPD; it can be unremarkable in patients with mild obstruction.

- In advanced COPD, and particularly during acute exacerbations, respiratory distress with expiratory wheezes, distant breath sounds, accessory muscle use, pulsus paradoxus >12 mm Hg, chest hyperinflation with increased anteroposterior dimensions, pursed lip breathing, active abdominal contractions during expiration, and peripheral and/or central cyanosis can be observed.

PULMONARY FUNCTION TESTS

- Spirometry is essential to diagnose COPD; it should be performed in all patients with persistent or progressive respiratory symptoms but particularly in those with active/previous histories of cigarette smoking. Serial spirometry measurements objectively document disease progression and/or response to treatment. COPD presumptively established by ambulatory spirometry is confirmed in the pulmonary function laboratory by inhaled bronchodilator testing. Incompletely reversible airflow limitation defined by a postbronchodilator FEV_1/FVC ratio of <70% confirms the diagnosis of COPD according to GOLD 2006 criteria,[1] with the severity of lung physiologic impairment based on the predicted FEV_1 percent (see Table 112–1).

- Classification of the severity of obstructive airflow limitation in COPD by different spirometric criteria has also been promulgated by consensus statements from the American Thoracic Society (ATS)/European Respiratory Society (ERS).[6] In contrast to the GOLD criteria for airflow obstruction in COPD, the ATS/ERS criteria emphasize the age-, gender-, race-specific lower limit of normal to guide interpretation of spirometric abnormalities. It is therefore important to be aware of device- and laboratory-specific reference standards for spirometric values.

- The ATS/ERS guidelines suggest that other measures, in addition to the degree of airflow obstruction, such as body mass index, degree of dyspnea, and exercise capacity measured by the 6-minute walk test, can also help predict outcomes including survival. These parameters, when combined, collectively predict a higher risk of death than lung function alone.[6]

- Because dyspnea on exertion can be related to arterial O_2 desaturation in patients with COPD, exercise pulse oximetry is indicated. Precise estimation of the flow rates of supplemental O_2 needed to prevent arterial O_2 desaturation during the patient's typical daily activities is best evaluated by exercise O_2 prescription treadmill testing.

- Determination of the relative contribution of COPD to symptom-limited exertion in patients with known or suspected cardiopulmonary comorbidities because of coronary artery disease or physical deconditioning is best accomplished by a cardiopulmonary exercise test with exhaled gas analysis.

- Patients with advanced COPD who otherwise do not require supplemental O_2 are at risk for dyspnea and hypoxemia with increasing altitude during air travel because aircraft cabins are pressurized to only approximately 8000 feet. Hence, they experience decreased inspired O_2 tensions contributing to hyperventilation, respiratory alkalosis, and increased work of breathing; at the same time, alveolar hypoxia can exacerbate pulmonary hypertension. Additionally, increased intrathoracic gas volumes occur that can expand bullae and predispose to pneumothorax. Similar problems can occur during visits to altitudes in excess of 8000 feet above sea level.

TABLE 112–3 Distinguishing Clinical Features of COPD Versus Asthma

	COPD	ASTHMA
Age	Onset in midlife	Onset early in life (often childhood)
Symptoms	Slowly progressive	Vary from day to day
Smoking	Almost invariable	Possible
Dyspnea	During exercise	Episodic
Nocturnal symptoms	Uncommon unless in severe disease	Worse at night, early morning
Family history	Uncommon unless family members also smoke May be positive α_1-antitrypsin deficiency	Common
Concomitant eczema or allergic rhinitis	Possible	Common
Airflow limitation	Largely irreversible	Largely reversible

COPD, chronic obstructive pulmonary disease.
SOURCE: From National Heart, Lung and Blood Institute (NHLBI)/World Health Organization (WHO) Workshop. Global strategy for the diagnosis and management and prevention of chronic obstructive pulmonary disease. 2006 update. http://www.goldcopd.org

• Provision of supplemental O_2 during air travel for COPD patients is recommended if the predicted partial pressure of arterial oxygen (PaO_2) is ≤50 mm Hg. The patient's predicted PaO_2 value at altitude can be performed by a high-altitude simulation test (HAST) in the pulmonary function laboratory before scheduled travel.

THORACIC IMAGING STUDIES

• Plain chest radiographs are relatively insensitive in detecting early stages of COPD and do not correlate well with its severity. Overt bullous disease and lung hyperinflation with low, flattened diaphragms and increased retrocardiac airspace on lateral projections are helpful findings. During acute exacerbations of COPD, pneumonia, pneumothorax, pleural effusions, or atelectasis can be prominent.
• Chest computed tomography (CT) scanning with or without intravenous (IV) contrast and the helical technique is useful when performed if the diagnosis is in question, when bullectomy or lung volume reduction surgery (LVRS) is contemplated,[1] or during acute exacerbations to evaluate the possibility of concomitant pulmonary embolism, pneumonia, or other lung parenchymal conditions.

LABORATORY MEASUREMENTS

• Arterial blood gas (ABG) measurement is indicated when the FEV_1 is <40% of predicted to quantify arterial hypoxemia and to detect possible hypercarbia and respiratory acidosis. An ABG is also recommended if the patient has signs of progressive respiratory limitation on exertion or decompensated cor pulmonale, manifested by increasing pedal edema or abdominal girth, a right-sided third heart sound, or hepatojugular venous distension.[1]
• Measurement of plasma α_1-antitrypsin is recommended if COPD develops in smokers at a younger age (ie, <40–45 years of age) or if there is a family history of emphysema, chronic bronchitis, or bronchiectasis.
• Dyspnea on exertion can reflect diverse cardiopulmonary conditions. Accordingly, echocardiography is useful in COPD patients to determine the presence of right ventricular hypertrophy/dilation, pulmonary hypertension, and tricuspid valve regurgitation, as well as to evaluate left ventricular contractility and valvular function.
• Sleep-disordered breathing including nocturnal O_2 desaturation is not uncommon in COPD and can coexist with obstructive sleep apnea. Determining the need for nocturnal O_2 supplementation or other sleep medicine treatments is best evaluated by an overnight polysomnography study, especially in patients complaining of poor sleep quality and daytime sleepiness.

THERAPEUTIC APPROACH

• Long-term supplemental O_2 therapy for >15 h/d is the only treatment shown to increase survival in COPD.[7] Accepted indications for O_2 therapy in COPD include a resting PaO_2 value ≤55 mm Hg or an arterial oxygen saturation (SaO_2) level ≤88% in the absence of acute complicating factors, or cor pulmonale and a PaO_2 value of 55 to 60 mm Hg or SaO_2 value ≤89% in patients with pulmonary hypertension, peripheral edema, or polycythemia.
• In patients with COPD, supplemental O_2 therapy improves pulmonary hemodynamics, reduces polycythemia, increases exercise capacity, and improves neurocognitive function. Supplemental O_2 therapy in COPD should be therapeutically targeted to maintain a SaO_2 saturation >90% during rest, sleep, and exertion.
• With respect to limiting the accentuated rate of annual FEV_1 decline in COPD, smoking cessation slows down the enhanced decline of lung function in patients susceptible to COPD to approximately normal levels within the year after quitting.
• In addition to smoking cessation, monthly IV enzyme augmentation therapy is indicated in COPD patients with AAT deficiency.
• The GOLD guidelines recommend a treatment approach based on the severity of obstruction (Table 112–4). Bronchodilators (inhaled β_2-adrenergic agonists, anticholinergic agents such as ipratropium) provide symptomatic relief, but have not been demonstrated to alter long-term decline in pulmonary function.
• Tiotropium, a new-generation long-acting anticholinergic that is an antimuscarinic M3 receptor agonist, has greater effects than short-acting anticholinergic agents in improving dyspnea, exacerbations, health-related quality of life, and lung function long term.
• Compared with placebo, the combination of β_2-agonist salmeterol and the inhaled corticosteroid (ICS) fluticasone reduces the annual rate of exacerbations of COPD and improves health status and spirometric values although not survival.[8] Such combinations of ICS and long-acting β_2-adrenergic agonist (eg, salmeterol/ fluticasone, budesonide/formoterol) provide greater improvements in dyspnea and lung function than either component alone.
• For acute exacerbations of COPD, equipotent doses of oral versus IV steroids generally yield similar responses. In this setting, steroid treatment for 2 weeks at 40 to 60 mg of prednisone once daily is associated with a lower rate of treatment failure, shorter hospital stays, and more rapid improvement in pulmonary function.[9]
• Pulmonary rehabilitation is recommended for patients with moderate COPD and breathlessness. Benefits of

TABLE 112–4   Therapy of Stable COPD Based on Severity

I: MILD	II: MODERATE	III: SEVERE	IV: VERY SEVERE
FEV_1:FVC <70% $FEV_1 \geq 80\%$ With or without symptoms	FEV_1:FVC <70% $50\% \leq FEV_1 \leq 80\%$ With or without symptoms	FEV_1:FVC <70% $30\% \leq FEV_1 \leq 50\%$	FEV_1:FVC <70% $FEV_1 <30\%$ or $30\% < FEV_1 <50\%$ plus chronic respiratory failure

Avoidance of risk factor(s); influenza vaccination.

Add short-acting bronchodilator when needed.

Add regular treatment with one or more long-acting bronchodilators.
Add pulmonary rehabilitation.

Add inhaled glucocorticosteroids if repeated exacerbations.

Add long-term oxygen if chronic respiratory
failure present.
Consider surgical treatments.

COPD, chronic obstructive pulmonary disease; FEV_1, forced expiratory volume at one second; FVC, forced vital capacity.

pulmonary rehabilitation include improvement in exercise capacity and quality of life, as well as reduction in dyspnea, anxiety and depression, and healthcare use.[1]

- Bullectomy can reduce dyspnea and improve lung function in selected patients with bullous disease.
- LVRS, when performed in the subset of COPD patients with severe disease (ie, FEV_1 <45% predicted), predominantly upper lobe emphysema, and low exercise capacity, provides a survival advantage over medical therapy. Beneficial effects of LVRS are not apparent in higher risk patients having FEV_1 and DLCO values of $\leq 20\%$ of predicted levels.[10]
- Lung transplantation does not confer clear-cut survival benefits in selected COPD patients but has been shown to improve functional capacity and quality of life. Criteria for referral of COPD patients for lung transplantation include a FEV_1 value of <25% predicted, a resting PaO_2 value of 55 to 60 mm Hg, a $PaCO_2$ level of >50 mm Hg, and secondary pulmonary hypertension, along with good performance capacity.

REFERENCES

1. National Heart, Lung and Blood Institute (NHLBI)/World Health Organization (WHO) Workshop. Global strategy for the diagnosis and management and prevention of chronic obstructive pulmonary disease. 2006 update. http://www.goldcopd.org.
2. Mannino DM, Homa DM, Akinbami LJ, Ford ES, Redd SC. Chronic obstructive pulmonary disease surveillance—United States, 1971–2000. *MMWR Surveill Summ*. 2002;51:1–16.
3. U.S. Department of Health and Human Services. The health consequences of smoking : A report of the Surgeon General. (electronic only) Call Number: HE 20.7002:2004021387 http://www.cdc.gov/tobacco/sgr/sgr_2004/index.htm
4. Hogg JC, Chu F, Otokaparch S, et al. The nature of small-airway obstruction in COPD. *N Engl J Med*. 2004;350: 2645–2653.
5. Broekhuizen R, Wouters EFM, Creutzberg EC, Schols AM. Raised CRP levels mark metabolic and functional impairment in advanced COPD. *Thorax*. 2006;61:17–22.
6. Celli, BR, MacNee W, ATS/ERS Taskforce. Standards for the diagnosis and treatment of patients with COPD. A summary of the ATS/ERS position paper. *Eur Respir J*. 2004;23:932–946.
7. Nocturnal Oxygen Therapy Trial Group. Continuous or nocturnal oxygen therapy in hypoxemic chronic obstructive lung disease: A clinical trial. *Ann Intern Med*. 1980;93:391–398.
8. Calverley PMA, Anderson JA, Celli B, et al, for the TORCH Investigators. Salmeterol and fluticasone propionate and survival in chronic obstructive pulmonary disease. *N Engl J Med*. 2007;356:775–789.
9. Niewoehner DE, Erbland ML, Deupree RH, et al. Effect of systemic glucocorticoids on exacerbations of chronic obstructive pulmonary disease. Department of Veterans Affairs Cooperative Study Group. *N Engl J Med*. 1999;340:1941–1947.
10. National Emphysema Treatment Trial Research Group. A randomized trial comparing lung-volume-reduction-surgery with medical therapy for severe emphysema. *N Engl J Med*. 2003;348:2059–2073.

113 INTERSTITIAL LUNG DISEASE

George M. Matuschak and Ravi P. Nayak

DEFINITION

- Interstitial lung disease (ILD) represents a diverse spectrum of more than 100 different pulmonary conditions that are characterized by a common pattern of diffuse inflammatory injury or infiltration as well as abnormal fibrotic proliferation and repair within alveolar walls and the lung's interstitial structures. ILD may have an acute presentation, simulating infectious pneumonia, but more conventionally develops over many weeks or months. Many ILDs not only cause thickening of alveolar walls and the pulmonary interstitium, but also the lumina and walls of small airways (ie, alveolar ducts, respiratory bronchioles, and terminal bronchioles) as well as the pulmonary capillary network.

- Regardless of the specific etiology of an ILD and its pathophysiological mechanisms, presenting clinical presentations are usually typified by three hallmark clinical features: (1) progressive dyspnea on exertion, (2) restrictive physiology on pulmonary function tests, and (3) diffuse reticular infiltrates and/or ground glass opacities on chest radiographs or thoracic CT scan imaging studies.

- To facilitate a comprehensive differential diagnosis of ILD, it is helpful to view this condition as being associated with 10 broad categories of diseases affecting the respiratory system

  1. The idiopathic interstitial pneumonias (Table 113–1), comprised of idiopathic pulmonary fibrosis (IPF), nonspecific interstitial pneumonia, cryptogenic organizing pneumonia, acute interstitial pneumonia (AIP) (Hamman-Rich syndrome), respiratory bronchiolitis-interstitial lung disease, desquamative interstitial pneumonia, and lymphoid interstitial pneumonia.[1]

  2. Sarcoidosis, a multisystem disorder of granulomatous inflammation characterized by the formation of nonnecrotizing granulomas

  3. Connective tissue diseases, especially systemic lupus erythematosus (SLE), polymyositis-dermatomyositis, and mixed connective tissue disease, with a lesser occurrence in rheumatoid arthritis (RA), progressive systemic sclerosis (PSS; either the diffuse form or CREST [calcinosis, Raynaud phenomenon, esophageal dysmotility, sclerodactyly, telangiectasia] variant), Sjögren syndrome, and ankylosing spondylitis

  4. Eosinophilic lung disorders, typified by chronic eosinophilic pneumonia and much less commonly, Churg-Strauss syndrome

  5. Hypersensitivity pneumonitis

  6. Pulmonary involvement by vasculitides such as microscopic angitis

  7. Pneumoconioses, typified by asbestosis, silicosis, and chronic beryllium disease

  8. Alveolar hemorrhage syndromes, including Goodpasture syndrome and diffuse alveolar hemorrhage following allogeneic bone marrow transplantation

  9. Drug-induced pulmonary disease, as exemplified by the adverse reactions to chemotherapeutic agents bleomycin, busulfan, and cyclophosphamide; antibiotics such as nitrofurantoin; antiinflammatory agents including gold, penicillamine, and methotrexate; antiarrhythmic drugs such as amiodarone; and other agents

  10. Miscellaneous rare disorders, including pulmonary histiocytosis X (eosinophilic granuloma), lymphangioleiomyomatosis (LAM), pulmonary alveolar proteinosis (PAP), and pulmonary hemosiderosis.

EPIDEMIOLOGY

- The prevalence and incidence of ILD of all causes are uncertain, mostly because of the large diversity of conditions that can culminate in ILD. Overall, ILD has an estimated prevalence of approximately 80.9 per 100,000 for men compared with 67.2 per 100,000 for women. The incidence of ILD is 31.5 per 100,000 per year in men versus 26.1 per 100,000 in women.[2]

- IPF, an important chronic and usually fatal ILD, is associated with a 5-year mortality rate of approximately 50%. Once thought to be relatively rare, it is

TABLE 113–1 Idiopathic Interstitial Pneumonias: American Thoracic Society (ATS)/European Respiratory Society (ERS) Classification of Idiopathic Interstitial Pneumonias

HISTOLOGIC PATTERN	CLINICAL/RADIOLOGIC/PATHOLOGIC DIAGNOSIS
Usual interstitial pneumonia (UIP) - Temporal heterogeneity: normal areas of lung alongside inflammatory and/or fibrotic areas, fibroblastic foci.	Idiopathic pulmonary fibrosis (IPF)/cryptogenic fibrosing alveolitis
Nonspecific interstitial pneumonia	Nonspecific interstitial pneumonia (NSIP)
Organizing pneumonia (OP)	Cryptogenic organizing pneumonia (COP)
Diffuse alveolar damage (DAD) - Uniformity of lung inflammation, fibrotic scarring; all areas look of similar age - Hyalin membrane formation	Acute interstitial pneumonia (AIP); Hamman-Rich syndrome)
Respiratory bronchiolitis	Respiratory bronchiolitis-interstitial lung disease (RB-ILD)
Desquamative interstitial pneumonia	Desquamative interstitial pneumonia (DIP)
Lymphoid interstitial pneumonia	Lymphoid interstitial pneumonia (LIP)

SOURCE: ATS/ERS International Multidisciplinary Consensus Classification of the Idiopathic Interstitial Pneumonias. *Am J Respir Crit Care Med.* 2002;165:277–304.

TABLE 113–2   ILD-Like Conditions with Mid-Upper Lung Involvement

CONDITION	DIFFERENTIAL DIAGNOSTIC FEATURES
Sarcoidosis	-Hilar/mediastinal lymphadenopathy common -Lymphocyte predominance in BALF (CD4+ cells; CD4+/CD8+ T-cell ratio >3.5) -Noncaseating, well-formed granulomas on lung biopsy -Multiorgan involvement, hypercalcemia, skin lesions

BALF, bronchoalveolar lavage fluid; ILD, interstitial lung disease.

now diagnosed with greater frequency; five million people worldwide are affected. Because of misdiagnoses, the actual number of IPF patients may be significantly higher. In the United States, approximately 200,000 patients are estimated to have IPF; of these, more than 40,000 die annually from its relentless progression.

- The incidence of IPF increases significantly with age, being most common between the ages of 50 and 70 years.
- About two-thirds of patients with IPF have a cigarette smoking history; smoking is thought to play a pathophysiological role in respiratory bronchiolitis-associated ILD, desquamative interstitial pneumonia, and pulmonary histiocytosis X (eosinophilic granuloma)
- Increasingly, acute exacerbations of IPF are recognized in which rapid progression of lung disease culminates in irreversible respiratory failure within a few weeks or months.
- Sarcoidosis is a relatively common cause of ILD in young or middle-aged adults, with a predilection for the mid- and upper lung zones. Pulmonary histiocytosis X also has a predilection for mid-upper lung zone involvement along with silicosis and cystic fibrosis (although the latter is not an ILD per se) (Table 113–2).
- Epidemiological data for sarcoidosis are imprecise because of varying case definitions, diagnostic criteria, and referral bias among reports. Not all patients with sarcoidosis have pulmonary symptoms despite incidental radiographic evidence of lung involvement (Table 113–3).

TABLE 113–3   Chest Radiographic Stages of Sarcoidosis

STAGE	INTRATHORACIC MANIFESTATIONS
I	Bilateral hilar lymphadenopathy
II	Bilateral lymphadenopathy + reticulonodular infiltrates/opacities
III	Bilateral reticulonodular infiltrates/opacities
IV	Fibrocystic changes with bullae, upper lobe fibrotic scarring, and upward hilar retraction

- Population-based surveys suggest an age-adjusted incidence of approximately 5.9:100,000 in males and 6.3:100,000 in females.[3]
- The incidence of sarcoidosis in African Americans is about 3.8-fold higher than whites, as is the lifetime risk between races (ie, 2.4% versus 0.85%, respectively).
- Because of the variable natural history of sarcoidosis, patient presentation with higher radiographic stages does not necessarily mean progression of disease from lower stages.
- The spectrum of histopathology in ILD associated with connective tissue diseases encompasses all of the patterns observed in idiopathic interstitial pneumonia. Development of ILD in patients with connective tissue disease may precede rheumatological symptoms and signs; alternatively, ILD may occur during or after the onset of overt rheumatic disease. No specific risk factors for pulmonary involvement in the form of ILD have been identified among connective tissue diseases, with the possible exception of antitopoisomerase antibodies in the diffuse form of PSS.
- Nonspecific interstitial pneumonia is the most common form of ILD found in the setting of connective tissue diseases, occurring in up to 80% of patients of PSS, Sjögren syndrome, and polymyositis/dermatomyositis (PM/DM).
- However, a usual interstitial pneumonia (UIP)-like pattern frequently predominates in ILD associated with RA. Previously approximately 5% of patients with RA were considered to have ILD; more recent estimates using high-resolution chest CT (HRCT) suggest a higher incidence of nearly 20%.[4] In addition to ILD, other pulmonary manifestations of RA include rheumatoid lung nodules, bronchiectasis, pleural effusion, and diffuse bronchiolitis resulting in an obstructive ventilatory pattern; laryngeal inflammatory involvement of the synovia of the cricoarytenoid joints may predispose to occult pulmonary aspiration and infectious pneumonia, even as immunomodulatory therapy such as corticosteroids or anti–tumor necrosis factor-α treatments predispose to opportunistic infections.
- Acute, rapidly progressive presentations of ILD may complicate connective tissue diseases, especially SLE and PM/DM. Such rapid-onset ILD, typified by acute lupus pneumonitis, may simulate infectious pneumonia and/or acute lung injury/acute respiratory distress syndrome (ARDS).
- Pulmonary involvement as ILD in PM/DM occurs in 5% to 30% of patients and adversely affects prognosis; anti–Jo-1 antibodies against transfer (t)RNA have been reported as a marker of increased risk.[5]
- Diffuse alveolar hemorrhage (DAH) associated with either alveolar inflammatory capillaritis or *bland*

DAH simulates ILD clinically by causing dyspnea and radiographically by producing interstitial infiltrates and/or increased ground glass attenuation on chest CT scans. DAH is a common interstitial process in SLE, frequently presenting in patients with established SLE and concomitant renal dysfunction from active glomerulonephritis. Other important pulmonary-renal syndromes in which DAH occurs include mixed connective tissue disease, pulmonary vasculitides such as microscopic angiitis, and Goodpasture syndrome. However, bland DAH without histological features of capillaritis can occur with SLE and related conditions, and also as a longer term complication of allogeneic bone marrow transplantation.

- DAH may occur with minimal or absent hemoptysis in as many as one-third of affected patients, since the bleeding may be confined to the respiratory (eg, alveolar) zone of the lungs. The diagnosis of DAH is supported by progressively greater bloody recovery of bronchoalveolar lavage fluid (BALF) during fiberoptic bronchoscopy in the absence of overtly bleeding large airway pathologies (eg, acute severe bronchitis or tumor).

- Connective tissue disease-related ILD with lymphocytic interstitial pneumonia occurs most commonly in patients with Sjögren syndrome and RA.

- ILD from chronic hypersensitivity pneumonitis (eg, extrinsic allergic alveolitis) results from inhalation of diverse organic antigens including those related to specific bacteria as typified by farmer's lung, mushroom worker's lung, and bagassosis involving moldy sugar cane in which thermophilic bacteria (eg, *Thermoactinomyces* and *Micropolyspora* spp.) play a role, animal proteins from feathers or avian droppings as in bird breeder's disease, or chemicals including isothiocyanates and trimellitic anhydride in industrial workers. Especially noteworthy is humidifier lung, in which inhalation of multiple microorganisms (eg, bacteria, fungi, and amebae) in bioaerosol mists from standing humidifier water causes disease. The development of chronic hypersensitivity pneumonitis may be occult and slowly progressive over time until symptoms occur, or may follow episodes of acute hypersensitivity pneumonitis which typically occur 4 to 12 hours after acute exposures.

- Although prevalence data for hypersensivity pneumonitis are limited, epidemiological data for farmers suggest an at-risk population ranging between 0.5% and 7%. The estimated prevalence of disease among bird breeders or fanciers varies widely (eg, 20–20,000 cases per 100,000 persons).

- Occupational and environmental inhalational exposures to inorganic dusts are the primary causes of pneumoconioses manifesting as ILD. The majority of patients with pneumoconioses are men. There are five groups of inorganic dusts of relevance: (1) silicates, typified by asbestos; (2) silica (crystalline silica dust); (3) coal dust; (4) beryllium and related compounds (eg, titanium, aluminum); and (5) hard metal dusts.

- Asbestosis is a form of chronic diffuse interstitial pneumonia principally involving the bilateral lower lung zones caused by prolonged inhalational exposure to asbestos fibers (especially chrysotile and amphibole fibers) in occupations such as mining, pipefitting, insulation workers, plumbers, and boilermakers. Disease is associated with a prolonged latency interval (eg, 15–20 y following exposure). ILD associated with asbestosis may coexist with other forms of asbestos-related respiratory disease, including calcific and non-calcific pleural plaques, exudative pleural effusion, and nonresolving rounded atelectasis in the lower lobe regions. Notably, asbestos exposure increases the risk of lung cancer by approximately sixfold, whereas smoking and asbestos exposure synergistically increases cancer risk to between 60- and 80-fold.

- Chronic silicosis occurs following a prolonged (eg, ≥20 y) occupational history of mining, ceramics work, sandblasting, and related trades, especially in the absence of respiratory protective devices. Chronic silicosis is unique among pneumoconioses with respect to its radiological distribution of nodular coalescing infiltrates in the mid-upper lung zones. Patients with silicosis are particularly susceptible to *Mycobacterium tuberculosis* infections (eg, silicotuberculosis)

- Because of the toxic effects of silica on alveolar macrophages, such individuals require prolonged antituberculosis chemotherapy.

- Berylliosis, also known as chronic beryllium disease, is a chronic hypersensitivity response of the lungs to beryllium fumes or dust resulting in granulomatous inflammation. Lung histopathological specimens in berylliosis showing noncaseating granulomas are in themselves, indistinguishable from specimens of patients with sarcoidosis and occasionally tuberculosis. Occupations associated with beryllium exposures are scrap metal working, automotive or aircraft electronics, and some oil and gas industries.

- Drug-induced pulmonary disease covers a broad spectrum of reactions of the lungs including eosinophilic pneumonia, cryptogenic organizing pneumonia (eg, bronchiolitis obliterans with organizing pneumonia), noncardiogenic pulmonary edema, and asthma-like symptoms, as well as parenchymal scarring culminating in ILD. Multiple drugs are associated with pulmonary toxicities causing pulmonary fibrosis/ILD (Table 113–4).

TABLE 113–4 Drugs Associated with Diffuse ILD

DRUG CLASS	DRUG
Chemotherapeutic agents	Bleomycin
	Busulfan*
	Cyclophosphamide
	Chlorambucil
	Nitrosoureas
	Vinca alkaloids (with mitomycin)
Antiinflammatory agents	Methotrexate*
	Gold salts
	Penicillamine
	Infliximab
	α-interferon
Cardiovascular agents	Amiodarone
	ACE inhibitors
	Flecainide
Antibiotics	Nitrofurantoin
	Sulfasalazine
	Amphotericin B
Anticonvulsants	Carbamazepine
	Diphenylhydantoin
Miscellaneous	Cocaine
	Methadone
	Heroin
	Silicone
	Mineral oil
	Radiation
	Oxygen (toxicity)

*May also cause acute pulmonary hypersensitivity reactions.
ACE, angiotensin-converting enzyme; ILD, interstitial lung disease.

- Among nonchemotherapeutic agents, the antiarrhythmic agent amiodarone is an important cause of pulmonary fibrosis and ILD, given the frequency of its use, very long half-life, and lack of significant metabolism by the liver or kidneys. Besides amiodarone-induced pulmonary toxicity manifesting as ILD, acute lung injury/ARDS, patchy lung opacities with organizing pneumonia, and solitary mass lesions have been reported. Serum amiodarone levels have no correlation with pulmonary toxicity.
- Amiodarone use is associated with foamy alveolar macrophages on lung biopsy specimens; however, this finding is not specific for pulmonary toxicity and only signifies drug exposure. Pulmonary amiodarone toxicity can occur at any time following initiation of therapy; patients receiving higher doses of amiodarone (eg, 400 mg/d) are more predisposed but toxicity has also been reported following lower dose therapy (eg, 200 mg/d). Concurrent use of high fractional inspired O_2 concentration and preexisting lung disease have been reported as predisposing factors.
- Among newer drugs, the anti–tumor necrosis factor-α agent infliximab has been associated with worsening of preexisting interstitial fibrosis in patients with RA.
- Chemotherapeutic agents associated with ILD include the antineoplastic agents bleomycin, busulfan, and

methotrexate. Pulmonary toxicity associated with bleomycin derives from its free radical-promoting ability; risk of life-threatening bleomycin-induced pulmonary injury is significantly increased by cumulative doses >500 mg/m,[2] concurrent or subsequent radiation, or high concentrations of inspired O_2, even when administered well after bleomycin. This latter effect is termed a recall phenomenon and can give rise to rapidly progressive ILD. Interstitial pneumonitis and fibrosis result in ground-glass opacities on chest CT scans, as well as focal areas of consolidation and irregular linear opacities that involving the lower lung zones.
- Busulfan-related pulmonary injury culminating in ILD occurs in <5% of patients treated for underlying myeloproliferative disorders. Apart from a history of receiving this agent, there are no unique clinical findings, radiographic features, or physiological abnormalities.
- Like busulfan, methotrexate may cause both an acute pulmonary hypersensitivity reaction as well as chronic ILD.
- Lymphangioleiomyomatosis (LAM) is a rare form of ILD caused by abnormal smooth muscle proliferation involving the alveolar septae, bronchioles, and lymphatic vessels that occurs sporadically in females of child-bearing age. The pathophysiology of LAM results in small airways obstruction; characteristic radiographic features are the combination of bilateral interstitial opacities and generalized pulmonary cyst formation. Recurrent pneumothorax is not uncommon and lymphatic obstruction may cause chylous pleural effusion. Despite the apparent ILD in LAM, an obstructive ventilatory pattern on pulmonary function testing is typically observed.

PATHOPHYSIOLOGY

- Overall, the primary causes of ILD associated with the idiopathic interstitial pneumonias or specific underlying conditions are unknown. Diverse pathophysiological features are responsible for differing manifestations ILD depending on the underlying condition and type of interstitial pneumonia/fibrosis (IPF).
- In IPF, the underlying usual interstitial pneumonia results from augmented fibrogenesis with varying degrees of inflammation.[1] An insult of unknown origin initiates and perpetuates IPF by injury to the alveolar epithelium, pulmonary capillary endothelium, and alveolar basement membrane throughout the lungs in a scattered, patchy manner. Reparative mechanisms are also deranged; an intra-alveolar exudative process occurs and macrophages, fibroblasts, and other inflammatory cells infiltrate alveoli and interstitial spaces.

- Repeated cycles of injury, aberrant repair, and fibrotic remodeling lead to neovascularization of intraalveolar structures and buds of granulation tissue associated with enhanced collagen deposition that eventually obliterate alveolar spaces and pulmonary capillaries. Collectively, these processes account for the characteristic histopathological finding in IPF lung specimens of temporal inhomogeneity, in which normal lung, alveolar inflammation, collagen-related fibrosis, and fibroblastic foci may all be seen it occur in one low power microscopic field.
- Whereas differential cell counts in BALF normally show ≤3% to 5% neutrophils (PMNs) in nonsmokers, significantly increased BALF PMN numbers (eg, ≥20%) are found in IPF.
- The cytokine transforming growth factor-(TGF) β is considered a causal cytokine mediator of stimulated fibrogenesis in IPF and other fibrotic lung disorders; increased TGF-β levels are found in the lungs and BALF of IPF patients. TGF-β signaling in the lungs to create a profibrotic milieu occurs via the SMAD transcription factor pathway, whose activity promotes fibroblast proliferation and differentiation, eventuating in abnormally increased rates of collagen synthesis and deposition.
- There is additional evidence for cytokine dysregulation in IPF and related fibrosing lung disease, that involves abnormal overexpression and elevations of type 2 (Th-2) cytokines (eg, IL-4, IL-5, IL-6, IL-10, and IL-13) and reduction of type 1 (Th-1) cytokines (eg, IL-2, interferon (IFN)-α, IL-12, and TNF-β).
- In contrast to IPF, AIP is characterized histopathologically by a uniform, homogenous pattern of injury and repair to alveolar structures; all lesions appear to be of the same age and diffuse alveolar damage is especially prominent. The initiating cause of AIP is unknown.
- Sarcoidosis is characterized by a CD4+ (helper) T-cell predominance in the lungs (eg, BALF and pulmonary interstitium), whereas peripheral blood mononuclear cells in this condition exhibit a predominant CD8+ (suppressor) T-cell phenotype. No specific cause of sarcoidosis has been identified; exposure of a genetically susceptible host to specific environmental agents that the immune system is unable to clear effectively has been proposed as a general mechanism.
- A unifying pathophysiological explanation for ILD associated with the diverse connective tissue diseases has not been proposed.
- Eosinophilic ILD and pneumonia are a diverse group of disorders with multiple etiologies sharing the common pathophysiology of enhanced eosinophil recruitment and trafficking into the lung parenchyma. Key eosinophil chemotactic factors such as IL-5 and various neuropeptides are elevated in BALF and lung specimens of such patients. IL-5 also stimulates eosinophil secretion and prolongs eosinophil survival; eosinophil basic protein released from cell granules has cytotoxic properties.
- Pathological features of hypersensitivity pneumonitis may include poorly formed, noncaseating interstitial granulomas, along with giant cells and mononuclear cell infiltration in a peribronchial distribution. Although precipitating IgG antibodies or positive skin tests are usually found to the suspected triggering antigen(s), this finding is itself not diagnostic, because similarly exposed individuals without evidence for lung disease may also have elevated precipitin concentrations or positive skin tests.
- In the pneumoconioses, the size and cumulative dose of inhaled material as well as its inherent fibrogenicity predispose to ILD. Thus, asbestos fibers ≤3 microns in diameter that penetrate to the respiratory (alveolar) zone of the lungs have increased fibrogenic potential. Asbestosis fibers as well as crystalline silica are ingested but not degraded by alveolar macrophages; these cells are then activated to secrete cytotoxic O_2 free radicals (eg, superoxide anion, hydrogen peroxide, and hydroxyl radical), peroxynitrite (as the product of superoxide anion and nitric oxide), and a variety of cytokines, chemokines, and profibrogenic growth factors.
- The pathophysiology of PAP is unique, involving increased secretion and abnormal processing by alveolar macrophages of surfactant-derived phospholipids, which accumulate in alveolar spaces and stain positive by the periodic acid-Schiff (PAS) reagent. Deficiency or inactivation of the cytokine granulocyte-macrophage colony-stimulating factor (GM-CSF) appears to play a causal role. Because host defense functions of alveolar macrophages are impaired in PAP, opportunistic lung infection may occur, especially with *Nocardia asteroides*.
- A central pathophysiological feature of ILD is restrictive lung impairment owing to decreased lung compliance secondary to interstitial fibrosis. Because the transpulmonary pressure (eg, airway pressure minus the pleural pressure) is the distending pressure of the lung during inspiration, a greater positive airway pressure is required for lung inflation in ILD. Consequently, inspiratory muscle work and O_2 consumption are greater, particularly during exertion, when higher levels of ventilation and increased respiratory muscle blood flow are required. Development of respiratory muscle fatigue then progressively limits exercise tolerance and predisposes to dyspnea on exertion.

- Besides an increased O_2 cost of breathing in ILD, exertional dyspnea results from three other mechanisms: (1) O_2 diffusion disequilibrium, (2) reduction in the volume of the pulmonary capillary bed because of fibrotic scarring, and (3) pulmonary hypertension.
- Diffusion disequilibrium in ILD occurs when the alveolar PO_2 (ie, PAO_2) does not equilibrate with end-capillary blood in pulmonary capillaries (eg, PaO_2) because of the abnormally thickened alveolar-capillary membrane. In normal lungs, equilibration between the PAO_2 in alveolar gas and the PaO_2 in pulmonary capillary blood is complete within about 0.25 seconds, and the transit time of red blood cells in pulmonary capillaries is approximately 0.75 seconds at rest. Although O_2 equilibration at rest is postulated to take longer in patients with ILD, it is still largely completed within the 0.75 seconds transit time. However, the combination of a longer equilibration time plus significantly increased red blood cell transit time during exertion (eg, because of increased right ventricular output and pulmonary blood flow) result in incomplete O_2 saturation in end-capillary blood, manifested clinical as exertional O_2 desaturation.
- Consistent with this concept, reductions in the diffusing capacity for carbon monoxide (DL_{CO}) characterize the various forms of ILD, since the DL_{CO} is a measure of the conductance of CO from alveolar gas to hemoglobin in pulmonary capillary blood.
- In addition to alveolar capillary loss and destruction in ILD causing exertional hypoxemia by a diffusion limitation mechanism, exercise-related falls in the PaO_2 (or SpO_2 by pulse oximetry) may also result from right-to-left shunting through a patent foramen ovale as pulmonary artery pressure pathologically increases. There is also an increase in dead space ventilation resulting from alveolar ventilation without corresponding alveolar capillary perfusion.
- Arterial hypoxemia along with metabolic acidosis during exercise or respiratory acidosis from the increased dead space ventilation are potent stimuli for pulmonary vasoconstriction, which over time results in abnormal vascular remodeling and luminal narrowing. The associated increases in pulmonary vascular resistance predispose to progressive secondary pulmonary hypertension, right ventricular (RV) hypertrophy (cor pulmonale), and progressive dyspnea on exertion.
- Up to 66% of patients with IPF have accompanying gastroesophageal reflux disease (GERD); reflux can occur in both the upright and supine positions, extend to the proximal esophagus, and be clinically silent.[6] Occult pulmonary aspiration and additional lung inflammatory scarring may ensue.

DIAGNOSIS

- The cardinal symptom of ILD is dyspnea on exertion, usually progressive. Chronic nonproductive or minimally productive cough is next in frequency; intermittent wheezing is less common, but may be present if there is coexisting asthma or tobacco abuse. Many individuals with ILD present after failed empiric treatment for presumed infectious pneumonia.
- Constitutional symptoms typified by fever, malaise, and unintentional weight loss may be prominent.
- The clinical presentation of different forms of ILD may vary significantly; ILD is frequently overlooked as a differential diagnostic possibility when disease onset is relatively acute. However, in AIP (ie, Hamman-Rich syndrome), acute exacerbations of IPF, flares of chronic hypersensitivity pneumonitis, alveolar hemorrhage syndromes, or drug-induced pulmonary disease, rapidly progressive dyspnea culminating in respiratory failure occurs, requiring emergent intubation and mechanical ventilatory support. Differentiation from acute infectious pneumonia may be difficult and require fiberoptic bronchoscopy if the patient cannot expectorate sputum for analysis.
- Obtaining a careful medical history is the single most helpful diagnostic procedure in patients with ILD in view of the large number of differential diagnostic possibilities. A detailed occupational history is especially crucial in the diagnosis of pneumoconiosis.
- Physical examination, including chest findings, may be normal in patients with ILD, except when preexisting conditions associated with ILD are present (eg, connective tissue diseases). When present, abnormal chest findings include dry inspiratory crackles at the lung bases (*velcro* crackles) or expiratory wheezes secondary to bronchial hyperreactivity or small airway obstruction. When ILD is associated with pulmonary hypertension, an accentuated pulmonic component of the second heart sound may be auscultated, along with a holosystolic murmur increasing on inspiration compatible with tricuspid regurgitation, or right ventricular third heart sound. Peripheral lymphadenopathy is uncommon; when present it may signify involvement by sarcoidosis. Digital clubbing is occasionally observed but lacks diagnostic specificity.
- Prolonged expiratory wheezing in a patient with ILD should raise the suspicion for eosinophilic lung disease (especially Churg-Strauss syndrome) respiratory bronchiolitis-ILD, airway involvement in sarcoidosis or hypersensitivity pneumonitis, lymphangioleiomyomatosis, or preexisting/concomitant asthma.

- Diagnostic biopsy should be performed of any skin lesion in a patient with ILD, with the exception of erythema nodosum which is sufficiently characteristic for sarcoidosis. Maculopapular, popular, or purpuric lesions suggest the possibility of sarcoidosis, vasculitis, or malignancy.

PULMONARY FUNCTION TESTS

- The classic spirometric finding of ILD on pulmonary physiologic testing is a restrictive ventilatory pattern, characterized by parallel reductions in the forced vital capacity (FVC) and the forced expiratory volume in one second (FEV_1), resulting in a normal or elevated FEV_1/FVC ratio on spirometry. The slow vital capacity is similarly reduced, while the expiratory flow-volume curve demonstrates an increased slope and reduced area.
- Respiratory muscle weakness is not uncommon in ILD, particularly in patients with connective tissue diseases such as SLE and those receiving long term corticosteroid treatment. Maximal inspiratory and expiratory pressure measurements are useful to specifically assess the contribution of respiratory muscle weakness to spirometric abnormalities and dyspnea.
- Reductions in the total lung capacity (TLC) to $\leq 80\%$ of predicted values are confirmatory, which as usually accompanied by decreases in the residual volume (RV). Considering the frequent association of ILD with fibrotic thickening of the alveolar-capillary membrane, decreases in the single breath DL_{CO} are also common.
- Gas exchange in ILD as determined by arterial blood gases may be normal at rest. In advanced ILD, respiratory alkalosis with hypocapnia and mild-to-moderate arterial hypoxemia and widening of the (alveolar-arterial) $A\text{-}aO_2$ gradient are frequent. Exercise tests usually show an increase in the ratio of dead space to tidal volume (Vd/Vt), increase in the respiratory rate, $A\text{-}aO_2$ gradient and hypoxemia.
- Overnight pulse oximetry and/or polysomnographic testing are indicated to exclude sleep-disordered breathing and nocturnal O_2 desaturation in patients with nocturnal dyspnea or those with pulmonary hypertension by transthoracic echocardiography or right heart catheterization.

CHEST RADIOGRAPHY

- A hallmark feature of ILD is an abnormal plain chest radiograph (CXR) showing reticular or nodular opacities, singly or combined with interstitial infiltrates. However, the CXR may be normal in up to 10% of patients with symptomatic ILD. Review of all prior chest radiographs is important to establish chronology and disease activity.
- The diagnosis of sarcoidosis in subjects with bilateral hilar lymphadenopathy and normal lung fields (ie, Stage I disease) along with acute erythema nodosum of the lower extremities may be made on clinical grounds; this presentation is most frequent in young adult female patients. Overall, plain chest radiographs are abnormal in nearly 90% of patients with sarcoidosis.
- The chest radiographic staging of sarcoidosis implies, but does not indicate, temporal progression of disease. Moreover, correlation is poor between radiographic stage of sarcoidosis and clinical symptoms, pulmonary function test abnormalities, or chest CT scan involvement.
- ILD with predominant involvement of the mid-upper lung zones should raise the possibility of sarcoidosis, pulmonary histiocytosis X, silicosis, and cystic fibrosis (CF) lung disease (although CF is not an interstitial lung disease per se), and hypersensitivity pneumonitis.
- Plain chest radiographs showing the *photographic negative of pulmonary edema*, in other words, bilateral peripheral infiltrates with relative sparing of the perihilar regions, have been associated with chronic eosinophilic pneumonia (CEP), although this pattern is not seen in up to one-third of cases of established CEP.
- Overt pleural abnormalities including pleural effusion in a patient with ILD should raise the suspicion of asbestosis, drug-induced ILD, malignancy (eg, lymphangitic spread of cancer), and connective tissue diseases, including RA.
- Spontaneous pneumothorax occurring in the setting of an ILD suggests the possibility of underlying sarcoidosis, pulmonary histiocytosis X, and lymphangioleiomyomatosis, the latter condition may also be distinguished by hyperinflated lungs due to gas trapping.

COMPUTED TOMOGRAPHY OF THE CHEST

- Conventional chest computed tomography (CT) scans that typically use 10-mm slices may not meaningfully improve detection of ILD in patients with negative findings on plain chest radiographs. However, high-resolution chest CT (HRCT) scanning employs tissue slices of 1 to 3 mm and significantly improves detection of airspace filling or interstitial opacities. As for plain chest radiograph, review of all previous chest CT imaging studies is important in establishing a diagnosis of ILD as well as following the response to treatment.
- HRCT performed in both prone and supine views is recommended for evaluation of ILD, because the radiographic density of dependent lung regions may simulate interstitial changes. Likewise, vascular engorgement of dependent lung zones may mimic

septal thickening on supine-only views. Thus, radiographic abnormalities that persist on the prone view support the presence of ILD.

- Specific distribution patterns of opacities on HRCT scan can suggest specific types of ILD, or assist in limiting the list of differential diagnostic possibilities, especially in conjunction with clinical findings. Thus, homogeneous linear fibrosis is characteristic of nonspecific interstitial pneumonia.
- The characteristic HRCT pattern in UIP associated with IPF or RA is a bilateral, predominantly peripheral (eg, subpleural) fibrosis in a patchy pattern with architectural distortion, cystic changes including basilar honeycombing and traction bronchiectasis, without significant nodules or ground glass attenuation.
- Small, generalized, multinodular opacities that are randomly distributed throughout the lungs along bronchovascular bundles, the pleural surfaces, as well as the lung parenchyma (ie, as nodules unattached to specific lung vascular or pleural structures) represent a miliary distribution and typically result from either infection or sarcoidosis.

FIBEROPTIC BRONCHOSCOPY WITH TRANSBRONCHIAL LUNG BIOPSY

- Fiberoptic bronchoscopy has a limited but important role in the diagnostic approach to patients suspected of having ILD. It is relatively safe to perform in patients with diffuse infiltrative/interstitial lung diseases; its main utility is to exclude the relatively limited number of other conditions that either simulate ILD, or have sufficiently pathognomonic or characteristic pathological findings (Table 113–5).
- Because the lungs are involved in ≥95% of patients with sarcoidosis, the diagnosis is otherwise best established by fiberoptic bronchoscopy with transbronchial lung biopsy. The hallmark of sarcoidosis is nonnecrotizing granulomas with epithelioid histiocytes and multinucleated giant cells, along with negative smears and cultures for microorganisms, particularly acid-fast bacilli and fungi.
- Chronic beryllium disease of the lungs simulates the histopathological (as well as the clinical and radiographic) features of sarcoidosis.

TABLE 113–5   Utility of Fiberoptic Bronchoscopy in ILD

CONDITION	PRIMARY DIAGNOSTIC QUESTION(S)	KEY DIAGNOSTIC FINDING(S)
Idiopathic interstitial pneumonia, ILD related to connective tissue diseases or other conditions already being treated with corticosteroid or other immune suppressive therapy	Infectious pneumonia vs. progression of underlying ILD	-Gram stain of BALF showing microorganisms and WBCs; -Quantitative bacterial culture of BALF with ≥10^4 CFU/mL, or protected brush catheter with ≥10^3 CFU/mL; -Transbronchial lung biopsy with positive results on special stains and/or cultures for microorganisms
Suspected sarcoidosis, radiographic stage II or III	Differentiation from other ILDs, lymphoma, mycobacterial infection	-Lymphocytic predominance on BALF differential count; -Noncaseating epithelioid granulomas on transbronchial lung biopsy with negative results on special stains and/or cultures for microorganisms
Diffuse interstitial infiltrates with peripheral blood eosinophilia	Chronic eosinophilic pneumonia vs. drug induced pulmonary disease, other ILD	-Eosinophilic predominance on BALF; -Transbronchial lung biopsy showing abundant tissue eosinophils
Interstitial pulmonary infiltrates with known or suspected lung cancer	Lymphangitic carcinomatosis vs. infectious pneumonia	-Tumor cells in BALF; -Cytology brush or transbronchial lung biopsy specimens positive for tumor
Established SLE with new-onset diffuse bilateral pulmonary infiltrates	Diffuse alveolar hemorrhage vs. infectious pneumonia	-Recovery of progressively more bloody BALF on serial aliquots; -Lack of microbial infection on BALF or protected brush specimens; -Transbronchial lung biopsy
Suspected pulmonary alveolar proteinosis	Infectious pneumonia, diffuse alveolar hemorrhage	-Recovery of milky-appearing, PAS-positive material from BALF; -Transbronchial lung biopsy findings showing proteinaceous, PAS-positive material in alveolar spaces with minimal inflammation or fibrosis

BALF, bronchoalveolar lavage fluid; CFU, colony-forming unit; ILD, interstitial lung disease; PAS, periodic acid-Schiff; SLE, systemic lupus erythematosus; WBC, white blood cell.

SURGICAL LUNG BIOPSY

- When transbronchial biopsy is inconclusive and a definitive diagnosis is required, surgical lung biopsy is indicated (Fig. 113–1). Advantages of surgical lung biopsy for the diagnosis of ILD include the ability to obtain larger specimens for pathological analysis and better control of oxygenation as well as biopsy-related bleeding.
- Surgical lung biopsy is best guided by the distribution of disease on HRCT images and after discussion with the thoracic surgeon. Video-assisted thoracoscopic surgery (VATS) biopsy causes less morbidity than open thoracotomy and is better tolerated, whereas patients with marginal oxygenation receiving mechanical ventilatory support secondary to acute respiratory failure and/or severe coexisting pleural disease may be better managed during open thoracotomy.
- Lung tissue specimens from surgical lung biopsy are ideally ≥2 cm in size, obtained from several separate sites, and include specimens from visually and radiographically normal lung as well as from areas with mild-to-moderate disease. Sampling from the right middle lobe and lingular segments is not recommended

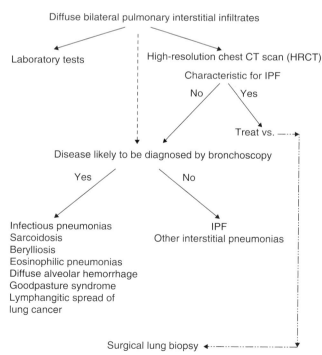

FIG. 113–1 General diagnostic algorithm for ILD after a comprehensive medical history, physical examination, and plain chest radiography. Dashed line reflects option of proceeding directly to fiberoptic bronchoscopy in the event that conditions such as infectious pneumonia or diffuse alveolar hemorrhage are suspected.

considering the frequency of modest nonspecific fibrosis in these areas.
- The need for a surgical biopsy to establish a diagnosis of IPF is undergoing reevaluation; a correct noninvasive diagnosis may be made in up to 85% to 90% of patients by integrating clinical and typical HRCT findings.

LABORATORY MEASUREMENTS

- Routine laboratory data are of limited diagnostic utility in most forms of ILD. Leukopenia is observed with sarcoidosis as is hypercalcemia in about 10% of patients. Peripheral eosinophilia should raise the suspicion of eosinophilic lung disorders, drug-induced ILD, and sarcoidosis.
- Serological studies including rheumatoid factor (RF), antinuclear antibodies (ANA), antineutrophil cytoplasmic antibody (ANCA), and other tests are be useful in supporting a diagnosis of connective tissue-related ILD. However, low-level positive serum titers of RF and ANA and/or an elevated erythrocyte sedimentation rate are common in a variety of ILD conditions and are not diagnostic.
- There are no specific diagnostic tests for drug-induced ILD; a high clinical index of suspicion is therefore necessary.
- Tuberculin skin testing and controls should be performed in patients with ILD; however, impaired delayed-type immune reactions are common because of the underlying condition or from anti-inflammatory therapy including corticosteroids. Up to two-thirds of patients with sarcoidosis have cutaneous anergy.
- Serum angiotensin-converting enzyme (ACE) levels have overall poor sensitivity and specificity for sarcoidosis; they correlate poorly with either the radiographic stage of sarcoidosis or with prognosis.
- In addition to an occupational history of beryllium exposure, the diagnosis of chronic berylliosis is facilitated in vitro lymphocyte transformation testing of peripheral blood mononuclear cells or alveolar macrophages harvested from BALF.
- Serum precipitin testing and/or skin tests along with clinical features and chest imaging results may be useful in supporting a diagnosis of hypersensitivity pneumonitis, if there is presumptive knowledge of the offending antigen(s).
- Dyspnea on exertion can reflect diverse cardiopulmonary conditions. Accordingly, echocardiography is useful in ILD patients to determine the presence of right ventricular hypertrophy/dilation, pulmonary hypertension, and tricuspid valve regurgitation, as well as to evaluate left ventricular contractility and valvular function.

THERAPEUTIC APPROACH

- ILD is not a single disease, but encompasses many different pathological conditions. Therefore, the therapeutic approach is different for each disease.
- Dyspneic patients with ILD may have several coexisting causes of breathlessness, such as atypical angina, congestive heart failure, pulmonary edema, infectious pneumonia, anemia, physical deconditioning, and other conditions. As noted, pulmonary hypertension related to ILD or to other causes (eg, obstructive sleep apnea, left ventricular dysfunction) may result in nonspecific symptoms and determine the level of exercise tolerance more than lung parenchymal involvement per se.
- The general approach to ILD patients involves determining the need for supplemental O_2 therapy at rest, during exertion, and during sleep to improve dyspnea and avoid arterial hypoxemia which may contribute to secondary pulmonary hypertension. Patients with advanced ILD are also at risk for dyspnea and hypoxemia with increasing altitude during air travel because aircraft cabins are pressurized to only about 8000 feet. Decreased inspired O_2 tensions at altitude may cause tachypnea with respiratory alkalosis and alveolar hypoxia. Provision of supplemental O_2 during air travel is recommended if the predicted PaO_2 by high-altitude simulation test (HAST) is ≤50 mm Hg.
- Optimal treatment of the idiopathic interstitial pneumonias typified by IPF is unknown. Since IPF and related conditions represent fibroproliferative disorders rather than inflammatory disease per se, the response to antiinflammatory treatment yields inconsistent results, depending on the degree of lung inflammation in individual patients. Initial treatment with oral prednisone therapy at 0.5 mg/kg/day is recommended, along with immunosuppressive drugs such as azathioprine or cyclophosphamide.[1] The efficacy of therapy in terms of symptom improvement as well as by thoracic imaging studies and pulmonary function testing should be reevaluated at 3 to 6 months. A recent phase 3 trial of interferon γ 1-b for IPF found no benefit.[7]
- Prognosis in IPF is better for patients 50 years of age or younger, those with a shorter history of respiratory symptoms and/or chest radiographic abnormalities (eg, ≤1 y), and subjects with less severe restrictive ventilatory impairment and lung parenchymal disease on HRCT.
- NSIP will generally respond to this pharmacological approach whereas UIP frequently does not. In respiratory bronchiolitis-ILD, smoking cessation is particularly important.

- For severe presentations of acute interstitial pneumonia associated with respiratory failure or acute exacerbations of IPF (eg, a relentlessly progressive, rapidly fatal deterioration over ≤4 wk or several mo), even in patients with mild-to-moderate disease, anecdotal evidence supports a trial of pulsed intravenous methylprednisolone, (1 g/d for 3–4 d) followed by oral prednisone therapy at 40 to 60 mg/day and a prolonged tapering course over several months.
- For subjects with IPF 60 years of age or younger, lung transplantation extends life and enhances its quality. Because approximately 30% of IPF patients currently listed for pulmonary transplantation will die waiting for a donor organ, this treatment option should be discussed with patients as early as possible followed by appropriate referral.
- In patients with sarcoidosis, up to two-thirds have spontaneous remissions of disease and do not require treatment. The likelihood of spontaneous remission varies with radiographic stage; remission occurs in up to 90% of patients with Stage I disease versus 10% to 20% of those with Stage III disease. Treatment with corticosteroid therapy starting at 0.5 mg/kg day (eg, 30–40 mg/d) is indicated for patients with cardiac, neurological, ocular, or hypercalcemic manifestations of sarcoidosis, Stage II disease with symptoms, and Stage III disease. Treatment with a tapering course of steroids for at least 12 months is recommended to avoid relapse. Steroid-sparing treatment with azathioprine or methotrexate is useful for steroid resistant disease or intolerable steroid-related side effects. Sarcoidosis patients with wheezing and evidence of obstructive ventilatory dysfunction on pulmonary function testing may benefit from inhaled β_2-agonists or treatment with combined inhaled long-acting salmeterol and fluticasone.
- The etiologies of eosinophilic ILD generally respond well to treatment with corticosteroids. However, relapses of chronic eosinophilic pneumonia following steroid withdrawal occur in up to 50% of cases if initial therapy is too abbreviated; despite rapid initial improvement, a 6- to 9-month course of treatment is recommended.
- The primary treatment of hypersensitivity pneumonitis is physical removal from the suspected offending antigen; corticosteroids accelerate the rate of recovery.
- Suspected drug-induced ILD is generally treated by systematic discontinuation of potential toxic agents; for severe or progressive disease, a trial of corticosteroid therapy is undertaken with serial monitoring of symptoms as well as chest imaging results and pulmonary physiologic testing.
- Treatment of pulmonary hypertension secondary to connective tissue-related ILD is FDA approved, although

the regimen varies with the acuity of presentation and degree of symptomatic impairment reflected by New York Heart Association (NYHA) functional status.

- For patients with severe disease (eg, NYHA Class IV with dyspnea at rest), epoprostenol administered by continuous intravenous infusion is the therapy of choice. Epoprostenol therapy is commenced in the inpatient setting and usually only after definitive confirmation of pulmonary hypertension severity by right heart catheterization. Other treatment options include non-specific endothelin receptor blockade with bosentan (Tracleer) beginning at 62.5 mg twice daily increasing to 125 mg twice daily, and phosphodiesterase inhibition with sildenafil (Revatio) 20 mg three times daily. Liver function test abnormalities occur in up to 10% of patients receiving bosentan and monthly testing is recommended.
- Pulmonary rehabilitation is recommended for patients with moderate ILD and breathlessness. Benefits of pulmonary rehabilitation include improvement in exercise capacity and quality of life, as well as reduction in dyspnea, anxiety and depression, and health care utilization.

REFERENCES

1. ATS/ERS International Multidisciplinary Consensus Classification of the Idiopathic Interstitial Pneumonias. *Am J Respir Crit Care Med.* 2002;165:277–304.
2. Coultas DB, Zumwalt RE, Black WC, Sobonya RE. The epidemiology of interstitial lung disease. *Am J Respir Crit Care Med.* 1994;150:967–972.
3. Henke CE, Henke G, Elveback LR, Beard CM, Ballard DJ, Kirland LT. The epidemiology of sarcoidosis in Rochester, Minnesota: A population-based study of incidence and survival. *Am J Epidemiol.* 1986;123:840–845.
4. Dawson JK, Fewins HE, Desmond J, Lynch MP, Graham DR. Fibrosing alveolitis in patients with rheumatoid arthritis as assessed by high resolution computed tomography, chest radiography, and pulmonary function tests. *Thorax.* 2001;56: 622–627.
5. Marie I, Hachulla E, Cherin P, et al. Interstitial lung disease in polymyositis and dermatomyositis. *Arthritis Rheum.* 2002;47: 614–622.
6. Sweet MP, Patti MG, Leard LD, et al. Gastroesophageal reflux in patients with idiopathic pulmonary fibrosis referred for lung transplantation. *J Thorac Cardiovasc Surg.* 2007;133: 1078–1084.
7. Raghu G, Brown K K, Bradford W Z, et al.; the Idiopathic Pulmonary Fibrosis Study Group. A placebo-controlled trial of interferon gamma 1-b in patients with idiopathic pulmonary fibrosis. *N Engl J Med.* 2004;350:125–133.

114 VENOUS THROMBOEMBOLISM

Wilman Ortega and George M. Matuschak

DEFINITION

- Deep venous thrombosis (DVT) and pulmonary embolism (PE) are considered differing clinical manifestations of the same underlying disorder of vascular biology, that is, venous thromboembolism (VTE), which is characterized by abnormal intravascular coagulation and formation of clots within the venous system. Pulmonary emboli originate from thrombi in the deep veins of the legs (75 to 90% of cases), renal, pelvic, and upper extremity veins. Thus, PE is not a disease per se, but rather a complication of DVT.

EPIDEMIOLOGY

- Venous thromboembolism is a common condition that affects 7.1 persons per 10,000 person-years in community residents. Incidence rates for VTE are higher in men and in African-Americans. Rates rise with increasing age, with an approximate doubling of risk over each 10-year interval.[1]
- Pulmonary embolism originating from VTE affects more than 600,000 people each year in the United States and contributes to 100,000 to 200,000 deaths annually.
- Pulmonary embolism is the third most common cause of death in hospitalized patients. Approximately 10% of patients with acute PE die within the first hour, and 30% of patients without treatment die subsequently from recurrent embolism. In patients with hemodynamic instability and shock associated with massive PE, mortality rates exceed 20% and 30%.
- Accurate diagnosis and effective treatment of PE reduces mortality rates to between 2% and 8%.
- Patients experiencing a PE have an approximate 8% 1-year risk of recurrence if effective initial treatment and secondary preventive therapy are not given.
- The incidence of DVT in hospitalized patients not receiving effective thromboprophylaxis varies between 20% and 70%.
- Deep venous thrombosis can occur in any venous bed of the body, including the upper or lower extremities. However, the main sites of origin of clinically significant thromboemboli (>70%) of arise in the proximal deep veins of the lower extremities, including the iliac,

femoral, superficial femoral veins, as well as the pelvic veins. In patients genetically predisposed to VTE, DVT within the renal or hepatic veins may also occur.

- In critically ill patients, the incidence of upper extremity DVT is increased owing to the frequency of central venous catheterizations. Pulmonary embolism may complicate upper extremity DVT in up to 15% of such patients.
- The most common risk factors for VTE are a prior history of VTE, advancing age, prolonged immobilization, pregnancy and the postpartum period (which are associated with a fivefold increased risk of VTE), estrogen therapy including oral contraceptive use, recent surgery (especially orthopedic procedures involving the hip or knee), congestive heart failure, obesity, severe trauma, critical illness, malignancy, and hospitalization (Table 114–1).
- Venous thromboembolism during or shortly after air travel is also associated with relative immobilization on flights covering >3100 miles (~5000 km).
- Several genetic/familial abnormalities of coagulation (thrombophilias) are associated with increased VTE risk (Table 114–2). These hereditary thrombophilias by themselves predispose to VTE but also synergistically interact with common medical, surgical, obstetric, and other conditions to amplify the risk of venous thromboembolic events.[2]
- Inherited thrombophilia should be suspected when a patient has recurrent or life-threatening VTE, a family history of VTE, is younger than 45 years of age, and has no overt medical or surgical risk factors.
- An inherited thrombophilia should also be suspected if the patient is a woman with a history of multiple spontaneous abortions, stillbirth, or both.

TABLE 114–1 Acquired Risk Factors for Venous Thromboembolism

Common acquired medical conditions:

Prior VTE
Advancing age, especially >60 years
Prolonged immobilization
Pregnancy and the postpartum period
Estrogen therapy including oral contraceptive use
Recent surgery, especially hip and knee replacement
Congestive heart failure
Obesity
Severe trauma
Critical illness
Malignancy
Inpatient hospitalization

Uncommon acquired medical conditions:

Nephrotic syndrome
Antiphospholipid antibody syndrome
Lupus anticoagulant
Inflammatory bowel disease
Paroxysmal nocturnal hemoglobinuria
Behçet syndrome

VTE, venous thromboembolism.

TABLE 114–2 Hereditary Risk Factors for Venous Thromboembolism

Common hereditary abnormalities of coagulation (familial thrombophilias):

Factor V Leiden mutation
 Homozygous
 Heterozygous
Prothrombin 20210A gene mutation
Homozygous C677T mutation in the methylenetetrahydrofolate reductase gene

Rare hereditary abnormalities of coagulation (familial thrombophilias):

Antithrombin III deficiency
Protein S deficiency
Protein C deficiency
Hyperhomocysteinemia
Homozygous homocystinuria

- Homocystinuria, a rare thrombophilia, is associated with both venous and arterial thromboses.
- Factor V Leiden, the G20210A prothrombin gene mutation, and deficiencies of protein C or protein S lead to increased thrombin generation; antithrombin III deficiency is associated with decreased neutralization of thrombin already generated.[2]
- The most important and common hereditary thrombophilia associated with VTE (up to 40% of cases) is the factor V Leiden mutation, in which the mutated activated factor V (eg, factor Va) is resistant to the anticoagulant effects of protein C, thereby inducing protein C resistance.
- The heterozygous carrier state occurs in approximately 5% of whites and to a lesser extent in other races. Heterozygosity for the factor V Leiden mutation elevates the risk of VTE by 5- to 10-fold, whereas the homozygous state increases VTE risk by nearly 80-fold.
- The factor V Leiden mutation specifically amplifies VTE risk associated with oral contraceptive use, pregnancy, or the postpartum state; these conditions plus the gene mutation enhance overall risk for venous thromboembolic events by 30-fold. Venous thromboembolism risk in these settings are further accentuated by coexisting mutations in the prothrombin 20210A gene.

PATHOLOGIC FEATURES

- Initial formation of venous thrombi in the lower extremities usually occurs as a progressively enlarging aggregation of platelets within the deep veins of the calf, primarily around valve cusps. However, thrombi can also initially arise in the ileofemoral deep venous system; femoral venous catheters predispose to VTE in this area. Mural thrombi in the right heart chambers can be an additional source of pulmonary thromboemboli.

- Microscopically, venous thrombi are composed of platelets and fibrin with variable amounts of enmeshed red blood cells (red thrombus).
- Organization of thrombi in the calves is accompanied by proximal extension and growth as more platelets, fibrin, and red blood cells are progressively deposited.
- Approximately 60% to 80% of venous thrombi in the calves resolve within weeks or months as a result of natural thrombolytic mechanisms. The remaining thromboemboli become adherent to the vessel wall, undergo organization, and are converted into fibrous masses. The venous valves of the calf veins are frequently irreversibly injured during this sequence of events.
- Spontaneous resolution of an established DVT in the ileofemoral deep venous system and full restoration of blood flow occurs in <10% of patients.
- Pulmonary thromboemboli are bilaterally distributed to both lungs in approximately 65% of cases. Because of the relatively greater perfusion to the lung bases, pulmonary emboli are four times more likely to be found in the pulmonary arteries of the lower lobes.
- In massive PE, defined as thromboembolic occlusion of two or more lobar pulmonary arteries, the main pulmonary arterial trunk and/or right and left main pulmonary arteries are blocked by a large mass of clot material that sometimes extends into the right ventricle.
- Pulmonary infarction complicating pulmonary embolization is uncommon, occurring approximately 10% of the time. Embolic infarction of peripheral lung segments is more common with submassive pulmonary emboli, especially when lung perfusion is already compromised, eg, decompensated congestive heart failure.

PATHOPHYSIOLOGY

- The three major pathophysiologic events that give rise to clots within the venous system are described by Virchow triad:
  1. Venous stasis, as might occur during prolonged immobilization
  2. Endothelial injury caused by trauma
  3. Hypercoagulability, reflecting inherited thrombophilias, increased levels of coagulation proteins including factor VIII and fibrinogen, or de novo abnormalities (eg, the antiphospholipid antibody syndrome and development of the lupus anticoagulant, etc).

The hemodynamic affect of PE is proportional to the degree of obstruction of the pulmonary arterial tree.

Pulmonary hypertension, defined as a resting mean pulmonary artery pressure >25 mm Hg, occurs when more than 50% of the pulmonary arterial circulation becomes occluded by thromboembolic material.

- Acute right ventricular (RV) failure leading to cardiac arrest is the principal cause of death from an initially massive thromboembolic event or recurrent PE. As embolic occlusion of the pulmonary arterial tree exceeds 50% to 70% of its cross-sectional area, pulmonary vascular resistance increases exponentially, and is charcterized by elevations in mean pulmonary artery pressures that exceed 40 mm Hg. The normal thin-walled right ventricle is incapable of acutely generating systolic pressures to overcome this increase in afterload. Right ventricular systolic dysfunction and dilation ensue, which reduce left ventricular (LV) compliance, LV diastolic filling, and cardiac output. Concomitant reductions in systemic blood pressure and RV coronary diastolic perfusion further impair RV contractility.
- Recurrent, clinically occult VTE may occur and gradually obstruct the pulmonary vasculature, ultimately leading to chronic thromboembolic pulmonary hypertension and cor pulmonale.
- Pulmonary gas exchange abnormalities as determined by arterial blood gas analysis are surprisingly variable in VTE complicated by PE. The Pao_2 is usually reduced and the alveolar-arterial O_2 gradient increased, primarily because of ventilation/perfusion ($\dot{V}/\dot{Q}$) mismatching; however, normal values for the Pao_2 and arterial O_2 saturation (Sao_2) by pulse oximetry are observed in up to 18% of patients with documented PE.
- Intrapulmonary reflexes during PE cause variable degrees of bronchoconstriction and vasoconstriction owing to the release of humoral mediators, which further contribute to $\dot{V}/\dot{Q}$ mismatching. Also, surfactant depletion in embolized lung segments predisposes to atelectasis.
- Acute hypoxemic respiratory failure following even massive PE is rare, unless there is significant preexisting lung disease, or when it arises in the presence of a patent foramen ovale (PFO). A PFO can acutely increase with elevated pulmonary artery pressure secondary to thromboembolic occlusion of the lung's vasculature and produces significant right-to-left shunting and corresponding reductions in Pao_2 values.
- An acute respiratory alkalosis with mild-moderate reductions in the $Paco_2$ value is a frequent but nonspecific finding in PE.
- In patients on mechanical ventilation receiving supplemental O_2 for other respiratory conditions, significant changes in Pao_2 or Sao_2 values may not be observed after a PE. Because significant and/or recurrent PE

increases dead space ventilation (ie, the fraction of ventilated alveoli without perfusion), increasing $PaCO_2$ levels may signal PE in this setting.

- The timing of resolution of pulmonary emboli in patients receiving anticoagulant therapy is variable; larger thromboemboli usually lyse within 4 weeks, whereas subsegmental abnormalities on lung perfusion scans may persist for longer periods of time, or only partially resolve.

CLINICAL PRESENTATION

- Acute unexplained dyspnea or gradually progressive dyspnea on exertion or at rest are hallmark features of VTE with PE.
- Nonetheless, the clinical presentation of a patient with VTE tends to be nonspecific and variable, although the size of the DVT and the anatomic extent and acuity of the pulmonary arterial occlusion are contributory factors.
- Because the symptoms and signs of VTE are nonspecific, a high index of suspicion followed by appropriate diagnostic testing are required to establish the diagnosis.
- Leg pain or objective findings on physical examination occur in only half the patients with subsequently documented DVT. Also, asymptomatic PE develops in more than 50% of patients with DVT.
- In patients with established PE, up to 70% have no concurrent leg symptoms or signs.
- The most common symptoms of acute PE in the initial Prospective Investigation of Pulmonary Embolism Diagnosis study were unexplained dyspnea (73%), pleuritic chest pain (66%), cough (37%), and hemoptysis (13%).[3] Pleuritic chest pain generally signifies peripheral lung embolization with infarction associated with submassive emboli and is caused by inflammation of the visceral/parietal pleura.
- Venous thromboembolism causing PE is common in geriatric patients, yet the diagnosis is often not considered because of coexisting chronic respiratory symptoms or impaired communication.
- Syncope (with or without seizures) or near syncope occurs in approximately 15% of patients with massive PE.
- Physical findings in patients with VTE and PE are also variable and nonspecific. In submassive or massive acute PE, tachypnea is the most frequent finding, followed by tachycardia. Fever, wheezes, or substernal chest discomfort may also be elicited. A pleural friction rub is characteristic of pulmonary infarction. A right-sided second heart sound, ventricular gallop, fourth heart sound, loud pulmonic second heart sound, or systolic murmur reflecting tricuspid regurgitation may be audible after massive PE or in subjects with recurrent multiple pulmonary emboli in whom pulmonary hypertension has developed.

- Massive and/or recurrent PE should be included in the differential diagnosis of syncope, near syncope, or acutely developing circulatory shock. The patient may appear weak, pale, sweaty, and/or oliguric with impaired mentation. The hypotension accompanying such obstructive shock may respond to fluids.
- New-onset cardiac arrhythmias, especially supraventricular atrial arrhythmias including atrial fibrillation, has been considered suggestive of PE. However, this is not a sensitive finding, occurring in only approximately 5% of cases.
- When present, physical findings of a DVT in an extremity include an increased circumference relative to the uninvolved side, tenderness, warmth, and erythema.

LABORATORY EVALUATION

- Initial laboratory tests:
  - Initial laboratory evaluation of patients with suspected VTE and PE should include an arterial blood gas determination, chest radiograph, electrocardiogram (ECG), complete blood count, and D-dimer blood test.
  - Arterial blood gas results may be normal, but hypocapnia and respiratory alkalosis are common. Hypercapnia and lactic acidosis occur when obstructive shock supervenes during massive PE.
  - The chest radiographs (either portable or standard posteroanterior and lateral films) are not uncommonly normal in patients without preexisting lung disease. There are no diagnostic features of PE on the plain radiographs. In certain patients, focal oligemia of the lung is visualized as a localized increase in radiographic lucency, along with an abrupt tapering of the vessel(s) because of thromboembolic obstruction (Westermark sign). This sign may be suggestive of the diagnosis but is of limited sensitivity.
  - Focal segmental or lobar atelectasis may be present owing to surfactant depletion and/or pulmonary infarction; in the latter case, a wedge-shaped peripheral opacity abutting the pleural surface (ie, Hampton hump) may be visualized, although chest imaging by computed tomography (CT) scan has superior sensitivity for this finding.
  - Pulmonary embolism is the fourth leading cause of pleural effusions; the possibility of a pulmonary embolus should considered in all patients who have undiagnosed pleural effusions.

◦ Effusions associated with PE may be transudative but are usually exudative, and rarely are larger than one-third of the hemithorax. The degree of dyspnea may be disproportionate to the size of the effusion. A bloody exudative effusion is more common after pulmonary infarction.

◦ The ECG is neither sensitive nor specific for PE. Its chief value is in excluding cardiac etiologies for dyspnea such as acute myocardial infarction. Sinus tachycardia and nonspecific changes in the ST segment and T wave are common. Anterior T-wave inversions with tachycardia, plus a new incomplete right bundle-branch block pattern are the ECG findings most compatible with the diagnosis of PE in the appropriate clinical setting.

◦ The S1Q3T3 (right heart strain) pattern is an uncommon ECG sign of acute cor pulmonale that may be seen in massive and/or recurrent PE. However, other respiratory causes for acute cor pulmonale such as pneumothorax and severe bronchospasm may also give rise to this pattern.

◦ D-Dimer is formed during acute VTE when crosslinked intravascular fibrin is lysed by plasmin. To distinguish such circulating crosslinked fibrin originating from VTE versus fibrinogen and/or non-crosslinked fibrin, testing should be carried out using sensitive monoclonal antibodies.

◦ Elevated levels usually occur with VTE and PE. The chief value of the D-dimer test is to exclude the diagnosis of VTE.

◦ When combined with other diagnostic testing, patients with a normal D-dimer test have a low probability of PE.[3,4]

◦ Other conditions that elevate D-dimer levels include disseminated intravascular coagulation, severe sepsis/septic shock, recent surgery, liver disease, and malignancy.

DIAGNOSIS

DEEP VEIN THROMBOSIS

• Duplex venous ultrasonography uses real-time ultrasound with Doppler flow studies. It is the most accurate means for diagnosing DVT regardless of patient care setting, having >95% sensitivity and specificity for lower extremity proximal vein DVT as well as a negative predictive value exceeding 96%. Failure to compress the vascular lumen (because of an occluding thrombus) is the ultrasonographic criterion for DVT. Doppler flow signals are normally phasic; loss of phasicity supports the diagnosis of venous occlusion.

• Normal results of duplex ultrasonography do not rule out PE if clinical suspicion is moderately high. Studies of the lower extremities are negative in up to 30% of patients with PE confirmed by helical CT angiography. False-negatives are usually caused by embolization of the entire venous thrombus or origination of the VTE in the iliac, pelvic, or other deep venous structures.

• Limitations of duplex ultrasonography include decreased sensitivity for calf vein DVT (approximately 70%), inability to visualize VTE above the inguinal ligament, and difficulty in distinguishing new versus old or nonocclusive thrombi.

• Normal results for duplex ultrasonography and D-dimer measurements exclude VTE in ambulatory patients.

CLINICAL PROBABILITY MODEL FOR DIAGNOSIS OF PULMONARY EMBOLISM

• Establishing a priori (pretest) clinical probability for PE during initial evaluation of risk factors, physical findings, and laboratory data is crucial to interpreting the significance of imaging results from $\dot{V}/\dot{Q}$ scanning or helical CT angiography. Explicitly determining clinical probability also guides further diagnostic testing when needed.

• A high clinical probability is assigned in approximately 60% to 70% of patients because of underlying risk factors (see Tables 114–1 and 114–2), a clinical presentation consistent with VTE, and no apparent alternate diagnosis.

• A low clinical probability is assigned to approximately 10% of patients without identifiable risk factors in whom an alternate or coexisting diagnosis accounts for the clinical findings.

• An intermediate clinical probability is assigned to approximately 20% to 30% of the remaining patients.

• Clinical probability alone is insufficient to confirm or exclude PE. Diagnostic imaging is always necessary.

• The combined use of estimated clinical probability and one or more noninvasive diagnostic tests significantly increases the accuracy of diagnosis, compared to either approach alone.

SPECIFIC TESTS

VENTILATION–PERFUSION SCAN

• The $\dot{V}/\dot{Q}$ scan is the most sensitive screening test for PE.[3,4] A normal ventilation study with lobar or segmental perfusion filling defects resulting in a $\dot{V}/\dot{Q}$ mismatch is the most characteristic finding. Even so, coexisting lung diseases such as pneumonia, chronic obstructive pulmonary disease, or interstitial disease may limit interpretation. Almost all patients with PE have abnormal scans of high, intermediate, or low probability, but many without PE have similar findings; the specificity of the $\dot{V}/\dot{Q}$ scan is therefore low (~10%).

- Prediction rules for establishing the probability of PE based on image interpretation differ from prediction rules to establish the pretest clinical probability. Thus, the positive predictive value of a $\dot{V}/\dot{Q}$ scan is based on the clinical pretest probability of PE, not on the scintigraphic characteristics of the imaging study per se.
- Several guidelines apply when interpreting a $\dot{V}/\dot{Q}$ scan. Clinical assessment combined with the $\dot{V}/\dot{Q}$ scan established the diagnosis PE for a minority of patients— those with clear and concordant clinical and ventilation/perfusion scan findings.
- A high-probability scan showing a $\dot{V}/\dot{Q}$ mismatch and lobar/segmental perfusion defects is diagnostic of PE in the presence of a high or intermediate pretest clinical probability. A normal $\dot{V}/\dot{Q}$ scan (or perfusion scan alone in ventilated patients) excludes the diagnosis of PE.[3,4] A $\dot{V}/\dot{Q}$ scan with low probability for PE such as subsegmental perfusion defects with or without mismatched ventilation abnormalities may still be associated with a positive predictive value approaching 40% in patients having a high pretest clinical probability. Most $\dot{V}/\dot{Q}$ scans are interpreted as having either low or intermediate probability, in which case the patient requires additional evaluation.

D-DIMER

- The combination of normal D-dimer levels and a low pretest clinical probability accurately excludes acute VTE, even after taking into account the type of D-dimer assay used.[4]

HELICAL COMPUTED TOMOGRAPHIC ANGIOGRAPHY

- This method can directly visualize intravascular thrombi as well as parenchymal abnormalities that may otherwise account for dyspnea and other symptoms. Its overall sensitivity ranges between 60% and 100%, especially for VTE involving the main or lobar pulmonary arteries, and its specificity between 75% and 100%. Newer multidetector scanners have improved diagnostic accuracy.
- Helical CT angiography of the chest is less accurate for peripheral lung thromboemboli in segmental and, particularly, subsegmental vessels, with sensitivity rates as low as 70%.
- The incidence of isolated subsegmental PE varies between 5% and 30%. Accordingly, negative CT angiography results do not completely exclude PE in patients having a high pretest clinical probability. At least 5% of such patients have had embolism subsequently confirmed by pulmonary angiography.

- Technically limited CT imaging resulting in suboptimal visualization of thromboemboli may also occur in another 10% of patients because of body habitus, patient movement artifact, or incomplete opacification of vessels.
- A negative helical CT scan significantly reduces the likelihood of PE but cannot definitely exclude the possibility to the same degree as a negative $\dot{V}/\dot{Q}$ scan.

PULMONARY ANGIOGRAPHY

- It is the gold standard for establishing a diagnosis of PE. Complications during catheter insertion, arrhythmias, and reactions to radiographic contrast media account for morbidity approximately 5% of the time; mortality from the procedure in experienced centers is <0.5%.
- A noninvasive diagnostic strategy combining clinical assessment, D-dimer measurement, duplex ultrasonography, $\dot{V}/\dot{Q}$ scanning, and/or helical CT angiography yield a diagnosis in most patients with suspected VTE without the need for pulmonary angiography.

OVERALL DIAGNOSTIC ALGORITHM

- In patients having a high clinical probability of PE, $\dot{V}/\dot{Q}$ scanning or helical CT angiography are equally suitable diagnostic approaches.
- Patients with negative results on CT angiography or with low-intermediate interpretations on $\dot{V}/\dot{Q}$ scanning should also undergo duplex ultrasonography.
- Patients with a high clinical probability of PE but who have negative results on duplex ultrasonography and helical CT scan as well as low-intermediate interpretations on $\dot{V}/\dot{Q}$ scans are candidates for pulmonary angiography.

TREATMENT

- Therapy for VTE is aimed at inhibiting the proximal extension of deep vein thrombi and preventing PE. Additional goals are to reduce the incidence of recurrent VTE and limit bleeding risks associated with anticoagulant therapy.

DEEP VEIN THROMBOSIS

- Unfractionated heparin (UFH) has been traditionally used to treat DVT, but this approach has limitations: Its variable dose-response relationship can result in subtherapeutic anticoagulation over the first 24 to 48 hours of treatment, which predisposes to clot propagation and/or embolization. Variable bioavailability may also cause supratherapeutic anticoagulation and increased risk of bleeding. Multiple laboratory determinations of the activated partial thromboplastin time (APTT) are necessary for dosage adjustments, and UFH is more frequently associated with development of heparin-induced thrombocytopenia (HIT).

• When used, UFH should be administered by a weight-based nomogram using an initial intravenous bolus of 80 units/kg, followed by a continuous intravenous infusion rate of 18 units/kg/h. The infusion rate is adjusted thereafter to result in prolongation of the APTT to 1.5 to 2.5 of control values.

• Low-molecular-weight heparin (LMWH) is superior to UFH for the initial treatment of DVT; mortality as well as risk of major bleeding are both reduced. Other advantages of LMWH include simplicity of fixed, weight-based dosages, minimal need for laboratory monitoring, and decreased incidence of HIT. Therefore, LMWH rather than UFH should be used when possible for the initial treatment of DVT.[5]

• Thrombolytic therapy for massive iliofemoral thrombosis complicated by severe swelling of the leg and signs of developing arterial insufficiency (phlegmasia cerulea dolens) is an accepted indication for thrombolytic therapy with tissue plasminogen activator (tPA; alteplase), streptokinase, or urokinase. Dosage regimens for tPA; 100 mg intravenous infusion delivered over 2 hours; for streptokinase, 250,000 units intravenously over 30 minutes followed by 100,000 units/h over 24 hours; and for urokinase, 4400 units/kg intravenously over 10 minutes followed by a continuous infusion of 2200 units/kg/h over 12 hours.

• After any form of thrombolytic therapy for acute VTE, standard doses and courses of LMWH or UFH therapy are indicated.

• The risk of intracranial hemorrhage (up to 3%) and other serious bleeding is higher with thrombolytic therapy than with heparin compounds or vitamin K antagonists.

• In hospitalized patients, an oral vitamin K antagonist such as warfarin should be started at the same time as parenteral LMWH or UFH when possible. An overlap of 5 days is needed in which LMWH or UFH and vitamin K antagonists are coadministered because of incomplete inhibition of all vitamin K–dependent coagulation factors (II, VII, IX, and X) and early prothrombotic effects of warfarin caused by inhibition of the natural anticoagulants proteins S and C.

• The initial dose of warfarin in VTE is usually 5 mg/day for 3 days; dosages are subsequently adjusted to obtain an international normalized ratio (INR) of 2 to 3 (conventional-intensity warfarin therapy).[5]

• In patients with acute lower extremity DVT who cannot receive acute anticoagulation because of strong contraindications, placement of an inferior vena cava (IVC) filter is recommended.

• Unlike vitamin K antagonists, neither UFH nor LMWH cross the placenta to cause embryopathy or fetal bleeding. Therefore, one of these agents is the treatment of choice for pregnant women with VTE.

• The postthrombotic syndrome involving venous insufficiency of the involved lower extremity with pain, edema, and hyperpigmentation complicates DVT in up to 50% of patients. Compression stockings should be used routinely to prevent postthrombotic syndrome, beginning within 1 month of diagnosis of proximal DVT and continuing for a minimum of 1 year after the diagnosis.[5]

• Outpatient treatment of DVT and, in certain instances, PE with LMWH is safe and cost effective for carefully selected patients, especially those with underlying malignancy it should be considered if the required support services are in place.[5]

PULMONARY EMBOLISM

• Weight-based intravenous UFH therapy has been traditionally used for initial treatment of PE. However, either weight-based LMWH in appropriate patients or UFH (using the same weight-based protocol as for DVT) may be used to treat hemodynamically stable patients with PE.[5]

• Thrombolytic therapy is effective in accelerating the rate of resolution of pulmonary embolic obstruction. Existing studies of thrombolytic therapy have been underpowered to demonstrate reduced mortality compared with heparin therapy. Even so, massive PE complicated by persistent shock and signs of acute RV failure is an accepted indication for thrombolytic therapy.

• In patients with massive PE (eg, a saddle thromboembolism demonstrated on chest CT angiography) but in which there is no shock, hemodynamic instability, or significant RV dysfunction or pulmonary hypertension by echocardiography, conventional anticoagulation with LMWH or UFH is appropriate.

• Patients with acute VTE and PE unable to receive anticoagulation because of strong contraindications should undergo placement of an IVC filter.

• Patients with documented recurrence of PE despite otherwise appropriate and therapeutic anticoagulation with LMWH or UFH should receive an IVC filter.

• Complications of IVC filters include a higher incidence of postthrombotic syndrome and recurrent DVT; selected patients in whom anticoagulation is acutely contraindicated may benefit from subsequent oral anticoagulation with a vitamin K antagonist when clinically appropriate.

- Hypoxemia from massive PE in subjects with normal underlying lung function is mostly from $\dot{V}/\dot{Q}$ mismatch and responsive to supplemental O_2 with nasal cannulae at flow rates of 2 to 5 L/min (corresponding to fractional inspired oxygen concentration [FIO_2] value of approximately 35%) or a Venturi mask at FIO_2 levels between 0.4 and 0.6. Refractory hypoxemia from supervening PE in patients with abnormal underlying lung function or right-to-left shunting through a PFO is an indication for intubation and mechanical ventilatory support, as is persistent tachypnea and increased work of breathing during circulatory shock from a massive embolism.
- The acute increase in RV afterload during massive PE causes RV dilation and increased RV myocardial oxygen consumption by the law of LaPlace; simultaneously, coronary diastolic perfusion pressure to the RV falls owing to reduced cardiac output. Preservation of RV diastolic perfusion pressure is achieved using combined α-adrenergic and β_1-adrenergic receptor stimulation with norepinephrine.
- Low cardiac output without accompanying arterial hypotension render RV ischemia unlikely and α-adrenergic stimulation unnecessary. Dobutamine is clinically effective in this setting.

DURATION OF ANTICOAGULATION FOR ACUTE VENOUS THROMBOEMBOLISM

- A first episode of VTE (DVT and/or PE) with transient risk factors is treated with 3 to 6 months of a vitamin K antagonist such as warfarin.[5] Recurrent VTE is treated for at least 12 months and idiopathic VTE optimally for up to 4 years.
- In patients with acute VTE and cancer, anticoagulant therapy is administered indefinitely or until the cancer resolves. For patients with malignancy LMWH is the preferred initial approach and may be more efficacious in preventing recurrences than oral anticoagulants.[5]
- In patients with VTE associated with antiphospholipid antibody syndrome, a first episode of VTE is treated with at least 12 months of anticoagulation; if additional risk factors are present, treatment is continued indefinitely.
- A first episode of VTE associated with factor V Leiden, deficiency of antithrombin III, protein C or S, or hyperhomocysteinemia is treated for 6 to 12 months; patients having 2 or more episodes of VTE should be anticoagulated indefinitely.

PREVENTION

- Several approaches using different anticoagulant drugs, varying dosages of each drug based on risk factor stratification, and physical methods such as graduated compression stockings and intermittent pneumatic compression devices can achieve effective thromboprophylaxis.
- A useful framework for deciding on a specific approach is as follows:
  1. Distinguishes between medical and surgical patients
  2. Takes into account the type of surgical procedure (eg, orthopedic surgery of the lower extremities involving hip or knee replacement vs. other surgical procedures)
  3. Considers underlying comorbidities including congestive heart failure, significant obesity, or other conditions
  4. Notes the special circumstances of VTE risk inherent in critically ill medical and trauma patients[4]
- Aspirin alone is not an effective thromboprophylaxis in any patient population.[6]
- For moderate-risk general surgery patients, prophylaxis with low-dose unfractionated heparin (LDUH; 5000 U subcutaneously twice daily) or LMWH ($\leq$3400 U subcutaneously once daily) is recommended.
- For higher-risk general surgery patients, evidence based data support thromboprophylaxis using LDUH (5000 U subcutaneously three times daily) or LMWH (>3400 U subcutaneously once daily).
- For high-risk general surgery patients with multiple risk factors for VTE, a combination of methods is useful, including LDUH subcutaneously three times daily or LMWH, >3400 U subcutaneously once daily, plus graduated compression stockings and/or intermittent pneumatic compression devices.[6]
- For patients undergoing elective total hip or knee arthroplasty that are at especially high risk for VTE, LMWH, fondaparinux, or adjusted-dose vitamin K antagonist with warfarin to an INR target of 2.5 (range: 2.0–3.0) are equally effective.
- In acutely ill medical patients with congestive heart failure or severe respiratory disease, or who are confined to bed and have one or more additional risk factors, prophylaxis with LDUH, LMWH, or the synthetic pentasaccharide fondaparinux which inhibits anti-factor Xa activity (dosage: 2.5 mg subcutaneously once daily), are effective.

REFERENCES

1. Horlander KT, Mannino DM, Leeper KV. Pulmonary embolism mortality in the United States, 1979–1998: An analysis using multiple-cause mortality data. *Arch Intern Med.* 2003;163:1711–1717.
2. Seligsohn U, Lubetsky A. Genetic susceptibility to venous thrombosis. *N Engl J Med.* 2001;344:1222–1231.

3. The PIOPED Investigators. Value of the ventilation/perfusion scan in acute pulmonary embolism. Results of the Prospective Investigation of Pulmonary Embolism Diagnosis (PIOPED). *JAMA*. 1990;263:2753–2759.

4. Kruip MJHA, Leclercq MGL, van der Heul C, Prins MH, Buller HR. Diagnostic strategies for excluding pulmonary embolism in clinical outcome studies: A systematic review. *Ann Intern Med*. 2003;138:941–951.

5. American College of Physicians, American Academy of Family Physicians. Management of venous thromboembolism: a clinical practice guideline from the American College of Physicians and the American Academy of Family Physicians. *Ann Intern Med*. 2007;146:204–210.

6. Geerts WH, Pineo GF, Heit JA, et al. Prevention of venous thromboembolism. The Seventh ACCP Conference on Antithrombotic and Thrombolytic Therapy. *Chest*. 2004;126: 338S–3400S.

115 PLEURAL DISEASES

*Patricia A. Dettenmeier and
George M. Matuschak*

DEFINITION

- A pleural effusion is an abnormal accumulation of fluid in the space between the parietal pleura lining the inner thoracic cage and the visceral pleura covering the outermost surfaces of the lungs. Normal pleural fluid is alkaline with a pH ranging between 7.60 and 7.64, and represents an ultrafiltrate derived from microvessels in the parietal pleura governed by hydrostatic capillary pressure (approximately 25 mm Hg). The pleural space normally contains only a few milliliters of fluid—approximately 10 to 20 mL in a 70 kg individual—that lubricates the parietal and visceral pleura during respiratory motion.

- The vascular supply of the parietal pleura is derived from the intercostal arteries, whereas the visceral pleura receives blood from the bronchial arteries.

- Differentiation of the type of pleural effusion into transudative versus exudative categories relates to the principal mechanism of fluid accumulation, which in turn accounts for the distinct biochemical profile that defines each type of effusion (Tables 115–1 and 115–2).

- Transudative pleural effusions are characterized by low pleural fluid concentrations of constituent plasma proteins (principally albumin) as well as other plasma biomarkers (eg, lactate dehydrogenase, cholesterol); by extension, pleural fluid/serum ratios for these substances are also low.

- Exudative effusions are characterized by increased pleural fluid and pleural fluid/serum ratios of protein, lactate dehydrogenase (LDH), cholesterol, and other substances normally confined to the intravascular space.

- Light's criteria[1–3] for classifying pleural effusions into exudative versus transudative collections consists of three elements: (1) a pleural fluid/serum protein concentration > 0.5, (2) a pleural fluid/serum concentration of LDH > 0.6, and (3) an absolute serum LDH concentration more than two-thirds of the upper normal limit of the testing laboratory (see Table 115–1).

- A pseudoexudative pleural effusion refers to a misclassified pleural effusion that is initially transudative, typically associated with congestive heart failure, but in which the protein and LDH concentrations become artificially increased over time secondary to augmented pleural water resorption during diuretic therapy.

- A hemothorax refers to blood in the pleural space, most commonly the result of penetrating or nonpenetrating trauma, excessive anticoagulation, or rarely, thoracic endometriosis.

- Yellow nail syndrome is a rare disorder of lymphatic vessels characterized by recurrent exudative pleural effusions, lymphedema, and yellowish discoloration of the nails.

- Chylous pleural effusions are defined as lipid-rich fluid collections with high triglyceride concentrations secondary to disruption of the thoracic or accessory thoracic ducts; alternatively, chylothorax results from central compression or effacement of lymphatic channels (eg, from lymphomatous tumor involvement of hilar/mediastinal lymph nodes).

- Parapneumonic pleural effusions are categorized into three groups: (1) uncomplicated parapneumonic effusions, (2) complicated parapneumonic effusions, and (3) thoracic empyema.

- An uncomplicated parapneumonic effusion is an exudative, culture-negative, free-flowing pleural effusion that develops in conjunction with pneumonia. The effusions are generally small and resolve completely following antimicrobial therapy directed at the pneumonia. Complicated parapneumonic effusions are defined as those that require pleural space drainage for resolution; they are associated with significant morbidity and mortality if not managed appropriately because of intrapleural adhesions, persistently infected loculated fluid collections, and development of trapped lung.[4,5] Thoracic empyema represents overt pus in the pleural space and is the end result of a complicated parapneumonic effusion. Pleural space drainage is mandatory in empyema.

- Trapped lung refers to restriction of lung expansion because of fibrous thickening of the visceral pleura,

TABLE 115–1 Laboratory Features for Differentiation Between Transudative and Exudative Pleural Effusions

TRANSUDATIVE EFFUSION	EXUDATIVE EFFUSION
Pleural fluid/serum protein ratio ≤0.5	Pleural fluid/serum protein ratio >0.5
Pleural fluid/serum LDH ratio ≤0.6	Pleural fluid/serum LDH ratio >0.6
Pleural LDH concentration less than two-thirds of the upper limit of laboratory normal value	Pleural LDH concentration greater equal to two-thirds of the upper limit of laboratory normal value
Pleural fluid cholesterol ≤45 mg/dL	Pleural fluid cholesterol >45 mg/dL
Serum albumin-pleural fluid gradient >1.2 g/dL	Serum albumin—pleural fluid gradient ≤1.2 g/dL

LDH, lactate dehydrogenase.
SOURCE: Light RW. *Pleural Diseases*. 4th ed. Philadelphia, PA: Williams & Wilkins; 2001. Light RW. Pleural effusion. *N Engl J Med*. 2002;346:1971–1977.

usually as a result of pleural infection, inflammation, or bleeding.

- A pneumothorax is defined as air or gas in the pleural cavity. It can occur spontaneously (eg, primary spontaneous pneumothorax), follow trauma of the parietal or visceral pleura, or arise from the presence of gas-forming organisms in the pleural space.
- A bronchopleural (BP) fistula is an abnormal connection between the tracheobronchial tree or lungs and the pleural space, resulting in pneumothorax. A characteristic feature of BP fistulae is continued intrapleural air leakage following chest-tube insertion.
- Tension pneumothorax is a medical emergency in which progressive elevations in intrapleural pressure secondary to an enlarging, trapped gas collection culminate in arterial O_2 desaturation, reduced venous return, decreased cardiac output, and a precipitous decrease in arterial blood pressure.
- Re-expansion pulmonary edema is a rare unilateral lung complication associated with pulmonary edema and alveolar consolidation that occurs following the rapid re-expansion of a chronically collapsed lung, eg, typically occurring after the removal of a large amount of air or fluid from the pleural space.
- Malignant mesothelioma is a tumor of the parietal or visceral pleura caused by asbestos exposure; the two main histologic subtypes of this tumor are the epithelioid or sarcomatoid variants; a mixture of the two is common.

EPIDEMIOLOGY

- The commonest cause of a pleural effusion is congestive heart failure (CHF); effusions in CHF are bilateral (right greater than left) in ≥85% of patients, transudative in nature, and usually accompanied by clinically overt symptoms and signs of left ventricular dysfunction such as bilateral lung crackles and an S_3 gallop. In approximately 5% of patients, isolated left pleural effusions occur.
- The nephrotic syndrome is associated with small to moderate pleural effusions in approximately 20% of patients; effusions are transudative and are directly related to the severity of hypoalbuminemia, particularly when serum albumin concentrations are <1.5 g/dL.
- The most frequent cause of an exudative pleural effusion is a parapneumonic effusion, which occurs in approximately 40% to 50% of bacterial pneumonias.[1,2,4,5] Annually, between 250,000 and 500,000 parapneumonic effusions develop in hospitalized patients in the United States.[4,5]
- The majority of parapneumonic pleural effusions are uncomplicated; approximately 10% to 15% of parapneumonic effusions become complicated, and 5% progress to empyema.[4] Clinical features predisposing to or indicative of complicated parapneumonic effusions include protracted symptoms (eg, >7–10 days to several weeks) despite antimicrobial therapy, large effusions (eg, >40%–50% of the hemithorax), loculated or multiloculated fluid collections on chest computed

TABLE 115–2 Causes of Transudative Versus Exudative Pleural Effusions

TRANSUDATIVE EFFUSION	EXUDATIVE EFFUSION
Congestive heart failure[a]	Pneumonia
Cirrhosis	Complicated parapneumonic effusion
-Hepatic hydrothorax	Empyema
Pulmonary thromboembolism	Malignancy
Nephrotic syndrome	Pulmonary thromboembolism
Hypothyroidism	Benign asbestos pleural effusion
Urinothorax	Connective tissue disease
Peritoneal dialysis fluid	Postcardiac injury (Dressler) syndrome
	Pancreatitis or pancreatic pseudocyst
	Tuberculous pleurisy
	Esophageal rupture
	Drug reaction
	Yellow nail syndrome
	Meigs syndrome

[a]Effusions are bilateral although not necessarily of equal size in approximately 80% of patients.

tomography (CT) scan with a thickened or enhancing visceral pleura, intrapleural air–fluid levels, or anaerobic pulmonary infections accompanied by pleural effusion.[3]

- Pulmonary thromboembolism can cause either transudative or exudative pleural effusions; pulmonary infarction and associated pleural inflammation generally causes an exudative effusion.

- The postcardiac injury syndrome has a relatively acute presentation with dyspnea, fever, symptoms of pericarditis, pleuritic chest pain, and an exudative pleural effusion (typically left sided), developing in the setting of previous cardiac surgery or instrumentation such as percutaneous coronary intervention, pacemaker implantation, or radiofrequency ablation procedures. The condition is also termed Dressler syndrome when it persists for several weeks to months and is associated with auto-antibodies directed against cardiac tissue.

- Hepatic hydrothorax is observed in 5% to 10% of patients with cirrhotic liver disease and portal hypertension. Effusions are typically transudative unless spontaneous bacterial peritonitis supervenes, and generally (but not uniformly) associated with clinically overt ascites. Hepatic hydrothorax is unilateral and right sided in approximately 50% to 70% of patients; bilateral and isolated left effusions occur in approximately 15% of patients. Patients usually have other stigmata of chronic liver disease such as jaundice, spider angiomata, and liver-function test abnormalities.

- Benign asbestos pleural effusion (BAPE) is an exudative fluid collection resulting from prior asbestos exposure; it is characterized by a long latency period (eg, 20–25 years).

- Pleural effusions associated with malignancy have multiple potential causes: (1) pleural inflammation and fibrin deposition from metastatic tumor involvement, (2) atelectasis from central bronchial obstruction in lung cancer, (3) postobstructive pneumonia, (4) decreased colloid osmotic pressure from malnutrition and hypoalbuminemia, (5) pulmonary thromboembolism, and (6) cardiotoxic effects of chemotherapy resulting in increased pleural fluid formation from elevated microvascular hydrostatic pressure. Pleural effusion(s) developing in the context of confirmed lung or extrathoracic neoplasms should not therefore be automatically equated with a malignant (eg, cytology-positive) effusion.

- Primary spontaneous pneumothorax is usually not associated with clinically overt pulmonary disease; even so, ≥80% to 90% of patients have ipsilateral subpleural bullae visualized on chest CT scans or thoracscopically. It is most common in young thin males, 10 to 30 years of age. Cigarette smoking strongly predispose

to primary spontaneous pneumothorax; the risk is increased up to 20-fold compared with nonsmokers.

- An increased risk of spontaneous pneumothorax is also seen with interstitial lung diseases including sarcoidosis, pulmonary histiocytosis X, and lymphangioleiomyomatosis. Women with thoracic endometriosis are also at risk for catamenial pneumothorax.

- Pneumothorax of any size in a patient undergoing or about to undergo positive-pressure ventilation requires tube thoracostomy to minimize the risk of tension pneumothorax.

- Re-expansion pulmonary edema as a complication of the rapid evacuation of fluid or gas from the pleural space characteristically manifests as sudden onset respiratory distress and hypoxemia, despite otherwise successful resolution of the initial pleural space issue (eg, large pleural effusion or pneumothorax). More than half of patients with this complication develop it within 1 hour of the pleural procedure; the reminder do so within 24 h. A new unilateral alveolar filling pattern by chest radiography on the involved side is characteristic.

- The most common pleural tumor is metastatic disease, especially from primary neoplasms of the lung, breast, and ovary.

- There are no laboratory tests to diagnose benign asbestosis pleural effusion; it is a diagnosis of exclusion.

- The rising worldwide incidence of malignant mesothelioma is not expected to peak for another 10 to 20 years.[6]

- The lifetime risk of developing malignant mesothelioma with a history of heavy asbestos exposure is 7% to 10%; its occurrence is typified by a long latency period (eg, 25–45 years following asbestos exposure). Occupations with asbestos exposure and increased risk of benign asbestos pleural effusion and malignant mesothelioma include boilermakers, carpenters, electricians, insulation workers, janitors, laborers, pipefitters, plumbers, steamfitters, and welders/cutters.

PATHOPHYSIOLOGY

- There are seven mechanisms by which pleural effusions can develop; they can occur singly or in combination: (1) increased hydrostatic pressure in parietal pleural microvessels (eg, CHF); (2) decreased serum colloid osmotic pressure (eg, hepatic cirrhosis, nephrotic syndrome); (3) increased permeability of pleural microvessels caused by inflammation, infection, or neoplasm (eg, parapneumonic pleural effusion, empyema, pleural metastatic tumor); (4) decreased or impaired lymphatic drainage of the pleural space (eg, lymphoma, yellow nail syndrome); (5) decreased peri-microvascular pressure in the pleural space from incomplete lung expansion favoring pleural fluid accumulation (eg, atelectasis, endobronchial obstruction, trapped lung); (6) enhanced transdiaphragmatic movement of peritoneal fluid (eg, hepatic hydrothorax, peritoneal dialysis); and (7) iatrogenic instillation of fluid into the pleural space, generally with accompanying pneumothorax (eg, misdirected central venous catheters, enteral feeding tubes).

- The forces regulating pleural fluid formation by the parietal pleura are summarized by the Starling equation:

$$Q = Kf\,(Pmv - Ppl) - \sigma\,(\pi mv - \pi pl),$$

where Q = fluid flow, Kf = the filtration coefficient, a function of the surface area and permeability of microvessels, Pmv = microvascular hydrostatic pressure, Ppl = pleural pressure, σ = the reflection coefficient for protein movement across the pleura, πmv = colloid osmotic pressure in parietal pleural microvessels, and πpl, colloid osmotic pressure in the pleural space. Notably, the protein reflection coefficient defines the barrier function of the parietal pleural microvessels and membrane, such that decreases in α, typified by inflammatory conditions, correlate with increased permeability to protein. The intravascular concentration of albumin (mol wt ~65-kD) is the primary determinant of serum colloid osmotic pressure.

- Pleural fluid reabsorption is accomplished by parietal pleural lymphatics in dependent regions of the pleural cavity, especially on the diaphragmatic surface and in the mediastinal regions. Under normal circumstances, rates of pleural fluid formation and reabsorption are tightly balanced; fluid accumulation occurs when the rate of pleural fluid formation exceeds that of reabsorption.

- Transudative pleural effusions are caused by two primary mechanisms, occurring singly or in combination: (1) increases in the hydrostatic pressure of the parietal pleural microvessels, and (2) decreases in serum colloid osmotic pressure.

- Exudative pleural effusions primarily result from increased permeability of microvessels in the parietal pleura.

- There are three stages in the development of complicated parapneumonic effusions with important patient care implications: (1) the early exudative or capillary leak stage lasting 2 to 5 days following the onset of the pleural effusion, during which time the effusion is mostly free-flowing and amenable to simple pleural drainage by tube thoracostomy, (2) the fibrinopurulent or bacterial invasion stage extending for 3 to 14 days; and (3) the organizational or empyema stage of between 10 and 21 days.[4,5]

- Atelectasis and trapped lungs predispose to development of pleural effusions by promoting a negative regional intrapleural pressure, which favors fluid formation along a pressure gradient from the parietal pleural interstitium.

- Enhanced transdiaphragmatic movement of peritoneal fluid into the pleural space through anatomic defects or enlarged lymphatic vessels in the diaphragm is the principal mechanism of pleural effusion development in hepatic hydrothorax. A similar process can occur with pleural effusions associated with pancreatic ascites, or more rarely, peritoneal dialysis.

- The mechanisms of dyspnea related to pleural effusions and its resolution following thoracentesis are complex. By themselves moderate to large pleural effusions have only modest effects on pulmonary mechanics (eg, the vital capacity, forced vital capacity, and forced expiratory volume at 1 second); despite often significant improvements in the sensation of dyspnea following thoracentesis, such parameters of pulmonary mechanics typically increase by an average of only 10%. Chest wall afferent vagal nerve fibers are involved in the sensation of dyspnea.

- An acute increase in the alveolar-arterial O_2 gradient of approximately 10 to 20 mm Hg is common after thoracentesis because of increased ventilation/perfusion mismatching in the expanding but still partially atelectatic lung.

- BAPE as well as malignant mesothelioma are initiated by inhalation and deposition of asbestos fibers within respiratory bronchioles and bifurcations of the alveolar ducts. Because of their straight, linear structure and peripheral lung deposition, amphibole asbestos fibers are most associated with benign asbestos pleural effusion and mesothelioma. Following asbestos fiber inhalation, an ensuing macrophage-driven inflammatory reaction extends outward to the pleural space; cytokines including tumor necrosis factor α are released along with growth factors, proteases, and reactive oxygen and nitrogen species, eventuating in oxidative DNA damage. Mesothelioma is characterized by chromosomal deletions, especially those involving p53; other deletions include 1p, 3p, 6q, 9p, and 22q.[6]

- The resolution rate of a pneumothorax is mainly dependent on the pleural–venous-blood-nitrogen (N_2) gradient. The average rate of resolution of a pneumothorax in a subject breathing ambient air without pleural aspiration or drainage is approximately 5% per day. In such subjects pneumothorax resolution rate is enhanced by breathing enriched O_2 mixtures (eg, high fractional inspired oxygen concentration [FIO_2]).

- Clinically apparent iatrogenic pneumothorax caused by puncture of the pleura during diagnostic procedures (eg, thoracentesis, lung, or pleural biopsy) or central vascular catheter insertion can be delayed for up to 24 hours post-procedure.

- The pathophysiology of tension pneumothorax involves a progressively falling pressure gradient for systemic venous return, which is defined as the difference between right atrial pressure and mean systemic pressure. An enlarging intrapleural gas collection caused by continuing gas entry from pleural disruption plus a check valve mechanism that prevents its decompression generates escalating intrapleural pressures. Such increases in intrapleural pressure create right atrial underfilling, followed by decreases in right ventricular stroke volume, pulmonary blood flow, left ventricular preload, and ultimately, arterial blood pressure.

DIAGNOSIS

- A comprehensive medical history and physical examination are critical elements in guiding the diagnostic workup of a patient with a pleural effusion and interpreting the results of pleural testing.
- The commonest symptoms of pleural disease are dyspnea and chest pain. The degree of dyspnea depends on the size of the pleural effusion and on underlying pulmonary function; smaller effusions are associated with more severe dyspnea in patients with preexisting obstructive or restrictive lung conditions, or with concomitant pneumonia.
- Acute or subacute dyspnea out of proportion to the size of the effusion should immediately raise the suspicion of coexisting pulmonary thromboembolism.
- The initial symptom of a pneumothorax is usually the sudden onset of acute, sharp chest pain on the side of the pneumothorax along with dyspnea.
- Chest discomfort associated with pleural effusion can be pleuritic or nonpleuritic; pleuritic discomfort is usually associated with exudative effusions from pneumonia, cancer, pulmonary infarction, viral pleurisy, or following coronary artery bypass graft surgery (eg, postpericardiotomy syndrome). Thoracic pain associated with pleural mesothelioma is characteristically progressive, localized, and of a dull-aching quality.
- The clinical presentation of a pleural effusion can be dominated by other respiratory symptoms and chest findings if there is coexisting asthma, chronic obstructive pulmonary disease (COPD), or pneumonia.
- Physical findings indicative of pleural effusion are unequal dullness of the hemithoraces to percussion, decreased tactile and vocal fremitus, and diminished breath sounds. Egophony is common near the upper levels of large pleural effusions. Lung compression from moderate to large effusions can modify physical

findings to include bronchial breath sounds; the reductions in fremitus can be offset by atelectasis as well. Very large pleural effusions can cause bulging in intercostal spaces or contralateral mediastinal shift.

- The physical examination can be normal in patients with a small (eg, <15%) pneumothorax. With larger pneumothoraces, percussion can reveal hyperresonance on the affected side along with diminished breath sounds.
- Tension pneumothorax is a clinical diagnosis made at the bedside. Tracheal deviation to the opposite side can be palpated in the suprasternal notch, in addition to muffled heart tones, progressive hypotension, tachycardia, and cyanosis that progress to pulseless electrical activity (PEA) cardiac arrest.
- In patients receiving mechanical ventilation, peak airway pressures often acutely increase during an enlarging pneumothorax, particularly with development of tension pneumothorax.

PLAIN CHEST RADIOGRAPHY

- Radiographic evaluation is central in confirming the presence of a pleural effusion as well as in formulating the most likely differential diagnostic possibilities. Distinguishing pleural effusions occurring alone (eg, without other chest radiographic abnormalities) versus those accompanying other intrathoracic manifestations of disease is a key initial step.
- Pleural effusions not associated with other lung parenchymal abnormalities include those caused by pulmonary thromboembolism, connective tissue disease (eg, rheumatoid pleurisy or lupus pleuritis), viral pleurisy, pleural metastases, drug reactions (especially bromocriptine, methotrexate, and cyclophosphamide), tuberculous pleurisy, chylothorax, and subphrenic inflammation or infectious processes.
- A pleural effusion on upright films is typified by a characteristic meniscus-like configuration in the costophrenic angle, requiring at least 300 to 500 mL of fluid in the pleural space for visualization. Lateral views are useful for confirmation. On supine portable anteroposterior films, free-flowing effusions are suspected by unilateral increases in radiographic density through which pulmonary vascular structures are readily visible, generally in the absence of air-bronchograms or other evidence of alveolar consolidation.
- The main value of lateral decubitus films is to confirm the existence of a pleural effusion as well as to evaluate the possibility of loculated fluid collections. In contrast to free-flowing pleural effusions with

accumulation that is gravity dependent and thus layer horizontally at least 10 mm on decubitus views, pleural opacification associated with loculated effusions is constant in location regardless of upright to decubitus repositioning.

- Pleural fluid can also collect in the major and minor fissures of the lungs; characteristically the appearance of these collections is that of a homogeneous, lens-shaped opacity without internal air bronchograms. In the minor (horizontal) fissure separating the right upper and middle lobes, such collections appear as a mid-lung opacification.

- Subpulmonic pleural effusions can appear only as a unilateral or bilateral elevated hemidiaphragm; the otherwise characteristic meniscus-like configuration of pleural fluid accumulation in the costophrenic angles is lacking. Ultrasonography or chest CT scan is confirmatory.

- The ease of visibility of a pneumothorax varies with its size and position as well as with preexisting lung conditions. A pneumothorax is usually identifiable by radiographic visualization of the white visceral pleural stripe within the involved hemothorax, in conjunction with apical or peripheral radiolucent areas in which pulmonary vascular structures are absent. Very small pneumothoraces may be visible only on expiratory radiographs.

- In critically ill patients receiving mechanical ventilation, pneumothorax may be associated with a deep sulcus sign, in which an anterior, basal pneumothorax simulates a unilateral inordinately deep sulcus that is disproportionate to the opposite side.

- Previous asbestos exposure suggesting the possibility of BAPE is commonly manifested as calcific or noncalcific parietal plaques in the mid-thoracic regions or involving the diaphragmatic pleura. Asbestos-related parenchymal abnormalities can coexist, such as nodular or reticular opacities or rounded atelectasis.

CHEST CT SCAN

- Chest CT scan is the most sensitive method to detect pleural disease and pleural fluid collections. Its main usefulness lies in the detection of unsuspected lung disease (eg, interstitial disease, parenchymal nodules). CT scans also assist in the management of complicated parapneumonic effusions and empyema by localizing all pleural fluid collections and confirming their resolution with intrapleural drainage.

- Consideration should always be given to the possibility of malignant mesothelioma for a pleural effusion with a pleural-based mass.

THORACENTESIS

- The main indication for thoracentesis is a clinically significant pleural effusion of unknown or unclear etiology by chest imaging studies.[2]

- Thoracentesis should be performed if symptoms are present and there is ultrasonographic confirmation of the effusion, including ≥10 mm of free-layering fluid on a lateral decubitus chest film, or chest CT scan evidence of effusion.

- Not all effusions require diagnostic thoracentesis. In a patient with bilateral pleural effusions and overt clinical evidence of CHF without fever, chest pain, or dyspnea out of proportion to the size of the pleural fluid collections, transudative effusions are most likely, especially if they regress during the first 3 days of diuretic therapy.[2] In this setting, lack of partial resolution of the pleural effusion despite diuretic treatment, unilateral effusions, or the presence of fever and/or chest pain are indications for thoracentesis.

- In general, up to 1500 mL of pleural fluid can be safely withdrawn during a thoracentesis procedure without inducing re-expansion pulmonary edema.

- The color of pleural fluid can assist in characterizing the effusion:[2]
  ◦ Bloody pleural effusions are associated with cancer, trauma, pulmonary thromboembolism with infarction, pneumonia, post-pericardiotomy syndrome, or benign asbestos pleural effusion.
  ◦ Clear yellow or straw-colored fluid is typical of a transudative effusion.
  ◦ Milky white fluid suggests a chylothorax, cholesterol effusion, or empyema.
  ◦ Brownish "anchovy paste" fluid can represent old hemothorax or rupture of an amebic liver abscess into the pleural space.
  ◦ Yellow-green fluid can be observed in rheumatoid pleurisy.
  ◦ Clear fluid or fluid of similar color as central venous catheter infusions can be caused by extravascular catheter migration into the pleural space.

- Light's criteria are the most sensitive (98%) criteria for distinguishing between transudative and exudative pleural effusions; however their specificity is approximately 77%, resulting in an overall accuracy of 90%.[2]

- Adjunctive use of the serum–pleural effusion albumin gradient (see Table 115–1) helps to improve the specificity and overall accuracy of diagnosing exudative effusions in patients with borderline pleural fluid values by Light's criteria.[2] However, it should not be used in isolation because it will misclassify approximately 13% of exudates as transudates.[2]

- For pH measurements of pleural fluid, specimens should be collected in an arterial blood gas syringe anaerobically and placed on ice prior to analysis on a blood gas machine for optimal accuracy. Transudative effusions usually have pH values ranging between 7.4 and 7.5; exudative effusions (with the exception of complicated parapneumonic effusions and empyema) typically have more acidic pH values of 7.30 to 7.45.

- Pleural fluid analysis showing a low pH (eg, <7.30), high LDH (eg, >1000 IU/L), and low pleural glucose (eg, <40 mg/dL) support the diagnosis of complicated parapneumonic effusion.
- The number of nucleated cells (eg, white blood cells) in pleural fluid is not diagnostic of specific pleural processes. Greatly elevated cells counts (eg, >50,000/μL) are frequently observed in complicated parapneumonic effusions and empyema.
- Differential pleural fluid cell count can assist in narrowing the differential diagnosis. Lymphocytic pleural effusions (eg, those containing >80% lymphocytes) are typically observed in lymphoma, sarcoidosis, tuberculosis, carcinoma, rheumatoid pleurisy, chylothorax, or yellow nail syndrome.
- Pleural fluid eosinophilia (eg, >10% by differential cell count) helps to narrow the differential diagnosis of effusions but lacks specificity. The most frequent causes include hemothorax or pneumothorax, pleuropulmonary drug reactions, pulmonary infarction, BAPE, fungal disease, and parasite involvement.
- Pleural fluid amylase should be measured if pancreatic disease such as chronic pancreatitis or pseudocyst, esophageal rupture, or malignancy are suspected.[7] Pleural fluid amylase concentrations can be elevated to extreme levels with pancreatic pseudocyst (eg, >50,000–100,000 IU/L).
- Pleural fluid glucose concentrations are of diagnostic value only if they are low (eg, <60 mg/dL, or <50% of concomitant serum values). Low pleural fluid glucose concentrations suggest empyema or complicated parapneumonic effusion, rheumatoid pleurisy, malignancy, tuberculous pleuritis, lupus-related pleural inflammation, or esophageal rupture.
- An adenosine deaminase (ADA) measurement is useful in the evaluation of lymphocytic effusions in which tuberculous infection is suspected but acid-fast smears are negative and/or pleural biopsy is nonrevealing for either acid-fast organisms or granuloma; ADA values <40 IU/L have a high negative predictive value for tuberculous pleural infections.
- A presumptive diagnosis of hepatic hydrothorax can be confirmed by a radionuclide scan in which tracer injected into the pleural space appears within 2 hours in the peritoneal compartment.
- Cytokeratin staining of pleural tissue in malignant mesothelioma helps to distinguish this pleural tumor from sarcoma and melanoma; mesothelioma

is distinguished from adenocarcinoma by specific antibodies.[6] Thus, mesothelioma is characterized by positive staining for calretinin, Wilm tumor 1, cytokeratin 5-6, or mesothelin; ≥85% of epithelioid mesotheliomas are positive for mesothelin.[6]

THERAPEUTIC APPROACH

- The approach to pleural effusions should employ a Bayesian analysis in which the pretest (eg, thoracentesis) probability of specific disorders based on the clinical presentation should be considered, after which the results of pleural fluid analysis (eg, posttest results) should be integrated to arrive at a focused list of differential diagnostic possibilities.
- Regardless of this Bayesian approach and the likelihood of a transudative effusion, thoracentesis should be performed in patients with dyspnea or respiratory compromise, with the intent to remove as much fluid as possible (eg, ≤1500 mL of fluid per procedure).
- Pleural effusions associated with CHF are proportional to the severity of pulmonary edema and similarly respond to diuretic therapy, angiotensin-converting enzyme inhibition, spironolactone, and other targeted cardiac therapies. Lack of improvement of a pleural effusion presumptively secondary to CHF despite other clinical evidence of therapeutic response such as decreasing pulmonary edema should trigger reevaluation of the effusion, including thoracentesis.[1,2]
- Antibiotic therapy for the underlying pneumonia generally resolves uncomplicated parapneumonic effusions without the need for pleural drainage by a chest tube. The chest tube can usually be removed when less than 100 mL of fluid accumulates in a 24-hour period.
- A positive Gram stain of pleural fluid for microorganisms or positive pleural fluid microbial culture in a patient with an exudative pleural effusion is an indication for chest tube thoracostomy and pleural drainage.[4,5] Antimicrobial therapy alone is never adequate treatment of a closed pleural space infection. The finding of pus on thoracentesis mandates immediate pleural space drainage.
- Loculated pleural fluid collections can frequently be successfully accessed by ultrasound-guided thoracentesis; smaller and/or multiple loculations are addressed by CT-guided percutaneous drainage. Thoracoscopy and/or video-assisted thoracoscopic surgery (VATS) may be required to lyse extensive intrapleural adhesions. Intrapleural instillations of streptokinase in an attempt to resolve loculated infected pleural effusions do not improve the rate of decortication surgeries, length of hospital stay, or mortality.[8]

- The most common error with respect to parapneumonic effusions is failure to integrate the patient's clinical features and pleural fluid results to diagnose a complicated parapneumonic effusion and/or empyema. Definitive drainage of the pleural space by tube thoracostomy in the earlier exudative phase of effusion is thereby delayed, necessitating an operative pleural decortication procedure for the fibrous, organizational stage of empyema and a lengthy recovery period.
- Following pleural decortication for empyema, a chest tube (eg, empyema tube) is usually left in place for several months attached to a dressing or bag drainage system; removal is via progressive outward advancement by approximately 1 cm per month. Because the tube is in a walled-off area of the pleural space, water (H_2O)-seal drainage is not necessary.
- Hemothorax requires drainage with larger caliber chest tubes (eg, $\geq$32 F) to avoid a fibrinous visceral pleural peel from developing and causing trapped lung. In trauma or postoperative patients, both the patient's clinical status and drainage should be monitored frequently for clotting or excessive bleeding (eg, $\geq$200 mL/h), which can result in hypovolemia and cardiopulmonary compromise.
- Chemotherapy or radiation therapy can reduce or eliminate pleural effusions including chylothorax associated with lymphoma, small-cell lung cancer, breast cancer, and other neoplasms without the need for pleurodesis.
- Recurrent cytology-positive malignant pleural effusions associated with dyspnea generally require chemical pleurodesis with tetracycline or talc. In some patients, placement of an indwelling catheter, such as Pleurx, allows intermittent home evacuation by the patient or home care agency.
- Small pneumothoraces (eg, <15%) in asymptomatic patients can be observed for progression or resolution; administering supplemental O_2 will facilitate resolution as along as there is no underlying BP fistula. In ambulatory patients use of a one-way Heimlich valve without underwater seal drainage can be appropriate.
- Larger pneumothoraces require the insertion of smaller caliber chest tubes (eg, $\leq$28 F) placed to underwater seal drainage with suction. In selected patients not receiving mechanical ventilation, placement of a small bore pneumothorax catheter in the second/third intercostal space in the midclavicular line is an acceptable initial approach.
- The first episode of primary spontaneous pneumothorax is treated conservatively by chest tube thoracostomy and lung re-expansion. Recurrent episodes are an indication for chemical pleurodesis or VATS-mediated obliteration of the pleural space by talc poudrage. Smoking cessation is critical to prevent relapses of primary spontaneous pneumothorax.
- Because of the life-threatening nature of tension pneumothorax, there is usually insufficient time for radiographic confirmation. If suspected, immediate decompression of the pleural space is indicated by needle thoracostomy; the therapeutic efficacy of this procedure is generally confirmed by rapid improvement in blood pressure and arterial O_2 saturation. Insertion of a chest tube is definitive treatment in all cases.
- Chest tubes placed for pneumothoraces are left in place until at least 24 hours after the leak has sealed as confirmed radiographically.
- Refractory hepatic hydrothorax occurs in approximately 10% of patients with this condition, characterized by persistence and/or recurrence of moderate to large pleural effusions and dyspnea despite sodium restriction and maximal diuretic therapy. The condition generally improves after a transjugular intrahepatic portosystemic shunt (TIPS). Selective patients may be candidates for VATS and repair of diaphragmatic defects. Chemical pleurodesis by intrapleural instillation of sclerosant materials such as tetracycline has limited success owing to the difficulty of maintaining pleural membrane contiguity during the procedure.
- Surgery is most useful in malignant mesothelioma for palliation of recurrent pleural effusions; the tumor is typically resistant to radiotherapy.

REFERENCES

1. Light RW. *Pleural Diseases*. 4th ed. Philadelphia, PA: Williams & Wilkins; 2001.
2. Light RW. Pleural effusion. *N Engl J Med.* 2002;346: 1971–1977.
3. Heffner JE, Brown LK, Barbieri CA. Diagnostic value of tests that discriminate between exudative and transudative pleural effusions. *Chest.* 1997;111:970–980.
4. Sahn S. Management of complicated parapneumonic effusions. *Am Rev Respir Dis.* 1993;148:813–817.
5. Colice G, Curtis A, Deslauriers J, Heffner J, Light R, Littenburg B. Medical and surgical treatment of parapneumonic effusions: An evidence based guideline. *Chest.* 2000; 118:1158–1171.
6. Robinson BWS, Lake RA. Advances in malignant mesothelioma. *N Engl J Med.*, 2005;353:1591–1603.
7. Joseph J, Viney S, Beck P, Strange C, Sahn S, Basran G. A prospective study of amylase-rich pleural effusion with special reference to amylase isoenzyme analysis. *Chest.* 1992;102: 1455–1459.
8. Maskell NA, Davies CWH, Nunn AJ, et al, and the First Multicenter Intrapleural Sepsis Trial (MIST1) Group. U.K. controlled trial of intrapleural streptokinase for pleural infection. *N Engl J Med.* 2005;352:865–874.

116 ACUTE RESPIRATORY FAILURE AND ACUTE LUNG INJURY/ARDS

George M. Matuschak

INTRODUCTION

- Acute respiratory failure has been defined using several approaches. The most useful, albeit simplified, conceptual approach divides acute respiratory failure into two categories: (1) acute hypoxemic respiratory failure, which is present when the partial pressure of arterial oxygen (PaO_2) is acutely decreased to <60 mm Hg, and (2) acute hypercapnic respiratory failure, characterized by an acute elevation of the $PaCO_2$ to >44 mm Hg in conjunction with a reduced arterial pH <7.36 (eg, a respiratory acidosis).

- The alveolar-arterial O_2 gradient (P_A-PaO_2 difference or A-a gradient) is a measure of lung oxygenation that takes into account arterial $PaCO_2$ levels and the respiratory exchange ratio (the ratio of carbon dioxide production to oxygen consumption):

$$P_A O_2 - PaO_2 \text{ difference} = (FIO_2/100 \times Patm - 47 \text{ mm Hg}) - PaCO_2/0.8 - PaO_2,$$

where Patm = atmospheric (or barometric) pressure and 47 mm Hg = H_2O vapor pressure in normally humidified air at 37°C. Alternatively, the alveolar gas equation can be used to arrive at a $P_A O_2$ and is calculated as follows: $P_A O_2 = FIO_2 (Patm - 47 \text{ mm Hg}) - 1.2 (PaCO_2)$. The P_A-PaO_2 difference is normally 10 to 12 mm Hg. There is no net alveolar exchange of either nitrogen or H_2O vapor.

- Because the P_A-PaO_2 difference can vary with inspired oxygen tension (FIO_2) it is of greatest diagnostic utility when the subject is either breathing ambient air (eg, $FIO_2 = 0.21$) or 100% oxygen ($FIO_2 = 1.0$). The normal P_A-PaO_2 gradient averages 8 to 12 mm Hg in young healthy individuals. The gradient in healthy people is due to nonuniform ventilation/perfusion ($\dot{V}/\dot{Q}$) matching; it increases with age, rising to approximately 24 mm Hg by 70 to 80 years of age.

- The PaO_2/FIO_2 ratio is a useful index of the efficiency of the lungs' oxygenating capacity across varying percentages of supplemental O_2, and is calculated independent of the $PaCO_2$. The FIO_2 is expressed as a value between 0.21 and 1.00. As an example, the normal PaO_2/FIO_2 ratio is calculated as follows: $PaO_2 = 100$ mm Hg while breathing room air and the ambient $FIO_2 = 0.21$. Therefore, the normal PaO_2/FIO_2 ratio = 100/0.21 = 476.

- The PaO_2/FIO_2 ratio detects significant reductions in the oxygenating efficiency of the lungs that may be masked by increased FIO_2 concentrations. Thus, a patient with a PaO_2 of 100 mm Hg while receiving an FIO_2 of 50% has a PaO_2/FIO_2 ratio of 200 (100/0.5).

- Venoarterial admixture or right-to-left shunting produces arterial hypoxemia because the systemic venous return bypasses or does not otherwise perfuse aerated alveoli and mixes with arterial blood. Shunt physiology does not respond (defined as an increase in PaO_2) to increases in FIO_2, including 100% oxygen. A small degree of shunting exists under normal circumstances but does not exceed 3% to 5%.

- Hypoxic vasoconstriction is a homeostatic mechanism in which reductions in the oxygenation of blood perfusing poorly ventilated alveoli causes shunting of blood flow away from these units.

- Dead space ventilation refers to alveolar ventilation that does not participate in pulmonary CO_2 clearance owing to nonperfused or underperfused alveolar structures and as such, is an index of the CO_2 exchanging efficiency of the lungs. Dead space ventilation consists of two elements: (1) the anatomic dead space, comprising the conducting airways of the tracheobronchial tree, which represent about 150 mL per 500 mL inspiratory tidal volume (in a 70-kg subject), and (2) the so-called *physiologic dead space*, that normally exists in the superior regions of the lungs in an upright individual (eg, West zone I condition). In this region, alveolar pressure (P_A) exceeds the driving pressure for lung perfusion; calculated as the difference between the pulmonary arterial pressure (Pa) and pulmonary venous pressure (Pv).

  ○ **Acute lung injury**
    ▪ ALI is defined as a syndrome of acute and persistent lung inflammation with increased vascular permeability. It is characterized by four clinical features: (1) acute onset, (2) diffuse, bilateral, acutely developing radiographic infiltrates, (3) a ratio of PaO_2 to the fraction of inspired oxygen (eg, PaO_2/FIO_2) of ≤300 mm Hg, regardless of the level of positive end-expiratory pressure (PEEP), and (4) no clinical evidence of increased left atrial pressure to suggest cardiogenic pulmonary edema; if a pulmonary artery catheter is in place the pulmonary artery occlusion pressure (Paop) is ≤18 mm Hg.

  ○ **Acute respiratory distress syndrome**
    ▪ ARDS criteria are similar to acute lung injury, except that ARDS is characterized by severe derangements in oxygenation, such that the PaO_2/FIO_2 is ≤200 regardless of the level of PEEP.

- ARDS is classified into two phases to underscore differing pathophysiological processes over time; however, there is considerable clinical overlap depending on underlying patient risk factors, etiology of lung injury, ongoing fluid balance, and other modifying variables: (1) an initial acute, exudative phase extending from days 1 through 7 to 10, characterized by increased extravascular lung H_2O (eg, noncardiogenic pulmonary edema) and hypoxemia responsive to fluid restriction, diuretic therapy, and positive end-expiratory pressure (PEEP); and (2) a fibroproliferative phase starting from days 7 to 14. The fibroproliferative phase is characterized by enhanced stimulation of fibroblasts and de novo collagen synthesis, which may lead to fibrotic thickening of the alveolar capillary membrane, derangement of airspace architecture, progressive reduction of lung compliance (change in lung volume per unit change in the lungs' distending pressure), rising airway pressures, increased shunt and dead space ventilation, and diminished response to fluid restriction, diuretic therapy, or PEEP.

- The arterial O_2 content (CaO_2) reflects the total number of O_2 molecules in arterial blood, and is defined as: (Hgb concentration $\times$ 1.36 mL O_2/g of Hgb $\times$ SaO_2) + (PaO_2 + 0.031), where Hgb = hemoglobin concentration, 1.36 = amount of O_2 carried per gram of hemoglobin, SaO_2 = percent saturation of Hgb by O_2; eg, arterial O_2 saturation expressed in decimal form (eg, 0.99 instead of 99%), and 0.031 = the solubility coefficient of hemoglobin-free O_2 dissolved in plasma.

- Tissue O_2 delivery (DO_2) per minute is the product of the arterial O_2 content (CaO_2) and blood flow (eg, cardiac output, CO), such that $DO_2 = CaO_2 \times CO$. Accordingly, tissue O_2 delivery can be increased in one of three ways: (1) increasing CaO_2; (2) augmenting CO; or (3) increasing elements of both.

- Multiple organ dysfunction syndrome (MODS) develops in up to 15% of patients requiring intensive care unit (ICU) admission. It is defined as severe, acutely evolving (within 48–72 hours) decreased function of at least two organ systems in critically ill patients that persists for longer than 48 hours, and that requires medical intervention to achieve and sustain homeostasis.

- The lungs are the most commonly affected organ system in MODS, manifesting as ALI or ARDS. Although definitions differ, typical organ-specific indicators of MODS (reflecting impaired organ perfusion as occur during severe sepsis/septic shock[1]) that can progress to established organ dysfunction include:

- Cardiovascular system: systolic blood pressure ≤90 mm Hg, or mean arterial pressure ≤70 mm Hg for at least 1 hour, despite adequate fluid resuscitation, adequate intravascular volume, or vasopressors for hemodynamic support (eg, any dose of norepinephrine or epinephrine, or dopamine infused at concentrations that exceed 5 µg/kg/min)
- Renal system: urinary output less than 0.5 mL/kg/h for 1 hour despite adequate fluid resuscitation, usually progressing to persistent oliguria and accompanied by an elevation in the serum creatinine;
- Metabolic system: lactic acid level 1.5 > than the upper limit of laboratory normal with an otherwise unexplained base deficit ≥5 mmol/L and an arterial pH < 7.3
- Hematologic system: platelet count <100,000/µL, or a decrease by ≥ 50% during the preceding 3 days.
- Gastrointestinal system: acute liver dysfunction with increased serum bilirubin

- Because organ dysfunction in MODS represents a continuum of change from normal rather than an all-or-nothing phenomenon, several scoring systems have been developed to quantify organ-specific derangements, including the Sepsis-Related Organ Failure Assessment Score (SOFA)[2], MODS score[3], and the Acute Physiologic and Chronic Health Evaluation Score (APACHE) III.

EPIDEMIOLOGY

- Acute respiratory failure is common in hospitalized patients, occurring in more than 30% of patients on admission, especially in those admitted to an intensive care unit; in whom new-onset acute respiratory failure develops in another 30%.[4]
- Each year in the United States, there are 190,600 cases of ALI requiring mechanical ventilation, which are associated with 3.6 million hospital days and a mortality rate of approximately 38%, or 74,500 deaths annually.[5]
- There are factors that directly cause injury to the lungs in acute hypoxemic respiratory failure, as well as systemic or indirect risk factors involving blood-borne mediators of injury (Table 116–1). After exposure to a risk factor(s), if ALI/ARDS develops, it is clinically apparent within 24 to72 hours.
- In addition to the specific factors which induce ALI/ARDS, clinical outcomes are influenced by additional events that delay or prevent the resolution of acute respiratory failure. Age is a significant independent risk

TABLE 116–1 Initiating Risk Factors for ALI/ARDS

RISK FACTORS OF DIRECT LUNG INJURY	RISK FACTORS FOR INDIRECT LUNG INJURY
-Pulmonary aspiration	-Bacteremic or nonbacteremic sepsis
-Diffuse pulmonary infection (eg, pneumonia)	-Fungal, viral, protozoal, or mycobacterial sepsis
-Traumatic lung contusion	-Severe nonthoracic trauma
-Near-drowning	-Multiple blood transfusions
-Smoke/toxic gas inhalation	-Severe acute pancreatitis
-Neurogenic pulmonary edema	-Severe burn injury
-Reexpansion pulmonary edema	-Chronic liver disease/cirrhosis
-Pulmonary O_2 toxicity	-Transfusion-associated acute lung injury

ALI, acute lung injury; ARDS, acute respiratory distress syndrome.

factor for ALI/ARDS mortality, which increases from approximately 24% for adolescent patients to 60% or greater in patients older than 70 to 80 years of age.[5] Further, chronic liver disease doubles the mortality rates.

- Approximately 15% of deaths in patients with ALI/ARDS are the consequence of progressive respiratory failure with intractable hypoxemia, usually during the fibroproliferative phase. In the remaining 85% of patients, the main cause of death is MODS. These patients die *with* ALI/ARDS but not necessarily because of lung involvement per se.

- A major complication of ALI/ARDS or other forms of acute or acute-on-chronic respiratory failure that significantly increases mortality in mechanically ventilated patients is late-onset ventilator-associated pneumonia (VAP). This condition carries a superimposed mortality rate of 30% to 50% despite antimicrobial therapy. Late-onset VAP refers to pneumonia that develops more than 48 hours after intubation in patients without clinically apparent pneumonia at the time of intubation, and is more frequently caused by multidrug-resistant (MDR) bacteria including methicillin-resistant *Staphylococcus aureus*, *Pseudomonas aeruginosa*, and *Acinetobacter baumannii*. Overall, *Pseudomonas aeruginosa* is the most common gram-negative MDR microorganism causing VAP. By contrast, VAP that develops within the first 48 hours of intubation is more frequently the result of aspiration and usually yields a better prognosis due to a higher rate of infection with non-MDR bacteria.

- The cumulative risk of developing VAP rises from about 7% on day 3 of mechanical ventilation to approximately 20% by day 14.

- Each additional nonpulmonary organ dysfunction or failure in MODS is associated with an approximate 20% to 30% increase in mortality rate.

- There are several acutely acquired neuromuscular problems that can impair ventilator weaning in the critically ill: peripheral neuropathies, typified by critical illness polyneuropathy and acute motor neuropathy; and myopathies, including disuse atrophy and type II muscle fiber atrophy. These conditions are important to consider because failure to recognize them may lead to erroneous conclusions regarding weaning patients from the ventilator.

- Critical illness polyneuropathy is a syndrome characterized by acute limb and respiratory weakness observed in patients with sepsis-induced MODS. It is an axonal sensory-motor neuropathy in which deep tendon reflexes are often preserved. Critical illness polyneuropathy may develop within 7 days in ventilated patients with acute respiratory failure, but more commonly correlates with longer durations of illness, severe sepsis/septic shock, MODS, and/or the use of neuromuscular paralyzing agents. Rarely, patients may develop severe quadriplegia requiring months of ventilatory support until resolution permits weaning. Residual peripheral nerve impairment is common.

- Survivors of acute respiratory failure and particularly those with ALI/ARDS develop significant losses of lean body mass during their critical illness averaging between 15% and 20% of their original baseline. Muscle weakness and fatigue rather than impaired lung function per se are common following hospital discharge.

- Long-term prognosis for recovery of lung function following ALI/ARDS is reasonably good; within approximately 6 months, spirometry (forced vital capacity [FVC], forced expiratory volume at 1 second [FEV_1], and FEV_1/FVC ratio) and lung volumes return to premorbid or predicted values.

- By 12 months after hospital discharge, the most common pulmonary sequela of ALI/ARDS is a mild-to-moderate reduction in the single-breath diffusion capacity for carbon monoxide (DLCO); exertional O_2 desaturation is also seen in up to 6%.

- Cognitive dysfunction manifested as memory loss, difficulty concentrating, and abnormalities on neuropsychological tests are increasingly recognized in survivors of ALI/ARDS. In addition, ICU posttraumatic stress disorder is characterized by ICU flashbacks, sleep disorders, anxiety, and depression. These problems are evident at 3 months following hospital discharge, and are persistent in more than 30% at 12 months.

PATHOPHYSIOLOGY

- Ventilation and perfusion are highest at the lung bases in the upright position and posteriorly in the supine position.

- There are five primary mechanisms responsible for arterial hypoxemia (1) hypoventilation, (2) ventilation/perfusion

$(\dot{V}/\dot{Q})$ mismatch, (3) shunt, (4) diffusion limitation, and (5) decreased FIO_2 (eg, high altitude). Of these, shunt is the primary mechanism responsible for hypoxemia in ALI/ARDS.

- A widened P_A-PaO_2 difference is observed in $\dot{V}/\dot{Q}$ mismatch, venoarterial admixture or true shunt, and diffusion limitation.

- Ventilation/perfusion $(\dot{V}/\dot{Q})$ mismatching is the most common mechanism responsible for arterial hypoxemia in non-ARDS acute hypoxemic respiratory failure and acute hypercapnic respiratory failure, the latter typified by exacerbations of chronic obstructive pulmonary disease (COPD).

- An intact neural transmission pathway from the brain to the respiratory muscles is required for normal ventilation. Acute respiratory failure can theoretically occur when neural transmission is perturbed at virtually any level from the CNS to the respiratory muscles. For example, the respiratory center in the midbrain can be impaired by sedative-hypnotic agents; transmission of neural impulses from the midbrain and pons can be altered after spinal cord trauma; the motor nerves themselves can be injured in critical illness polyneuropathy; synaptic transmission of neural impulses to skeletal muscle is altered in myasthenia gravis or as the result of neuromuscular blocking agents; and skeletal muscle contraction may be decreased as the result of critical illness myopathies or steroid-induced myopathy.

- A central pathophysiological feature of ALI/ARDS is increased lung extravascular H_2O secondary to increased microvascular permeability that culminates in noncardiogenic pulmonary edema.

- Fluid accumulation in the lungs can be determined using the Starling relationship, as follows:

$$Q = Kf\,(Pmv - Ppmv) - \sigma\,(\pi mv - \pi pmv)$$

where Q = fluid flux, Kf = the filtration coefficient, a function of the surface area and permeability of the microvessels; Pmv = microvascular hydrostatic pressure; Ppmv = perimicrovascular pressure; σ = the reflection coefficient for proteins across the lung microvasculature and ranges between 0 (freely permeable) to 1.0 (impermeable), normal values are estimated at approximately 0.5; πmv = microvascular colloid osmotic pressure; and πpmv, interstitial colloid osmotic pressure. The serum albumin concentration (mol. wt., ~ 65-kD) is the main determinant of microvascular colloid osmotic pressure, which is typically 25 mm Hg.

- Removal of pulmonary edema fluid is dependent on 2 mechanisms: (1) active Na^+ and H_2O transport from the alveolar space by the Na^+-K^+ ATPase in alveolar type I and type II epithelial cells, and (2) lung lymphatic drainage.

- During acute alveolar injury, decreases in the reflection coefficient coupled with augmented microvascular hydrostatic pressure (often because of fluid resuscitation during severe sepsis/septic shock) promote accumulation of a protein-rich fluid in the alveoli. Alveolar fluid inactivates surfactant, which in turn promotes end-expiratory alveolar collapse and reduces functional residual capacity (FRC) and lung compliance. Collapsed, but perfused, alveoli contribute to right-to-left shunting of venous blood and arterial hypoxemia.

- These changes are amplified by bronchial epithelial sloughing, apoptosis and necrosis of Type I alveolar epithelial cells (which compromise active removal of alveolar fluid), and simultaneous activation of alveolar macrophages. Activated macrophages contribute to alveolar injury via the synthesis and secretion of reactive O_2 species, proteases, pro-inflammatory cytokines such as TNF-α, IL-1β, polymorphonuclear neutrophil (PMN) chemoattractant signals such as IL-8, CXC chemokines, complement, and leukotriene B_4. Whereas the number of PMNs in bronchoalveolar lavage fluid (BALF) in nonsmokers is normally <5%, PMN numbers in patients with ALI/ARDS may exceed 50%. Activated PMNs promote oxidant damage and recruitment of additional inflammatory cells leading to neutrophilic alveolitis.

- Collectively, these complex cascades induce diffuse alveolar injury, which can be amplified by ventilator-associated lung injury, and O_2 toxicity. Thus, pulmonary edema, neutrophilic alveolitis, varying degrees of alveolar hemorrhage, and hyaline membrane formation are common histopathological findings. In protracted ARDS, transforming growth factor-β (TGF-β), promotes interstitial collagen deposition and irreversible scarring.

- As alluded to above, an abundance of inflammatory mediators, chemokines, growth factors, and proteases have been characterized in the BALF from patients with ALI/ARDS. Importantly, there is overlap in the BALF concentrations of many of these mediators in patients at hisk for developing ALI/ARDS (critically-ill patients) but who do not develop it as compared to patients with ALI/ARDS.

VENTILATOR-ASSOCIATED LUNG INJURY

- There are four types of ventilator-associated lung injury (VALI) which are summarized in Table 116–2. The mechanism of VALI is incompletely understood, but is thought to reflect the heterogeneous distribution of ALI/ARDS. Accordingly, scattered throughout the lungs are normal alveoli lying in close proximity to edematous or atelectatic units.

TABLE 116–2 Types of Ventilator-Associated Lung injury (VALI)

CONDITION	CONSEQUENCE
-Alveolar overdistention (volutrauma)	-Increased lung microvascular permeability, increased lung extravascular H_2O (pulmonary edema)
-Cyclic stress/strain injury to alveolar walls (atelectrauma) as lung units collapse and re-open repeatedly	-Fracture of alveolar capillary basement membranes, PMN influx, activation of inflammatory cytokines
-Excessively increased alveolar pressure (barotrauma)	-Alveolar wall rupture, pneumomediastinum, pneumothorax including tension pathophysiology, cardiovascular collapse
-Biotrauma	-Pulmonary and nonpulmonary organ injury caused by release of inflammatory mediators from improperly-ventilated lungs

PMN, polymorphonuclear neutrophil.

- Mechanical ventilation tends to overexpand normal alveolar units (which are relatively compliant). Overexpansion is believed to injure these normal alveoli and is referred to as *volutrauma*.
- Atelectrauma is thought to occur when recurrent cycles of alveolar recruitment/de-recruitment creates stress/strain failure of alveolar walls secondary to loss of surfactant.
- The generation of transiently elevated peak and mean airway pressures is responsible for barotrauma in ventilated patients, a potentially life-threatening condition. Barotrauma is characterized by rupture of perivascular alveoli, followed by the tracking of air along bronchovascular sheaths to the mediastinum. The accumulation of air within the mediastinum (pneumomediastinum) can be complicated by rupture of the mediastinal pleura, causing a pneumothorax. This condition should be suspected if the patient deteriorates quickly, manifested by arterial O_2 desaturation, respiratory distress, and hypotension. In additon, barotrauma may be associated with subcutaneous emphysema or rarely, free air trapped under the diaphragm simulating a ruptured intra-abdominal viscus.
- Biotrauma refers to lung and nonpulmonary organ inflammation during positive-pressure ventilation secondary to mechanical inflation of damaged lung units.
- Several mechanisms have been proposed to explain the development of critical illness polyneuropathy: alterations in the microcirculation; increased release of inflammatory cytokines such as TNF-α and IL-1β causing increased microvascular permeability; axonal

degeneration due to phosphate depletion; impaired transport of axonal proteins; and endoneural edema and/or hypoxia.

DIAGNOSIS

- Accurate diagnosis of acute respiratory failure relies on a comprehensive review of the medical history and a thorough physical examination. Indeed, hypoxemia is often associated with more than one underlying risk factor or disease.
- Besides dyspnea, the commonest symptoms and signs of acute hypoxemic respiratory failure are anxiety, nonproductive cough, nonspecific chest discomfort, and tachypnea. Wheezing is prominent in patients with preexisting obstructive lung diseases such as COPD and asthma, as well as anaphylactic or anaphylactoid reactions complicated by edema of the upper airway.
- The diaphragm, innervated by the phrenic nerve at spinal levels C3-C5, is the primary force-generating muscle of inspiration. In the supine position, spontaneous breathing is associated with contraction and downward displacement of the diaphragm, resulting in compression of the abdominal viscera and outward movement of the abdominal wall.
- The earliest sign of inspiratory muscle (eg, diaphragmatic) fatigue at the bedside of a spontaneously breathing patient is a paradoxical inward movement of the abdominal wall. This occurs because the intrapleural pressure falls incident to the use of the accessory muscles of respiration (scalene, sternocleidomastoid, trapezius, and pectoralis muscles) resulting in the passive movement of the diaphragm upward toward the thorax.
- Progressively greater muscle fatigue indicates impending respiratory failure and/or arrest characterized by sustained respiratory rates exceeding 35/min and respiratory paradox in which alternating contraction of the diaphragm and accessory muscles along with active contraction of the muscles of expiration give rise to inspiratory chest expansion and expiratory abdominal expansion.
- Bilateral pulmonary infiltrates on the chest radiograph and noncontrast chest CT support the diagnosis of ALI/ARDS. Chest CT scans, in particular, demonstrate the patchy nature of alveolar opacities and not infrequently reveal evidence of atelectasis because of dimished lung volumes and/or pleural effusions. A number of other lung conditions are associated with acute respiratory failure and bilateral pulmonary infiltrates (Table 116–3), which may simulate ALI/ARDS.

- Continuous monitoring of O_2 saturation by pulse oximetry (SpO_2) is useful to detect hypoxemia associated with acute respiratory failure and guide mechanical ventilatory support. Although usually correlating relatively well with PaO_2 levels, SpO_2 values are not reliable in the presence of molecular derangements of hemoglobin (Hb) that alter oxyhemoglobin dissociation. The two most frequent dyshemoglobinemias associated with acute respiratory failure include carboxyhemoglobinemia associated with smoke inhalation and carbon monoxide exposure (HbCO) and methemoglobin (metHb). In these settings, the pulse oximeter does not differentiate Hb with bound CO from Hb with bound O_2; the current devices report the sum of both values as oxyhemoglobin and therefore may overestimate true arterial oxygen saturation.
- The optimal method for the diagnosis of VAP during acute respiratory failure is controversial, especially in the presence of ALI/ARDS. ALI/ARDS can be accompanied by fever, increased bronchopulmonary secretions, change in oxygenation, and new radiographic infiltrates, thus rendering these features nonspecific.
- Bronchoscopy employing quantitative microbial cultures (to exclude contamination or colonization) are commonly used to diagnose VAP. Bronchoscopy employing a protected specimen brush (PSB) collects 0.001 mL of distal lower respiratory tract secretions and has a diagnostic threshold of $\geq 10^3$ CFU/mL. Alternatively, BAL can be employed which theoretically samples approximately one million of the lungs 300 million alveoli and has a diagnostic threshold of $\geq 10^4$ CFU/mL. Detection of $\geq 5\%$ PMNs with intracellular organisms on a smear of cytocentrifuged BAL fluid is also strongly suggestive of VAP.
- Echocardiography is useful to exclude coexisting cardiac dysfunction during the evaluation of acute respiratory failure.

- A high index of suspicion is required to diagnose critical illness polyneuropathy. This condition should be suspected in patients unable to tolerate even short periods of ventilator weaning after optimization of respiratory and cardiac factors. Electrophysiologic testing with electromyography (EMG) and nerve conduction studies usually suggest the diagnosis.

THERAPEUTIC APPROACH

- In patients with acute respiratory failure, the priority is normalize gas exchange and minimize hemodynamic derangements in order to prevent hypoxic organ damage, progressive respiratory muscle fatigue from increased work of breathing, and cardiopulmonary arrest.
- Patients with acute hypoxemic respiratory failure may respond to supplemental O_2 via Venturi or partial non-breather masks, although the use of these devices is of limited benefit in patients with significant right-to-left shunt physiology.
- Depending on the mechanism of acute respiratory failure, a trial of noninvasive positive-pressure ventilation (NPPV) by full face mask in conscious patients may be used to provide inspiratory positive airway pressure (IPAP) and assist failing respiratory muscles, as well as promote alveolar recruitment.
- Most studies of NPPV have been performed in two patient populations: those with acute respiratory failure from cardiogenic pulmonary edema (eg, flash pulmonary edema), and acute-on-chronic hypercapnic respiratory failure secondary to COPD exacerbations.
- NPPV is contraindicated in patients with coma and impaired reflexive airway protection or circulatory shock; results of arterial blood gas analysis alone should not be used to exclude otherwise appropriate patients. Titration at the bedside in such patients may obviate the need for endotracheal intubation and

TABLE 116–3 Conditions Inducing Acute Respiratory Failure with Diffuse Bilateral Infiltrates Simulating ALI/ARDS

CONDITION	DIAGNOSTIC STRATEGY
-Acute interstitial pneumonia (Hamman-Rich syndrome)	-Exclude infectious cause by bronchoscopy → Surgical lung biopsy
-Acute exacerbation of IPF	-Exclude infectious cause by bronchoscopy ±→ Surgical lung biopsy
-*Pneumocystis jiroveci* pneumonia	-HIV antibody test, bronchoscopy with BAL and microbial brushings ± lung biopsy
-Diffuse alveolar hemorrhage in vasculitic or pulmonary-renal syndromes	-Bronchoscopy, progressively bloody BAL fluid
-Acute eosinophilic pneumonia	-Bronchoscopy, ↑ eosinophils in BAL fluid, lung biopsy
-Cryptogenic organizing pneumonia	-Clinical and radiographic features, surgical lung biopsy

ALI, acute lung injury; ARDS, acute respiratory distress syndrome; BAL, bronchoalveolar lavage; HIV, human immunodeficiency virus; IPF, idiopathic pulmonary fibrosis.

attendant increases in hospital length of stay. An effective response is defined as an acute reduction in the respiratory rate and increase in SpO_2 within 10 to 15 minutes. The usual settings for NPPV are as follows; 12 to 14 cm H_2O IPAP and 5 to 7 cm H_2O EPAP. In approximately 25% of patients, NPPV will be unsuccessful in reversing symptoms (sometimes because of patient intolerance).

• Indications for endotracheal intubation and mechanical ventilation include: noncorrectable persistant arterial hypoxemia (eg, SpO_2 values <88% and/or PaO_2 values <55 mm Hg); progressive obtundation with rising $PaCO_2$ levels; voluminous bronchopulmonary secretions requiring frequent suctioning to reduce dyspnea and hypoxemia; stupor or coma with loss of protective upper airway reflexes; and sustained increased work of breathing during circulatory shock states.

• Initial ventilator settings for acute respiratory failure typically include an FIO_2 of 1.0, a V_T of 8 mL/kg of predicted body weight, a volume-cycled mode such as assist-control, a backup respiratory rate of 12 to 14 breaths/minute, and a PEEP of 5 cm H_2O. Further titration of ventilatory therapy is based on SpO_2 and arterial blood gas results.

• Only one specific treatment among multiple randomized clinical trials has been proven to be beneficial for ALI/ARDS—a **lung protective ventilatory strategy** with tidal volumes of 6 mL/kg of predicted (ideal) body weight.[6] This strategy is associated with a 22% reduction in 28-day mortality compared to ventilation with a V_T of 12 mL kg of predicted body weight,

as well as a reduced number of days spent on the ventilator. Guidelines for implementation of this strategy and amelioration of VALI are summarized in Fig. 116–1.

• The primary therapeutic objective of protective lung ventilation during ALI/ARDS is to avoid VALI. In particular, maintenance of normocarbia is not considered essential to successfully managing ALI/ARDS; hypercapnia is therefore tolerated as are reductions in the arterial pH, a strategy termed permissive hypercapnia. In this setting, supplemental bicarbonate therapy is administered to maintain the arterial pH ≥ 7.25.

• Plateau pressure (Pplat) measurements in ventilated patients with ALI/ARDS or those with other forms of acute hypoxemic respiratory failure reflect the static distending pressure of the lungs when airflow (and thus, frictional resistance to that flow) is zero. As such, Pplat represents an index of lung compliance, and is best measured during a 0.5 sec inspiratory hold in a relaxed, sedated patient. VALI is minimized when the Pplat is kept below 30 cm H_2O.

• The development of acute respiratory distress and agitation in a patient receiving mechanical ventilation requires immediate evaluation, including a chest examination, since an increase in respiratory rate, elevated O_2 consumption, and patient–ventilator dyssynchrony can result in barotrauma, hypoxemia, and hemodynamic derangements including hypotension. Ventilator malfunction should always be excluded by disconnecting the patient from the ventilator and initiating bagmask ventilation with an FIO_2 of 1.0. The differential

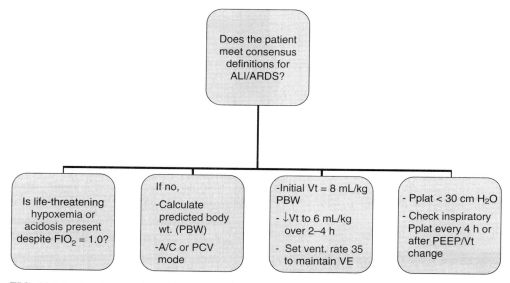

FIG. 116–1   Implementation of lung protective ventilation in ALI/ARDS. FIO_2, inspired oxygen tension; A/C, assist control; PCV, pressure-cycled ventilation; PEEP, positive end expiratory pressure; Vt, tidal volume; Pplat, ventilator plateau pressure; VE, minute ventilation.

diagnosis includes pain, delirium, bronchospasm, pneumonia, advancing pulmonary edema, pulmonary thromboembolism, and pneumothorax.

- The transmural pressure of the lung during positive pressure ventilation is calculated as the pressure difference between alveolar pressure (Palv) and intrapleural pressure (Ppl). Elevations in Ppl and thus, intrathoracic pressure occur with all forms of positive-pressure ventilation (especially when PEEP is applied). The right atrial pressure (Pra) reflects the systemic venous return, and the transmural right atrial pressure (effective RV preload) is dependent on the difference between Pra and Ppl. Thus positive-pressure ventilation with PEEP can adversely effect cardiac preload and hemodynamics (Table 116–4).

- Pulmonary artery catheters (PACs) provide physiological data concerning pulmonary hemodynamics, parameters of right and left ventricular function, and estimates of biventricular filling (eg, the Pra and the pulmonary artery occlusion pressure, respectively). Use of PACs to guide management and improve outcomes in ALI/ARDS has received considerable attention. Importantly, a recent NIH trial evaluated the benefits versus risks of PAC in 1000 patients, comparing hemodynamic management guided by a PAC versus a central venous catheter (CVC) using an explicit management protocol.[7] Neither the primary endpoint (60-day mortality) or secondary endpoints including days off the ventilator (as an index of faster weaning) were improved by PACs, indicating that they are not required in the routine management of ALI/ARDS.

- Because of increased microvascular permeability in ALI/ARDS, a conservative fluid management strategy has been advocated to limit the number of ventilator days and thereby reduce the incidence of superimposed VAP. A recent large clinical trial found no significant difference in mortality between a conservative and a more liberal fluid management strategy; however, the conservative strategy of fluid management improved lung function and shortened the duration of mechanical ventilation and ICU care without increasing nonpulmonary-organ failures including renal dysfunction.[9] Therefore a conservative strategy of fluid management is recommended.

- There is no benefit to the use of methylprednisolone or other steroids to prevent or treat lung inflammation associated with sepsis-induced ALI/ARDS. With specific reference to persistent (eg, fibroproliferative) ARDS of at least 7 days duration, high-dose methylprednisolone therapy (eg, 2 mg/kg predicted body weight IV, followed by 0.5 mg/kg IV every 6 h for 14 d and a tapering over 21 d) was not effective in reducing mortality, and actually increased mortality at 60 and 180 days if initiated more than 2 weeks after onset of ALI/ARDS.[8]

- The ideal method of weaning from mechanical ventilation following acute respiratory failure is controversial. In most patients, conversion to a partial ventilatory support mode such as PSV allows gradual recovery of lung function until spontaneous breathing can be sustained for 30 to 60 minutes, after which an extubation trial is performed.

- Tracheostomy is performed in subjects with prolonged ventilator dependence; it is associated with a 15% reduction in the anatomic dead space as well as improved tracheobronchial suctioning and oral care. Weaning of patients with acute-on-chronic respiratory failure, particularly those with underlying COPD, generally involves sequential and progressive spontaneous breathing trials with a high humidity tracheostomy collar until successful decannulation.

- Supportive treatment of acute respiratory failure is critically important in preventing secondary septic and nonseptic complications. Prophylaxis for deep venous thrombosis using unfractionated or low-molecular weight heparin, prevention of stress ulceration using H_2 receptor antagonists or proton pump inhibitors, continuous IV insulin therapy to minimize hyperglycemia, and physical therapy are standard approaches.

TABLE 116–4 Mechanisms By Which Positive-Pressure Ventilation with PEEP Affects Cardiovascular Function

MECHANISM	CONSEQUENCE
-Decreased pressure gradient for systemic venous return	-Decreased right atrial filling and right ventricular (RV) preload, fall in cardiac output; reduced tissue O_2 delivery
-Increased end-expiratory lung volume, elevates pulmonary vascular resistance	-Increased RV afterload, RV dilation, right-to-left septal shift, -decreased LV geometry and compliance, artifactually increased estimates of LV filling pressure (eg, Paop[a])

[a]Pulmonary artery occlusion pressure
LV, left ventricular; PEEP, positive end-expiratory pressure.

REFERENCES

1. Bernard GR, Vincent J-L, Laterre P-F, et al.; The Recombinant Human Activated Protein C Worldwide Evaluation in Severe Sepsis (PROWESS) Study Group. Efficacy and safety of recombinant human activated protein c for severe sepsis. *N Engl J Med.* 2001;344:699–709.

2. Vincent JL, Moreno R, Takala J, et al. The SOFA (Sepsis-related Organ Failure Assessment) score to describe organ dysfunction/failure. *Intensive Care Med.* 1996;22:707–710.

3. Marshall JC, Cook DJ, Christou NV, Bernard GR, Sprung CL, Sibbald WJ. Multiple Organ Dysfunction Score: A reliable descriptor of a complex clinical outcome. *Crit Care Med.* 1995;23:1638–1652.

4. Vincent JL, Acka S, Mendonca A, et al.; SOFA Working Group. The epidemiology of acute respiratory failure in critically ill patients. *Chest.* 2002;121:1602–1609.

5. Rubenfeld GD, Caldwell E, Peabody E, et al. Incidence and outcomes of acute lung injury. *N Engl J Med.* 2005;353:1685–1693.

6. The Acute Respiratory Distress Syndrome Network. Ventilation with lower tidal volumes as compared with traditional tidal volumes for acute lung injury and the acute respiratory distress syndrome. *N Engl J Med.* 2000;342:1301–1308.

7. The National Heart, Lung and Blood Institute Acute respiratory Distress Syndrome (ARDS) Clinical Trials Network. Pulmonary-artery versus central venous catheter to guide treatment of acute lung injury. *N Engl J Med.* 2006;354:2213–2224.

8. The National Heart, Lung, and Blood Institute Acute Respiratory Distress Syndrome (ARDS) Clinical Trials Network. Efficacy and safety of corticosteroids for persistent acute respiratory distress syndrome. *N Engl J Med.* 2006;354:1671–1684.

9. The National Heart, Lung, and Blood Institute Acute Respiratory Distress Syndrome (ARDS) Clinical Trials Network. Comparison of two fluid-management strategies in acute lung injury. *N Engl J Med.* 2006;354:2564–2575.

10. Kress JP, Pohlman AS, O'Connor MF, Hall JB. Daily interruption of sedative infusions in critically ill patients undergoing mechanical ventilation. *N Engl J Med.* 2000;342:1471–1477.

117 SLEEP-RELATED BREATHING DISORDERS

Joseph Roland D. Espiritu

NORMAL SLEEP PHYSIOLOGY

- Sleep is an active process; at times the brain is more electrically and metabolically active during sleep than during the awake state.
- Sleep is normally comprised of non-rapid eye movement sleep (non-REM sleep) and rapid eye movement (REM) sleep.
- Non-REM sleep occurs in three stages (I through III), with stage III often referred to as *slow-wave sleep.* Slow-wave sleep is considered the deepest level of sleep, constitutes approximately 25% of total sleep time, and decreases with age.
- Rapid eye movement sleep is associated with dreaming and loss of muscular tone. It constitutes approximately 20% to 25% of total sleep time.

- Sleep normally occurs in recurring 90- to 110-minute cycles repeating four to six times each night.
- As sleep progresses, REM sleep periods become longer and non-REM sleep becomes shorter.

OBSTRUCTIVE SLEEP APNEA SYNDROME

DEFINITION

- Obstructive sleep apnea syndrome (OSAS) is a sleep disorder characterized by repetitive nocturnal episodes of complete upper airway obstruction/closure, resulting in cessation of respiratory airflow (apnea) for ≥10 seconds, accompanied by a ≥4% oxygen (O_2) desaturation on pulse oximetry. Partial upper airway obstructions (hypopneas) frequent coexist with apneic events, and result in respiratory airflow that is diminished by at least 30%, last at least 10 seconds per episode, and are likewise accompanied by a ≥4% O_2 desaturation.
- These upper airway obstructive events frequently induce oxyhemoglobin desaturations of <90% by pulse oximetry and are terminated by brief central nervous system (CNS) arousals of which the patient is usually unaware.

EPIDEMIOLOGY

- The prevalence of OSAS is 6% in men and 3% in women in the United States when defined by symptoms of excessive daytime sleepiness and fatigue, in conjunction with an apnea-hypopnea index (AHI) averaging ≥5 episodes per hour of sleep during an overnight sleep study (polysomnography).
- Major clinical features that predispose to OSAS include male gender, obesity, increasing age, the postmenopausal state, neck circumference >40 cm (ie, approximately 16 in), hypothyroidism, acromegaly, and craniofacial abnormalities associated with decreased oro-hypopharyngeal space as well as certain congenital developmental disorders (Table 117–1).

TABLE 117–1 Risk Factors for Obstructive Sleep Apnea Syndrome

Male gender	Narrow mandible or maxilla
Obesity	Dental overjet/retrognathia
Menopause	Crossbite and dental malocclusion
Increasing age	High and narrow hard palate
Neck circumference > 40 cm	Elongated and low-lying uvula
Hypothyroidism	Prominent tonsillar pillars
Acromegaly	Enlarged tonsils and adenoids
Macroglossia	Smoking
Enlarged nasal turbinates	Down syndrome
Deviated nasal septum	

PATHOPHYSIOLOGY

- Obstructive sleep apnea syndrome is caused by dynamic upper airway closure or narrowing resulting from the interaction of two primary mechanisms: (1) decreased tone of the pharyngeal dilator muscles during sleep and (2) excessive hypopharyngeal tissue volume caused by obesity, adenotonsillar hypertrophy, macroglossia, craniofacial anatomy, and other miscellaneous factors.
- The recurrent episodes of nocturnal O_2 desaturations, negative swings in intrathoracic pressure during inspiratory efforts against a closed or partly closed upper airway, and CNS arousals in response to the resulting hypoxia lead to chronically increased activation of the sympathetic nervous system, augmented catecholamine secretion, and abnormal arterial baroreceptor reflexes.
- The pathophysiology of OSAS culminates in cardiovascular, endocrinologic, and neurocognitive derangements.
- Generalized panendothelial cell injury from chronically increased activation of the sympathetic nervous system has been implicated in the pathogenesis of vascular dysfunction in OSAS.
- Left untreated, OSAS can be associated with six major types of cardiovascular dysfunction: (1) systemic hypertension, (2) coronary artery disease, (3) systolic left ventricular dysfunction (ie, congestive heart failure), (4) secondary pulmonary hypertension with resultant right ventricular hypertrophy/failure, (5) atrial as well as ventricular arrhythmias, (6) and cerebrovascular disease.
- Endocrine abnormalities associated with augmented catecholamine and stress hormone secretion during untreated OSAS include reduced insulin sensitivity, which causes or exacerbates glucose intolerance.
- Other endocrinologic abnormalities include reductions in plasma insulin-like growth factor I (IGF-I), a key anabolic and antiapoptotic peptide that has wide-ranging effects on multiple cells and tissues, and diminished total testosterone as well as sex hormone-binding globulin-1 levels.
- Multiple neurocognitive impairments owing to repetitive nocturnal sleep fragmentation may occur with OSAS, such as excessive daytime sleepiness and inattention, reduced memory and vigilance, mood disturbances, and increased risk for motor vehicle accidents.

DIAGNOSIS

- The likelihood of detecting underlying OSAS is facilitated by taking an abbreviated sleep history in all patients and obtaining more detailed information if poor sleep quality is reported.
- The diagnosis of OSAS requires the combination of several key clinical features plus characteristic findings on overnight polysomnographic testing. Additional diagnostic requirements are that the symptoms are not explained by another sleep disorder, medical or neurologic disorder, medication use, or substance abuse disorder.
- The main clinical features of OSAS include loud snoring, apneas witnessed by a bed partner, excessive daytime sleepiness (frequently with unintentional sleep episodes), unrefreshing sleep, fatigue, and insomnia.
- Patients with OSAS may complain of awakening with gasping or choking sensations, or a feeling of breath holding.
- A definitive diagnosis of OSAS in patients with characteristic clinical features is established by an overnight polysomnographic recording showing ≥5 abnormal respiratory events (ie, apneas or hypopneas) per hour of sleep. Apneas and hypopneas lasting more than 10 seconds during sleep studies are combined into a Respiratory Disturbance Index (RDI); patients with OSAS have an RDI (5 per hour of sleep).
- In the absence of typical clinical features of OSAS, an RDI ≥ 15 per hour of sleep is required (Table 117–2).
- The possibility of underlying hypothyroidism should be investigated in patients with symptoms and signs of OSAS by measuring serum concentrations of thyroxine (T4) and thyrotropin-stimulating hormone.

TABLE 117–2 Definition of Respiratory Events in Obstructive Sleep Apnea Syndrome

Respiratory disturbance index[a]: average number of episodes of apnea, hypopnea, and respiratory-related arousal per hour of sleep

Apnea-hypopnea index (AHI)[b]: average number of episodes of apnea and hypopnea per hour and must be based on a minimum of 2 hours of sleep recorded by polysomnography using actual recorder hours of sleep (ie, the AHI may not be extrapolated or projected).

Apnea[b]: a cessation of airflow for at least 10 seconds

Hypopnea[b]: an abnormal respiratory event lasting at least 10 seconds with at least a 30% reduction in thoracoabdominal movement or airflow as compared to baseline, and with at least a 4% oxygen desaturation

Respiratory related arousal[a]: an abnormal respiratory event characterized by a clear drop in inspiratory airflow, an increased inspiratory effort (best seen by esophageal manometry), associated with an arousal but not with a discernible drop in oxyhemoglobin saturation

SOURCES: [a]Modified from Collop N, Badr S, Bradley D, et al. Sleep related breathing disorders. In: Sateia MJ, ed. *International Classification of Sleep Disorders.* 2nd ed. Westchester, IL: American Academy of Sleep Medicine; 2005:33–77.
[b]Centers for Medicare & Medicaid Services (CMS) Medicare. *Coverage Issues Manual*, Transmittal 150, December 26, 2001;60–17.

- In obese patients, evaluation should be considered for obesity-hypoventilation syndrome and chronic respiratory acidosis by an arterial blood gas determination, especially in the presence of an elevated serum bicarbonate concentration.

THERAPEUTIC APPROACH

- Continuous positive airway pressure (CPAP) delivered by nasal mask during sleep is the mainstay of treatment for OSAS in adults.
- The level of CPAP required to splint open the upper airway during sleep varies among patients and is usually determined during a *split-function* overnight sleep study, in which the first part of the study characterizes the OSAS and the second part determines the optimal CPAP level to relieve the obstruction.
- Nasal CPAP therapy has beneficial effects on sleep, as well as on neurocognitive, cardiovascular, and endocrinologic function (Table 117–3).
- Weight loss for obese patients has been shown to decrease the AHI and improve nocturnal oxygenation in patients with OSAS.[1]
- Positional therapy (sleeping in the lateral decubitus position) can decrease the AHI and respiratory-related arousal index in patients with positional obstructive sleep apnea, in which the supine AHI is twice the lateral decubitus AHI.[2]

Table 117–3 Beneficial Effects of Continuous Positive Airway Pressure Therapy for Obstructive Sleep Apnea Syndrome

Improved sleep quality
- □   ↓ Arousal index, ↓ stage 1 sleep
- □   ↑ Stage 3 sleep, ↑ sleep efficiency

Decreased daytime somnolence
Improved neurocognitive function
- □   Driving simulator performance
- □   ↑ Vigilance

Improved subjective work performance
Improved self-reported health status
Improved cardiovascular function
- □   ↑ LV systolic function
- □   ↓ Systemic hypertension
- □   ↓ Pulmonary hypertension
- □   ↑ Exercise performance
- □   ↓ Endothelial dysfunction

Improved glycemic control and insulin sensitivity
Endocrinologic homeostasis
- □   ↑ Plasma IGF-1
- □   ↑ Serum testosterone, ↑ sex-hormone binding globulin-1
- □   ↓ TSH

IGF, insulin-like growth factor; LV, left ventricular; TSH, thyroid-stimulating hormone.

- Oral or dental devices that advance the mandible (ie, mandibular advancement splints) to increase the oro-hypopharyngeal space in patients with mild to moderate OSAS can modestly decrease the AHI and improve systemic blood pressure.[3]
- Tonsillectomy and adenoidectomy is the treatment of choice for children with OSAS resulting from adeno-tonsillar hypertrophy.[4]
- Patients intolerant of CPAP therapy or those for whom CPAP produces suboptimal results owing to nasal septal deviation and/or obstruction should be referred for otolaryngologic evaluation.
- Uvulopalatopharyngoplasty, the most commonly performed surgical procedure for adults with OSAS, involves the surgical removal of the tonsils and redundant soft palate and tonsillar pillars. Uvulopalatopharyngoplasty has an overall success rate of 40% for correcting OSAS.[5]
- Other surgical procedures for OSAS may help correct specific anatomic abnormalities causing upper airway obstruction. These procedures include, but are not limited to nasal reconstruction, mandibular osteotomy with genioglossus advancement, bariatric surgery, and tracheotomy.
- Patients with OSAS and chronic respiratory acidosis benefit the most from noninvasive nocturnal bilevel positive airway pressure. During bilevel positive airway pressure, the expiratory positive airway pressure splints open the upper airway, whereas the inspiratory positive airway pressure enhances carbon dioxide (CO_2) clearance from the blood by increasing alveolar ventilation.

CENTRAL SLEEP APNEA SYNDROMES

DEFINITION

- Central sleep apnea (CSA) is a condition defined by recurrent cessation of respiration during sleep, with the apnea characterized by the absence of ventilatory effort.[6]
- A multitude of conditions may result in CSA syndromes. Central sleep apnea may be idiopathic or associated with multiple clinical disorders; alternatively, CSA may result from medical or neurological conditions, drugs, or high altitude (Table 117–4). Therefore, the clinical context in which CSA syndromes occur has important diagnostic and therapeutic implications.
- An important subtype of CSA is the Cheyne-Stokes periodic breathing pattern, characterized by recurrent apneas, hypopneas, or both, where the hypopneas reflect minimal respiratory efforts cyclically alternating

TABLE 117–4 Classification of Central Sleep Apnea Syndromes

PRIMARY/IDIOPATHIC	SECONDARY CAUSES
Primary central sleep apnea (adult)	Cheyne-Stokes breathing pattern
	• Congestive heart failure
Primary sleep apnea of infancy	• Cerebrovascular disease
	• Renal failure
	High-altitude periodic breathing
	Drug or substance
	• Long-acting opioids
	Medical condition not Cheyne-Stokes

SOURCE: Collop N, Badr S, Bradley D, et al. Sleep related breathing disorders. In: Sateia MJ, ed. *International Classification of Sleep Disorders.* 2nd ed. Westchester, IL: American Academy of Sleep Medicine; 2005:33–77.

with prolonged hyperpneas during accentuated respiratory efforts. Thus thoracic and abdominal respiratory efforts at the bedside and, by extension, tidal volume and alveolar ventilation wax and wane in a gradual crescendo-decrescendo pattern.[6] This periodic breathing is caused by failure of brain respiratory centers to compensate quickly for changing $PaCO_2$ levels owing to CNS damage, neuronal depression, or prolonged circulation time associated with decreased cardiac output.

- Cheyne-Stokes respiration can be transient or sustained and is observed in a variety of medical conditions including congestive heart failure, stroke, brain neoplasms, coma, and carbon monoxide poisoning.
- Cheyne-Stokes respiration may also be transiently observed in otherwise healthy subjects following rapid ascent to high altitude ($\geq$4000 m). The main cause is considered to be disequilibration between reduced blood $PaCO_2$ levels secondary to altitude-related hyperventilation versus the slower pH adaptation of brain respiratory centers.

EPIDEMIOLOGY

- Primary CSA most commonly occurs in patients greater than the age of 40.
- Central sleep apnea caused by Cheyne-Stokes respirations most often occurs in subjects at least age 60 years in which congestive heart failure, cerebrovascular disease with stroke, and renal insufficiency are more common. There is a modest male predominance. Notably, the presence of Cheyne-Stokes periodic respirations is associated with a worse cardiac transplant free survival.[7]
- Long-acting opioids (eg, methadone, time-released morphine, and hydrocodone) are the most common drugs associated with CSA. Alcohol potentiates the respiratory depressive effects of these opioids and other medications such as benzodiazepines and tranquilizers.

PATHOPHYSIOLOGY

- The predisposing factor for CSA is thought to be a high ventilatory chemoresponsiveness to arterial $PaCO_2$.[8]
- Patients with CSA caused by Cheyne-Stokes periodic breathing during sleep are thought to have an unstable respiratory control system at the transition from wakefulness to non-REM sleep, which may be responsible for the crescendo-decrescendo respiratory pattern. In this context apneas of central origin are common in subjects with clearcut OSAS, where they may constitute up to 10% of apnea events in the latter condition.

DIAGNOSIS

- The diagnosis of CSA requires clinical features (excessive daytime sleepiness, frequent arousals and awakenings during sleep, insomnia complaints, or awakenings caused by dyspnea) plus an overnight polysomnogram showing a central apnea index of 5 or more per hour of sleep.[6] The diagnosis of the Cheyne-Stokes breathing pattern can be established at the bedside and is confirmed by a nocturnal polysomnogram showing at least 10 central apneas and hypopneas per hour of sleep, in which the hypopnea has a crescendo-decrescendo pattern of tidal volume accompanied by frequent arousals from sleep and derangement of sleep structure.[6]

THERAPEUTIC APPROACH

- Depending on the underlying cause of CSA, treatment options addressing Cheyne-Stokes periodic breathing include optimizing treatment of underlying conditions such as congestive heart failure. Other treatments include O_2 therapy to minimize arterial PaO_2 reductions,[9] CPAP and/or bilevel positive airway pressure,[10] theophylline as a respiratory stimulant owing to its inhibitory effects on adenosine deaminase,[11] and atrial pacing in selected patients.[12]
- In patients with Cheyne-Stokes respirations and acute altitude sickness, descent by only 500 to 1000 m, supplemental O_2 therapy, and acetazolamide[13] are effective therapies for high-altitude pulmonary edema.
- Nifedipine and inhaled salmeterol have been demonstrated to be effective in preventing high-altitude pulmonary edema.[14,15]
- Discontinuation of long-acting opioid medications and reduction of alcohol use may help ameliorate drug-related CSA.

SLEEP-RELATED HYPOVENTILATION SYNDROMES

DEFINITION

- Sleep-related hypoventilation is a pathophysiological disturbance and sleep-related breathing disorder associated with varied causes (excluding OSAS), all of which have as a common denominator decreased nocturnal alveolar ventilation that results in sleep-related arterial oxygen desaturation and, commonly, CO_2 retention.[6]
- Sleep-related hypoventilation may be idiopathic, congenital (Ondine curse), or secondary to pulmonary, vascular, neuromuscular, or skeletal abnormalities, often occurring in combination (Table 117–5).

EPIDEMIOLOGY

- The demographics of patients with secondary sleep-related hypoventilation syndromes parallel those of the underlying medical condition.
- Little is known about the epidemiology of idiopathic and congenital sleep-related hypoventilation syndromes, both of which rarely occur.

PATHOPHYSIOLOGY

- The idiopathic and congenital forms of sleep-related hypoventilation syndromes are characterized by decreased ventilatory responsiveness to hypercapnia or hypoxia during wakefulness and sleep caused by a lesion in the medullary chemoreceptors (idiopathic) or abnormality in the brainstem integration of chemoreceptor afferents (congenital).
- Conversely, sleep-related hypoventilation/hypoxemia caused by medical conditions occur because of ventilation-perfusion abnormalities or mechanical ventilatory insufficiency.

TABLE 117–5 Classification of Sleep-Related Hypoventilation/Hypoxemic Syndromes

Sleep-related nonobstructive alveolar hypoventilation, idiopathic
Congenital central alveolar hypoventilation syndrome (Ondine curse)
Sleep-related hypoventilation caused by medical conditions:
- Pulmonary parenchymal abnormalities (eg, interstitial lung disease)
- Pulmonary vascular conditions (eg, pulmonary embolism)
- Lower airways obstruction (eg, chronic obstructive pulmonary disease)
- Neuromuscular disorder (eg, amyotrophic lateral sclerosis)
- Chest wall disorders (eg, kyphoscoliosis)

SOURCE: Modified from Collop N, Badr S, Bradley D, et al. Sleep related breathing disorders. In: Sateia MJ, ed. *International Classification of Sleep Disorders*. 2nd ed. Westchester, IL: American Academy of Sleep Medicine; 2005:33–77.

DIAGNOSIS

- Congenital central alveolar hypoventilation syndrome is suspected in a newborn who presents with shallow breathing, cyanosis, and apnea during sleep.
- The idiopathic form is diagnosed only after excluding medical conditions that can result in sleep related hypoventilation/hypoxemia in the adult.
- In sleep-related hypoventilation/hypoxemia caused by medical conditions in which the lungs or respiratory muscles are affected (see Table 117–5), the diagnosis may be suspected by the finding of a chronic respiratory acidosis on arterial blood gas analysis, supported by evidence of nocturnal arterial O_2 desaturations (<90% during overnight pulse oximetry), and confirmed by polysomnographic testing or a sleep arterial blood gas showing persistent nocturnal hypoxemia and/or hypercapnia in the absence of obvious obstructive apneas or periodic breathing.
- Specific criteria verifying the presence of sleep related hypoventilation and hypoxemia include one of the following:
- Arterial oxyhemoglobin saturation (SpO_2) values during sleep of <90% for more than 5 minutes, with a nadir of at least 85%
- Greater than 30% of total sleep time with SpO_2 values less than 90%
- Asleep arterial blood gas in which there is an elevated $Paco_2$ level that is disproportionately higher than $Paco_2$ values during wakefulness during the day

THERAPEUTIC APPROACH

- Optimal therapy of the underlying medical condition may ameliorate the secondary forms of sleep-related hypoventilation/hypoxemia. Examples include nocturnal oxygen supplementation,[16] long-acting bronchodilators and inhaled steroids for chronic obstructive pulmonary disease, and thyroid hormone replacement for hypothyroidism.
- Drugs intended to improve ventilatory drive per se such as theophylline, progesterone, and acetazolamide are not uniformly effective, nor are agents to improve muscular strength such as anabolic steroids, growth hormone, and insulin-like growth factor I.
- Noninvasive positive pressure ventilation via a nasal interface or orofacial mask and a bilevel positive airway pressure device or a mechanical ventilator is the mainstay of treatment for symptomatic patients complaining of fatigue, dyspnea, or morning headache, especially when frequent episodes of acute-on-chronic respiratory failure supervene.[17] Thus, maintaining daytime arterial CO_2 homeostasis by such nocturnal ventilation strategies

avoid the deleterious effects of chronic respiratory acidosis on respiratory muscle excitation-contraction coupling, strength, and endurance.

REFERENCES

1. Collop N, Badr S, Bradley D, et al. Sleep related breathing disorders. In: Sateia MJ, ed. *International Classification of Sleep Disorders.* 2nd ed. Westchester, IL: American Academy of Sleep Medicine; 2005:33–77.

2. Young T, Palta M, Dempsey J, et al. The occurrence of sleep-disordered breathing among middle aged adults. *N Engl J Med.* 1993;328:1230–1235.

3. Kajaste S, Brander PE, Telakivi T, et al. A cognitive-behavioral weight reduction program in the treatment of obstructive sleep apnea syndrome with or without initial nasal CPAP: A randomized study. *Sleep Med.* 2004;5:125–131.

4. Kushida CA, Littner MR, Hirshkowitz M, et al. Practice parameters for the use of continuous and bilevel positive airway pressure devices to treat adult patients with sleep-related breathing disorders. *Sleep.* 2006;29:375–380.

5. Jokic R, Klimaszewski A, Crossley M, et al. Positional treatment vs. continuous positive airway pressure in patients with positional obstructive sleep apnea syndrome. *Chest.* 1999; 115:771–781.

6. Gostopoulos H, Kelley JJ, Cistulli PA. Oral appliance reduces blood pressure in obstructive sleep apnea: A randomized, controlled trial. *Sleep.* 2004;27:934–941.

7. Shintani, T, Asakura K, Kataura A. The effect of adenotonsillectomy in children with OSA. *Int J Pediatr Otorhinolaryngol.* 1998;44:51–58.

8. Sher AE, Schectman KB, Piccirillo JF. The efficacy of surgical modifications of the upper airway in adults with obstructive sleep apnea syndrome. *Sleep.* 1996;19:156–177.

9. Lanfranchi P, Braghiroli A, Bosimini E, et al. Prognostic value of nocturnal Cheyne-Stokes respiration in chronic heart failure. *Circulation.* 1999;99:1435–1440.

10. Javaheri S. A mechanism of central sleep apnea in patients with heart failure. *N Engl J Med.* 1999;341:949–954.

11. Sasayama S, Izumi T, Seino Y, et al. Effects of nocturnal oxygen therapy on outcome measures in patients with chronic heart failure and Cheyne-Stokes respiration. *Circ J.* 2006; 70:1–7.

12. Javaheri S. Acetazolamide improves central sleep apnea in heart failure: A double-blind, prospective study. *Am J Respir Crit Care Med.* 2006;15; 173:234–237.

13. Javaheri S, Parker TJ, Wexler L, et al. Effect of theophylline on sleep-disordered breathing in heart failure. *N Engl J Med.* 1996 335:562–567.

14. Garrigue S, Bordier P, Jaïs P, et al. Benefit of atrial pacing in sleep apnea syndrome. *N Engl J Med.* 2002;346:404–412.

15. Andreas S, Weidel K, Hagenah G, Heindl S. Treatment of Cheyne-Stokes respiration with nasal oxygen and carbon dioxide. *Eur Respir J.* 1998;12:414–419.

16. Bartsch P, Maggiorini M, Ritter M, Noti C, Vock P, Oelz O. Prevention of high-altitude pulmonary edema by nifedipine. *N Engl J Med.* 1991;325:1284–1289.

17. Sartori C, Allemann Y, Duplain H, et al. Salmeterol for the prevention of high altitude pulmonary edema. *N Engl J Med.* 2002;346:1631–1636.

118 APPROACH TO THE PATIENT WITH KIDNEY DISEASE

Kevin J. Martin

INTRODUCTION

The presence of kidney disease comes to the attention of the treating physician for any one of the following reasons:
- An abnormality has been detected on routine clinical or laboratory studies that suggest an underlying kidney disease (eg, hematuria, proteinuria, elevated creatinine).
- The patient has symptoms or physical signs that suggest the presence of kidney disease (eg, nocturia, frequency, edema).
- The patient has a systemic disease, which is known to be associated with kidney involvement (eg, diabetes mellitus).
Once kidney disease is suspected the clinician must
- Ascertain the underlying cause of the kidney disease.
- Identify reversible factors that might contribute to renal dysfunction (eg, medications).
- Assess risk factors that are known to contribute to the progression of kidney disease (eg, hypertension).
- Assess the patient for complications of kidney disease (eg, metabolic acidosis, hyperkalemia, anemia, renal osteodystrophy).
- Initiate specific therapy for the kidney disease, if possible.
- Initiate therapy to prevent the complications of kidney disease or its progression.

PHYSICAL FINDINGS

The following are physical findings or laboratory studies suggestive of kidney disease in asymptomatic patients:

- Hypertension
- Proteinuria
- Hematuria (>5 RBCs/HPF)
- Pyuria (>5 WBCs/HPF)
- Elevated blood urea nitrogen (BUN) or creatinine
- Metabolic acidosis
- Abnormal kidney size or contour on an abdominal ultrasound
- Edema

INITIAL EVALUATION

- Obtain a detailed medical history, both current and past, including prior laboratory data, that can provide a clue to the diagnosis (eg, family history of polycystic kidney disease) or duration of the problem.
- Perform a detailed physical examination to uncover clues to the diagnosis (malar rash consistent with lupus, palpable kidneys consistent with polycystic kidney disease)
- Obtain relevant laboratory studies to quantitate glomerular filtration rate (GFR), which will also permit staging of the kidney disease (Table 118–1).
- Analyze the urine for protein and blood and perform a microscopic examination of the urine sediment for cells, cast, and crystals.
- Obtain laboratory tests to assess the complications of kidney disease, such as measurements of hemoglobin, serum calcium and phosphorus, albumin, carbon dioxide (CO_2), parathyroid hormone, 1,25-dihydroxyvitamin D, and a fasting lipid profile.

URINALYSIS

Examination of the urine sediment is an essential step in the evaluation of a patient with suspected kidney disease. The urine dipstick is readily performed in the office and can detect and estimate proteinuria and hematuria. The urine dipstick also screens for the presence

TABLE 118–1   Stages of Chronic Kidney Disease

STAGE	DESCRIPTION	GFR (mL/min/ 1.73 m²)
1.	Kidney damage with a normal GFR	>90
2.	Mild decrease in GFR	60–89[a]
3.	Moderate decrease in GFR	30–59
4.	Severe decrease in GFR	15–29
5.	Kidney failure	<15 or dialysis

GFR, glomerular filtration rate.
[a]Can be normal for age

of glucose, leucocytes and bacteria. An estimate of urine concentration (specific gravity) can also be obtained. This initial screen can direct more definitive testing. For example, proteinuria should be quantitated; the 24-hour excretion of protein can be reliably approximated in most patients (excluding very large patients or those at the extremes of life) by calculating the ratio of urinary protein to urine creatinine in mg/dL (the ratio is roughly equivalent to grams of protein per 24 hours). Normal subjects excrete between 50 and 150 mg of protein per day. Additionally, the nature of the protein in the urine can be characterized with a urine protein electrophoresis (predominately albuminuria versus light chains). Urine sodium, chloride, and creatinine determinations will allow calculation of the fractional excretion of sodium or chloride, which is useful in the differential diagnosis of acute kidney injury (see Chap. 120).

Further information can be gained by careful examination of the urinary sediment, which can reveal the presence of casts, such as hyaline casts, red blood cell casts, white blood cell casts, crystals, or the presence of red blood cells, white blood cells or bacteria. The urinary findings, although not specific, are more commonly associated with certain renal diseases as follows:

Proteinuria → Glomerular disease.

Hematuria → Dysmorphic red blood cells suggest glomerular disease.

Absence of dysmorphic cells suggest a lower urinary tract pathology.

Hyaline casts	→	Usually associated with dehydration or decreased renal perfusion (heart failure).
Granular casts	→	Usually accompany acute tubular injury.
White cell casts	→	Pyelonephritis, allergic interstitial nephritis.
Red cell casts	→	Acute glomerulonephritis, renal vasculitis.
Pyuria	→	Urinary tract infection or interstitial disease.
Crystals	→	Kidney stones

Thus, the urinary sediment is extremely useful in the initial evaluation of kidney disease as summarized in Fig. 118–1. An elevated serum creatinine without proteinuria or cells in the urine sediment should suggest a hemodynamically-mediated decrease in kidney function induced by volume contraction, congestive heart failure, hepatorenal syndrome, renovascular disease, or obstruction of the urinary tract. The presence of isolated hematuria without proteinuria should suggest (lower tract pathology nephrolithiasis or bleeding from the ureters or bladder) and lead to appropriate investigations such as cystoscopy and retrograde pyelography. The presence of proteinuria with or without other cellular elements usually indicates intrinsic kidney disease (especially glomerular disease) and often requires a percutaneous renal biopsy.

IMAGING OF THE GENITOURINARY TRACT

A variety of imaging studies are useful in the evaluation of suspected kidney disease.

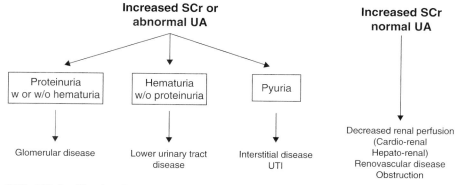

FIG. 118–1   Simple scheme to classify suspected renal disease. SCr, serum creatinine; UA, urinalysis; UTI, urinary tract infection.

These include the following:
- Evaluation of kidney size by ultrasonography intravenous pyelography (IVP), or computed tomography.
- Evaluation of the renal vasculature by angiography or magnetic resonance imaging.
- Evaluation of potential or suspected kidney masses by IVP, computed tomography, or magnetic resonance imaging.

Of these tests, the renal ultrasound is the most widely used, as it is noninvasive and provides useful information with regard to kidney size and the presence of cysts, stones or masses. Moreover, when coupled with Doppler interrogation of the renal arteries renal ultrasonography provides a noninvasive alternative to renal angiography. Plain radiographs of the abdomen are useful for detecting the presence of radioopaque kidney stones. Renal masses can be evaluated by intravenous pyelography, although computed tomography and magnetic resonance imaging are generally preferred. Magnetic resonance imaging is also useful for the evaluation of suspected renal artery stenosis. The relative function of each kidney can be assessed by radionuclide scanning (using technetium-99), and lower urinary tract disease can be assessed by retrograde pyelography and cystoscopy.

QUANTITATING GFR

The standard parameter used for the assessment of kidney function and determining progression of disease is the glomerular filtration rate (GFR). Classically, GFR is measured using the clearance relationship, UV/P, where P is the plasma concentration of a filterable marker, U is the urine concentration of the marker, and V is the urine flow rate. Most often, this is calculated in clinical practice using creatinine as the marker. Creatinine clearance is a useful estimate of GFR; however, creatinine is not an ideal marker, as tubular secretion of creatinine can increase (and, thus overestimate GFR) when kidney function is reduced. In addition, creatinine secretion is altered by a variety of commonly used drugs, such as cimetidine and trimethoprim. The serum creatinine concentration also reflects muscle mass, so that the absolute value for serum creatinine in a muscular individual are necessarily higher.

In recent years, several formula have been developed that permit a more accurate estimation of GFR from the serum creatinine. The most frequently used formula for the estimation of GFR is the abbreviated Modification in Diet and Renal Disease Study (MDRD) equation, which is calculated as follows:

$$GFR = 186 \times creatinine^{-1.154} - age^{-0.203} - 1.210 \text{ (if black)} - 0.742 \text{ (if female)}$$

Alternate calculations such as the Cockroft-Gault relationship is also widely used:

$$C_{Cr} = (140\text{-age}) \times body\ weight\ in\ kg\ /\ (72 \times S_{Cr}) \times 0.85 \text{ (if female)}$$

Although these estimations are not ideal they do provide reasonably accurate estimates of GFR. Importantly, the MDRD equation is the currently accepted method used to classify chronic kidney disease into the clinical stages described in Table 118–1. Although the Cockroft-Gault formula is easily calculated by hand, the more widely used and reliable MDRD equation is available for downloading into most handheld computing platforms directly via the Internet (www.kdoqi. org).

ACUTE VERSUS CHRONIC KIDNEY DISEASE

The first step in the evaluation of the patient with decreased kidney function is aimed at determining whether the kidney DISEASE is acute or chronic in nature. Acute decreases in kidney function require urgent evaluation and treatment, whereas the evaluation of chronic kidney disease can take a more deliberate course. Acute decreases in kidney function can also arise in patients with preexisiting chronic kidney disease (acute on chronic kidney disease). The cause of the acute decline in renal function in this setting must also be evaluated with urgency so that reversible factors are correctly identified and eliminated. If no previous history or laboratory test results are available it can be challenging to determine whether the kidney disease is acute or chronic. However, as the evaluation proceeds, and laboratory testing and imaging results become available, the nature of the kidney insult is usually apparent. For example, small kidneys (<9 cm in length) on an ultrasound examination indicate that a chronic process has caused the decrease in kidney function.

ACUTE KIDNEY DISEASE

The initial approach to the evaluation of the patient with acute kidney injury should include the following:
- Establish that the injury is acute and the nature of the injury:
  - History (previously normal kidney function)
  - Clinical circumstances (new medication)
  - Prior laboratory data (serum creatinine)

- Identify potential factors that can precipitate or exacerbate kidney disease.
  - Hypotension
  - Volume contraction
  - Nephrotoxic drugs, such as aminoglycosides and radio-contrast agents
  - Sepsis
  - Congestive heart failure
  - Renal vascular disease
  - Renal vein thrombosis
- Examine the urinary sediment.
  - Identification of casts or cells
- Obtain a renal ultrasound to exclude urinary tract obstruction.
- Obtain a urine sodium, chloride, creatinine, and calculate the fractional excretion of sodium.

Often acute kidney failure occurs in the hospital setting, and background information is readily available. The most common cause of acute kidney failure in this setting is *acute tubular necrosis* (ATN). Conversely, the presence of = red blood cell casts together with proteinuria would suggest the possibility of an acute glomerular process such as rapidly progressive glomerulonephritis or vasculitis. The presence of eosinophils in the sediment should lead to consideration of an allergic interstitial nephritis.

Urine biochemistries to obtain fractional excretion of sodium, chloride, urea, and uric acid are helpful in oliguric patients. Further details of the evaluation of cases of acute kidney failure are found in Chap. 120.

Once a diagnosis is established, further evaluation and therapy is directed toward the following:
- Therapy and/or elimination of precipitating factors.
- Careful monitoring for complications.
  - Volume overload
  - Hyperkalemia
  - Acidosis
  - Anemia
- Careful attention to appropriate drug dosing.
- Evaluation for renal replacement therapy.

CHRONIC KIDNEY DISEASE

The initial evaluation of the patient with chronic kidney disease should include the following:
- Define and confirm the stage of kidney disease (see Table 118–1).
- Establish the extent and severity of the chronic kidney disease.
  - History
  - Symptoms
  - Laboratory abnormalities
  - Kidney size
- Identify potential factors that can exacerbate kidney disease.
  - Volume contraction
  - Drugs
  - Congestive heart failure
  - Renal vein thrombosis
  - Hypercalcemia
  - Hyperuricemia
  - Hypertension
- Assess for complications of chronic kidney disease
  - Anemia
  - Hypertension
  - Abnormalities in bone and mineral metabolism
  - Hypocalcemia
  - Hyperphosphatemia
  - Hyperparathyroidism
  - Vitamin D insufficiency or deficiency
- Assess risk factors which contribute to progression of chronic kidney disease
  - Hypertension
  - Magnitude of proteinuria
  - Hyperlipidemia
  - Glucose control in diabetes
- Consider a renal biopsy for definitive diagnosis.

This evaluation will yield useful information and allow rationale institution of a treatment plan. Once this plan is in effect, the patient will need regular monitoring:
- The progression of the underlying kidney disease should be assessed with serial GFRs.
- Evaluate the effectiveness of general measures to slow progression of renal disease.
  - Control of hypertension (target blood pressure is <130/80 mmHg)
  - Control of proteinuria (target 24-hour protein is <1–2 gm)
  - Control of hyperlipidemia (target LDL cholesterol is <100mg/dL)
  - Control of blood glucose in diabetics (target HgbA1c is <7.0%)
- The complications of chronic kidney disease should be closely monitored.
  - Anemia should be managed with erythropoiesis stimulating agents (target Hgb is 11–13g/dL)
    - Iron status (target iron saturation is >25% in CKD patients)
- Renal bone disease should be treated early and aggressively (target parathyroid hormone level varies from 150–300 pg/dL depending on the kidney stage, see Chap. 121).
- Preparation for the management of end-stage renal disease (ESRD) (eg, placement of vascular access) should occur in stage 4.

BIBLIOGRAPHY

Cockcroft DW, Gault MH. Prediction of creatinine clearance from serum creatinine. *Nephron.* 1976;16(1):31–41.

Andrew S Levey, Josef Coresh, Ethan Balk, et al. National Kidney Foundation practice guidelines for chronic kidney disease: Evaluation, classification, and stratification. *Ann Intern Med.* 2003;139(2):137–147.

119 FLUID, ELECTROLYTE, AND ACID-BASE DISORDERS

Paul G. Schmitz

WATER DISORDERS

INTRODUCTION

Abnormalities in water homeostasis result in deranged plasma osmolality manifested as hyponatremia or hypernatremia. In contrast, disorders of sodium homeostasis are characterized by volume contraction or volume expansion. Absorption or excretion of sodium by the kidney induces passive water movement in an isoosmotic fashion; thus, changes in renal NaCl handling per se are not associated with disturbances in the plasma osmolality. In contrast, water absorption and excretion in the kidney can be altered independent of sodium via antidiuretic hormone (ADH). Water retention in excess of sodium (concentrated urine) lowers the plasma osmolality, whereas water loss in excess of sodium (dilute urine) raises the plasma osmolality. The circulating ADH level is the primary regulator of water excretion in the kidney. Importantly, water and sodium disorders often coexist.

HYPONATREMIA

- Hyponatremia is a common electrolyte disturbance in the hospitalized patient. The mean plasma sodium concentration obtained in randomly selected hospitalized patients is approximately 8 mEq/L less than that observed in the outpatient setting.
- Must distinguish a reduction in *effective* plasma osmolality from pseudohyponatremia or hypertonic hyponatremia.

- Hypertonic hyponatremia is secondary to an increase in the plasma glucose concentration.
- Pseudohyponatremia is a false positive reduction in the plasma sodium concentration; the plasma osmolality, when measured by standard freezing point depression, is unchanged. The decrease in plasma sodium concentration in pseudohyponatremia occurs when dilution-based methods are employed to measure the serum sodium. Dilution-based methods underestimate the true plasma sodium concentration because the same volume of diluent is used to prepare the sample regardless of the percentage of solid-phase particles in the sample. The most common cause of pseudohyponatremia is severe hyperlipidemia and multiple myeloma (increased plasma proteins).

SYMPTOMS

- Almost exclusively secondary to an increase in brain cell volume.
- Most cells can tolerate changes in volume (10%–20%) with little adverse consequence. However, significant intracranial hypertension may arise when brain cells swell.
- Intracranial pressure rises exponentially with as little as a 10% decrease in the plasma osmolality.
- The cardinal clinical manifestations of hyponatremia are secondary to a rise in intracranial pressure and include nausea, vomiting, lethargy, confusion, coma, and seizures.
- In the complete absence of adaptation, life-threatening cerebral edema may occur with as little as a 10% decrease in osmolality. Acute adaptation (<48 h), principally secondary to extrusion of cell salt and water, attenuates brain edema. Chronic adaptation (>48 h) is believed to depend on the extrusion of cell organic compounds referred to as osmolytes. Chronic adaptation may completely attenuate brain edema even with extreme reductions in plasma osmolality.

PATHOPHYSIOLOGY

Hyponatremia arises when there is an imbalance of water intake relative to water excretion:

$$Water_{in} > Water_{out}$$

- Rarely, excessive water intake alone (psychogenic polydipsia) may underlie the development of hyponatremia.
- Although it is theoretically possible to ingest sufficient water to induce a fall in plasma osmolality, most instances of hyponatremia are secondary to impaired renal free water excretion rather than excessive intake.

Renal free water excretion can be inferred from knowledge of two variables:

- The lowest achievable urine osmolality (urine dilution), which is approximately 50 mOsm of solute per liter of water.
- The average daily solute excretion (which is approximately 600 mOsm/day derived from excess NaCl, KCl, and urea from protein catabolism).

Therefore, the maximal urine free water excretion in an otherwise healthy individual is 12 L/day. Accordingly, water intake, in the absence of impaired free water excretion, must exceed 10 to 12 L to produce hyponatremia. Since the maximal urinary volume depends on the daily solute excretion, it is possible to dramatically limit free water excretion by restricting solute intake. Such a phenomenon has been described in the elderly and the alcoholic.

The primary factors, which regulate free water excretion in the kidney, include:

- Reabsorption of NaCl and water in the proximal tubule (reducing free water excretion).
- Reabsorption of NaCl in excess of water in the loop of Henle (generation of a dilute urine).
- The water permeability of the collecting duct which is governed exclusively by the circulating level of ADH.
- Solute intake.

The majority of hyponatremic states are caused by an increase in circulating ADH that, in turn, promotes water retention by the kidney. The prevailing level of ADH reflects the net effect of factors that stimulate or inhibit ADH secretion (Table 119–1).

CLINICAL APPROACH

The hyponatremic states can be classified into two major categories:

- Conditions associated with a low effective circulating volume (ECV).
- Conditions associated with a normal ECV.

TABLE 119–1   Common Factors That Change the Concentration of ADH

INCREASE	DECREASE
Hyperosmolality	Hypoosmolality
Hypovolemia	Hypervolemia
Pain	Ethanol
Nausea	Phenytoin
Pregnancy	
Hypoglycemia	
Carbamazepine	
Nicotine	

ADH, antidiuretic hormone.

CONDITIONS ASSOCIATED WITH A LOW EFFECTIVE CIRCULATING VOLUME

Four clinical conditions account for the majority of these states:

- Dehydration
- Congestive heart failure
- Nephrotic syndrome
- Cirrhosis

All of these disorders are characterized by a nonosmotic increase in circulating ADH (see Table 119–1).

While the pathophysiology of these disorders is similar, the management of each condition varies depending on the underlying cause. Dehydration responds to hydration (0.9% saline) regardless of the underlying cause. The management of hyponatremia in CHF, the nephrotic syndrome, and cirrhosis should be aimed at correcting the underlying disorder. In refractory cases restriction of free water intake is necessary.

CONDITIONS ASSOCIATED WITH A NORMAL EFFECTIVE CIRCULATING VOLUME

Hyponatremia in a euvolemic patient should alert the clinician to the presence of the syndrome of inappropriate antidiuretic hormone secretion (SIADH). This disorder is characterized by an increase in circulating ADH, however, there is no obvious physiologic stimulus to ADH secretion. Since these individuals are euvolemic, this disorder is also characterized by a urine Na^+ >20 mEq/L. Importantly, treatment with 0.9% saline only serves to aggravate the plasma Na^+ concentration (although there may be a transient increase in Na^+) and, hence, should be avoided. Unless the underlying etiology can be corrected, water restriction is the mainstay of therapy. Increasing solute intake (NaCl tablets or dietary protein supplementation) to facilitate free water excretion may also prove valuable. ADH-receptor antagonists (tolvaptan) may emerge as an important new therapy. Demeclocycline antagonizes the action of ADH, however, photosensitivity is a relatively common complication with its use.

The etiology of SIADH is diverse. Four major diagnostic entities are responsible for SIADH:

- Central nervous system lesions (bleeding, infection, and tumor).
- Malignancies (especially lung).
- Pulmonary disease (abscess, empyema, fungal, and tuberculosis).
- Drugs (carbamazepine).

Fig. 119–1 summarizes the approach to the patient with hyponatremia.

TREATMENT OF HYPONATREMIA

In general, the approach to managing hyponatremia is aimed at increasing free water excretion relative to intake.

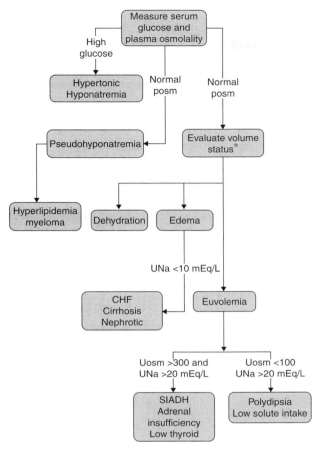

FIG. 119–1 Approach to the patient with hyponatremia. CHF, congestive heart failure; SIADH, syndrome of inappropriate antidiuretic hormone.

* Administer 0.9% saline in patients with reduced extracellular volume.
* If possible, correct the underlying cause (eg, improve cardiac output in CHF, plasma volume expansion in cirrhosis or the nephrotic syndrome, increased solute intake in malnourished patients); if not possible to increase free water excretion, restrict water intake to 500 to 1500 mL/day.
* Life-threatening hyponatremia (coma, seizures, profound CNS dysfunction): treat with intravenous furosemide to increase free water excretion and replace urine NaCl losses (measured hourly) with 3% to 5% saline. Avoid overcorrection and generally aim for sodium concentration of 125 mEq/L or less.

Rapid restoration of the plasma sodium concentration to normal can elicit injury to the myelin sheath of neurons precipitating the syndrome of osmotic demyelination.

This syndrome is also referred to as central pontine myelinolysis (CPM) or the osmotic cerebral demyelinating syndrome.

Features of the osmotic cerebral demyelinating syndrome:

* Often linked to ethanol abuse.
* Pontine and extrapontine myelin injury is common.
* Flaccid quadriplegia and pseudobulbar palsies are the classic symptoms.
* Behavioral changes are common.
* Rapid correction in animal models of hyponatremia consistently results in demyelination.
* Appears to correlate with the rate as well as magnitude of correction.
* **Delayed onset is the rule rather than the exception.**

PRUDENT APPROACH TO MANAGEMENT OF HYPONATREMIA

* Manage asymptomatic patients conservatively.
* 10% increase in plasma sodium should reverse symptoms.
* Correction rate ~ 0.5–1.0 mEq/hour (never exceed 2.5 mEq/h).
* Absolute correction ~ 10–15 mEq/day (never exceed 20 mEq/d).
* Consider high-risk patients: female, alcoholic, previous CNS disease.

HYPERNATREMIA

PATHOPHYSIOLOGY

The pathophysiology of hypernatremia is conceptually analogous to the hyponatremic states since the prerequisite for developing this disorder is an imbalance in water homeostasis.

$$Water_{in} < Water_{out}$$

However, abnormalities in water intake (thirst) are effectively responsible for most cases of hypernatremia. The absence of hypernatremia in an otherwise healthy patient with diabetes insipidus underscores the importance of abnormal water intake in the pathogenesis of hypernatremia. Accordingly, diabetes insipidus (nephrogenic or central) is typically characterized by polyuria and polydipsia rather than hypernatremia. Impaired thirst is common in two clinical settings:

* The patient with altered CNS function for example, dementia or cerebrovascular disease.
* The patient who cannot express the need for water, such as the infant or patients with marked CNS depression.

APPROACH TO HYPERNATREMIA

The clinical examination coupled with a measured urine osmolality is quite helpful in the evaluation of hypernatremia (Fig. 119–2). Since most individuals presenting with hypernatremia possess normal or near normal renal function, the urine osmolality is often appropriately high (usually >800 mOsm/L).

In contrast, a urine osmolality of <150 mOsm/L is consistent with the diagnosis of diabetes insipidus. Administration of vasopressin will permit differentiation of nephrogenic from central diabetes insipidus (Fig. 119–2).

A urine osmolality between 200 and 800 mOsm/L is consistent with:
- Tubulointerstitial disease resulting in a partial defect in urine concentration (eg, papillary necrosis).
- Partial forms of diabetes insipidus (the majority of these patients do not exhibit marked polyuria/polydipsia)
- Osmotic diuresis (urine osmolality is usually fixed at 300 mOsm/L). An osmotic diuresis can usually be differentiated from partial forms of diabetes insipidus after careful analysis of the solute composition of the urine since most of these clinical disorders are characterized by excessive excretion of urea or glucose.

ETIOLOGY OF DIABETES INSIPIDUS
The etiology of diabetes insipidus is diverse; however, CNS disturbances such as trauma, infection, and tumors are relatively common causes of central diabetes insipidus. In contrast, drugs, metabolic disturbances, and renal parenchymal injury are often responsible for the nephrogenic forms of diabetes insipidus.

Causes of central diabetes insipidus:
- Idiopathic
- S/P neurosurgery
- Head trauma
- Anoxic encephalopathy (cardiac arrest)
- Neoplasm (lung, metastatic, CNS tumors).
- CNS infections
- Miscellaneous (sarcoidosis, histiocytosis X)

Causes of nephrogenic diabetes insipidus:
- Reduced generation or effect of cAMP (the effector of ADH action) in the collecting duct (congenital, hypercalcemia, hypokalemia, lithium, demeclocycline, streptozotocin, amyloid, Sjögren syndrome).
- Interference with urine concentration (osmotic diuresis, loop diuretics, acute and chronic renal failure, hypercalcemia, hypokalemia, sickle cell trait or disease).
- Increased degradation of cAMP (pregnancy).
- Unknown (ifosfamide, propoxyphene overdose, methoxyflurane).

Diabetes insipidus typically presents with polyuria and polydipsia rather than hypernatremia, therefore, the differential diagnosis of polyuria overlaps with hypernatremia. Polyuria can be conveniently divided into three major groups based on the composition of the urine.

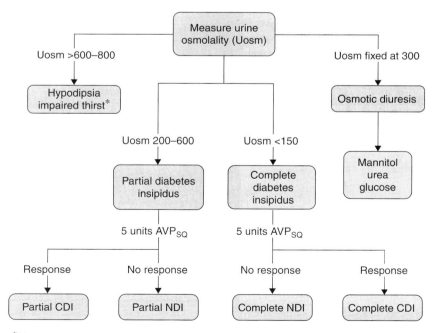

*Most common

FIG. 119–2 Approach to the patient with hypernatremia. All units in Osm/L of water. AVP, arginine vasopressin; CDI, central diabetes insipidus, NDI, nephrogenic diabetes insipidus; subQ, subcutaneous.

- Water diuresis
- Osmotic diuresis
- NaCl diuresis (salt-wasting nephropathies and diuretics)

Patients exhibiting a water diuresis will customarily present with a urine osmolality <150 mOsm/L. This group comprises patients with diabetes insipidus and psychogenic polydipsia. Patients with psychogenic polydipsia usually have a serum sodium concentration slightly above normal, whereas, patients with diabetes insipidus usually present with a slightly higher than normal sodium concentration. The urinary electrolyte composition will permit differentiation of a NaCl diuresis from an osmotic diuresis secondary to glucose, urea, or mannitol.

PRINCIPLES OF TREATMENT

The treatment of hypernatremia depends on the underlying cause. In the setting of normal renal function (eg, impaired thirst/hypodipsia), one need simply provide sufficient water to balance water losses. Aqueous vasopressin is useful in patients with central diabetes insipidus, whereas the use of thiazide diuretics may reduce free water excretion in patients with nephrogenic diabetes insipidus. Minimizing solute intake can be helpful in patients resistant to other forms of therapy and is the treatment of choice in the patient with an osmotic diuresis. The following strategies should be employed in all patients with hypernatremia:

- Restore the effective circulating volume with 0.9% saline.
- Correct the water deficit at a rate not to exceed 12 mEq/day or 0.5 mEq/h (rapid correction will produce cerebral edema and possibly precipitate seizures, permanent neurologic damage, and death).
- Remember to replace ongoing water losses (urine, insensible) with a salt solution of comparable tonicity (particularly important when the urine output is high, eg, osmotic diuresis).

POTASSIUM DISORDERS

PATHOPHYSIOLOGY

The total extracellular K^+ content is <80 mEq, thus, cellular redistribution plays an essential role in maintaining a stable plasma K^+ concentration following an oral or intravenous load of KCl. Indeed, changes in the serum K^+ concentration are attenuated rapidly (minutes) through cellular uptake. In contrast, renal elimination of a K^+ load requires hours to days to achieve maximal effect. Since all of the K^+ eliminated in the urine is derived from aldosterone-stimulated tubular secretion in the cortical collecting duct, changes in the circulating level or bioactivity of aldosterone are frequently responsible for disturbances of K^+ homeostasis.

Disorders of K^+ homeostasis can be broadly classified into three entities:

- Altered intake
- Altered distribution
- Altered renal elimination

The clinical symptoms of altered K^+ concentration are principally secondary to changes in the electrical potential of cardiac and skeletal muscle resulting in cardiac arrhythmias and muscle paralysis.

GENERAL APPROACH TO POTASSIUM DISORDERS

A reasonable initial step in the evaluation of potassium disorders is evaluation of the renal excretion of K^+. This allows differentiation of potassium disorders into two major categories:

- Disturbed extrarenal potassium homeostasis
- Disturbed renal elimination of potassium

While the 24-hour urine collection for K^+ is considered the gold standard to assess the renal elimination of K^+, the transtubular potassium gradient (TTKG) is a convenient bedside method of evaluating changes in the plasma K^+ concentration. The TTKG is calculated as the ratio of K^+ concentration at the end the cortical collecting duct to plasma K^+ concentration. The urine osmolality must exceed the plasma osmolality in order for the calculation to be reliable.

$$ TTKG = \frac{\left(\frac{Urine_{K^+}}{\left(\frac{U_{osm}}{P_{osm}} \right)} \right)}{Plasma_{K^+}} $$

The TTKG is a semi-quantitative reflection of the driving force for K^+ secretion in the kidney (effectively a bioassay of aldosterone action). Normally, the TTKG is increased in the hyperkalemic states and decreased in the hypokalemic states. Accordingly, abnormalities in the TTKG imply deranged renal elimination of K^+ as the basis for the plasma K^+ disturbance.

HYPOKALEMIA

PATHOPHYSIOLOGY

The principal factors involved in producing a fall in the serum potassium include poor oral intake or absorption (uncommon), cellular uptake, or increased renal loss. The evaluation of hypokalemia will depend on whether the urinary studies (TTKG or 24-hour urine collection for K^+) suggest a renal or extrarenal etiology of the hypokalemia (Fig. 119–3).

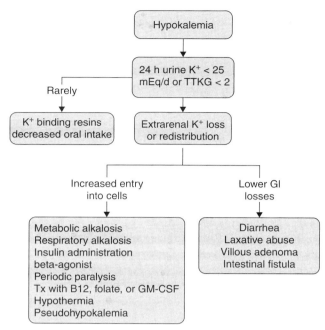

FIG. 119–3   Evaluation of extrarenal losses of potassium leading to hypokalemia.
GM-CSF, granulocyte-macrophage colony-stimulating factor; TTKG, transtubular potassium gradient.

Three mechanisms account for an extrarenal decrease in K^+

• Decreased oral intake (uncommon).
• Cellular uptake (induced by insulin, β-adrenergic activity, or an increase serum pH).
• Gastrointestinal losses.

When the urinary studies suggest increased renal elimination, assessment of the patient's blood pressure, arterial pH, and urinary chloride provide valuable clues to the differential diagnosis of hypokalemia (Fig. 119–4).

For example, when hypertension accompanies the hypokalemia, hyperaldosteronism (primary or secondary) is typically responsible for the renal loss of K^+. A systemic acidemia strongly suggests the presence of a renal tubular acidosis (RTA) whereas, an alkalemia suggests vomiting, diuretic use/abuse, Bartter syndrome, or Gitelman syndrome.

Bartter syndrome is caused by a mutation of the loop diuretic-sensitive pump in the thick ascending limb of the loop of Henle. Gitelman syndrome is caused by a mutation of the thiazide diuretic-sensitive pump in the distal convoluted tubule. The features of these genetic disorders parallel the symptoms and signs induced by overzealous use of loop or thiazide diuretics, respectively.

PRINCIPLES OF MANAGEMENT

Since most of the K^+ resides within cells, the plasma K^+ concentration is a poor predictor of the total body K^+ deficit.

• Plasma K^+ concentration of 3.0–3.5 mEq/L is associated with a K^+ deficit of 100 to 300mEq.
• Plasma K^+ concentration of 2.5 to 3.0 mEq/L is associated with a deficit of 300 to 800 mEq.
• A plasma K^+ concentration of < 2.5 mEq/L is almost always associated with a total deficit in excess of 600 mEq.

If possible, treat with oral not intravenous K^+ preparations (oral preparations are absorbed well and safer). Since the deficit is difficult to predict on the basis of the plasma K^+ concentration, it is essential to monitor the plasma K^+ concentration frequently during replacement. The maximal rate of administration of intravenous KCl is 20 to 40 mEq/h. The risk of transient hyperkalemia and cardiotoxicity is considerable at rates that exceed this.

HYPERKALEMIA

PATHOPHYSIOLOGY

The hyperkalemic disorders are divided into extrarenal versus renal causes by analyzing the 24-hour urine K^+ or calculating the TTKG. When the urinary studies suggest an extrarenal etiology of the hyperkalemia, two mechanisms account for the majority of such cases (Fig. 119–5).
• Increased oral intake
• Cellular release

In contrast, when the urinary studies suggest a renal etiology of the hyperkalemia, a decrease in circulating aldosterone underlies many of these conditions, with one notable exception; patients with chronic renal failure (Fig. 119–6). The latter constitute the largest group of patients presenting with an increase in the plasma K^+ concentration.

TREATMENT OF HYPERKALEMIA

The management of hyperkalemia involves two primary strategies:
• Promote cellular uptake.
• Promote renal or gastrointestinal loss.

Agents, which promote the cellular uptake of K^+, include:
• Insulin/glucose (10 U of regular insulin IV + 50 mL of 50% glucose; a continuous infusion of glucose may be necessary to prevent hypoglycemia).
• Sodium bicarbonate (1 ampule of 7.5% solution over 5 min; particularly valuable in patients with a metabolic acidosis).
• Administration of β-adrenergic agonist (albuterol 0.05 mg IV; avoid in patients with coronary artery disease).

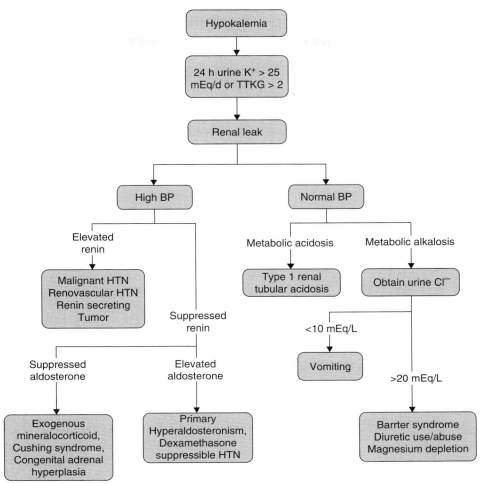

FIG. 119–4   Evaluation of renal losses of potassium leading to hypokalemia. BP, blood pressure; HTN, hypertension; TTKG, transtubular potassium gradient

The immediate management of life-threatening hyperkalemia involves the rapid administration of intravenous calcium. Calcium restores membrane excitability to normal and minimizes the neuro and cardiotoxicity of severe hyperkalemia. The usual dose of calcium is 10 mL of calcium gluconate (10% solution) given over 5 minutes while monitoring the ECG. This dose can be repeated as necessary to stabilize the ECG.

Agents which promote K+ loss from the body, include:
- Oral cation exchange resins (30 g of sodium polystyrene sulfonate orally or 50 g as a retention enema; intestinal necrosis has been reported with the retention enema)
- Loop diuretics (furosemide 1 mg/kg of body weight)
- Dialysis

In conditions associated with hypoaldosteronism, the use of mineralocorticoids may be helpful, but they may precipitate edema and hypertension.

EDEMATOUS DISORDERS

PATHOPHYSIOLOGY

Adjustments in sodium intake and excretion are the principle homeostatic mechanisms responsible for maintenance of the total body volume. The effective circulating volume (ECV) can be operationally defined as that volume which is necessary for effective perfusion of the tissues. Maintenance of a stable ECV is coordinated through vascular volume and pressure sensors, which, in turn, are coupled to a variety of effectors of salt homeostasis, including hemodynamic, hormonal, and local factors, which influence renal salt and water handling. Volume expansion arises when the intake of salt and water exceeds its output:

$$NaCl_{in} > NaCl_{out}$$

The kidney plays an essential role in maintaining the extracellular volume by altering the excretion of salt and

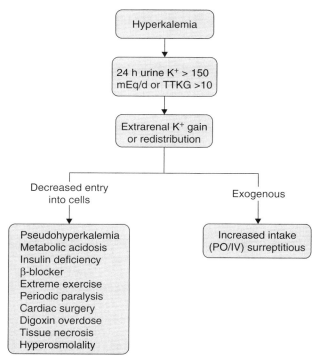

FIG. 119–5 Evaluation of the patient with hyperkalemia secondary to a nonrenal accumulation.
CKD, chronic kidney disease; TTKG, transtubular potassium gradient.

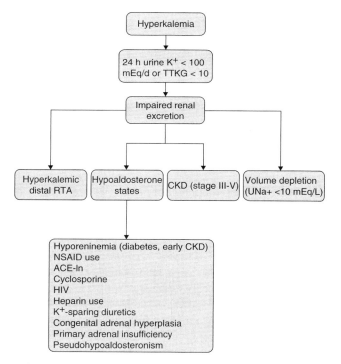

FIG. 119–6 Evaluation of the patient with hyperkalemia secondary to impaired renal elimination of potassium.
ACE-In, angiotensin-converting enzyme inhibitor; CKD, chronic kidney disease; HIV, human immunodeficiency virus; RTA, renal tubular acidosis; TTKG, transtubular potassium gradient.

water. Volume sensors have been classified into three groups: (1) vascular (cardiac atria, pulmonary vessels, carotid sinus, aortic arch, and the afferent arteriole of the juxtaglomerular apparatus); (2) central nervous system and (3) hepatic. The mechanism(s) whereby these sensors detect changes in ECV remains incompletely understood. The effectors of this response include:
• Natriuretic peptides.
• Antidiuretic hormone.
• The renin-angiotensin-aldosterone system.
• The sympathetic nervous system.

Edema-forming states are characterized by a disruption of the normal relationship between NaCl intake and excretion, such that a higher extracellular fluid is necessary (at a given NaCl intake) to maintain steady-state excretion of NaCl. However, edema per se is a clinical finding, which results from the accumulation of NaCl and water in the interstitial space. Ultimately the accumulation of interstitial fluid results from an imbalance in the hydrostatic and oncotic pressures, which govern fluid movement across the capillary bed (Fig. 119–7). In general, two fundamental mechanisms must occur simultaneously for clinically detectable edema formation:
• Salt and water retention.
• Perturbed capillary hemodynamics, favoring fluid movement from the plasma compartment into the interstitium (Fig. 119–7).

An increase in hydrostatic pressure (Pc) promotes fluid movement into the interstitium. An increase in Pc occurs when the plasma volume expands (salt retention), venous pressure rises (venous thrombosis) or the arteriole dilates (vasodilator drugs).

Salt retention occurs in settings characterized by a low effective circulating volume such as congestive heart failure. In cirrhosis or the nephrotic syndrome, the capillary oncotic pressure (Po) decreases favoring fluid

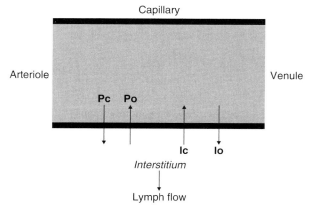

FIG. 119–7 Hemodynamic basis of interstitial edema formation.
Pc, capillary hydrostatic pressure; Po, capillary oncotic pressure; Ic, interstitial hydrostatic pressure; Io, interstitial oncotic pressure.

translocation into the interstitial space. The attendant fall in plasma volume promotes NaCl retention that, in turn, contributes to interstitial volume expansion as the retained fluid is sequestered in the interstitial space. A decrease in lymph flow may also promote edema formation when the lymphatics are mechanically obstructed (tumor) or surgically severed. An increase in venous pressure secondary to venous outflow obstruction (stenosis or thrombosis) may also promote edema formation by increasing Pc. The most common causes of edema formation in the clinical setting include:
- Congestive heart failure
- Cirrhosis
- Nephrotic syndrome
- Arterial vasodilators (calcium channel blockers)

Interestingly, several edema-forming states are characterized by an increase in cardiac output. These disorders include:
- High-output cardiac failure
- Cirrhosis
- Sepsis
- Pregnancy
- Arteriovenous fistulas
- Drugs that promote arterial vasodilatation.

These disorders are believed to promote NaCl and water retention via *arterial underfilling*. The mechanism of arterial underfilling in these conditions is the result of a relative imbalance in arterial capacitance versus cardiac output. Thus, arterial vasodilatation obligates an increase in cardiac output sufficient to *fill* the expanded arterial circuit. Presumably, when cardiac index is insufficient to compensate for the dilated arterial circuit, a state of relative hypoperfusion exists, analogous to that observed with frank reductions in cardiac output and ECV.

PRINCIPLES OF MANAGEMENT

Three general therapeutic strategies may be employed to limit expansion of extracellular fluid volume in the edema forming states:
- Reduce NaCl intake (usually <100 mEq/d).
- Correct the underlying pathophysiology that contributes to NaCl retention by the kidney.
- Diuretic use.

CLINICAL PHARMACOLOGY OF DIURETICS

Diuretics are classified into four major groups based on their site of action:
- Proximal tubule (carbonic anhydrase inhibitors, eg, acetazolamide)
- Loop of Henle (furosemide, bumetanide, torsemide)
- Distal convoluted tubule (thiazide diuretics)
- Cortical-collecting duct (triamterene, spironolactone, and amiloride)

CARBONIC ANHYDRASE INHIBITORS

These agents inhibit the brush border carbonic anhydrase of the proximal tubule. CA inhibitors are generally quite weak because the distal segments of the nephron are capable of increasing NaCl reabsorption in response to increased delivery. They are rarely used in clinical practice; however, they may prove valuable in treating edema associated with a metabolic alkalosis.

LOOP DIURETICS
- Most potent diuretics available (often referred to as high-ceiling diuretics).
- Rapid onset of action (5–10 min after IV administration).
- Peak effect in 30 minutes.
- Estimated half-life of 1 to 3 hours (torsemide 4–6 h).
- Inhibit Na^+ transport by blocking the Na^+ transporter in the loop of Henle.
- Side effects include hypokalemia, hyperuricemia, hypocalcemia, volume contraction, metabolic alkalosis, nephrotoxicity, and ototoxicity.

THIAZIDE DIURETICS
- Inhibit NaCl transport by blocking the Na^+ transporter in the distal convoluted tubule.
- Facilitate calcium reabsorption at this site.
- All thiazides are similar and merely differ on the basis of half-life and potency.
- Side effects include hypokalemia, hyperuricemia, hypercalcemia, volume contraction, metabolic alkalosis, and hyperglycemia.
- Rapid onset of action (5–10 min after IV administration, 1 h after oral administration).
- Peak effect in 30 to 120 minutes.
- Estimated half-life of 6 to 12 hours (depends on the specific thiazide).

DIURETICS ACTING IN THE COLLECTING DUCT
- Amiloride and triamterene block the Na^+ channel in the cortical collecting duct.
- Spironolactone blocks the aldosterone receptor.
- All diuretics in this class inhibit renal excretion of K^+ (K^+ sparing diuretics).
- Usually weak diuretics given the limited delivered load of NaCl to the collecting duct.
- Hyperkalemia and metabolic acidosis are the principal side effects.

CLINICAL PHARMACOTHERAPEUTICS OF DIURETICS

SITE OF ACTION

All diuretics are highly protein bound and require secretion into the renal tubule to exert their effects (the exception is spironolactone which acts on the basolateral side of the tubular cell). Diuretics require active secretion into the tubular lumen via organic anion transporters. The activity of these transporters varies directly with the GFR. Thus when the GFR falls, the secretion of diuretics into the lumen falls. This can be overcome with progressively higher doses of diuretics; however, there is a limit to dose escalation.

ORAL BIOAVAILABILITY
- Thiazide diuretics: 70% to 90%.
- Furosemide: 30% to 90%.
- Bumetanide and torsemide: >80%.

Importantly, poor oral bioavailability of some diuretics (furosemide) may limit their effectiveness. Therefore, in patients responding poorly to an oral diuretic, switching to a diuretic with greater bioavailability, such as torsemide, or giving the diuretic intravenously may dramatically improve the dose-response.

PHARMACODYNAMICS
Diuretics must achieve a *threshold* concentration in the lumen to elicit a diuresis (Fig. 119–8).

Increasing the dose of diuretic above the threshold will elicit a dose-dependent increase in salt excretion until saturation of the receptor occurs (ceiling dose). Approximate plateau or *ceiling* doses for currently available loop diuretics (assuming a normal GFR and > 80% oral bioavailability) are:
- Furosemide, 60 to 80 mg.
- Bumetanide, 1 to 2 mg.
- Torsemide, 50 to 100 mg.

Rational application of the pharmacodynamic and pharmacokinetic principles elucidated above avoids the usual pitfalls in the use of the diuretic drugs. Several clinical conditions deserve special commentary:

- Kidney failure
- Congestive heart failure
- Nephrotic syndrome
- Post-diuretic NaCl retention

KIDNEY FAILURE

Since retained organic acids in kidney failure competitively inhibit the transport pathway responsible for diuretic secretion, an increase in diuretic dose is essential to elicit an effective diuresis. In stage IV and V chronic kidney disease (eg, when the GFR <20 mL/min) only one-fifth of the administered dose of furosemide reaches its site of action.

CONGESTIVE HEART FAILURE

The dose of a loop diuretic necessary to achieve a diuresis in patients with congestive heart failure is complex. For example, while the dose-response relationship is similar in normal individuals versus those with CHF, the maximal response is greatly impaired. In end-stage heart failure, the relationship of dose to response may be sufficiently impaired as to preclude an effective diuresis. In addition, while the bioavailability may be similar between normal individuals and those with CHF, the absorption profile in the patient with decompensated CHF is flattened because of delayed absorption. Delayed absorption results in lower peaks but may actually prolong the action of the diuretic. Because of these uncertainties, it is generally advisable to treat decompensated CHF with intravenous diuretics. An additional factor that commonly accompanies severe CHF and necessitates dosing adjustments is the coexistence of kidney failure.

NEPHROTIC SYNDROME

Diuretics are delivered to the proximal tubule bound to plasma proteins. Thus, hypoalbuminemia limits the delivery of diuretic to the proximal tubule secretory pathway. Moreover, proteinuria binds diuretic in the lumen and, therefore, reduces free (active) diuretic concentration. In addition, sodium retention in the nephrotic syndrome flattens the diuretic dose-response relationship.

POSTDIURETIC NACL RETENTION

The pathophysiology of loop diuretic resistance is believed to be secondary to compensatory mechanisms induced in the distal nephron, which result in a phenomenon known as post-diuretic NaCl retention. Blockade of

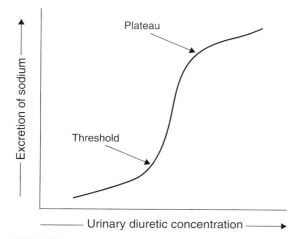

FIG. 119–8 Diuretic dose-response relationship.

solute reabsorption in the loop augments NaCl reabsorption in the distal nephron. Chronic furosemide increases the size and the number of NaCl transporters in the distal convoluted tubular cells. Strategies to ameliorate postdiuretic NaCl retention could include: increasing the frequency of the dosing interval; using diuretics with an extended half-life; adding thiazide diuretics; and reducing NaCl intake.

APPROACH TO THE DIURETIC-RESISTANT PATIENT

- Assess compliance with the medical regimen (diet and drugs).
- Measure 24-hour Na^+ excretion (if >100 mEq/d reduce oral intake of salt).
- Assess status of underlying diseases (CHF). Does the patient really need further reduction of extracellular volume? Can treatment of the underlying disease be improved?
- Discontinue drugs (NSAIDs) that promote NaCl retention.
- Intravenous diuretics to circumvent poor bioavailability.
- Consider continuous infusion of diuretics to maintain the steady-state threshold concentration of diuretic.
- Consider diuretic combinations.
- Disease-specific maneuvers: intravenous albumin (for nephrotic syndrome, may be mixed with loop diuretic), dopamine 1 to 3 mcg/min to induce renal vasodilatation (especially in low-output cardiac failure).

ACID-BASE DISORDERS

PATHOPHYSIOLOGY

The clinical acid-base disorders are classified by analyzing the products and reactants of the carbon dioxide/bicarbonate buffer system.

$$pCO_2 \leftrightarrow CO_{2(dis)} + H_2O \leftrightarrow H_2CO_3 \leftrightarrow H^+ + HCO_3^-$$

Although, theoretically, analysis of any buffer system would permit classification of the acid-base disorders (all buffer systems being in equilibrium), analysis of the carbon dioxide/bicarbonate system is invaluable because:

- The products and reactants (P_{CO_2}/HCO3) are easily measured using standard laboratory assays.
- It is the most abundant buffer system in the extracellular space.
- The system is homeostatically regulated through alterations in minute ventilation and renal function.

In this context, the metabolic acid-base disturbances are characterized by changes in the systemic HCO3 concentration, whereas, the respiratory acid-base disturbances are characterized by changes in the arterial P_{CO_2}.

DEFENSE AGAINST CHANGES IN THE SYSTEMIC PH

Three systems provide protection against fluctuations in systemic pH:

- Chemical buffers (maximal effect in min to h)
- Respiratory regulation (effective in h, full effect may require 1–2 d)
- Renal regulation (several d to achieve maximal effect)

Since these systems are primarily driven by changes in the systemic pH, they do not completely correct the underlying pH disturbance to normal. Indeed, normalization of the systemic pH implies a mixed acid-base disturbance.

The Henderson equation provides a useful framework to appreciate compensatory changes designed to protect against alterations in the systemic pH.

$$H^+ = 24 \frac{pCO_2}{HCO_3}$$

Thus, changes in the H^+ ion concentration (and, accordingly, pH) can be offset by parallel changes in the P_{CO_2} or HCO3. For example, an increase in P_{CO_2} raises the H^+ concentration (decreasing the pH); while an increase in renal bicarbonate generation would tend to compensate for the change in systemic pH.

EXAMPLE OF RESPIRATORY ADAPTATION

The respiratory system has a remarkable capacity to buffer otherwise life-threatening changes in systemic pH. Changes in minute ventilation are activated by chemoreceptors in the midbrain and pons. These receptors increase minute ventilation following an acid load or, conversely, decrease minute ventilation following an alkali load. The efficiency of respiratory buffering can be illustrated using the Henderson equation. For example, assume after an acid load, the plasma bicarbonate decreases to 10 mEq/L. If left uncompensated, the new H^+ ion concentration is 96 nM and pH = 7.0:

$$H^+ = 24 \frac{40}{10} = 96$$

However, the fall in systemic pH increases minute ventilation. Assume a doubling of the minute ventilation (eg, reduce the arterial P_{CO_2} to 20 mm Hg). The new H^+ ion concentration is 48 nM or a pH of 7.32.

RENAL REGULATION OF ACID-BASE HOMEOSTASIS

The kidney contributes to acid-base homeostasis by regulating two processes:

- Reclamation of filtered bicarbonate (proximal tubule).
- Excretion of the daily fixed acid load (distal tubule).

Ammonium ($NH4+$) is the principal acid excreted in the urine comprising more than 80% to 90% of the net acid excreted.

SIMPLE ACID-BASE DISTURBANCES

METABOLIC ACIDOSIS

The clinical hallmark of this disturbance is a decrease in serum bicarbonate concentration, which is the consequence of either an increase in the generation of protons (such as ketoacids or lactic acid) or loss of bicarbonate (which can either be of renal origin, as in a proximal RTA or gastrointestinal origin as in diarrhea).

METABOLIC ALKALOSIS

The hallmark of this disturbance is an increase in serum bicarbonate concentration, which is usually the consequence of proton loss, either extrarenal (vomiting) or renal (hyperaldosteronism), but can also occur as a consequence of exogenous intake of bicarbonate (uncommon).

RESPIRATORY ACIDOSIS

This acid-generating state is characterized by an increase in the partial pressure of carbon dioxide and occurs as a consequence of impaired respiratory mechanics.

RESPIRATORY ALKALOSIS

This alkali-generating state is characterized by a fall in the partial pressure of carbon dioxide. This disorder is commonly seen in patients with anxiety but can occur in a variety of other clinical settings which stimulate the respiratory center.

CLINICAL APPROACH TO METABOLIC ACID-BASE DISORDERS

Initial characterization of clinical acid-base disorders can be accomplished by analyzing the arterial blood gas systematically:

1. Measure the arterial pH.
2. Determine whether the change in arterial pH is secondary to a metabolic (HCO3) or respiratory disturbance (P_{CO_2}).
3. Determine whether the compensation for the disorder is in the expected direction and appropriate (Table 119–2).

TABLE 119–2 Expected Compensations for Simple Acid-Base Disturbances

DISORDER	COMPENSATION
Metabolic acidosis	$\Delta PCO2 = 1.2 \times \Delta HCO3$
Metabolic alkalosis	$\Delta PCO2 = 0.6 \times \Delta HCO3$
Acute respiratory acidosis	$\Delta HCO3 = 0.1 \times \Delta PCO2$
Chronic respiratory acidosis	$\Delta HCO3 = 0.5 \times \Delta PCO2$
Acute respiratory alkalosis	$\Delta HCO3 = 0.2 \times \Delta PCO2$
Chronic respiratory alkalosis	$\Delta HCO3 = 0.5 \times \Delta PCO2$

If the compensation falls outside of the expected range, a mixed acid-base disorder must be considered.

METABOLIC ACIDOSIS

In general, two mechanisms are responsible for the development of a metabolic acidosis:

- H^+ ion generation (eg, increased ketoacid or lactic acid production)
- HCO3 loss (eg, diarrhea or renal tubular loss).

Once established, the differential diagnosis of a metabolic acidosis can be further analyzed by an assessment of the serum and urine anion gap (Fig. 119–9). Additional laboratory analysis may include measurement of specific organic anions, toxins or evaluation of renal acidification.

THE SERUM ANION GAP

The serum anion gap is normally assessed as the difference between the routinely measured serum cations and anions.

$$\text{Anion Gap} = Na^+ - (HCO_3 + Cl^-)$$

The normal anion gap is 6 to 12 mEq/L because the measured cation Na^+ is slightly higher than the sum of the major measured anions (Cl^- and HCO3). Importantly, there are over 40 unmeasured anions and cations in plasma, many of which are not readily available as routine laboratory studies. Therefore, determination of the etiology of a change in the anion gap represents a challenge. Nevertheless, an increase in organic acid production is typically responsible for an increase in the measured gap. A serum anion gap that exceeds 20 to 25 mEq/L indicates the presence of an unmeasured organic anion such as:

- Ketoanions (acetoacetic acid and β-hydroxybutyric acid) produced from the metabolism of fatty acids when the ratio of insulin to glucagon is sufficiently reduced (diabetes, starvation, and alcoholism)
- Lactic acid derived from nonoxidative metabolism (hypoxia) or deranged utilization (severe liver disease)
- Miscellaneous organic acids produced from the metabolism of certain toxins (salicylates, ethylene glycol, methanol)

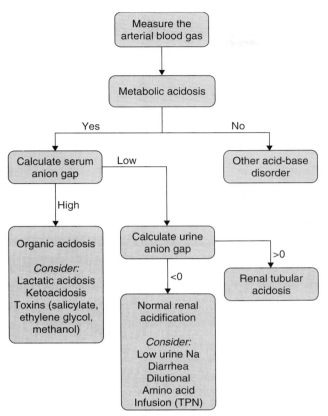

FIG. 119–9 Evaluation of the patient with simple metabolic acidosis.
TPN, total parenteral nutrition.

The most common cause of a normal anion gap metabolic acidosis is either diarrhea or RTA (Fig. 119–9).

In diarrhea, the colonic transit is hastened resulting in loss of a HCO3 rich, Cl⁻ poor fluid. Ureteral diversion can result in a hyperchloremic metabolic acidosis if the ileal loop is particularly long or constricted. The abundance of urinary Cl⁻ augments Cl⁻:HCO3 exchange, thus, increasing HCO3 excretion. Parenteral nutrition may cause either a metabolic acidosis (secondary to the metabolism of infused amino acids) or a metabolic alkalosis (if acetate is used instead of Cl⁻ as the anion for the cations infused). Unusual causes of a normal anion gap acidosis include administration of ammonium and arginine HCl.

Renal Tubular Acidosis
An understanding of the kidney's role in acid-base homeostasis permits the classification of renal tubular acidosis (RTA) on a physiologic basis. In general, RTA can be caused by a decrease in bicarbonate reclamation (proximal RTA) or abnormal distal acidification (distal renal tubular acidosis, dRTA).

An important caveat in the evaluation of a RTA is that proximal RTA is uncommon in adults, occurring in <10% of all cases. Moreover, proximal RTA is usually characterized by diffuse proximal tubular dysfunction resulting in glucosuria, phosphaturia, and aminoaciduria (eg, Fanconi syndrome). A notable exception is the use of acetazolamide. This drug inhibits carbonic anhydrase and, thus, selectively impairs bicarbonate reabsorption.

Utility of the Urine Anion Gap in the Diagnosis of dRTA
All of the dRTAs are characterized by a defect in net renal acidification. Importantly, the urine pH is only dependent on the concentration of free (unbound) protons. Nonetheless, free protons account for less than 1% of the total acid excreted. The majority of acid excreted in the urine is complexed with a buffer (primarily ammonium). Accordingly, the urine pH is often misleading when used to diagnose dRTA. A more accurate method of determining net acid excretion would be through direct measurement of urine ammonium. However, this test is cumbersome and not readily available. A surrogate index of ammonium excretion can be derived from calculation of the urine anion gap (UAG). The UAG is calculated using the routinely measured urine ions:

$$UAG = (Na^+ + K^+) - Cl^-$$

An acid load should cause a negative UAG because the acid stimulates renal synthesis of ammonia that leads to an increase in ammonium excretion. Increased excretion of ammonium is accompanied by a parallel increase in the excretion of the measured anion Cl⁻. Thus, the measured UAG becomes increasingly negative after an acid load. In contrast, all dRTAs are characterized by a decrease in net acid excretion (NAE), which results in a positive UAG. The UAG is a sensitive and readily available test for the bedside determination of NAE. Thus, calculation of the serum and UAG provides two critical branching points in the clinical evaluation of a metabolic acidosis (Fig. 119–9).

METABOLIC ALKALOSIS

Three clinical scenarios account for the majority of cases of metabolic alkalosis:
• Vomiting or nasogastric suctioning
• Diuretic use
• Primary or secondary hypermineralocorticoidism (eg, aldosterone or other mineralocorticoid-like hormones produced in excess)

The first two conditions are associated with volume contraction and respond well to the administration of NaCl containing solutions (they are often referred to as

Cl⁻ responsive alkalosis). The hypermineralocorticoid states are usually associated with volume expansion and do not respond to the infusion of NaCl (Cl⁻ unresponsive). In metabolic alkalosis, the urinary Cl⁻ provides a better guide to volume assessment as compared to the urinary Na⁺. This paradox arises because an increase in plasma HCO3 concentration above the tubular threshold for its reabsorption results in bicarbonaturia. Loss of HCO3 in the urine obligates cation loss (electroneutral loss of ions). Since the most abundant cation in the urine is Na⁺, it usually accompanies HCO3. Hence, the urinary Na⁺ may not reflect the patients underlying volume status, whereas the urinary Cl⁻ will accurately reflect the underlying volume status of the patient.

Normally as the plasma HCO3 increases above 25 to 27 mEq/L the kidney promptly excretes the excess HCO3 in the urine. Therefore, perpetuation of a metabolic alkalosis requires diminished HCO3 excretion in the urine in conjunction with net synthesis of HCO3 (Fig. 119–10).

Several factors appear to participate in augmenting the net renal reabsorption of HCO3 in these clinical syndromes including:

• Decreased effective circulating volume
• Renal insufficiency
• Chloride depletion
• Hypokalemia
• Hyperaldosteronism

VOMITING AS A PARADIGM OF METABOLIC ALKALOSIS

Two phases (generation and maintenance) are necessary to produce a sustained metabolic alkalosis after vomiting.

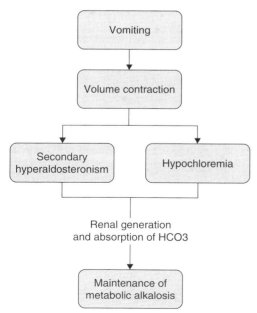

FIG. 119–10 Factors that sustain metabolic alkalosis.

Net generation of HCO3 derived from the parietal epithelial cell is normally counterbalanced by the excretion of HCO3 via pancreatic secretion, which, itself, is stimulated by entry of HCl into the proximal duodenum. Gastric emptying prevents acid from entering the duodenum and, hence, the stimulus for pancreatic secretion is removed. Therefore, the absorption of HCO3 by the gastric circulation is unopposed by pancreatic secretion of HCO3. Normal renal function would mitigate the transient rise in plasma HCO3 by rapidly excreting the excess HCO3 in the urine. However, the attendant volume contraction and chloride depletion induced by vomiting activates neurohumoral mechanisms that augment HCO3 reabsorption by the nephron, thus, perpetuating the alkalosis.

RESPIRATORY ACID-BASE DISORDERS

The respiratory acid-base disorders result from either hyperventilation or hypoventilation. Moreover, these disorders elicit acute as well as chronic compensation. The complete renal response to changes in acid-base status induced by altered ventilation requires several days to reach steady state. Thus, calculation of the expected compensation requires knowledge of the chronicity of the process. If the onset is unknown, a mixed acid-base disturbance cannot be reliably excluded. A careful history may disclose the true acid-base disturbance. The etiological factors involved in the pathogenesis of disturbed minute ventilation are summarized in Table 119–3.

TABLE 119–3 Etiology of Perturbed Minute Ventilation

DECREASED VENTILATION	INCREASED VENTILATION
CNS depression (sedatives, primary or secondary lesions involving the respiratory centers)	Anxiety
Neuromuscular disorders (myopathies and neuropathies)	CNS disorders (CVA, tumor, infection)
Thoracic cage disorders (kyphoscoliosis, scleroderma)	Cancers
Impaired lung mechanics (pleural effusion, pneumothorax)	Hormones/drugs (salicylates, catecholamines, progesterone, analeptics, hypothyroidism)
Severe acute and chronic lung disease (COPD, asthma, aspiration, tumor, laryngospasm, pneumonia, pulmonary edema, pulmonary embolus)	Mild-moderate acute and chronic lung disease (COPD, asthma, aspiration, tumor, laryngospasm, pneumonia, pulmonary edema, pulmonary embolus)
Miscellaneous (ventilator malfunction)	Miscellaneous (sepsis, cirrhosis)

CNS, central nervous system; COPD, chronic obstructive pulmonary disease; CVA, cerebrovascular accident.

BIBLIOGRAPHY

Adrogué HJ, Madias NE. Hypernatremia. *N Engl J Med.* 2000; 342:1493–1499.

Adrogué HJ, Madias NE. Hyponatremia. *N Engl J Med.* 2000; 342:1581–1589.

Batlle DC, Hizon M, Cohen E, et al. The use of the urine anion gap in the diagnosis of hyperchloremic metabolic acidosis. *N Engl J Med.* 1988;318:594–599.

Berl T. Treating hyponatremia: Damned if we do and damned if we don't. *Kidney Int.* 1990;37:1006.

Brater DC. Diuretic therapy. *N Engl J Med.* 1998;339:387–389.

Ethier JH, Kamel KS, Magner PO, et al. The transtubular potassium concentration in patients with hypokalemia and hyperkalemia. *Am J Kidney Dis.* 1990;15:309.

Gabow PA, Kaehny WD, Fennessey PV, et al. Diagnostic importance of an increased anion gap. *N Engl J Med.* 1980;303:854.

Gabow PA. Disorders associated with an altered anion gap. *Kidney Int.* 1985;27:472.

Greenberg A, Verbalis JG. Vasopressin receptor antagonists. *Kidney Int.* 2006;69:2124.

Kurtz I. Molecular pathogenesis of Bartter's and Gitelman's syndromes. *Kidney Int.* 1998;54:1396.

Rodriguez Soriano J. Renal tubular acidosis: The clinical entity. *J Am Soc Nephrol.* 2002;13:2160.

Rose BD, Post TW. *Clinical Physiology of Acid-Base and Electrolyte Disorders.* 5th ed. New York: McGraw-Hill; 2001.

120 ACUTE KIDNEY INJURY
Zhiwei Zhang

DEFINITION

- Acute kidney injury (AKI) is defined as a loss of renal function, measured by a decline in glomerular filtration rate (GFR), developing over a period of hours to days. It occurs in a variety of settings with varied clinical manifestations that range from a minimal but sustained elevation in serum creatinine (SCr) to anuric renal failure.
- The Acute Dialysis Quality Initiative group has proposed the RIFLE (**r**isk of kidney injury, **i**njury to the kidney, **f**ailure of kidney function, **l**oss of kidney function, **e**nd-stage disease) system (Table 120–1), to classify acute kidney injury into three severity categories (risk, injury, and failure) and two clinical outcome categories (loss and end-stage renal disease).

EPIDEMIOLOGY

- Acute kidney injury is common, with a reported incidence of 1% to 25% depending on the definition used and the population being studied.
- Hospital mortality for patients with acute kidney injury has been reported to vary from 28% to 90% depending on comorbidities.
- Acute kidney injury is associated with an adjusted prolongation of hospital length of stay by 2 days and an adjusted odds ratio of 2.0 for discharge to short- or long-term care facilities.

PATHOPHYSIOLOGY

Glomerular filtration rate is the sum of the filtration rates in all functioning nephrons and therefore serves as an index of the functioning renal mass. A decrease in GFR may reflect intrinsic renal disease with a reduction in the number of functioning nephrons. However, the GFR can also be reduced if there is a decline in renal perfusion (prerenal) or if there is obstruction to urine flow in the urinary tract (postrenal). As a result, all causes of acute kidney injury can be classified into three broad categories: (1) prerenal, (2) intrinsic, and (3) postrenal (Table 120–2).

PRERENAL ACUTE KIDNEY INJURY

- Prerenal AKI implies that the decrease in GFR is secondary to renal hypoperfusion and not directly involving the renal parenchyma. It is usually reversible if the offending factors are eliminated, but protracted prerenal states may ultimately lead to ischemic acute tubular necrosis. The causes of renal hypoperfusion are diverse but can be broadly classified into those conditions that elicit a fall in renal perfusion pressure

TABLE 120–1   RIFLE Criteria for Classification of Acute Kidney Injury

	SERUM CREATININE (SCr)	URINE OUTPUT
Risk of kidney injury	1.5 × baseline	<0.5 mL/kg/h for >6 h
Injury to the kidney	2 × baseline	<0.5 mL/kg/h for >12 h
Failure of kidney function	3 × baseline or SCr >4 with an acute rise >0.5 mg/dL	<0.3 mL/kg/h for >24 h or anuria for >12 h
Loss of kidney function	Persistent renal failure for >4 wk	
End-stage disease	Persistent renal failure for >3 mo	

TABLE 120–2 Major Causes of Acute Kidney Injury

Prerenal: Reduced Renal Perfusion
1. **True volume depletion**
   Hemorrhage
   Renal or extrarenal losses (GI, skin)
2. **Decreased effective blood volume (EBV)**
   Congestive heart failure
   Hepatorenal syndrome
   Third-space fluid accumulation
3. **Increased renal vascular resistance**
   Hypercalcemia
   NSAIDs
   Calcineurin inhibitors: cyclosporine, tacrolimus
   ACE inhibitors or ARBs

Intrinsic Injury to the Kidney
1. **Glomerular or microvascular disease**
   Rapid progressive glomerulonephritis (RPGN)
   • Granular immune complex deposition (eg, postinfectious GN)
   • Linear immune complex deposition (anti-GBM disease)
   • Pauciimmune/ANCA-associated vasculitis (eg, Wegener granulomatosus)
   Thrombotic microangiopathy (TMA)
   • Hemolytic-uremic syndrome (HUS)
   • Thrombotic thrombocytopenic purpura (TTP)
   • Malignant hypertension
   • Scleroderma renal crisis
2. **Acute tubular necrosis (ATN)**
   Ischemic
   • Hypotension
   • Prolong prerenal state
   • Sepsis syndrome
   Nephrotoxic
   • Nephrotoxin: radiocontrast, antibiotics, anticancer drugs
   • Intratubular pigments: heme proteins (rhabdomyolysis, hemolysis)
   • Intratubular proteins: light chains (myeloma)
   • Intratubular crystals: uric acid, oxalate, drugs (eg, acyclovir, sulfonamide)
3. **Acute interstitial nephritis (AIN)**
   Allergic interstitial nephritis: antibiotics, NSAIDs, allopurinol, diuretics
   Infections: viral, bacterial, fungal
   Infiltration: lymphoma, leukemia, sarcoidosis
4. **Vascular disease**
   Renal artery: stenosis, thrombosis, atheroembolism, vasculitis
   Renal vein: thrombosis, compression

Postrenal: Obstruction of Urine Flow
1. **Intraurinary tract**
   • Intraluminal: stone, blood clot, sloughed papillae, crystal
   • Intramural: tumor, infection, neurogenic drugs, stricture
2. **Extraurinary tract**
   • Prostate: hypertrophy, cancer
   • Retroperitoneal fibrosis, lymphoma

ACE, angiotensin-converting enzyme; ANCA, antineutrophilic cytoplasmic antibody; ARBs, angiotensin receptor blockers; GBM, glomerular basement membrane; GI, gastrointestinal; GN, glomerulonephritis; NSAIDs, nonsteroidal anti-inflammatory drugs.

versus conditions that elicit changes in renal vascular resistance (see Table 120–2).

• A fall in renal perfusion pressure, which reflects the aortic pressure perfusing the kidneys, may occur as a consequence of volume depletion or a decrease in effective arterial blood volume. Conversely, an increase in renal vascular resistance secondary to intrarenal vasoconstriction reduces the renal perfusion pressure transmitted to the glomerular capillaries, and GFR falls.

• The glomerular capillaries are interposed between two arterioles: the afferent or precapillary arteriole and the efferent or postcapillary arteriole. As a result, the GFR is also determined by the *relative* change of the afferent versus efferent arteriolar resistance. A decrease in afferent arteriolar resistance or an increase in efferent arteriolar resistance maintains GFR within fairly narrow limits in response to a decrease in renal perfusion pressure. This phenomenon is referred to as *autoregulation,* and is mediated by three factors:
   1. Myogenic stretch reflex in the afferent arteriole
   2. Tubuloglomerular feedback
   3. Generation of intrarenal vasodilators (eg, prostaglandins, nitric oxide)

• These autoregulatory systems provide intrinsic protection against ischemic injury to the kidneys. When the renal autoregulatory system is maximized and the conditions causing the renal hypoperfusion remain uncorrected, GFR decreases.

• Angiotensin II contributes to renal autoregulation by preferentially increasing the resistance at the efferent arteriole. Blocking the effects of angiotensin by either angiotensin-converting enzyme (ACE) inhibitors or angiotensin receptor blockers decrease GFR in conditions where angiotensin plays a crucial role in maintaining GFR, such as:
   ◦ Volume depletion
   ◦ Bilateral renal artery stenosis
   ◦ Unilateral renal artery stenosis in a solitary kidney
   ◦ Congestive heart failure
   ◦ Cirrhosis
   ◦ Diuretic administration
   ◦ Chronic kidney disease, especially diabetic nephropathy

POSTRENAL ACUTE KIDNEY INJURY

• Postrenal AKI is caused by obstruction of the urine flow in the urinary tract, including the renal pelvis, ureter, bladder, or urethra. The GFR falls as a result of elevated pressure within Bowman space. The causes of the obstruction can be further divided into the following conditions (see Table 120–2):
   ◦ Intraurinary tract obstruction (intraluminal or intramural, eg, stone, tumor)
   ◦ Extraurinary tract obstruction (outside the wall, eg, compression by a mass)

• Acute kidney injury arises only if both kidneys are obstructed, or the obstruction involves a solitary functioning kidney. The elevated pressures incident to obstruction result in adaptive dilatation (hydroureter, hydronephrosis), and progressive renal parenchymal injury (tubular atrophy, interstitial fibrosis, and glomerular scarring) if unrelieved.

INTRINSIC ACUTE KIDNEY INJURY

- Intrinsic AKI occurs when the renal parenchyma is damaged. The parenchymal structures involved (glomeruli, tubules, blood vessels, or interstitium) determine the clinical and laboratory characteristics observed. Unlike prerenal and postrenal causes, the fall in GFR secondary to intrinsic AKI is directly linked to the extent of kidney structural damage. Importantly, the urinalysis is usually abnormal and may reflect the type of renal parenchymal injury.
- Acute tubular necrosis (ATN) is the most common type of AKI (at least 45% of all cases of AKI). The term ATN is sometimes used interchangeably with AKI. As illustrated in Table 120–2, however, ATN represents only one type of intrinsic AKI.
- Acute tubular necrosis may be precipitated by an ischemic event or from toxic effects of endogenous or exogenous compounds (see Table 120–2). The S$_3$ segment of the proximal tubule and the thick ascending limb of Henle loop are particularly susceptible to injury because of relative hypoxia in this region. This occurs in part because of the high metabolic activity required for various transport processes in this segment of the nephron along with countercurrent flow in the vasa recta. The hairpin configuration of the vasa recta capillaries results in the exchange of oxygen between the oxygen-rich blood entering the descending capillary limb from the cortex and the oxygen-poor blood leaving the ascending capillary limb from inner medulla. The net effect is that the P$_{O_2}$ bathing the tubular cells of the outer medulla is as low as 10 to 20 mm Hg, thus rendering cells in this region susceptible to ischemic injury.
- Three factors are important in the pathogenesis of ATN (see Fig. 120–1):

  ○ Vascular abnormalities: loss of autoregulation and increased renal vasoconstriction, and vascular congestion in the outer medulla eventually lead to critical decreases in renal perfusion.
  ○ Tubular injury: cytoskeletal abnormalities, loss of cell polarity, and apoptosis/necrosis of the lining tubular epithelial cells (cell sloughing and clumping obstruct the tubular lumens).
  ○ Inflammation: release of inflammatory cytokines, increased neutrophil adhesion, and increased oxygen radicals; intrarenal inflammation decreases renal perfusion and contributes to tubular injury.
- Several pathways are believed to contribute to the fall in GFR which is the hallmark of ATN (see Fig. 120–1):
  ○ Obstruction of the tubules secondary to sloughed cellular debris, proteins, or crystals (eg, uric acid) is responsible in some instances of ATN (this effectively decreases clearance).
  ○ Backleak of tubular fluid secondary to disruption of the tubular basement membrane has also been noted in ATN (this effectively decreases clearance).
  ○ Injury to the medullary thick ascending limb of Henle loop increases sodium chloride delivery to the macular densa which, in turn, promotes the release of compounds that decrease renal perfusion via constriction of the afferent arteriole (tubuloglomerular feedback).

CLINICAL FEATURES

- Acute kidney injury may impair the excretory, regulatory, and endocrine functions of kidneys and is characterized by retention of nitrogenous waste products in the blood (azotemia), and changes in urine volume.

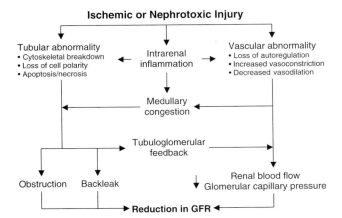

FIG. 120–1 Pathophysiology of acute tubular necrosis. GFR, glomerular filtration rate.

BLOOD UREA NITROGEN

- Blood urea nitrogen (BUN) is derived from the degradation of proteins that can be of exogenous or endogenous origin. It is completely filtered at the renal glomerulus but reabsorbed by the proximal tubule. Blood urea nitrogen is not a reliable marker of GFR, but it tends to correlate with the symptoms of uremia.
- Spurious or nonrenal elevations in BUN must be distinguished from changes in BUN occurring as a consequence of a change in GFR. Nonrenal elevations of BUN include the following:
  ○ Hypercatabolic state (protein degradation)
  ○ Corticosteroid use (increased protein catabolic rate)

○ Excessive protein intake (catabolized to urea nitrogen)
○ Gastrointestinal bleeding (metabolism of red blood cells to urea nitrogen)

SERUM CREATININE

- Serum Cr derives from nonenzymatic hydrolysis of creatine released from skeletal muscle. It is completely filtered at the renal glomerulus with some degree of tubular secretion. The serum Cr is a good marker of GFR at steady state but correlates poorly with uremic symptoms. Moreover, the Cr is affected by age, sex, muscle mass, diet, and volume of distribution. It does not accurately reflect GFR in the non–steady-state condition of acute kidney injury.
- Spurious or nonrenal elevations in Cr must be distinguished from changes in serum Cr occurring as a consequence of a change of GFR. Nonrenal elevations may occur because of a laboratory error or a change in tubular secretion of Cr:
  ○ Laboratory interference with the assay (eg, ketones, cephalosporins)
  ○ Inhibition of tubular Cr secretion (eg, cimetidine, trimethoprim)

CHANGE IN URINE VOLUME

- The minimum amount of urine that a stable patient must excrete to eliminate the daily solute load is approximately 500 mL. Acute kidney injury may be subdivided according to the urine output:
  ○ Nonoliguric (>500 mL/day)
  ○ Oliguric (100–500 mL/day)
  ○ Anuric (<100 mL/day)
- Changes in urine output can occur before biochemical changes are apparent. Prerenal AKI nearly always presents with oliguria, although nonoliguric prerenal AKI can be seen in the following settings:
  ○ Renal concentrating defects (eg, diabetes insipidus)
  ○ Osmotic diuresis (eg, glucose)
  ○ Administration of angiotensin-converting enzyme inhibitor or angiotensin receptor blocker
- Intrinsic or postrenal AKI may present with any pattern of urine volume ranging from anuria to nonoliguria.

COMPLICATIONS OF ACUTE KIDNEY INJURY

- Various complications associated with acute kidney injury are outlined in Table 120–3.

TABLE 120–3   Common Complications of Acute Kidney Injury

Metabolic	• Metabolic acidosis • Hyperkalemia • Hyponatremia • Hypocalcemia • Hyperphosphatemia • Hypermagnesemia • Hyperuricemia
Cardiovascular	• Pericarditis • Arrhythmias • Pulmonary edema • Hypertension
Neurologic	• Asterixis • Neuromuscular irritability • Mental status change • Seizure
Hematologic	• Anemia • Coagulopathies
Gastrointestinal	• Nausea, vomiting • Gastrointestinal bleeding
Infectious	• Pneumonia • Urinary tract infection • Septicemia

DIAGNOSTIC APPROACH

- A stepwise approach to the evaluation of acute kidney injury is summarized in Fig. 120–2.

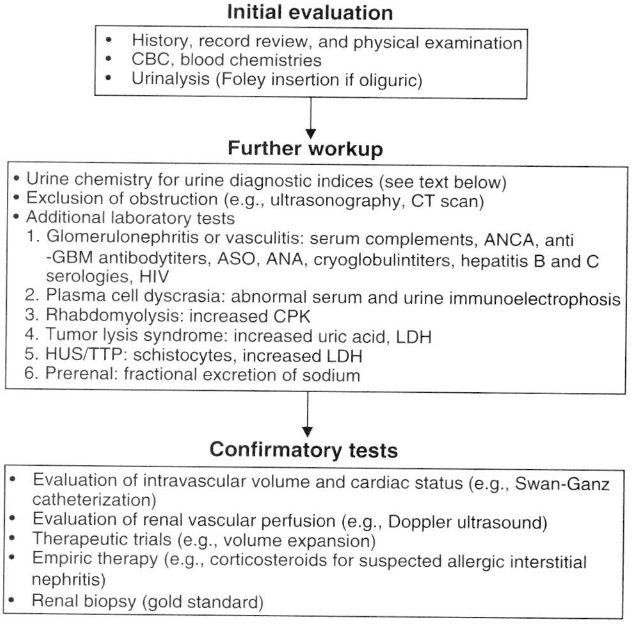

Initial evaluation

- History, record review, and physical examination
- CBC, blood chemistries
- Urinalysis (Foley insertion if oliguric)

Further workup

- Urine chemistry for urine diagnostic indices (see text below)
- Exclusion of obstruction (e.g., ultrasonography, CT scan)
- Additional laboratory tests
  1. Glomerulonephritis or vasculitis: serum complements, ANCA, anti-GBM antibodytiters, ASO, ANA, cryoglobulintiters, hepatitis B and C serologies, HIV
  2. Plasma cell dyscrasia: abnormal serum and urine immunoelectrophosis
  3. Rhabdomyolysis: increased CPK
  4. Tumor lysis syndrome: increased uric acid, LDH
  5. HUS/TTP: schistocytes, increased LDH
  6. Prerenal: fractional excretion of sodium

Confirmatory tests

- Evaluation of intravascular volume and cardiac status (e.g., Swan-Ganz catheterization)
- Evaluation of renal vascular perfusion (e.g., Doppler ultrasound)
- Therapeutic trials (e.g., volume expansion)
- Empiric therapy (e.g., corticosteroids for suspected allergic interstitial nephritis)
- Renal biopsy (gold standard)

FIG. 120–2 Stepwise approach to the diagnosis of acute kidney injury.
ANA, antinuclear antibody; ANCA, antineutrophilic cytoplasmic antibody; ASO, antistreptolysin-O antibody; Ca, calcium; CPK, creatine phosphokinase; CT, computed tomography; GBM, glomerular basement membrane; HIV, human immunodeficiency virus; HUS, hemolytic uremic syndrome; LDH, lactate dehydrogenase; TTP, thrombotic thrombocytopenic purpura.

HISTORY, RECORD REVIEW, AND PHYSICAL EXAMINATION

- Helpful hints to establish the diagnosis of acute kidney injury are outlined in Table 120–4. A variety of medications associated with AKI are listed in Table 120–5.

URINALYSIS

- Examination of the urine is an essential step in the differential diagnosis of acute kidney injury. Urine specific gravity, pH, glucose, and protein should be recorded; and the urine sediment should be inspected for the presence of cells, casts, and crystals. Table 120–6 summarizes the urine findings in various causes of AKI.

URINARY INDICES

- Clinically, differentiation between prerenal AKI and ATN in oliguric patients may be difficult, but it is very important to render the appropriate therapy and avoid complications including fluid overload with resultant pulmonary congestion and hypoxia. Urinary indices

TABLE 120–4   Helpful Hints for Diagnosis of Acute Kidney Injury

Chronic kidney disease	• Baseline Cr • Normocytic normochromic anemia • Small kidney (<10 cm)
Prerenal AKI	• Evidence of volume depletion • Decompensated CHF or cirrhosis • NSAIDs, diuretics, ACE inhibitors, ARBs, calcineurin inhibitors
Postrenal AKI	• Abdominal and frank pain • Bladder distension • History of kidney stone or prostate disease
Acute tubular necrosis	• Hypotension • Nephrotoxin (see Table 120–5) • Sepsis • Cardiac surgery • AAA repair
Acute interstitial nephritis	• Fever, rash • Medications (see tubulointerstitial disease) • Pyelonephritis
Glomerulonephritis/vasculitis	• Infection (skin, shunt, throat) • Hypertension, edema, dyspnea, oliguria • Skin rash, arthritis • Pulmonary-renal syndrome

AAA, abdominal aortic aneurysm; ACE, angiotensin-converting enzyme; AKI, acute kidney injury; ARBs, angiotensin receptor blockers; CHF, congestive heart failure; Cr, creatinine; NSAIDs, nonsteroidal anti-inflammatory drugs

TABLE 120–5   Commonly Used Medications Associated With Acute Kidney Injury

Prerenal	• Diuretics • Antihypertensive agents • Interleukin 2 • NSAIDs • Cyclosporine, tacrolimus • Amphotericin • ACE inhibitors, ARBs
Tubular toxicity	• Antibiotics: aminoglycosides, vancomycin, amphotericin, pentamidine, foscarnet • Chemotherapeutic agents: cisplatin, ifosfamide • Antiretroviral agents: cidofovir, tenofovir, adefovir • Radiocontrast • Interferon-α
Crystalluria	• Sulfonamides • Methotrexate • Acyclovir • Triamterene • Protease inhibitors: indinavir, saquinavir, ritonavir • Ethylene glycol
Glomerulopathy	• Gold • Penicillamine • NSAIDs • Interferon-α
TTP/HUS	• Cyclosporine, tacrolimus • Mitomycin C • Ticlopidine
Interstitial nephritis	• Multiple, see tubulointerstitial disease

ACE, angiotensin-converting enzyme; ARBs, angiotensin receptor blocks; HUS, hemolytic uremic syndrome; NSAIDs, nonsteroidal anti-inflammatory drugs; TTP, thrombotic thrombocytopenic purpura.

are a series of diagnostic tests which facilitate this differentiation (Table 120–7).
- Assuming tubular function remains intact, renal hypoperfusion should elicit sodium and water retention. As a

TABLE 120–6   Urinalysis in Acute Kidney Injury

URINALYSIS	CAUSES OF ACUTE KIDNEY INJURY
Normal	• Prerenal • Postrenal
Granular casts	• Acute tubular necrosis • Interstitial nephritis
RBCs or RBC casts	• Glomerulonephritis or vasculitis • Malignant hypertension
WBCs or WBC casts	• Interstitial nephritis • Pyelonephritis
Eosinophiluria	• Allergic interstitial nephritis • Atheroembolic disease
Crystaluria	• Uric acid • Calcium oxalate • Drugs (see Table 120–5)
Proteinuria	• Glomerulonephritis or vasculitis • Renal vain thrombosis • Plasma cell dyscrasia

RBC, red blood cell; WBC, white blood cell

TABLE 120–7 Urinary Diagnostic Indices

	PRERENAL	ACUTE TUBULAR NECROSIS
Urine osmolality, mOsm/kg H_2O	>500	<350
Urine sodium, mEq/L	<20	>40
Fractional excretion of Na	<1%	>2%
Fractional excretion of urea	<35%	>50%
Serum BUN/creatinine	>20:1	<20:1

BUN, blood urea nitrogen; Na, sodium.

result, a low urine sodium concentration, low fractional excretion of sodium (FE_{Na}), and high urine osmolality will usually be seen in patients with prerenal AKI. In contrast, an elevated urine sodium concentration, high FENa, and an isotonic urine would be expected in patients with ATN, since tubular injury impairs the ability of the kidney to reabsorb sodium and water (see Table 120–7).

• Of these tests, the FE_{Na} is the most sensitive with a diagnostic specificity of approximately 80%. The FE_{Na} represents the fraction of filtered sodium that is excreted in the urine and is calculated as follows:

$$FE_{Na} = \frac{Urine\ Na \times Plasma\ Cr}{Urine\ Cr \times Plasma\ Na} \times 100$$

$$FE_{Na} = \frac{Urine\ Na \times Plasma\ Cr}{Urine\ Cr \times Plasma\ Na} \times 100$$

• Limitations of FE_{Na} include the following:
  ○ Conditions associated with prerenal AKI that may increase the FE_{Na}
    ▪ Diuretic administration
    ▪ Tubular adaptation in patients with established chronic kidney disease
    ▪ Saline infusion
  ○ Conditions other than prerenal AKI that are associated with a low FE_{Na} include
    ▪ Ten percent of patients with nonoliguric ATN, presumably because of persistent renal ischemia and adjustments in tubular sodium handling
    ▪ Acute tubular necrosis superimposed on a chronic prerenal state (congestive heart failure or cirrhosis)
    ▪ Contrast-induced nephropathy
    ▪ Pigment nephropathy (especially early)
    ▪ Some cases of acute interstitial nephritis
    ▪ Intrinsic AKI that do not primarily affect tubular function (glomerular and vascular injury)
    ▪ Postrenal AKI

• Urea reabsorption is also increased in response to renal hypoperfusion provided tubular function is intact. As a result, the ratio of BUN to Cr is usually increased in prerenal AKI. Recent studies have revealed that the fractional excretion of urea (FE_{Urea}) is a more sensitive and specific index than the FE_{Na} in

differentiating between prerenal AKI and ATN especially when patients are receiving diuretics.

$$FE_{Urea} = \frac{Urine\ Urea \times Plasma\ Cr}{Urine\ Cr \times Plasma\ Urea} \times 100$$

$$FE_{Urea} = \frac{Urine\ Urea \times Plasma\ Cr}{Urine\ Cr \times Plasma\ Urea} \times 100$$

RADIOLOGY

• Imaging of the kidney and the urinary tract is recommended for most patients with AKI to distinguish between acute and chronic kidney disease and to exclude obstruction. Occasionally, assessment of the renal vascular anatomy may yield useful information (renal vein thrombosis).

RENAL ULTRASONOGRAPHY

• Kidney and bladder size (especially to exclude chronic kidney disease).
• Hydronephrosis or dilatation of the urinary tract (obstruction).
• Renal vascular stenosis and renal vein thrombosis (Doppler interrogation).

COMPUTED TOMOGRAPHY SCAN
• Obstruction without dilatation (eg, retroperitoneal fibrosis).
• Kidney stones.

RENAL BIOPSY

• A renal biopsy provides tissue that can be used to determine the etiology of renal parenchymal injury, predict the prognosis, and direct or monitor treatment. General indications for a renal biopsy include:
  ○ Prerenal and postrenal causes have been excluded.
  ○ Intrinsic AKI that cannot be explained by noninvasive tests.
  ○ Suspicion of rapidly progressive glomerulonephritis, systemic disease (eg, vasculitis), or interstitial nephritis as the cause of acute kidney injury these diseases are amenable to specific therapies.

NEW BIOMARKERS

• The search for new biomarkers to establish AKI is evolving rapidly with advancement in modern technologies. Newer markers are urgently needed to:

- Detect injury earlier (and render earlier therapy) and identify subclinical injury
- Provide prognostic information on the course of renal impairment
- Establish unambiguous markers of AKI for clinical trial design
- Guide timing of therapy and assess response to therapy
- Screen patients at risk for renal injury
- Examples of promising biomarkers include the following:
  - Cystatin C
  - Kidney injury molecule 1 (KIM-1)
  - Neutrophil gelatinase-associated lipocalin (NGAL)

PRINCIPLES OF TREATMENT

GENERAL MANAGEMENT

- Search for and correct underlying disorders.
- Review medications and discontinue known nephrotoxins.
- Adjust the dose of medications for the degree of renal impairment.
- Optimize cardiac output and renal perfusion.
- Search for and aggressively treat infection.
- Monitor blood pressure, intake/output, and daily weights.

FLUID AND ELECTROLYTES

- Avoid volume overload or depletion.
- Restrict potassium and phosphate.
- Correct metabolic acidosis.
- Monitor the polyuric phase of ATN to prevent volume. and electrolyte disturbances.
- Monitor and manage postobstructive diuresis.

NUTRITIONAL SUPPORT

- At least 100 g of carbohydrate should be administered to avoid catabolism of endogenous protein.
- Up to 1.5g/kg/day of high biological quality protein should be administered.
- Enteral feeding is the preferred means of delivering nutrients.
- Total parenteral nutrition should only be administered to patients who are severely malnourished or those unable to tolerate enteral feeding for more than 14 days.

DIURETICS

- Although of limited use in the treatment of AKI, diuretics may convert oliguric patients to nonoliguric patients and render fluid management easier. Importantly, the use

TABLE 120–8   Proposed Criteria for Initiation of Renal Replacement

1. Oliguria or anuria not responsive to diuretics
2. Hyperkalemia (especially when coupled with electrocardiographic changes)
3. Severe acidosis
4. Symptomatic uremia
   - Encephalopathy
   - Pericarditis
   - Neuropathy/myopathy
5. Fluid overload
6. Drug overdose with a dialyzable toxin

of diuretics per se does not improve prognosis. However, patients who convert from an oliguric state to a nonoliguric state have been shown to have less severe renal injury and, accordingly, their prognosis is improved.

RENAL REPLACEMENT THERAPY

GOAL

- Maintain fluid, electrolyte, and acid-base homeostasis.
- Limit the adverse consequences of the uremic state by removing toxins.
- Permit optimal nutritional support.
- These goals should be accomplished without potentiating renal injury or preventing repair.

PROPOSED CRITERIA FOR INITIATION OF RENAL REPLACEMENT THERAPY

- If one criterion is met, renal replacement therapy is strongly recommended; if more than one criterion is met, renal replacement is mandatory (Table 120–8).

MAIN MODALITIES

- Renal replacement therapies are presently comprised of intermittent hemodialysis (IHD) and continuous renal replacement therapy (CRRT). Table 120–9 summarizes the advantages and disadvantages of IHD and CRRT. Importantly, clinical studies have not revealed a difference in mortality between these two modalities; therefore, they are largely based on hospital/center expertise.

SPECIFIC CLINICAL EXAMPLES OF AKI

NONSTEROIDAL ANTIINFLAMMATORY DRUGS

- Administration of nonsteroidal antiinflammatory drugs (NSAIDs) including COX-2 inhibitors has been implicated in several renal abnormalities, including:
  - Acute kidney injury
  - Acute interstitial nephritis
  - Hyperkalemia
  - Hyponatremia

TABLE 120–9   Advantage and Disadvantages of Intermittent versus Continuous Renal Replacement Therapy

	INTERMITTENT RENAL REPLACEMENT THERAPY	CONTINUOUS RENAL REPLACEMENT THERAPY
Advantage	Lower risk of systemic bleeding Lower cost Patient mobility Minimal technical difficulties	Greater hemodynamic stability Unrestricted alimentation Improved fluid and metabolic control Elimination of inflammatory cytokines
Disadvantage	Hemodynamic instability Inadequate dialysis dose Poor fluid control Limited nutritional support Limited removal of cytokines	Vascular access problems Continuous anticoagulation is necessary Immobilization of the patient Technical problems with the equipment Greater cost

- ○ Nephrotic syndrome (minimal change nephropathy)
- ○ Chronic kidney disease (interstitial scarring)
- Acute kidney injury associated with NSAID use is characterized by prerenal features including oliguria, salt and water retention, edema, and improvement in renal function on discontinuation of these agents. It usually occurs in conditions that promote intrarenal vasoconstriction, such as:
  - ○ Volume depletion
  - ○ Congestive heart failure
  - ○ Cirrhosis
  - ○ Nephrotic syndrome
  - ○ Chronic kidney disease
  - ○ Diabetes mellitus
  - ○ Diuretic use

CONTRAST-INDUCED NEPHROPATHY

- Contrast-induced nephropathy is a relatively common cause of acute kidney injury but is rarely associated with irreversible loss of renal function. It can present as oliguria or nonoliguria, and the FE_{Na} is usually low (<1%) in this syndrome. The onset occurs within 24 to 48 hours after exposure, reaches a peak within 3 to 5 days, and subsides within 7 to 10 days. A variety of risk factors have been implicated in the development of contrast-induced nephropathy including:
  - ○ Age older than 55 years
  - ○ Preexisting renal insufficiency
  - ○ Diabetic nephropathy
  - ○ Volume depletion
  - ○ Low cardiac output
  - ○ Multiple myeloma
  - ○ Large volume of contrast
  - ○ Coadministration with NSAIDs, ACE inhibitors, or other nephrotoxins
- Importantly, renal atheroemboli may also occur after arteriography; thus a rise in Cr following contrast

administration must be differentiated from atheroembolic renal disease. The clinical features of renal atheroembolic disease that differentiate it from contrast-induced nephropathy include the following:
  - ○ Delayed onset (3–5 days) and progressive renal insufficiency
  - ○ Severe hypertension (renin mediated)
  - ○ Livedo reticularis
  - ○ Ischemic necrosis of the digits
  - ○ Eosinophiluria and eosinophilia
  - ○ Hypocomplementemia and an elevated erythrocyte sedimentation rate
- In up to 30% of cases, renal atheroemboli occurs spontaneously. Renal atheroemboli may also present weeks to months following an invasive procedure.
- Strategies to prevent contrast-induced nephropathy include the following:
  - ○ Minimize contrast volume and repeated exposure.
  - ○ Avoid nephrotoxic drugs.
  - ○ N-acetylcysteine (Mucomyst®) is of questionable value.
  - ○ Intravenous hydration with normal saline is the most widely accepted preventive intervention.
  - ○ Sodium bicarbonate may be of value, but larger multicenter studies are needed to determine its true effectiveness.
  - ○ Newer contrast agents (nonionic and of lower osmolality than conventional contrast) are less nephrotoxic.

AMINOGLYCOSIDES

- Acute kidney injury occurs in 10% to 25% of patients receiving aminoglycosides even with careful dosing and monitoring therapeutic plasma levels. The pathophysiology of aminoglycoside nephrotoxicity remains poorly understood. However, cationic aminoglycosides are attracted to anionic megalin present in the apical membrane of the proximal tubular epithelial cells and are subsequently endocytosed. As a result the concentration of intracellular aminoglycoside may exceed 100-fold that of the plasma concentration. The latter explains the persistence of AKI following aminoglycoside withdrawal.

- A variety of risk factors have been characterized, which appear to increase the risk of aminoglycoside nephrotoxicity including the following:
  ○ Advanced age
  ○ Coadministration with other nephrotoxins
  ○ Volume contraction
  ○ Liver disease
  ○ Preexisting renal insufficiency
  ○ Hypokalemia
  ○ Prolonged course of treatment (>10 days)
  ○ Gentamicin > amikacin > tobramycin
- The clinical course of aminoglycoside nephrotoxicity is usually gradual in onset and is related to the dose and duration of drug exposure. In the absence of preexisting renal disease, overt aminoglycoside nephrotoxicity is uncommon in the first 5 to 6 days of therapy. Moreover, a cumulative dose of >1000 mg is usually a prerequisite. Clinical features of aminoglycoside nephrotoxicity include the following:
  ○ Nonoliguria
  ○ Potassium and magnesium wasting
  ○ Urine concentrating defect
- Although recovery is the rule, the course may be protracted (weeks) because of accumulation of drug in the renal cortex.

PIGMENT NEPHROPATHY

- The kidney is vulnerable to the toxicity of heme proteins such as myoglobin or hemoglobin. Heme proteins may induce oliguric acute kidney injury through several mechanisms:
  ○ Renal vasoconstriction secondary to increased vasoactive peptides (stimulated by heme proteins) and decreased nitric oxide (scavenged by heme proteins)
  ○ Tubular toxicity through oxidative pathways (liberation of Fe^{2+} from the metabolism of filtered pigments believed to promote free radical formation and subsequent tubular injury)
  ○ Pigment cast formation
- Although hemoglobinuria is an uncommon cause of AKI (ABO incompatibility), rhabdomyolysis (muscle necrosis) has been described in a number of clinical settings:
  ○ Excessive muscle activity (eg, seizure activity and vigorous exercise)
  ○ Physical trauma to the muscle (eg, crush injury)
  ○ Ischemia (eg, compartment syndrome)
  ○ Drugs (eg, statins, fibrates) and toxins (eg, ethanol, cocaine abuse)

- Electrolyte and metabolic disturbances (eg, hypophosphatemia)
- Inflammation (eg, vasculitis)
- Infection (eg, toxic shock syndrome, hemolytic streptococcal infection)
- The clinical features of rhabdomyolysis include the following:
  ○ Disproportionate increase in Cr relative to BUN (Cr is liberated from injured muscle cells)
  ○ Red/brown urine and dipstick positive for blood (pigments) but absence of red blood cells from the urine sediment
  ○ Increased muscle enzymes in the serum such as creatine phosphokinase (usually >10,000)
  ○ Disproportionate increase in potassium, phosphorous, and uric acid relative to the degree of renal injury (liberated from injured muscle cells)
  ○ Hypocalcemia (deposited at the site of myonecrosis)
- Strategies to limit renal injury in pigment nephropathy include the following:
  ○ Vigorous hydration with normal saline.
  ○ Maintain adequate urine output (>100 mL/h).
  ○ The usefulness of bicarbonate and mannitol administration is controversial.

ACUTE KIDNEY INJURY IN PATIENTS WITH ACQUIRED IMMUNODEFICIENCY SYNDROME

- Acute kidney injury may develop in up to 20% of hospitalized patients with acquired immunodeficiency syndrome. Most cases of AKI are related to hypovolemia or drug toxicity.
- Prerenal causes include the following:
  ○ Hypovolemia (eg, diarrhea)
  ○ Decreased effective blood volume (eg, hypoalbuminemia)
  ○ Salt wasting
- Intrinsic causes include the following:
  ○ ATN: sepsis, hypotension, antibiotics, antiretroviral drugs (see Table 120–5)
  ○ Intraluminal crystals: acyclovir, sulfadiazine, indinavir, saquinavir, ritonavir
  ○ Acute interstitial nephritis: allergic (drugs) or infectious (cytomegalovirus, *Candida,* tuberculosis)
  ○ Thrombotic thrombocytopenic purpura and hemolytic uremic syndrome have been well characterized in patients with HIV
  ○ Human immunodeficiency virus–associated nephropathy
- Postrenal causes include the following:
  ○ Intraurinary tract: crystals, fungus balls
  ○ Extraurinary tract: tumors, adenopathy

ACUTE KIDNEY INJURY IN CANCER PATIENTS

- Most cases of AKI in patients with cancer are caused either by prerenal mechanisms (hypovolemia or NSAIDs) or nephrotoxic ATN triggered by chemotherapeutic drugs or the products of tumor lysis.
- Prerenal causes include the following:
  - Hypovolemia (eg, poor oral intake, vomiting, diarrhea)
  - Nonsteroidal antiinflammatory drugs
  - Hypercalcemia (eg, myeloma, parathyroid-related peptide)
- Intrinsic causes include the following:
  - Exogenous toxins: chemotherapeutic drugs (see Table 120–5)
  - Endogenous toxins: hyperuricemia, light chains, tumor lysis
  - Thrombotic thrombocytopenic purpura and hemolytic uremic syndrome
  - Glomerulonephritis associated with cancer
  - Interstitial nephritis: infiltration with tumor cells
- Postrenal causes include the following:
  - Ureteric or bladder neck obstruction
- Retroperitoneal fibrosis

ACUTE KIDNEY INJURY IN PREGNANCY

- AKI during pregnancy or after delivery is rare in industrialized nations, occurring in <1 of 10,000 deliveries. The marked decline over the past 50 years is the result of improved prenatal care and obstetric practice. Most cases of AKI in pregnancy occur between gestational week 35 and the puerperium and are primarily due to preeclampsia and bleeding complications.
- First trimester:
  - Hyperemesis gravidarum (volume contraction)
  - Septic abortion
  - Direct toxicity of illegal abortifacients
- Late pregnancy:
  - Preeclampsia or eclampsia
  - Hemolysis, elevated liver enzymes, low platelet count (HELLP) syndrome
  - Bilateral renal cortical necrosis: abruptio placentae, amniotic fluid embolus
  - Acute fatty liver of pregnancy
  - Thrombotic thrombocytopenic purpura (TTP)
  - Urinary tract obstruction
  - Pyelonephritis
- Postpartum:
  - Postpartum hemorrhage
  - Hemolytic uremic syndrome (HUS)

BIBLIOGRAPHY

Bellomo R, Ronco C, Kellum JA, et al. Acute renal failure-definitions, outcome measures, animal models, fluid therapy and information technology needs: The Second International Consensus Conference of the Acute Dialysis Quality Initiative (ADQI) Group. *Crit Care.* 2004;8:R204.

Liangos O, Wald R, O'Bell JW, et al. Epidemiology and outcomes of acute renal failure in hospitalized patients: A national survey. *Clin J Am Soc Nephrol.* 2006;1:43.

Schrier RW, Wang W, Poole B, et al. Acute renal failure: Definitions, diagnosis, pathogenesis, and therapy. *J Clin Invest.* 2004;114:5.

Thadhani R, Pascual M, Bonventre JV. Acute renal failure. *N Engl J Med.* 1996;334:1448.

121 CHRONIC KIDNEY DISEASE

Marie D. Philipneri

DEFINITION

- Chronic kidney disease is defined as either kidney damage or a glomerular filtration rate (GFR) less than 60 mL/min/1.73 m^2 for 3 months or longer. Kidney damage is defined as pathologic abnormalities or markers of damage, including abnormalities in blood or urine tests or imaging studies."[1]
- Acute renal failure (ARF) or ARF superimposed on chronic kidney disease must be distinguished from stable or progressive chronic kidney disease. When multiple serum creatinine measurements are available on a patient, and a plot of the reciprocal of the creatinine versus time is linear, the patient has slowly progressive chronic kidney disease. Conversely, if there is considerable deviation from linearity, superimposed ARF is likely and potentially reversible causes must be explored.
- A variety of clinical, laboratory, and radiologic tests can be useful to differentiate ARF from chronic kidney disease. The features that suggest chronic kidney disease include the following:
  - Chronic symptoms (albeit, these are nonspecific)
  - Band keratopathy
  - Chronic anemia that is otherwise unexplained
  - Sustained increase in serum creatinine
  - Kidneys measuring <10 cm in length on renal ultrasonography
  - Radiologic evidence of subperiosteal erosions consistent with advanced renal osteodystrophy

EPIDEMIOLOGY

- Chronic kidney disease is a growing public health problem both in the United States and worldwide. Based on the third National Health and Nutrition Examination Survey (NHANES III) involving 18,723 individuals aged 12 years and older, from 1988 to 1994 and a more recent study of roughly 200,000 patients enrolled in a large health maintenance organization, the prevalence of chronic kidney disease is estimated to be 8.3 million (4.7%) of the US population.[2]
- There are significant racial and ethnic differences in the prevalence of chronic kidney disease, particularly at advanced stages. African Americans and Hispanics tend to have a higher incidence and prevalence of chronic kidney disease compared to whites.[3–4]

ETIOLOGY

- The etiology of chronic kidney disease can be either caused by primary renal disease or secondary to a systemic process or external factors. Diabetes mellitus is the most common secondary cause of end-stage renal disease (ESRD) across various racial and ethnic groups. However, hypertension is the most frequent cause of ESRD among African Americans in the United States.[4]
- Additional risk factors for chronic kidney disease include family history of chronic kidney disease, advancing age, chronic use of nephrotoxic agents, particularly nonsteroidal antiinflammatory drugs (NSAIDs), obesity, and smoking. The National Kidney Foundation (NKF) recommends risk assessment for all individuals at their routine clinic visits.[1]
- Screening for chronic kidney disease is recommended for individuals with known diabetes mellitus, hypertension, and/or family history of chronic kidney disease. Screening procedures for these patients involve urinalysis, a random urine sample for protein and creatinine measurements, and a serum creatinine level.[1]

DIAGNOSIS

- Patients with chronic kidney disease are often asymptomatic (Fig. 121–1). Moreover, if clinical features are present they are often variable and nonspecific. Symptoms caused by chronic kidney disease can be either attributable to the kidney itself (flank pain and hematuria) or secondary consequences resulting in extrarenal symptoms (edema and pruritus).
- Routine laboratory testing can reveal an elevated serum creatinine or an abnormal urinalysis. Although the serum creatinine level had been in routine use as a marker of renal function for many years, it has several limitations (eg, influenced by muscle mass). Therefore, estimation of GFR had been advocated, and many laboratories calculate the estimated GFR in their reporting of chemistry panel results.
- There are a number of ways to estimate GFR. The abbreviated Modification of Diet in Renal Disease (MDRD) study equation is commonly used today.[5] An electronic GFR calculator is available at the NKF Web site (www.kidney.org/professionals/kdoqi/gfr_calculator.cfm).
- If a patient is noted to have decreased GFR and/or any markers of kidney damage, the next step is to assess for the presence of secondary causes of chronic kidney disease. History taking should disclose the use of nephrotoxic agents including the over-the-counter NSAIDs and use of herbal supplements that have been linked to kidney damage. In addition, the patient should be questioned regarding urinary tract infections or stones, previous kidney disease including during childhood years, recent travel, and a family history of chronic kidney disease. In addition to blood pressure (BP) measurement and physical examination, a series of tests that are commonly employed to uncover the etiology of chronic kidney disease include the following:
  - Screening for diabetes mellitus if symptoms or risk factors are present
  - Antinuclear antibody titers (autoimmune disorders, particularly systemic lupus erythematosus)
  - Hepatitis B surface antigen, hepatitis C antibody, and human immunodeficiency virus antibody (especially, if risk factors such as intravenous drug use, multiple sexual partners, or exposure to blood products are identified).
  - Serum and urine protein electrophoresis, if older than 50 years of age and/or accompanied by bone pain, hypercalcemia, elevated total protein level, and unexplained anemia

  In addition, retroperitoneal renal ultrasound is very helpful in establishing kidney size, ruling out congenital anomalies, excluding hydronephrosis and identifying renal stones.
- If the etiology of chronic kidney disease remains uncertain after a thorough history, physical and laboratory evaluation and the kidneys are not atrophic, a renal biopsy is usually indicated. Renal histology often provides the definitive diagnosis of the underlying kidney disease. Importantly, it is not uncommon to uncover an unexpected diagnosis on renal biopsy.
- Since a renal biopsy is an invasive procedure, a detailed discussion with the patient and family, including the potential benefits and risks of the biopsy, and alternate options should take place prior to the procedure.

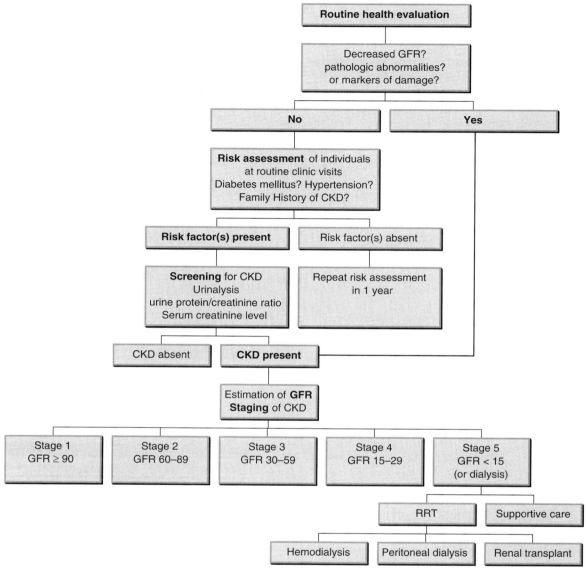

FIG. 121–1 An outline of diagnosis and management of chronic kidney disease.
CKD, chronic kidney disease; GFR, glomerular filtration rate; RRT, renal replacement therapy.
SOURCE: Adapted from National Kidney Foundation Kidney Disease Outcomes Quality Initiative (NKF KDOQI) clinical practice guidelines for chronic kidney disease: Evaluation, classification, and stratification. *Reference 1.*

MANAGEMENT

- At each stage of chronic kidney disease, the clinician should establish optimal therapy for the underlying disease, monitor disease progression and development of complications, and initiate therapies to delay progression of chronic kidney disease and its complications. In addition, medications should be reviewed to ensure optimal renal dosing, and measures should be employed to prevent and treat cardiovascular disease, given its extraordinary incidence in chronic kidney disease (Table 121–1).

- Reversible factors which can complicate and/or contribute to the progression of chronic kidney disease including, extracellular volume depletion, urinary tract obstruction, renal vascular disease, use of nephrotoxic agents, and metabolic derangements (for example, hypercalcemia) should be corrected promptly.

- Management to slow chronic kidney disease progression includes optimal glycemic and blood pressure control in patients with diabetes and hypertension respectively, lowering of intraglomerular hypertension via administration of an angiotensin-converting enzyme (ACE) inhibitor and/or an angiotensin II

TABLE 121–1 Stages and Characteristics of Chronic Kidney Disease

CHARACTERISTICS	STAGE OF CHRONIC KIDNEY DISEASE				
	1	2	3	4	5
GFR (mL/min/1.73 m^2)	≥90	60–89	30–59	15–29	<15 (or dialysis)
Description	Kidney damage with normal or high GFR	Kidney damage with mild decrease in GFR	Moderate decrease in GFR	Severe decrease in GFR	Kidney failure
Prevalence[a]	2.8	2.8	3.7	0.13	0.2
Symptoms	−	−	±	+	++
Complications	−	±	+	++	+++
Action[b]	Diagnosis and treatment of kidney disease and comorbid conditions. Slowing progression and CV disease risk reduction	Estimating progression	Evaluating and treating complications	Preparations for renal replacement therapy	Dialysis (if indicated)

CV, cardiovascular; GFR, glomerular filtration rate; NHANES, National Health and Nutrition Examination Survey.
[a]Estimation based on the NHANES 1999–2000 and represents percent of the total US population.
[b]Includes actions from earlier stages.
SOURCE: Adapted from National Kidney Foundation Kidney Disease Outcomes Quality Initiative (NKF KDOQI) clinical practice guidelines for chronic kidney disease: Evaluation, classification, and stratification. *Reference 1.*

receptor blocker (ARB), treatment of dyslipidemia, and perhaps dietary protein restriction (0.8 g/kg/d). The beneficial effects derived from these measures are maximized when they are initiated early and adhered to strictly.[6] Recently, there has been interest in lowering the serum uric acid as another measure to retard the progression of chronic kidney disease. Therefore, it is valuable to obtain serum uric acid levels in patients with chronic kidney disease and treat it, particularly if the levels exceed 8–9 mg/dL.

RENAL REPLACEMENT THERAPY

• Renal replacement therapy options include hemodialysis, peritoneal dialysis, and kidney transplantation. The timing of renal replacement therapy is critical, as the patients who initiate renal replacement therapy with adequate preparation tend to cope better and experience fewer complications. It is recommended that renal replacement therapy options be discussed with the patients during stage 4 of chronic kidney disease or perhaps even earlier. Arteriovenous (AV) fistula creation, which typically is an outpatient surgical procedure, is best performed during stage 4 so that sufficient time is available for fistula maturation.

• Indications for initiation of renal replacement therapy include uremic encephalopathy, pericarditis, other persistent symptoms or signs attributable to uremia (nausea, vomiting, anorexia, and weight loss), uremic bleeding and fluid overload refractory to routine medical management, suboptimal correction of critical electrolyte and acid-base disturbances with medical management, and uncontrolled hypertension.

HEMODIALYSIS

• In the United States, hemodialysis (HD) is the most frequently performed renal replacement therapy, and it is commonly performed at a dialysis center. Typically, the patients receive three HD sessions a week; each session is usually 4 hours in duration. A small number of patients choose to perform HD at home. Recently, more frequent HD (daily but shorter sessions, for example) has received attention among the renal community and further clinical trials are in progress to assess the effectiveness of this approach.

• During an HD procedure, the patient's blood is accessed via insertion of a large bore catheter into an AV native fistula or an AV synthetic graft. Blood is then circulated through a filter (known as a *dialyzer*) that serves to partition uremic solutes from the blood. Dialysis solutions (known as *dialysate*) also circulate through the dialyzer in a countercurrent fashion. Blood and dialysate circulate in their own compartments that are separated by a semipermeable membrane, thus establishing a blood/membrane/dialysate interface for diffusion of uremic solutes.

PERITONEAL DIALYSIS

• Peritoneal dialysis (PD) is a less common, yet effective, renal replacement therapy option. The patients or their caregivers perform PD at home. The peritoneal membrane of the patient serves as a semipermeable membrane rather than an external filter used in HD. PD could be performed either manually or with the use of an automated machine. The majority of the patients on PD in the United States opt for the latter. A history of multiple abdominal surgeries can pose difficulty with peritoneal catheter placement and/or limit the efficiency of dialysis (because of extensive adhesions and fibrosis). Thus, it is important to explore past medical and surgical histories of patients when renal replacement therapy options are addressed.

- An indwelling dialysis catheter is placed in the peritoneal cavity by an interventional nephrologist or a surgeon, frequently under laparoscopic guidance. The catheter can be accessed in 2 to 4 weeks or earlier if necessary, under close supervision. A dialysis exchange involves instillation of a special dialysis solution (known as *Dianeal*) in the peritoneal cavity, via the catheter, and drainage after 2 to 4 hours. On average, the patients perform four to six of these exchanges daily. PD can also be performed at night using an automated machine (known as *cycler*).

RENAL TRANSPLANT

- A third renal replacement therapy option is renal transplantation, either from a living donor or a deceased donor. A living donor need not be a blood relative. Thus, a suitable kidney donor could be a spouse, friend, or even someone who is anonymous. Interestingly, on November 14, 2006, five patients with ESRD received kidney transplants from five living but unrelated donors (a five-way *domino-donor* simultaneous kidney transplant) at a single institution.[7] It is worth noting that anyone who considers kidney donation needs to undergo appropriate testing and counseling by an experienced renal transplant team for determination of suitability.

- Finally, renal replacement therapy options may not be appropriate in all cases. Both dialysis and transplantation involve surgical procedures, frequent visits to clinics and hospitals, regular intake of multiple medications, dietary and other lifestyle modifications. Therefore, when a patient with ESRD has significant incapacities warranting care by others or another terminal illness, a detailed discussion involving the patient (if possible) along with immediate family members or a legal representative is very helpful. In other words, under relevant circumstances, an informed decision by a patient or a legal representative to decline renal replacement therapy (ie, dialysis or transplant) should be respected. Alternatively, if dialysis is already undertaken but because of subsequent medical conditions, overall quality of life is poor, periodic discussions with the patient and/or family regarding the continuation of renal replacement therapy is advised.

REFERRAL TO NEPHROLOGISTS

- The management of chronic kidney disease (particularly stage 3 and higher) is challenging and timely referral to a nephrologist is imperative. The nephrologist is skilled in effectively managing chronic kidney disease and its complications, including counseling of patients, with regards to available renal replacement therapy options.[8–9] In addition, when the etiology of chronic kidney disease is uncertain, evaluation by a nephrologist, with or without a renal biopsy could be valuable in defining the diagnosis and rendering the appropriate therapy.

COMPLICATIONS OF CHRONIC KIDNEY DISEASE

- The complications of chronic kidney disease can be classified into two major groups:[1] fluid, electrolyte, and acid-base disturbances; and disorders of metabolism and specific organ/system function.[2]
  - Fluid, electrolyte, and acid-base complications
    - Volume overload
    - Hyponatremia or hypernatremia
    - Hyperkalemia
    - Hypocalcemia
    - Hyperphosphatemia
    - Hypermagnesemia
    - Metabolic acidosis
  - Disorders of metabolism and organ/system function
    - Renal osteodystrophy
    - Anemia
    - Uremic coagulopathy
    - Cardiovascular complications including: pericarditis, severe vascular calcification, coronary artery disease, and cardiomyopathy
    - Encephalopathy
    - Peripheral neuropathy
    - Sleep disorders
    - Sexual dysfunction
    - Psychologic disorders
    - Immune disorders
    - Dermatologic complications (pruritus)

RENAL OSTEODYSTROPHY

- Renal osteodystrophy, characterized by either osteitis fibrosa, osteomalacia, adynamic bone disease, or a combination of these, is present in nearly all patients with chronic kidney disease and can occur early in the course of renal disease (stage 3 or earlier). Therefore, a therapeutic strategy to manage renal bone disease is often required before the creatinine has increased.

- Renal osteodystrophy is usually attributed to secondary hyperparathyroidism, precipitated by the combined effects of phosphorus retention, hypocalcemia, and vitamin D deficiency. It is to be noted that these factors can contribute to bone disease independently. Regardless, the mechanism of renal osteodystrophy remains incompletely understood.
- The clinical features of renal osteodystrophy include bone pain, fractures, and avascular necrosis, tendon rupture, tumoral calcinosis, soft tissue calcification (blood vessels, skin, eye), and proximal muscle weakness.
- The management of renal osteodystrophy is challenging, and its success depends on implementing management strategies in a rational, stepwise manner. These strategies include dietary restriction of phosphorus, use of phosphate binders, judicious correction of hypocalcemia (soft tissue calcification may occur with indiscriminate use of calcium supplements), administration of vitamin D analogues, and/or calcimimetics and correction of metabolic acidosis.

METABOLIC ACIDOSIS

- Metabolic acidosis is common in patients with chronic kidney disease, particularly at its advanced stages and among patients taking sevelamer (Renagel®) as a phosphate binder. Deleterious effects of untreated metabolic acidosis include bone resorption, accelerated skeletal muscle breakdown, and impaired albumin synthesis. Administration of exogenous alkali to correct serum bicarbonate levels to 22–24 mEq/L is generally advocated to minimize these undesired consequences.[10]

ANEMIA

- Anemia of chronic kidney disease is typically a normocytic normochromic anemia mainly secondary to decreased production of erythropoietin by the diseased kidneys. Other reasons include inhibition of erythropoiesis by uremic toxins and a shorter lifespan of erythrocytes.
- The mainstay of therapy for anemia of chronic kidney disease is administration of recombinant human erythropoietin (rh-EPO). The goal of therapy using rh-EPO is to achieve a target hemoglobin and hematocrit level of 11 to 12 g/dL and 33% to 36% respectively per the National Kidney Foundation Kidney Disease Outcomes Quality Initiative (NKF KDOQI) guidelines. Overcorrection of anemia to normal or near normal levels, found in healthy individuals, is *not* advocated for patients with chronic kidney disease.
- Additional management approaches include correction of iron, vitamin B$_{12}$, and folate deficiencies, if present, avoidance of medications and toxins that could potentially inhibit erythropoiesis, diagnosis and

prompt management of occult gastrointestinal blood loss, and delivery of adequate dialysis.
- Potential complications of rh-EPO include hypertension caused by increased red blood cell mass, premature thrombosis of vascular access, antibody mediated pure red cell aplasia, and iron deficiency secondary to iron consumption.

INCREASED BLEEDING RISK

- An increased bleeding tendency is also frequently noted in patients with chronic kidney disease. The mechanism for this common complication include inhibition of platelet function because of circulating uremic toxins, decreased platelet thromboxane synthesis, circulating aberrant multimeric factor VIII von Willebrand protein (VIII:vWP) and anemia.
- Therefore, management of a patient with uremic bleeding is aimed at correcting the underlying platelet dysfunction and includes the following: (1) administration of the vasopressin analogue, 1-deamino-8-D-arginine vasopressin (dDAVP) 0.3 mcg/kg intravenously every 4–8 hours. dDAVP promotes endothelial release of normal VIII:vWP from Weibel-Palade bodies (tachyphylaxis can occur after two to three doses); (2) cryoprecipitate (a rich source of VIII:vWP) 10 units intravenously every 12 to 24 hours; (3) conjugated estrogens 0.6 mg/kg/d for 5 days; (4) aggressive dialysis for patients with uremia; and (5) correction of anemia.

INCREASED CARDIOVASCULAR RISK

- There is mounting clinical evidence that chronic kidney disease is associated with an increased risk of cardiovascular (CV) disease, independent of the underlying disease.[11] In addition to the traditional CV risk factors such as hypertension and dyslipidemia, chronic kidney disease itself has been shown to be associated with development of premature coronary artery disease and a poorer prognosis of CV disease outcomes overall. Therefore, prompt diagnosis and treatment of chronic kidney disease is crucial in the management of patients with established risk factors for CV disease.

REFERENCES

1. National Kidney Foundation Kidney Disease Outcomes Quality Initiative (NKF KDOQI) clinical practice guidelines for chronic kidney disease: Evaluation, classification, and stratification. *Am J Kidney Dis.* 2002;39:S1.
2. Jones CA, McQuillan GM, Kusek JW. Serum creatinine levels in the US population: Third national health and nutrition examination survey. *Am J Kidney Dis.* 1998;32:992.

3. Nissenson AR, Pereira BJ, Collins AJ, Steinberg EP. Prevalence and characteristics of individuals with chronic kidney disease in a large health maintenance organization. *Am J Kidney Dis.* 2001;37:1177.

4. Coresh J, Astor BC, Greene T, et al. Prevalence of chronic kidney disease and decreased kidney function in the adult US population: Third National Health and Nutrition Examination survey. *Am J Kidney Dis.* 2003;41:1.

5. Levey AS, Greene T, Kusek JW, Beck GJ, and MDRD study group. A simplified equation to predict glomerular filtration rate from serum creatinine [abstract]. *J Am Soc Nephrol.* 2000; 11:155A.

6. Jafar TH, Stark PC, Schmid CH, et al. Progression of chronic kidney disease: The role of blood pressure control, proteinuria, and angiotensin-converting enzyme inhibition: a patient-level meta-analysis. *Ann Intern Med.* 2003;139:244.

7. Johns Hopkins Medicine. Hopkins performs historic "domino donor" "quintuple" kidney transplant. http://www.hopkinsmedicine.org/Press_releases/2006/Transplant/11_20_06.html.

8. Kinchen KS, Sadler J, Fink N, et al. The timing of specialist evaluation in chronic kidney disease and mortality. *Ann Intern Med.* 2002;137:479.

9. Pereira BJ. Optimization of pre-ESRD care: The key to improved dialysis outcomes. *Kidney Int.* 2000;57:351.

10. Uribarri J. Acidosis in chronic renal insufficiency. *Semin Dial.* 2000;13:232.

11. Sarnak MJ, Levey AS, Schoolwerth AC, Coresh J. Kidney disease as a risk factor for development of cardiovascular disease: A statement from the American Heart Association Councils on Kidney in Cardiovascular Disease, High Blood Pressure Research, Clinical Cardiology, and Epidemiology and Prevention. *Circulation.* 2003;108:2154.

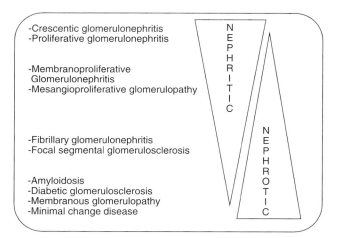

FIG. 122–1 Nephrotic and nephritic manifestation of different glomerular diseases and their overlap.

- The clinical hallmark of glomerular disease is proteinuria and/or hematuria. With rare exception, the golden rule, *no proteinuria, no glomerulonephritis,* holds true. Nephrotic range proteinuria or the presence of red blood cell casts in the urine sediment is virtually pathognomonic for glomerular disease. Thus, examination of the urine is a crucial initial step in the clinical evaluation of glomerular disease.
- Regardless of the initial workup, a renal biopsy is generally required to establish the diagnosis, and/or for staging the glomerular pathology (eg, lupus nephritis).

122 GLOMERULAR DISEASE

Rizwan A. Qazi and Bahar Bastani

INTRODUCTION

- Various inflammatory and noninflammatory diseases can alter glomerular physiology and anatomy, leading to a host of glomerular pathologies. Glomerular diseases are the most common cause of chronic kidney disease.
- Glomerular diseases can be classified on the basis of histology or clinical presentation. Since many of the etiologies share common histological patterns, it is convenient from a clinical standpoint to classify glomerular pathologies into those presenting with a nephritic or nephrotic clinical picture, although overlap does occur (Fig. 122–1).

PATHOPHYSIOLOGY OF THE NEPHROTIC SYNDROME

- *Nephrotic* syndrome is characterized by a urine protein excretion in excess of 3.5 g/24 hours coupled with hypoalbuminemia, edema, and hyperlipidemia. Conversely, *nephritic* syndrome is characterized by hypertension, proteinuria (sometimes in the nephrotic range) and hematuria.
- The pathophysiologic mechanisms underlying the nephrotic syndrome remain poorly understood; however, an abnormality of glomerular permeability is the hallmark of this disorder. Altered glomerular permeability may be secondary to injured epithelial cells and loss of glomerular anionic sialoglycoproteins (eg, minimal change disease) and/or physical disruption of the glomerular filtration barrier (eg, necrotizing glomerulonephritis).
- Recent detailed studies of congenital nephrotic syndrome of the Finnish type has greatly expanded our understanding of the nature of the glomerular filtration barrier. Congenital nephrotic syndrome of the Finnish type is caused by a mutation in the NHPS1

gene which encodes for a protein referred to as nephrin. Nephrin is an adhesion-like protein that promotes the formation of a zipper like structure between glomerular podocytes eg, the slit diaphragm. The slit diaphragm, is a crucial component of the glomerular protein filtration barrier. Since the discovery of Nephrin, a variety of other proteins have been characterized in the slit diaphragm. Mutations in many of these proteins leads to heavy proteinuria. Accordingly, it is now believed that the protein filtration barrier resides predominantly in the slit diaphragm and not in the basement membrane as was previously thought.

- The concept of a circulating permeability factor has also received attention. The primary evidence in favor of a circulating "proteinuric factor" is derived from renal transplant studies in patients that develop recurrence of focal segmental glomerulosclerosis (FSGS). Recurrent disease can occur in a matter of hours or days, and has been successfully treated with plasma exchange, or elution with protein A or anti-IgG columns. Importantly, the eluates from these columns when injected into animals cause heavy proteinuria.

- Various theories have been proposed to explain the anasarca or generalized edema formation, which is a hallmark of the nephrotic syndrome. The two widely accepted theories are: (1) The *underfill theory* in which a low serum albumin leads to low plasma oncotic pressure and extravasation of plasma into the interstitial space which, in turn decreases effective circulating volume, and (2) The *overfill theory*, in which kidneys are avidly salt-retaining before a noticeable decline in the plasma oncotic pressure. These two pathways may not be mutually exclusive and may depend on the stage and type of glomerular injury.

- Since hepatic synthesis of albumin can normally increase several fold (exceeding 30 g/d), the mechanism of hypoalbuminemia in the setting of nephrotic syndrome continues to generate much debate. Possible factors contributing to hypoalbuminemia include: enhanced degradation of albumin by the kidney; impaired hepatic synthesis of albumin; and extrarenal changes in albumin catabolism.

- Hyperlipidemia also accompanies urinary loss of protein and is thought to be secondary to increased hepatic synthesis of very low-density lipoproteins (VLDL). An increase in low-density lipoproteins (LDLs) is also common in patients with the nephrotic syndrome and is probably the result of VLDL catabolism. The increased incidence of cardiovascular disease noted in patients with the nephrotic syndrome is believed to be induced by changes in serum lipids.

- There is an increased incidence of arterial and venous thrombosis in patients with nephrotic syndrome. Urinary loss of endogenous anticoagulants, particularly antithrombin III, protein C, and protein S, may account for the hypercoagulable state. Plasma levels of these factors are often decreased in patients with nephrotic syndrome. Whether systemic anticoagulation should be initiated prophylactically in all patients with severe proteinuria remains controversial.

- There is an increased incidence of infection associated with nephrotic syndrome. This is believed to be secondary to loss of immunoglobulins in the urine. Also important for host defense are zinc, transferrin, and complement factor B, all of which are lost in the urine in proteinuric patients. Serum IgG levels that remain persistently <600 mg/dL portend a high risk of infection which may be amenable to treatment with intravenous IgG (10–15 gm IV per month).

HISTORY AND PHYSICAL EXAMINATION

- A detailed history is essential; for example, childhood nephrotic syndrome is most likely secondary to minimal change disease, whereas adult nephrotic syndrome is often due to membranous glomerulopathy.

- Intravenous drug abuse has been associated with nephrotic syndrome secondary to FSGS.

- Use of drugs like nonsteroidal antiinflammatory drugs (NSAIDs), gold, penicillamine, or calcineurin inhibitors may point to a specific glomerular pathology associated with those drugs.

- An important component of the history is directed toward establishing the chronicity of the disease process.

- The presence of comorbid conditions such as diabetes, cancer, systemic lupus erythematosus (SLE), or viral hepatitis may also provide an important clue to the underlying renal pathology.

- Obtaining a detailed family history is also helpful, for example, when considering hereditary nephritis, reflux uropathy, or some familial forms of FSGS.

- The presence of hypertension, edema, and generalized fatigue are all important, albeit nonspecific findings observed in a variety of renal diseases.

- Hemoptysis and hematuria should suggest a pulmonary renal syndrome (vasculitis).

- Periorbital and facial edema, especially in the mornings, is characteristic of nephrotic syndrome as compared to other causes of edema formation.

- Other specific physical findings are as follows
  ○ The presence of a malar rash in a patient with renal insufficiency, proteinuria, and hematuria strongly suggests renal involvement secondary to SLE.
  ○ Peripheral neuropathy in an elderly patient with proteinuria, macroglossia, and an elevated serum globulin suggests systemic amyloidosis.

○ Livedo reticularis in a patient who has recently undergone cardiac catheterization should raise the possibility of cholesterol atheroembolization.

○ Abdominal pain and a purpuric rash in an adolescent with new-onset renal failure would strongly support the diagnosis of Henoch-Schönlein purpura.

LABORATORY STUDIES AND RADIOLOGICAL PROCEDURES

URINALYSIS

• Microscopic examination of the urine is sometimes referred to as the *poor man's kidney biopsy*. Patients with clinically significant renal disease most often present with an abnormal urinalysis (hematuria, proteinuria, casts, etc.) and/or a decline in glomerular filtration rate (GFR). Therefore, examination of a freshly voided urine specimen and determination of serum creatinine are the first steps in the evaluation of a patient with renal disease.

• Isolated or transient abnormalities in the urinalysis must be distinguished from abnormalities secondary to glomerular pathology. Transient proteinuria may occur in up to 10% of otherwise healthy individuals. The magnitude of proteinuria is typically mild but can rarely be severe. Transient proteinuria is particularly common in patients with congestive heart failure, infection, and other stress-related illnesses. The mechanism responsible for transient proteinuria in these settings in poorly understood but may involve changes in the circulating levels of stress hormones (angiotensin II, epinephrine). These hormones alter glomerular permeability for protein and modulate intrarenal blood flow and glomerular pressure. Importantly, transient episodes of proteinuria are not associated with the presence of significant glomerular pathology, and thus are considered benign.

• Postural or orthostatic proteinuria is noted only with upright posture during daily activity, and not during recumbence. The magnitude of proteinuria is generally mild (less than 1g/d) but can rarely exceed 3 g/day. It is much more common in adolescents and is rare in patients older than 30 years of age. The diagnosis rests on establishing the relationship between posture and the presence of protein in the urine. However, postural changes in urine protein excretion may also occur in serious renal disease. Therefore, benign orthostatic proteinuria should only be diagnosed when recumbent protein excretion rate is less than 50 mg/day.

• In contrast to proteinuria, hematuria can arise anywhere within the urogenital tract. The most common cause of hematuria in an adult is urinary tract disease (eg, prostatitis, renal calculi, cystitis). In the absence of red blood cell casts or a rising creatinine, a thorough urologic evaluation (CT scan of abdomen/pelvis, intravenous pyelography, renal ultrasonography, and/or cystoscopy) should be performed. Noncontrast computed tomography (CT) scan of the abdomen/pelvis is the preferred radiologic examination for evaluation of kidney stones as a cause of hematuria.

• Red blood cell (RBC) morphology has been used to distinguish renal parenchymal from lower urinary tract causes of hematuria. Typically, extrarenal hematuria is characterized by >80% isomorphic RBCs, whereas glomerular hematuria is usually accompanied by >80% dysmorphic RBCs. Dysmorphic RBCs arise as a result of their passage through the renal tubules and the hypertonic medullary interstitium. RBC morphology is best visualized under phase contrast microscope.

• An algorithm useful in the evaluation of proteinuria is depicted in Fig. 122–2.

MEASUREMENT OF GLOMERULAR FILTRATION RATE

• A hallmark of renal disease is a reduction in glomerular filtration rate (GFR). Different formulas have been used to estimate GFR:
  ○ Cockcroft-Gault formula.

  Creatinine clearance = (140-age) × weight in kg/ (72 × serum creatinine in mg/dl).

  ○ Multiply by 0.85 for females.
  ○ Modification of Diet in Renal Disease (MDRD), and modified MDRD equations are the most widely used and accepted estimates.

• All of the formulas utilize the serum creatinine as the basis for calculating GFR. It is important to recognize that creatinine only provides an estimate of the absolute GFR.

• The endogenous creatinine clearance tends to overestimate GFR since with normal renal function approximately 10% of the urine creatinine is derived from proximal tubular secretion. The endogenous creatinine clearance may grossly overestimate the GFR when renal function is reduced by more than 75%. Under these conditions the percentage of creatinine undergoing tubular secretion may exceed 60%.

• New kidney injury markers such as kidney injury molecule-1 (KIM-1) and neutrophil gelatinase-associated lipocalin (NGAL) are emerging as sensitive markers of impending or early renal disease.

• Alternate methods of measuring GFR using plasma disappearance curves of iohexol or technetium-99 DTPA can also be used.

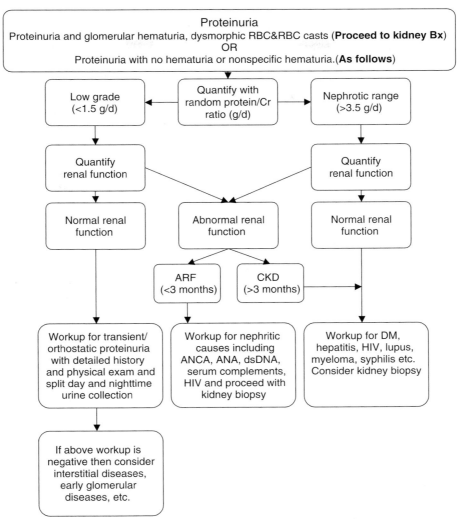

FIG. 122–2 Workup of a patient with proteinuria with and without glomerular hematuria. ARF, acute renal failure; ANCA, antineutrophil cytoplasmic antibody; ANA, antinuclear antibody; CKD, chronic kidney disease; Cr, creatinine; DM, diabetes mellitus; dsDNA, double-stranded DNA; HIV, human immunodeficiency virus; RBC, red blood cell.

BLOOD AND SEROLOGIC STUDIES

A variety of laboratory tests may prove useful in guiding further evaluation of suspected renal disease. These include:

- Serum complement components (C_3, C_4, CH_{50}), which aid in differentiating the nephritic syndromes and also serve as markers of disease activity.
- Serum cryoglobulins to aid in the diagnosis of essential mixed cryoglobulinemia.
- Hepatitis serologies in membranous glomerulopathy and MPGN secondary to viral hepatitis.
- Human immunodeficiency virus (HIV) serologies in collapsing FSGS.

- Serum and urine immunoelectrophoresis to aid in the diagnosis of myeloma kidney and amyloidosis.
- Quantitative determination of antinuclear antibodies in lupus nephritis and other connective tissue disorders that alter renal function.
- Anti-GBM antibodies in anti-GBM disease, Goodpasture syndrome/pulmonary renal syndromes.
- Serum RPR in syphilis.
- Blood cultures, erythrocyte sedimentation rate (ESR), and C-reactive protein (CRP) in infective endocarditis associated glomerulonephritis. The inflammatory markers are relatively nonspecific, however.
- Antineutrophil cytoplasmic antibodies (c-ANCA and p-ANCA) have been associated with systemic vasculitis

and rapidly progressive glomerulonephritis (RPGN). Antibodies with a cytoplasmic pattern of staining (c-ANCA) are directed toward proteinase-3 (PR3) and are commonly found in Wegener granulomatosis. In contrast, antibodies with specificity to myeloperoxidase (MPO) demonstrate a perinuclear staining pattern (p-ANCA). The p-ANCA is often noted in patients with microscopic polyangiitis, and in several nonrenal diseases, such as inflammatory bowel disease and primary biliary cirrhosis, and therefore is not specific for renal disease.

RADIOLOGICAL STUDIES

- Renal ultrasonography is a valuable study to rule out hydronephrosis and to evaluate the size of the kidneys. Small echogenic kidneys with loss of corticomedullary distinction should suggest advanced chronic kidney disease. Large kidneys (>12 cm) suggest diabetes, amyloidosis, or HIV nephropathy.
- Contrast-enhanced CT scan is helpful when cortical necrosis, renal vein thrombosis or renal infarction is suspected. Noncontrast CT scan can identify nephrocalcinosis and nephrolithiasis.
- Radionuclide scanning is helpful in assessing renal perfusion and calculation of split renal function.
- Magnetic resonance angiography (MRA) or CT angiography are used for evaluation of renal artery stenosis.

RENAL BIOPSY

Cortical renal tissue examination (renal biopsy) remains the *gold standard* for establishing the diagnosis of glomerular disease. Often, the clinical and laboratory features of renal diseases may be insufficient to arrive at a definitive diagnosis. In these circumstances, a renal biopsy is necessary to delineate the underlying disease. Examination of the renal biopsy involves:(1) light microscopy with several unique stains, (2) immunofluorescence (particularly to identify antibody deposition), and (3) electron microscopy. Special collagen stains are also performed if Alport syndrome is suspected. Kappa and lambda light chain stains are crucial to diagnose light chain deposition disease and amyloidosis.

DIFFERENTIAL DIAGNOSIS OF GLOMERULAR DISEASES

Classifying glomerular pathology according to the urinary findings (nephrotic versus nephritic) is a useful clinical strategy to formulate a differential diagnosis.

GLOMERULAR DISEASES ASSOCIATED WITH NEPHROTIC SYNDROME

Five clinical entities account for most cases of the nephrotic syndrome in the adult: (1) diabetic nephropathy, (2) membranous glomerulonephritis (MGN), (3) focal segmental glomerulosclerosis (FSGS), (4) amyloidosis, and (5) minimal change disease (MCD).

The general supportive treatment useful in the management of all nephrotic patients are as follows.
- Maintain BP <130/85 using preferably angiotensin-converting enzyme (ACE) inhibitors and/or angiotensin receptor blockers (ARBs). Nondihydropyridine calcium channel blockers (verapamil and diltiazem) are second line agents that modestly reduce proteinuria. *The target 24-hour urine protein excretion rate in these patients is < 1–2g.*
- Administer statins to lower cholesterol (target LDL-cholesterol is <100mg/dL).
- Judicious use of diuretics for edema.
- Provide adequate dietary protein (1 g/kg body weight) along with carbohydrates to minimize negative nitrogen balance.
- Consider deep venous thrombosis (DVT) prophylaxis in high-risk patients.
- Consider intravenous immunoglobulins (IVIG) if the patent is experiencing recurrent infections and the serum IgG level is less than 600 mg/dL.
- Correct metabolic acidosis, if present.

DIABETIC NEPHROPATHY

- Is responsible for the majority of cases of end-stage renal disease worldwide (particularly developed nations).
- The earliest sign of diabetic nephropathy is the presence of hyperfiltration (GFR greater than 140 mL/min) which is followed by microalbuminuria (30–300 mg/d of urinary albumin).
- Poor glycemic control, abnormal intrarenal hemodynamics, and hyperlipidemia have been implicated in the progression of latent hyperfiltration to overt proteinuria.
- Microalbuminuria progresses over 15 to 20 years to end-stage renal disease. Uncontrolled hypertension and poor glycemic control accelerate this progression.
- Nephropathy is strongly associated with other complications of diabetes (retinopathy, neuropathy). Indeed, in the absence of retinopathy, one should question the diagnosis of diabetic nephropathy.
- Aggressive blood pressure control is as important, if not more important, than tight glycemic control in patients with diabetic nephropathy.
- ACE inhibitors (type I diabetes) and angiotensin-receptor blocking agents (type 2 diabetes) ameliorate

renal injury and proteinuria independent of alterations in systemic blood pressure.

- A protein-restricted diet (0.6–0.8 g/kg/d) has also been shown to slow the rate of progressive renal disease in diabetic nephropathy, although the effects are likely modest.
- Since diabetic nephropathy cannot be cured, the complications of CKD should be sought and aggressively managed, particularly when the patient reaches stage 3 CKD (GFR less than 60 mL/min). The major complications that arise early in the course of CKD include renal osteodystrophy and anemia (Chap. 121).

MEMBRANOUS GLOMERULOPATHY (MGN)

- 25% to 40% of adult patients with idiopathic nephrotic syndrome have MGN.
- Associated diseases include hepatitis B and C, systemic lupus (lupus nephritis class V), malignancies, and some drugs (gold, penicillamine).
- The glomerular basement membrane typically appears thick and has characteristic spikes when stained with silver-methenamine and examined under light microscopy. Also, subepithelial electron dense antibody deposits are visible on electron microscopy.
- Glomerular hematuria and RBC casts are very unusual with idiopathic MGN. Their presence in a patient with previously diagnosed MGN should prompt a repeat kidney biopsy and serum testing for anti-glomerular basement membrane antibodies.
- Complement levels are usually normal in idiopathic MGN. When present, hypocomplementemia usually suggests MGN secondary to SLE or viral hepatitis.
- The incidence of thrombotic events, especially renal vein thrombosis, is inexplicably more common in MGN than other causes of the nephrotic syndrome.
- Typically one-third of patients progress to end-stage kidney disease, another third spontaneously remit, and the remainder follow a slowly progressive course.
- Corticosteroids, cyclophosphamide, or chlorambucil have been used for patients with heavy proteinuria and a rising serum creatinine.
- Older patients with idiopathic MGN should undergo cancer surveillance with mammography, chest x-ray, and colonoscopy.

FOCAL SEGMENTAL GLOMERULOSCLEROSIS

- Focal segmental glomerulosclerosis (FSGS) accounts for 10% to 30% of cases of the adult nephrotic syndrome.
- Incidence is rising especially in the African American population.

- FSGS can be primary (idiopathic), secondary (HIV-related), or rarely familial.
- Sclerosis of glomeruli is focal in nature (less than 50% of the glomeruli are involved), and segmental (only affecting a part of the glomerulus). However, FSGS can progress to diffuse and global glomerulosclerosis.
- Secondary FSGS has been associated with HIV infection (some patients can present with nephrotic syndrome), hepatitis B, intravenous heroin use, and drugs such as pamidronate. It may also develop in patients with pre-existing nephron loss or a relative deficiency of nephron mass compared to body mass (eg, subtotal nephrectomy, unilateral renal dysgenesis/agenesis and morbid obesity). In these individuals, the mechanisms of FSGS is thought to depend on maladaptive changes in the remaining (remnant) nephrons (hyperfiltration) which promote renal fibrosis.
- Unfortunately, most patients with FSGS progress to end-stage renal disease within 10 years of the diagnosis.
- Aggressive forms of FSGS, for example collapsing FSGS, that are associated with HIV, may progress within months to advanced renal disease requiring dialysis.
- Highly active antiretroviral therapy (HAART) is effective in the treatment of HIV-associated nephropathy.
- Recent studies recommend a course of high-dose steroid administration in patients with idiopathic FSGS for at least a period of 4 to 6 months. Up to 50% of patients may respond to such a regimen.
- Recent evidence suggest that steroid-resistant patients may respond to daily cyclosporine, mycophenolate mofetil, or cyclophosphamide administration.
- Treatment with corticosteroids and other immunosuppressive agents can induce partial or complete remission rates in up to 70% of patients.
- FSGS can recur after renal transplantation. This type of FSGS responds well to plasmapheresis, suggesting that a circulating permeability factor is involved in its pathogenesis.

AMYLOIDOSIS

- Plasma cell dyscrasias (multiple myeloma) may cause primary (AL type) amyloidosis which is characterized by glomerular deposits of amyloid composed of light chains.
- Chronic inflammatory disorders, such as rheumatoid arthritis, may occasionally be complicated by renal deposition of amyloid (secondary or AA amyloidosis). The amyloidogenic protein in these disorders is distinct from light chains and appears to be derived from a circulating protein synthesized in the liver.

- Treatment for secondary amyloidosis is directed at the underlying infectious/inflammatory disease process.
- The renal disease in amyloidosis often accompanies a variety of other systemic symptoms that arise from amyloid deposits at remote sites (heart, nerve, liver). Accordingly, the clinical manifestations include: nephrotic proteinuria, enlarged kidneys, hepatosplenomegaly, congestive heart failure, peripheral neuropathy, macroglossia, and carpal tunnel syndrome.
- Monoclonal proteins are almost always identified on serum and urine protein electrophoresis and/or immunoelectrophoresis in patients with AL amyloid.
- Tissue is necessary to confirm the diagnosis. Gingival, rectal, abdominal fat pad, and kidney are common biopsy sites. A bone marrow biopsy must be performed in patients with AL amyloid to exclude myeloma.
- The overall prognosis is poor, and the mean survival is less than 1 year, with most patients succumbing to renal failure or infection.
- Light chain deposition disease (LCDD) can cause acute renal failure in patients with multiple myeloma; however, the fibrils detected on electron microscopy are distinct from amyloid fibrils.
- More than 80% of patients with renal amyloidosis or LCDD demonstrate a circulating or urinary monoclonal protein.
- Treatment of primary amyloidosis is unclear unless secondary to myeloma. Melphalan, steroids, and vincristine have shown some survival benefit.

MINIMAL CHANGE DISEASE

- The most common cause of nephrotic syndrome in childhood.
- 20% of adults with nephrotic syndrome may have steroid-responsive minimal change disease (MCD).
- MCD can be idiopathic or can occur in association with NSAIDs or Hodgkin disease.
- Light microscopy reveals normal histology, but on electron microscopy there is diffuse effacement of the foot processes.
- Renal failure is rare in MCD.
- MCD is steroid responsive, especially in children. Most children respond after 2 to 12 weeks of steroid therapy. Adults require longer duration therapy and are more likely to be resistant.
- Steroid-resistant patients or those with frequent relapses may benefit from cyclophosphamide, chlorambucil, or cyclosporine administration.

GLOMERULAR DISEASES ASSOCIATED WITH THE NEPHRITIC SYNDROME

HEREDITARY NEPHRITIS

- Hereditary nephritis or Alport syndrome is characterized by ocular abnormalities, renal insufficiency, and sensorineural hearing loss.
- Three modes of inheritance with different phenotypes have been described
  - X-linked (renal insufficiency and deafness, less severe in females)
  - Autosomal dominant (renal insufficiency with no auditory or eye involvement)
  - Autosomal recessive (renal insufficiency with no auditory or eye involvement)
- Urinary findings include hematuria and proteinuria (usually nephrotic).
- Most males with this disorder progress to end-stage renal disease (ESRD) by age 40. Females typically follow a less virulent course, although some may progress to ESRD by age 30.
- Unfortunately, no specific therapy exists for hereditary nephritis.

POSTINFECTIOUS GLOMERULONEPHRITIS

- Poststreptococcal glomerulonephritis (PSGN) is the most common form of postinfectious glomerular injury.
- Certain *nephritogenic* strains of streptococci are associated with glomerular inflammation. Typically caused by group A (pyogenes) and less commonly group C (Zooepidemicus) streptococci.
- Nephritic picture typically manifests 1 to 3 weeks after a pharyngeal or skin infection with a nephritogenic strain of streptococci.
- Affected glomeruli usually show diffuse proliferation with inflammatory cells (exudative) and in some cases crescent formation.
- Glomerulonephritis may occur in up to 25% of patients infected with nephritogenic strains of β-hemolytic streptococci.
- Serum complement components, particularly C3, are low (Table 122–1).
- Circulating antibodies, for example, antistreptolysin O (ASO) and anti-DNAse B are usually elevated. The Streptozyme panel which measures four different antigens is more sensitive than either ASO or anti-DNAse B alone.
- Clinical manifestations range from acute renal failure or florid nephrotic syndrome to asymptomatic hematuria and proteinuria.

TABLE 122–1   Nephritic Syndrome Segregated on the Basis of Normal or Low Serum Complements

NEPHRITIC SYNDROME WITH LOW C3 AND C4	NEPHRITIC SYNDROME WITH NORMAL C3 AND C4
Lupus nephritis	Rapidly progressive glomerulonephritis
Membranoproliferative glomerulonephritis	IgA nephropathy
Cryoglobulinemia	Renal vasculitis (ANCA associated)
Poststreptococcal glomerulonephritis	Hereditary nephritis
Renal atheroembolic disease	
Subacute bacterial endocarditis	

- Most patients recover spontaneousuly, although some may exhibit mild urinary abnormalities for years. Sporadic reports of patients with CKD and severe renal scarring occurring 30 to 40 years after an acute episode have been described.

MEMBRANOPROLIFERATIVE GLOMERULONEPHRITIS

- Membranoproliferative glomerulonephritis (MPGN) is often associated with a combination of nephrotic range proteinuria and hematuria.
- The clinical course of MPGN ranges from acute renal failure (ARF) with rapidly progressive glomerulonephritis (RPGN) to a slowly progressive indolent course dominated by symptoms and signs of the nephrotic syndrome.
- Type 1 MPGN is characterized by activation of the classic complement pathway (low C3 and C4, see Table 122–1). On electron microscopy, there are extensive subendothelial dense deposits.
- Type II MPGN is characterized by activation of the alternate complement pathway (low C3, but normal C4). On electron microscopy there is increased density of the glomerular basement membrane diffusely.
- Type II MPGN is thought to occur as a consequence of persistent activation of C3 via an antibody (C3 nephritic factor, C3NeF), which stabilizes and prolongs the half-life of C3 convertase.
- Most cases of childhood Type I MPGN are idiopathic. Adult forms of the disease are usually secondary to hepatitis C. Other associations include: SLE, hepatitis B, chronic lymphocytic leukemia, cryoglobulinemia, IV drug abuse, and transplant rejection.
- The treatment of idiopathic MPGN is controversial, although many patients respond to alternate day steroid administration.

SYSTEMIC LUPUS ERYTHEMATOSUS

- Renal disease in the setting of systemic lupus erythematosus (SLE) is extremely common.

- Patients with SLE that present with an active urine sediment, rise in serum creatinine, or proteinuria almost always undergo a renal biopsy. Virtually 100% of such patients will have abnormalities on renal biopsy. Interestingly, pathologic abnormalities may be present even in the absence of clinical or urinary findings.
- Five histologic subtypes of lupus nephritis have been described
  - Class 1: Normal histology.
  - Class II: Mesangial proliferation. Low probability of renal failure.
  - Class III: Focal segmental proliferative glomerulonephritis (<50% of glomeruli are partially involved). About 30% of these patients have nephrotic syndrome.
  - Class IV: Diffuse proliferative glomerulonephritis (>50% of glomeruli are globally involved). Crescents may also be observed. Electron microscopy typically reveals large subendothelial and mesangial deposits. More than 50% will have the nephrotic syndrome, and >50% will ultimately develop advanced renal disease.
  - Class V: Diffuse membranous nephropathy.
- Hypocomplementemia frequently accompanies active lupus nephritis.
- Serum complement levels may be used to follow disease activity and response to treatment.
  - Spontaneous conversion from one histologic subtype to another is often the rule rather than the exception.
  - Treatment has been best defined for diffuse proliferative lupus nephritis (lupus nephritis class IV), where response to combined prednisone and cyclophosphamide are clearly superior to placebo, steroids or cyclophosphamide alone. Mycophenolate mofetil (MMF), may offer a reasonable alternative to cyclophosphamide, although long-term investigations remain inconclusive.
  - Patients with class V lupus nephritis (membranous lupus nephritis) have a prognosis comparable to that of idiopathic membranous nephropathy.

RAPIDLY PROGRESSIVE GLOMERULONEPHRITIS

- Rapidly progressive glomerulonephritis (RPGN) should be viewed as a medical emergency, as irreversible scarring may occur in a matter of weeks.
- The clinical features include a nephritic urinary sediment with an acutely rising creatinine.
- All patients with RPGN *must* exhibit cellular crescents (involving greater than 60% of the glomeruli) on the renal biopsy.
- Three major subtypes of RPGN have been described based on the pathologic distribution of immune deposits.
- Type 1 RPGN, is characterized by linear deposits of immunoglobulin G (IgG) along the glomerular

capillary basement membrane (anti-glomerular basement membrane disease [anti-GBM disease]). If there is concomitant pulmonary alveolar hemorrhage due to IgG antibodies against the alveolar basement membrane, the disease is referred to as Goodpasture's syndrome.

- Type 2 RPGN is characterized by immune complex deposition along the glomerular capillary basement membrane. Theoretically, any condition that gives rise to immune-complex formation can produce this syndrome (eg, lupus nephritis, cryoglobulinemia, postinfectious).

- Type 3 RPGN (pauci-immune) is characterized by the absence of immune deposits in glomeruli. Most of these patients have an underlying vasculitis (eg, Wegener granulomatosis, microscopic polyangiitis, Churg-Strauss syndrome). Importantly, type 3 RPGN is frequently associated with the presence of circulating ANCAs.

- Treatment of all subtypes of RPGN involves a combination of high-dose corticosteroids and cyclophosphamide (plasmaphesis is useful in anti-GBM disease). The response rate is quite good (>90%) if the diagnosis is established before the serum creatinine exceeds 5 mg/dL. If the diagnosis is delayed the prognosis for renal recovery is significantly worse (<20%).

IGA NEPHROPATHY

- Most common cause of glomerulonephritis worldwide.
- Clinical presentation can vary from asymptomatic hematuria and/or proteinuria to a rapidly progressive course.
- Elevated plasma IgA levels are found in as many as 50% of these patients, although the levels do not correlate with disease activity.
- The pathogenesis of this disorder is thought to depend on abnormal glycosylation causing qualitative alterations in circulating IgA which promote renal deposition.
- Gross or microscopic hematuria is the most common presenting feature of IgA nephropathy and is often preceded by a viral syndrome.
- Most patients have normal renal function and follow a benign course. However, progression to ESRD with nephrotic range proteinuria may occur in up to 20% of the affected individuals.
- Omega-3 fatty acids and ACE inhibitors ameliorate progression of the renal disease.
- Heavy proteinuria portends a poor prognosis and these patients usually receive a course of steroids, although the data supporting this approach is controversial.
- IgA nephropathy can recur in 50% of renal transplant recipients; however, it is the cause of graft failure in only 10% of these patients.

SYSTEMIC VASCULITIS

- Vasculitis is classified based on the caliber of the vessels involved: large, medium or small vessel vasculitis, however renal vasculitis usually involves the small arteries (See also Chap. 127, Vasculitis). Therefore, the most common causes of renal vasculitis are microscopic polyangiitis, Wegener granulomatosis and Henoch-Schönlein purpura.

- **Wegener granulomatosis** is associated with necrotizing granuloma formation in the upper and lower respiratory tract. The clinical manifestations usually include nonspecific features such as arthralgias, myalgias, weight loss, sinusitis, and fever.
  ○ Other features such as hemoptysis, hematuria, renal insufficiency, and proteinuria should prompt an immediate evaluation to confirm the diagnosis. Untreated Wegener granulomatosus is a uniformly fatal disease.
  ○ The renal biopsy reveals segmental necrotizing glomerulonephritis with or without crescent formation.
  ○ Immune deposits are conspicuously absent. Notwithstanding, most patients with active disease will exhibit circulating C-ANCA (anti-proteinase 3 antibodies).
  ○ Affected patients may either have renal-limited disease or may present with involvement of the upper and lower respiratory tract (sinusitis and pulmonary hemorrhage).
  ○ Response rates as high as 90% are obtained with a combination of cyclophosphamide and prednisone (if initiated early).
  ○ Patients with massive hemoptysis may benefit from plasmapheresis.

- **Microscopic polyangiitis** is a systemic vasculitis that typically involves the small arterioles and capillaries.
  ○ cANCA (anti-PR3) and/or pANCA (anti-MPO) is positive in 40% to 50% of the cases (>90% are positive in active disease).
  ○ The clinical features are similar to those of Wegener granulomatosis, with the notable exception of granuloma formation and sinus involvement.
  ○ Treatment and prognosis are also similar to Wegener granulomatosus.

RENAL ATHEROEMBOLIC DISEASE

- Suspected in patients who have had invasive arterial vascular procedures.
- In 30% of the cases it occurs spontaneously, especially in elderly patients on chronic anticoagulation.
- Livedo reticularis and/or *blue toe* are often seen on physical examination.
- Course is indolent but progressive, with the serum creatinine rising in a step ladder fashion.

- Most patients have severe vascular disease with ulcerative plaques involving the large vessels such as the aorta and its major branches.
- Eosinophilia and hypocomplementemia have been reported in as many as 90% of cases.
- A renal biopsy will reveal microthrombi and pathognomonic needle-shaped cholesterol crystals in arterioles and glomerular capillaries, as well as an interstitial inflammatory reaction with giant cell formation. Cholesterol crystals are sometimes visible as refractile bodies on ophthalmological examination.
- No definitive therapy exists other than to avoid invasive procedures.

THROMBOTIC MICROANGIOPATHIES

- The thrombotic microangiopathies (TMs) are characterized by thrombocytopenia, microangiopathic hemolytic anemia, and renal insufficiency. In adults, neurologic complications secondary to thrombotic occlusion of the cerebral vessels may also occur (thrombotic thrombocytopenic purpura [TTP]).
- Renal insufficiency is typically severe in the childhood form of the disease (hemolytic uremic syndrome [HUS]).
- Indices of disseminated intravascular coagulation (elevated prothrombin time (PT), partial thromboplastin time (PTT), and fibrin split products) are usually *not* increased in these syndromes.
- Thrombotic microangiopathy may occur spontaneously or in association with calcineurin inhibitors, chemotherapy, malignant hypertension, vasculitis, postpartum acute renal failure, and HIV infection.
- Schistocytes are visible on the peripheral blood smear.
- Outbreaks of hemolytic uremic syndrome have been associated with verotoxin-producing *Escherichia coli* (serotype 0157:H7)
- The pathogenesis remains poorly understood, but recent studies suggest that acquired or congenital abnormalities in von Willebrand cleaving protease (ADAMTS13) predispose to platelet aggregation.
- Treatment must be initiated without delay because the mortality rate can exceed 90%.
- Infusion of fresh frozen plasma coupled with plasmapheresis is remarkably effective at inducing a remission in idiopathic TTP.

BIBLIOGRAPHY

Contreras G, Pardo V, Leclercq B, et al. Sequential therapies for proliferative lupus nephritis. *N Engl J Med.* 2004;350(10): 971–980.

Donadio JV Jr, Grande JP, Bergstralh EJ, Dart RA, Larson TS, Spencer DC. The long-term outcome of patients with IgA nephropathy treated with fish oil in a controlled trial. Mayo Nephrology Collaborative Group. *J Am Soc Nephrol.* 1999;10(8): 1772–1777.

Ginzler EM, Dooley MA, Aranow C, et al. Mycophenolate mofetil or intravenous cyclophosphamide for lupus nephritis. *N Engl J Med.* 2005;353(21):2219–2228.

Jayne D, Rasmussen N, Andrassy K, et al. A randomized trial of maintenance therapy for vasculitis associated with antineutrophil cytoplasmic autoantibodies. *N Engl J Med.* 2003;349(1):36–44.

Johnson RJ, Feehally J, eds. *Comprehensive Clinical Nephrology.* 2nd ed. New York: Mosby; 2003.

Smith AC, Molyneux K, Feehally J, Barratt J. O-Glycosylation of serum IgA1 Antibodies against Mucosal and Systemic Antigens in IgA Nephropathy. *J Am Soc Nephrol.* 2006;17(12):3520–3528.

Troyanov S, Wall CA, Miller JA, Scholey JW, Cattran DC. Focal and segmental glomerulosclerosis: Definition and relevance of a partial remission. *J Am Soc Nephrol.* 2005;16(4):1061–1068.

123 TUBULOINTERSTITIAL DISEASE

Alejandro C. Alvarez

INTRODUCTION

- Tubulointerstitial disease refers to a miscellaneous group of renal disorders that features inflammation of the tubules and interstitium. These disorders may develop acutely or follow a slowly progressive course.

HISTOLOGY

- The renal interstitium is comprised of connective tissue enveloping the tubules and vasculature.
- It is rich in type I and type III collagen, and proteoglycans.
- Type I cells in the cortical interstitium produce erythropoietin and regulate extracellular matrix synthesis and degradation.
- Medullary type I cells secrete prostaglandins via cyclooxygenase-2 and do not produce erythropoietin.
- Type II interstitial cells are derived from circulating monocytes and are involved in antigen recognition and presentation.

GENERAL OVERVIEW

- Acute interstitial nephritis (AIN) presents as acute renal failure with a predominant lymphocytic and monocytic cellular infiltrate in the interstitium.
- Chronic interstitial nephritis (CIN) is characterized by progressive loss of renal function and subtle tubular defects with a predominance of tubular atrophy and fibrosis.

- Proteinuria is not prominent in these disorders and is usually less than 1.5 g/day. The proteins in the urine are derived from low molecular weight proteins that escape tubular reabsorption, eg, light chains in multiple myeloma or β_2 microglobuline.
- The urinary sediment is often normal; but mild abnormalities including low-grade hematuria, pyuria, or occasionally casts may be observed.
- Heavy proteinuria, red blood cell casts or dysmorphic red blood cells, lipiduria, or oval fat bodies should suggest a glomerular etiology rather than tubulointerstitial nephritis (Fig. 123–1).

ACUTE INTERSTITIAL NEPHRITIS

- Acute interstitial nephritis (AIN) is characterized by abundant T-cells, monocytes/macrophages, eosinophils, and neutrophilic granulocytes in the interstitium coupled with interstitial edema.
- Although AIN is uncommonly observed in renal biopsy specimens (1% to 3%), it may actually account for up to 30% of patients with acute renal failure, as many of these patients are not subjected to a kidney biopsy.

PATHOPHYSIOLOGY

- Acute interstitial nephritis is secondary to either an immune-mediated hypersensitivity reaction to an antigen generated outside the kidney (usually a drug) or less frequently by an infectious agent (bacterial or viral) (Fig. 123–2).
- Some antigens trigger the immune response through molecular mimicry, binding to renal structures (planted antigens), modifying the immunogenicity of the renal structures (haptens), or precipitating as immune complexes.
- Regardless, this process activates complement, and induces macrophage and lymphocyte chemotaxis causing these cells to secrete cytokines and growth factors as well as promote direct cytotoxic injury.
- Cytokines (transforming growth factor β, endothelin 1, RANTES, osteopontin, and monocyte chemotactic peptide-1), amplify the inflammatory response, and increase cellular adhesion.
- Sustained inflammation may lead to irreversible interstitial fibrosis and tubular atrophy.

CLINICAL FEATURES

- AIN becomes clinically apparent within 2 to 30 days after exposure to the offending agent.
- Although this is usually a drug, occasionally it is the result of a bacterial or viral infection.
- Sudden onset of nonoliguric ARF, abnormal urinalysis, and flank pain is most suggestive of AIN. However

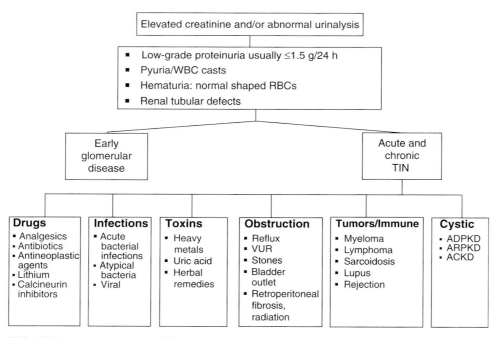

FIG. 123–1 Approach to the differential diagnosis of suspected tubulointerstitial diseases. ACKD, aquired cystic diseases: ADPKD, autosomal dominant polycystic kidney disease; ARPKD, autosomal recessive polycystic kidney disease; RBC, red blood cell; TIN, tubulointerstitial nephritis; VUR, vesicoureteral reflux; WBC, white blood cell.

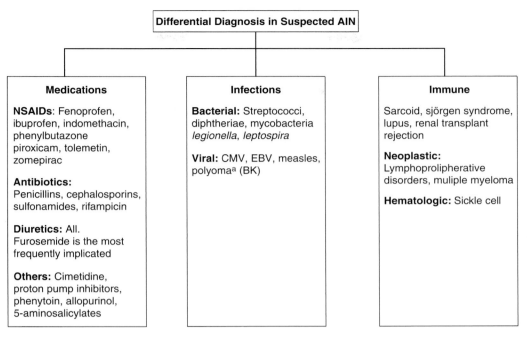

Differential Diagnosis in Suspected AIN

Medications	**Infections**	**Immune**
NSAIDs: Fenoprofen, ibuprofen, indomethacin, phenylbutazone piroxicam, tolemetin, zomepirac	**Bacterial:** Streptococci, diphtheriae, mycobacteria *legionella*, *leptospira*	Sarcoid, sjörgen syndrome, lupus, renal transplant rejection
Antibiotics: Penicillins, cephalosporins, sulfonamides, rifampicin	**Viral:** CMV, EBV, measles, polyoma[a] (BK)	**Neoplastic:** Lymphoproliperative disorders, muliple myeloma
Diuretics: All. Furosemide is the most frequently implicated		**Hematologic:** Sickle cell
Others: Cimetidine, proton pump inhibitors, phenytoin, allopurinol, 5-aminosalicylates		

[a]It is particularly seen in renal transplant recipients.

FIG. 123–2   Common causes of AIN.
AIN, acute tubulointerstitial nephritis; CMV, cytomegalovirus; EBV, Epstein-Barr virus; NSAID, nonsteroidal antiinflammatory drug.

these clinical features are noted in less than a fourth of the cases.

• Although low-grade proteinuria (<1.5 g/d) is noted in the majority of patients, AIN secondary to nonsteroidal antiinflammatory drugs is accompanied by nephrotic range proteinuria (80%). The glomerular histology reveals minimal change disease in addition to interstitial inflammation.

• Microscopic hematuria is present in more than 90% of cases.

• Sterile pyuria and white blood cell casts are present in more than 80% of cases.

• Extrarenal manifestations include low-grade fever (20%– 80%), skin rash (30%–50%), eosinophilia (50%), and arthralgias (15%) reflecting a hypersensitivity reaction. However, they are simultaneously present in less than 5% of the cases.

DIAGNOSIS

• It may be inferred from a suggestive clinical history and presentation (Fig. 123–3).

• Removal of the suspected offending agent and observing for clinical improvement while providing supportive care is a reasonable indirect method of inferring the diagnosis.

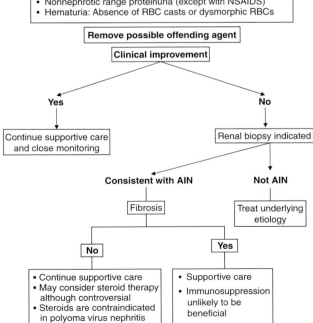

FIG. 123–3   Diagnostic and therapeutic approach to AIN.
AIN, acute tubulointerstitial nephritis; RBC, red blood cell; WBC, white blood cell.

- Renal biopsy for histologic confirmation is indicated if renal failure is rapidly progressive, advanced, or if conservative treatment fails.
- Gallium scintigraphy may be helpful in the absence of a renal biopsy (strongly positive uptake is consistent with the diagnosis of AIN).
- Eosinophiluria is consistent with, but not diagnostic of, AIN because urinary eosinophils may also be observed with urinary tract infections, acute glomerulonephritis, and atheroembolic renal disease.

TREATMENT

- Prompt removal of the offending agent is critical.
- Supportive care including renal replacement therapy is indicated.
- There is meager support from small uncontrolled trials that corticosteroid therapy may facilitate renal recovery, particularly when administered early in the course of the disease. Steroids are unlikely to be effective with advanced interstitial fibrosis and tubular atrophy.
- Corticosteroids are contraindicated in BK virus (polyoma virus) nephropathy. This entity most often occurs after renal transplantation.

CHRONIC INTERSTITIAL NEPHRITIS

- In contrast to AIN, chronic interstitial nephritis (CIN) is an indolent process that develops over months or years.
- Tubular defects such as renal tubular acidosis (RTA), urinary concentrating defects, glycosuria, aminoaciduria, or phosphaturia are relatively common.
- CIN is characterized by a mononuclear inflammatory cell infiltrate, interstitial fibrosis, and tubular atrophy.
- The myriad causes of CIN include anatomic abnormalities such as reflux nephropathy; exposure to toxins such medications, heavy metals, or herbal remedies; metabolic disorders such as hyperuricemia, hyperoxaluria, or chronic hypokalemia; hematologic abnormalities such as multiple myeloma or sickle cell disease; and infiltrative disorders such as sarcoidosis or lymphoma.
- CIN may also be seen in the advanced stages of a wide variety of pathologic processes that involve the glomerulus.

PATHOGENESIS

- Regardless of the inciting event, a mononuclear cell infiltrate ensues with tubular cell proliferation, dilatation, cast formation, and tubular atrophy.
- Fibroblast numbers increase via reverse differentiation of tubular epithelial cells (tubular epithelial cell–myofibroblast transition).
- Epithelial cell–myofibroblast transition is particularly aggressive in states of sustained injury and inflammation.
- Proliferation and activation of fibroblasts leads to expansion of the interstitium through increased secretion of interstitial collagens (types I, II, and VI), thickening of the tubular basement membrane, and eventually interstitial fibrosis.
- These events are amplified by local growth factors such as transforming growth factor beta-1 (TGF-β1), angiotensin II, and increased expression of adhesion molecules.
- Glomerulosclerosis also occurs in advanced disease characterized by severe tubular damage and extensive interstitial fibrosis.

CLINICAL PRESENTATION

- Loss of renal function over months to years.
- Nonnephrotic range proteinuria.
- Anemia disproportionate to the degree of renal dysfunction due to damage of type I cortical cells.
- Bland urinary sediment.
- Tubular dysfunction manifested as a non–anion gap metabolic acidosis (renal tubular acidosis), concentrating defects, or Fanconi syndrome.
- The kidneys are usually small and hyperechoic by ultrasonography. The exceptions to the rule are infiltrative and cystic disorders.
- Although interstitial fibrosis and tubular atrophy are irreversible, therapy is aimed at the underlying disease process in an attempt to halt or delay progression of the disease.

TREATMENT

- Aimed at removing the insulting agent if possible.
- Supportive care includes management of metabolic abnormalities and slowing progression of chronic kidney disease (CKD).
- Control of hypertension and hyperlipidemia slows progression of the disease.

- A low-protein diet in an attempt to reduce ammonia-genesis which accelerates renal injury.
- Angiotensin-converting enzyme (ACE) inhibitors and angiotensin receptor blockers (ARBs) reduce systemic and intraglomerular pressures, decrease proteinuria and slow progression of CKD. Their effectiveness in the setting of CIN is not known, although both agents can exert an antifibrotic effect.

DRUGS, TOXINS, AND HERBAL REMEDIES

ANALGESIC-INDUCED NEPHROPATHY

- Most common form of drug-induced CKD.
- There is wide geographic variation in the incidence of analgesic nephropathy.
- End-stage renal disease (ESRD) caused by analgesic nephropathy is as high as 18% in Germany, 3% in Australia, and less than 1% in the United States.
- The combination of aspirin, caffeine, and phenacetin seems particularly deleterious.
- Analgesics are believed to induce ischemic injury via inhibition of local prostaglandin synthesis and generation of oxygen radicals through the depletion of glutathione.
- The renal medulla is the main site of injury because the concentration of toxic radicals is high and the oxygen tension is low.
- The characteristic feature of analgesic nephropathy is papillary necrosis, which is present in more than 90% of the cases.
- It is more common in women than men by a ratio of approximately 6:1.
- A history of peptic ulcer disease or gastrointestinal bleeding is usually elicited.
- A history of cumulative ingestion greater than 1000 mg is usually present.
- Renal abnormalities include tubular defects characterized by urinary concentrating defects, salt wasting syndromes or classic distal RTA.
- The UA is usually benign but may reveal sterile pyuria.
- Computed tomography (CT) may demonstrate medullary microcalcifications usually in the papillary tip, along with small kidneys, and a *bumpy* contour.
- Therapy is directed at stopping the offending agent(s). Otherwise no specific treatment is available.

CALCINEURIN INHIBITOR NEPHROTOXICITY (CYCLOSPORINE OR TACROLIMUS)

- The calcineurin inhibitors include cyclosporine and tacrolimus. These agents are standard of care in solid organ transplantation and are also frequently used in the treatment of autoimmune diseases.
- The typical pathology is characterized by striped interstitial fibrosis of the cortical and medullary interstitium, arteriolar hyalinosis, and tubular vacuolization and atrophy. This is the result of chronic ischemic injury, induction of TGFβ, and connective tissue growth factor leading to epithelial cell–myofibroblast transition.
- Clinical manifestations include progressive renal failure, hypertension, hyperkalemic metabolic acidosis, magnesium wasting, hypercalciuria, hypophosphatemia, and hyperuricemia.
- Treatment is directed at discontinuation of the calcineurin inhibitor and switching to an alternative agent if possible, otherwise reducing the dose to maintain levels within the lower therapeutic range is indicated.
- If used cautiously, ACE inhibitors or ARBs may delay progression of fibrosis.

LITHIUM-INDUCED CHRONIC INTERSTITIAL NEPHRITIS

- The prevalence of CIN with lithium therapy has been reported as high as 20%.
- Renal tissue shows interstitial fibrosis and 1 to 2 mm microcystic dilatations of the distal tubules lined with enlarged columnar epithelium. Microcysts can sometimes be seen via magnetic resonance imaging (MRI).
- Patients with decreased glomerular filtration rate should have the lithium therapy withdrawn if possible and switched to valproic acid or carbamazepine. Otherwise, closely monitor and maintain the lithium levels within the lower level of the therapeutic range.

LEAD NEPHROTOXICITY

- Lead nephrotoxicity is associated with environmental (lead pipes, consumption of crops grown in lead-contaminated soil, ingestion of lead paint scraps or moonshine) and occupational lead exposure (manufacturing industry, lead containing batteries, radiators, etc.).
- Chronic exposure to lead can produce interstitial fibrosis, with a modest interstitial infiltrate, low-grade proteinuria, proximal tubule inclusion bodies, and eventually small kidneys.
- Given the slow progression of the disease, patients usually present with advanced symptoms and signs such as an elevated creatinine and hypertension. Many patients also experience gouty attacks and have an elevated uric acid. The relationship of these findings to lead exposure remains incompletely understood.

- The diagnosis of chronic lead intoxication is established by measuring a 24-hour urine lead excretion rate following the administration of ethylenediaminetetraacetic acid (EDTA) IV.
- The therapy also involves the adminstration of intramuscular EDTA to chelate lead. The urine chelatable lead levels are monitored and therapy continued until lead excretion returns to normal.

CADMIUM NEPHROTOXICITY

- Cadmium nephrotoxicity is characterized by renal dysfunction and bone disease (*Ouch Ouch* disease).
- The first reported cases occurred in the 1950s in Japan. Cadmium nephrotoxicity was caused by contamination of the Jinzu River with cadmium as a result of gold and silver mining during World War II.
- Environmental exposure is rare but may occur with ingestion of contaminated food (shellfish/mushroom) or through the respiratory tract (particularly smoking).
- Occupational hazards are also rare but may occur as a result of zinc smelting, mining, battery handling, and burning of household waste.
- Cadmium is bound by metallothionein in the liver (cadmium- and zinc-binding protein in the liver). This cadmium/metallothionein complex is absorbed by pinocytosis in the S1 segment of the proximal tubule where lysosomal enzymes release free cadmium (Cd^{2+})
- Free cytosolic cadmium induces the release of reactive oxygen species (O_2 free radicals) leading to disruption of sodium/potassium adenosine triphosphatase and mitochondrial swelling and cell necrosis.
- Cadmium causes irreversible proximal tubular dysfunction manifested as tubular proteinuria (especially low molecular proteins), renal tubular acidosis, hypercalciuria, and nephrolithiasis.
- Osteoporosis and osteomalacia are caused by impairment of vitamin D hydroxylation in the kidney.
- No specific treatment is available other than discontinuation of toxic exposure and supportive care.

CHINESE HERB–ASSOCIATED NEPHROPATHY

- First described in a group of nine Belgian women who developed rapidly progressive fibrosing interstitial nephritis in association with a slimming regimen containing Chinese herbs at a weight loss clinic in Brussels.
- In 1990, the manufacturer accidentally substituted *Aristolochia fangchi* for the Chinese herb *Stephania tetrandra* (also known as *fangji*).
- Since the original description more than 100 cases have been described worldwide; it should be suspected in patients who develop renal disease while taking herbal supplements.

PATHOGENESIS
- Aristolochic acid binds covalently to the exocyclic amino acid group of purine nucleotides to form irreversible adducts with DNA.
- This altered DNA eventually leads to dysfunction of the P53 suppressor gene leading to an increased incidence of uroepithelial malignancies.
- The DNA adducts are also believed to underlie the cellular apoptosis and eventual fibrosis seen in CIN.

PATHOLOGY
- Pathologically, the disease is characterized by hypocellular cortical interstitial fibrosis.
- Uroepithelial malignancy occurs in up to 40% to 50% of patients with ESRD.

CLINICAL PRESENTATION
- Progressive renal insufficiency.
- Proximal tubular dysfunction is manifested as nonnephrotic range tubular proteinuria.
- Bland urinary sediment is characteristic.
- Anemia is also a frequent feature.
- Most patients are normotensive.

TREATMENT
- There is no proven effective therapy.
- Regular surveillance for abnormal urinary cytology is indicated, given the high incidence of uroepithelial atypia.

REFLUX NEPHROPATHY AND CHRONIC PYELONEPHRITIS

- Reflux nephropathy results from the abnormal backflow of urine from the bladder to the renal parenchyma because of a defect at the vesicoureteral junction.
- This often is secondary to incompetence of the vesicoureteral valves.
- It is unclear weather interstitial scarring is the direct consequence of infected refluxed urine or repeated episodes of high pressure sterile reflux.
- Reflux nephropathy is characterized by scarring and tubulointerstitial fibrosis of renal tissue in association with the involved calyces.
- Children with chronic reflux present with signs and symptoms of urinary tract infection (UTI): dysuria, pyuria, flank pain, and/or fever.
- In later stages, glomerular involvement is manifested by nephrotic range proteinuria ($\geq 3.5g/24$ h). At this stage, the renal biopsy reveals focal segmental glomerulosclerosis.
- The diagnosis must be established early because advanced fibrosis can develop in childhood with high-grade vesicoureteral reflux (VUR).

TABLE 123–1 International Classification of Vesicoueretreral Reflux

GRADE	FINDINGS AND CLINICAL COURSE
I	Reflux into the ureter without dilatation. It resolves by age 5 in most cases, independent of laterality.
II	Reflux into ureter and collecting system without dilatation. It resolves by age 5 in most cases, independent of laterality.
III	Reflux and dilatation of ureter and collecting system with mild blunting of the calyces. If unilateral, spontaneous resolution occurs in most patients.
IV	Moderate dilatation of the ureter and collecting system with blunting of the calyces. Papillary contour preserved in most calyces. If unilateral, spontaneous resolution occurs in the majority of patients.
V	Intrarenal reflux may be present. Significant dilatation and tortuosity of the ureter, blunted calyces, and loss of papillary contour. Spontaneous resolution unlikely.

- Screening for VUR is indicated in childhood if a sibling or parent has a history of VUR or reflux nephropathy; otherwise screen after the child's first UTI.
- The diagnosis and grading is established through voiding cystourethrography (Table 123–1).
- Technetium-99 (^{99}Tc)-labeled dimercaptosuccinic acid (DMSA) renal scan provides excellent cortical imaging. It is the study of choice in adults with suspected reflux nephropathy.

- Reflux grades I through III usually resolve spontaneously.
- Surgery may be required in grades IV and V if reflux is bilateral particularly in pediatric patients.
- In adults with VUR, the only indication for surgery is recurrent acute pyelonephritis or persistent loin pain while voiding.

OBSTRUCTIVE NEPHROPATHY

- Chronic interstitial damage is associated with partial or intermittent long standing obstruction.
- The etiology of obstruction differs with age; in infants and children, it is usually caused by congenital abnormalities such as VUR, and in adults it is usually acquired.
- In acquired obstruction, the location reflects the etiology:
  - Intraparenchymal: crystals (uric acid, drugs, light chains)
  - Ureteral: stones, tumors, papillary necrosis, retroperitoneal fibrosis, tuberculosis, and sarcoid
  - Bladder: functional reflux in diabetes and spinal injury, stone, tumor
  - Urethra: stricture, prostate (hypertrophy, tumor), stone, anterior urethral valves (Fig. 123–4)

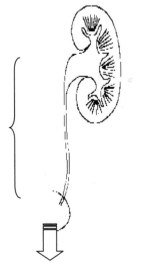

- Nephrolithiasis
- Tumors
- Irradiation fibrosis
- Papillary necrosis
- TB and sarcoidosis
- Congenital (VUR)
- Clots
- Extrinsic: tumors, retroperitoneal fibrosis, pregnancy

Intraluminal crystals:
- Urate, oxalate
- Medicines: acyclovir, indinavir
- Light chains

- Neurogenic bladder dysfunction: (autonomic dysfunction, spinal cord injury)
- Bladder stone
- Cancer

Bladder outlet obstruction:
- Prostatic hypertrophy (BPH), prostate cancer
- Urethral stricture
- Anterior urethral valves
- Stones

FIG. 123–4 Etiology of obstruction based on site. BPH, benign prostatic hyperplasia; TB, tuberculosis; VUS, vesicoureteral reflux.

CLINICAL FEATURES

- Clinical manifestations are determined by the location, time course, and etiology of the obstruction.
- Chronic obstruction usually becomes symptomatic after permanent renal damage has occurred.
- Acute obstruction presents with acute renal failure and anuria (if the obstruction is complete and bilateral).
- Patients may present with tubular dysfunction manifested as hyperkalemic renal tubular acidosis and concentrating defects.
- Hypertension is a common long-term complication of obstructive nephropathy.
- Hematuria may occur in the presence of uroepithelial tumors or nephrolithiasis.
- Crystalluria, hematuria, and flank pain are common in nephrolithiasis.
- Urinary urgency, frequency, and hesitancy is observed with prostate enlargement.
- Papillary necrosis is occasionally observed in diabetics with pyelonephritis.

DIAGNOSIS

- Renal ultrasound reveals hydronephrosis or hydroureter. Intravenous pyelography is useful to localize the level of obstruction but carries the risk associated with contrast.
- Cystoscopy and retrograde cystography are generally considered the gold standard to establish the etiology of urinary tract obstruction.
- CT or MRI may be useful to further characterize tumors, adenopathy, or retroperitoneal fibrosis.

TREATMENT

- Expeditious relief of obstruction is crucial to prevent permanent damage.
- Bladder outlet obstruction requires catheterization of the bladder without delay.
- Ureteral stenting or percutaneous nephrostomy are used to relieve upper tract obstruction. These techniques may be used as a bridge until the underlying etiology is established, or they may be employed as a palliative measure in patients with a contraindication to definitive therapy.
- Renal stones may be treated conservatively with analgesia and fluids. Larger stones may require extracorporeal shock wave lithotripsy or transurethral retrieval.

- Postobstructive diuresis refers to the increased urine output following obstruction relief. It is believed to be secondary to increased circulating natriuretic peptides, osmotic diuresis (caused by increased urea), salt wasting caused by impaired renal tubular reabsorption, and volume expansion.

CYSTIC RENAL DISEASE

- This is a group of renal diseases characterized by the development of renal cysts.
- The cysts may be acquired or hereditary (Fig. 123–5).

ACQUIRED CYSTIC DISEASE

- Acquired cystic disease is commonly identified in the presence of chronic kidney disease.
- African American men are more frequently affected.
- The incidence increases with age.
- Cysts tend to be bilateral, generally ≤4 per kidney and usually ≤0.5 cm in diameter; but occasionally they may be as large as 3 cm.

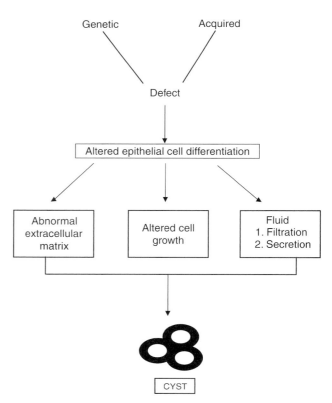

FIG. 123–5 Pathogenesis of cyst formation.

- Cysts are the result of proximal tubular epithelial hyperplasia and hypertrophy caused by nephron loss.
- For the most part, acquired cystic disease is asymptomatic. However, radiologic studies have demonstrated that cysts continue to grow in size and number, and they may be complicated by bleeding and infection. Rarely, they progress to renal cell carcinoma.
- Patients who develop hematuria or perinephric hematomas should have a CT scan or MRI to evaluate for the presence of renal cell carcinoma.

AUTOSOMAL RECESSIVE POLYCYSTIC KIDNEY DISEASE

- This is a genetic disorder that affects 1 in 6000 to 1 in 50,000 births and is characterized by increased renal size and the presence of *microcysts* in the renal parenchyma.

PATHOLOGY

- The abnormal gene (PKHD 1) is located on chromosome 6. The gene product is known as fibrocystin, a transmembrane protein localized in tubular epithelial cells of the ascending limb of the loop of Henle and collecting tubule.
- The cysts are usually 2 to 3 mm in size and are derived from ecstatic dilatation of the collecting tubule and flattening of the epithelium.

CLINICAL FEATURES

- The clinical presentation is unpredictable and determined by the severity of renal or liver involvement.
- Patients diagnosed in early infancy usually present with enlarged kidneys and renal failure.
- Tubular dysfunction is manifested by impaired urinary concentration and dilution and decreased urinary acidification giving rise to RTA.
- Hypertension and liver fibrosis are almost universal.
- Patients in their teens usually present with hepatosplenomegaly, hypersplenism, and/or variceal bleeding secondary to portal hypertension as a result of hepatic fibrosis.

DIAGNOSIS

- The diagnosis can be established with antenatal ultrasonography after the 24th gestational week. The ultrasound reveals enlarged kidneys with increased echogenicity.
- Postnatal ultrasonography reveals enlarged kidneys that are more than two standard deviations from normal.
- CT and MRI are more sensitive and may reveal microcystic dilatation of the collecting ducts.

TREATMENT

- Supportive care. Definitive therapy involves liver and kidney transplantation.

AUTOSOMAL DOMINANT POLYCYSTIC KIDNEY DISEASE

- Autosomal dominant polycystic kidney disease (ADPKD) is the most common monogenic disease affecting 1 in 500 to 1000 live births.
- It is characterized by cyst formation in the kidney, liver, and pancreas.
- The cysts eventually replace the normal renal parenchyma resulting in progressive renal dysfunction.
- The natural history of the disease is influenced by both environmental and genetic factors, and many patients may not present until the 6th decade of life.

PATHOGENESIS

- In 85% of the cases, the affected gene (PKD1) is located on the short arm of chromosome 16. It is adjacent to the gene responsible for tuberous sclerosis (TSC2) which encodes for tuberin.
- The gene product of PKD1 is known as polycystin 1 (PC1), an integral membrane protein localized to the base and tip of the primary cilium of epithelial cells in the renal tubules, bile duct, and pancreatic ducts.
- PKD1 may play a role in epithelial cell differentiation, maturation, cell–cell interactions, polarity, and extracellular matrix formation.
- The remaining cases of ADPKD are secondary to an abnormal gene (PKD2) localized to chromosome 4.
- The gene product of PKD2 (known as polycystin 2) is a voltage-activated calcium channel. It colocalizes with PC1 in the luminal membrane of tubular epithelial cells.
- Recent studies suggest that PC1 interacts with tuberin (the gene product of TSC2), and Rheb G protein to form a complex leading to the inactivation of the mammalian target of rapamycin (mTOR) a phosphatidylinositol kinase.
- In the presence of a defective PC1, mTOR is not inhibited leading to cyst formation and cellular proliferation.
- Interestingly, experimental models have demonstrated increased mTOR activity in cystic epithelial cells with defective PC1.
- In addition, cystogenesis is believed to depend on inactivation of the normal PKD1 or PKD2 allele via a *"second hit"* during fetal development or later in life. This implies a high mutagenesis rate for the PKD gene, a theory supported by the relatively high rate of sporadic cases of ADPKD.
- The phenotype of PKD1 is more severe than that observed with PKD2. Patients with PKD1 tend to develop ESRD at approximately age 55 years compared

to PKD2 patients, who tend to develop ESRD in their late 60s or early 70s.
- Cysts begin as small tubular dilatations. Their initial growth is the result of fluid accumulation and epithelial cell proliferation. As they enlarge, the cysts encroach on normal tissue resulting in compression and scarring. Eventually the surrounding fibrosis separates the cysts from the functioning nephrons. At this stage, cyst growth is the result of intrinsic cyst cell secretion of fluid.
- Progressive renal dysfunction is secondary to interstitial fibrosis and the cystic burden.

CLINICAL FEATURES
- In up to 40% of the patients, hematuria is the presenting symptom.
- Pain is a frequent complaint. Acute pain may be the result of cyst rupture, infection, or a stone.
- Chronic pain may occur in patients with severely distorted and enlarged kidneys.
- Urinary tract infection is frequent and should be treated promptly because of the increased risk of cyst infection and pyelonephritis.
- Nephrolithiasis occurs in approximately 20% of the cases. It should be entertained in the differential diagnosis of hematuria and flank pain.
- Tubular dysfunction may be manifested as concentrating and acidification defects.
- Once established, the rate of progressive renal dysfunction is approximately 5mL/min/y. It is more rapid in males requiring renal replacement therapy at an earlier age.

EXTRARENAL MANIFESTATIONS

- Liver cysts are present in approximately 75% of cases. Liver cysts are exceedingly rare before the age of 30 and increase with age.
- Colonic diverticuli occur in up to 70% of patients.
- Hypertension is present in up to 75% of patients before the development of renal dysfunction.
- Hypertension and target organ involvement, particularly left ventricular hypertrophy, occurs earlier in affected patients compared to matched controls.
- Mitral valve prolapse is the most common valvular abnormality affecting up to 25% of patients, followed by aortic regurgitant lesions affecting anywhere from 8% to 19% of patients.
- Valvular disease may progress with age as a result of myxomatous degeneration of the valve and eventually require surgical intervention.
- The incidence of intracerebral artery (ICA) berry aneurysms increases with age, on average 8% per year. ICA appears to cluster in families, occurring in up to 22% of patients with a family history of ICA or subarachnoid hemorrhage. Rupture is the most dreaded complication, occurring in approximately 4% of patients.

DIAGNOSIS AND SCREENING
- The diagnosis of ADPKD is confirmed by renal ultrasonography.
- In approximately 40% of the cases, the diagnosis is established during an evaluation of hematuria and/or progressive renal insufficiency of unknown etiology.
- In patients with a family history of a berry aneurysm, presymptomatic screening by ultrasound is not recommended before the age of 20 years, because cystic involvement of the kidney may not be apparent yet.
- Diagnostic criteria for patients with an affected parent includes at least two cysts present in one or both kidneys before the age of 30 years, at least two cysts in each kidney between the ages of 30 to 59 years, and at least four cysts after the age of 60 years.
- Screening for a berry aneurysm is recommended in those patients with a family history of ICA or subarachnoid hemorrhage.

TREATMENT
- There is no specific therapy for the disease, but recent animal studies suggest promising results through the inactivation of mTOR.
- Treatment is otherwise supportive and geared toward the management of complications.
- Optimal blood pressure control to delay progression of renal insufficiency and target organ involvement is recommended. Usually, ACE inhibitors and angiotensin receptor blockers are employed because they are believed to attenuate renal fibrosis.
- Urinary tract infections should be treated promptly to prevent pyelonephritis and cyst infection.
- Chronic flank pain may require surgical intervention (cyst debulking) if medical management has failed and infection, stone, or tumor have been ruled out.
- An annual magnetic resonance angiography is appropriate for asymptomatic aneurysms less than 5 mm. Surgical clipping is appropriate for aneurysms ≥10 mm or if the size increases. Optimal management for aneurysms between 6 and 9 mm is controversial.

BALKAN ENDEMIC NEPHROPATHY

- Balkan nephropathy is a chronic tubulointerstitial disease of unclear etiology. Environmental and genetic factors have been implicated.
- It typically affects those living in the confluence of the Danube River.
- Balkan endemic nephropathy progresses over more than 20 years; the kidneys are usually small with a smooth contour. There is minimal cellular infiltration, however, interstitial fibrosis, and tubular atrophy are extensive.

- In some of the Balkan regions, it accounts for up to 10% of patients with ESRD.
- There is an increased incidence of uroepithelial tumors.

BIBLIOGRAPHY

Bagnis CI, Deray G, Baumelou A, et al. Herbs and the kidney. *Am J Kidney Dis.* 2004;44(1):1.

Brenner BM. *Brenner and Rector's The Kidney.* Elsevier Saunders; 2004.

McMorrow T, Gaffney MM, Slattery C, et al. Cyclosporine A induced epithelial-mesenchymal transition in human proximal tubular epithelial cells. *Nephrol Dial Transplant.* 2005;20: 2215.

Rossert J. Drug-induced acute interstitial nephritis. *Kidney Int.* 2001;60:804.

Shillingford JM, Murcia NS, et al. The mTOR pathway is regulated by polycystin-1 and its inhibition reverses renal cystogenesis in polycystic kidney disease. *Proc Natl Acad Sci U S A.* 2006;103:5466.

Tahvanainen E, Tahvanainen P, Kääriäinen H, Höckerstedt K. Polycystic liver and kidney diseases. *Ann Med.* 2005;37(8): 546.

Van Vleet TR, Schnellmann RG. Toxic nephropathy: Environmental chemicals. *Semin Nephrol.* 2003;23(5):500.

124 PATHOPHYSIOLOGY AND TREATMENT OF KIDNEY STONES

Rizwan A. Qazi and Bahar Bastani

EPIDEMIOLOGY

- Nephrolithiasis affects nearly 500,000 people in the United States and accounts for 1:1000 hospital admissions.
- It is two to three times more common in males, and the incidence peaks between ages 30 and 50 years.
- It is uncommon in African American, Asian, and Native American populations.
- Of recurrent calcium stone formers, 60% to 80% have a first-degree relative with stone disease.
- The types of renal stones encountered clinically and their frequency is summarized in Table 124–1.
- Renal calculi, generated in the kidney, travel downstream until they become lodged in one of four sites:

TABLE 124–1 Types of Renal Stone and Their Frequency

STONE COMPOSITION	FREQUENCY(%)	CRYSTALS IN THE URINE
Calcium oxalate and calcium phosphate	37	Octahedrons or amorphous
Calcium oxalate	26	Octahedrons
Magnesium ammonium phosphate	22	Coffin lid
Calcium phosphate	7	Amorphous crystals
Uric acid	5–10	Diamonds or amorphous
Cystine	2	Hexagons

the renal calyx, ureteropelvic junction (UPJ), pelvic brim, and ureterovesical junction (UVJ).
- Recurrence of renal calculi is very common such that over a 20-year period almost 75% of the patients will have a recurrence. The recurrence rate is particularly high in the first two years (almost 40%).

PATHOPHYSIOLOGY

- Renal calculi develop when there is an imbalance in the conditions (pH, urine volume, concentration of stone forming elements such as calcium) favoring stone formation versus those that inhibit stone growth (solubilizers such as citrate).
- In general, stone-forming elements must exceed a threshold concentration and also exist in the optimum ionic form for stones to develop. The ionic state of stone-forming elements is dependent on the urine pH, citrate concentration, and urine volume. Importantly, these conditions can be manipulated to minimize stone formation and are the basis of many successful therapeutic approaches.
- A crucial step in the pathogenesis of nephrolithiasis is supersaturation of the urine with stone-forming elements and subsequent formation of solid-phase nuclei (stone nidus). For example, when the ionic concentration of calcium, phosphorus, oxalate, uric acid, and cystine is raised sufficiently, the solution becomes unstable and solid-phase nucleation (precipitation) of the element occurs. This mechanism is referred to as *homogenous nucleation*. The locus for homogenous nucleation is believed to be cellular irregularities in the urinary tract.
- Heterogeneous nucleation (the underlying mechanism of stone growth in humans) involves the precipitation of a crystal on a preformed nidus which lowers the level of supersaturation required for crystal formation in the urine. The factors that may serve as a nidus in heterogeneous nucleation include nidus solid-phase nuclei cellular debris, and proteinaceous material.

- The phenomenon of heterogeneous nucleation involving one solid-phase crystal serving as a nidus for another solid-phase crystal is also referred to as *epitaxy*.
- Because development of the initial template is essential for subsequent stone growth, it is important to consider therapies that can inhibit the template involved in heterogeneous nucleation. For example, lowering the urinary uric acid concentration (crystalline template), in stones predominately comprised of calcium phosphate or calcium oxalate may be beneficial in preventing epitaxy and stone growth.

LABORATORY TESTS AND RADIOLOGIC STUDIES

- Blood chemistries, calcium, phosphorus, and a routine urinalysis are usually done as part of the initial investigation of all patients with nephrolithiasis. Urine cultures should be obtained if there is clinical suspicion of urinary tract infection or pyuria on the urinalysis.
- The comprehensive workup of nephrolithiasis should include two or three 24-hour urine collections for: volume, pH, calcium, phosphorus, oxalate, citrate, sodium, uric acid, magnesium, sulfate, and creatinine excretion; along with a one-time urine screen for cystine, a serum uric acid, and a parathyroid hormone (PTH) level (if the serum calcium level is high).
- The comprehensive workup is typically delayed by at least 3 to 4 weeks after an acute stone and need not be performed in adult patients who are first time stone formers, and otherwise healthy with no family history of kidney stones.
- Noncontrast helical CT is 95% to 100% sensitive and specific for detection of renal calculi and, therefore, is the imaging modality of choice.
- Renal ultrasonography although very specific, is only 25% to 50% sensitive for detecting nonobstructing stones, especially involving the ureter.
- Calculi should, when available, be submitted for chemical analysis.

MAJOR CLASSES OF KIDNEY STONES AND THEIR MANAGEMENT

Calcium-based stones (calcareous stones) are the most common stones encountered. Other less common types of stones include struvite, uric acid, and cystine.

CALCIUM-CONTAINING STONES

- Calcium is solely or partly responsible for approximately 70% to 75% of all kidney stones.

- The urinary abnormalities encountered on a comprehensive workup of recurrent calcium stone formers are as follows:
  ○ Hypercalciuria (40%–50%)
  ○ Hypocitraturia (30%–40%)
  ○ Hyperuricosuria (30%–40%)
  ○ Hyperoxaluria (30%)
  ○ Hypomagnesuria (20%)
  ○ Urine volume of <1.5 L/24 h (60%)
  ○ No risk factors discovered (2%)

HYPERCALCIURIA

- Hypercalciuria is the most common metabolic disturbance associated with renal calculus formation. It is defined as a urinary calcium excretion of >300 mg/24 h in males and >250 mg/24 h in females.
- Hypercalciuria is idiopathic in 90% to 95% of patients, and secondary in 5% to 10% (Fig. 124–1).
- Secondary hypercalciuria can develop in the following conditions: primary hyperparathyroidism, malignancies associated with bony metastasis, granulomatous diseases (eg, sarcoidosis, histoplasmosis), lymphoma's, multiple myeloma, Paget disease, prolonged immobilization, Cushing syndrome, hyperthyroidism, distal renal tubular acidosis (dRTA), loop diuretic use, and milk-alkali syndrome.
- Primary hyperparathyroidism should be suspected when concomitant hypercalcemia and hypophosphatemia are present. It is important to recognize that a "normal" PTH level is considered inappropriately elevated in a patient with high, or high-normal serum calcium concentration.
- Hypercalcemia of malignancy is typically associated with very high levels of calcium, often greater than 14 mg/dL.
- The history is essential in ruling out overzealous calcium and vitamin D use or the milk-alkali syndrome.
- Urinary calcium excretion increases with increased protein intake, particularly meat protein. This effect is independent of dietary calcium content.
- The etiology of idiopathic hypercalciuria remains incompletely understood. Many of these patients (50%) have hyperabsorption of calcium from their gastrointestinal tract (absorptive hypercalciuria); some have renal phosphate leak (19%), or renal calcium leak, and a small number appear to mobilize excessive calcium from bone.
- Distal RTA is one of the secondary causes of hypercalciuria. Systemic acidosis that accompanies distal RTA induces bone resorption, which promotes hypercalciuria. The alkaline urinary pH that often accompanies dRTA causes calcium (Ca)-phosphate to precipitate in the urine. Distal RTA is also associated with hypocitraturia because of the presence of hypokalemia and intracellular acidosis in the proximal tubular epithelial cells. These two

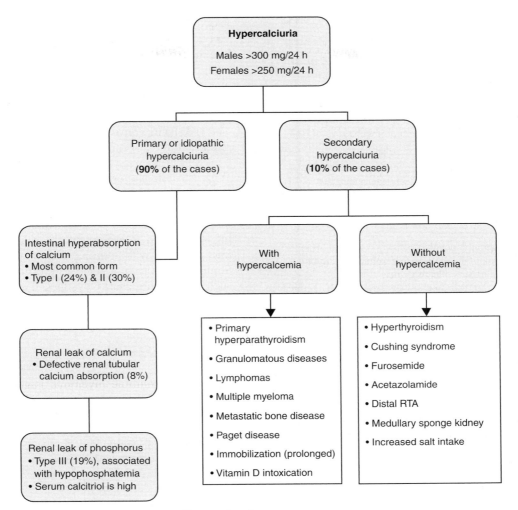

FIG. 124–1   Type and causes of hypercalcemia. RTA, renal tubular acidosis.

effects conspire to promote citrate reabsorption in the proximal tubule, and thus, promote hypocitraturia. Both hypocitraturia and hypercalciuria are important in the eventual development of renal calculi.

- Tubular calcium reabsorption is increased by thiazide diuretics or amiloride. Amiloride also maintains the serum potassium concentration. Thus, these two diuretics are useful in the management of renal calculus formation secondary to dRTA.

HYPOCITRATURIA

- Typically defined as a urinary citrate excretion of less than 300 mg/24 h.
- Various conditions are associated with hypocitraturia including:
  - Distal renal tubular acidosis
  - Chronic kidney disease with systemic acidosis
  - Acetazolamide therapy
  - Hypokalemia
  - Idiopathic (20%)
- Most of these conditions increase reabsorption of filtered citrate in the proximal tubule.
- Importantly, any condition that results in an intracellular acidosis in the proximal convoluted tubule (PCT) epithelial cells (eg, systemic acidosis, exercise, starvation, chronic kidney disease, infections, etc) will promote citrate reabsorption and hence lower the urinary concentration of citrate (Fig. 124–2).
- Therapy with potassium citrate can be employed to raise the urinary citrate concentration.

HYPEROXALURIA

- Hyperoxaluria occurs in up to 30% of calcium-containing stone formers.
- Hyperoxaluria can be primary, because of specific enzyme deficiencies, or secondary because of increased

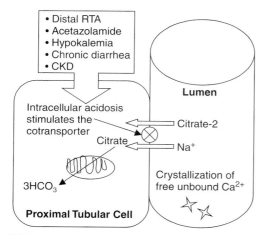

FIG. 124–2 Intracellular acidosis causing increased absorption of citrate in the proximal tubule with resultant precipitation of calcium and oxalate in the collecting duct.
Ca^{2+}, calcium ion; CKD, chronic kidney disease; $3HCO_3$, bicarbonate; Na^+, sodium ion; RTA, renal tubular acidosis.

delivery of uncomplexed oxalate to the colon which is then absorbed into the circulation (Fig. 124–3).

- Oral intake of calcium decreases the absorption of oxalate. Thus, if intestinal calcium content is reduced because of decreased oral intake or increased binding of dietary calcium to bile acids (pancreatic insufficiency, intestinal malabsorption, or jejunoileal bypass surgery) then additional oxalate is absorbed into the circulation resulting in hyperoxaluria. Therefore, stone formers should *not* markedly reduce their dietary calcium intake.

HYPERURICOSURIA

- The normal uric acid excretion in the urine is <800 mg/24 h in men and <750 mg/24 h in women.
- Hyperuricosuria can result in uric acid caculi, or can contribute to calcium-oxalate stones via heterogeneous nucleation with epitaxy (see above).
- Hyperuricosuria occurs when the production of uric acid is increased (eg, increased dietary purine intake, inborn errors of purine metabolism, or increased turnover of nucleic acids from leukemias, lymphomas, multiple myeloma, hemolytic anemia, and psoriasis).
- Other conditions associated with uric acid stone formation include gout, chronic diarrhea, and a low urine volume (<1.5 L/day) coupled with an acidic urine pH.

MAGNESIUM AMMONIUM PHOSPHATE STONES (STRUVITE STONES)

- Also known as *infection* or *triple phosphate stones.*
- Often secondary to an infection with a urease-producing bacteria such as Proteus, Klebsiella, Citrobacter,

Pseudomonas, and Enterococci. These bacteria convert urinary urea into carbon dioxide (CO_2) and ammonia; the latter alkalinizes urine and precipitates struvite (magnesium ammonium phosphate [$MgNH_4PO_4$]) crystals.

- The presence of urinary bacteria and leukocytes are required for the diagnosis of struvite stones.
- The risk factors involved in struvite stone formation include female gender and patients with chronic/recurrent urinary tract infections (paraplegia).
- When struvite stones involve more than one calyx, it is referred as a *staghorn calculus.*
- In addition to general supportive measures, optimal treatment of these stones requires removal of all existing stones and treatment of the underlying urinary tract infection with antimicrobial agents.
- Some patients have a coexisting urinary abnormality such as hyperuricosuria, cystinuria, or hypercalciuria that should be treated accordingly.

URIC ACID STONES

- Hyperuricemia and hyperuricosuria are found in up to 20% of patients.
- Dehydration can contribute to uric acid lithiasis in up to 10% of affected individuals.
- The most important factor promoting uric acid nephrolithiasis is an acidic urine pH, which is usually <5.5. Uric acid solubility decreases in a logarithmic fashion with a decrease in urine pH.
- Uric acid stones are radiolucent (not visible on plain radiography).
- Treatment is aimed at raising the urine pH by alkali administration, (or occasionally by using acetazolamide), decreasing protein intake, judicious use of allopurinol, and forced diuresis (>2.5 L/d).

CYSTINE STONES

- Cystinuria is a rare autosomal recessive disorder in which there is a tubular defect in the amino acid transport of dicarboxylic amino acids such as cystine, ornithine, arginine, and lysine. Homozygosity is usually necessary for stone formation.
- The disease usually manifests in the fourth or fifth decade of life.
- The associated risk factors include a low urine volume, urine pH of <7, and a diet rich in salt and methionine.
- Cystine is poorly soluble in urine with a saturation limit of approximately 240 to 480 mg/L. Therapy should be directed toward reducing the saturation of cystine in the urine to less than 200 mg/dL.

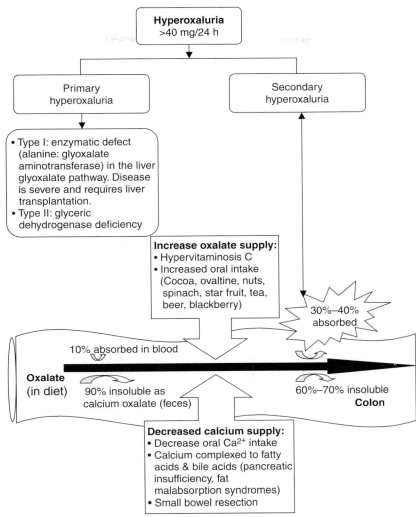

FIG. 124–3 Types and causes of hyperoxaluria.
Ca^{2+}, calcium ion.

• The addition of sodium nitroprusside to a urine sample with more than 75 mg of cystine per gram of creatinine results in a positive reaction and is a valuable screening test for cystinuria. A 24-hour urine cystine excretion rate can confirm the diagnosis.

HEREDITARY NEPHROLITHIASIS

Hereditary diseases involving specific enzymes, hormonal perturbations, and receptor abnormalities are associated with nephrolithiasis. These include: adenine/hypoxanthine phosphoribosyl transferase deficiency, hereditary hypomagnesemic hypercalciuria (paracellulin-1 mutation), hereditary hyperoxaluria, X-linked recessive nephrolithiasis with renal failure (Dent disease), cystinuria, and familial hyperparathyroidism. Distal renal tubular acidosis, which is an important risk factor for nephrolithiasis, can also be hereditary (autosomal dominant or recessive).

DRUG-INDUCED NEPHROLITHIASIS

• Indinavir, which is a protease inhibitor used to treat HIV infection, causes crystalluria in 20% of patients and renal stones in 4% to 43% of the patients.
• Ephedrine (Ma-Huang extract) is an energy supplement that is associated with kidney stones in 0.06% of patients.
• Star fruit (Chinese remedy) can cause acute oxalate nephropathy.
• Sulfonamide administration for an extended period (usually >4 weeks) can produce stones.
• Loop diuretics cause hypercalciuria, which is a risk factor for nephrolithiasis.

- Acetazolamide causes hypokalemia, metabolic acidosis, hypocitraturia, and hypercalciuria, all of which are important risk factors for stone formation.
- Probenecid, salicylates, and ablative chemotherapies are associated with hyperuricemia and uric acid stones.

MANAGEMENT OF ACUTE RENAL COLIC

The classic patient presents with acute colicky flank pain radiating to the groin and genitalia, with or without gross hematuria. A previous history of kidney stones should be sought. Acutely, these patients should be treated with a potent analgesic, for example, ketorolac 30 mg intravenous (IV) or 60 mg intramuscular (IM), or meperidine 50 to 150 mg IM, followed by aggressive hydration. Routine complete blood count, blood chemistries, urinalysis, and urine culture should be performed. Blood cultures can be obtained and IV antibiotics initiated if an infection is suspected. A noncontrast spiral CT scan of the abdomen and pelvis using a stone protocol is the imaging modality of choice. Once the stone has passed or been removed, additional studies may be performed to identify risk factors and prevent further stone formation.

Immediate urologic consult is usually recommended if the following exists:
- Urosepsis induced by an obstructing stone
- Kidney stones larger than 7 mm (it is unusual for these stones to spontaneously pass)
- Complete ureteral obstruction on imaging
- Solitary kidney with a kidney stone (high risk of renal injury)
- Acute renal failure and hydronephrosis
- Persistent colicky pain

Acute renal failure can be relieved by percutaneous nephrostomy and lithotripsy. Extracorporeal shock wave lithotripsy (ESWL) or retrograde basket are important nonsurgical interventions that successfully eliminate large or obstructing stones.

RISK FACTOR MODIFICATION TO PREVENT RECURRENCE OF KIDNEY STONES

GENERAL MEASURES

- Adequate fluid intake to ensure greater than 2.5 L of urine/ d, (approximately 4L in the case of cystine stones).
- Limit animal protein intake to 0.8 to 1.0 g/kg per day, and institute a low purine diet.

- Modest dietary calcium intake (ie, dairy products), but avoid calcium supplements.
- Correct electrolyte abnormalities such as a low serum potassium and magnesium.
- Specific measures based on urinary abnormalities:
  - Low salt diet (less than 3–4 g/d) in patients with hypercalciuria or cystinuria.
  - Low-oxalate diet in patients with hyperoxaluria.
  - Calcium carbonate, as an oxalate binder, in enteric hyperoxaluria.

PHARMACOLOGIC OPTIONS

- Chlorthalidone or thiazide diuretics to reduce hypercalciuria.
- Urocit K or Polycitra-K (potassium citrate) in doses of 20 mEq twice or three times daily, corrects acidosis, alkalinizes the urine, and corrects hypocitraturia. This is a valuable treatment option for most kidney stone formers regardless of the etiology.
- Calcibind (cellulose sodium phosphate) can bind dietary calcium and hence can diminish hypercalciuria, although it can exacerbate secondary hyperoxaluria and accelerate osteoporosis. This drug is very seldom used, and only in selected patients with severe absorptive hypercalciuria.
- D-penicillamine and tiopronin (Thiola) form soluble complexes with cystine and hence can be helpful in patients with hypercystinuria.
- The angiotensin-converting enzyme (ACE) inhibitor captopril reduces the cystine content of the urine.
- Allopurinol reduces hyperuricosuria.
- Pyridoxine can reduce urinary oxalate levels in some patients with type 1 primary hyperoxaluria.

BIBLIOGRAPHY

Borghi L, Schianchi T, Meschi T, et al. Comparison of two diets for the prevention of recurrent stones in idiopathic hypercalciuria. *N Engl J Med.* 2002;346:77–84.

Coe FL, Evan A, Worcester E. Kidney stone disease. *J Clin Invest.* 2005;115(10):2598–2608.

Frick KK, Bushinsky DA. Molecular mechanisms of primary hypercalciuria. *J Am Soc Nephrol.* 2003;14(4):1082–95.

Johnson RJ, Feehally J. *Comprehensive Clinical Nephrology.* New York, NY: Mosby; 2003.

Leumann E, Hoppe B. The primary hyperoxalurias. *J Am Soc Nephrol.* 2001;12:1986–1993.

Taylor EN, Curhan GC. Diet and fluid prescription in stone disease. *Kidney Int.* 2006;70(5):835–839.

125 CLINICAL HYPERTENSION

Paul G. Schmitz

EPIDEMIOLOGY

- Hypertension affects nearly 65 million Americans, yet less than 30% achieve the target or goal blood pressure (NHANES dataset).
- Age-adjusted mortality rates for stroke and coronary artery disease have declined in the past 20 years; however, the incidence of end-stage renal disease and congestive heart failure are increasing.
- The Seventh Report of the Joint National Committee on Prevention, Detection, Evaluation, and Treatment of High Blood Pressure (JNC VII) revised the classification scheme into four stages (Table 125–1).
- *White coat* or office hypertension may account for as many as 20% of elevated blood pressures and is associated with an increased cardiovascular risk.
- Isolated systolic hypertension (ISH), defined as a systolic blood pressure ≥160 mm Hg and a diastolic blood pressure ≤90 mm Hg, is a far greater risk factor for the development of cardiovascular disease than is the diastolic blood pressure.

The systolic blood pressure increases in a linear fashion throughout life, whereas, the diastolic blood pressure increases until 50 years of age and falls thereafter. This phenomenon is thought to reflect a gradual decrease in arterial compliance over time (due to remodeling and calcification of the vessel wall). The decrease in compliance causes an increase in blood pressure during systole and a decrease during diastole (because of loss of the elastic recoil which augments pressure during diastole). Because a decrease in compliance in the vessel is related to vascular remodeling and calcification, ISH is a de facto clinical marker of injury in the vessel wall.

PATHOPHYSIOLOGY

While an increase in cardiac output has been described in some patients with hypertension, an increase in peripheral arterial resistance is the principal variable responsible for the persistence of hypertension. A number of theories have evolved to explain a sustained increase in blood pressure.

- Evidence for a genetic influence on blood pressure is derived from twin studies and population-based studies, which reveal a greater concordance between blood pressure in monozygotic twins and within families. Moreover, gene mutations have been described which alter renal sodium handling and are associated with hypertension in some families.
- Cardiovascular risk factors tend to cosegregate with hypertension; for example, 40% of patients with hypertension have hypercholesterolemia. Insulin resistance, which is associated with heightened sensitivity to vasoconstrictor compounds, may explain the relationship between dyslipidemia and hypertension.
- Stress leading to sympathetic nerve discharge promotes structural changes in the vessels, decreasing vessel wall compliance. An increase in sympathetic tone also promotes metabolic (insulin resistance), hemodynamic (vasoconstriction), and thrombotic (platelet activation) derangements which contribute to endothelial dysfunction.

TABLE 125–1   Classification of Blood Pressure for Adults ≥ 18 Years of Age[a]

CLASS	SYSTOLIC BLOOD PRESSURE (mm Hg)	DIASTOLIC BLOOD PRESSURE (mm Hg)
Normal	<120	<80
Prehypertension	120–139	80–89
Hypertension, Stage 1	140–159	90–99
Hypertension, Stage 2	≥160	≥100

[a]Not taking antihypertensive drugs and not acutely ill. When systolic and diastolic pressures fall into different categories, the higher category should be selected to classify the individual's blood pressure status. In addition to classifying the stages of hypertension on the basis of average blood pressure levels, the clinician should specify presence or absence of target-organ damage and additional risk factors. This specificity is important for risk classification and management. Optimal blood pressure with respect to cardiovascular risk is less than 120 mm Hg systolic and less than 80 mm Hg diastolic. Should be based on the average of 2 or more readings taken at each of 2 or more visits after an initial screening.
Source: Chobanian AV, Bakris GL, Black HR, et al. The Seventh Report of the Joint National Committee on Prevention, Detection, Evaluation, and Treatment of High Blood Pressure. *JAMA*. 2003;289:2560–2572.

- Tropic cytokines, peptides, and growth factors (angiotensin II, natriuretic hormone, catecholamines, insulin) have been shown to correlate with vascular hypertrophy and a decrease in vessel wall compliance.
- Angiotensin II increases systemic blood pressure by increasing vascular resistance and inducing vessel wall remodeling. Angiotensin II also promotes salt and water retention.

DIAGNOSIS

Blood pressure measurements should be obtained in the sitting position after 5 minutes of rest. The blood pressure should be obtained twice, 5 minutes apart and confirmed in the contralateral arm. Routine use of ambulatory blood pressure monitoring is not currently recommended. However, several situations in which 24-hour ambulatory blood pressure may prove useful are:

- Office or white coat hypertension (blood pressure repeatedly elevated in the office setting but repeatedly normal out of the office).
- Evaluation of multidrug resistance.
- Evaluation of nocturnal blood pressure.
- Episodic or labile hypertension.
- Hypotensive symptoms associated with antihypertensive medications or autonomic dysfunction.

CLINICAL AND LABORATORY FEATURES

- Assess family history.
- Assess risk factors and comorbidities; cardiovascular, renal disease, diabetes mellitus, dyslipidemia.
- Assess lifestyle: weight gain, leisure time, physical activities, smoking, and alcohol use.
- Dietary assessment, including sodium intake and intake of cholesterol and saturated fats.
- Funduscopic examination (with pupil dilation if necessary) for arteriolar narrowing, arteriovenous nicking, hemorrhages, exudates, or papilledema.
- Examination of the neck for carotid bruits, distended neck veins, or an enlarged thyroid gland.
- Examination of the heart for increased rate, increased size, precordial heave, clicks, murmurs, arrhythmias, and third (S3) and fourth (S4) heart sounds.
- Examination of the abdomen for bruits, enlarged kidneys, and abnormal aortic pulsation.
- Examination of the extremities for diminished or absent peripheral arterial pulsations, bruits, and edema.
- Obtain laboratory tests: urinalysis, blood glucose, hematocrit, lipid panel, serum potassium, creatinine, calcium, and urinary albumin/creatinine ratio (optional).

- Obtain electrocardiogram

Additional testing may be indicated in those patients with features suggestive of secondary hypertension such as:

- Age of onset younger than 20 years of age and older than 50 years of age.
- Presence of other features suggestive of secondary hypertension such as unprovoked hypokalemia, abdominal bruit, labile blood pressure with tachycardia, sweating, and tremor, and family history of renal disease.
- Refractory to combination (usually ≥3 drugs) therapy.

THERAPEUTIC APPROACH

The management of hypertension typically involves both lifestyle modifications and pharmacologic therapies (Fig. 125–1). Both are required to achieve target blood pressure. Lifestyle modifications are initiated before pharmacologic interventions unless the blood pressure is stage 2, target organ disease is present, or a comorbid condition exists which is favorably influenced by a specific antihypertensive drug.

LIFESTYLE MODIFICATIONS

- *Weight reduction.* Target body mass index of 18.5 to 24.9 kg/m^2. **Average systolic blood pressure (SBP) reduction of 5 to 20 mm Hg per 10 kg weight loss**.
- *Moderate alcohol intake.* Men: limit to ≤2 drinks (15 mL of ethanol). Women and lighter weight persons: limit to ≤1 drink per day. **Average SBP reduction of 2 to 4 mm Hg**.
- *Regular aerobic physical activity.* Brisk walking at least 30 minutes per day, most days of the week. **Average SBP reduction of 4 to 9 mm Hg**.
- *Reduce dietary sodium intake.* Decrease to ≤100 mmol/day (2.4 g of Na or 6 gm of NaCl). **Average SBP reduction of 2 to 8 mm Hg**.
- *Dietary Approaches to Stop Hypertension (DASH) diet.* Adopt a diet rich in fruits, vegetables, and low fat dairy products with reduced content of saturated and total fat. **Average SBP reduction of 2 to 8 mm Hg**.

PHARMACOLOGIC THERAPIES

A variety of drugs are available to manage the patient with hypertension. These agents can be classified into seven categories (prototypes)

- Diuretics (hydrochlorothiazide).
- Adrenergic inhibitors (α-blocker, prazosin; β-blocker, propranolol; mixed, labetalol; centrally acting, clonidine).
- Direct vasodilators (hydralazine).
- Calcium channel blockers (CCBs), such as nifedipine.

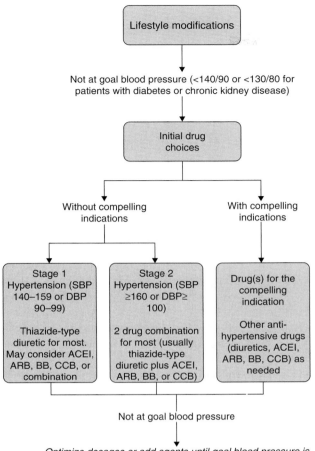

FIG. 125–1 Approach to the treatment of hypertension.
ACEI, angiotensin-converting enzyme inhibitor; ARB, angiotensin
receptor blocker; BB, β-blocker; CCB, calcium channel blocker.
SOURCE: Adapted from Chobanian AV, Bakris GL, Black HR, et al.
The Seventh Report of the Joint National Committee on Prevention,
Detection, Evaluation, and Treatment of High Blood Pressure.
JAMA. 2003;289:2560–2572.

- Converting-enzyme inhibitors (CEI) such as captopril.
- Angiotensin I (AT1)-receptor blockers (losartan).
- Direct inhibitors of renin (aliskiren)

Importantly, only diuretics, β-blockers, and CEI have
been proven to reduce morbidity and mortality in hypertension. In addition, it is important to base the initial
choice of therapy on a patients comorbid conditions. For
example, a patient with a history of cardiovascular disease will likely benefit from β-blocker therapy, whereas
these agents would be contraindicated in the setting of
chronic obstructive pulmonary disease.

β-BLOCKERS
- Decreased mortality from coronary artery disease
  (CAD) and congestive heart failure (CHF)
- Decreased incidence and progression of CAD

- Decreased mortality after a myocardial infarction
- Greater efficacy in high-renin hypertension
- Modest cost
- May lower high-density lipoprotein (HDL) cholesterol
- Sexual dysfunction in men is common

THIAZIDE DIURETICS
- Protection against cardiovascular events (equal or
  better than others)
- Inexpensive
- Greater efficacy in salt-sensitive hypertension
- May increase low-density lipoprotein (LDL) and total
  cholesterol (usually shortlived)
- May produce hypokalemia and hyperglycemia
- May worsen impotence and fatigue
- Likely to protect the elderly against hip fractures by
  decreasing urinary Ca2+ excretion

CALCIUM-CHANNEL BLOCKERS
- Greater efficacy in African Americans and the elderly
  (low-renin hypertension or ISH)
- Effective for symptomatic management of CAD, but
  little data to support a long-term beneficial effect on car-
  diovascular endpoints (except in the elderly with ISH).
- Sustained release (SR) formulations minimize side
  effects, improve compliance, and are more effective
- No adverse effects on lipids or glucose
- Little adverse effects on quality of life
- Often expensive

CONVERTING-ENZYME INHIBITORS
- Greater efficacy in high-renin essential hypertension
- No adverse effects on lipids or glucose
- May raise potassium and precipitate reversible acute
  renal insufficiency
- Cough is observed in more than 10%
- Excellent quality of life
- Retards progression and reduces the incidence of
  nephropathy in diabetes and perhaps other forms of
  chronic kidney disease.
- Often expensive

ANGIOTENSIN RECEPTOR ANTAGONISTS
- Block AT1 receptors selectively
- Recent clinical trials suggest similar efficacy in cardiac
  and renal disease as compared to ACE-inhibitors
- May engender unique properties by diverting angiotensin
  II to other angiotensin receptor subtypes (vasodilation
  and inhibition of vessel wall remodeling)
- Low incidence of cough

DIRECT RENIN INHIBITORS
- Aliskiren is the first high blood pressure drug approved
  by FDA that inhibits renin

- The effectiveness of aliskiren in lowering blood pressure has been demonstrated in six placebo-controlled 8 week clinical trials, which studied more than 2000 patients with mild to moderate hypertension.
- Aliskiren may prove especially useful in cardiovascular and renal disease (because of its effects on the renin-angiotensin system), although studies have not been published in these specific areas

SECONDARY CAUSES OF HYPERTENSION

- Renal vascular disease (5%– 8%)
- Primary hyperaldosteronism (1%–2%)
- Cushing's syndrome (<1%)
- Pheochromocytoma (<1%)
- Coarctation of the aorta (<1%)

RENOVASCULAR HYPERTENSION

The exact incidence of renovascular hypertension (RVH) is almost certainly underestimated in the vast population of patients with clinically detectable stage 1 or greater high blood pressure. Indeed, many cases of renal vascular disease are diagnosed at the time of an autopsy. Regardless, renovascular hypertension is the most common cause of secondary hypertension. The clinical and laboratory features of RVH include:

- Atherosclerotic vascular disease in 60% to 70% (usually men)
- Fibromuscular dysplasia in 20% to 30% (usually women)
- Age younger than 20 years of age or older than 50 years of age
- Familial occurrence of some fibromuscular dysplasias
- Acute deterioration of renal function is common after administering an ACE-I
- Abdominal bruits
- Unprovoked hypokalemia with metabolic alkalosis (secondary hyperaldosteronism)
- Unilateral small kidney on x-ray suggesting renal artery ischemia

On the basis of the above clinical clues, patients with suspected renovascular hypertension should be screened for the presence of renal artery stenosis. While no test at the present time completely satisfies the criteria as an ideal screening study (simple, safe, inexpensive, easy to perform, sensitive, and specific), magnetic resonance angiography appears to provide the best balance of sensitivity, specificity, performance, and safety.

A recent FDA alert, issued on December 22, 2006, reported 90 cases of nephrogenic systemic fibrosis (NSF) in patients with moderate to end-stage renal failure. NSF is a debilitating and potentially fatal condition, occurring within 2 days to 18 months of receiving gadodiamide. Therefore, caution should be exercised in patients with a serum creatinine >2.0 mg/dL when considering gadolinium based studies.

The principal goals of therapy in this disorder are:
- Preservation of renal function
- Amelioration of blood pressure (less likely in atherosclerotic vascular disease)

PRIMARY HYPERALDOSTERONISM

- The incidence of primary hyperaldosteronism ranges between 0.5% and 2.2% of all hypertensives.
- Causes include an aldosterone producing adenoma (30%–60%) or bilateral zona glomerulosa hyperplasia.
- Hypokalemia occurs with or without metabolic alkalosis accompanied by inappropriate potassium loss in the urine.
- Increased circulating plasma aldosterone coupled with suppressed plasma renin activity (because of volume expansion) are common.

Of the currently utilized readily available laboratory tests to screen for primary hyperaldosteronism, the following are particularly useful:
- Suppression of plasma renin activity to <5 ng/dL (not on diuretics or CEI) is highly sensitive but relatively nonspecific
- Ratio of plasma aldosterone to plasma renin of >30:1
- A 24-hour urinary aldosterone (>15 ng/24 h) on a high NaCl diet is highly suggestive of primary hyperaldosteronism, provided the patient is not volume contracted (eg, excreting approximately 200 mEq NaCl per day).

Surgery is the procedure of choice for unilateral adrenal adenoma. Spironolactone is very effective in controlling blood pressure and the plasma potassium in patients with hyperplasia. Amiloride and triamterene are alternate, albeit less effective, medical therapies.

PHEOCHROMOCYTOMA

This rare tumor is believed to occur in less than 1% of all patients with hypertension. It is most commonly diagnosed between the ages of 30 and 60 years. The clinical features suggestive of pheochromocytoma include:
- Hypertension (50% are paroxysmal)
- Hypermetabolism (tachycardia, anxiety, fever, and palpitations)
- Headache
- Sweating

- Hyperglycemia
- Orthostatic hypotension (not taking antihypertensive drugs)
- Malignant tumors are rare and metastasize at a surprisingly low rate

Because incidentally discovered adrenal masses are increasingly recognized, imaging studies such as computed tomography (CT) and magnetic resonance imaging (MRI) should be supplemented by biochemical tests of increased catecholamine production. The biochemical evaluation of catecholamine production can be affected by many drugs (labetalol and tricyclic antidepressants) and conditions (stress, anxiety).

- The best screening test is a 24-hour urinary metanephrine (especially when the blood pressure is increased).
- The clonidine suppression test has also been advocated in the diagnosis of pheochromocytoma. The rationale for this test is that clonidine suppresses plasma catecholamine release in normal patients but not in patients with pheochromocytoma.
- Recent studies have advocated the use of 131I-MIBG (metaiodobenzylguanidine) scanning to localize the tumor (rather than CT). The latter compound is extracted from plasma by neuronal tissue.
- Surgery, when possible, is the treatment of choice.
- Hypertension should be treated with α-blockade; ideally, phentolamine 2.5 to 10 mg every 5 to 10 minutes to control the blood pressure. Other α-blocking agents such as prazosin may be effective but are less potent. β-Blockade after α-blockade may be necessary in some patients with persistent tachycardia or tachyarrhythmias.
- β-Blocker therapy should never precede α-blockade because of the risk of unopposed α-mediated vasoconstriction.
- The α, β-blocker, labetalol, may also be effective in the treatment of pheochromocytoma.
- Preoperative treatment with phentolamine (10–20 per day until symptoms subside) is essential to prevent hypertensive crisis during and immediately after surgery.

HYPERTENSIVE EMERGENCIES

A hypertensive emergency exists when immediate reduction in blood pressure is necessary to prevent progressive target organ injury. Usually the systolic blood pressure exceeds 240 mm Hg and the diastolic blood pressure is greater than 140 mm Hg. Target organ dysfunction is usually present and includes

- Cardiac dysfunction associated with congestive heart failure and pulmonary edema.
- Renal dysfunction associated with oliguric acute renal failure often accompanied by a clinical pattern suggestive of thrombotic microangiopathy, for example, microangiopathic hemolytic anemia.
- Encephalopathy usually characterized by papilledema and/or hemorrhages.
- The drug of choice for the treatment of a hypertensive emergency varies depending on the type of emergency. Moreover, one must be cautious in lowering the blood pressure, since the autoregulatory range of the affected target organ is usually abnormal.

PHARMACOLOGIC TREATMENT OF HYPERTENSIVE EMERGENCIES

- Nitroprusside: 0.25 to 10 mcg/kg/min IV, proven in almost all hypertensive emergencies; caution with high intracranial pressure and azotemia; may cause nausea/vomiting and thiocyanate toxicity.
- Fenoldopam: 0.1 to 0.3 mg/kg/min IV, proven in most hypertensive emergencies; caution with glaucoma; may cause tachycardia, nausea/vomiting, and flushing; renal vasodilator.
- Nicardipine: 2 to 10 mg/h, proven in most hypertensive emergencies except CHF; caution in coronary ischemia; may cause tachycardia.
- Hydralazine: 10 to 20 mg IV every 20 to 30 min; safe in pregnancy; may cause tachycardia or aggravate angina.
- Labetalol: 20 to 80 mg IV bolus every 10 min; 0.5 to 2 mg/min IV infusion, useful in most emergencies except acute heart failure.

BIBLIOGRAPHY

ALLHAT Officers and Coordinators for the ALLHAT Collaborative Research Group. Major outcomes in high-risk hypertensive patients randomized to angiotensin-converting enzyme inhibitor or calcium channel blocker vs diuretic. *JAMA*. 2002;288: 2981–2987.

Chobanian AV, Bakris GL, Black HR, et al. The Seventh Report of the Joint National Committee on Prevention, Detection, Evaluation, and Treatment of High Blood Pressure. *JAMA*. 2003;289:2560–2572.

Hansson L, Zanchett A, Carruthers SG, et al. Effects of intensive blood-pressure lowering and low-dose aspirin in patients with hypertension: Principal results of the hypertension optimal treatment (HOT) randomised trial. *Lancet*. 1998;351:1755.

Safian RD, Textor SC. Renal artery stenosis. *N Engl J Med*. 2001;344:431.

Tight blood pressure control and risk of macrovascular and microvascular complications in type 2 diabetes: UKPDS 38 UK Prospective Diabetes Study Group. *BMJ*. 1998;317: 703–713.

126 CRYSTAL-INDUCED ARTHROPATHIES

Katherine K. Temprano

GOUT AND HYPERURICEMIA

EPIDEMIOLOGY

- Hyperuricemia is found exclusively in man since humans lack the enzyme urate oxidase. Hyperuricemia is associated with a variety of clinical conditions including asymptomatic hyperuricemia, acute gouty arthritis, chronic tophaceous gout, urate nephropathy, and uric acid nephrolithiasis.
- Hyperuricemia, usually defined as a serum urate concentration >7 mg/dL, has been identified in as many as 17.6% of individuals (range 2.3% to 17.6%), depending on the population studied. The overall prevalence is thought to be 1.6 to 13.6 per 1000 individuals.
- Serum urate values usually correlate directly with body weight and body mass index, therefore, gout has been referred to as *the disease of kings*.
- Gout has been reported as far back as the fifth century BC by Hippocrates. Accordingly, the epidemiology, clinical features, and natural history of gout have evolved over more than two thousand years.
- A number of risk factors for gout have been elucidated:
  - Hyperuricemia: Risk of gout directly correlates with the serum uric acid concentration.
  - Age: Prevalence and incidence of gout increases with age in men and women.
  - Obesity: Body mass index and waist-to-hip ratios are strong predictors of the subsequent development of gout, even after adjusting for confounding variables, such as diet.[1]
  - Diet: Purine-rich foods and high-protein diets are generally considered risk factors for the development of gout, but several well-designed prospective studies have called this association into question. Recent studies have shown that diets enriched with dairy products confer a protective role (relative risk reduction of 40%-50% in those consuming dairy products daily).
  - Alcohol: Beer confers a higher risk than other alcohol-containing beverages because beer contains a significant quantity of purine, mostly guanosine. Moderate wine drinking does not appear to increase risk.[2]
  - Medications and toxins: See Tables 126–1 and 126–2.
  - Other medical conditions: There appears to be a link between gout and other conditions including the metabolic syndrome, hypertension, renal insufficiency, hypertriglyceridemia, and cardiovascular disorders, but an exact causal link remains incompletely understood.

PATHOPHYSIOLOGY

- Uric acid in humans can originate exogenously from purines in the diet (meat/protein) or from synthesis and turnover of endogenous purines.
- Uric acid is eliminated from the body either through the kidney (70%) or by way of the gastrointestinal tract (30%) via intestinal tract bacteria that degrade uric acid.
- Uric acid is freely filtered at the glomerulus and is reabsorbed in the proximal tubule via active transport. Conditions that promote proximal tubular reabsorption of uric acid (volume contraction), reduce uric acid clearance, increase the serum uric acid concentration. Conversely, conditions that decrease proximal tubular reabsorption of uric acid (drugs, volume expansion), increase uric acid clearance and decrease serum uric acid concentration. In addition, uric acid also undergoes proximal tubular secretion, which accounts for most of the uric acid in the normal urine.

TABLE 126–1 Causes of Hyperuricemia

Increased Uric Acid Synthesis

Primary hyperuricemia (see Table 126–2)
Secondary hyperuricemia
  Increased dietary purine intake
  Increased nucleotide turnover
    Psoriasis
    Lymphoproliferative and myeloproliferative disorders
    Hemolytic anemia
  Ethanol
  Glycogen storage diseases
  Hypoxemia
  Tissue necrosis
  Seizures
  Exercise

Decreased Uric Acid Excretion

Primary hyperuricemia
  Idiopathic
  Familial juvenile hyperuricemic nephropathy
Secondary hyperuricemia
  Renal insufficiency
  Hypertension
  Diuretics
  Dehydration
  Diabetic ketoacidosis
  Lactic acidosis
  Lead nephropathy
  Hypothyroidism
  Hyperparathyroidism
  Salt restriction
  Diabetes insipidus
  Bartter syndrome
  Sarcoidosis
  Down syndrome
  Preeclampsia
  Chronic beryllium
  Medications
    Low-dose aspirin
    Diuretics
    Pyrazinamide
    Ethambutol
    Nicotinic acid
    Laxative abuse
    Cyclosporine
    Cytotoxic agents
    B_{12} (patients with pernicious anemia)
    Pancreatic extract

TABLE 126–2 Metabolic Causes of Primary Hyperuricemia Leading to Overproduction of Uric Acid

Hypoxanthine guanine phosphoribosyltransferase deficiency (X-linked)
Complete deficiency: Lesch-Nyhan syndrome (choreoathetosis, growth and mental retardation, spasticity, self-mutilation, marked hyperuricemia, uric acid crystalluria)
Partial deficiency: Kelley-Seegmiller syndrome (uric acid calculi or gouty arthritis but no neurological defects with gout onset usually before age 20 years)
Phosphoribosyl pyrophosphate synthetase overactivity (X-linked)
Glucose-6-phosphate deficiency (autosomal recessive)
Fructose-1-phosphate aldolase deficiency (autosomal recessive)

although the mechanism(s) responsible for resolution of the acute attack are poorly understood.
• Tophi are comprised of deposits of uric acid crystals surrounded by granulomatous inflammation. They are only seen in patients with recurrent episodes of gout with sustained hyperuricemia. Tophi can develop in and around joints leading to chronic synovitis and permanent joint injury.

CLINICAL FEATURES

• Gout is classified into four stages: (1) asymptomatic hyperuricemia, (2) acute gouty arthritis, (3) intercritical gout, and (4) chronic tophaceous gout.
  ○ Asymptomatic hyperuricemia:
    ▪ Characterized by an elevated serum uric acid level, but without evidence of urate deposition (arthritis).
    ▪ Most patients remain asymptomatic.
    ▪ This stage necessarily ends with the first attack of arthritis or urolithiasis. Several decades may pass before the first attack occurs.
  ○ Acute gouty arthritis:
    ▪ This usually develops between the fourth and sixth decades, and virtually all attacks that occur before the age of 50, arise in males. Attacks that develop in younger individuals (<25 years of age) require a thorough investigation to rule out a genetic enzyme defect (see Table 126–2).
    ▪ Between 85% and 90% of first attacks are monoarticular. The first metatarsophalangeal (MTP) joint is classically affected, and 90% of patients develop MTP involvement at some time during their disease course. Acute attacks more commonly involve the joints of the lower extremities.
    ▪ Polyarticular disease may also occur and involve the knees, feet, ankles, wrists, fingers, and elbows. Polyarticular involvement is more common in joints with preexisting injury from trauma or another type of arthritis such as rheumatoid arthritis. It is also seen with increasing frequency late in the course of gouty arthritis (after recurrent attacks).

• Gout may be divided into two categories: (1) primary or (2) secondary (drugs or other medical conditions). Primary gout is usually characterized by impaired renal excretion (90%), but occasionally occurs as a consequence of increased synthesis (10%).
• Monosodium urate (MSU), the final product of purine metabolism in humans, can crystallize in joints and tissues if the concentration exceeds 6.4 mg/dL. MSU crystals are phagocytosed by synovial lining cells and infiltrating neutrophils. These cells release proinflammatory cytokines (interleukin–1, 6, 8, and tumor necrosis factor) which promote recruitment of additional neutrophils and induce an intense inflammatory response. The joint inflammation is self-limited,

- Acute gouty bursitis commonly affects the prepatellar or olecranon bursa.
- Classically, the first attack occurs suddenly, often at night and is associated with a hot, erythematous, swollen joint that is exquisitely tender to even minimal contact. Systemic signs of inflammation such as fever, leukocytosis, and elevated inflammatory markers (sedimentation rate or C-reactive protein) are often present.
- Attacks may last from hours to weeks.
- Importantly, uric acid levels may be normal during an acute attack.
  ○ Intercritical gout:
    - Intercritical gout refers to the time period between acute attacks.
    - In asymptomatic patients, with a history of proven gout, up to 70% have MSU crystals identified in synovial fluid during this period.
    - After the first attack, most patients have a recurrence within the next 6 months to 2 years, although decades may separate attacks. The intercritical period shortens in untreated patients, and radiographic findings may develop or progress during this period.
  ○ Chronic tophaceous gout:
    - There is generally a long time frame (perhaps decades) from the initial attack to the development of tophaceous gout.
    - The rate of formation of tophi is related to the length and severity of hyperuricemia and accompanying renal disease (impairs uric acid excretion).
    - Tophi may appear as irregularly shaped, firm nodules with a shiny, yellowish appearance of the overlying skin. If tophi ulcerate or are aspirated, a thick-white chalky material composed of uric acid crystals is observed.
    - Tophi can develop in any joint or tendon as well as the ulnar surface of the forearm, the olecranon bursa, along the Achilles tendon, or the helix of the ear. Tophi have been known to produce peripheral nerve root or spinal cord compression; moreover tophi have been reported to occur in the myocardium, eye, and larynx. The nodular appearance can be confused with rheumatoid nodules.
    - Radiographic changes at this stage include erosions with sclerotic margins accompanied by a thin overhanging calcified edge (Figure 126–1 and Figure 126–2).

DIAGNOSIS

- The diagnosis of an acute attack should be suspected in patients that develop a painful, red, hot, and swollen

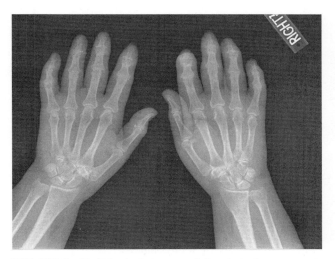

FIG. 126–1 Radiological changes of chronic tophaceous gout.

joint over a period a several hours. However, arthrocentesis is necessary to establish a definitive diagnosis as well as to differentiate gout from septic arthritis, which may appear clinically similar.
- A cell count, Gram stain, culture, and crystal analysis should be performed on the synovial fluid; and the clinician should be aware that gout and septic arthritis can coexist.

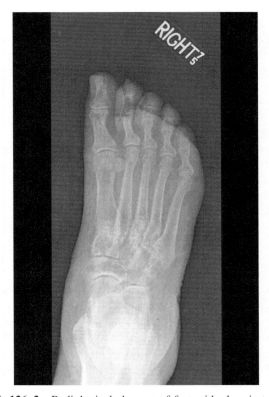

FIG. 126–2 Radiological changes of feet with chronic tophaceous gout.

• Aspiration of MSU crystals from joints during inter-critical periods may prove useful in difficult or mixed cases.
• Uric acid levels are monitored during gout management; however, they are less useful during an acute attack as the serum uric acid can be normal during that time.
• Although hyperuricemia is the most important risk factor for gout, serum uric acid levels do not confirm or exclude gout. One should be aware of the numerous states that can lead to hyperuricemia. Indeed, many patients with hyperuricemia never develop clinical gout (see Table 126–1).
• Radiographs may reveal characteristic changes in chronic gout but are likely to merely show soft tissue swelling in early or acute gout.
• Under polarized microscopy, MSU crystals appear as negatively birefringent needle-shaped crystals, which can also be observed within neutrophils. Crystal examination on aspirated synovial fluid should be performed promptly, because room temperature can modify the structure of crystals and cells may lyse. If there is a delay before microscopy, synovial fluid can be maintained at −20°C, however cell lysis will still occur.

MANAGEMENT

• The short-term goals of therapy is the treatment of the acute inflammatory episode. However, long-term goals include prevention of recurrent attacks, reducing serum urate to subsaturation levels of 6.0 mg/dL or less, preventing complications associated with uric acid crystal deposition (kidney stones), and modifying risk factors that predispose to gout.
• During the acute gout attack, treatment should be initiated as soon as possible as delays in treatment are accompanied by protracted acute attacks. Therapy consists of:
  ○ Colchicine:
    ▪ This is widely considered the drug of choice, particularly when the diagnosis of gout is in question, since relief with colchicine is diagnostic of a crystal-induced arthropathy.
    ▪ Administered as an initial dose of 0.5 or 0.6 mg by mouth or intravenously.
    ▪ The dose can be repeated hourly for 10 doses; or until the patient develops nausea, vomiting, or diarrhea; or until symptomatic relief.
    ▪ Because of intrinsic side effects and kinetic properties, colchicines should be avoided in patients with cytopenias, liver or renal disease.
    ▪ Although intravenous colchicine circumvents gastrointestinal toxicity, in general the intravenous route should be avoided because local extravasation can produce inflammation and necrosis of the extremity. If deemed necessary, 1 to 2 mg of intravenous colchicine diluted in 20 mL of normal saline can be administered through an established venous line. It may be repeated once in 6 hours if needed. However, if this route is utilized, no further colchicine should be administered, either intravenously or by mouth, for at least 1 week to avoid toxicity.
  ○ Nonsteroidal antiinflammatory drugs:
    ▪ Recently, these drugs have gained favor as the preferred treatment in patients with established gout unless gastrointestinal bleeding, peptic ulcer disease, or renal impairment, prohibit their use. Indomethacin was the first nonsteroidal antiinflammatory drug (NSAID) used in the management of acute gout; however, clinical studies of other NSAIDs confirm similar pain relief, efficacy, and tolerability. Accordingly, the choice of NSAID should largely be based on cost, convenience, and patient preference.
  ○ Corticosteroids:
    ▪ Intraarticular corticosteroid injections to single/few joints or bursa or intramuscular adrenocorticotropic hormone have also be used in the acute setting. These agents are generally reserved for patients unable to tolerate NSAIDs or colchicine.
• Several options exist for prophylactic therapy in gout:
  ○ Colchicine:
    ▪ This agent prevents acute gouty attacks at a dose of 0.6 mg once or twice daily. It is usually continued until there have been no acute attacks for 3 to 6 months.
    ▪ Caution should be exercised in patients with renal impairment because they are at risk for developing a reversible axonal neuromyopathy as well as myelosuppression.
    ▪ Ongoing crystal deposition occurs while on prophylactic colchicine; thus, urate-lowering therapy is also required to prevent relapses and ongoing joint destruction.
  ○ Allopurinol:
    ▪ This agent inhibits xanthine oxidase, which is involved in the conversion of purines to urate.
    ▪ This agent is administered to reduce uric acid to a subsaturation level in the joint and to prevent urate accumulation in the kidney and ureters (uric acid nephropathy and nephrolithiasis), and to prevent tumor lysis syndrome.
    ▪ Should neither be initiated nor discontinued during an acute flare.
    ▪ The goal of therapy with this agent is a decrease in the serum urate concentration to less than 6.0 mg/dL. The treatment is continued indefinitely.

○ Uricosuric Agents:

- Probenecid and sulfinpyrazone are both available in the United States.
- These agents are only used in patients with normal renal function, no history of renal calculi, and a uric acid excretion of <700 mg/24 h. They are ineffective in patients with a creatinine clearance of <30 mL/min. These agents can be combined with allopurinol to lower the urice acid below the saturation threshold (<6.0 mg/dL).

CALCIUM PYROPHOSPHATE DIHYDRATE DEPOSITION DISEASE

EPIDEMIOLOGY

- Calcium pyrophosphate dihydrate (CPPD) deposition disease or pseudogout can be asymptomatic or associated with a variety of musculoskeletal syndromes. The prevalence is approximately 0.9/1000 and is based mainly on radiographic data (accordingly, most patients are likely asymptomatic).
  ○ Although usually idiopathic, several clinical conditions have been described in association with CPPD. It is unclear whether there is causal link between these conditions and CPPD deposition. The conditions most commonly described are:
  - Aging, osteoarthritis, and joint trauma
  - Hyperparathyroidism
  - Hypothyroidism
  - Hemochromatosis
  - Hypomagnesemia
  - Hypophosphatasia
  - Inherited conditions (Gitelman syndrome, familial chondrocalcinosis)

PATHOPHYSIOLOGY

- Shares several similarities to gout, with crystals serving as the inciting event in the joint.
- CPPD crystals upregulate interleukin-8, which promotes neutrophil chemotaxis and joint inflammation leading to pseudogout.[3]
- CPPD crystals may also inhibit neutrophil apoptosis, which may sustain the response.
- CPPD crystals have also been shown to decrease the anabolic effect of osteoblasts on bone contributing to degenerative changes (pseudoosteoarthritis).

CLINICAL FEATURES

- The most frequent musculoskeletal manifestation of CPPD deposition is calcification of articular cartilage or chondrocalcinosis.

- An acute arthritis can occur with pain, swelling, redness, and warmth, usually involving one or only a few joints at onset. Recurrent disease or disease associated with endocrine or metabolic disease is associated with polyarticular involvement.
- The large joints (ie, knee) are most commonly affected, but other joints, such as wrists, metacarpal phalangeal hips, shoulders, elbows, and ankles, can be involved. It should be noted that the first MTP is rarely affected, unlike gout.
- Acute episodes can last from days to months and may be precipitated by surgery, trauma, arthroscopy, or after intraarticular sodium hyaluronate injections.
- Although CPPD can mimic a chronic arthritis resembling osteoarthritis (OA), arthralgias occur in unusual locations such as the wrists and MCPs. Rarely, CPPD deposition disease may mimic rheumatoid arthritis, ankylosing spondylitis or resemble a neurogenic arthropathy. Because patients develop wrist tenosynovitis, ulnar deviation, and interosseous atrophy, it can easily be confused with rheumatoid arthritis. Intervertebral disk calcification, syndesmophytes, and flowing osteophytes can be mistaken for ankylosing spondylitis. Also, soft tissue CPPD deposits can appear as tumorlike masses that may produce neurologic symptoms (ie, carpal tunnel syndrome).

DIAGNOSIS

- The current classification system is based on studies from McCarty.[4] The McCarty system emphasizes the multiple presentations of the disease that can mimic other forms of arthritis. In general, the disease is characterized by one of five clinical presentations: (1) asymptomatic; (2) pseudogout; (3) pseudorheumatoid arthritis: (4) pseudoosteoarthritis, with or without superimposed acute attacks; and (5) pseudoneuropathic joint disease.
- Diagnosis is confirmed by the presence of rhomboid or rod-shaped crystals with weakly positive birefringence in synovial fluid aspirates or articular tissue samples and accompanied by the presence of calcified deposits in the synovium, articular cartilage, or menisci.
- A common finding radiographically is a linear area of calcification in the knee menisci and articular cartilage, triangular ligaments of radiocarpal joint, and fibrocartilage of symphysis pubis.
- Radiographic changes can be confused with typical OA changes, however, CCPD involves the wrists, MCPs, elbows, or shoulders, which are unusual in OA. There may be isolated areas of joint space narrowing in the radiocarpal or patellofemoral joint. In addition, there can be subchondral cyst formation and progressive degenerative changes with subchondral

bony collapse and fragmentation with intraarticular radiodense bodies.[4]

- As in gout, pseudogout can coexist with rheumatoid arthritis or a septic joint.

MANAGEMENT

- Nonsteroidal antiinflammatory drugs are administered to relieve pain and treat acute attacks.
- Oral colchicine is less effective than in gout.
- Intraarticular or oral steroids, especially for monarticular involvement is effective.
- Surgery is an option if spinal stenosis develops.
- There is no effective therapy to remove the pyrophosphate deposits or inhibit disease progression.

BASIC CALCIUM PHOSPHATE CRYSTAL (APATITE) DISEASE

EPIDEMIOLOGY

- Basic calcium phosphate (BCP) deposition can be asymptomatic or can cause a range of musculoskeletal problems including calcific periarthritis, soft tissue calcification, or a destructive arthropathy (ie, Milwaukee shoulder).
- The prevalence of intraarticular BCP crystals in joints with OA may be as high as 67%.
- A wide variety of conditions can predispose or are associated with BCP deposition. Aging can lead to bursitis, tendonitis, destructive arthropathies, OA, or synovial osteochondromatosis. There are hereditary forms of tumoral calcinosis or bursitis/tendonitis. Enthesopathy can occur in X-linked hypophosphatemia. BCP deposition may occur in other diseases such as calciphylaxis, renal failure requiring dialysis, hypercalcemia (ie, hyperparathyroidism, sarcoid), foreign body synovitis, or connective tissue diseases (ie, dermatomyositis, scleroderma). In addition, hypervitaminosis D or milk-alkali syndrome can also lead to BCP deposition.

PATHOPHYSIOLOGY

- How calcium-containing crystals promote cartilage damage is poorly understood; however, several mechanisms have been proposed.
  - Crystals may induce synoviocyte proliferation and increase production of matrix metalloproteinases and cytokines that promote cartilage and joint damage. They may also stimulate cyclooxygenase–1 and −2 and prostaglandin E_2 production and possibly induce the synthesis of reactive oxygen metabolites, ultimately leading to cartilage damage.[3]

CLINICAL FEATURES

- Intraarticular involvement is associated with OA and the Milwaukee shoulder syndrome. Although poorly understood, deposition of these crystals may develop after recurrent flares of OA.
- Milwaukee shoulder syndrome is characterized by a destructive arthropathy that is associated with severe OA, subchondral bone collapse, and possibly soft tissue calcification.
- Extraarticular involvement is common and can present as calcific bursitis or tendonitis, periarticular calcifications, or severe OA. Crystal deposition, as in CPPD, can produce large nodular calcium deposits (tumoral calcinosis) or ligamentous calcification.
- Apatite deposits usually involve bursae and tendons around one or a few joints such as the shoulders, fingers, or hips. These deposits can be associated with chronic pain syndromes, especially if the patient had recurrent acute attacks in a particular joint. When the shoulder is affected, rotator cuff injury can occur.

DIAGNOSIS

- Typically, the diagnosis is established by plain radiographs. BCP crystals are not visible on light microscopy but rather require electron microscopy. The crystals stain red with alizarin red S stain.

MANAGEMENT

- Nonsteroidal antiinflammatory drugs.
- Colchicine.
- Glucocorticoid injections.
- Surgery is indicated if destructive arthropathy occurs. Debridement, synovectomy, and/or joint replacement may be required.
- For soft tissue calcinosis:
  - Treat underlying disease (ie, parathyroidectomy in primary hyperparathyroidism), which may promote mobilization of the deposits.
  - The role of bisphosphonates and calcium channel blockers have been utilized for calcinosis related to other diseases, such as dermatomyositis.

REFERENCES

1. Choi HK, Atkinson K, Karlson EW, et al. Obesity, weight change, hypertension, diuretic use, and risk of gout in men: The Health Professionals Follow-up Study. *Arch Intern Med.* 2005;165:742–748.
2. Choi HK, Atkinson K, Karlson EW, et al. Alcohol intake and risk of incident gout in men: A prospective study. *Lancet.* 2004;363:1277–1281.
3. Molloy ES, McCarthy GM. Calcium crystal deposition diseases: Update on pathogenesis and manifestations. *Rheum Dis Clin North Am.* 2006:32:383–400.
4. McCarty DJ. Crystal and arthritis. *Dis Mon.* 1994:6:253–300.

127 VASCULITIS

Gideon Nesher

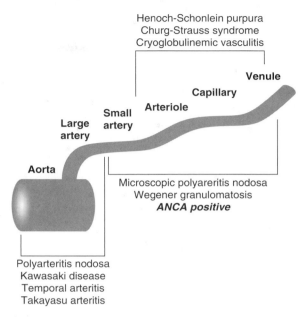

FIG. 127–1 Classification of vasculitis based on size of the vessel involved.

INTRODUCTION AND CLASSIFICATION

- Vasculitis comprises a heterogeneous group of inflammatory disorders involving blood vessel walls. Most of these disorders are considered to be autoimmune, although the precise pathogenesis remains incompletely understood.
- These disorders are classified according to the size of the blood vessel that is predominantly involved. However, some vasculitides can involve more than one size of blood vessel (Figure 127–1).
- Vasculitis is an important consideration in patients that present with a fever of undetermined origin (FUO).
- Since the vasculitis syndromes typically involve multiple organ systems (kidney, skin, joints and brain), the clinical presentation can easily be confused with other diseases. Nevertheless, there are a variety of clinical, laboratory, and histologic features which prove useful in the differential diagnosis of vasculitis (Table 127–1).

LARGE VESSEL VASCULITIS

GIANT CELL (TEMPORAL) ARTERITIS

- Giant cell arteritis (GCA) involves the major branches of the aorta with a predilection for the extracranial branches of the carotid artery, especially the temporal arteries. The aorta itself can also be involved.
- GCA is often associated with polymyalgia rheumatica (PMR).

EPIDEMIOLOGY

- GCA occurs in individuals older than 50 years of age, and the incidence gradually increases with advancing age (mean age at the time of diagnosis is 72 years of age). Women are more commonly affected.
- GCA is most common among people of North European descent. The annual incidence ranges between 16 to 25 per 100,000 people older than 50 years of age. It is less common among Mediterranean people (7–11 per 100,000), and rare among African Americans, Native Americans, and Asians.

CLINICAL FEATURES

- The signs and symptoms of GCA tend to be nonspecific, however, most patients present with one or more of the following: headache (60%), jaw claudication (50%), fever (50%), visual disturbances (40%), and musculoskeletal complaints (30%). The onset can be abrupt, but in most instances symptoms develop gradually over a period of several weeks. Patients with GCA appear ill and have a variety of physical ailments including, temporal artery tenderness and swelling, amaurosis fugax, diminished pulses, weight loss and bruits.
- PMR can occur in tandem with GCA (40% to 50%) but can also develop after a long interval, and either one can present first. PMR usually presents as an "isolated" disease, without evidence of GCA. Importantly, GCA is discovered in up to 15% of patients with PMR.

TABLE 127–1   Typical Features of the Major Vasculitides

VASCULITIS	TYPICAL FEATURES
Giant cell arteritis	Affects the elderly, headaches, polymyalgia rheumatica, jaw claudication, acute vision loss. Vasculitis in temporal arteries.
Takayasu arteritis	Affects mostly young women, intermittent claudication of upper extremities, absent brachial and radial pulses, renovascular hypertension. Imaging studies showing involvement of the aorta.
Cogan syndrome	Keratitis and hearing loss associated with Takayasu-like arteritis.
Polyarteritis nodosa	Abdominal angina, renovascular hypertension, livedo reticularis, tender subcutaneous nodules, mononeuritis multiplex. Angiography of visceral arteries shows alternating segmental widening and narrowing.
Kawasaki disease	Acute febrile disease in children. Rash, oropharyngeal inflammation, lymphadenopathy, hand edema, and coronary vasculitis.
Wegener granulomatosis	Granulomatous vasculitis primarily affecting the upper respiratory tract, lungs and kidneys. C-ANCA/anti-PR3 positive.
Microscopic polyangiitis	Nongranulomatous vasculitis predominantly affecting renal and pulmonary arterioles and capillaries, with rapidly progressive renal failure and alveolar hemorrhages. P-ANCA/anti-MPO positive.
Churg-Strauss syndrome	Asthma, fleeting lung infiltrates, prominent eosinophilia, P-ANCA positive. Biopsy showing vasculitis and tissue infiltration with eosinophils.
Leukocytoclastic vasculitis	Palpable purpura. Can be associated with other vasculitides or systemic diseases, or exposure to drugs.
Cryoglobulinemic vasculitis	Palpable purpura, cryoglobulinemia, hepatitis C, membranoproliferative glomerulonephritis.
Henoch-Schönlein purpura	Mostly in children. Palpable purpura, abdominal pain, glomerulonephritis, and arthralgia/arthritis of large joints. IgA deposits in affected vessel walls.
Behçet's disease	Oral and genital ulcers, uveitis, thrombophlebitis, positive pathergy test.

C-ANCA, cytoplasmic antineutrophil cytoplasmic antibody; IgA, immunoglobulin A; MPO, myeloperoxidase; P-ANCA, perinuclear antineutrophil cytoplasmic antibody; PR3, proteinase 3.

LABORATORY FEATURES AND DIAGNOSIS

- Erythrocyte sedimentation rate (ESR) and/or C-reactive protein (CRP) are increased in >95% of GCA patients. Thrombocytosis, anemia of inflammation, and modest elevation of alkaline phosphatase are also common.
- Temporal artery biopsy is the diagnostic procedure of choice. Arteries are affected in a segmental fashion, so the biopsy sample size should be at least 1 cm in length. Notwithstanding, approximately 15% of patients with GCA have "false-negative" biopsy results.
- The histopathologic findings consist of transmural mononuclear infiltrates. Multinucleated giant cells are often present, but their presence is not required for the diagnosis. The internal elastic lamina is fragmented.

Concentric intimal thickening can narrow or occlude the vessel (Fig. 127–2).
- Various imaging modalities can aid in the diagnosis of GCA. Duplex ultrasonography of the temporal arteries can disclose the pathognomonic hypoechoic halo around the artery. Magnetic resonance imaging (MRI), positron emission tomography, and angiography of the aortic arch and its branches can serve to diagnose large-vessel involvement.

TREATMENT AND PROGNOSIS

- Glucocorticoids are the mainstay of treatment for PMR and GCA. Symptoms typically begin to abate within 1 to 3 days.
- Prompt treatment is crucial, to prevent irreversible ischemic complications including stroke and visual loss. In patients suspected of GCA, empiric therapy should be initiated immediately while awaiting the results of an emergent temporal artery biopsy.
- Treatment guidelines for GCA and "isolated" PMR are summarized in Table 127–2.
- The duration of treatment varies. The average duration of therapy is 2 to 3 years, but in some cases it is necessary to continue low doses of prednisone for longer periods of time.
- Relapses are experienced by 25% to 65% of patients. In most cases disease flares are mild. However, vision loss or stroke can develop despite steroid therapy in some patients (distinctly unusual with prednisone doses greater than 15 mg/daily).
- Levels of ESR and CRP do not always correlate with disease activity, but remain a usual adjunct to monitor disease.

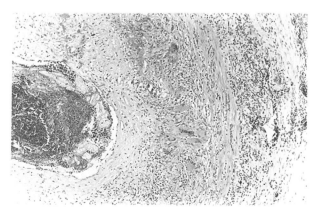

FIG. 127–2 Temporal artery biopsy of a patient with giant cell arteritis, showing transmural inflammatory mononuclear infiltrate, especially in the adventitia. Several multinucleated giant cells are seen in the media. The intima is thickened, and there is thrombus formation in the lumen of the artery.

TABLE 127–2   Suggested Guidelines for Steroid Therapy in GCA and Isolated PMR[a]

	GIANT CELL ARTERITIS	POLYMYALGIA RHEUMATICA[A]
Starting daily dose of prednisone	40–60 mg for 2–4 weeks[b]	15–20 mg for 2–4 weeks
Tapering and maintenance	Reduce by 5–10 mg every 2–4 weeks until dose is 20 mg, then reduce by 2.5–5 mg every 2–4 weeks until the dose is 10 mg, and then by 1 mg every month	reduce by 2.5–5 mg every 2–4 weeks until the dose is 10 mg, and then by 1 mg every month
Additional therapies	Aspirin 100 mg/d (decreases the rate of vision loss and CVA) Calcium, vitamin D, and bisphosphonates (prevent osteoporosis)	Calcium, vitamin D, and bisphosphonates (prevent osteoporosis)

CVA, cerebrovascular accident; GCA, giant cell arteritis; PMR, polymyalgia rheumatica.
[a] Individual cases vary greatly. The exact doses and the duration of treatment should be adjusted to the needs of the individual patient.
[b]Patients with vascular ischemic complications are treated initially with higher doses or 500–1000 mg/d of intravenous methylprednisolone for 3 consecutive days, in an attempt to prevent additional ischemic complications.

- While the adverse effects of glucocorticoids are common in this setting, no effective steroid-sparing agent has been found for GCA.
- GCA can cause serious irreversible ischemic complications (especially vision loss and stroke) and can rarely be fatal. The major cause of death includes, stroke, rupture of thoracic aortic aneurysms, and aortic dissection.

TAKAYASU ARTERITIS

- Takayasu arteritis (TA) is a granulomatous vasculitis, involving predominantly the aorta and its main branches. The pulmonary arteries can also be involved.
- Vessel inflammation results in stenosis, occlusion, or aneurysms which in turn leads to a wide variety of symptoms.

EPIDEMIOLOGY

- TA is more common in Asia and less common in Europe and North America, where the annual incidence is 1 to 2 per million.
- TA typically affects young women. The female-to-male ratio is approximately 9:1 and the age of onset is typically between 10 and 40 years of age.

CLINICAL FEATURES

- The course of TA is protracted. The initial manifestations can be nonspecific (low-grade fever, malaise, anorexia, weight loss) and without localizing signs. This can result in substantial delays in establishing the diagnosis of TA. A high index of suspicion is essential to establish the diagnosis at this early stage.

- Other initial manifestations can include headache, myalgia, postural dizziness, and blurring of vision.
- Symptoms of vascular stenosis or aneurysms are uncommon upon initial presentation and may only develop after several years. They are related to the affected vascular territory (eg, syncope secondary to subclavian artery stenosis). Bruits can be audible over the subclavian and carotid arteries, as well as the abdominal aorta. The carotid arteries can be tender to palpation.

LABORATORY FEATURES AND DIAGNOSIS

- Elevated acute-phase reactants (ESR and CRP) and anemia are often present.
- The diagnosis is confirmed by vascular imaging: arterial angiography or noninvasive angiography with computerized tomography (CT) or MRI. CT and MRI also allow evaluation of the arterial wall, thus permitting earlier diagnosis of TA, prior to luminal stenosis.
- Imaging characteristically reveals dilation of the vessel, alternating with stenotic and normal appearing segments in the thoracic and abdominal aorta, pulmonary artery, and the proximal large arteries.

TREATMENT AND PROGNOSIS

- Corticosteroids are the therapy of choice, starting with 40 to 60 mg/d. Tapering is tailored to the individual response. Low-dose aspirin can be beneficial in preventing ischemic events.
- Methotrexate, azathioprine, or cyclophosphamide have been successfully administered to patients with life-threatening and refractory disease. These drugs have also been used as steroid-sparing agents.

- Levels of ESR and CRP do not always correlate with disease activity, but are typically monitored. Repeat vascular imaging can help guide the duration of therapy.
- Vascular surgery and transluminal angioplasty should be considered in patients with ischemic symptoms and/or severely stenotic vessels. Surgery should ideally be performed during a period of disease remission.
- Hypertension, secondary to renal artery stenosis, is not uncommon. The blood pressure must be recorded using several arteries since measurements obtained from the brachial artery are not reliable. Hypertension is initially treated medically, however renal artery angioplasty should be considered in patients with refractory hypertension or severely stenotic renal vessels.
- The short term prognosis is generally quite good, with 5-year survival rates exceeding 80%. Not surprisingly, severe uncontrolled hypertension and cardiac involvement are predictors of increased mortality.

COGAN SYNDROME

- Ocular-vestibuloauditory inflammatory disease, consisting of interstitial keratitis, hearing loss and vestibular dysfunction. Ten to fifteen percent of the patients develop Takayasu-like arteritis.

EPIDEMIOLOGY

- Rare disease affecting young adults more commonly but can occur at any age.

CLINICAL FEATURES

- Ocular disease (primarily keratitis) is characterized by eye pain and redness, blurred vision, and photophobia. Other ocular lesions include conjunctivitis, scleritis, episcleritis, uveitis, and retinal vasculitis.
- Inner ear manifestations include vertigo, tinnitus, ataxia, and hearing loss. Bilateral deafness develops in one-half of the patients.
- Features of arteritis, when present, resemble those of TA.
- Systemic symptoms are present in >90% of the patients with vasculitis but only one-third of patients without vasculitis.

LABORATORY FEATURES AND DIAGNOSIS

- Increased acute-phase reactants, anemia, leukocytosis, and thrombocytosis are usually present. They are more prominent in patients with vasculitis.

- The diagnosis of vascular involvement is established using vascular imaging. Biopsy specimens are rarely available for diagnostic purposes, since the large arteries are involved. If obtained, the histology is similar to that observed in TA.

TREATMENT AND PROGNOSIS

- Patients with vasculitis respond to steroids, prescribed in a manner similar to that of TA. The efficacy of immunosuppressive steroid-sparing agents is not clear. Methotrexate, azathioprine, cyclophosphamide, and cyclosporine have been used with some success.

MEDIUM VESSEL VASCULITIS

POLYARTERITIS NODOSA

- Polyarteritis nodosa (PAN) is a necrotizing vasculitis primarily affecting medium-sized vessels, with a predilection for mesenteric, renal, dermal, and neuromuscular arteries, and sparing of pulmonary vessels.

EPIDEMIOLOGY
- The annual incidence is 4 to 9 per 1 million people.
- The age of onset in most cases is between 40 and 60 years of age.

CLINICAL FEATURES
- Nonspecific systemic symptoms are common including fever, chills, arthralgias, and weight loss. Since multiple arterial beds are often involved, the symptoms and signs may mimic a variety of other clinical syndromes (eg, acute kidney failure, heart failure, seizure disorders, gastrointestinal bleeding, and skin lesions).

LABORATORY FEATURES AND DIAGNOSIS
- Elevated acute-phase reactants (ESR and CRP), anemia, thrombocytosis, and leukocytosis are common. Studies which can prove useful in establishing an underlying etiology include: (1) antineutrophil cytoplasmic antibodies (ANCA), (2) antinuclear antibodies (ANA), (3) antibodies to nuclear antigens (anti-SSA, anti-SSB, anti-RNP, etc), (4) cryoglobulins, (5) complement determinations (C_3 and C_4). For example, an elevated titer of ANA would suggest systemic lupus rather than PAN.
- The diagnosis is confirmed by a biopsy of an affected organ, which reveals necrotizing arteritis and neutrophilic infiltration.
- Alternatively, angiography of renal or mesenteric arteries can show the typical pattern of alternating segmental widening (aneurysms) and narrowing.

TREATMENT AND PROGNOSIS

- Approximately 50% of patients respond to prednisone alone at a dose 60 mg/d. In severe or refractory cases, pulse therapy with intravenous methylprednisolone (1000 mg/d for 3 days), and/or oral cyclophosphamide (2 mg/kg/d) is associated with prolonged survival. The duration of therapy is controversial, however, a slow taper over 9–12 months is common practice.
- Addition of antiviral agents (lamivudine 100 mg/d) is indicated in patients with Hepatitis B-associated PAN.
- Treatment is associated with a 5-year survival rate of approximately 80%. Once remission is achieved, however, the relapse rate is low.

KAWASAKI DISEASE

- An acute self-limited febrile illness, predominantly described in children, involving the large to medium-sized blood vessels (often referred to as mucocutaneous lymph node syndrome). Rarely the coronary arteries are involved leading to life-threatening clinical manifestations including heart failure and malignant arrhythmias. Sequelae of coronary involvement can continue into adulthood.

EPIDEMIOLOGY

- In Japan, the annual incidence rate is 70 to 80 per 100,000 children younger than 5 years of age. In whites, the incidence is 17 to 18 per 100,000 children younger than 5 years of age.

CLINICAL FEATURES

- High fever is an invariable finding in Kawasaki disease (KD). Other symptoms which occur simultaneously or shortly after the onset of fever include a polymorphous rash, conjunctivitis, oropharyngeal inflammation (erythema of the oropharynx and lips, "strawberry" tongue), cervical lymphadenopathy, and edema of the hands and feet with palmar and plantar erythema. Skin desquamation develops 2 weeks after the initial skin manifestations.
- Transient carditis is a major complication of KD and likely develops in up to 40% of affected individuals. Coronary vasculitis with aneurysm formation, valvular insufficiency and pericarditis develops in 20% of untreated cases within 1 month.
- Other organ systems, such as the gastrointestinal (GI) and the central nervous system (CNS), can also be involved.

LABORATORY FEATURES AND DIAGNOSIS

- Elevated acute phase reactants (ESR and CRP), leukocytosis, thrombocytosis, anemia, and increased liver enzymes are common.

- Echocardiography can detect coronary aneurysms, and is recommended at weekly intervals for the first month. Coronary angiography is indicated in severe cases complicated by coronary ischemia or valvular regurgitation.

TREATMENT AND PROGNOSIS

- Intravenous gammaglobulin (IVIG) is recommended as a single dose of 2 g/kg. IVIG reduces the occurrence of coronary aneurysms to <5%, and of large aneurysms to <1%.
- Antiinflammatory doses of aspirin (80–100 mg/kg/d) are included until fever subsides, followed by low-dose aspirin to exert an antiplatelet effect. The benefit of anti-platelet therapy remains controversial.
- Small aneurysms tend to regress within several years, and are often asymptomatic. Large aneurysms are associated with stenosis, thrombosis, and infarction. In such cases, long-term anticoagulant therapy is indicated, and surgical repair should be considered.
- Myocardial infarction occurs more often during the first year after the onset, but infarctions occurring in young adults have been reported.

SMALL VESSEL VASCULITIS

ANTINEUTROPHIL CYTOPLASMIC ANTIBODY ASSOCIATED VASCULITIS

- This group of diseases is comprised of three clinically distinct syndromes predominantly involving the small vessels: (1) Wegener granulomatosis (WG), (2) Churg-Strauss syndrome, and (3) microscopic polyangiitis (MPA). All are associated with a high titer of serum ANCA.

WEGENER GRANULOMATOSIS (WG)

- WG is a small vessel vasculitis, primarily affecting the upper respiratory tract, lungs, and kidneys, associated with cytoplasmic antineutrophil cytoplasmic antibody (C-ANCA) and granuloma formation.

EPIDEMIOLOGY

- The age at diagnosis is usually between 40 to 60 years. The annual incidence is 2 to 10 per million people.

CLINICAL FEATURES

- Most patients present with respiratory manifestations including persistent rhinorrhea, bloody nasal discharge, cough, hoarseness, sinus pain, and dyspnea. In addition, nonspecific systemic symptoms including fever, chills, weight loss, myalgias, and arthralgias can be present. Renal involvement tends to occur later in the course of the disease and usually presents as a rapidly progressive glomerulonephritis. Nearly any organ system can be involved during the course of the disease and, accordingly, the initial and subsequent clinical features are diverse.

- Approximately 20% of patients present with "limited" WG, a disease confined to the upper respiratory tract and orbit. Many of these cases later develop involvement of other organs.

LABORATORY FEATURES AND DIAGNOSIS

- Leukocytosis, anemia, thrombocytosis, and acute phase reaction (increased ESR and CRP) are common.
- C-ANCA (specifically anti–proteinase-3, PR3-ANCA) antibodies are relatively specific for WG (specificity >90%). The sensitivity of PR3-ANCA ranges between 30% in patients with "limited" disease to >85% in patients with active generalized disease. Some patients are positive for perinuclear antineutrophil cytoplasmic antibody (P-ANCA).
- PR3-ANCA titers generally correlate with disease activity and, thus, are usually monitored during therapy and remission.
- The cranial CT can show evidence of sinusitis and rarely orbital involvement. The chest CT can show cavitary nodules, alveolar infiltrates and pleural densities.
- In all cases, a diagnosis should be confirmed by a tissue biopsy of an involved site, most often lung or sinuses. The classic histopathology reveals necrotizing granulomatous vasculitis. Unfortunately, many patients do not exhibit granuloma formation on biopsy and, therefore, the diagnosis of WG is often confused with microscopic PAN.
- Renal histology can show crescentic glomerulonephritis, with or without granuloma formation.
- Rarely, treatment is initiated without a confirmatory biopsy if the diagnosis of WG is highly likely (lung nodules, PR3-ANCA+, sinusitis) and the patient is acutely ill.

TREATMENT AND PROGNOSIS

- Initial therapy: oral cyclophosphamide, 2 mg/kg/d, and prednisone 1 mg/kg/d. In severe cases, pulse intravenous methylprednisolone 1000 mg/d for 3 days. An oral pulse of cyclophosphamide (4 mg/kg/d for 3 days) can also be considered in severely ill patients.
- Maintenance therapy: prednisone is tapered gradually over 3 to 6 months. Cyclophosphamide is discontinued after 3 to 6 months and the patient is converted to methotrexate (15–25 mg/wk) or azathioprine (2 mg/kg/d)

- In patients with renal failure the dose of cyclophosphamide and methotrexate should be reduced.
- *Pneumocystis carinii* prophylaxis with cotrimoxazole is also indicated during immunosuppressive therapy.
- Remission rates exceed 80% after 1 year, however, one-half of these patients relapse.
- During a mean follow-up of 8 years, a 13% mortality was reported. The principal cause of death was secondary to complications of the underlying disease or the immunosuppression regimen (infections, malignancy).

MICROSCOPIC POLYANGIITIS

- Microscopic polyangiitis (MP) is a necrotizing small vessel vasculitis predominantly affecting the renal and pulmonary vessels. There is considerable clinical overlap with WG, however, MP is not characterized by granulomatous inflammation. Moreover, some experts suggest that MP does not cause upper respiratory pathology (sinusitis). Whether WG and MP represent two distinct disease entities or are part of a clinical spectrum of small vessel vasculitis remains controversial. Notwithstanding, the treatment for either condition is similar.

EPIDEMIOLOGY

- Annual incidence rates are 2 to 8 per million. The mean age at diagnosis is 50 years of age.

CLINICAL FEATURES

- Pauci-immune glomerulonephritis occurs in almost all cases (however, the renal pathology is indistinguishable from WG) and is often the presenting manifestation. It leads to rapidly progressive renal failure in one-third of the cases. Early diagnosis and therapy can reduce the likelihood of progression to end stage renal disease. Multiple organ system involvement is common and, therefore, the symptom complex is similar to that observed with WG.

LABORATORY FEATURES AND DIAGNOSIS

- Elevated acute phase reactants (ESR and CRP), anemia, thrombocytosis, and depressed serum albumin are common.
- ANCA is present in 75% of the cases (especially in active disease) and is predominantly directed toward myeloperoxidase (MPO-ANCA).
- The urine sediment may reveal hematuria, nephrotic range proteinuria, and RBC casts.
- The renal biopsy shows crescentic glomerulonephritis and necrosis of the glomerular capillaries without immune deposits (pauci-immune necrotizing

glomerulonephritis). This histology is identical to that observed with WG. Fortuitously the treatment for WG and MP is similar.

TREATMENT AND PROGNOSIS
- Treatment guidelines are identical to those of WG.
- One-third of the patients relapse after a median time of 2 years. The clinical manifestations at the time of relapse are often less severe than those seen initially.
- Most deaths are related to pulmonary hemorrhage and complications of renal failure.

CHURG-STRAUSS SYNDROME

- The Churg-Strauss syndrome (CSS) is characterized by granulomatous vasculitis preceded by allergic rhinitis and asthma and is associated with peripheral eosinophilia.

EPIDEMIOLOGY
- Incidence rates are 1 to 4 per million per year. The mean age at onset is 40 years of age.

CLINICAL FEATURES
- Asthma is the initial symptom and usually precedes evidence of vasculitis by 5–10 years. Rapid progression from the asthma phase to the vasculitic phase is associated with a poor prognosis.
- Pulmonary involvement is manifested by cough, wheezing and dyspnea. Transient lung infiltrates are seen in 75% of patients on plain radiographs. Other, less common, chest x-ray findings include: lung opacities, cavitary lesions, and pleural effusions.

LABORATORY FEATURES AND DIAGNOSIS
- Elevations in CRP and ESR are common.
- Eosinophilia is prominent as are elevated levels of immunoglobulin E (IgE).
- ANCA are present in two-thirds of the patients, mostly MPO-ANCA.
- Confirmation of the diagnosis requires a biopsy of involved tissue (usually lung) which, in turn reveals vasculitis and tissue infiltration with eosinophils.

TREATMENT AND PROGNOSIS
- CSS is highly responsive to steroids, resulting in a dramatic decrease in symptoms coupled with regression of eosinophilia. Relapse of CSS may occur in up to 25% of cases.
- Cyclophosphamide and/or pulse therapy with methylprednisolone are useful for severe, progressive or refractory disease.
- Residual asthma can require maintenance therapy with low-dose prednisone.

- CSS has been reported in some asthma patients treated with leukotriene receptor antagonists. It is controversial as to whether the leukotriene receptor antagonists are directly responsible for CSS, or whether the tendency to develop CSS was unmasked by their steroid-sparing effect.
- The 6-year survival rate is nearly 90% but is considerably worse in patients with other organ system involvement (GI or myocardial involvement).

IMMUNE-COMPLEX ASSOCIATED VASCULITIS

- The immune-complex mediated vasculitides are a heterogenous group of disorders characterized by deposits of immune-complexes in the walls of blood vessels, and usually accompanied by marked reductions in serum levels of complement components. The etiopathogenesis of immune-complex formation and deposition is poorly understood, but could be precipitated by virtually any systemic autoimmune or inflammatory disease (eg, lupus, infectious endocarditis).

CUTANEOUS LEUKOCYTOCLASTIC (HYPERSENSITIVITY) VASCULITIS

- Cutaneous leukocytoclastic vasculitis is characterized by a palpable purpuric rash predominantly over the legs and histologically by granulocytes and their debris (leukocytoclasis) in the walls of affected small vessels.
- Cutaneous leukocytoclastic vasculitis can be primary or can be associated with other vasculitidies, drug reactions, infections, malignancies, or autoimmune diseases. Cutaneous leukocytoclastic vasculitis is by definition, confined to the skin.

EPIDEMIOLOGY
- Cutaneous leukocytoclastic vasculitis is believed to be very common, although the exact incidence is difficult to surmise since it is often confused with other clinical syndromes characterized by a rash (including systemic vasculitis). Notwithstanding, its estimated annual incidence approximates 30 per 1 million people.

CLINICAL FEATURES
- Typically, crops of palpable purpura appear on the legs and buttocks, sometimes a generalized rash occurs. Edema can develop in the involved areas, as well as vesicles, ulcers, necrosis, and urticaria.
- Urticarial vasculitis can be differentiated from common urticaria by the duration of lesions (>2 days), presence

of a purpuric component, and postinflammatory hyper-pigmentation of the involved skin. This subset of cutaneous leukocytoclastic vasculitis has been described in association with acute glomerulonephritis and obstructive lung disease.

LABORATORY FEATURES AND DIAGNOSIS

- Acute phase reactants such as CRP and the sedimentation rate can be unremarkable. However, low levels of complement (C3 and C4) are common. Anti-C1q antibodies are often present in urticarial vasculitis.
- Skin histology demonstrates leukocytoclastic vasculitis in the cutaneous microvasculature, primarily venules, with variable patterns of immunoglobulin and complement deposition.
- Importantly, a careful workup should be performed to rule out the presence of an underlying disorder (eg, lupus, WG, MP, etc).

TREATMENT AND PROGNOSIS

- Therapy of cutaneous leukocytoclastic vasculitis itself depends on the severity and extent of involvement. Any suspected offending agents (drugs, chemicals) should be avoided or discontinued. This often results in resolution within days or weeks.
- Mild cases can resolve without specific treatment. Otherwise, colchicine, nonsteroidal antiinflammatory drugs (NSAIDs), dapsone, and hydroxychloroquine can be effective. Antihistamines are useful in urticarial vasculitis.
- In severe or refractory cases steroids should be prescribed, often with steroid-sparing agents such as azathioprine. Cyclophosphamide is reserved for severe cases.
- The prognosis is generally excellent, since the disease is confined to the skin.

CRYOGLOBULINEMIC VASCULITIS

- Cryoglobulinemic vasculitis (CV) is characterized by cutaneous leukocytoclastic vasculitis and the presence of cryoglobulins in the serum. It is often associated with hepatitis C virus infection.

EPIDEMIOLOGY

- Cryoglobulins in the serum are present in 50% of patients with hepatitis C virus infection, but only a minority develop CV. An increase in circulating cryoglobulins has also been described in HIV infection. However, the existence of HIV or hepatitis C co-infection does not appear to influence the development of CV. Thus, the pathogenesis of this disorder remains incompletely understood.

CLINICAL FEATURES

- Skin manifestations, identical to those observed with cutaneous leukocytoclastic vasculitis, occur in almost all cases. Extracutaneous manifestations can include membranoproliferative glomerulonephritis, peripheral neuropathy, arthralgia, GI involvement (abdominal pain, bleeding, diarrhea), Raynaud phenomenon and Sjögren syndrome. The extracutaneous manifestions of CV may not appear for decades.

LABORATORY FEATURES AND DIAGNOSIS

- Liver enzyme abnormalities are present in approximately one-half of the cases.
- Depressed serum complement components, especially C4 levels, are found in most cases.
- The urine sediment can reflect the presence of glomerulonephritis (hematuria, proteinuria and RBC casts).
- Eighty to ninety percent of patients have anti-hepatitis C virus antibodies or hepatitis C virus RNA. Hepatitis B serology is positive in a small percentage of cases.
- Detection of mixed cryoglobulins in the serum is essential to confirm the diagnosis. Mixed cryoglobulins represent immune complexes, typically containing the precipitating antigen (mostly hepatitis C virus), an immunoglobulin G (IgG) antibody, immunoglobulin M (IgM) rheumatoid factor (polyclonal or monoclonal), and complement components.

TREATMENT AND PROGNOSIS

- Antiviral therapy (interferon-alfa and ribavirin) can be quite effective for mild cases. In severe or refractory cases, steroids and cyclophosphamide have been used successfully. Plasmapheresis has been effective as salvage therapy.
- More than one-half of the patients have a relatively benign course. The prognosis is significantly worsened by the presence of renal or liver involvement. Fifteen percent of the patients develop malignancies, most notably non-Hodgkin's lymphoma.

HENOCH-SCHÖNLEIN PURPURA

- Henoch-Schönlein purpura (HSP) is a small vessel vasculitis characterized by the tetrad of (1) cutaneous leukocytoclastic vasculitis, (2) arthralgia/arthritis of large joints, (3) abdominal pain (caused by mesenteric vasculitis) and (4) glomerulonephritis.
- Typically there is deposition of immunoglobulin A (IgA) in the affected vessel walls.

EPIDEMIOLOGY

- Children are most commonly affected. Among them, the annual incidence is 135 per 1 million, while in adults it is 14 per 1 million.

CLINICAL FEATURES

- Many patients describe a recent history of an upper respiratory tract infection.
- Fever can accompany the tetrad. The abdominal pain is often colicky and can exhibit features of abdominal angina. Vomiting and GI bleeding can also develop. Some children develop ileoileal intussusception.
- Renal involvement generally occurs within the first 3 months after disease onset. Adults tend to develop renal involvement more frequently than children.

LABORATORY FEATURES AND DIAGNOSIS

- Microscopic hematuria and proteinuria are common. Macroscopic hematuria occurs in some cases. Renal histology ranges from minimal disease to diffuse proliferative glomerulonephritis, however mesangial proliferation is most common, accompanied invariably by IgA deposition.
- A third of the adult patients have increased serum IgA levels, while C3 and C4 are normal or slightly depressed.

TREATMENT AND PROGNOSIS

- Most cases are self-limited and resolve within a few weeks. Low-dose steroids can alleviate the nonrenal manifestations, but are rarely indicated.
- In cases of significant renal involvement high-dose steroids and cyclophosphamide should be considered. The severity of renal disease at onset appears to predict outcome. Ten to twenty percent of adult patients develop sustained impairment in renal function.

MISCELLANEOUS VASCULITIDES

BEHÇET DISEASE

- Behçet disease is a systemic inflammatory disease, with mucocutaneous involvement and vasculitis that can affect all vessel types and sizes.

EPIDEMIOLOGY

- The age at the time of diagnosis is 20 to 35 years in most cases. Behçet disease is most prevalent in the Middle East, North Africa, and Far East. The prevalence in these areas is 10 to 300 per 100,000 people.
- There is familial clustering, probably related to an association with histocompatibility leukocyte antigen (HLA)-B51.

CLINICAL FEATURES

- The most common manifestation (>97% of the patients) is recurrent painful oral ulcers. Often these ulcers are the first manifestation of Behçet disease, and sometimes present years before the occurrence of other symptoms.
- Genital ulcers and skin lesions (folliculitis, papulo-pustular lesions and erythema nodosum) are also common (60%–80%).
- Uveitis and arthritis occur in approximately one-half of the patients. CNS manifestations (stroke, intracranial hypertension, aseptic meningitis) and gastrointestinal symptoms (resembling those of inflammatory bowel disease) are less common.
- Thrombophlebitis occurs in 25% of the patients. It most commonly involves the leg veins, but the upper extremity, thoracic, abdominal and cerebral veins can also be involved. Superior or inferior vena cava syndromes and Budd-Chiari syndrome can develop. Embolization from these thrombophlebitic lesions is rare.
- Arterial involvement occurs in <5% of the patients. All vessel sizes can be involved, including the pulmonary arterial bed. Aneurysms can develop in the large arteries and can rupture.

LABORATORY FEATURES AND DIAGNOSIS

- Elevated acute-phase reactants, anemia, and mild leukocytosis can be present. HLA-B51 is identified in approximately one-half of the cases. The pathergy test (formation of a papule or a sterile pustule 48 hours after a needle prick or intracutaneous injection of sterile saline) is positive in two-thirds of patients from the Middle East and Far East, but less common elsewhere.

TREATMENT AND PROGNOSIS

- In general, treatment in system-directed. Mucocutaneous lesions are treated with local measures and colchicine. In severe, unresponsive cases addition of azathioprine or thalidomide can be considered. Most cases of arthritis respond to NSAIDs. Eye involvement often requires initiation of immunosuppressive therapy with steroids, azathioprine, and cyclosporine.
- Anticoagulation is indicated for thrombophlebitis in the large vessels. However, this can significantly increase the incidence of major bleeding complications in patients with arterial aneurysms. Addition of azathioprine is indicated in patients with recurrent thrombophlebitis.
- Cyclophosphamide and steroids are the treatment of choice for arteritis.
- Most patients have mild disease. Behçet disease tends to be more severe in males. Severe uveitis can result in loss of vision. Mortality is related to involvement of the large arteries (especially the pulmonary artery) and CNS involvement.

PRIMARY ANGIITIS OF THE CENTRAL NERVOUS SYSTEM

- These rare syndromes are a collection of vasculitic conditions involving *only* the CNS. They are characterized by the presence of new and unexplained neurologic deficits, angiographic or histologic evidence of CNS vasculitis, and no evidence of systemic vasculitis elsewhere or other systemic diseases.

EPIDEMIOLOGY

- Primary angiitis of the central nervous system (PACNS) is rare, but should be considered in patients with unexplained neurologic symptoms.

CLINICAL FEATURES

- Granulomatous angiitis of the CNS (GACNS) is the best characterized variant. The symptoms are nonspecific and are usually slowly progressive with cumulative neurologic deficits and mental status changes arising, in association with chronic headaches.

LABORATORY FEATURES AND DIAGNOSIS

- Elevated acute phase reactants and anemia are often absent. Spinal fluid findings are consistent with chronic meningitis (mononuclear cells, elevated protein, normal glucose). The MRI is abnormal in most cases showing nonspecific multifocal vascular injury. Cerebral angiography can be normal in more than one-third of the cases, but often reveals segmental stenosis and ectasia. Unfortunately, these findings have also been observed in benign angiopathy of the CNS.
- Brain biopsy is the preferred diagnostic modality, although GACNS involves discontiguous areas of the brain leading to falsely negative brain histology.

TREATMENT AND PROGNOSIS

- Prompt diagnosis and therapy are critical to achieving improvement in outcome.
- GACNS is treated with prednisone (1 mg/kg/d) and cyclophosphamide (2 mg/kg/d). Steroids are tapered over several months, and cyclophosphamide is continued for at least 1 year.

BIBLIOGRAPHY

Abril A, Kalamia KT, Cohen MD. The Churg-Strauss syndrome (allergic granulomatous angiitis): Review and update. *Semin Arthritis Rheum.* 2003;33:106–114.

Ferri C, Sebastiani M, Giuggioli D, et al. Mixed cryoglobulinemia: demographic, clinical and serologic features and survival in 231 patients. *Semin Arthritis Rheum.* 2004;33: 355–374.

Gayraud M, Guillevin L, le Toumelin P, et al. Long-term followup of polyarteritis nodosa, microscopic polyangiitis, and Churg-Strauss syndrome: Analysis of four prospective trials including 278 patients. *Arthritis Rheum.* 2001;44:666–675.

Gonzalez-Gay MA, Garcia-Porrua C, Pujol RM. Clinical approach to cutaneous vasculitis. *Curr Opin Rheumatol.* 2005;17:56–61.

Reinhold-Keller E, Beuge N, Latza U, et al. An interdisciplinary approach to the care of patients with Wegener granulomatosis: Long term outcome in 155 patients. *Arthritis Rheum.* 2000;43: 1021–1032.

Salvarani C, Cantini F, Boiardi L, Hunder GG. Polymyalgia rheumatica and giant cell arteritis. *N Engl J Med.* 2002;347: 261–271.

128 THE SPONDYLOARTHRO-PATHIES

Rama Bandlamudi

ANKYLOSING SPONDYLITIS

EPIDEMIOLOGY

- The prevalence of ankylosing spondylitis (AS) is 197 cases per 100,000 individuals in the United States.
- A family history of AS is a strong risk factor for the development of the disease.
- The incidence of AS is approximately 7.3 per 100,000 person years.
- 90% of white patients with AS are HLA-B27 antigen positive.
- 50% of African Americans with AS are positive for HLA-B27 antigen.

ETIOLOGY

- AS is thought to occur when an external antigenic challenge activates autoreactive T cells that recognize endogenous peptides presented by macrophages.
- Tumor necrosis factor-α (TNF-α) promoter gene expression variability might also contribute to the development of AS.

PATHOPHYSIOLOGY

- Inflammation of the enthesis or the insertion of muscle tendons or ligaments into bones is the characteristic feature of AS.
- Changes engendered by enthesitis include syndesmophyte formation, squaring of the vertebral bodies,

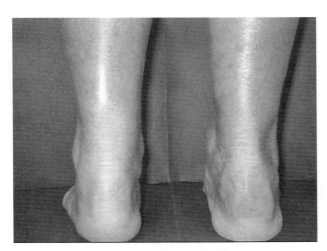

FIG. 128–1 Evidence of Achilles tendonitis.

vertebral end-plate destruction, and Achilles tendonitis (Fig. 128–1)
• CD4+, CD8+, T-cells, and macrophages are present in the inflamed sacroiliac joints.

CLINICAL MANIFESTATIONS

SKELETAL MANIFESTATIONS
• Back pain experienced deep in the gluteal region, is dull in character and insidious in onset.
• Morning stiffness may last up to three hours, but usually improves with physical activity.
• Chest pain can develop because of involvement of the costovertebral and costotransverse joints, which in turn, is thought to reflect enthesopathy at the costosternal and manubriosternal joints.
• Prevalent tender sites (incident to enthesitis) include the costosternal junctions, spinous processes, iliac crests, greater trochanters, tibial tubercles, and heels.
• The hips and shoulders are the most frequently involved extra-axial joints.

EXTRASKELETAL MANIFESTATIONS
• Acute anterior uveitis or iridocyclitis is the most common extraskeletal manifestation of AS. 20% to 25% are unilateral (more common in HLA-B27 patients). This finding should alert the astute clinician to the possibility of AS. The uveitis responds to therapy with local steroids and atropine, but may recur.
• Ascending aortitis, aortic valve incompetence, conduction abnormalities, cardiomegaly, and pericarditis have also been described. Aortic incompetence (because of scarring) and cardiac conduction defects occur twice as often in patients with AS.

PHYSICAL FINDINGS

• Limited motion of the vertebral spine, eventually leading to postural abnormalities (stooping).
  ◦ The modified Schober test measures the forward flexion of the spine (with the patient standing erect, make a mark over the spinous process of the 5th lumbar vertebra. Make another mark 10 cm above it in the midline. When the patient bends maximally forward, the distance between the two points normally exceeds 15 cm).
  ◦ Mild to moderate reduction of chest expansion.
• Enthesitis is common in the Achilles tendon, ischial tuberosities, greater trochanter, spinous processes, costochondral and manubriosternal junctions, and iliac crests.
• Direct pressure over the sacroiliac joints may elicit sacroiliac pain.

LABORATORY FINDINGS

• The erythrocyte sedimentation rate (ESR) or C-reactive protein (CRP) levels can be elevated during active inflammation.
• A mild normochromic normocytic anemia (anemia of chronic disease) has been characterized.

RADIOGRAPHY AND IMAGING

• Imaging of the sacroiliac joint invariably reveals sacroiliitis (particularly in long-standing cases) and the findings are typically symmetric.
  ◦ Subchondral sclerosis is common.
  ◦ The combination of destructive osteoiliitis and repair leads to "squaring" of the vertebral bodies and gradual ossification of the annular fibrosis and eventual bridging between involved vertebral syndesmophytes.
  ◦ Hip and shoulder joint imaging may reveal joint space narrowing with subchondral sclerosis.
• Spinal inflammation (spondylodiscitis) can be apparent with computerized tomography (CT).
• Magnetic resonance imaging (MRI) with gadolinium contrast reveals the early stages of sacroiliitis. MRI is considerably more sensitive than plain films in establishing the diagnosis of sacroiliitis. However, MRI should be reserved for patients in whom the suspicion for ankylosing spondylitis is high but plain radiographs are normal. MRI-STIR (short tau inversion recovery) sequences are very sensitive for the detection of sacroiliitis (usually described as "bone marrow edema"). MRI is also useful to visualize arachnoid

diverticula which may develop in AS and produce a cauda equina syndrome.

THERAPY

The goals of therapy include pain relief, restoration of function, decrease or prevent joint damage, prevent spinal fusion, reduce the incidence of extraarticular manifestations, and reduce complications associated with the disease. Importantly, the extent and severity of the disease (pain, spinal mobility, stiffness, etc) dictates the therapeutic approach. Several expert panels have proposed a core set of guidelines to utilize when assessing disease severity (www.spartangroup.org).

FIRST LINE
- Physical therapy, exercises, and anti-inflammatory medications are the mainstays of therapy. Specific exercises have been developed to minimize the complications associated with AS (www.nass.co.uk/exercises.htm)
- Nonsteroidal antiinflammatory drugs (NSAIDs), especially tolmetin, naproxen, meloxicam, or indomethacin are necessary to control pain and stiffness. The dose should be maximized and the agent should be administered continuously to minimize joint injury and deformity.

SECOND LINE
- Sulfasalazine up to 1 g three times daily is mostly helpful for patients with peripheral arthritis. Otherwise its effects on the clinical course of AS appear modest, at best.
- Methotrexate (MTX) may exert some effect in AS, especially if patients have failed to respond to NSAIDs or sulfasalazine. Overall, MTX should not be administered for prolonged periods of time unless there is clear and sustained improvement of disease activity.
- Anti-tumor necrosis factor (TNF) α agents have achieved superior results in AS and are now considered the most active drugs for the treatment of AS. Infliximab intravenously (5 mg/kg at 0, 2, and 6 weeks, and then every 4–8 weeks), etanercept 25 mg subcutaneously (SQ) twice weekly, or adalimumab 40 mg SQ every 2 weeks have all proven remarkably beneficial. Unless contraindicated these agents should be offered to all patients with a proven diagnosis of AS who have not responded to NSAIDS or sulfasalazine.

REACTIVE ARTHRITIS

DEFINITION AND CLASSIFICATION CRITERIA

- Characterized by the clinical triad of arthritis, urethritis, and conjunctivitis (Reiter syndrome). The syndrome is usually manifested by inflammatory spinal pain and asymmetric synovitis, predominantly in the lower limbs.
- The following bacteria have been associated with the development of reactive arthritis: *Chlamydia, Salmonella, Shigella, Yersinia,* and *Campylobacter.*
  - Associated with an acute inflammatory arthritis, low back pain, or enthesitis.
  - There must be clear evidence of an infection preceding this condition by approximately 4 to 8 weeks.

EPIDEMIOLOGY

Prevalence is 13.6% among HLA-B27 positive subjects and 0.8% among HLA-B27 negative subjects.

PATHOGENESIS

- The development and severity of reactive arthritis is associated with HLA-B27.
- HLA-B27 plays a modulatory role in the early signal transduction events induced by *Salmonella* invasion.
- Several in vitro studies suggest that HLA-B27 may induce a defect in the intracellular elimination of reactive pathogens, thus triggering the arthritis.
- Most of the bacteria that trigger reactive arthritis contain lipopolysaccharide (LPS). One hypothesis suggests that HLA-B27 confers an aberrant response in cells subjected to stimulation with LPS. Presumably this response manifests as inflammatory arthritis.

CLINICAL FEATURES

SKIN AND MUCOUS MEMBRANE
- Painless small, shallow ulcers of the glans penis and urethral meatus, termed *balanitis circinata* may precede the arthritis.
- The skin lesions are seen in 14% of affected patients.
- Keratoderma blennorrhagica is a hyperkeratotic skin lesion that begins as a clear vesicle on an erythematous base and progresses to maculopapular lesions with nodules. These are frequently seen on the soles of the feet, toes, scrotum, penis, palms, trunk, and scalp.
- The nails can become thickened and ridged. Keratotic material accumulates under the nail and lifts it from the nail bed.
- Erythema nodosum develops after some infections eg, post-*Yersinia* infections.

EYE MANIFESTATIONS
- The conjunctivitis is usually sterile and resolves in a week, but may persist for a month.

- Anterior uveitis is usually seen in HLA-B27 positive patients. The initial attack is typically unilateral and tends to spare the choroid and retina. It may be associated with photophobia, erythema, and pain. Uveitis resolves within 2 to 4 months.

MUSCULOSKELETAL MANIFESTATIONS

- Joint involvement is typically asymmetric and oligoarticular. The lower extremities are commonly involved (knees, ankles, and feet), however, upper limb arthritis may also occur. Joint erosions have been observed with chronic disease. Enthesitis commonly produces heel pain and metatarsalgia. It may also cause dactylitis (*sausage digits*) of the fingers and toes. Forty percent of patient with reactive arthritis may develop axial skeletal symptoms (sacroiliitis) and/or spondylitis.

LABORATORY FINDINGS

- During the acute illness:
  ○ Leukocytosis with an elevated ESR and CRP
- The prevalence of HLA-B27 in patients with reactive arthritis is approximately 50%. Thus, the clinician should only screen for HLA-B27 in the appropriate clinical setting. Accordingly, a positive test supports, but does not establish the diagnosis.
- Arthrocentesis with synovial fluid analysis is useful to exclude infectious and crystal induced arthritis.

RADIOGRAPHIC FEATURES

- Enthesopathy
  ○ Imaging reveals the signs of enthesitis including proliferation and bony reactivity at enthesis sites. Since enthesitis may be obvious on the clinical examination, imaging studies are not always indicated. Additional findings observed on radiographs include periostitis and calcification of the tendons.
- Sacroiliitis
  ○ Much like AS, sacroiliitis (which is unilateral and asymmetric) can be detected by plain radiographs, CT scan, and MRI. Imaging studies may prove valuable as a tool to document objective improvement during treatment.

THERAPY

- Antibiotics should be employed to eradicate the bacterial infection. The first line of therapy for all patients are the NSAID class of drugs, although there is little evidence that these agents alter the course of the disease. Nonetheless, they produce subjective improvement in pain and function.
- Local intraarticular injections of corticosteroids are helpful for monoarthritis and localized areas of inflammation. The sacroiliac joints respond especially well to local corticosteroid injections.

- Topical corticosteroids and keratolytic agents are useful for keratoderma blennorrhagica and circinate balanitis. For resistant skin lesions, methotrexate, retinoids, and phototherapy have proven beneficial.
- Anterior uveitis requires treatment with topical corticosteroids, mydriatics and cycloplegics.
- If the patient experiences persistent pain (arthritis) after receiving a minimum of 2 weeks of NSAID treatment, a disease modifying antirheumatic drug (DMARDs) should be considered.
  ○ Sulfasalazine is effective for peripheral arthritis, but has negligible effects on axial disease. A dose of 500 mg daily followed by a gradual increase to 3 g daily is necessary to control the disease. In patients resistant to NSAIDS or sulfasalazine, MTX has been utilized. The response is similar to that observed in AS and can also be used if patient shows no improvement in symptoms. While no randomized controlled trials have been published to support the use of TNF inhibitors, a trial of an anti-TNF agent, such as etanercept 50 mg subcutaneously weekly is reasonable based on a several small trials. These agents should be reserved for patients refractory to NSAIDS and sulfasalizine.

PSORIATIC ARTHRITIS (PsA)

Psoriatic Arthritis (PsA) is an inflammatory arthritis associated with psoriasis. PsA patients are seronegative for rheumatoid factor, although this disease was initially thought to be a variant of rheumatoid arthritis.

EPIDEMIOLOGY

- The prevalence in the general population is approximately 2% to 3%. In patients with an established diagnosis of psoriasis, PsA varies from 7% to 42%. It affects both the proximal and distal interphalangeal joints and differs from rheumatoid arthritis by lack of gender preference and asymmetric joint involvement.

GENETIC FACTORS

- First-degree relatives of patients with PsA are 50 times more likely to develop arthritis. HLA-B-38 and B-39 have been associated with peripheral arthritis.

CLINICAL FEATURES

- Patterns of PsA joint involvement:
  ○ Arthritis of the distal interphalangeal (DIP) joints.
  ○ Symmetric polyarthritis.

○ Destructive (mutilans) arthritis.
○ Asymmetric oligoarthritis.
○ Spondyloarthropathy—axial involvement.

The patterns of PsA joint involvement are not permanent. They may change from their original presentation. Spondyloarthropathy develops in 20% to 40% of patients. This tends to develop in men and older patients, and tends to begin later in the disease course and is characterized by asymmetric sacroiliitis and spinal disease similar to that observed with AS.

• Other features
  ○ Dactylitis occurs in more than 30% of patients. It is characterized by diffuse swelling of the entire digit accompanied by arthritis of the DIP, proximal interphalangeal and metacarpophalangeal joints. Enthesitis usually affects the Achilles tendon insertion area.
• Extraarticular manifestations
• Nail pitting, ridging, and onycholysis are common. For example, nail changes are seen in 90% of patients with PsA.
• Conjunctivitis or iritis occurs in 7% to 33% of patients.
• Aortic incompetence occurs in less than 4% of patients with PsA and usually develops later in the course.

LABORATORY FINDINGS

• An elevated ESR and WBC is seen in 40% to 60% of patients (more common with the polyarticular form, likely because of the associated inflammatory response). A small number of patients (<5%) have rheumatoid factor or antibodies to citrullinated cyclic peptides.

RADIOGRAPHIC FEATURES

• Radiographs reveal asymmetric distribution of joint involvement. The DIP joints are characterized by bony ankylosis with resorption of the distal phalanges. Bony erosions with new bone formation may also be seen. Some patients develop spondylitis and sacroiliitis.
• *Pencil-in-cup* type changes in the peripheral joints are unique to PsA, because of marked lysis of the distal phalanx with remodeling of the proximal end of the distal phalanx.
• Temporomandibular, sternoclavicular, and manubriosternal joint involvement are also seen in PsA. Enthesopathy results in the formation of bone spurs and is accompanied by a periosteal reaction. Marginal syndesmophytes and paramarginal syndesmophytes may also be seen in the spine.

CLINICAL COURSE AND OUTCOME

• The course of PsA is characterized by a series of flares and remissions. Destructive arthritis develops in 25% of patients with oligoarthritis and 64% of patients with polyarticular arthritis.

THERAPY

• The first-line therapy is usually an NSAID for pain control and suppression of the inflammatory response. In patients with persistent arthritis or involvement of multiple joints, the DMARDs should be considered. In general, methotrexate up to 20 mg/wk or azathioprine up to 150 mg/d have been used in these patients. Sulfasalazine up to 1 g three times daily is also useful. Leflunomide (20 mg/day) and cyclosporin-A is effective for the skin lesions as well as arthritis. The toxicity of these agents (hepatoxicity and nephrotoxicity) must be weighed against their benefits.
• Several randomized-controlled trials have shown significant improvement in symptoms and signs with the anti-TNF agents (infliximab intravenously, etanercept, or adalimumab in the same dosages as used for reactive arthritis). These agents are typically reserved for patients not responding to NSAIDs and/or MTX.

ENTEROPATHIC ARTHRITIS

Gastrointestinal diseases have been linked to the development of arthritis (enteropathic arthritis). The gastrointestinal pathologies associated with inflammatory arthritis include:
• Inflammatory bowel disease (Crohn disease and ulcerative colitis)
• Bypass arthritis
• Celiac disease
• Whipple disease
• Collagenous colitis and lymphocytic colitis

INFLAMMATORY BOWEL DISEASE

• Symptoms of arthritis tend to coincide with disease activity in ulcerative colitis. Peripheral arthritis is seen in up 5% to 10% of these patients. The peripheral arthritis is usually acute in onset, oligoarticular, asymmetric, and migratory, and resolves within 6 weeks. If polyarticular arthritis develops, the patient may experience persistent symptoms. The arthritis is generally of a nondestructive and reversible nature. Spinal involvement has been characterized in approximately

10% to 20% of patients with peripheral arthritis. Sacroiliitis may also occur. Radiographs may reveal squaring of the vertebrae.
- Other manifestations include
  - Clubbing of the fingers.
  - Pyoderma gangrenosum (a painful ulcerating skin lesion associated with systemic disease).
  - Acute anterior uveitis.
  - Erythema nodosum.
  - Aphthous stomatitis.
  - Achilles tendonitis/plantar fasciitis.
  - Septic arthritis of the hip.
  - Vasculitis.
  - Amyloidosis.
- Pathogenesis
  - Genetic factors such as HLA associations have been associated with the development of arthritis, especially spinal involvement. HLA-B27 is thought to modulate cytokine expression in the gut mucosa, and coupled with increased gut permeability may produce arthritis.
- Laboratory abnormalities
  - Elevated ESR (nonspecific)
  - Negative antinuclear antibody (ANA) and rheumatoid factor serologies. Although, the P-anti-neutrophil cytoplasmic antibody (ANCA) is positive in most of these patients.
- Therapy
  - Generally directed toward treating the underlying inflammatory bowel disease. For pain control and suppression of inflammation, the cyclooxygenase (COX)-II inhibitors should be used with caution as they have been shown to paradoxically exacerbate inflammation. Miscellaneous agents useful in other spondyloarthropathies have been used with some success in patients with polyarticular involvement (sulfasalazine, azathioprine, methotrexate, mycophenolate mofetil, and the anti-TNF agents).

BYPASS ARTHRITIS AND DERMATITIS SYNDROME

- This arthritis is only seen in patients after undergoing intestinal bypass surgery.
- The arthritis is inflammatory, polyarticular, symmetric, and migratory. It can affect both upper and lower extremity joints and be associated with flares and spontaneous remission. A maculopapular or papulo-pustular rash has been observed in some patients.
- The pathogenesis is believed secondary to bacterial overgrowth in the blind loop, which induces immune complex formation and deposition in the skin and joints.
- The therapy typically involves the use of NSAIDs and antibiotics which usually improve the symptoms.

Surgical reanastomosis of the blind loop may eliminate the symptoms.

CELIAC DISEASE AND ARTHRITIS

- The arthritis is symmetric and involves multiple, predominantly large joints (hips, knees, ankles, and shoulders), although monarticular disease may also occur. The changes are nondestructive and there is a strong association with HLA-DQ2. The diagnosis is usually established by documenting the presence of IgA or IgG antibodies against gliadin, transglutaminase, and endomysium. Jejunal biopsy reveals villous atrophy. The patients typically respond to institution of a gluten-free diet.

WHIPPLE DISEASE

- This disorder is caused by the microorganism *Tropheryma whippleii*. 15% of patients present with articular symptoms, usually involving the knee. Other peripheral joints and spinal involvement may also occur. The therapy consists of benzyl penicillin and streptomycin for 2 weeks, followed by trimethoprim and sulfamethoxazole for 1 to 2 years.

COLLAGENOUS COLITIS AND LYMPHOCYTIC COLITIS

- This disease is characterized by thickening of the collagen layer beneath the intestinal epithelium. Lymphocytic colitis or lymphocytic infiltration is seen in the upper colon. Both diseases are associated with autoimmune thyroid disease. Joint symptoms occur in 40% to 60% of cases. Collagenous colitis is associated with Sjögren's syndrome, nondestructive oligoarthritis, migratory arthralgias, sacroiliitis, and rheumatoid arthritis. The therapy consists of NSAIDs, sulfasalazine, antibiotics such as metronidazole, glucocorticoids, and in resistant cases, colonic resection.

BIBLIOGRAPHY

Anandarajah A, Ritchlin CT. Treatment update on spondyloarthropathy. *Curr Opin Rheumatol.* 2005;17:247–256.

De Keyser F, Baeten D, Van den Bosch F, et al. Gut inflammation and spondyloarthropathies. *Curr Rheumatol Rep.* 2002;5: 525–532.

François RJ, Braun J, Khan MA. Entheses and enthesitis: A histopathologic review and relevance to spondyloarthropathies. *Curr Opin Rheumatol.* 2001;13:255–264.

Gladman DD. Current concepts in psoriatic arthritis. *Curr Opin Rheumatol.* 2002;14:361–366.

Helliwell PS. Relationship of psoriatic arthritis with the other spondyloarthropathies. *Curr Opin Rheumatol.* 2004;16:344–349.

Höhler T, Märker-Hermann E. Psoriatic arthritis: Clinical aspects, genetics, and the role of T cells. *Curr Opin Rheumatol.* 2001; 13:273–279.

Penttinen MA, Liu Y, Granfors K. The role of infection in the pathogenesis of spondyloarthropathies with special reference to human leukocyte antigen-B27. *Curr Rheumatol Rep.* 2002;4: 518–524.

Turner MJ, Colbert RA. HLA-B27 and pathogenesis of spondyloarthropathies. *Curr Opin Rheumatol.* 2002;14:367–372.

Van der Linden S, Van der Heijde D, Braun J. Spondyloarthropathies, In: Harris ED, Budd RC, Genovese MC, et al, eds. *Kelley's Textbook of Rheumatology.* 7th ed. Philadelphia, PA: Elsevier Saunders; 2005:1125–1173.

Wollheim FA. Enteropathic arthritis: How do the joints talk with the gut? *Curr Opin Rheumatol.* 2001;13:305–309.

129 OSTEOARTHRITIS

Peri Hickman Pepmueller

DEFINITION

- Osteoarthritis (OA), sometimes referred to as *osteoarthrosis* or *degenerative joint disease,* is the most common form of arthritis. Prior to 1986, no standard definition of OA existed; OA was described as a disorder of unknown etiology that primarily affects the articular cartilage and subchondral bone. Since then, various workshops of national and world experts proposed new definitions. The current definition was developed in 1994 at a consensus workshop sponsored by the American Academy of Orthopedic Surgeons and the National Institutes of Health and emphasized the concept that OA may not represent a single disease entity.

OA is the result of both mechanical and biologic events that destabilize the normal coupling of degradation and synthesis of articular cartilage and subchondral bone. Although it may be initiated by multiple factors including genetic, developmental, metabolic and traumatic; OA involves all of the tissues of the diarthrodial joint. Ultimately, OA is manifested by morphologic, biochemical, molecular, and biomechanical changes of both cells and matrix which lead to a softening, fibrillation, *ulceration and loss of articular cartilage, sclerosis and eburnation of subchondral bone, osteophytes and subchondral cysts. When clinically evident, OA is characterized by joint pain, tenderness, limitation of movement, crepitus, occasional effusion, and variable degrees of local inflammation. (Brandt K.D. et al., 1986.)*

CLASSIFICATION

- OA is usually classified as idiopathic (primary) or secondary (Table 129–1).
- When OA is related to previous trauma, metabolic or inflammatory disease, crystal deposition, or other underlying medical/surgical conditions, patients are classified as having secondary OA.
- When no precipitating cause can be identified, the disorder is referred to as primary or *idiopathic.*
- This classification is helpful for instructional purposes, but necessarily suffers from the current lack of understanding of the precise pathogenesis of the disorder.

EPIDEMIOLOGY

- OA is the most common joint disorder in the United States and the world.
- OA is the leading cause of long-term disability among adults in the United States and the most common cause of lost workdays.
- Advanced age is considered one of the strongest risk factors in the development of OA. The prevalence and severity of OA parallels advancing age in most individuals. Greater than 50% of patients older than 65 years

TABLE 129–1 Classification of Osteoarthritis

Idiopathic

Localized (hands, feet, knee, hip, spine, other)
Generalized (includes three or more areas listed above)

Secondary

Trauma (acute, chronic)
Congenital or developmental
  Localized (eg, congenital hip dislocation, slipped epiphysis)
  Mechanical (eg, unequal lower extremity length, valgus/varus deformity)
Metabolic (eg, ochronosis, hemochromatosis)
Endocrine (eg, acromegaly, diabetes mellitus, hyperparathyroidism)
Calcium deposition diseases (eg, calcium pyrophosphate dihydrate deposition)
Other bone and joint diseases
  Localized (fracture, avascular necrosis, gout)
  Diffuse (eg, inflammatory arthritis, Paget disease)
Other (eg, neuropathic arthropathies, frostbite, hemoglobinopathies)

SOURCE: Modified from Brandt KD, Mankin HJ, Shulman LE. Workshop on etiopathogenesis of osteoarthritis. *J Rheumatol.* 1986;13:1126–1160.

have radiographic changes of OA, and virtually all have compatible radiographic changes in at least one joint after age 75.

- A familial pattern of inheritance has long been recognized in the development of Heberden nodes. Further evidence for hereditary factors includes twin studies demonstrating heritability for radiographic features of OA at the knee and hip. Moreover, genome-wide scanning and haplotype association data has suggested multiple potential loci associated with the development or progression of OA. Nonetheless, candidate genes have yet to be identified, although the field is evolving rapidly.
- Obesity is the strongest modifiable risk factor associated with OA, especially OA of the knee.
- Mechanical stresses (such as with certain occupations), which subject weight-bearing joints to repetitive trauma, or a previous history of joint trauma correlate with OA in the injured joints. Baseball pitchers tend to develop osteoarthritis in the shoulder, whereas ditch diggers and pneumatic drill workers experience an increased incidence of elbow and wrist OA.
- Miscellaneous risk factors include congenital and developmental diseases of bone and cartilage. Congenital dysplasias, history of slipped capital femoral epiphysis, history of inflammatory arthritis, and muscle weakness have been associated with OA as well. Some metabolic and endocrine disorders also predispose patients to OA (eg, hemochromatosis, acromegaly).

PATHOLOGY

- On gross examination, early OA is characterized by articular irregularities. This is followed by ulceration of the cartilage and eventually by frank cartilage loss.
- Microscopically, the surface layers flake off while deeper layers develop longitudinal fissures, a process termed fibrillation. Eventually the cartilage thins and becomes denuded. At this time there is loss of extracellular cartilage matrix and chondrocytes, with noticeable clefts in the cartilage surface.
- Reactive changes are seen in the subchondral bone including bony sclerosis in the areas underlying denuded cartilage, subchondral bone cysts, and osteophytes (bony outgrowths) seen near the margin of the joint.

PATHOGENESIS

- Articular cartilage has two primary functions: to provide a smooth load-bearing surface to permit motion of the joint with minimal friction and to cushion the stress within the joint by deforming under mechanical loading.

- Normal articular cartilage is primarily composed of water, collagen, and proteoglycans. The network of collagen fibrils provides a strong three-dimensional framework to constrain the proteoglycan molecules; the negative charge of the proteoglycans provides a strong hydrophilic force. Water molecules are released with compression of cartilage and recaptured when compression is released, thus permitting smooth joint motion and cushioning impact. Chondrocytes synthesize matrix proteins and enzymes that degrade the extracellular matrix proteins, allowing for gradual turnover of the cartilage constituents.
- Arthritis develops when mechanical stressors promote degradation of the bone and cartilage, that exceeds its synthesis. Production of matrix degrading enzymes (eg, matrix metalloproteases) and inflammatory cytokines (eg, interleukin-1) decreases the quantity and quality of proteoglycans, which perturbs the normal viscoelastic properties of cartilage.
- The subchondral bone changes observed in OA may be secondary to the development of OA, rather than the consequence of cartilage injury.

CLINICAL FEATURES

SIGNS AND SYMPTOMS

- Pain accompanied by limitation of function in one or several joints is usually the presenting complaint for patients with degenerative arthritis.
- The patients are often overweight, middle-aged, or elderly.
- Onset of pain is gradual, over years.
- The pain is worsened by activity and relieved by rest. As the disease advances, the pain may occur even at rest.
- Morning stiffness usually lasts less than 30 minutes.
- Limitation of function is a common complaint.
- The pain is often worse when the weather changes.
- The gel phenomenon is characterized by morning-like stiffness after periods of rest or inactivity, but resolves within a few minutes of normal activity.

JOINT INVOLVEMENT

- The joints most commonly involved include the following:
  - Hand: Involvement in the distal interphalangeal joints of the hands may be asymptomatic, whereas involvement of proximal interphalangeal and first carpometacarpal joints cause stiffness and difficulty with manual dexterity.

- Knee: Involvement of the the tibiofemoral joint and the patellofemoral joint are common. The patients may complain of instability or buckling, especially when descending stairs or stepping off curbs. Symptoms that develop or worsen while ascending stairs are common with patellar disease.
- Hip: OA of the hip may result in pain referred to the thigh, knee, or groin and often interferes with ambulation.
- Foot: The first metatarsophalangeal joint is the most commonly affected joint. This is associated with bony swelling and deformity (bunion) and is usually accompanied by pain while walking.
- Spine: Patients may exhibit symptoms in the neck and lower back when the disease affects the apophyseal or facet uncovertebral joints. Irritation of adjacent nerve roots produces radicular pain. Spinal osteophytes may narrow the foramen and compress the adjacent nerve roots. Radiographic changes are insensitive, particularly with early disease, and correlate poorly with symptoms.
- Other joints: Involvement of other joints, such as the metacarpophalangeal joints, wrists, elbows and ankles are unusual in OA and should prompt an evaluation for other conditions, such as trauma, congenital joint abnormalities, and for evidence of a metabolic (hemosiderosis) or crystalline (calcium pyrophosphate deposition) disease.

PHYSICAL EXAMINATION

- Typical findings are as follows:
  - Bony hypertrophy or enlargement (eg, Heberden nodes at the distal interphalangeal joints, Bouchard nodes at the proximal interphalangeal joints) (Figure 129–1).
  - Decreased range of motion.
  - Crepitus, felt on passive range of motion, is caused by irregularities in the opposing cartilage surfaces.
  - Gait disturbance.
  - Malalignment.
  - Signs of local inflammation with warmth and swelling are atypical. Effusions are occasionally seen in the knee. The presence of inflammatory signs such as warmth, erythema, and marked swelling suggest a confounding diagnosis of septic arthritis or a superimposed process such as gout or a crystalline-induced arthritis.

RADIOGRAPHIC ABNORMALITIES

- Classically characterized by bony proliferation at the joint margins (osteophytes).

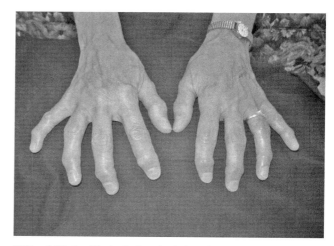

FIG. 129–1 Typical hand deformities in osteoarthritis. Heberden nodes at the distal interphalangeal joints and Bouchard nodes at the proximal interphalangeal joints are seen.

- Asymmetric joint space narrowing.
- Subchondral sclerosis.
- Subchondral cysts (Figure 129–2).

LABORATORY FINDINGS

- Results of routine laboratory tests are normal unless a comorbid condition exists.
- Laboratory tests are useful primarily to screen for associated conditions and to establish a baseline for monitoring therapy.
- Synovial fluid analysis usually reveals a white blood cell count less than 1000.

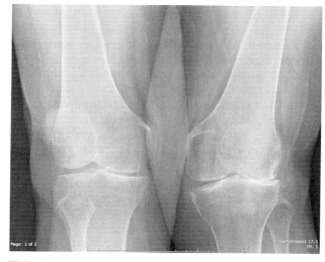

FIG. 129–2 This radiograph shows many changes commonly seen in osteoarthritis. An osteophyte, medial joint space narrowing (mild to moderate), lateral joint space narrowing (severe), and subchondral sclerosis are present.

THERAPEUTIC APPROACH

PRINCIPLES

- The management of OA is directed toward symptom relief and maintaining (or improving) functional status.
- Currently, there is no approved therapy that definitively arrests or retards the disease process (eg, cartilage degradation and synthesis).
- Both nonpharmacologic and pharmacologic therapies are helpful in the management of OA.

NONPHARMACOLOGIC MODALITIES

- Nonpharmacologic therapies are often overlooked, yet show equal or greater efficacy than some commonly recommended pharmacologic therapies.
- Patient educational materials such as those published by the Arthritis Foundation provide basic information which allows the patient to better understand the disease process. Some information is available online at www.arthritis.org.
- Occupational therapy provides valuable information about the patients functional status, educates the patient regarding joint protection techniques, and provides assistive devices when needed.
- Physical therapy educates the patient regarding optimal local measures such as therapeutic heat and massage techniques and customized exercise plans.
- Exercise programs stressing range of motion and muscular strengthening are helpful for reducing pain and lessening the stress placed on joints (especially quadriceps strengthening for knee OA). Low-impact aerobic exercise has also been shown to decrease pain.
- Weight loss, especially if combined with exercise has been shown to diminish pain.
- Wedged insoles may help correct malalignment across the knee.
- Corrective footwear may diminish foot pain.
- Patellar taping or bracing may help alleviate pain in patellofemoral disease.
- The use of canes or crutches in appropriate patients is helpful to maintain independence.

PHARMACOLOGIC THERAPY

- Acetaminophen (500–1000 mg up to four times daily) is the first-line recommended therapy.
- Traditional nonsteroidal antiinflammatory drugs (NSAIDs) or cyclooxygenase-2 inhibitors are reasonable options for pain relief; however, their toxicities such as gastric and duodenal ulceration, gastrointestinal bleeding (traditional NSAIDs), renal toxicity, and recently, cardiovascular complication, must be weighed against their benefits.
- Topical compounds such as capsaicin have been shown to be helpful for modest pain relief in patients with OA.
- Intraarticular corticosteroid injections can relieve pain for an average of 1 to 3 weeks; however, they should not be used for long-term management. Corticosteroid injections are best reserved for special events or occasions (weddings, travel, etc).
- Glucosamine and chondroitin sulfate are widely used for the treatment of OA. Several randomized controlled clinical trials report greater pain relief than with placebo and relatively little toxicity; however, publication bias has been noted in many of these trials. A multicenter study funded by the National Institutes of Health did not observe a reduction in pain in patients receiving these supplements. Subgroup analysis suggested that the combination of glucosamine and chondroitin sulfate relieved pain in patients with moderate-to-severe OA.
- Injections of hyaluronic acid into the knee joint has been approved by the Food and Drug Administration for the treatment of OA. Nonetheless, the data on efficacy remain controversial.
- Opioid analgesics are more efficacious than placebo in controlling pain, but side effects and drug dependence are major concerns.

SURGICAL MANAGEMENT

- Some experts believe that total joint arthroplasty has been the single most significant advance in the treatment of OA in the past 50 years.
- The patients whose symptoms are not adequately controlled with medical therapy and who have moderate-to-severe pain and functional impairment are candidates for orthopedic surgery.
- Total joint arthroplasty almost always provides significant pain relief; however, functional status is less consistently improved. The most satisfying results are obtained when the surgery is performed for pain relief.
- The ideal patient is otherwise healthy with good muscle mass and tone and is greater than 60 years of age. Younger patients are usually not considered because of the small but real occurrence of joint instability.
- Other surgical treatments that attempt to preserve or restore articular cartilage include joint debridement, penetration of the subchondral bone, osteotomy, and replacement of damaged cartilage with grafts or soft tissue; however, the efficacy of these procedures has not been demonstrated by prospective, controlled randomized studies.

BIBLIOGRAPHY

Altman RD. Structure/disease-modifying agents for osteoarthritis. *Semin Arthritis Rheum.* 2005;34(suppl 2):3.

American College of Rheumatology Subcommittee on Osteoarthritis Guidelines. Recommendations for the medical management of osteoarthritis of the hip and knee: 2000 update. *Arthritis Rheum.* 2000;43:1905–1915.

Brandt KD, Doherty M, Lohmander LS. *Osteoarthritis.* New York, NY: Oxford Press, 2003.

Brandt KD, Mankin HJ, Shulman LE. Workshop on etiopathogenesis of osteoarthritis. *J Rheumatol.* 1986;13:1126–1160.

Dieppe P, Brandt KD. What is important in treating osteoarthritis? Whom should we treat and how should we treat them? *Rheum Dis Clin North Am.* 2003;29:687.

Felson, DT. Osteoarthritis of the knee. *N Engl J Med.* 2006;354:841.

Keuttner KE, Goldberg VM. In: Keuttner KE, Goldberg VM, eds. *Osteoarthritic Disorders.* Rosemont, IL: American Academy of Orthopedic Surgeons; 1995:xxi–xxv.

130 SYSTEMIC LUPUS ERYTHEMATOSUS

Terry L. Moore

EPIDEMIOLOGY

- Systemic lupus erythematosus (SLE) is the most common cause of systemic illness in young females between the ages of 15 and 40 years. It is by far the most common disease in young African American females. It is estimated between 250,000 and 500,000 cases of SLE occur in the United States alone with an overall prevalence of approximately 100 per 100,000 women.

- Lupus affects all age groups with the age of onset being younger than 10 years of age in approximately 4% of patients and up to 12% occurring before the age of 20 years. The majority of the patients are between the ages of 15 and 40 years.

PATHOGENESIS

- The pathogenesis of SLE is a complex process. SLE is the classic autoimmune disease manifested by type III hypersensitivity. Target tissue damage is caused primarily by pathogenic autoantibodies, and immune complex formation that induces a vasculitis in many organ systems. The abnormal immune response also permits persistence of pathogenic B and T cells, hyperactivation of T and B cells, and failure to interrupt this process.

- The immunologic abnormalities are thought to be secondary to lupus susceptibility genes which engender abnormalities in complement, apoptosis, and cell surface receptors.

- Environmental stimuli including ultraviolet light promotes apoptosis in dermal cells which releases RNA protein, DNA protein, and phospholipid self-antigens resulting in the proliferation of autoantibodies including antinuclear antibodies (ANA) and antiphospholipid antibodies (APLA).

- Multiple genetic defects appear to contribute to the development of pathogenetic autoantibodies.

- General characteristics that favor the induction of pathogenic autoantibodies are the capacity of the antibody to bind directly to target tissues, such as red cells, white cells, and platelets. The antibodies can also bind to glomerular antigens and activate complement. Autoantigens, which are present in target tissues, produce immune complexes and activate inflammatory pathways that, in turn, give rise to a wide range of systemic manifestations. Immune complex formation overwhelms the clearance mechanisms of the macrophage-monocyte system resulting in immune complex deposition. The relatively small size of the immune complex enable them to escape phagocytosis and the physicochemical characteristics of the complex allow it to bind to anions in tissues. Subsequently, decreased immune complex clearance (also related to acquired and genetically determined low levels of crystallizable fragment, [Fc] gamma receptors and complement receptors), coupled with decreased solubilization of immune complexes as complement levels fall or are genetically low, produce the ideal milieu for further immune complex mediated injury.

CLINICAL FINDINGS

SLE is a systemic disease that can present with multiple-organ involvement.

- The most common presenting clinical features in SLE are arthralgias or arthritis in 55%, skin involvement in 20%, nephritis, fever, and miscellaneous manifestations in 5% to 15% of patients.

- In patients younger than the age of 20 years, the most common presentation is renal disease.

TABLE 130–1   Systemic Lupus Erythematosus Criteria

1. Malar rash
2. Discoid rash
3. Photosensitivity
4. Oral ulcers
5. Arthritis
6. Serositis
7. Renal abnormalities
8. Neurologic abnormalities
9. Hematologic disorder
10. Immunologic manifestations
11. Positive antinuclear antibody

- Over time, SLE involves the joints in 90% of cases, the skin in up to 70%, and the kidneys in almost all patients; with 50% developing diffuse proliferative glomerulonephritis. Thirty percent of patients develop pleural or pericardial involvement, and up to 50% develop central nervous system manifestations.

- The American College of Rheumatology (ACR) has established criteria for the diagnosis of SLE (Table 130–1) which include malar rash, photosensitivity, oral ulcers, arthritis, serositis, renal, neurologic and hematologic disorders, and immunologic manifestations.

- The classic skin finding of SLE is the malar rash sparing the nasolabial folds, but almost any skin manifestation can occur including painful nail fold lesions and urticaria. On skin biopsy, there is thinning of the epidermis with a lymphocytic infiltrate and increased deposition of connective tissue. Immunofluorescence staining of the skin reveals a positive lupus band test with immunoglobulin and complement deposition at the dermal/epidermal junction.

- Other manifestations of SLE include mucous membrane involvement with oral or nasopharyngeal ulcerations and possible vaginal ulcerations. The ulcerations are usually painless but can become infected and painful. Oral lesions usually occur on the soft palate.

- The arthritis of SLE is a nonerosive arthritis involving two or more peripheral joints characterized by tenderness, swelling, or effusion. The classic finding of nonerosive ulnar deviation of Jaccoud arthritis can be seen in lupus patients.

- SLE patients can also develop multiple organ system manifestations including serositis, which can involve both pleura and pericardium. A computed tomogram of the chest and echocardiogram may prove useful in these patients.

- Renal disease, usually manifests as proteinuria (often greater than 500 mg/24 hours) or by hematuria, pyuria, and cellular casts. A renal biopsy is indicated to render the appropriate therapy in these patients. The World Health Organization (WHO) classification of kidney disease in patients with SLE include class I, which is normal; class II, which is characterized by mesangial proliferation (class IIa indicates normal light microscopy with mesangial immune deposits, whereas, class IIb is characterized by mesangial proliferation plus mesangial immune deposits); class III is characterized by focal proliferation and typically involves less than 50% of the glomeruli; class IV is characterized by diffuse proliferation in more than 50% of the glomeruli; class V is characterized by membranous changes including diffuse basement membrane thickening; and class VI is characterized by chronic scarring (glomerulosclerosis).

- Immunofluorescence of kidney biopsy specimens shows the classic immune complex lesions (lumpy, bumpy pattern) and on electron microscopy immune complexes are visible in the subendothelial and subepithelial space.

- Involvement of the central nervous system results in significant long-term morbidity associated with multiple neuropsychiatric symptoms and may mimic a variety of neurologic diseases. These include confusion, anxiety, aseptic meningitis, cerebrovascular injury, cognitive dysfunction, demyelinating syndromes, headaches, mood disorders, movement disorders, myelopathy, psychosis, and most commonly, seizures. In addition, peripheral nervous systemic involvement may also occur and include autonomic neuropathy, cranial nerve injury, mononeuritis, and peripheral neuropathy. The evaluation of nervous system involvement should include lumbar puncture, electroencephalography (EEG), and magnetic resonance imaging (MRI) with both T1- and T2-weighted images, which can reveal changes at the white-gray matter border indicating immune complex disease.

LABORATORY EVALUATION

- Laboratory evaluation is essential in patients with SLE, and includes a complete blood count (CBC), urinalysis, erythrocyte sedimentation rate (ESR), C-reactive protein (CRP), comprehensive metabolic panel, and the muscle enzymes, creatine phosphokinase (CPK), aldolase, and lactate dehydrogenase (LDH), as well as a comprehensive antibody panel.

- The CBC reveals anemia of inflammatory disease, but in some cases a hemolytic process characterized by a positive Coombs test for immunoglobulin G (IgG) results in a marked fall in red cell count. While leukocytosis can occur with steroid administration, the most common finding in SLE is leukopenia. Leukopenia or thrombocytopenia is generally seen in patients younger than age 30, and is usually secondary to anti-white cell and/or anti-platelet antibodies.

- ESR and CRP are inflammatory markers that are normally less than 15 mm/h or less than 0.4 mg/dL, respectively in healthy patients. An elevated sedimentation rate and CRP almost always occurs with active SLE. The normal ratio of ESR to CRP is 10:1. If the CRP is disproportionately high, an underlying infection should be considered.

- Urinalysis can reveal proteinuria with various cellular elements including white and red cells; red cell casts are pathognomonic for acute glomerulonephritis (often class IV). Additional studies should include a 24-hour urine for creatinine clearance and total protein. Importantly, a renal biopsy is almost always indicated in patients with an abnormal sediment. The biopsy provides essential information to render the appropriate therapy in lupus nephritis.

- The evaluation must also exclude other connective tissue diseases and, thus includes testing for rheumatoid factor (RF), antinuclear antibodies (ANA), complement levels, and cryoglobulin levels. Clotting studies should also be obtained for lupus anticoagulant.

- RF is a classic 19S immunoglobulin M (IgM) molecule that is found in all immunoglobulin classes and is by definition an anti-IgG globulin for the Fc fragment of IgG. It is found more commonly in patients with rheumatoid arthritis, but can be found in 30% to 40% of patients with SLE and other connective tissue diseases. Anticyclic citrullinated peptide antibodies are usually not found in patients with SLE.

- The best screening test for SLE is an ANA; a diverse array of antibodies directed against numerous macromolecules and normal constituents of the cell nucleus. The presence of ANA is a hallmark of connective tissue disease but not diagnostic. Low titers of ANA (less than or equal to 1:320) can be found in up to 30% of the healthy, females. Viral infections such as Epstein-Barr, cytomegalovirus, and parvovirus can transiently increase the ANA. In young females, and patients with autoimmune thyroiditis, the ANA can also be positive.

- Importantly, when the ANA is positive, highly-specific antibodies can be further characterized to establish a particular underlying connective tissue disorder (eg, antibodies to double-stranded DNA) or serve as markers of disease activity. However, the titer of ANA (increasing or decreasing) is generally not a reliable index of disease activity or response to therapy, with a few notable exceptions (antibodies to double-stranded DNA [dsDNA] and antibodies to ribonucleoprotein).

- The most widely used technique for the detection of ANA is indirect immunofluorescence using human epithelial 2 (HEp-2) cells as substrate. The standard assay can detect antibodies that are present in abundance, however antibodies in low concentration (especially those to nuclear antigens) such as antibodies to SS-A may require specific enzyme-linked immunoabsorbent assays (ELISAs) for identification.

- Five common ANA patterns have been characterized including homogeneous, speckled, discrete speckled, rim, and nucleolar; however, these patterns are relatively nonspecific. Therefore, specific autoantibodies must also be screened for in patients with a suspected connective tissue disorder.

- Autoantibodies occur in greater than 99% of patients with SLE.

- Antibodies to dsDNA are discovered frequently in patients with SLE. Titers of anti-dsDNA antibodies correlate with renal disease, central nervous system disease, vasculitis, and low complement levels. They usually correlate with active disease as well. Two assays are commonly employed to detect anti-dsDNA antibodies. The *Crithidia luciliae* assay is very specific for SLE and tends to correlate with disease activity. In contrast, while the ELISA assay is more sensitive, it is less specific since it may also detect single-stranded DNA antibodies.

- Other ANAs include antichromatin, antihistone, and antinucleosome antibodies, which are identified in 75% of the patients (via ELISA) but can also be identified in drug-induced syndromes which mimic SLE.

- Anti-Smith (anti-Sm) antibodies are discovered in 30% to 40% of patients with SLE and correlate well with pleural disease, vasculitis, and central nervous system disease. Patients with anti-Sm antibodies should be evaluated and followed for restrictive lung disease.

- Antibodies to (U1)-ribonucleoprotein (anti-U1nRNP) also occur in 30% to 40% of patients with SLE but may also be identified in patients with mixed connective tissue disease.

- Antibodies to Ro/SS-A occur in 30% to 60% of patients and correlate with subacute cutaneous lupus, neonatal lupus, sicca complaints, and occur in patients with complement deficiencies. Antibodies to La/SS-B occur in 20% to 30% of patients with SLE and also correlate with sicca complaints. Anti-Ro/SS-A and anti-La/SS-B can cross the placenta and bind to the cardiac tissue in the fetus and produce the neonatal lupus syndrome.

- Lastly, antiribosomal-P antibodies occur in 10% to 20% of patients with SLE and tend to correlate with central nervous system vasculitis and cerebritis. For example, they have been identified in approximately

60% to 90% of patients with SLE and symptoms of psychosis.

- Further workup in patients with SLE includes measurement of complement levels, which also serve as a reasonable measure of disease activity. The total hemolytic complement (CH_{50}), is obtained to rule out a general decrease in complement activity. Specific measurements of C3 and C4 by nephelometry, reveal evidence of complement activation. Depleted levels of C3 (less than 60) and C4 (less than 10) are consistent with active immune complex mediated disease. C4 is more sensitive and thus can detect subtle episodes of complement activation.
- Other products of the complement cascade such as C3a or C5a, the membrane attack complex (MAC), or direct assays of circulating immune complexes may prove useful in the future.
- Cryoglobulins, which are cold precipitable proteins, correlate well with immune complex disease.
- These patients may also develop an antiphospholipid antibody syndrome, which is characterized by an increase in prothrombin time and a hypercoagulable state. This syndrome predisposes the SLE patient to migraine headaches, miscarriages, and deep venous thrombosis. The evaluation of this syndrome involves determination of anticardiolipin antibodies, lupus anticoagulant, and anti-β_2-glycoprotein-I antibodies.
- All patients with lupus should undergo chest imaging. If the patient has antibodies to Sm or ribonucleoprotein (RNP), they should be followed carefully for the development of restrictive pulmonary disease (measure the diffusing capacity for carbon monoxide, DLCO). An echocardiogram should also be obtained in patients with antibodies to Sm or RNP, since there is a high prevalence of right ventricular hypertrophy and pulmonary hypertension in these individuals. Importantly, patients with lupus tend to develop cardiovascular disease at an early age, therefore cardiovascular risk factors should be identified and treated (eg, hypercholesterolemia).

THERAPY

- With advances in treatment of the disease, the morbidity and mortality of lupus has decreased greatly over the last 20 years.
- The first-line therapy is to reduce all sun exposure since more than 70% of patients with SLE are photosensitive. Using a sunblock at all times with at least a skin protection factor (SPF) of 35 without a preservative or 50 with preservatives is indicated.
- The arthritis is treated with antiinflammatory agents. Cyclooxygenase-1 (COX-1) inhibitors such as sulindac,

a nonspecific prostaglandin inhibitor, at 200 mg twice daily, naproxen at 375 mg to 500 mg twice daily, or diclofenac at 50 mg to 75 mg twice daily, are excellent. However, renal status must be monitored closely. COX-2 inhibitors such as celecoxib or meloxicam also can be used.

- Collectivelly, patients with SLE have been shown to stabilize their disease when treated with hydroxychloroquine, an antimalarial, at 200 mg once or twice daily. This approach is particulary helpful for skin manifestations and arthralgias. Patients receiving hydroxychloroquine require a complete eye examination every 6 months to 1 year to rule out retinal toxicity or pigment deposition.
- Class III to IV lupus glomerulonephritis should be treated with a combination of prednisone and intravenous cyclophosphamide (500 mg/m² for six doses and then every 3 months for 18 months).
- For rapidly progressive glomerulonephritis or cerebral vasculitis, pulse methylprednisolone (1 g daily for 3 days) is also indicated.
- In cases of acute vasculitis or cerebritis, oral cyclophosphamide at a dose of 4 mg/kg for 2 days followed by 2 mg/kg for 2 days, and then 1 mg/kg/d is indicated. Once the patient has stabilized, the long-term morbidity and side effects of steroids must be weighed against their benefits.
- Steroid-sparing agents such as oral azathioprine up to 200 mg per day in divided doses, methotrexate up to 30 mg per week, mycophenolate mofetil up to 1 g orally two to three times a day, or leflunomide up to 20 mg per day may also prove useful.
- Plasmapheresis for 5 to 7 consecutive days concurrent with IV immunosuppression should be considered, particularly in refractory cases or in patients with severe vasculitis or lupus cerebritis.
- Recently, the biologic response modifier, rituximab, an anti-CD20 monoclonal antibody, has been shown to be effective in patients with very high antibody titers. The dose of rituximab is 375 mg/m² weekly for 4 weeks to reduce the immune complex burden and inhibit B cell proliferation.

BIBLIOGRAPHY

Edworthy SM. Clinical manifestations of systemic lupus erythematosus. In: Harris ED, Budd RC, Genovese MC, et al, eds. *Kelley's Textbook of Rheumatology*. 7th ed. Philadelphia, PA: Elsevier Saunders; 2005:1201.

Hahn BH. Management of systemic lupus erythematosus. In: Harris ED, Budd RC, Genovese MC, et al, eds. *Kelley's*

Textbook of Rheumatology. 7th ed. Philadelphia, PA: Elsevier Saunders; 2005:1225.

Hahn BH, Karpouzas GA, Tsao BP. Pathogenesis of systemic lupus erythematosus. In: Harris ED, Budd RC, Genovese MC, et al, eds. *Kelley's Textbook of Rheumatology.* 7th ed. Philadelphia, PA: Elsevier Saunders; 2005:1174.

Kamat SS, Pepmueller PH, Moore TL. Triplets with systemic lupus erythematosus. *Arthritis Rheum.* 2003;48:3176.

Kurien BT, Schofield RH. Autoantibody determination in the diagnosis of systemic lupus erythematosus. *Scand J Immunol.* 2006;64:227.

Temprano KK, Bandlamudi R, Moore TL. Anti-rheumatic drugs in pregnancy and lactation. *Semin Arthritis Rheum.* 2005; 35:112.

131 MISCELLANEOUS CONNECTIVE TISSUE DISEASES

Thomas G. Osborn

SJÖGREN'S SYNDROME

- Autoimmune disorder characterized by exocrine gland dysfunction.
- Common features include dry eyes, mouth, and skin; arthralgias, neuropathies, and fatigue.

EPIDEMIOLOGY

- Prevalence: 2.5% of the population.
- Gender: female-to-male, 9:1.
- Age: predilection, 20 to 40 years, but seen in all age groups.

PATHOPHYSIOLOGY

- Strict criteria established.[1,2] These include
  ○ Gritty or dry eyes, dry mouth for over 3 months
  ○ Require liquids to swallow dry food, frequent sips of water, obvious swelling of the salivary glands.
- If seen by an ophthalmologist/optometrist, the patient may have a positive Schirmer test, rose bengal staining, or lissamine green staining.
- A lip biopsy, if performed, may show inflammation of the salivary glands.

- Sjögren patients develop hypergammaglobulinemia and are positive for antinuclear antibodies, especially antibodies to SS-A (Ro) or SS-B (La), or rheumatoid factor.
- Less likely to be performed, but helpful is a positive salivary scintigraphy, parotid sialography, or an unstimulated salivary flow assessment.
- Autoreactive lymphocytes infiltrate the tissue of exocrine glands. Thus, lacrimal glands, salivary glands, sweat glands, mucosal epithelial glands in the bronchial tree and vaginal epithelium may be injured with loss of function. This causes the major features of the disease: dry eyes (xerophthalmia), dry mouth (xerostomia), dry skin, chronic bronchitis, and dyspareunia. The cause of the lymphocytic infiltration is unknown, but it has been suggested that it is initiated by a virus. Epstein-Barr virus and Hepatitis C virus have been implicated in a small number of cases. Similarly, human immunodeficiency virus, and human lymphotrophic virus type 1 have been implicated in a small number of cases.
- There is a familial risk for those with a first-degree relative with Sjögren syndrome. HLA-DR3 is the most common gene association, and is present in up to 50% of patients.
- Among the diagnostic criterion a positive lip biopsy showing a localized lymphocytic infiltrate in the minor salivary glands is quite useful. A majority of these cells are T-cells; however, B-cells may comprise up to 25% of this infiltrate. It is thought that glandular epithelial cells participate in antigen presentation There is considerable interest in the biology of antigen presentation from these tissues.
- It is not uncommon for the diagnosis to be established retrospectively, as the presenting symptoms may include neuropathy, renal tubular acidosis, or recurrent/persistent bronchitis.

EXTRAGLANDULAR INVOLVEMENT

ARTHRITIS
- Common, seen in >50%
- Characterized by arthralgias, intermittent joint swelling, or synovitis
- Usually not associated with deformities

NEUROLOGIC
- Common, seen in >50%
- Sensory or motor peripheral neuropathy
- Cranial neuropathy
- Central nervous system (CNS) involvement has been characterized by paralysis, seizures, transverse myelopathy, encephalopathy, meningitis, or dementia

ENDOCRINE
- Common, seen in >50%
- Antithyroid antibodies
- Altered thyroid function

GASTROINTESTINAL
- Common, seen in >50%
- Dysphagia
- Atrophic gastritis
- Acute or chronic pancreatitis
- Elevated liver enzymes

DERMATOLOGIC
- Common, seen in >50%
- Dryness
- Palpable purpura
- Nonpalpable purpura

RENAL
- Uncommon, seen in <10%
- Glomerulonephritis
- Interstitial nephritis
- Distal or proximal renal tubular acidosis
- Nephrogenic diabetes insipidus

DIAGNOSIS

- When suspected, the patient should be questioned about symptoms and appropriate laboratory screening should be performed. Four of the classic findings should be present. Most commonly the symptoms will consist of dry eyes, dry mouth, and positive laboratory tests for antibodies to SS-A and SS-B. Secondary Sjögren syndrome should be considered in the presence of other connective tissue diseases, such as rheumatoid arthritis, systemic lupus erythematosus, scleroderma, or polymyositis.
- Many patients develop arthralgias and fatigue along with severe sicca symptoms but do not strictly meet criteria for the diagnosis. The term *partial* or *incomplete* Sjögren's syndrome is applied in these settings. These patients should be seen periodically by their care provider to monitor for further evidence of classic Sjögren's syndrome.
- Lymphomas have been characterized in patients with Sjögren (7% of patients). Lymphomas are more common when extraepithelial involvement is present.

THERAPEUTIC APPROACH

- Ocular
  - Moisture replenishment: saline, methylcellulose, hydroxyethylcellulose, carboxymethylcellulose, hydroxyethylcellulose, polyvinyl alcohol, polyethylene glycol, and petroleum jelly have all been used.
    - Avoid wind, breezes, ventilation ducts, and dry air
    - Use of clear glasses or sunglasses to protect the eyes
    - Avoiding drugs with anticholinergic effects; tricyclic antidepressants, antispasmodics, and phenothiazines
    - Avoid irritants such as smoke, powders, sprays, and makeups
    - Pilocarpine, 5 mg four times per day
    - Cyclosporine ophthalmic drops, 0.05%
    - Tear duct ablation or plugging
- Oral dryness
  - Encourage water intake
  - Lozenges
  - Fastidious dental care/hygiene
  - Topical stannous fluoride treatments
  - Pilocarpine HCL, 5 mg four times per day or cevimeline tablets, 30 mg three times per day
- Vaginal lubricants
- Skin dryness
  - Minimize bathing
  - Utilize oil, moisturizers, and lotions
  - Maintain a higher humidity
- Arthralgias/arthritis
  - NSAIDs
  - Hydroxychloroquine, 100 to 400 mg per day
  - Methotrexate 10 to 25 mg per week
  - Corticosteroids, bursts with high dose or continuous low dose
  - Azathioprine, 50 to 200 mg per day
  - Mycophenolate mofetil, 250 to 2000 mg per day
  - Anti-TNF inhibitors such as infliximab
- Organ-specific and constitutional symptoms
  - Corticosteroid bursts or continuous azathioprine or mycophenolate mofetil
- Bronchitis
  - Corticosteroids, azathioprine, mycophenolate mofetil, and consider prophylactic antibiotics

INFLAMMATORY MYOPATHIES

- Polymyositis, dermatomyositis, inclusion body myositis
- These three illnesses are characterized by inflammatory lesions in the muscles. They are all associated with weakness.

EPIDEMIOLOGY

- The annual incidence of polymyositis and dermatomyositis is approximately five per million persons.
- The mean age at diagnosis of adult polymyositis is 45 years, adult dermatomyositis is 40 years, childhood

myositis is 10 years, inclusion body myositis is greater than 65 years.

- The ratio of females-to-males is generally 2:1;the exception to this is inclusion body myositis where it is 1:2.
- The disease onset is more frequent in the winter and spring months. This suggests viral or bacterial infections as a cause.
- Antibodies to coxsackie B have been found more frequently in dermatomyositis in childhood than in other children with arthritis.
- Other factors thought to play a role may be physical activity and emotional stress.
- Medications associated with myositis including D-penicillamine and, more recently, the statin agents.
- While myositis can accompany other connective tissue diseases such as lupus or rheumatoid arthritis, vasculidities, scleroderma, Sjögren syndrome, or antiphospholipid antibody syndrome, it is not usually a major component of those diseases. The exception to this may be mixed connective tissue disease with positive anti-RNP antibodies which is characterized by overlapping symptoms of lupus, myositis, and scleroderma.
- Genetic factors are involved as suggested by monozygotic twin and first-degree relative studies.
- HLA-DQA1 has been associated with familial myositis. This relationship is in keeping with many of the connective tissue diseases where there is a higher familial incidence of inflammatory connective tissue diseases in patients who are first degree relatives.

PATHOPHYSIOLOGY

POLYMYOSITIS
- Proximal muscle weakness, often progressive to medial then distal muscle weakness without treatment
- Muscle enzymes are high including creatinine kinase (CK), aldolase, and lactic dehydrogenase (LDH)
- Abnormal EMG, which reveals characteristic changes of inflammation
- Characteristic muscle biopsy—endomysial inflammation, mononuclear cell infiltrate, lymphocytes, macrophages, polymorphonuclear leukocytes, T-cell CD8 cells, and plasma cells in the paramysial area
- Necrosis of muscle fibers
- Regeneration of muscle fibers
- Fibrosis replacing muscle fibers
- Loss of capillaries

DERMATOMYOSITIS
- Presumed viral etiology
- Muscle weakness similar to polymyositis
- Inflammation of the skin

 ○ Heliotrope rash—bluish hue around eyes
 ○ Gottron papules—over joint extensor surfaces
 ○ Diffuse vasculitic skin rash
 ○ Macrophages and lymphocytes found in inflammatory skin lesions near vessels
 ○ Immune complexes and complement deposition is also present
- Muscle inflammation is slightly different than in polymyositis—more paramysial and perivascular versus endomysial in polymyositis

INCLUSION BODY MYOSITIS
- More common in elderly males
- Distal muscle weakness is more common, although proximal muscle weakness also occurs
- Often less severe weakness initially, but eventually persistent and progressive
- Muscle biopsy shows inclusion bodies, endomysial inflammation, and vacuoles
- Inclusion bodies often show evidence of amyloid and other reactive proteins such as Tao protein and ubiquitin
- Presumed viral etiology, variable (generally poor) response to steroids and other immunosuppressive agents

DIAGNOSIS

POLYMYOSITIS/DERMATOMYOSITIS
The classic criteria published in 1975[5] by Bohan and Peter remain unchanged. These criteria include proximal muscle weakness in the arms, legs, and neck, inflammation, necrotic muscle biopsy, muscle enzyme elevations in the serum, and EMG abnormalities.

INCLUSION BODY MYOSITIS
- No established criteria for diagnosing this condition
- Generally requires a muscle biopsy which reveals classic inclusion bodies
- Presumed diagnosis can be established based on male gender, advanced age, distal (hand and finger) involvement, and poor response to therapy
- Laboratory testing should reveal an elevation of creatine kinase and aldolase levels, as in polymyositis and dermatomyositis

DIAGNOSTIC TESTS

- Elevated CK (CPK) and/or aldolase
- Elevated nonspecific test include lactate dehydrogenase (LDH), aspartate aminotransferase (AST), alanine aminotransferase (ALT), and C-reactive protein
- Positive anti-nuclear antibody (ANA) with antibodies to Jo-1, PM-Scl, Mi-2, PL-7, PL-12, SRP, and OJ have been observed.

- EMG reveals classic findings in all inflammatory myopathies, including insertional irritation, fibrillations, positive sharp waves, and small polyphasic motor activity
- The muscle biopsy is the definitive test revealing an inflammatory pattern, muscle fiber necrosis, and loss of muscle mass, regeneration and scarring fibrosis. In inclusion body myositis, vacuolization is seen along with inclusion bodies in the muscle biopsy
- Vasculitis and perivascular inflammation may also be seen, especially in dermatomyositis

SKIN BIOPSY

DERMATOMYOSITIS

- Vasculitis is often seen in the skin biopsy, and immune complex deposition is commonly described in the lesions.

THERAPEUTIC APPROACH

- Early aggressive treatment in collaboration with a provider with expertise in the treatment of polymyositis and dermatomyositis is desirable. The earlier the inflammation is suppressed, the better the long-term prognosis.
- Corticosteroids are considered first-line. Usually the starting dose is prednisone, 1 mg/kg body weight per day. The duration of therapy depends upon clinical response, as well as the laboratory markers of disease activity.
- If severe respiratory weakness, dysphagia, or cardiac involvement is seen, higher dose steroids given intravenously should be considered (1000 mg IV methylprednisolone per day for 3 d).
- Steroids should not be tapered until there is an unequivocal clinical response and a reduction in serum muscle enzymes. Ideally, the CK has normalized before steroids are discontinued. Objectively, patients should experience improved strength, if treated aggressively and early.
- If there is a partial response, consider adding an additional immunosuppressive agent. If there is no response, the diagnosis is called into question eg, consider inclusion body myositis. In addition, the clinician should consider steroid-induced myopathy with prolonged use of steroids, particularly if the CK normalize but muscle strength does not.
- Other immunosuppressive drugs that have been used include:
  - Methotrexate
  - Azathioprine
  - Cyclophosphamide
  - Cyclosporine A
  - Mycophenolate mofetil
  - Hydroxychloroquine–dermatomyositis rash
  - Intravenous immunoglobulin (IVIG)—Unproven newer medications but, nonetheless promising including TNF inhibitors: etanercept, adalimumab, and infliximab. Also currently under investigation is rituximab. Various dosage schedules have been suggested for IVIG, but it is frequently administered daily for 2 to 5 days and then repeated weekly, monthly, or every 2 months depending on the response. IVIG is sometimes associated with a dramatic response. It is especially useful in refractory dermatomyositis and may offer promise in inclusion body myositis.

If Jo-1 antibodies are present or the patient has interstitial lung disease associated with the myositis, the prognosis is significantly worse. Such patients may respond to initial therapy with improvement both in muscle strength and lung disease; only to relapse with lung involvement.

SCLERODERMA

- Classically presents as skin tightness with deposition of collagen in the dermis

EPIDEMIOLOGY

- Prevalence
  - Recent estimates
    - 250 cases per 1,000,000 population in the United States.
    - 4000 per 1,000,000 population in Choctaw Indians, Oklahoma
- Recent studies indicate that the geographic and cultural distribution may be secondary to mutations in fibrillin-1 or antibodies to fibrillin-1
- Gender
  - Female-to-male 4:1
- Mortality
  - 9-year survival rate, 38% to 72%
  - Depending upon organ involvement and severity
- Onset
  - All ages
  - Midlife more likely; most common, 40 to 50 years of age
- Heredity
  - No clear pattern from major histocompatibility complex allele analysis
  - 1% risk of developing scleroderma if a first-degree relative has scleroderma

MAJOR DISEASE MANIFESTATIONS

- Two major patterns of skin thickening
  - Systemic, diffuse
  - Limited, with involvement distal to the elbows and knees, may also involve the face and neck
    - Limited subtype-CREST syndrome
      - Subcutaneous calcinosis
      - Raynaud syndrome
      - Esophageal dysmotility
      - Sclerodactyly–skin tightness just over the fingers
      - Telangiectasias (predominantly face and hands)

PATHOPHYSIOLOGY

- Raynaud syndrome often precedes the onset by years
- Higher familial incidence, especially evident in specific populations (see above)
- In most cases, there is no known risk or events associated with the development of this disease
- Chemicals or medications may produce a similar pattern of fibrosis: vinyl chloride, trichloro- or perchloroethylene, toluene, benzene, silicas, rape seed oil toxin, L-tryptophan, bleomycin.
- Classical stages
  - Edematous (early), fibrotic (most commonly recognized stage), atrophic (late stage)
- Early findings
  - Warm, edematous, erythematous, skin (usually in the distal extremities)
  - Appears inflammatory
  - Sometimes difficult to distinguish from other early onset connective tissue diseases
  - Lymphocytic and monocyte infiltrate in areas of recent involvement
  - Mast cells are increase in number and activity in areas of involvement
  - Cytokine production, particularly TGF-β and interleukin-4 have been characterized at sites of activity
  - Fibroblasts promote collagen and glycosaminoglycan (matrix) deposition
  - Endothelial activation has been described
  - Elevated circulating levels of cytokines, interleukins, platelet aggregates, growth factors, and endothelin
- Subsequent events
  - The epidermis thins while the dermis thickens
  - These changes migrate slowly up the extremities, producing a classic scleroderma appearance.
  - Massive collagen and glycosaminoglycan deposition is observed in the dermis

- The matric deposits may also occur in the lungs, heart, kidney, and gastrointestinal tract to varying degrees.
  - Microvascular occlusion and endothelial cell activation has been described
  - Vascular insufficiency, especially the digits, with slow-healing digital ulcers
- Long-term or late
  - The skin, especially the dermis, becomes thinner
  - Contractures occur, particularly around the distal joints (fingers, hands, wrists)
  - Tightness of the skin, ligaments, and joint capsule often produces a fixed, immobile flexion contractures of the joint
- Internal organ involvement
  - Lungs—fibrotic lesions in the bases gradually becoming diffuse; an inflammatory component has also been described.
  - Pulmonary hypertension may develop
  - Vascular lesions, intimal proliferation, medial thickening is common
  - Since the lesions have an inflammatory component, if treated with immunosuppression the signs and symptoms may improve
- Heart
  - Pericarditis and pericardial fibrosis
  - Myocardial lesions and vascular intimal proliferation
  - Contraction band necrosis in the heart with a typical ischemic appearance
  - Pulmonary hypertension
- Gastrointestinal tract
  - The entire digestive tract may be involved
  - Tight mouth secondary to skin tightness, decreased oral aperture
    - Esophagus
      - Esophageal dysmotility with reflux is very common. Dysphagia and reflux due to inflammation and fibrosis of the lamina propria, submucosa, and muscularis layers
      - Usually begins distally and evolves proximally
      - Loss of peristalsis and massive dilatation of the esophagus is a later finding
      - Strictures in the distal esophagus are common
    - Stomach and bowel
      - Gastroparesis, *watermelon stomach*, gastritis
      - Small bowel bacterial overgrowth because of stasis
      - Slowing of peristalsis is secondary to muscularis involvement
      - Large bowel bacterial overgrowth, constipation alternating with diarrhea, and wide-mouth diverticula, are characteristic of scleroderma
- Kidney
  - Narrowing of the arteries/arterial tree with microvascular occlusion

- Thickening of the lamina propria, thinning of the media, and reduplication of the elastic lamina in the media (characteristic findings on renal biopsy)
- Fibrinoid necrosis on a renal biopsy, particularly fibrinoid deposition in the glomerular loops
- Tendon
  - Tendon rubs are characteristic of scleroderma, particularly around the wrists and ankles
  - Flexion contractures occur secondary to fibrosis
- Laboratory or serologic abnormalities
  - Positive antinuclear antibodies
  - Positive anticentromere antibody (especially with pulmonary hypertension)
  - Positive antibody to Scl-70 (topoisomerase 1) (seen with pulmonary fibrosis)
  - Positive antibody to U1-RNP
  - Numerous other autoantibodies have been identified but are not commonly tested for such as: antibodies to PM-Scl, U3RNP, CENT A and B, Th, and RNA polymerase I and III

DIAGNOSIS

- Criteria
  - Proximal scleroderma with symmetrical thickening of the skin over the fingers, dorsum of the hands, forearms, upper arms, face, neck, trunk, abdomen, legs, ankles, and feet. This may be limited to sclerodactyly. There may also be digital pitting, scars, loss of substance in the finger pads, and pulmonary fibrosis.[4]

THERAPEUTIC APPROACH

- It is absolutely essential to determine the extent and severity of organ involvement.
- Skin
  - No known anti-fibrotic medications exist. Many open-label trials and anecdotal case reports have been described using a wide variety of medications.
  - Stretching of the skin may reduce the development of flexion contractures
  - Hand warmers are important during cold exposure, not just mittens, as the digits will not rewarm without external heat.
  - Avoiding prolonged cold exposure is important.
- Digital ulcers
  - Prevention of vasospasms by avoiding cold and triggering situations
  - Vasodilators, calcium channel blockers, anti-endothelin medications (bosentan),
  - phosphodiesterase inhibitors

- Diligent wound care
- Early edematous stage may symptomatically respond to nonsteroidal antiinflammatory medications or steroids, but should be used with caution due to renal and cardiac risks.
- Calcinosis: no effective medication
- Surgical removal is uncommonly performed, except for persistent ulcerations and/or recurrence

Scleroderma sine scleroderma: 1% to 2% of patients with scleroderma have visceral abnormalities without skin involvement.

- Pulmonary
  - Symptoms usually begin with dyspnea on exertion or fatigue
  - Physical findings: bibasilar rales
  - Pulmonary function tests with carbon monoxide diffusion capacity often show remarkable abnormalities early on. These should be followed periodically, based on symptoms.
  - Six-minute walk distance, definitive method to assess progress
  - Chest x-ray
  - High-resolution CT scan of the chest, looking for ground-glass appearance, may be an indication for treatment with immunosuppressive agents
  - Bronchoalveolar lavage to detect inflammatory cells.
  - Medications used when inflammation is present usually include cyclophosphamide, azathioprine, mycophenolate mofetil, steroids, and cyclosporine
- Cardiac
  - Yearly Doppler echocardiogram to assess for pulmonary hypertension, as recommended by the World Health Organization
  - Cardiac catheterization, if right ventricular systolic pressure elevation is detected; if greater than 50 mm Hg or rapidly rising values. Also may be performed if symptoms do not correlate with echocardiogram results.
- Renal
  - Check blood pressure every visit and/or every six months
  - Check creatinine yearly or if blood pressure rises
  - Check urinalysis
  - Early use of angiotensin-converting enzyme (ACE) inhibitors is crucial and has clearly decreased the mortality with renal involvement
- Gastrointestinal
  - Yearly history, physical examination
  - Accurate weight; unexplained loss should trigger further evaluation to include upper and lower endoscopies.
  - Anemia is an indication for upper endoscopy to rule out gastritis or search for other digestive tract involvement.

- Oral aperture tightness
  - Meticulous oral hygiene and dental visits
  - Change the diet to a mechanically soft diet
  - Add multivitamins
- Emergencies described with scleroderma
  - Hypertensive crisis with renal failure (ACE-inhibitors are the drugs of choice)
  - Esophageal stricture with obstruction (endoscopy with dilatation)
  - Absence of bowel motility (endoscopy to rule out obstruction)
  - Rapid escalation of dyspnea (consider immunosuppression)
  - Pulmonary hypertension (consider immmunosuppression and pulmonary vasodilators)

REFERENCES

1. Vitali C, Bombardieri S, Moutsopoulos HM, et al. Preliminary criteria for the classification of Sjögren's syndrome. *Arthritis Rheum.* 1993;36:340–347.
2. Vitali C, Bombardieri S, Jonsson R, et al. Classification criteria for Sjögren's syndrome: A revised version of the European criteria proposed by the American-European Consensus Group. *Ann Rheum Dis.* 2002;61:554–558.
3. Bohan A, Peter JB. Polymyositis and dermatomyositis. *N Engl J Med.* 1975;292:344–347.
4. Preliminary criteria for the classification of systemic sclerosis (scleroderma). *Arthritis Rheum.* 1980;23:581–590

RECOMMENDED READING

Preliminary criteria for the classification of systemic sclerosis (scleroderma). *Arthritis Rheum* 1980;23:581–590.

Cherin P, Pelletier S, Teixeira A, et al. Results and long-term follow-up of intravenous immunoglobulin infusions in chronic, refractory polymyositis. *Arthritis Rheum.* 2002;46:467–474.

Derk CT, Jimenez SA. Systemic sclerosis: Current views of its pathogenesis. *Autoimmun Rev.* 2003;2:181–191.

Fox RI, Michelson P. Approaches to the treatment of Sjögren's syndrome. *J Rheumatol.* 2000;61(Suppl):15–21.

Schnabel A, Reuter M, Biederer J, et al. Interstitial lung disease in polymyositis and dermatomyositis: Clinical course and response to treatment. *Semin Arthritis Rheum.* 2003;32:273–284.

Witte T, Matthias T, Arnett FC, et al. IgA and IgG autoantibodies against α fodrin as markers for Sjögren's syndrome. *J Rheumatol.* 2000;27:2617–2620.

Zhou X, Tan FK, Milewicz DM, Guo X, Bona C, Arnett FC. Autoantibodies to fibrillin-1 activate normal human fibroblasts in culture through the TGF-β pathway to recapitulate the "scleroderma phenotype." *J Immunol.* 2005;175:4555–4560.

132 RHEUMATOID ARTHRITIS

Terry L. Moore

EPIDEMIOLOGY

- Rheumatoid arthritis (RA) is the most common inflammatory arthritis affecting from 0.5% to 1% of the general population worldwide. The prevalence spans the globe regardless of geographic location or race; however, there are some notable exceptions (rural Africans have a low incidence of the disease).
- A chronic systemic autoimmune inflammatory disorder, RA is characterized by synovial tissue inflammation, proliferation and pannus formation, which invades adjacent bone, cartilage, and ligaments.
- Although RA is primarily considered a disease of the joints, it can cause a variety of extraarticular manifestations underscoring the systemic nature of the disease.
- The incidence of RA rises dramatically through adulthood. Women are affected 2–3 times more frequently than men and peaks at age 35 to 45 years with one-third of the patients affected after age 60.
- RA is an important cause of functional limitation, highlighted by frequent lost work days (roughly 2 days in 5 lost) during the first 5 years after diagnosis.
- The American College of Rheumatology (ACR) 1987 classification criteria is used to define RA. A patient must exhibit four of the seven criteria:
  1. Morning stiffness lasting at least 1 hour and present for at least 6 weeks
  2. Swelling in three or more joints for at least 6 weeks
  3. Swelling in hand joints for at least 6 weeks
  4. Symmetrical joint swelling for at least 6 weeks
  5. Erosions or decalcification on x-ray of the hands
  6. Presence of rheumatoid nodules
  7. Elevated level of serum 19S immunoglobulin M (IgM) rheumatoid factor (RF)
- The disease usually presents as a slow, progressive disease with moderate activity interspersed with short episodes of acute arthritis (polycyclic or palindromic), however one third of all patients undergo complete and permanent remission within 2 years of disease onset (monocyclic), and 10% develop an unrelenting, progressive, and destructive form of RA with deformity, disfigurement and extraarticular manifestations. When it involves multiple joints, extraarticular features such as nodules may occur early.

PATHOPHYSIOLOGY

- The sinovial pathology in the early stages is characterized by edema, angiogenesis or formation of new blood vessels, hyperplasia of the synovial lining, and inflammatory infiltrates.
- As the disease progresses, hyperplasia of the synovial cells occurs coupled with a subintimal mononuclear cell infiltrate. In the later stages, there is extensive infiltration of plasma cells, macrophages, and lymphocytes with pannus formation and erosion of the adjacent bone. The cellular infiltrate is comprised of CD4-$^+$ T lymphocytes, B cells, and plasma cells.
- The inflammatory process is aggravated by the generation of pro-inflammatory cytokines, chemokines, growth factors, enzymes, and other soluble mediators. The most common inflammatory mediators include interleukin (IL)-1; IL-6; tumor necrosis factor (TNF) α; and colony-stimulating factor 1, which stimulates production of other proinflammatory cytokines such as IL-8,12,15,17, and 18. Antiinflammatory cytokines have also been identified, including IL-4, 10, 11, and 13.
- Two antibodies are commonly discovered in the synovium or serum of patients with RA. The most common is RF; which is a 19S IgM molecule, that binds the crystallizable portion of immunoglobulin (IgG) G. Rheumatoid factor is found in up to 90% of patients with RA using a standard enzyme-linked immunoabsorbent assay (ELISA). However, rheumatoid factors have been associated with all Ig classes; with the IgA RF being associated with disease activity. Rheumatoid factors have been shown to be locally produced in synovial tissue and are associated with severe erosive disease, poor functional outcome, rheumatoid nodules, extraarticular manifestations, and HLA-DR4 positivity.
- Recently, antibodies to citrulline containing proteins (anti-CCP) have been described in RA. They are found in approximately 75% of patients with RA and possess high specificity for RA (90% to 95%). Since anti-CCP are IgG antibodies they are believed to indicate acute disease activity. Importantly, RF is not specific for RA and can be found in 30% of patients with unrelated connective tissue diseases and in a high percentage of patients with hepatitis C.

CLINICAL FINDINGS

- Rheumatoid arthritis is a polyarticular disease that most commonly involves the peripheral nonweight-bearing joints (Table 132–1). The most common joints

TABLE 132–1 Most Common Joints Involved During the Course of Rheumatoid Arthritis

JOINT	PERCENTAGE INVOLVEMENT (%)
Metacarpophalangeal	90–95
Wrist	80–90
Proximal interphalangeal	70–90
Knee	60–80
Metatarsophalangeal	50–90
Ankle	50–80
Shoulder	50–60

involved are the metacarpophalangeal joints (MCPs) of the hands (90% to 95%); the proximal interphalangeal joints (90%); and the wrists (90%). In the lower extremities, the metatarsophalangeal joints may be involved (50% to 90%). The knee is involved in 60% to 80%, as is the shoulder and ankle; and to a lesser extent the cervical spine, hip, elbow, and temporomandibular joints may be involved. Involved hands may develop ulnar styloid prominence; ulnar deviation with subluxation of the MCP joints; fusiform swelling and boutonnière deformity, which is caused by a weakening of the central slip of the extensor tendon and palmar displacement of the lateral bands; and finally, swan neck deformities as a result of contraction of the flexors of the MCPs. The foot deformities include claw toe or hammer toe deformity, flattening of the arch, and hind-foot valgus deformity.

- Early on, the radiographic features of RA include soft tissues swelling, abnormal alignment, and periarticular demineralization. If the disease is progressive, symmetric uniform joint space narrowing and marginal erosions may occur. The first manifestation of the disease is usually soft tissue swelling, indicating inflammation, which then promotes periarticular demineralization with erosions and joint space narrowing.
- The systemic manifestations of RA include the development of rheumatoid nodules. Biopsies of nodules reveals a central area of fibrinoid necrosis surrounded by palisading histiocytes and a peripheral layer of cellular connective tissue. Between 20% and 30% of RF-positive patients may develop rheumatoid nodules, which usually accompany active and severe disease. The nodules are located on the elbows, finger joints, Achilles tendon, and occipital regions. Other systemic manifestations include eye involvement such as iritis, scleritis, and episcleritis. Twenty percent of patients, especially older age males with a smoking history, may develop pleural disease characterized by exudative pleural effusions. Also, solitary or multiple pulmonary nodules have been observed. Rheumatoid involvement of the lung may produce interstitial fibrosis

with fibrosing alveolitis. Cardiac manifestations are rare but may include pericarditis, and nodules can arise within the cardiac conduction system. Occasionally, coronary arteritis and myocarditis may occur. Rheumatoid vasculitis may also occur and be associated with nailfold infarcts, evidence of panarteritis with mononuclear cell infiltrates, and obliterative endarteritis of the fingers and toes. The vascular injury is secondary to the deposition of immune complexes and cryoglobulins and most commonly occurs in the lower extremities around nailfold beds.

• Two common syndromes that are somewhat unique to RA, include Sjögren syndrome (dry eyes and dry mouth), and Felty syndrome, (leukocytopenia and splenomegaly). Neurologic manifestations include peripheral entrapment neuropathies and, in severe cases, spinal cord injury from atlantoaxial subluxation.

LABORATORY FEATURES

• Laboratory studies in patients with longstanding RA may reveal a normochromic, normocytic anemia of inflammatory disease. White blood cell counts and platelet counts are usually normal. Urinalysis and the comprehensive metabolic panel should also be within normal limits unless complicated by extrarenal RA.

• 19S IgM RF is present in approximately 80% to 90% of patients, and anti-CCM antibodies are present in up to 75% to 80% of the patients. When, both antibodies are present, the disease is typically more severe.

• Inflammatory markers such as the erythrocyte sedimentation rate and C-reactive protein (CRP) are elevated with flares of the disease; the sedimentation rate remains elevated longer than the CRP which gradually returns to normal as the disease remits. Both are reasonable markers of disease activity and, accordingly, prove useful in the follow-up and management of patients.

• The antinuclear antibody is positive in 30% of the patients, but specific antibodies observed in other connective tissue diseases should be negative.

• Synovial fluid findings reveal inflammatory fluid with white blood cell counts of 5000 to 25,000/mm^3, although it is not uncommon for the count to exceed 100,000. Most of the cells are polymorphonuclear leukocytes (85%). Synovial glucose is low, while the protein concentration is high in RA.

THERAPY

• The treatment of RA should involve multiple domains including physical therapy, occupational therapy, social work, dietary and nursing. The patient must receive

education regarding the longstanding nature and anticipated course of the disease.

• Nonpharmacologic modalities such as physical therapy should be offered to all patients. The use of moist heat, hot packs, Hubbard tank, and paraffin baths for the hands and feet, as well as muscle-strengthening exercises of muscles surrounding the joints are important to minimize functional disability and pain. Muscle strengthening and toning reduce impact loading on the joints. Occupational therapists provide joint protection strategies and instructions in posture, body mechanics, and activities of daily living to reduce joint impact. Physical therapy should be aggressively pursued because most damage occurs within the first 2 years of the diagnosis.

• While nonpharmacologic strategies are essential in all patients, the vast majority require pharmacologic therapy to control disease activity. First-line agents include the nonsteroidal antiinflammatories drugs (NSAIDs), which have intrinsic analgesic and antiinflammatory effects. The NSAIDS also promote rapid pain relief and accelerate functional improvement. The disadvantages of NSAID use include, gastrointestinal erosions/ulcers, impaired platelet function, nephrotoxicity, and hepatic toxicity. Moreover, a fair number of patients have a poor or variable response to the administration of NSAIDS. While receiving NSAIDs, patients should undergo regular blood work including a CBC, urinalysis, and comprehensive metabolic panel every four months. There are multiple NSAIDs (Table 132–2) available for use in RA including the cyclooxygenase (COX) 1 inhibitors (diclofenac sodium, naproxen, fenoprofen, and nabumetone) and the COX-2 inhibitors such as celecoxib and meloxicam.

TABLE 132–2   Nonsteroidal Antiinflammatory Medications for Use in Rheumatoid Arthritis

NONSTEROIDAL ANTIINFLAMMATORY MEDICATION	DOSAGE
COX-1 inhibitors:	
Diclofenac sodium	50 mg tid–75 mg bid
Naproxen	250–500 mg bid
Ibuprofen	600–800 mg tid
Fenoprofen calcium	600 mg tid
Nabumetone	500–1000 mg bid
Sulindac	200 mg bid
Tolmetin sodium	600 mg tid
COX-2 inhibitors:	
Celecoxib	100–200 mg bid
Meloxicam	7.5–15 mg once daily

bid, twice a day; COX 1, cyclooxygenase 1; tid, three times a day.

- The use of intraarticular glucocorticoids may be indicated in monoarticular joint involvement (rare) or when one joint is disproportionately affected. Intrarticular steroids promote a local antiinflammatory effect and provide significant symptomatic relief. The large joints (knee) may be injected with 20 to 40 mg of triamcinolone hexacetonide, and 10 to 20 mg may be injected into smaller joints (MCPs).
- First-line therapy (in addition to NSAIDS) should also include two or more disease-modifying antirheumatic drugs (DMARDs). In the United States, the most common combination employed is an NSAID and methotrexate (MTX) in doses from 7.5 to 25 mg once weekly by mouth, subcutaneous injection, or intramuscular injection. Methotrexate is a purine antagonist with potent immunosuppressive effects. Importantly, MTX is the most effective DMARD for RA eg, it is considered the gold standard of care in patients with RA. However, MTX administration has been associated with hepatotoxicity and bone marrow suppression; therefore, a CBC, urinalysis, and comprehensive metabolic panel should be monitored every 4 to 6 weeks. Up to 20 mg can be administered orally. If more than 20 mg is required, subcutaneous or intramuscular administration is preferred because of erratic oral absorption. Folic acid (1 to 2 mg/day) appears to reduce the incidence of oral/nasal ulcers and decrease gastrointestinal symptoms including nausea and vomiting and liver toxicity.
- Hydroxychloroquine, an antimalarial, is also employed in the initial management of RA. This agent stabilizes lysosomal membranes at a dose of 200 to 400 mg/day, the dose should never exceed 6 mg/kg because of the risk of ocular toxicity.
- Other agents which are active in RA include sulfasalazine (500 to 1000 mg three time daily) and intramuscular gold sodium thiomalate.
- Leflunomide, a pyrimidine antagonist, given as a loading dose of 100 mg per 3 days, and then 20 mg/daily has also been effective, especially in patients refractory to other agents. This drug is teratogenic and also causes liver injury, therefore liver function studies must be obtained regularly in these patients (4- to 6-week intervals).
- Older immunosuppressives such as azathioprine, 100 to 200 mg/day and cyclophosphamide, 50 to 200 mg/day may also be used (especially in refractory patients), however they have largely been replaced with triple therapy combinations and the new biologics.
- Several important new biologics are approved for the use in RA including etanercept, infliximab, adalimumab, anakinra, abatacept, and rituximab.
- Etanercept is a dimeric fusion protein consisting of the extracellular ligand binding portion of the human p75 TNF receptor linked to the Fc-fragment, crystallizable portion of human IgG-1. This agent binds soluble and cell-bound TNF, rendering it biologically inactive and promoting a potent anti-inflammatory effect. The drug is administered as a subcutaneous 25 mg injection twice weekly or 50 mg once weekly. It has a rapid onset of action with a half-life of approximately 115 hours. Etanercept has been shown to be effective in combination with triple drug therapy in reducing erosions and joint space narrowing. Adverse effects include injection site reactions and an increased incidence of upper respiratory tract infections. Therefore, it should be discontinued temporarily if an infection is suspected. Occasionally, an autoantibody is generated to the protein rendering it inactive. Because TNF inhibitors can aggravate indolent tuberculosis infection, a purified protein derivative (PPD) skin test and chest x-ray should be performed yearly. In addition, recent studies have suggested an association of biologics with the development of lymphomas.
- Infliximab is a chimeric mouse/human monoclonal antibody which targets free and cell-bound TNF. It lyses TNF-expressing cells in vitro and has an extended half-life of 9.5 days. It is administered by intravenous infusion. It can be immunogenic, forming human antichimeric antibodies (HACA), and usually requires concomitant use of methotrexate to suppress HACA formation. It is dosed as an intravenous infusion in doses from 3 to 10 mg/kg, at 0, 2, and 6 weeks and then every 4 to 8 weeks depending on the clinical response. Dosages may be tapered up or intervals shortened pending response. Adverse reactions include infusion-related reactions, and autoantibody formation. Biologics should be withheld in patients with suspected infections, and yearly PPD and chest x-ray should be performed. Infliximab therapy has been shown to decrease joint erosions and joint space narrowing. Similar to etanercept, the incidence of lymphomas may be increased in patients receiving Infliximab.
- Adalimumab is a fully humanized recombinant monoclonal antibody to TNF-α with a half-life of 10 to 20 days. It is administered as a subcutaneous injection (20 to 40 mg) every other week. Adverse effects include injection site reactions and infections. Adalimumab, like the other biologics, improves erosions and joint space narrowing.
- The tumor necrosis factor inhibitors should not be used in patients with systemic lupus, multiple sclerosis, optic neuritis, active infections, history of tuberculosis or untreated positive PPD, or congestive heart failure.
- Anakinra is an IL-1 receptor antagonist with a half-life of 4 to 6 hours and, thus, must be given daily at a dose of 100 mg subcutaneously. Importantly, IL-1

stimulates macrophages and lymphocytes to produce proinflammatory cytokines. The most common side effects associated with this medication include reactions at the site of the injection, which are usually mild but can be serious with erythema, swelling, and pain. Also, the risk of infection appears similar to that observed with the TNF inhibitors.

- A recent agent approved for use in RA is the fusion protein, abatacept. In rheumatoid synovium, antigen presenting cells are activated and express both class II major histocompatability complex and costimulatory molecules such as CD80 and CD86. Abatacept (recombinant CTLA-4 fusion protein with a fragment of the Fc domain of human IgG1) is constructed by genetically fusing the external domain of human CTLA4 to the heavy chain constant region of human IgG-1; CTLA4Ig binds both CD80 and CD86 on antigen presenting cells, thereby preventing these molecules from engaging CD28 on T cells. This blocks T cells from proliferating and producing inflammatory cytokines. Patients receiving this agent are treated with 10 mg/kg intravenously over 30 minutes on days 1, 15, and 30 and then monthly along with methotrexate.

- Rituximab is a chimeric anti-CD20 monoclonal antibody directed at the CD20 antigen on developing B cells. It induces long-term B-cell depletion when administered in dosages of 375 mg/m^2 for four doses a week apart or 1000 mg every 2 weeks for 2 doses. Side effects include infusion reactions and infections, which occur in 30% of the patients. It is usually given in combination with methotrexate. The treatment can be repeated at 6 months if immunoglobulin levels return to normal and the patient has had a partial response.

BIBLIOGRAPHY

Breedveld FC, Kalden JR, Smolen JS, eds. Advances in targeted therapies. *Ann Rheum Dis.* 2005;64(suppl IV):1.

Firestein GS. Etiology and pathogenesis of rheumatoid arthritis. In: Harris ED, Budd RC, Genovese MC, et al, eds. *Kelley's Testbook of Rheumatology.* 7th ed. Philadelphia, PA: Elsevier Saunders; 2005:996.

Genovese MC, Harris ED Jr. Treatment of rheumatoid arthritis. In: Harris ED, Budd RC, Genovese MC, et al, eds. *Kelley's Testbook of Rheumatology.* 7th ed. Philadelphia, PA: Elsevier Saunders; 2005:1079.

Moore TL. Disease of the joints. In: Pathy MSJ, Sinclair AJ, Morley JE. eds. *Principles and Practices of Geriatric Medicine.* 4th ed. West Sussex, England: John Wiley and Sons; 2006:1347.

Nowak UM, Newkirk MM. Rheumatoid factors: Good or bad for you? *Int Arch Allergy Immunol.* 2005;138:180.

van Gaalen F, Ioan-Facsinay A, Huizinga TW, Toes REM. The emerging role of anticitrulline autoimmunity in rheumatoid arthritis. *J Immunol.* 2005;175:5575.

INDEX

Page numbers followed by a *t* or *f* indicate that the entry is in a table or figure.